D1592888

Sleep Medicine

Sudhansu Chokroverty • Michel Billiard
Editors

Sleep Medicine

A Comprehensive Guide to Its Development, Clinical Milestones, and Advances in Treatment

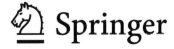 Springer

Editors
Sudhansu Chokroverty
Professor of Neuroscience, Seton Hall University,
South Orange, NJ;
Clinical Professor of Neurology, Rutgers Robert
Wood Johnson Medical School,
New Brunswick, NJ;
Director of Sleep Research & Co-Chair emeritus
of Neurology,
JFK New Jersey Neuroscience Institute, Edison,
NJ, US

Michel Billiard
Honorary Professor of Neurology
School of Medicine
University Montpellier I
Honorary Chair
Department of Neurology
Gui de Chauliac Hospital
Montpellier, France

ISBN 978-1-4939-2088-4   ISBN 978-1-4939-2089-1 (eBook)
DOI 10.1007/978-1-4939-2089-1

Library of Congress Control Number: 2015936923

Springer New York Heidelberg Dordrecht London
© Springer Science+Business Media, LLC 2015

Printed on acid-free paper

Springer is part of Springer Science+Business Media (www.springer.com).

Preface

Sleep medicine is now accepted as an independent medical specialty. Therefore, it is important for sleep specialists practicing sleep medicine to know its roots and historical evolution. Despite a remarkable progress and development of the field of sleep medicine there are no books whatsoever addressing the evolution of the development of this tremendous endeavor. In addition to the need for carefully documenting this fascinating evolution from the rudimentary concepts of the ancient prehistoric and the early classical periods to our contemporary knowledge, it is essential for young sleep clinicians and researchers entering the field to have access to a comprehensive, highly readable account of the evolution of sleep medicine, chosen by these aspiring physicians as their professional career.

Within the past two decades there has been at least a tenfold increase of volume on sleep disorder textbooks. There are now many tens of thousands of individuals involved in clinical sleep medicine and sleep research in addition to an explosion of sleep laboratories and sleep centers worldwide spanning from East to the West and from North to the South along with the growth of national and international sleep societies. A new and rapidly emerging field needs its own specialty journals and societies. Beginning with the first in the field, the journal *Sleep* followed by the *Journal of Sleep Research* and *Sleep Medicine*, now there are a significant number of journals exclusively devoted to sleep medicine and sleep research both as print and online versions.

Despite the exponential growth of the field including the number of societies and participants involved, there has been little documentation of its historical development and its challenges until recently. Some early books on sleep provide a good account of the historical aspects including the early French volumes "Le Sommeil et les Reves" by Alfred Maury (1861), "Le Probleme Physiologique du Sommeil" (1913) by Henri Pieron, "Le Sommeil" (see the last chapter) by Dr. J. Lhermitte (1931), and "Les Troubles du Sommeil: Hyersomnies, Insomnies and Parasomnies" by Henri Roger (1932). These were followed by "Sleep and Wakefulness" (1939 and 1963) by Nathaniel Kleitman, "Sleep and Waking" by Ian Oswald (1962), "Le Sommeil de Nuit Normal et Pathologique" edited by Henri Fischgold (1965) and "The Abnormalities of Sleep in Man" edited by Lugaresi et al. (1968). Much information of historical interest is also in the volume "Sleep and its Disorders" by J. David Parkes (1985). However, all these volumes are either on sleep or sleep disorders in general rather than on the overall historical development of the field. There have been a number of historical articles on individual breakthroughs in our understanding of the basic sleep–wake mechanism and discovering new sleep disorders but there are no books on the historical milestones in this fascinating field. The time is now not only ripe but overdue to document the remarkable progress on a state approaching rapidly "At Day's close" (nighttime sleep) in which we spend one third of our existence.

The purpose of this book is to provide a comprehensive, balanced, fair, and easily readable account of the history of developmental milestones of sleep medicine. The book will be of interest not only to individuals working in the field but also the physicians in general. As such the book is directed at internists (especially those specializing in pulmonary, cardiovascular,

gastrointestinal, renal and endocrine medicine), neurologists, neurosurgeons, family physicians, psychiatrists, psychologists, otolaryngologists, dentists, pediatricians, neuroscientists,
as well as those technologists, nurses, and other paraprofessionals with an interest in sleep and
its disorders. We believe that this book could attract significant interest in the general public
as well.

Sudhansu Chokroverty
Michel Billiard

Acknowledgements

We thank all the contributors for their lucid, scholarly, informative, and eminently readable contributions. We also wish to thank all authors, editors, and publishers who granted us permission to reproduce illustrations that were published in other books and journals. We are particularly indebted to Gregory Sutorius, editor of Clinical Medicine at Springer Science, New York for his professionalism, thoughtfulness, and for efficiently moving forward various stages of production. We must also acknowledge with appreciation the valuable support of Jacob Gallay, developmental editor and all the other staff at the Springer production office for their dedication and care in the making of the book.

The editors would like to acknowledge Roger Broughton, MD (author of Chap. 29 and co-author of Chap. 11), for encouraging them to write a book on the historical developmental of sleep medicine and in fact some of his thoughts and justifications have been incorporated in this preface. SC would also like to acknowledge the splendid help of Samantha Staab and Toni Bacala, editorial assistants to the journal *Sleep Medicine* for correspondence with the contributors and making appropriate track changes and also Jenny Rodriguez for typing some materials for the book.

Last but not the least the editors would like to thank their wives. Dr. Chokroverty expresses his love, appreciation, and gratitude to his wife, Manisha Chokroverty, MD, for inspiring and encouraging him during all stages of production of the book while he had been stealing precious weekends from her for continuing to work in order to finish the book in a timely manner; Dr. Billiard expresses his appreciation for his wife, Annick Billiard, for tolerating long hours spent in reviewing all the chapters.

Sudhansu Chokroverty
Michel Billiard

Contents

Contributors

Torbjörn Åkerstedt Stockholm University, Stockholm, Sweden; Clinical Neuroscience, Karolinska Institute, Stockholm, Sweden

Richard P. Allen Department of Neurology, Johns Hopkins University, Baltimore, MD, USA

Sonia Ancoli-Israel Departments of Psychiatry and Medicine, University of California, San Diego, CA, USA

Tarek Asaad Ain Shams University Hospital, Institute of Psychiatry-Psychophysiology & Sleep Research Unit, Nasr City, Cairo, Egypt

Joseph Barbera The Youthdale Child and Adolescent Sleep Centre, Toronto, ON, Canada

Ruth M. Benca Departments of Psychiatry and Psycology, Center for Sleep Medicine and Sleep Research, University of Wisconsin-Madison, Madison, WI, USA

Francesco Benedetti Department of Clinical Neurosciences, Scientific Institute and University Vita-Salute San Raffaele, Milano, Italy

Sándor Beniczky Department of Clinical Neurophysiology, Danish Epilepsy Centre, Dianalund, Denmark; Department of Clinical Neurophysiology, Aarhus University, Aarhus, Denmark

Sushanth Bhat JFK New Jersey Neuroscience Institute, Edison, NJ, USA; Seton Hall University, South Orange, NJ, USA

Michel Billiard Department of Neurology, Gui de Chauliac Hospital, Montpellier Cedex 5, France; School of Medicine, University Montpellier I, Montpellier, France

Kyoung Bin Im Department of Neurology, Sleep Disorders Center, University of Iowa, Roy J and Lucille A Carver College of Medicine, Iowa, IA, USA

Bradley F. Boeve Mayo Center for Sleep Medicine, Department of Neurology, Mayo Clinic and Foundation, Rochester, MN, USA

Bernard Bouteille Laboratory of Parasitology, Dupuytren University Hospital of Limoges, Limoges, France

Roger Broughton Division of Neurology, Department of Medicine, University of Ottawa, Ontario, Canada

Oliviero Bruni Department of Developmental and Social Psychology, Center for Pediatric Sleep Disorders, Sapienza University, Rome, Italy

Alain Buguet Polyclinic Marie-Louise Poto-Djembo, Pointe-Noire, Congo

Scott S. Campbell Chappaqua, NY, USA

Richard J. Castriotta Division of Pulmonary and Sleep Medicine, University of Texas Medical School at Houston, Houston, TX, USA; Sleep Disorders Center, Memorial Hermann Hospital—Texas Medical Center, Houston, TX, USA

Raymond Cespuglio Centre de recherche en neuroscience de Lyon, University of Lyon, Lyon, France

Sarah L. Chellappa Cyclotron Research Centre, University of Liège, Liège, Belgium

Sudhansu Chokroverty JFK New Jersey Neuroscience Institute, Edison, NJ, USA; Seton Hall University, South Orange, NJ, USA

Georges Copinschi Laboratory of Physiology and Physiopathology, Université Libre de Bruxelles, Brussels, Belgium

Sara Dallaspezia Department of Clinical Neurosciences, Scientific Institute and University Vita-Salute San Raffaele, Milano, Italy

Mark Eric Dyken Sleep Disorders Center, University of Iowa Hospitals and Clinics, Iowa, IA, USA; University of Iowa, Roy J and Lucille A Carver College of Medicine, Iowa, IA, USA

Jack D. Edinger National Jewish Health, Denver, CO, USA

A. Roger Ekirch Department of History, Virginia Tech, Blacksburg, VA, USA

M. E. Estep Lynn Health Science Institute, Oklahoma City, OK, USA

Wang Fang Psychology Department (Sleep Medicine Clinic), Guang'anmen Hospital, China Academy of Chinese Medical Sciences, Beijing, China

Fabio Ferrarelli Department of Psychiatry, School of Medicine and Public Health, University of Wisconsin-Madison, Madison, WI, USA

Raffaele Ferri Department of Neurology, Sleep Research Centre, I.C., Oasi Institute for Research on Mental Retardation and Brain Aging (IRCCS), Troina, Italy

Carmen Garcia Interdisciplinary Sleep Medicine Center, Charité—Universitätsmedizin Berlin, Berlin, Germany

Paul B. Glovinsky Department of Psychology, The City College of the City University of New York, New York, NY, USA; St. Peter's Sleep Center, Albany, NY, USA

Munish Goyal Department of Neurology, University of Missouri Hospitals & Clinics, Columbia, MO, USA

Michael A. Grandner University of Pennsylvania, Philadelphia, PA, USA

Christian Guilleminault Sleep Medicine Division, Stanford University Outpatient Medical Center, Redwood City, CA, USA

Mary E. Gunther The University of Tennessee, College of Nursing, Knoxville, TN, USA

Kristyna M. Hartse Sonno Sleep Centers, El Paso, TX, USA

Max Hirshkowitz Department of Medicine and Menninger, Baylor College of Medicine, Houston, USA; Department of Psychiatry, Baylor College of Medicine, Houston, USA; Sleep Disorders & Research Center, Michael E. DeBakey Veterans Affairs Medical Center, Houston, TX, USA; Michael E. DeBakey Veterans Affairs Medical Center, Houston, Linkwood, TX, USA

Jean-Rosaire Ibara Department of Gastroenterology and Medicine, University Hospital of Brazzaville, Brazzaville, Congo

Alex Iranzo Neurology Service, Hospital Clínic de Barcelona, Barcelona, Spain; Institut d'Investigació Biomèdiques August Pi i Sunyer (IDIBAPS), Barcelona, Spain; Centro de Investigación Biomédica en Red sobre Enfermedades Neurodegenerativas (CIBERNED), Barcelona, Spain

Takashi Kanbayashi Department of Neuropsychiatry, Akita University, Akita, Japan

Akihiro Karashima Biomodeling Lab, Graduate School of Information Sciences, Tohoku University, Sendai, Japan

Norihiro Katayama Biomodeling Lab, Graduate School of Information Sciences, Tohoku University, Sendai, Japan

V. Mohan Kumar SA, Heera Gate Apartments, Thiruvananthapuram, Kerala, India; Sree Chitra Tirunal Institute for Medical Sciences & Technology, Thiruvananthapuram, Kerala, India

Suresh Kumar Department of Neurology, Sree Balajee Medical College and Hospital, Chennai, India; Chennai Sleep Disorders Centre, Chennai, India

Carol A. Landis Department of Biobehavioral Nursing and Health Systems, University of Washington, Seattle, WA, USA

Kathryn A. Lee Family Health Care Nursing, University of California, San Francisco, San Francisco, CA, USA

Teofilo Lee-Chiong Department of Medicine, National Jewish Health, University of Colorado Denver, Denver, CO, USA

Rachel Leproult Unité de Recherches en Neuropsychologie et Neuroimagerie Fonctionnelle (UR2NF), Université Libre de Bruxelles, Campus du Solbosch, Brussels, Belgium

√**Erik K. St. Louis** Mayo Center for Sleep Medicine, Department of Neurology, Mayo Clinic and Foundation, Rochester, MN, USA

Shahira Loza Cairo Centre for Sleep Disorders, Mohandessin, Cairo, Egypt

Serge Lubin Former Medical Director of L. Lafon Laboratory, Maisons-Alfort, France

Elio Lugaresi Department of Biomedical and Neuromotor Sciences, University of Bologna, Bologna, Italy

Julien Q. M. Ly Cyclotron Research Centre, University of Liège, Liège, Belgium

Vipin Malik Department of Medicine, National Jewish Health, University of Colorado Denver, Denver, CO, USA

Pierre Maquet Cyclotron Research Centre, University of Liège, Liège, Belgium

Mari Matsumura Stanford University Sleep and Circadian Neurobiology Laboratory, Department of Psychiatry and Behavioral Sciences, Stanford University School of Medicine, Palo Alto, CA, USA

√ **Stuart J. McCarter** Mayo Clinic and Foundation, Rochester, MN, USA

Harvey Moldofsky Department of Psychiatry, Faculty of Medicine, University of Toronto, Toronto, ON, Canada; Toronto Psychiatric Research Foundation, North York, Canada; Centre for Sleep and Chronobiology Research, Toronto, ON, Canada

Jaime M. Monti Department of Pharmacology and Therapeutics, School of Medicine, Clinics Hospital, Montevideo, Uruguay

Donatien Moukassa Medical and Morphology Laboratory, Loandjili General Hospital, Pointe-Noire, Congo

Mitsuyuki Nakao Biomodeling Lab, Graduate School of Information Sciences, Tohoku University, Sendai, Japan

Sona Nevsimalova Department of Neurology, 1st Faculty of Medicine, Charles University, Prague 2, Czech Republic

Seiji Nishino Stanford University Sleep and Circadian Neurobiology Laboratory, Department of Psychiatry and Behavioral Sciences, Stanford University School of Medicine, Palo Alto, CA, USA

Obengui Department of Infectious Diseases, University Hospital of Brazzaville, Congo

Ruth O'Hara Department of Psychiatry and Behavioral Sciences, Stanford University, Stanford, CA, USA; VA MIRECC Fellowship Program, VA Palo Alto, Palo Alto, CA, USA

Masako Okawa Department of Sleep Medicine, Shiga University of Medical Science, Otsu, Japan

W. C. Orr Lynn Health Science Institute, Oklahoma City, OK, USA

Edgar S. Osuna Department of Morphology, School of Medicine, National University of Colombia, Bogotá, Colombia; Department of Neurology, University Hospital Fundacion Santa Fe de Bogota, Bogotá, Colombia

David Parkes Clinical Neurology, The Maudsley Hospital and King's College Hospital, London, UK

Markku Partinen Helsinki Sleep Clinic, VitalMed Research Centre, Helsinki, Finland; Department of Clinical Neurosciences, University of Helsinki, Helsinki, Finland

Thomas Penzel Interdisciplinary Sleep Medicine Center, Charité—Universitätsmedizin Berlin, Berlin, Germany

Brendon Richard Peters Stanford Sleep Medicine Center, Stanford School of Medicine, Redwood City, CA, USA

Pierre Philip Université de Bordeaux, Sommeil, Attention et Neuropsychatrie, Bordeaux, France

Kenneth D. Phillips The University of Tennessee, College of Nursing, Knoxville, TN, USA

Mark R. Pressman Sleep Medicine Services, Lankenau Medical Center/Lankenau Institute For Medical Research, Wynnewood, Pennsylvania, USA; Jefferson Medical College, Philadelphia, Pennsylvania, USA; Lankenau Institute For Medical Research, Wynnewood, Pennsylvania, USA; Villanova School of Law, Villanova, Pennsylvania, USA

Michelle M. Primeau Department of Psychiatry and Behavioral Sciences, Stanford University, Stanford, CA, USA; VA MIRECC Fellowship Program, VA Palo Alto, Palo Alto, CA, USA

Federica Provini IRCCS Istituto delle Scienze Neurologiche di Bologna, University of Bologna, Bologna, Italy; Department of Biomedical and Neuromotor Sciences, University of Bologna, Bologna, Italy

George B. Richerson The Roy J. Carver Chair in Neuroscience, Roy J and Lucille A Carver College of Medicine, University of Iowa, Iowa, IA, USA

Brady A. Riedner Psychiatric Institute, University of Wisconsin-Madison, Madison, WI, USA

Broughton Roger Division of Neurology, Department of Medicine, University of Ottawa, Ottawa, ON, Canada

Pradeep Sahota Department of Neurology, University of Missouri Hospitals & Clinics, Columbia, MO, USA

Piero Salzarulo Trento, Italy

María Montserrat Sánchez-Ortuño Facultad de Enfermería, Campus de Espinardo, Universidad de Murcia, Murcia, Spain

Joan Santamaria Neurology Service, Hospital Clínic de Barcelona, Barcelona, Spain; Institut d'Investigació Biomèdiques August Pi i Sunyer (IDIBAPS), Barcelona, Spain; Centro de Investigación Biomédica en Red sobre Enfermedades Neurodegenerativas (CIBERNED), Barcelona, Spain

Masatoshi Sato Stanford University Sleep and Circadian Neurobiology Laboratory, Department of Psychiatry and Behavioral Sciences, Stanford University School of Medicine, Palo Alto, CA, USA

Carlos H. Schenck Minnesota Regional Sleep Disorders Center, Minneapolis, USA; Department of Psychiatry, Hennepin County Medical Center, Minneapolis, USA; Department of Psychiatry, University of Minnesota Medical School, Minneapolis, MN, USA

Markus H. Schmidt Ohio Sleep Medicine Institute, Dublin, OH, USA

Hartmut Schulz Erfurt, Germany

Li Shasha Information Institute, China Academy of Chinese Medical Sciences, Beijing, China

Niranjan Singh Department of Neurology, University of Missouri Hospitals & Clinics, Columbia, MO, USA

Arthur J. Spielman Department of Psychology, The City College of the City University of New York, New York, NY, USA; Center for Sleep Medicine, Weill Cornell Medical College, Cornel University, New York, NY, USA

Naoko Tachibana Center for Sleep-related Disorders, Kansai Electric Power Hospital, Fukushima, Osaka, Japan

Joshua Z. Tal Department of Psychiatry and Behavioral Sciences, Stanford University, Stanford, CA, USA; VA MIRECC Fellowship Program, VA Palo Alto, Palo Alto, CA, USA

Michael Thorpy The Saul R. Korey Department of Neurology, Albert Einstein College of Medicine, Yeshiva University, Bronx, NY, USA

Mark C. Wilde Department of Physical Medicine and Rehabilitation, University of Texas Medical School at Houston, Houston, TX, USA

Peter Wolf Department of Neurology, Danish Epilepsy Centre, Dianalund, Denmark

Yan Xue Psychology Department (Sleep Medicine Clinic), Guang'anmen Hospital, China Academy of Chinese Medical Sciences, Beijing, China

Liu Yanjiao Psychology Department (Sleep Medicine Clinic), Guang'anmen Hospital, China Academy of Chinese Medical Sciences, Beijing, China

Hou Yue Department of Neurology, Xuanwu Hospital, Capital Medical University, Beijing, China

Wang Yuping Department of Neurology, Xuanwu Hospital, Capital Medical University, Beijing, China

Juergen Zulley Regensburg, Germany; Department of Psychology, University of Regensburg, Regensburg, Germany

Introduction

Sudhansu Chokroverty and Michel Billiard

The evolution of history of sleep medicine from the antiquity to modern time is a fascinating reading. Since the dawn of civilization, sleep has fascinated and inspired religious scholars, poets, philosophers, playwrights, artists, historians, and scientists as reflected in numerous mythological, poetic, dramatic, and scientific writings [1].

Preserved Babylonian and Assyrian clay tablets, recording dreams and their interpretations, date back to 5000 BC Egyptians erected temples to Serapis, god of dreams, where people would sleep in the hope of inducing fortuitous dreams.

There are references to sleep and dream in Indian and Greek mythologies. For example, *Upanishad* (c. 1000 BC), the great ancient Indian textbook of philosophy sought to divide human existence into four states: the waking, the dreaming, the deep dreamless sleep, and the super conscious ("the very self") [2]. This description is a reminiscent of modern classification of sleep–wakefulness. In Greek mythology, one finds reference to famous sleeping characters, e.g., Endymion falling asleep, forever, after receiving a kiss from the moon [3]. Nyx, the Greek god of night, has twin sons: Hypnos, the god of sleep; and Thanatos, the god of death.

One of the greatest Chinese (Taoist) philosophers (300 BC), Chuang-Tzu (Zhuangzi) stated [4]:

Everything is one;
During sleep the soul, undistracted, is absorbed into the unity;
When awake, distracted
It sees the different beings.

The ancient Chinese believed in two basic principles of life: *Yang,* the active, light, and positive; and *Yin,* the passive, dark, and negative. The Yin–Yang concept, originated with *Fu Hsi* (c. 2900 BC), has since become the symbol for sleep and wakefulness [4].

There are many references to a close relationship between sleep and death in poetic, religious, and other writings, such as the following quotations: "There she (Aphrodite) met sleep, the brother of death" (Homer's *Iliad*, c. 700 BC); "Sleep and death are similar…sleep is one sixtieth (i.e., one piece) of death (The Talmud, Berachoth 576)"; "The deepest sleep resembles death" (The Bible, I Samuel 26:12); "Each night, when I go to sleep, I die. And the next morning, when I wake up; I am reborn" (Mahatma Gandhi, the greatest proponent of nonviolence and about whom Einstein stated that such a man will never again walk this planet in another century). The Islamic literature also indicates some similarities between sleep and death [5] as noted in this Qur'anic verse: "It is Allah who takes away the souls (Wafat) at the time of their death, and those that die not during their sleep" [39.42].

William Shakespeare, the great English literary figure in the Elizabethan era (seventeenth century) evoked themes about sleep throughout his writings. One referring to sleep and death appeared in *Macbeth, Act II, Scene ii:*

Sleep that knits up the ravell'd sleave of care,
The death of each day's life, sore labour's bath,
Balm of hurt minds, great nature's second course,
Chief nourisher in life's feast.

There are many other memorable quotes from Shakespeare referring to sleep and dream. Iago after attempting to poison Othello's mind about Desdemona stated:

Not poppy, nor mandragora,
Nor all the drowsy syrups of the World,
Shall ever medicine thee to that sweet sleep
Which thou owed'st yesterday. (William Shakespeare, Othello, Act iii, Scene 3)

It is interesting to note about opium and mandragora as sleeping aids (see Chap. 2) and the interpretation here is that despite using the best sleep medicine in the world, suspicious Othello will never again have a good night's sleep.

S. Chokroverty (✉)
JFK New Jersey Neuroscience Institute, 65 James Street,
Edison, NJ 08818, USA
e-mail: schok@att.net

M. Billiard
School of Medicine, University Montpellier I, Montpellier, France

Department of Neurology, Gui de Chauliac Hospital, 70 allée James
Anderson, 34090 Montpellier, France

S. Chokroverty, M. Billiard (eds.), *Sleep Medicine,* DOI 10.1007/978-1-4939-2089-1_1,
© Springer Science+Business Media, LLC 2015

Another famous Shakespearean quotation often used in sleep literature in reference to sleep, death, and dream is the following one:

To die: to sleep;

....

....

To Sleep: perchance to dream:ay, there's the rub;
For in that sleep of death what dreams may come
When we have shuffled off this mortal coil,
Must give us pause. (Hamlet, Act 3, Scene i)

The English romantic poet John Keats in his 1817 poem "sleep and poetry" touches on the soothing softer side of sleep as reflected in the following excerpt from that poem:

What is gentler than a wind in summer?

What is more tranquil than a musk-rose blowing?

What, but thee Sleep? Soft closer of our eyes!

Thee for enlivening all the cheerful eyes
That glance so brightly at the new sun-rise.

In contrast, the contemporary English poet Lord Byron touches on the reality of sleep:

Sleep hath its own world,
And a wide realm of wild reality,
And dreams in their development have breath,
And tears, and tortures, and the touch of joys.

Prior to the twentieth century, views about sleep were not based on solid scientific foundation. However, remarks by some of the astute physicians and scientists proved to be strikingly similar to the contemporary views about sleep. For example, the opinion of Paracelsus, a sixteenth-century physician, that "natural" sleep lasted 6 h, and the suggestion that individuals should not sleep too much or too little are similar to modern thinking (see [1]). The nineteenth-century physicians like Humboldt and Pfluger began to use principles of physiology and chemistry to explain sleep. The observations of Ishimori from Japan, in 1909 [6], and Legendre and Pieron from France, in 1913 [7], of sleep-promoting substances in the cerebrospinal fluid of animals during prolonged wakefulness were the beginnings of scientific research in the twentieth century. The table (Table 1.1) lists some milestones in the history of sleep medicine and sleep research. The discovery of the electroencephalographic (EEG) activity in rabbits and dogs by the English physician Caton, from Liverpool, England, in 1875, and, finally, documentation of EEG activity from the surface of human brain by Hans Berger (Fig. 1.1), the German physician from Jena, in 1929 [8], provided the scientific framework for contemporary sleep research. It is notable that the nineteenth-century German physiologist, Kohlschutter, thought that sleep was deepest during the first few hours based on his construction of classical depth-of-sleep curve, using auditory thresholds at different hours of

the night [9]. Modern sleep laboratory studies have generally confirmed this observation.

The description of sleep staging (stages A–E) based on the EEG changes in 1937 by the American physiologist Loomis et al. [10] followed by the discovery of rapid eye movement (REM) sleep by Aserinsky and Kleitman [11] at the University of Chicago, in 1953, propelled sleep research to the forefront of neuroscience (Fig. 1.2). Later observations of muscle atonia in cats by Jouvet (Fig. 1.2) and Michel, from Lyon, France, in 1959 [12], and human laryngeal muscles by Berger, from the USA, in 1961 [13], completed the discovery of all major components of REM sleep. In addition to phasic eye movements, later investigators observed other important phasic components of human REM sleep: middle ear muscle activity (MEMA) [14]; periorbital integrated potentials (PIPs) [15]; phasic tongue movements [16]; transient myoclonic muscle bursts; phasic penile erections; phasic blood pressure; heart rate variability. It is interesting to note that Griesinger, in 1868, observed REMs under closed eyelids concomitant with twitching movements of the body in sleeping humans, and he commented that these were connected to dreams [17]. In 1892, Ladd, a professor of Psychiatry at Yale University in the USA, distinguished between fixed eye position in dreamless sleep as opposed to moving eyes in dreaming sleep [18]. In 1930, Jacobson also observed eye movements during dreaming sleep [19]. Freud, in 1895, observed that body muscles became relaxed during dreaming [20]. These findings of seemingly paralyzed body, REMs, and transient body muscle twitching during dreaming sleep before the advent of polysomnographic recordings are remarkable and astute clinical observations. Another developmental milestone in the history of sleep medicine research is the publication of a paper by Dement (Fig. 1.2) and Kleitman [21] documenting cyclic variation of EEG during sleep in relation to eye movements, body motility, and dreaming. Subsequent production by Rechtschaffen and Kales [22], of the standard sleep scoring technique monograph, in 1968, remained the gold standard until the American Academy of Sleep Medicine published the Manual for the Scoring of Sleep and Associated Events in 2007 [23].

Before outlining further clinical milestones in the history of sleep medicine, we briefly mention about the progress and evolution of some basic science research in sleep medicine. As early as 1920, before the discovery of EEG, McWilliam observed changes in blood pressure (BP), heart rate (HR), respiration, and other autonomic changes (e.g., penile erections) episodically during sleep [24]. He also distinguished between "disturbed" and "undisturbed" sleep by noting that during "disturbed" sleep there was an increase in BP and HR [25].

In the first quarter of the last century, Von Economo (see Fig. 20.1 an astute young Austrian neurologist, cleverly observed that those patients with encephalitis lethargica, suf-

Table 1.1 Some milestones in the history of sleep medicine

Willis T (AD 1672): Description of RLS like symptoms
de Mairan J-J D (AD 1729): Discovery of a circadian clock in plants
Parkinson J (AD 1817): Description of Parkinson's disease with sleep dysfunction
Gelineau E. (AD 1880): Description of narcolepsy
Ishimori K (AD 1909) from Japan, and Legendre R and Pieron H (AD 1913) from France independently described sleep-inducing factors ("hypnotoxin") in the brain of sleep-deprived dogs
Von Economo (AD 1926–1929): The concept of a wakefulness centre in the posterior and a hypnogenic centre in the anterior hypothalamus
Hans Berger (AD 1929): First report of EEG activity on the surface of the scalp of human
Bremer F (AD 1935): Feline preparations of midbrain transection causing cerveau isole and spinomedullary transection causing encephale isole
Loomis AL, Harvey EN, Hobart G (AD 1937): EEG Sleep staging A-E
Kleitman N (AD 1939): Considered "father of sleep medicine research" wrote "Sleep and Wakefulness," a comprehensive tome on all past and present sleep research citing 4337 references
Hess WR (AD 1944): Sleep, a well-coordinated active process and induced sleep in animals by stimulating the thalamus
Ekbom KA (AD 1945): Modern description of RLS
Moruzzi G, Magoun H (AD 1949): Discovery of the ascending reticular activating system (ARAS) in the upper brain stem as an arousal system
Aserinsky E, Kleitman N (AD 1953): Discovery of rapid eye movements
Burwell CS, et al. (1956): Pickwickian syndrome (obesity-hypoventilation syndrome)
Dement W, Kleitman N (AD 1957): Described cyclic variation of sleep body, and eye movements throughout the night
Jouvet M, Michel M (AD 1959): REM muscle atonia in cat
Oswald I (1959): Hypnic jerks at sleep onset
Aschoff J (1960): Discovery of circadian rhythms in human
Severinghaus JW, Mitchell RA (AD 1962): Described Ondine's curse or central hypoventilation, syndrome
Jouvet M, Delorme JF (AD 1965): Animal model of RBD in cat
Jung R, Kuhlo W (AD 1965): Obstructive sleep apnea syndrome (OSAS) called Pickwickian syndrome in those days)
Gastaut H, et al. (AD 1965): First PSG recording in OSAS
Gastaut H, Tassinari C, Duron B (1965): Discovery of the site of obstruction in upper airway obstructive sleep apnea syndrome (OSAS)
Lugaresi E, et al. (AD 1965): First Polygraphic recording in RLS
Broughton R (1968): Disorders of arousal (sleepwalking, sleep terror, confusional arousal)
Rechtschaffen A, Kales A (AD 1968): Sleep stage scoring techniques
Khulo W, Doll E, Franck MC (AD 1969): Tracheostomy for OSAS
Fujita S, et al. (AD 1981): Uvulopalatopharyngoplasty (UPPP) for OSAS
Lydic R, Schoene WC, Czeisler C, Moore-Ede MC (1980); Discovery of human circadian clock in the suprachiasmatic nucleus
Coleman RM (AD 1980): Periodic limb movements in sleep (PLMS)
Sullivan C, Issa F, Berthon-Jones, et al. (1981): Introduction of CPAP to reverse OSA
Honda Y (AD 1983): Association of HLA-DR2 in narcolepsy
Lugaresi E, et al. (AD 1986): Nocturnal paroxysmal dystonia (NPD)
Schenck C, Mahowald M (AD 1986): Description of human RBD
Lugaresi E, et al. (1986): Fatal familial insomnia
de Lecea L, Kilduff T, Peyron C, et al. (1998): Indentification of two neuropeptides independently (hypocretin 1 and 2)
Sakurai T, Amemiya A, Ishii M, et al. (1998): Indentification of two neuropeptides independently (orexin A and B)
Lin L, Faraco J, Li R, et al. (1999) Animal models of narcolepsy-cataplexy with mutation of hypocretin receptor 2 gene
Chemelly R, Willie J, Sinton C, et al. (1999): Prepro-orexin knockout mice causing narcolepsy-cataplexy phenotype
Allen R P, Barker P B, Wehrl F, Song HK, Earley CJ (2001): Identified decreased iron acquisition in substantia nigra and iron-dopamine connection in RLS (Willis–Ekbom Disease) patients
Winkelmann J, et al. (2007); Stefansson H, et al. (2007): Genome-wide association studies identified novel RLS susceptibility genes

RLS restless legs syndrome, *EEG* electroencephalography, *PSG* polysomnography, *RBD REM* sleep behavior disorder

fering from excessive sleepiness, had extensive lesions in the posterior hypothalamus at autopsy, whereas those having severe insomnia had prominent lesions in the anterior hypothalamus. Based on these observations, he predicted that sleep-and-wake-promoting neurons reside in the anterior and posterior hypothalamus, respectively [26]. These findings propelled further research into generating fundamental theories about sleep and wakefulness. It is interesting to note

that in 1809, Luigi Rolando produced a permanent state of sleepiness after removing the cerebral hemispheres in the birds, and Marie Jan Pierre Flourens, in 1822, repeated the same experiment in pigeons producing similar results. Experiments by Ranson, Hess, and Dikshit, during 1930-1934, and later, Nauta, in 1946, (see [27]) confirmed Economo's conclusion of existence of sleep center in the anterior hypothalamus. However, the emphasis shifted toward passive

Fig. 1.1 Hans Berger

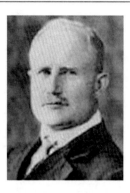

theory of sleep following publication by the Belgian physiologist Bremer [28] of two preparations in cats: Cerveau isole and encephale isole. Bremer (Fig. 1.3) found that midcollicular transection (cerveau isole) produced somnolence in the acute stage and that transection at the spinomedullary junction (encephale isole) showed EEG fluctuations between wakefulness and sleep, indicating that, in cerveau isole preparation, all specific sensory stimuli were withdrawn from the brain facilitating sleep. This conclusion was modified later to reflect the role of nonspecific ascending reticular activating system (ARAS) in maintenance of wakefulness, following the discovery by Moruzzi and Magoun [29], in 1949, of the existence of reticular formation in the center of the brain stem. The passive theory was subsequently challenged by the findings of persistent EEG and behavioral signs of alertness after midpontine pretrigeminal brain stem transection experiments by Batini et al. in 1959 [30]. This preparation was only a few millimeters below the section that produced

somnolence in the cerveau isole preparation. These observations implied that structures at the mesopontime junctions between these two preparations (cerveau isole and midpontial pretrigeminal) are responsible for wakefulness. It has been demonstrated that cholinergic neurons in the peduncedupontine (PPT) and laterodorsal tegmental (LDT) nuclei in the mesopontine junction and their projections to cerebral hemispheres through thalamus and forebrain regions in addition to ascending aminergic, hypocretinergic, and dopaminergic neurons maintain alertness. There is clear scientific evidence, based on discrete lesion, ablation, stimulation, extracellular and intracellular studies, as well as immunohistochemical studies using c-fos activation, that sleep is not just a passive but an active state. The contemporary theory for sleep includes both active and passive mechanisms. Hypothalamic sleep/wake switch theory proposed by Saper et al. in 2001 [31] is currently the most popular theory of nonrapid eye movement (NREM) sleep. Briefly, there is a reciprocal interaction between two groups of antagonistic GABAergic and galaninergic sleep-promoting neurons in the ventrolateral preoptic (VLPO) region of the anterior hypothalamus and wake-promoting neurons in the tuberomammillary histaminergic neurons of the posterior hypothalamus, lateral hypothalamic hypocretinergic, basal forebrain, and mesopontine tegmental clolinergic, dopaminergic and brain stem noradrenergic and serotonergic neurons. Sleep–wake is thus self-reinforcing; when one end of the switch is on (firing actively), the other end is "off" (disfaciliation). Disruption of one side of the switch will cause instability due to destabilization of

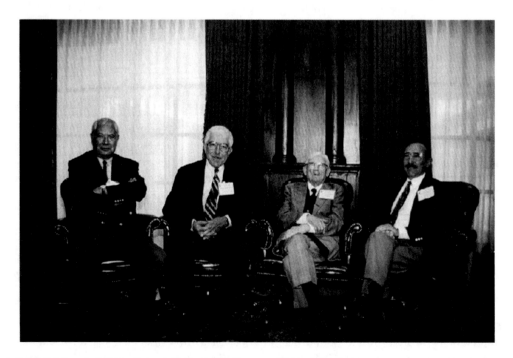

Fig. 1.2 From left, Michel Jouvet, William Dement, Nathaniel Kleitman, and Eugene Aserinsky

Fig. 1.3 Frédéric Bremer

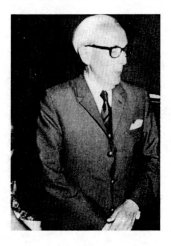

the switch. For REM sleep, currently, there are three models available. The earliest one proposed, in 1975, is the McCarley–Hobson model of reciprocal interaction between brain stem "REM-on" cholinergic and "REM-off" aminergic neurons initiated by GABAergic interneurons through pontine reticular formation (PRF) effector neurons [32]. This model stood the test of time until challenged by Saper's group in 2006 [33] who proposed a "flip–flop" switch model, with sublaterodorsal (SLD) GABAergic neurons in the pons ("REM-on"), initiating REM sleep through glutamatergic mechanism, and, at the same time, inhibiting "REM-off" GABAergic neurons in the ventrolateral periaqueductal grey and lateral pontine tegmentum. Ventral SLD through glutamatergic neurons activates glycine–GABA interneurons causing motor neuron hyperpolarization and muscle atonia, whereas dorsal SLD-ascending glutamatergic system of neurons activates forebrain to cause EEG desynchronization. The latest model is that proposed by Luppi et al. [34] in which, during REM sleep, SLD glutamatergic "REM-on" neurons are activated with deactivation of "REM-off" GABAergic ventrolateral periaqueductal grey and mesopontine tegmentum. Ventral SLD glutamatergic neurons, using both a direct pathway to spinal cord and an indirect one through ventromedial medulla, activate glycinergic and GABAergic inhibitory interneurons, causing hyperpolarization of motor neurons and causing REM atonia, a hallmark of REM sleep state. The dorsal SLD glutamatergic neurons project upward to activate thalamocortical system and subsequent EEG desynchronization. The spectacular advances in basic science research in sleep in the twentieth and twenty-first centuries stimulated tremendous growth of clinical sleep medicine, giving rise to "sleep disorders medicine" as a separate specialty recognized by the American Medical Association, as such, in 1996. In the following sections, we summarize a part of this sleep medicine revolution.

Before elaborating on some clinical milestones in the evolution and history of sleep medicine, we should like to mention that famous novelists of the past centuries gave colorful descriptions of characters, seemingly having distinctive symptoms of primary sleep disorders, before these entered the scientific literature. We cite the following examples: The American novelist Edgar Alan Poe in *Premature Burial* describing narcoleptic-like symptoms in a character published in 1844 (36 years before Gelineau's descriptions of narcolepsy); sleep paralysis of the character Ishmael in the American novelist Herman Melville's *Moby Dick* [35] published in 1851 (25 years before the description of night palsy by Mitchell in 1876 [36]); sleep walking (somnambulism) of Lady Macbeth described by the famous English playwright William Shakespeare (c. 1603–1607) long before the description of this entity in the medical literature; REM sleep behavior disorder (RBD)-like symptoms in the *Ingenious Gentleman Don Quixote of La Mancha* by the famous Spanish author Miguel de Cervantes Saavedra in 1605 [37], centuries before description of RBD, in 1986, by Schenck et al. [38]; vivid nightmares in Shakespeare's *Macbeth, A Midsummer Night's Dream,* and *Richard III,* Tolstoy's *War and Peace* and *Anna Karenina,* and Dostoevsky's *Crime and Punishment* and *The Brothers Karamazou;* and sleep paralysis and nightmare of the protagonist in *The Horla* written by one of the greatest short storytellers, Guy de Maupassant of France, in 1887. Perhaps, the most famous of all these fictional characters is "The fat boy Joe" (Fig. 1.4) in *The Posthumous Papers of the Pickwick Club* [39] written, in 1836, by the famous British novelist Charles Dickens ("The object that presented itself to the eyes of the astonished clerk, was a boy—a wonderfully fat boy—habited as a serving lad, standing upright on the mat, with his eyes closed as if in sleep"). Joe was indeed fat, excessively sleepy, and snoring. One hundred and twenty years after Dickens' description of the somnolent "fat boy Joe," Burwel et al. [40] published a paper entitled "Extreme obesity associated with alveolar hypoventilation: A Pickwickian Syndrome." As pointed out by Comroe [41] and Lavie [42], this title created both literary and scientific errors. All members of Pickwick Club did not have this syndrome. There was also no evidence of apnea in Dickens' description of Joe. Furthermore, Burwel and coworkers erroneously attributed their patient's extreme somnolence to chronic hypercapnia related to hypoventilation. It is notable that, prior to Burwel et al.'s publications, Auchincloss et al. [43] and Siekert and coworkers [44] published similar cases in 1955. However, 50 years before Burwel et al.'s description, Osler, in 1906 [45], referred to Dickens' description of "the fat boy Joe": "An extraordinary phenomenon in excessively fat young persons is an uncontrollable tendency to sleep–like the fat boy in Pickwick." The first polygraphic recording of a Pickwickian patient was performed by Gerardy et al. [46] from Germany in 1960 showing repeated apneas during sleep, and the authors erred in attributing the patient's daytime somnolence to carbon dioxide poisoning similar to that by Burwel et al. In 1962, Drachman and Gumnit [47] in

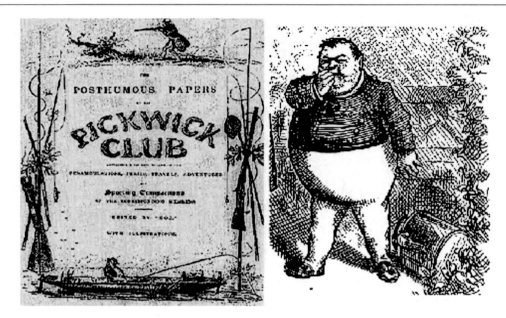

Fig. 1.4 Joe, the fat boy

Bethesda, Maryland, USA, recorded repeated sleep-related apneas and awakenings from a Pickwickian patient, and, like Gerardy et al., attributed excessive sleepiness to carbon dioxide poisoning. Two neurologists from Germany, Jung and Kuhlo [48] performed nighttime polygraphic sleep recordings for the first time in Pickwickian patients demonstrating recurrent sleep-related apneas and awakenings, and they correctly attributed their patients' excessive daytime sleepiness to sleep fragmentation and not to carbon dioxide poisoning, but they erred in ascribing the problem of breathing to disruption of brain stem respiratory center activity. It was, however, Gastaut (Fig. 1.5), Tassinari, and Duron, three neurologists from Marseilles, France [49], in 1965, who pointed out, for the first time, that the recurrent apneas and awakenings were related to upper airway obstruction during sleep. Lugaresi et al. [50], in a publication in the same year, confirmed the astute observations and conclusions of Gastaut et al., and described three types of apneas: central, mixed, and obstructive. They also made a very important observation of periodic fall of BP during apnea and rise on resumption of breathing. The next milestone in the evolution of the story of sleep apnea syndrome was the demonstration of dramatic relief of symptoms in these patients following tracheostomy (which bypasses the upper airway obstruction) by Kuhlo et al. [51], in 1969. In a brief report, published in the *Transactions of the American Neurological Association Journal,* in 1969, Chokroverty et al. [52], from the USA, made the following important observations after polygraphic study in four patients with obesity hypoventilation syndrome: Recurrent episodes of apneas–hypopneas associated with relative bradycardia followed by awakenings and relative tachycardia; systolic BP dropped by 20–30 mmHg during apnea–hy-

popnea; on many occasions EEG changes preceded respiratory alterations; oxygen inhalation produced more prolonged and frequent episodes of apneas indicating the importance of peripheral chemoreceptor-driven hypoxemia causing respiratory stimulation and arousal in presence of chronic daytime hypercapnia (these findings were confirmed by Guilleminault et al. [53] in a later publication). Another important observation was that in two patients, following weight loss of 100–150 pounds, symptoms improved, daytime arterial carbon dioxide tension normalized but apneas–hypopneas persisted, though these were less frequent (implying that obesity played a secondary aggravating and not a primary factor). Subsequently, numerous papers were published by Guilleminault et al. when he came to Stanford, California, USA, in 1972, and Guilleminault coined the term *sleep apnea syndrome* [53–55]. Then came the seminal paper by Sullivan et al. in 1981 [56] showing reversal of obstructive sleep apnea following continuous positive airway pressure (CPAP) delivered through the nose which revolutionized the treatment of this common condition associated with many adverse consequences to health. Subsequently, there was further development of positive pressure titration in terms of bi-level delivery (BiPAP), assisted servo ventilation (ASV), intermittent positive pressure ventilation (IPPV), and others. There was an explosion of growth in publication of papers on sleep apnea syndrome since 1990, and it is still continuing. The other developments in the continuing saga of evolution of sleep apnea syndrome include uvulopalatopharyngoplasty (UPPP) surgery by Fujita et al. [57], in 1981, and the use of dental appliance for treating upper airway obstructive sleep apnea. In 1962, in an abstract, Severinghaus and Mitchell [58] described two patients with failure of automatic control

Fig. 1.5 Henri Gastaut

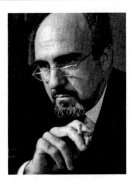

of ventilation following surgery in the medullospinal junction under the eponym *Ondine's curse* named after the water nymph in Giraudaux's play *Ondine* (see [41]). As pointed out by Comroe [41], the use of this term is full of literary and scientific errors.

Finally, to conclude the introductory section on clinical milestones in sleep medicine research, we must include one of the greatest clinical contributions in sleep medicine—Gelineau's description of *narcolepsy* in 1880 [59]. The term was derived from the Greek words *narkosis* (meaning "benumbing") and *lepsis* (meaning "overtake"). Gelineau (Fig. 1.6) also mentioned about atonic attacks (referring to these as "astasia") as essential features in addition to excessive sleepiness for diagnosis of this entity. Prior to Gelineau's classic paper, Westphal, in 1877 [60], described a familial form of excessive sleepiness associated with the waking episodes of loss of muscle tone, but Westphal unfortunately did not get any credit as he did not introduce the term narcolepsy which caught the imagination of the medical community, and the condition remained known as Gelineau's disease in France and Narcolepsy in the rest of the world. The waking atonic episodes were later defined by Lowenfeld (see [61]), in 1902, who called these spells *Kataplectische Starre* (German for cataplectic attacks). Redlich in 1915 (see [61]) used the terms *plotzlicher Tonusvertust* for sudden loss of muscle tone and *Korper Schlaf* to mean body sleep. Adie, in 1926 (see [62]) calling narcolepsy a specific disease, sui generis,

Fig. 1.6 Jean-Baptiste-Édouard Gélineau

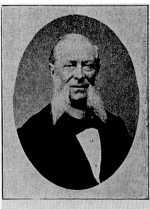

D' JEAN-BAPTISTE-ÉDOUARD GÉLINEAU

brought the entity to general recognition. Sleep paralysis was added to excessive sleepiness and cataplexy to symptom combination in this condition by Wilson in 1928, and this was later confirmed by Lhermitte and Daniels (see [61]). The fourth symptom "vivid hypnagogic hallucination" was added by Alajouaninine and Baruk, Redlich and Wenderowic (see [61]), and finally, Yoss and Daly [62] from Mayo Clinic coined the term *narcoleptic tetrad*. In fact, two other common symptoms should be added coining *narcoleptic hextad*: automatic behavior related to *microsleeps* (see [61]) and disturbed night sleep with repeated spontaneous arousals. Vogel, in 1960, described the characteristic sleep-onset REM periods (SOREMs) [63]. The multiple sleep latency test (MSLT) documenting pathologic sleepiness and SO-REMs were applied to the diagnosis of narcolepsy by Richardson et al. in 1978 [64]. The discovery by Honda et al. of a strong association of narcolepsy–cataplexy with the histocompatability antigen HLA-DR2 haplotype in both Asians and Caucasians [65] propelled narcolepsy research another step further toward autoimmune theory. Finally, the new and exciting era of sleep research began with the identification of two neuropeptides, in 1998, in the lateral hypothalamus and perifornical regions independently by two groups of neuroscientists. De Lecea et al. [66], from California, named these hypocretin 1 and 2, whereas Sakurai et al. [67], from Texas, called the same peptides orexin A and B. Within one year of this discovery, Lin et al. [68] produced a canine model of a human narcolepsy phenotype by mutation of hypocretin 2 receptors, and Chemelly et al. [69] created a similar phenotype in pre-prohyprocretin knockout mice. Shortly thereafter, Hara et al. [70] used transgenic mice to produce narcoleptic phenotype. Research progressed rapidly with documentation of the decreased hypocretin 1 in the cerebrospinal fluid of human narcolepsy–cataplexy syndrome followed by autopsy confirmation of the marked depletion of lateral hypothalamic orexin neurons in human narcolepsy patients [71, 72]. These findings confirm that human narcolepsy is a hypocretin deficiency disorder, thus providing proof for the prophetic prediction of young Austrian neurologist Von Economo made in 1930 that the cause for the disease described by Westphal and Gelineau resides in the lateral and posterior hypothalamic region [26]. The dramatic development and remarkable progress in basic and clinical research in sleep medicine are described in the following chapters of this book.

References

1. Borbely A. Secrets of sleep. New York: Basic Books; 1984.
2. Wolpert S. A new history of India. New York: Oxford University Press; 1982. p. 48.
3. Urandg L, Ruffner FG Jr., editors. Allusions-cultural literary, biblical and historical: a thematic dictionary. Detroit: Gale; 1986.

4. Thorpy M. History of sleep medicine. In: Montagna P, Chokroverty S, editors. Handbook of clinical neurology: sleep disorders, part 1, vol. 98 (3rd series), Amsterdam: Elsevier; 2011. pp. 3–25.

5. Bahamman AS, Gozal D. Qur'anic insights into sleep. Nat Sci Sleep. 2012;4:81–7.

6. Ishimori K. True causes of sleep—a hypnogenic substance as evidenced in the brain of sleep-deprived animals. Igakkai Zasshi (Tokyo). 1909;23:429.

7. Legendre R, Pieron H. Recherches sur le besoin de sommeil consecutif a une veille prolongée. Z Allerg Physiol. 1913;14:235.

8. Berger H. Uber das Elektroenkephalogramm des Menschen. Arch Psychiatr Nervenber. 1929;87:527.

9. Kohlschutter E. Messungen der Festigkeit des Schlafes. Z ration Med. 1862;17:209–53.

10. Loomis AL, Harvey EN, Hobart GA. Cerebral states during sleep, as studied by human brain potentials. J Exp Physiol. 1937;21:127.

11. Aserinsky E, Kleitman N. Regularly occurring periods of eye motility and concomitant phenomena during sleep. Science. 1953;118:273.

12. Jouvet, M, Michel F. Correlatios electromyographique du sommeil chez le chat decortique et mesencephalique chronique. CR Soc Bil (Paris). 1959;153:422–5.

13. Berger RJ. Tonus of extrinsic laryngeal muscles during sleep and dreaming. Science. 1961;134:840.

14. Pessah M, Roffwarg H. Spontaneous middle ear muscle activity in man: a rapid eye movement sleep phenomenon. Science. 1972;178:773–776.

15. Rechtschaffen A, Molinari S, Watson R, Wincor MZ. Extra-ocular potentials: a possible indicator of PGO activity in the human. Psychophysiology. 1970;7:336.

16. Chokroverty S. Phasic tongue movements in human rapid-eye-movement sleep. Neurology. 1980;30:665–8.

17. Griesinger W. Berliner medizinich-psycologische Gesellschaft. Arch Psychiatr Nervenkr. 1868;1:200–4.

18. Ladd GT. Contribution to the psychology of visual dreams. Mind. 1892;1:299–304.

19. Jacobson E. Electrical measurements of neuromuscular states during mental activities. III. Visual imagination and recollection. AM J Physiol. 1930;95:694–702.

20. Freud S. Die Traumdeutung. Liepzig: Franz Deuticke; 1900. (The interpretation of dreams, translated by James Strachey. New York: Basic Books; 1955).

21. Dement W, Kleitman N. Cyclic variations in EEG during sleep and their relation to eye movements, body motility, and dreaming. Electroencephlogr Clin Neurphysiol. 1957;9:673.

22. Rechtschaffen A, Kales A. A manual of standardized terminology, techniques and scoring systems for sleep stages of human subjects. Los Angeles: UCLA Brain Information Service/Brain Research Institute, Techniques and Scoring Systems for Sleep Stages of Human Subjects; 1968.

23. The AASM Manual 2007 for the scoring of sleep and associated events. Rules, terminology and technical specifications. American Academy of Sleep Medicine, Westchester, IL, USA, 2007.

24. Mc William JA. Some applications of physiology to medicine. III. Blood pressure and heart action in sleep and dreams. Br Med J. 1920;II:1196–200.

25. McWilliam JA. Some applications of physiology to medicine. III. Blood pressure and heart action in sleep and dreams: their relation to hemorrhages, angina and sudden death. Brit Med J. 1923;II:1196–200.

26. von Economo C. Sleep as a problem of localization. J Nerve Ment Dis. 1930;71:249.

27. Kleitman N. Sleep and wakefulness. Chicago: University of Chicago Press; 1939.

28. Bremer F. Cerveau "isole" et physiologie du sommeil. C R Soc Biol. 1935;118:1235.

29. Moruzzi G, Magoun H. Brainstem reticular formation and activation of the EEG. Electroencephalogr Clin Neurophysiol. 1949;1:455–73.

30. Battini C, Magni F, Paletini M, Rossi GF, Zanchetti M. Neuronal mechanisms underlying EEG and behavioral activation in the mid-pontine pretigeminal cat. Arch Ital Biol. 1959;97:13–25.

31. Saper CB, Scammell TE, Lun J. Hypothalamic regulation of sleep and circadian rhythms. Nature. 2005;437:1257–63.

32. McCartey RW, Hobson JA. Neuronal excitability modulation over the sleep cycle: a structural and mathematical model. Science. 1975;189:58–60.

33. Lu J, Sherman D, Devor M, Saper CB. A putative flip-flop switch for control of REM sleep. Nature. 2006;441:589–94.

34. Luppi PH, Clement O, Sapin E, et al. The neuronal network responsible for paradoxical sleep and its dysfunction causing narcolepsy and rapid eye movement (REM) behavior disorder. Sleep Med Rev. 2011;15:153–63.

35. Herman J. An instance of sleep paralysis in Moby-Dick. Sleep. 1997;20:577–9.

36. Weir Mitchell S. Some disorders of sleep. AM J Med Sci. 1890;100:190–227.

37. Iranzo A, Santamaria J, de Riquer M. Sleep and sleep disorders in Don Quixote. Sleep Med. 2004;5:97–100.

38. Schenck CH, Bundlie SR, Ettinger MG, Mahowald MW. Chronic behavioral disorders in human sleep: a new category of parasomnia. Sleep. 1986;9:293–308.

39. Dickens C. The posthumous papers of the pickwick club. London: Chapman and Hall; 1837.

40. Burwell CS, Robin ED, Wahley RD, Bickelmann AG. Extreme obesity with alve-olar hypoventilation: a Pickwickian syndrome. Am J Med. 1956;21:811–8.

41. Comroe JH Jr. Frankenstein, Pickwick and Ondine. AM Rev Respir Dis. 1975;111:689–92.

42. Lavie P. Who was the first to use the term Pickwickian in connection with sleepy patients? History of sleep apnea syndrome. Sleep Med Rev. 2008;12:5–17.

43. Auchincloss JH Jr., Cook E, Renzetti AD. Clinical and physiolgical aspects of a case of obesity, polycythemia and alveolar hypoventilation. J Clin Invest. 1955;34:1537–45.

44. Sieker HO, Estes EW Jr., Kesler GA, Mcintoch HAD. Cardiopulmonary syndrome associated with extreme obesity. J Clin Invest. 1955;34:1955.

45. Osler W. The principles and practice of medicine. New York: Appleton; 1906.

46. Gerardy W, Herberg D, Khun HM. Vergleichende Untersuchungen der Lungenfunktion und des Elektroencephalogramms bei zwei Patienten mit Pickwickian Syndrome. Z Klin Med. 1960;156:362–80.

47. Drachman DB, Gumnit RJ. Periodic alteration of consciousness in the Pickwickian syndrome. Arch Neurol. 1962;6:471–7.

48. Jung R, Kuhlo W. Neurophysiological studies of abnormal night sleep and the Pickwickian syndrome. In: Albert K, Baly C, Stradl JP, editors. Sleep mechanisms. Amsterdam: Elsevier; 1965. pp. 140–59.

49. Gastaut H, Tassinari CA, Duron B. Etude polygraphique des manifestations, épisodiques (hypniques et respiratoires) du syndrome de Pickwick. Rev Neurol. 1965;112:568–79.

50. Lugaresi E, Coccagna G, Tassinari GA, Ambrosetto C. Particularites cliniques et polygraphiques du syndrome d'impatience des membres inferieurs. Rev Neurol. 1965;113:545.

51. Kuhlo W, Doll E, Franck MC. Erfolgreiche Behandlung eines Pickwick-syndromes durch eine Dauertrachealkanule. Deut Med Wochenschr. 1969;94:1286–90.

52. Chokroverty S. Hypoventilation syndrome and obesity: a polygraphic study. Trans Am Neurol Assoc. 1969;94:240–2.

53. Guilleminault C, Eldridge FL, Dement CW. Insomnia with sleep apnea: a new syndrome. Science. 1973;181:856–8.

54. Guilleminault C, Dement WC. Two hundred and thirty-five cases of excessive daytime sleepiness. Diagnosis and tentative classification. J Neurol Sci. 1977;31:13–27.

55. Guilleminault C, Tilkian A, Dement WC. The sleep apnea syndrome. Annu Rev Med. 1976;27:465–84.

56. Sullivan CE, Berthon-Jones M, Issa FG, et al. Reversal of obstructive sleep apnea by continuous positive airway pressure applied through nose. Lancet. 1981;1:862–5.

57. Fujita S, Conway W, Zorick F, Roth T. Surgical-correction of anatomic abnormalities in sleep-apnea syndrome-uvulopalatopharyngoplasty. Otolaryngol-Head Neck Surg. 1981;89:923–34.

58. Severinghaus JW, Mitchell RA. Ondine's curse-failure of respiratory automaticity while awake. Clin Res. 1962;10:122.

59. Gelineau J. De la narcolepsie. Gaz des Hop (Paris). 1880;53:535–637.

60. Westpal C. Eigenthumlich mit einschlafen verbundene Anfalle. Arch Psychiatr Nervenkr. 1877;7:631–5.

61. Broughton RJ. Narcolepsy. In: Thorpy MJ, editor. Handbook of sleep disorders. New York: Marcel Dekker; 1990. pp. 197–216.

62. Yoss RE, Daly DD. Criteria for the diagnosis of the narcolepsy syndrome. Proc May Clin. 1957;3:320–8.

63. Vogel G. Studies in psychophysiology of dreams III. The dream of narcolepsy. Arc Gen Psychiatry. 1960;3:421–8.

64. Richardson G, Carskadon M, Flagg W, van den Hoed J, Dement W, Mitler M. Excessive daytime sleepiness in man: multiple sleep measurement in narcolepsy and control subjects. Electroencephalogr Clin Nuerophysiol. 1978;45:621–37.

65. Juji T, Satake M, Honda Y, Doi Y. HLA antigens in Japanese patients with narcolepsy: all the patients were DR2 positive. Tissue Antigens. 1984;24:316–9.

66. DeLecea L, Kilduff TS, Peyron C, et al. The hypocretins: hypothalamus-specific peptides with neuroexcitatory activity. Proc Natl Acad Sci U S A. 1998;95:322–7.

67. Sakurai T, Amemiya A, Ishii M, et al. Orexins and orexin receptors: a family of hypothalamic neuropeptides and G protein-coupled receptors that regulate feeding behavior. Cell. 1998;92:573–85.

68. Lin L, Faraco J, Li R, et al. The sleep disorder canine narcolepsy is caused by a mutation in the hypocretin (orexin) receptor 2 gene. Cell. 1999;98:365–376.

69. Chemelly RM, Willie JT, Sinton CM, et al. Narcolepsy in orexin knockout mice: molecular genetics of sleep regulation. Cell. 1999;98:437–51.

70. Hara J, Beuckmann CT, Nambu T, et al. Genetic ablation of orexin neurons in mice results in narcolepsy, hypophagia, and obesity. Neuron. 2001;30:345–54.

71. Thannical TC, Moore RY, Nienhuis R, et al. Reduced number of hypocretin neurons in human narcolepsy. Neuron. 2000;27:469–74.

72. Peyron C, Faraco J, Rogers W, Ripley B, Overeem S, Charnay Y, et al. A mutation in a case of early onset narcolepsy and a generalized absence of hypocretin peptides in human narcoleptic brains. Nat Med. 2000;6:991–1007.

Part I

Evolution of Sleep Medicine by Historical Periods

Sleep in Ancient Egypt

2

Tarek Asaad

Introduction

Despite being the oldest civilization in history, there is still an increasing fascination for everything Egyptian, something which was referred to as *Egyptomania* [1]. Regarding sleep medicine, the contribution of ancient Egypt dates back to 4000 BC and it tackles various aspects concerning the nature of sleep and dreaming, dream interpretation, use of sleep as therapy, description of sleep problems like insomnia, description of treatments for sleep disorders, and others.

How Were the Words "Sleep" and "Dream" Expressed in *Hieroglyphics* (Ancient Egyptian Language)?

The ancient Egyptians used the word *qed* (symbolized by a bed) to denote sleep, and the word *rswt* or *resut* (depicted as an open eye) to refer to dream. The literal translation of *rswt* means *to come awake*; thus, a dream is expressed in hieroglyphics by the symbol of *bed,* combined with the symbol of *open eye*. Such a combination makes the word dream to be read as *awaken within sleep,* which is an early description of the physiologic similarity of dreams to wakefulness, despite being asleep [2].

Dream =" *rswt*" (**awaken**) (**open eye**) +" *qed*" (**sleep**) (**bed**)

This symbol may be pointing also to the state of consciousness that we call today *lucid dreaming* [3].

T. Asaad (✉)
Ain Shams University Hospital, Institute of Psychiatry-
Psychophysiology & Sleep Research Unit, 14 Aly El-Gendy Street,
PO Box 11371, Nasr City, Cairo, Egypt
e-mail: dr.tarekasaad@yahoo.com

What Is the Meaning (Concept) of Sleep in Ancient Egyptian Culture?

Ancient Egyptians believed each person has five bodies [4]:
1. *ka* = creative or divine power or the living physical body
2. *ba* = soul, able to travel beyond the physical body
3. *akh* or *Shat* = body of the deceased in the afterlife (the corpse body) which means the union of the *ka* and *ba*
4. *the name* = living part of the person
5. *the shadow* = another living part of the person

This description of multidimensional levels of the self has something to do with sleep, as the ancient Egyptians believed in the ability of the *ba* (soul) to travel beyond the physical body during sleep. The *ba* was represented in hieroglyphics as a human-headed bird floating above the sleeping body. In that sense, sleep was viewed to be similar, in some aspect, to death, in which the person is in a different state or a different world. Being strong believers in the afterlife, sleep was considered as a way or outlet to that mysterious world and a means through which a person can communicate with the dead as well as his *gods*. For this reason, it is not surprising to find some rituals related to sleep to resemble what is adopted in preparation for death [5].

The headrests used for the act of sleeping during life were most probably of a symbolic nature and were essential requirement for funeral—to be kept with the dead in his burial chamber, acting as a pillow for eternal sleep, ensuring the head remained physically intact with the body in the afterlife (Fig. 2.1). Thus, if the tomb represented the home for the deceased, the burial chamber represented the bedroom [6].

The idea that the dead were sleeping or that they occupied another dimension not totally disconnected from the living is indicated in letters to the dead written on *papyrus* or *ostraca*, including Coffin Texts. These Coffin Texts functioned as ritually protective spells and instructions, intended to ensure safe passage to the afterlife. In Coffin Text (CT) 74, it was written "Oh sleeper, turn about in this place which you do not know, but I know it. Come that we may raise his head. Come that we may reassemble his bones" [6].

S. Chokroverty, M. Billiard (eds.), *Sleep Medicine,* DOI 10.1007/978-1-4939-2089-1_2, 13
© Springer Science+Business Media, LLC 2015

Fig. 2.1 Two headrests from the tomb of Tutankhamun [6]

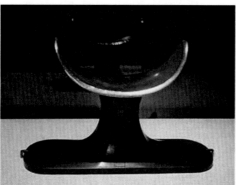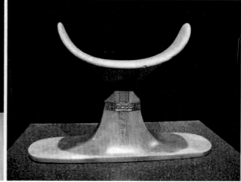

How Were Dreams Dealt with by Ancient Egyptians?

The Importance of Dreams

Like many ancient cultures, the Egyptians put quite a bit of emphasis on dreams. They believed the gods could show themselves in dreams, delivering messages that could guide them in their lives, i.e., the received messages might cure an illness or help them make important decisions, to the point of deciding where to build a new temple or when to wage a war.

The Egyptians also believed that their dreams could serve as a window to see the activities of the dead. However, they often feared these types of dreams, being afraid that this could bring about unwanted evil spirits [7].

Types of Dreams

The records list three main types of dreams [8]:
1. Those in which the gods would demand some pious act
2. Those that contained warnings (perhaps about illness) or revelations
3. Those that came about through ritual

Dream Incubation

Like other Near Eastern people, the Egyptians believed that the dreams could serve as oracles, bringing messages from the gods. The best way to get the desired answer, especially in sickness, was to induce or "incubate" dreams (Incubate comes from the Latin *incubare*, meaning *to lie down upon*). To incubate dreams, Egyptians would travel to a sanctuary or shrine, where they slept overnight on a special *dream bed* in the hope of receiving divine advice, comfort, or healing from their dreams. There were dream or sleep temples built specifically for this reason. The temples were open to everyone who believed in the god the temple was dedicated to, as long as they were considered pure. To achieve this, the person often went through a ritual of cleansing that included

fasting and abstinence for several days prior to entering the temple to assure their purity. The name of the god the person hoped to contact at the temple was written on a piece of linen and that linen cloth was burned in a lamp while at the temple. To help call the god, the dreamer would often recite a special prayer to him or her. Once they visited the ancient Egyptian dream temple, the person would often go to a priest or dream interpreter for dream analysis [7].

Dream Analysis in Ancient Egypt (The Dream Book)

Because they put so much stock into dreams, it was important for Egyptians to be able to understand the significance and meaning of their dreams. Like many others, some Egyptians kept a dream book—a book that chronicled their dreams and the interpretation of them. One such dream book, written on papyrus, dates all the way back to approximately 1275 BC, during the reign of Ramesses II [9, 10] (Fig. 2.2).

It is believed that the ancient Egyptian dream book kept in the British Museum in London had many owners as it was passed down for more than a century. All in all, the dream book included 108 different dreams, which included such activities as weaving, stirring, seeing, eating, and drinking.

The dreams were categorized into good (*auspicious*) dreams and bad (*inauspicious*) dreams, with the bad dreams being written in red, a color of bad omens. In this book, there are hieratic signs that state such interpretations, as that it is good when a man dreams he sees himself looking out of a window. Even a man seeing himself dead was seen as a good sign, meaning that he would live a long life. However, if a man dreamed he saw his own face in a mirror it was a bad omen. Also, dreaming of putting your own face to the ground was seen as a bad omen. It was believed that that particular dream meant that the dead wanted something.

Qenherkhepshef's dream book was a family affair; penned by his grandson, the scribe Amen-nakht, who was the son of Kha-em-nun, Qenherkhepshef's oldest child. The texts allow insight, not only into the dreams of these ancient people but also into the everyday experiences of their lived lives.

Fig. 2.2 Qenherkhepshef's dream book, BM 10683,3 [10]

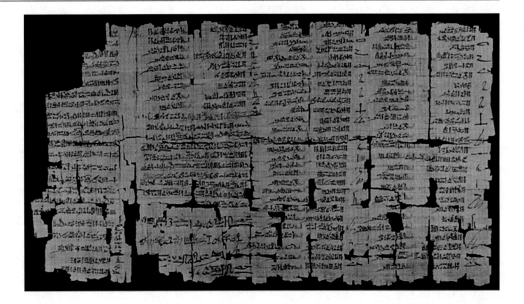

Listing of Dreams in the Dream Book [9]:

The dream book is divided into lists of auspicious and inauspicious dreams:

a. Auspicious dreams (good dreams)

- If a man sees himself eating crocodile meat, it is good, meaning that he becomes an official among his people.
- If a man sees himself burying an old man, it is good, meaning prosperity.
- If a man sees himself sawing wood, it is good, meaning his enemies are dead.
- If a man sees himself seeing the moon shining, it is good, meaning a pardon from God.
- If a man sees himself in a dream slaying a hippopotamus, it is good, meaning that a large meal from the palace will follow.
- If a man sees himself in a dream plunging into the river, it is good, meaning purification from all evil.

b. Inauspicious dreams (bad dreams)

- If a man sees himself in a dream seizing one of his lower legs, it is bad, meaning a report about him by those who are yonder (the dead).
- If a man sees himself measuring barley in a dream, it is bad, meaning the rising of worlds against him.
- If a man sees himself bitten by a dog in a dream, it is bad, meaning that he is touched by magic.
- If a man sees himself in a mirror in a dream, it is bad, meaning that he will find another wife.
- If a man sees himself in a dream making love to a woman, it is bad, because it means mourning.

- If a man sees himself in a dream looking at an ostrich, it is bad, meaning that harm will befall him.
- If a man sees himself in a dream feeding cattle, it is bad, because it means wandering the earth.
- If a man sees himself in a dream casting wood into water, it is bad, meaning bringing suffering to his house.
- If a man sees himself removing the nails of his fingers, it is bad, because this means removal of the work of his hands.
- If a man sees the gods making cessation of tears for him in a dream, it is bad, because it means fighting.

It is not known to what extent these interpretative guides were used in daily life. Few people would have had access to such texts; few were literate and able to read them. There are indications that many villages may have had a priest, or a local scribe, or else who could interpret dreams in which deceased relatives or gods might appear. Some later New Kingdom Deir el Medina texts refer to "the wise woman" of the village who supplied advice. Such *seers* were consulted not only concerning dreams, but also on other issues affecting daily life including disputes with neighbors, or concerns over failing crops. Dreams could be powerful experiences and revelatory dreams in particular, were taken seriously [11].

Most Prevalent Dreams

Like today, the ancient Egyptians had some dreams that were more prevalent than others were. People often dreamed of breaking stones, which the Egyptians interpreted as having one's teeth fall out. Dreaming of your teeth falling out is still a common dream today [11].

Many often dreamed of drowning in the Nile or climbing to the top ship's mast. However, some other common dreams seem to defy explanation. Dreaming that your face turned into a leopard was a common dream in ancient Egypt [11].

Reading Dreams in Different Ancient Cultures, Compared to Egypt

Dream interpretation differed in various ancient cultures. The symbolic meaning of items in a dream might even have contradictory explanations. Table 2.1 is an illustration of how four different common items are symbolically interpreted in the ancient Egyptian culture, compared to other ancient cultures, namely the Assyrian, the Greek, and the Hebrew [8].

How Did Ancient Egyptian Medicine Deal with Sleep Disorders?

The medicine of ancient Egypt is one of the oldest documented scientific disciplines. It is said that, "If one had to be ill in ancient times, the best place to do so would probably have been in Egypt."

The Egyptian priest–physicians served a number of important functions, discovering and treating a lot of diseases, through some powerful magic (rituals, spells, incarnations, talismans, and amulets), deities, scripture, herbal medicine, and some other methods.

Unfortunately, only a few papyri have survived, from which one could learn about Egyptian Medicine [12]:

1. The *Edwin Smith Papyrus* describing surgical diagnosis and treatments (Fig. 2.3)

Table 2.1 Dream symbols in different ancient cultures [8]

Item	Pot	Tree	Snake	Bird
Egyptian	Filling a pot=bad omen Beer poured from a pot=robbery	Sitting in a tree=troubles could be overcome	Good omen, indicating that the dreamer would soon settle some dispute	Catching birds=loss of something precious
Assyrian	Empty pot=poverty Full goblet=children and fame	Cutting date palm trees=solution of problems	Seizing a snake=protection from angels	Meeting a bird=return of lost property
Greek	Wine poured from pots=serenity Drinking a cup dry was lucky	Trees for making ships=unlucky sign (except for carpenters and seamen)	Ill omen (illness, enemies)	Eagles=rulers Wild pigeons=immoral women
Hebrew	Cooking pots=peace and domestic calm	Palm trees=punishment for past sins	Snakes=secure livelihood Snake bite=doubled income	Good omen, except owls (bad luck)

Fig. 2.3 Edwin Smith Papyrus [12]

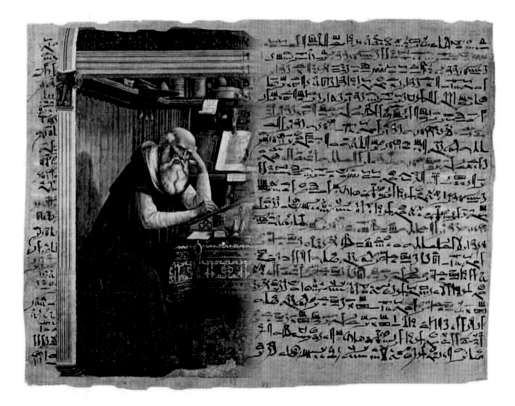

2. The *Ebers Papyrus* (dates from the sixteenth century B.C.) on ophthalmology, diseases of the digestive system, the head, the skin and specific maladies like aAa, which some think may have been a precursor of aids and others, perhaps more reasonably, consider to have been a disease of the urinary tract, a compilation of earlier works that contains a large number of prescriptions and recipes (Fig. 2.4)
3. The *Kahun Gynaecological Papyrus*
4. The Berlin Medical Papyrus
5. The London Medical Papyrus
6. The *Hearst medical papyrus* repeats many of the recipes found in the Ebers papyrus
7. The *Demotic Magical Papyrus of London and Leiden* contains a number of spells for treating physical ailments

Insomnia

The Egyptian medical papyri mentioned for the first treatment in history that the ancient Egyptians described use of poppy seed (*opium*) as hypnotic to relieve insomnia, headache, and also as an anesthetic [12].

Lavender, which is considered *herbal sleep remedy,* was used by the Egyptians to preserve their mummies, which has something to do with their belief about death as an *eternal sleep* [13].

Chamomile was considered a sacred plant by the ancient Egyptians, being offered to the gods. It was used for different purposes as a cosmetic treatment, anesthetic, and antiseptic. It was known to induce a state of quiet and serenity foreword for sleep [14].

Snoring

Ebers Papyrus mentioned that *Thyme*—a herb used by the Egyptians for embalming—was thought to be beneficial in reducing snoring [15].

An interesting story about snoring was mentioned in one of the famous myths about "Isis" (the mother of goddess of ancient Egypt). According to this story, *Isis* found *Ra* (*the sun god*), asleep one day, snoring loudly, and saliva dripping from his mouth. She collected the saliva and mixed it with earth to form *poisonous serpent,* which she later used to force *Ra* to disclose his secret name to her! [16]

Narcolepsy

The Edwin Smith Papyrus referred to epilepsy without clear description of narcolepsy, as described in the translated Babylonian texts [17].

Hypnosis

The ancient civilizations of Egypt, China, and Tibet used hypnosis in one way or another, with reference to deep sleep. Sleep temples are regarded by some as an early instance of hypnosis, over 4000 years ago, under the influence of *Imhotep*, who served as chancellor and high priest of the sun god *Ra*. Such sleep temples were like hospitals of sorts, healing a variety of ailments, perhaps many of them psychological in nature. The treatment involved chanting and placing the patient in a trancelike or hypnotic state, before analyzing his dreams, to determine the treatment [18].

Conclusion

As in any other field of science, the ancient Egyptians did have their own fingerprint in the area of sleep medicine. They linked sleep to death (and afterlife), and practiced dream interpretation in a rather systematized and constructive way. Their medical papyri included mentioning of some sleep disorders and their treatments. However, more research and studying are still needed to clarify some of the many undiscovered secrets of the miraculous Egyptian civilization regarding the mysterious world of sleep.

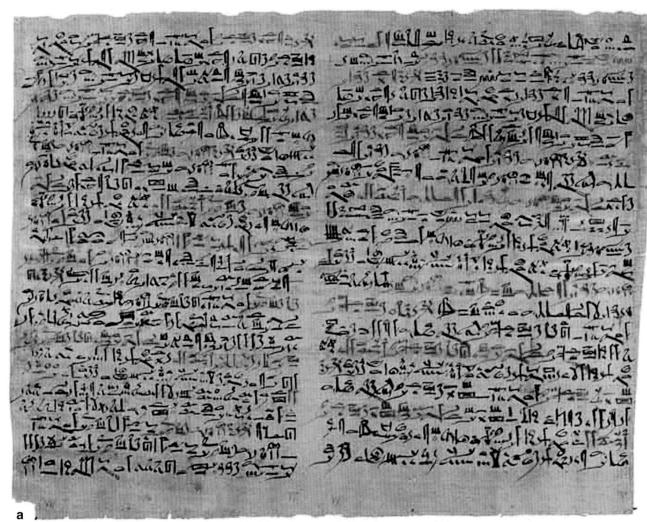

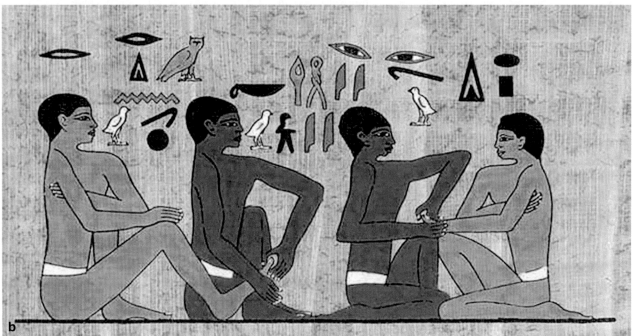

Fig. 2.4 Ebers Papyrus [12]

References

1. Humbert JM, Pantazzi M, Ziegler C. Egyptomania: Egypt in Western art,1730–1930 (exhibition catalog). Paris: Musée du Louvre; 1994.
2. Allen J. Middle Egyptian: an introduction to the language and culture of hieroglyphs. Cambridge: Cambridge University Press; 2000.
3. Szpakowska K. Behind closed eyes: dreams and nightmares in ancient Egypt. Swansea: Classical Press of Wales; 2003.
4. Lucy G. And now a word from ancient Egypt—the lucid dream exchange. 2009. http://www.dreaminglucid.com/issues/LDE50.pdf
5. Assmann J. Death and salvation in ancient Egypt. Ithaca: Cornell University Press; 2006.
6. Barbara O'Neill. Sleep and the sleeping in ancient Egypt. Published on magazine articles on egyptological. 2012. http://www.egyptological.com/2012/04/sleep-and-the-sleeping-in-ancient-egypt-8146. Accessed 3 April 2012.
7. Gotthard GT. Dreams as a constitutive cultural determinant—the example of ancient Egypt. Int J Dream Res. 2011:4(1):24–30.
8. Diagram Visual Information Limitcd. Understanding dreams. Collins: HarperCollins; 2005. pp. 220–23 (1).
9. Gardiner AH, Litt D, editors. Hieratic papyri in the British museum, 3rd series: Chester Beatty gift (Vol. I. Text, pp. 7–23; No. III (Brit.Mus.10683), Plates 5–12a, Recto, The Dream Book). London: British Museum;1935.
10. British Museum. The dream book. http://www.britishmuseum.org/search_results.aspx?searchText=Dream+book.
11. Libby Pelham BA. Ancient Egypt and dream analysis. Updated 16 Aug 2012. http://www.analysedreams.co.uk/ancient-egypt-dream-analysis.html. Aug 2012.
12. Ancient Egyptian medicine—smith papyrus—ebers papyrus. http://www.crystalinks.com/egyptmedicine.html.
13. An herbal sleep remedy for Egyptians. http://www.sleeppassport.com/herbal-sleep-remedy.html.
14. Ancient Egypt. Herbal secrets. Chamomile. http://::www.angelfire.com/ut2/egyptherb/chamomille.html.
15. Sleep and snoring—non-drug and non-surgical approaches. http://www.breathing.com/articles/sleeping-snoring.htm.
16. Isis—Myth encyclopedia. http://www.mythencyclopedia.com/Ho-Iv/Isis.html.
17. A brief history of sleep medicine. http://www.talkaboutsleep.com/sleep-disorders/archives/history.htm.
18. Ancient hypnosis—hypnosis in history. https://hypnosisinhistory.com/ancient-hypnosis.

Sleep Medicine in the Arab Islamic Civilization

3

Shahira Loza

> Medicine is a science from which one learns the states of human body with respect to what is healthy and what is not, in order to preserve good health when exists and restore it when it is lacking. (Ibn Sina Avicenne Canon 1.3, 1025 AD) [1]

Islamic civilization covers a time frame between the seventh century and the fifteenth century spreading to a vast area from Spain in the West, to China in the East and encompassing the whole of northern Africa including Egypt as well as Syria, Palestine, Transjordan, Central Asia, and parts of western India. Later, it was spread by Muslim merchants to the Far East: Malaysia and Indonesia [2].

The two sources of Islamic jurisprudence are the Quran and Hadith. The Holy Quran is the basis of Islamic religion and Hadith the teachings of Prophet Muhammad (Peace be upon him, PBUH) as recorded by his followers. Among Hadiths are rules pertaining to personal hygiene, bathing, drinking, marriage, circumcision, sanitation, and sleep posture [3].

Muslim medicine has an important theological basis, with reference to taking care of the body, a religious obligation for the Muslims. Quranic verses and Hadith played an important role in creating the Islamic frame of mind of the future physicians.

Sleep specifically is mentioned in the Quran as a miracle and a sign of Allah.

Surat Al-Room (30:23)

وَمِنْ آيَاتِهِ مَنَامُكُم بِاللَّيْلِ وَالنَّهَارِ وَابْتِغَاؤُكُم مِّن فَضْلِهِ ۚ إِنَّ فِي ذَٰلِكَ لَآيَاتٍ لِّقَوْمٍ يَسْمَعُونَ

And among His Signs is the sleep that ye take by night and by day, and the quest that ye (make for livelihood) out of His Bounty: verily in that are signs for those who listen.

Surat Al-Room (30:23)

وَمِنْ آيَاتِهِ مَنَامُكُم بِاللَّيْلِ وَالنَّهَارِ وَابْتِغَاؤُكُم مِّن فَضْلِهِ ۚ إِنَّ فِي ذَٰلِكَ لَآيَاتٍ لِّقَوْمٍ يَسْمَعُونَ

"And He it is Who makes the Night as a covering for you, and Sleep as Repose, and makes the Day (as it were) a Resurrection."

With the rise of the Abbasid dynasty during AD 750–1158 known as the Islamic golden age, a great deal of development occurred in science, philosophy, and medicine. Physicians occupied a high social position in the Arab culture [4]. Prominent physicians served as ministers or judges and were appointed as royal physicians, not only to Caliphs but also in foreign courts. Khubilai, the founder of the Yuan dynasty in China, appointed a Moslem physician [5]. The title of "Hakim" was bestowed upon physicians, which translates to "wise" as they were acknowledged for their great wisdom as well as their medical knowledge. This title is still used today in most Arab countries.

During the reign of caliph Haroun Al Rashid AD 830, "Bait ul Hikma" or the House of Wisdom was built representing an educational institute devoted to translation and research [6]. Hunayn Ibn Ishaq d.c. AD 873–877, Yuhanna Ibn Masawyh AD 777–857, and Al Kindi were among the most famous translators of the period [2]. It is through these Arabic translations that medieval Europe rediscovered Greek medicine. Specifically, some works of Galen that had been lost in Greek medicine were only found in Arabic translations [2, 7].

Among many physicians who contributed to medicine in Islamic civilization is Avicenna or Abu Ali Al Hussain Bin Ali Ibn Sina AD 980–1037. He is considered to be the most legendary physician of the Middle Ages [8]. His Canon of Medicine (Kitab Al Qanun fi al tibb), an encyclopedia of medicine in five books, completed in AD 1025 and considered to be one of the most famous books in the history of medicine, presents the medical knowledge of the time. It supports the ancient theory of four humors and four temperaments and extended it to encompass emotional aspect,

S. Loza (✉)
Cairo Centre for Sleep Disorders, 55 Abdel Moneim Riad, Mohandessin, Cairo, Egypt

Fig. 3.1 Text and painting, Avicenne's Canon of Medicine, 1632 AD

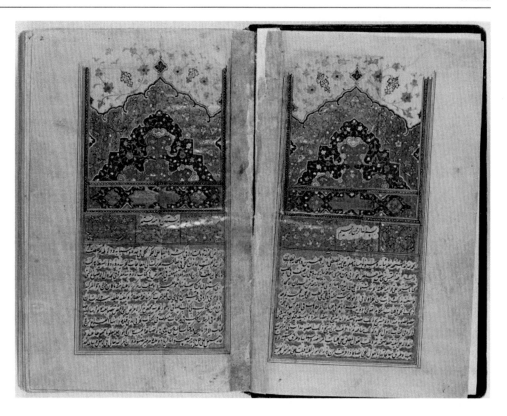

mental capacity, moral attitudes, self-awareness, movements, and dreams. He dedicated a chapter in this book to sleep and vigilance (Chap. 9 in the first book) [1]. (Fig. 3.1)

Avicenna describes several aspects of sleep and its benefits in this chapter. He states that sleep in moderation assists and renews bodily functions and comforts the psyche. "Sleep arrests the dissipation of breath," which he considers to be the vital power. The effects of sleep are recognized as restoring the equilibrium in quantity and quality of humors. He mentions that sleep also remedies the weakness due to dispersal of breath attributed to bodily fatigue, coitus, anger, or violent disturbance (Fig. 3.2).

Another interesting aspect mentioned in the Canon is the subject of sleep and the elderly; that sleep provides a humectant and warm action which is specially advantageous to those advanced in age. Galen is quoted in the Canon saying "I am now careful to obtain sleep as I am an old man, the humidity which sleep brings is beneficiary to me" and that he consumes every evening lettuce leaves with aromatics—the lettuce to help him sleep; the aromatics to rectify the coldness of the lettuce.

In the same chapter, there is a description of how to obtain sleep: "A bath taken after the digestion of a meal, plenty of hot water poured over the head." He also makes a note of the possibility of using more potent treatments, the details of which, he specifies, would be in the section of the book under medicaments. He therefore had a behavioral as well as a pharmacological approach to treat insomnia. The timing of sleep is also mentioned: the good qualities of night

sleep, as it is deep and continuous. He also mentioned that if one is used to sleeping during daytime, the change to night sleep should be gradual and not abrupt. This is an example of a behavioral approach to circadian rhythm problems, a rule that is used today. He also suggests sleep hygiene rules: "Healthy persons should pay attention to sleep. It must be moderate, properly timed, and excess must be avoided. They must avoid remaining awake too long, that might result in injuring mental faculty." He therefore associated lack of sleep and insomnia to mental health. He gives a description of the best sleep being "the deep sleep after the passage of food from the stomach and after ridding off flatulences and eructations, for to sleep on this is detrimental in many ways; it keeps the person turning from side to side, bringing harm to the person. Thus a walk before sleeping to ensure digestion is recommended. It is also bad to go to sleep on an empty stomach." Today, we know that hunger will interfere with sleep, that sleeping after a heavy meal could lead to gastroesophageal reflux and disturb sleep.

An interesting part of this chapter is the description of daytime sleepiness as related to illnesses: "Depending on humidity and catarrhal states resulting in bad color of health, heavy spleen, nerves losing their tone, lethargy, lack of libido, and leading to tumors and inflammatory conditions." Avicenna explains that among reasons for these injurious effects is the sudden interruption of sleep causing natural faculties to be dulled. This description could well be symptoms of obstructive sleep apnea syndrome.

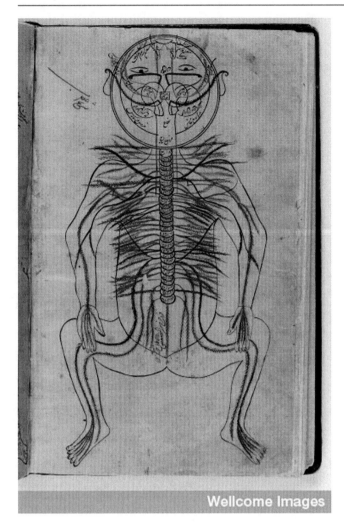

Fig. 3.2 Nervous system, Avicenne's Canon of Medicine, 1632 AD

Finally, Avicenna recommends that the posture of sleep is best if started on the right and then turning to the left. This, in the author's view, is according to medical and Islamic law, probably on account of earlier Prophetic Hadith. He continues by explaining that the prone position helps digestion but considers sleeping on the back or supine position bad practice that leads to stroke, paralysis, and nightmares. He attributes the problem to accumulation of excreted matter in the tissues of the back preventing them from entering the natural channels like the nostrils and the palate. He considered the supine position to be a weakness due to weakness of the muscles and the limbs; they are unable to support themselves on either side, as the back is stronger. The consequence is that such individuals sleep with their mouth open as the muscles, which keep the jaws closed, are too weak to maintain them in the open position. Again he describes mouth breathing in individuals with upper airway obstruction [9, 10].

Avicenna also discusses respiratory diseases in volume three of the Canon of Medicine covering the functional anatomy and pathophysiology of the pulmonary diseases known in his time. One of the important symptoms he discusses is dyspnea during sleep that leads to awakening [11].

Many other physicians contributed to medicine during the Middle Ages. Contributions of a few might be indirectly related to the science of Sleep Medicine.

Ali Ibn al Tabary AD 838–870 wrote "The Paradise of Wisdom" with nine discourses including diseases and conditions affecting the head and nervous diseases. Abu Bakr al Razi (Razes) AD 865–925 mentioned and counseled against over prescribing Hashish [12].

Ali Ibn Abbas al Majusi (Haly Abbas) AD 949–983 wrote "The Complete Art of Medicine" (Kitab Kamel As Sinaa al Tibbiya) and "Royal Book" (Kitab al Maliki). His writings deal with medical ethics, scientific research methodology, neuroscience, and psychology [13]. Al Zahrawi AD 936–1013 used gold and silver tubes to overcome laryngeal obstruction and keep the upper airway patent. He surgically removed laryngeal tumors and performed tonsillectomies. He used opium and hashish as anesthetics [14]. Ibn al Nafis AD 1213–1288 was the first to discover the pulmonary circulation (the lesser circulation) [7].

Abu Marwan Ibn Zohr (Avenzoar) AD 1091–1161, an Arab physician born in Seville, wrote on preparation of drugs, reported on tracheotomy, and gave an accurate description of neurological disorders including meningitis and intracranial thrombophlebitis [2].

Another important contribution to medicine is the development of hospitals or Bimaristans. The word Bimaristan is Persian in origin; Bimar is a disease and Stan is a place. A large number of hospitals were developed in the Islamic world in the eighth century, an institutional place for the caring of the sick as opposed to the areas attached to temples where patients were attended by priests, and they attended a therapy which consisted of prayers and sacrifices [6].

The first Bimaristan was built in Damascus by Caliph Al Walid bin Abdel Malik circa AD 707 [14]. According to Ibn Batuta, a fourteenth-century traveler from Tangier to China, there were 34 hospitals in the east; some can still be visited in Baghdad, Aleppo, and Cairo. These establishments were divided into quarters for the insane, pharmacy, library, mosque, and Quranic school. Construction of these establishments was regarded as holy work. Caliph al Mugtadir made preliminary examination compulsory before practicing medicine and gave one of his doctors the task of organizing the tests, making them into an early model of teaching hospitals [4].

The most renowned of Medieval Islamic hospitals is Al Mansouri hospital built in Cairo AD 1284–85 by Sultan Al Mansour Qalawun. There were specialized wards for general medicine, surgery, and those dealing with fractures, fever, eye diseases, and with separate sections for males and females. Admission to the Bimaristan was regardless of race, color, or religion and there was no limited time for inpatient treatment. Patient stayed till they fully recovered, when they were able to eat a full chicken [2, 6, 14]. Special care is noted in the archives of Sultan Qualawun trust: points pertaining to cleanliness, food, and music therapy to help patients fall asleep. Also, there is a description of the teaching facility and notably the time shifts of caregivers [14].

Medieval Islamic medicine emerged as an intense cross-pollination with other cultures, by translation, trade, and travel. The Arab Islamic period formed an important link in the chain of scientific advancement between the Greek civilization and late medieval and renaissance Europe. Unfortunately, much of this rich culture has been lost as a result of the Mongol invasion in AD1258 [15]. Ibn el Nadim's Fihrist (Catalogue), AD 938, lists many of those works and gives an indication of the losses sustained [6, 7, 15]. It has been estimated that less than one in thousand books listed has survived. It is remarkable that in the eleventh century, a chapter in the medical textbook, the Canon, considered a reference, which was dedicated to sleep covering topics for many centuries that are still being researched today.

References

1. Wikipedia Contributors. Wikipedia, the free encyclopedia. [Online]. 2012. http://en.wikipedia.org/w//index.php?title=The_Canon_of_Medicine&oldid=511971595. Accessed 20 Aug 2012.
2. Lyons AS, Petrucelli RJ. Medicine under Islam Arabic medicine. In: Rawls W, editor. Medicine an illustrated history. New York: Abrams; 1987. pp. 294–317.
3. Bukhari HS. Abu Abdallah Mohamed bin Ismail el Bukhari 854 AD. Riyadh K.S.A: Risalah Press; 2009.
4. Sournia JC. The muslem digression. In: Sournia JC, editor. The illustrated hisotry of medicine. England: Harold Starke; 1992. pp. 122–37.
5. Clements J. A brief history of Khubilai Khan, Lord of Xanadu Emperor of China. Philadelphia, Pennsylvania: Running Press; 2010.
6. Nagamia HF. Islamic medicine history and current practice. International Institute of Islamic Medicine (IIIM). 1995 April 30.
7. Pormann PE, Savage-Smith E. The emergence of Islamic medicine in medieval Islamic medicine. Edinburgh: Edinburgh University Press; 2007.
8. Abdel Rehim S. Al Tibb Al Nafsi Fi Al Islam (Psychiatry in Islam). Damascus: Al Faraby; 1997.
9. Ibn Sina AHA. Al Qanun Fi Al Tibb (Avicenna Canon of Medicine). Beirut Lebanon (arabic): Ezz el Din Press; 1987. pp. 980–1037.
10. Gruner OC. Chapter 9 in the Second Thesis, The regimen proper for the physically matured, in Part 3 Preservation of health. In: A treatise on the Canon of Medicine of Avicenna—incorporating a translation of the first book. London: Luzak; 1930. pp. 417–9.
11. Hashemi SM, Raza M. Science Daily. [Online]. 2009. http://www.sciencedaily.com/releases. Accessed 19 Aug 2012.
12. Nahas GG. Hashish in Islam. Bulletin NY Academy of Medicine. 1982 December. pp. 814–30.
13. Wikipedia Contributors. Wikipedia, the free encyclopedia. [Online]. 2012. http://en.wikipedia.org/w/index.php?title=%27Ali_ibn_al-%27Abbas_al-Majusi&oldid=511933070. Accessed 21 Aug 2012.
14. El Haddad MHI. Al Mogmal Fi Al Athar We Al Hadara Al Islamia (Comprehensive text in antiquities and civilization). Egypt: Zahran Al Shark; 2006.
15. Prioreschi PA. A history of medicine: byzantine and Islamic medicine, 2nd edn. Omaha: Horatius; 2001.

Sleep Medicine in Ancient and Traditional India

V. Mohan Kumar

Many centuries before the advent of the Aryans into India, the Indus Valley civilization flourished in this region as is evident from the excavations at Mohenjo-Daro and Harappa. Most of these regions are now in Pakistan. The knowledge of the original inhabitants about body function and medicine must have been based on magical, religious, and empirical practices [1]. When the Aryans entered the Indus Valley, they brought with them their knowledge of gods, medicine, and physiology. The chief sources of their culture and knowledge were the four *Vedas*. Four *Vedas* (books of knowledge), twelve *Upanishadas* (brief catechistical treatises) and various *Smritis* (canons of law) are the principal sources of knowledge of ancient Indian Philosophy. Though these scriptures are believed to have been brought to India by the Aryans, there is definitive evidence to assume that many elements of the Indus Valley civilization were assimilated by the Aryans [1].

According to traditional Indian belief (or Hindu religious belief) the Vedas were told to the sages by Brahma, the creator of man, probably about 6000 years before Christ. But according to most scholars, even the Rig Veda, which is the oldest among Vedas, is not older than 2000 years before Christ [1]. The four *Vedas* are *Rig Veda, Sama Veda, Yajur Veda,* and *Atharva Veda.* They contain hymns and prayers addressed to different deities. Even in these purely religious texts we find a reflection of anatomical, physiological, psychological, pathological, and therapeutic views, which may have some symbolic origin and which had found their reflection in the traditional Indian medicine, called *Ayurveda.* The meaning of the term *Ayurveda* is knowledge of life [2, 3, 4]. Though the word *Ayurveda* sounds as if it is related

to the *Vedic* period, it was derived much later. According to traditional Indian belief, Brahma, the creator, also provided the knowledge contained in the *Ayurveda.* Unfortunately, *Ayurveda* in its original form is not available now, but most of its contents are revealed in the *Samhitas* (encyclopedia) written by Charaka and Sushruta in 1000 BC [5, 6].

Charaka has dealt with sleep and sleep disorders in more detail. *Charaka Samhita* gives details about his approach to sleep. According to *Ayurveda,* there are three *Dhatus* (basic factors) which decide the health or ill health of an individual. They are called *Vata, Kapha*, and *Pitta.* They cannot be translated into any other language, as they do not have any equivalent terminology either in modern physics or in physiology and medicine. When they are in their natural state they provide the individual with strength, happiness, and long life. On the other hand, if these *Dhatus* are altered they bring about health problems. According to Ayurvedic concepts *nidradhikya* (excessive sleep) is caused by disturbance in *Kapha*, and *asvapna* (sleeplessness) is caused by disturbance in *Vata.*

According to *Charaka Samhita* "When the mind gets tired, when the senses get dulled and incapable, the man goes to sleep." In *Ayurveda* sleep is classified into seven types on the basis of its causative factors. Sleep can be either physiological or pathological [2, 1]. Thus seven types of sleep are produced as a result (or consequence) of night time (physiological sleep), *tamas* (ignorance), *kapha* (one of the basic factors or *Dhatus*), mental exertion, physical exertion, bad prognosis of disease or as a side effect of disease (e.g. fever). The night sleep is considered good, and it is described as that which "nurses all the living beings." The sleep which is caused by *tamas* is considered as "the root cause of sinful acts."

Proper or improper sleep would decide whether you are happy, miserable, obese, emaciated, strong, weak, virile, sterile, knowledgeable or ignorant, long-lived, or short-lived. The *Charaka Samhita* goes on to say that if the sleep is proper it brings about happiness and longevity. The consequences of both deficient and excess sleep will be just the

V. M. Kumar (✉)

8A, Heera Gate Apartments, D.P.I. Junction, Jagathy, 695014 Thiruvananthapuram, Kerala, India
e-mail: wfsrs2005@rediffmail.com

V. M. Kumar
Sree Chitra Tirunal Institute for Medical Sciences & Technology, Thiruvananthapuram, Kerala, India
e-mail: wfsrs2005@rediffmail.com

S. Chokroverty, M. Billiard (eds.), *Sleep Medicine,* DOI 10.1007/978-1-4939-2089-1_4,
© Springer Science+Business Media, LLC 2015

opposite. Sleeping during the day time, in all seasons, is advocated for the young, weak, tired, and those suffering from various diseases. During summer season (when nights become shorter) some sleep during the day is advocated for all. In other seasons, daytime sleep is not advocated. Although any comfortable position of the body may be regarded as suitable for sleep, sleeping on one's right side (daksirasana) is considered the most favorable position for sleep. According to them sleeping in sitting posture does not produce any harm. Keeping awake during night causes roughness in the body. Obesity and emaciation are specially mentioned as two conditions caused by improper sleep and diet.

For some reason, if one does not get sleep, it can be achieved by massage, bath or by consuming milk, rice with curd, alcohol, meat soup or by listening to some agreeable music [2, 4]. In addition, the following medicinal preparations are suggested for curing insomnia [2]:

1. Root of *kaka jangha (Peristrope bicalyoulata)* tied onto the head produces sleep.
2. Application of *til oil* (gingelly oil) and sour fermented drink called *kanjika* on the head, legs, and heels produce sleep.
3. Powder of *pippali mula* (*Piper longum)* boiled with *guda* (jaggery) can be used as linctus to cure even chronic sleeplessness.
4. Soup of *Sali parni(Oryga sativa), bala (Sida Cordifolia), Eranda (Ricnus communis), yava (Solanum melongeva),* and *mudga parni (Phaseolus mungo)* produce instantaneous sleep.
5. *Vrntaka (Solanum melongeva)* boiled at night and mixed with honey when consumed produces immediate sleep.

On the other hand, excess sleep can be dealt with by eliminating *dosas* from the body and head through various means like purgation, emesis, etc. Application of paste prepared from *nilotpala (Nymphaea stlellata)*, seeds of *sigru (Moringa oleifera)*, and *naga kesara (Masua ferrea)* prevents excessive sleep [2].

Sushruta had devoted one complete chapter on the analysis of dreams. He considered them as omens. According to him, a favorable or unfavorable termination of a disease could be predicted from the dreams. Though Charaka fully recognized the lack of meaning in most of our dreams, *Charaka Samhita* deals, at length, with the theories of dream. Charaka, Sushruta, and Vagbhatta, the great medical scientists of ancient India, did believe that the dreams are produced when the vital equilibrium between the three *dhatus* is disturbed. These are seven types of significant dreams [7]. They are dreams about objects seen earlier, things which we have heard earlier, past experience, wish fulfillment, imagination, premonition, and morbid things.

Ayurveda does recognize prayer as one form of treatment. The goddess of sleep *Nidra devi* is invoked to get sleep for the patient suffering from insomnia [2]. The following *mantra* should be chanted:

"Om shuddhe yu yogini maha nidre svaha." Along with chanting of this *mantra,* white *tila* should be put on the body of the patient. By this procedure he is expected to get sleep.

The subsequent writings like the *Yoga Sutras* of Patanjali (second century BC) give an account of the manner in which a healthy body can be prepared for higher states of mental function like *Samadhi* (meditation) [8]. Though *Ayurveda* and *Yoga* are still practiced in India, the scripts on *Yoga* provided the most interesting information regarding the functioning of brain, consciousness, and sleep [9].

Yoga is popularly considered as a physical exercise *(Asana)*, the practice of which maintains a healthy body. But traditional Indian philosophy considers physical exercise as only a step towards that mystical experience, which is achieved by physical and mental practice. Various treatises on *Tantric Yoga* shed some light on the supposed neural basis of many of these Yogic phenomena [10]. According to this, there are six to eight nerve centers located at different levels in the human body. These are called *Chakras* (or centers).

The lowest one, which is located at the level of the anus and sex organs, is the *Muladhara chakra*. This center controls the sexual activities. Similarly, different *chakras* are assigned various functions. The biological energy which resides at the level of the *chakra* has been referred to as *Kundalini Shakti* (Serpent power). The practitioner of yoga successfully channels his *Kundalini Shakti* through the successive *chakras* (nerve centers) till he can activate the *chakra* of the highest level. Once he learns, by practice, to control the *chakras* he can not only control all the autonomic functions but he can also acquire skills and powers, which are super normal. In order to understand the concept of sleep and wakefulness in Yogic terminology, one has to understand or appreciate the concept of consciousness in Yoga.

In modern understanding, consciousness is considered as a by-product of the proper functioning of the brain, and it ceases to exist with death or with damage to the brain, but according to Yogic concept consciousness is an expression of God and it is within every human being. In fact, everything in the universe is derived from and is the expression of God. So, the consciousness, mind, and matter are the three basic derivatives of God (or the Ultimate Reality). These three basic derivatives of reality exist in many subtleties and they also function at different levels. What we know of these derivatives of reality on the physical plane is their crudest expression at the lowest level. It is claimed that consciousness, through various intermediary states gives rise to the five elements (*Panchabhutas*) [11]. These elements, under the influence of the three *gunas* (or energies), bring into existence the universe and all its constituents including man himself. The three *gunas* are the *sattava, rajas*, and *tamas*. The *sattava* represents intelligence, knowledge, cognition, etc. whereas *rajas* represents energy, activity, change, etc. The *tamas* stands for inertia, ignorance, etc. These three energies are symbolized in the *Puranas* as three goddesses namely Saraswati, Lakshmi, and Kali, respectively [12]. Depending on the permutations and combinations of the influence of these three energies man goes into states of sleep, dreaming, and waking.

After appreciating a bit about the concept of consciousness in Yogic philosophy, we can try to understand the four states of consciousness. The four states are termed and interpreted differently by different authors. When they are described as different stages through which a yogi passes during his meditation, it is given one type of interpretation. It has been dealt with in some detail in the *Mandukya Upanishad*. According to them the four states of consciousness are *Jagrat, Svapna, Sushupti*, and *Turiya* [13]. *Jagrat* is the waking state in which consciousness is in touch with objects around. Though the word meaning of *Svapna* is dream, it is considered as that state in which there is some mental image as a result of recall of memory or imagination. In this state he is not asleep. The state of *Sushupti* resembles dreamless sleep, but it is considered as totally different from sleep. In this state there is no mental image, and his mind is totally blank. A yogin is said to derive great pleasure after going through this state while practicing meditation. The yogin passes from *Jagrat* through *Svapna* and *Sushupti* before reaching the fourth and final state called *Turiya*. The word meaning of *Turiya* is "fourth." This is the highest spiritual state of consciousness, where one is in union with the ultimate reality. During this state an individual is said to be oblivious of the internal and external world. A voluntary control over thought process is essential for obtaining this state of consciousness.

According to a more radical interpretation, sleep and dreaming are two different states of consciousness [14]. In this interpretation *Jagrat* (or *Vaisvanara*) is the waking state, whereas *Svapna* (or *Taijasa*) is the dreaming state. In India, as in other countries, people have shown deep interest in the interpretation of dreams. The *Puranas* have numerous stories of dreams and dreamers. One of the *slokas* on *Yoga* when translated into English, states that "man sees his waking desires fulfilled while asleep." The statement is very close to the theory of Freud. The *Sushupti* (or *Prajana*) is the dreamless sleep, equivalent to slow wave sleep. According to *Chhandogya Upanishad*, man gets united with the pure Being during sleep [15]. In other words, people go to Brahma during sleep, though they do not realize it. One can always find the emphasis laid on deep sleep throughout the ancient literature.

According to *Sushruta Samhita* ten nerves control the various functions of the body. Man goes to sleep by using two of them and with the help of two others he wakes up. Curiously enough, at many places in the ancient literature it is mentioned that one dreams when the nerve center "*Svapnavha nadi*" is functioning.

Several studies were undertaken during the last several years to understand and analyze scientifically the various claims made on yogic achievements. The first scientifically documented investigation on Yoga was initiated in 1924 at Lonavala (Poona, India) by a yogin named Swami Kuvalayananda. He and his colleagues studied many psycho-physiological functions during yogic practices [16]. Then came a period during which scientific proofs were provided for many of the claims by yogins like stopping the heart. These findings by some Western and Indian scientists were later proved incorrect [22]. But systematic scientific research showed that the yogin does possess the ability to control his autonomic nervous system, in a remarkable way. It is claimed that the fall in respiration, blood pressure, and heart rate, during yogic relaxation postures, are nearly 10 % more than that achieved during deep sleep. Das and Gastaut [17] were possibly the first to study the electroencephalographic (EEG) changes during meditation. They observed high voltage, high frequency waves during the early stages of meditation, and sleep-like EEG in the later stages. But their subjects were those who had practiced meditation for a short period only. Several studies were undertaken on renowned yogins at All India Institute of Medical Sciences in 1960's by Anand, Chhina, and Baldev Singh [18, 18–21]. The inferences arrived at by them, by and large, remain valid even today, in spite of studies undertaken in various laboratories of the world during the past several years. It can be summarized that during the practice of Yoga and also as a result of this practice, there is an increase in the amplitude of alpha activity, more synchronization and spread of synchronized waves to the anterior regions of the brain. There were differences in the EEG pattern observed in different individuals during the later stages of meditation. Some yogins had predominant theta waves, and some others showed spurts, of short EEG desynchronizations in between [11]. The EEG pattern observed during meditation is less prone to alteration by external stimuli. In this state, sound and other peripheral stimuli do not produce desynchronization of the EEG. It does produce EEG desynchronization, in the same subject, when he is not doing meditation.

Many of the statements regarding Yoga and its effect on sleep need confirmation, particularly the relationship between the state of meditation and sleep. Can meditation in any way compensate for normal sleep? There is some suggestive evidence which has shown the absence of compensatory increase of sleep in the sleep-deprived yogi. More systematic research is required in this field. It is claimed that yogins can exercise a control over all states of consciousness including sleep. They are said to be capable of eliminating the dream phase of sleep (a claim which needs substantiation by scientific studies). It is also claimed that a Yogi passes through a special kind of sleep called yogic sleep (*Yog-ni-dra*), and he is capable of controlling its progress, including elimination of dreams.

After having taken the liberty of looking into the yogic practice from a scientific angle, we should be also prepared to listen to what the yogins have to say about scientific investigations. They really do not think very highly of the scientific investigation. According to them, consciousness, which is the penultimate reality of existence, and the source of mind and matter, cannot be investigated with a physical apparatus, however elaborate and imposing it may be. A yogin living in the foothills of Himalayas was approached by a team of scientists who wanted to investigate him during his meditation. He subjected himself to their tests. They did their tests and thanked him profusely before leaving the place. The yogin was never told about the results of their test, nor was he interested in knowing about it. He did not want to offend the scientists by telling it to their faces. According to him the ultimate secrets of existence cannot be investigated using physical means. Only physical data can be verified by physical means.

Though the scientific approach in various ancient beliefs has not proved all the claims, it is certainly worth looking into these aspects as seen by the ancient people. Thomas Henry Huxley said in 1881 "It is easy to sneer at our ancestors—but it is much more profitable to try to discover why they, who were really not one whit less sensible persons than our own excellent selves, should have been led to entertain views which strike us as absurd." It is in this spirit that we should build a borderless mind, which connects the past with the present. The idea is not to "recreate" the past but "understand" the past by using new science.

References

1. Anand BK. Yoga and medical sciences. Ind J Physiol Pharmacol. 1991;35:84–7.
2. Keswani NH. Medical heritage of India. In: Keswani NH, editor. The science of medicine and physiological concepts in ancient and medieval India. New Delhi: National Book Trust; 1974. pp. 3–52.
3. Dash VB, Kashyap VL. Diagnosis and treatment of diseases in ayurveda. New Delhi: Concept; 1981. p. 626.
4. Kurup PNV, Raghunathan K. Human physiology in Ayurveda. In: Keswani NH, editor. The science of medicine and physiological concepts in ancient and medieval India. New Delhi: National Book Trust; 1974. pp. 67–78.
5. Sharma RK, Dash VB. Agnivesa's Charak Samhita. Varanasi: Chowkhamba Sanskrit Series office; 1976. p. 619.
6. Bhishagratna KKL. The Sushruta Samhita—an English translation based on original texts. Calcutta: Kaviraj Kunja Lal Bhishagratna; 1916. (Year Printed By M. Bhattacharyya, At The Bharat Mihir Press, 25, Roy Bag An Street).
7. Kaviratna, AC, Sharma P. The Charaka Samhita 5 vols., Indian medical science series. Delhi: Sri Satguru; 1997.
8. Bagchi AK. Concept of neurophysiology in ancient India. In: Keswani NH, editor. The science of medicine and physiological concepts in ancient and medieval India. New Delhi: National Book Trust; 1974. pp. 99–106.
9. Wood E. Practical yoga, ancient and modern. Being a new, independent translation of Patañjali's yoga aphorisms, interpreted in the light of ancient and modern psychological knowledge and practical experience. London: Rider; 1951.
10. Kumar VM. Ancient concept of sleep in India. In: Liu S, Inoue S, editors. Sleep: ancient and modern. Shanghai: The Shanghai Scientific and Technological Literature; 1995. pp. 25–33.
11. Manchanda SK, Keswani NH. The yoga and the scientist. In: Keswani NH, editor. The science of medicine and physiological concepts in ancient and medieval India. New Delhi: National Book Trust; 1974. pp. 107–18.
12. Singh B, Chhina GS. Changing concepts of human consciousness from ancient to modern times. In: Kothari DS, Brahmachari D, Joshi SK, Chhina GS, Kurup PNB, editors. Seminar on yoga, science and man. New Delhi: Central Council for Research in Indian Medicine and Homoeopathy; 1976. pp. 284–9.
13. Pal K. Yoga and psycho-analysis. New Delhi: Bhagavan Das Memorial Trust; 1966. p. 180.
14. Taimni IK. Glimpses into the psychology of yoga. Madras: Theosophical Publishing House; 1976. p. 409.
15. Chhina GS, Singh B. Whither scientific research on yoga. In: Kothari DS, Brahmachar D, Joshi SK, Chhina GS, Kurup PNV, editors. Seminar on yoga, science and man. New Delhi: Central Council for Research in Indian Medicine and Homoeopathy; 1976. pp. 290–302.
16. Krishnananda S. Chhandogya Upanishad. Rishikesh: The Divine Life Society, Sivananda Ashram; 1984.
17. Das NN, Gastaut H. Variations de l'activité du coeur, de la méditation et de l'extase yoguique. Electroenceph Clin Neurophysiol. 1955;Suppl 6:211–9.
18. Singh B, Chhina GS. Some reflections on ancient Indian physiology. In: Keswani NH, editor. The science of medicine and physiological concepts in ancient and medieval India. New Delhi: National Book Trust; 1974. pp. 79–98.
19. Anand BK, Chhina GS. Investigations on yogis claiming to stop their heart beats. Ind J Med Res. 1961;49:90–4.
20. Anand BK, Chhina GS, Singh B. Studies on Shri Ramanand Yogi during his stay in an airtight box. Ind J Med Res. 1961a;49:82–9.
21. Anand BK, Chhina GS, Singh B. Some aspects of electroencephalographic studies in yogis. Electroencephalogr Clin Neurophysiol. 1961b;13:454–6.
22. Wenger MA, Bagchi BK, Anand BK. Experiment in India on "voluntary" control of the heart and pulse. Circulation. 1961;24:1319–25.

Sleep Medicine in Ancient and Traditional China

Liu Yanjiao, Wang Yuping, Wang Fang, Yan Xue, Hou Yue
and Li Shasha

The Discovery and Understanding of Circadian Rhythm, Sleep, and Sleep Disorders in TCM in Ancient China

The Theory and Practice of Circadian Rhythm of TCM

Deeply affected by Chinese traditional ancient philosophy, traditional Chinese sleep medicine (TCM) has placed great importance on the relations between nature and humans. It looks at the changes of human body from the standpoint of changes of "yin–yang". Thus, a unique understanding of circadian rhythm of TCM has formed. From the view point of ancient philosophy, sleep is not only a physiological phenomenon but also a kind of nature treatment or therapy.

The Discovery of Circadian Rhythm in TCM and Chinese Philosophy

In ancient China, through observing the changes in nature, such as the contradiction between earth and sky, day and night, sun and moon, cloudy and clear, cold and hot, water and fire, men and women, etc., people realized the characteristics of "yin–yang" changes and summed them up to form certain theories [1]. At the end of the Western Zhou Dynasty (AD eleventh century–771 BC), the concept of yin–yang was gradually concluded from contradictions in nature. People explained the reason for causing things to change by

"yin–yang" changes. Laozi (《老子》) said, though yin and yang was mutually contradictory, they were actually in unity. The contradiction between yin and yang exists everywhere in the world. Yizhuan (《易传》) first put forward that Tao means the combination of yin and yang, which means that yin–yang plays the most important part in Chinese Philosophy. On the one hand, yin–yang emphasizes the differences and opposites between contradiction in movements; on the other hand, it emphasizes the combination and unification in the formation of objects. Yin and yang achieve relative balance in alternations. On the basis of traditional philosophy, TCM developed the theory of circadian rhythm.

Suwen (《素问》), which is one of the most important books in TCM, said yin–yang is the principle of nature, the routine of all things, the source of changes, and the beginning of growth. TCM associates all kinds of human life activities with the natural phenomena and also correlates them to the physiological functions of viscera. Then the rhythm of viscera, diseases, cure, acupuncture, and so on were formed.

According to the theory of TCM, the changes of viscera rhythm follow the changes of yang in nature. The changes of human body follow the alternation of day and night. *Suwen–Shengqi Tongtian Lun* (《素问·生气通天论》) said "yang qi hosts the exterior in day time, beginning ascending at dawn, being prosperous at noon and being weak at sunset."

The ancients used 12 Earthly Branches (di-zhi 地支) for timing. The 12 Earthly Branches divide a day and a night together into 12 sections, which are also called 12 double-hour (Shichen 时辰). Qi and blood flowed through the 12 regular channels into 5 zang viscera and 6 fu viscera according to certain sequence from 3 a.m. (Yinshi 寅时). When the functions of zang viscera or *fu* viscera were poured by *qi* and blood, it reached its functional peak period. So the functional peak period of 5 *zang* viscera and 6 fu viscera was determined as follows: 11 p.m.–1 a.m. (Zishi 子时) to 1–3 a.m. (Choushi 丑时) for liver and gallbladder, 3–5 a.m. (Yinshi 寅时) to 5–7 a.m. (Moushi 卯时) for lung and large intestine, 7–9 a.m. (Chenshi辰时) to 9–11 a.m. (Sishi 巳时) for stomach and spleen,11 a.m. to –1 p.m. (Wushi午时) to

W. Yuping (✉) · H. Yue
Department of Neurology, Xuanwu Hospital, Capital Medical University, Beijing, China
e-mail: wangyupi@public.bta.net.cn, ywang@xidian.edu.cn

L. Yanjiao · W. Fang · Y. Xue
Psychology Department (Sleep Medicine Clinic), Guang'anmen Hospital, China Academy of Chinese Medical Sciences, Beijing, China

L. Shasha
Information Institute, China Academy of Chinese Medical Sciences, Beijing, China

S. Chokroverty, M. Billiard (eds.), *Sleep Medicine,* DOI 10.1007/978-1-4939-2089-1_5,
© Springer Science+Business Media, LLC 2015

1–3 p.m. (Weishi 未时) for heart and small intestine,3–5 p.m. (Shenshi申时) to 5–7 p.m. (Youshi 酉时) for bladder and kidney, 7–9 p.m. (Wushi戊时) to 9–11 pm (Haishi亥时) for pericardium and sanjiao.

The Practice of Circadian Rhythm of TCM

Circadian rhythm greatly affects our work and life. The rhythm of time has been put to use in TCM. In Suwen–Sanbu Jiuhou Lun (《素问·三部九候论》), Huangdi asked "winter belongs to yin and summer belongs to yang, how does pulse correspond to this?" Qibo answered "if the pulses of nine sub-parts are all deep and thready, and being much different than normal, the patient will die at midnight. Winter belongs to yin. Midnight which corresponds to winter for a day also belongs to yin." "If the pulses of nine sub-parts are all large and fast, and patient can hardly breathe and being restless, he or she will die at noon. Summer belongs to yang. Noon which corresponds to summer for a day also belongs to yang. Patient suffering from illness with dramatic alternation between cold and hot syndrome will die at dawn, which corresponds to the time yin and yang make alternation…" The above examples demonstrate how to judge the prognosis of diseases or time of death by pulse according to certain circadian rhythm.

The relationship between the rhythm of time and occurrence, and development of diseases are also mentioned in some books of TCM, such as Beiji Qianjin Yao Fang (《备急千金要方》) which said the following: "If the position of disease locates in liver, it will improve at dawn and get better at midnight." "If there is food retention in the small intestine, patient will get fever at night and get better the next day." "If the position of disease locates in spleen, it will improve at dusk, get serious at noon and get better at night." "If the position of disease locates in kidney, it will improve at midnight, get serious at daytime and get better in the afternoon." Yizong Jinjian–Sizhen Xinfa Yao Jue (《医宗金鉴·四诊心法要诀》) said the disease was stable at daytime, improved at dawn, got serious at dusk, and critical at night. Spirit plays an important role in the recovery of disease when the vital—qi and pathogenic factors are fighting with each other. The rhythm of time for different diseases also differs from each other, some of which have been proved by the western and Chinese clinical medicine, some of which also need to be further proved.

In terms of the relationship between disease and season, Zhouli·Tianguan·Zhongzai (《周礼·天官·冢宰》) said, "the epidemic disease can occur in all seasons, headache in spring, skin disease in summer, malaria in autumn, and cough in winter."

In Tang Dynasty (AD 618—907), people treated epilepsy and anxiety by improving sleep. They helped insomnia patients to regain natural sleep by taking herbs. This treatment is called sleep therapy, which is one of the most important therapies of TCM psychology.

The Application of Rhythm of Time in TCM Practice

In TCM, there are three theories about sleep including yin–yang sleep theory, nourishing-defensive sleep theory and soul-inferior spirit sleep theory, summarized from the book of Huangdi Neijing (《黄帝内经》). The brain theory of sleep in TCM was formed at the end of Ming Dynasty (AD 1368–1644) and Qing Dynasty (AD 1616–1911). Taking yawn for example, Lingshu-Kouwen(《灵枢·口问》) said "yin and yang host night and daytime respectively. Yang is related to ascent and is pertaining to above. Yin is related to descent and pertaining to below. When people go to sleep at night, yin qi will accumulate below; yang qi will go down and enter into the yin portion gradually. The still running up yang qi and going down yin qi cause yawn." So, yawn is the result of crisscross between yin and yang, which is the signal of the shift of sleep and wake.

Moreover, it says, in TCM, that yang qi is on a rise from morning to 2:00 p.m., and then falls to the lowest point at midnight. Based on this theory, patients suffering from insomnia are asked to take drug twice everyday, an hour after lunch and an hour after supper, to improve the clinical curative.

In brief, the theory of circadian rhythm in TCM has the characteristics of Chinese philosophy which directly influenced the development of TCM. Today, when we study the related theories of sleep medicine in TCM, we have to confirm them through modern measurements. Maybe we can find more useful knowledge to guide study and treatment in the near future.

Application and Development of Sleep Medicine in Ancient TCM

There has been a long history of TCM research in sleep and sleep disorders. Thirty kinds of treatment methods were recorded in ancient TCM books to treat sleep disorders. China may be the first country in the world to give an account of sleepwalking. The dream analysis of TCM had become the important part of TCM clinic. The explanations of dream can be found early in Huangdi Neijing (《黄帝内经》), which had been an important reference to diagnose and treat diseases. Sleep health science originated in Tang dynasties. It obtained good effect to use sleep therapy to treat epilepsy disease during that period. TCM prescriptions created by ancient doctors in past dynasties are still widely used in clinic.

Sleep disorders recorded in *Huangdi Neijing* (《黄帝内经》) (403 BC–AD 220) were relatively rich, such as insomnia, somnolence, and different kinds of dream diseases, such as dream fly, dream fall, dream diet, night terror. The sleep theories include Ying and Wei theory, Yin and Yang theory, which have an important influence in the realization of TCM to sleep disorders.

Insomnia in elders and its mechanism as well as somnolence were recorded early in the book of Nan Jing (407–310 BC).

Shang Han Lun (Treatise on Febrile Diseases), written by Zhang Zhongjing (AD 150–219), recorded snore during sleep, such as "insomnia caused by febrile disease" and "sleepiness caused by febrile disease." Jinkui Yaolue, written by Zhang *Zhongjing* (AD 150–219), recorded insomnia caused by consumptive disease and dysphoria, as well as Baihe disease accompanied with insomnia.

Huatuo Shenfang, may be written by Hua Tuo (AD 145– 208), recorded sleep disorders which include dream sexual intercourse, night sweat, insomnia, dream spermatorrhea, child night cry, and so on. (The author of this book is not clear). The sleep disorders recorded in Zhong Zang Jing (AD 145–208) included insomnia, pavor nocturnus during sleep and dream disorder related with deficiency and excess of Zang and Fu.

Zhenjiu Jiayi Jing (A-B Classic of Acupuncture and Moxibustion; AD 259) recorded the acupuncture treatment for insomnia and the *prescription of moxibustion* to treat lethargy.

Sleep disorders in Zhu Bing Yuan Hou Lun (*General Treatise on the Cause and Symptoms of Diseases*), written by Cao Yuanfang (AD 610), included insomnia caused by consumptive disease, insomnia due to serious illness, dreaminess caused by consumptive disease, insomnia caused by febrile disease, temper and insomnia due to cholera, somnolence, night terror, and night cry.

Sleep disorders recorded in *Prescriptions Worth Thousand Gold for Emergencies,* written by Sun Simiao (AD 652), included insomnia, dream terror, dream cry, nightmare, dream fear, dream pavor, dream singing, dream waist soreness, and so on. Sleep disorders recorded in Qian Jin Yi Fang (AD 682) included dream pavor, dream supernatural beings, insomnia, sleepiness and their relative prescriptions, and herbs.

Shi Zhai Zhi Fang, written by Shi Kan (AD 1127–1279) recorded women with insomnia which was diagnosed through pulse.

Sleep disorders recorded in Sheng Ji Zong Lu, written by Zhao Zhe (AD 1117), included insomnia caused by febrile disease, insomnia due to cholera, sleepiness due to heat in gall-bladder, sleep lack, sleep terror, and restless sleep due to cold in gall-bladder, and insomnia caused by consumptive disease.

Sleep disorders recorded in *Taiping Huimin Heji Ju Fang,* written by the government of Song dynasty (AD 1078–1085), included sleep disorder due to different causes, such as strange dream accompanied by lack of vigor during day time, dream terror, sleepiness, nightmare, restless sleep accompanied by spermatorrhea, dream pavor, restless sleep accompanied by dream dangerous experience, and so on, and their different prescriptions and herbs have also been recorded.

Pujing Benshi Fang, written by Xu Shuwei (AD 1132), recorded the manifestations of night terror which included being terrified, unable to sleep alone, worrying about being arrested, and head discomfort.

Ji Sheng Fang, written by Yan Yonghe (AD 1253), recorded dream terror, many strange dreams during the night, dream pavor, sleeplessness during the night, restless sleep and dream, restlessness and sleeplessness, and so on. The causes and relative diseases of these sleep disorders have also been mentioned.

Su Wen Xuan Ji Yuan Bing Shi, written by Liu Hejian (AD 1152), first put forward sleep talking.

Pi Wei Lun, written by Li Dongyuan (AD 1249), put forward somnolence diseases related with spleen and stomach such as sleepiness, sleepiness after eating, and so on. *Yi Xue Fa Ming* recorded sweat during sleep, sleep terror, and feeling hot during sleep.

Zhang Cong Zheng (AD 1156–1228) who learned from Liu Wan Su, corrected the current malpractice of warming and tonifying therapy. He, guided by Nei Jing and Nan Jing, and by using the sweating, vomiting, and purgative method made by Zhang Zhongjing, created the theory which took attacking evil as the core and took insomnia as one kind of disease alone. Based on generation and restriction theory in Nei Jing, he used psychotherapy to treat different kinds of emotion diseases such as insomnia.

Shi Yi De Xiao Fang, written by Wei Yilin (AD 1345), has recorded sleeplessness during night, nightmare, dreaming ominous things, and sleeplessness due to dysphoria.

Ben Cao Gang Mu, written by Li Shizhen (AD 1590) recorded sleeplessness, sleepiness, hallucination, night cry, dream talking and their relative prescriptions, and herbs. It has also put forward the important theory that brain is the fu-viscera of mental activity.

Ming Yi Zhi Zhang, written by Huang Puzhong (AD 1368–1644), has put forward that phlegm stagnating in meridian could result in restless sleep and strange dream.

Dong Yi Bao Jian, written by Xu Jun (Korea, AD 1610) recorded "mind pillow method," dream ejaculation, murkiness and sleepiness, sleepless due to dysphoria, restless sleep, feeling heaviness in body and sleepiness, night sweat, drowsiness after eating, nightmare, night cry, night teeth chattering, grinding of teeth, and so on. The book has also mentioned about the theory of sleep physiology such as dream, "Yang Qi is the key of sleep and wake," "differences between elder and youth," sleep method and "Yin, Yang, deficiency and excess differentiations of sleep."

Qi Fang Lei Bian, written by Wu Shichang (AD 1644–1911), has mentioned the therapy to suddenly falling asleep without natural waking as biting the patient's foot thumb and spitting on his face; if the patient is still not waking, filling Chinese chive in the patient's nose. The therapy for sleep paralysis has also been suggested, such as using the powder mixed with Xiong Huang, Niu Huang, Zhu Sha to burn under the bed, and then pouring warm wine into patient's mouth.

Yi Xue Yuan Shi, written by Wang Honghan (AD 1692), is the book which had relatively more descriptions of sleep such as in the chapter "wake and sleep." It stated the relationship between wake and sleep, dream, "positive dream," "drunken person without dream," nightmare, "dreaming is the soul getting out of the body," and so on, which had not been mentioned before.

Chang Sheng Mi Jue, written by Shi Chengjin (AD 1697), had mentioned that a drunken person should not sleep outdoors, if suffering from apoplexia, tinea, and rheumatism caused by the deficiency of Zheng Qi and suffering from Xie Qi.

Zun Sheng Dao Yang Bian, written by Zhang Yinhan (AD 1823), put forward the recuperate method for insomnia in elders. "Elders are susceptive to sleepless. At that time, it is best to sit up and action, calm thoughts, and keep unobstructive of blood circulation."

Yang Sheng Mi Zhi (AD 1644–1911), emphasized the method to keep essence was that sleep as a cat, essence would not run away; sleep as a dog, essence would not go away. It is a method important to keep Yuan Qi.

Lu Di Xian Jing, written by Ma Qi (AD 1644–1911), has put forward three sleep postures which help to calm, such as sickness dragon sleep, fist of the knee; sleep as ape, embrace of the knee; and sleep as turtle, bend of the hand and foot.

After the ending of feudal society in China (AD 1911), the medicine development laid particular stress on the prevention and treatment of epidemical diseases, which are the results of many factors such as war and so on. A hundred years passed since then, and Chinese economical situation also changed greatly, the incidence of sleep disorders gradually increased following the development of economy.

The Development of Sleep Medicine of TCM in Modern China

The China Academy of Chinese Medical Science did the initial work for the development of sleep medicine using TCM. It has been in a leading position in this field. The research group and center for sleep medicine of TCM founded here is the earliest one in modern China.

Research on Sleep Medicine in TCM

In AD 1994, researchers from the Theoretical Research Institute of China Academy of Chinese Medical Sciences first put forward the idea to carry out researches on sleep medicine in TCM. Sleep medicine specialty clinic was founded there. The first seminar of sleep medicine in TCM was held during that time. Until now, this seminar has been held five times. The scientific research cooperation network to preventing and treating sleep disorders was founded in Shanghai. Since AD 2005, the research direction of China Academy of Chinese Medical Sciences has been changed from theoretical investigation to clinical practice. The sleep medicine specialty clinic, which has sleep monitoring rooms and related equipments, has become one of the typical clinical research centers. It promotes the development of sleep medicine in TCM.

Academic Organizations of Sleep Medicine in TCM

In AD 2008, Traditional Chinese Medicine Committee, Chinese Sleep Research Society was founded in Shanghai. Sleep Medicine Specialty Committee, World Federation of Chinese Medicine Societies was founded in Beijing. These two typical organizations of sleep medicine of TCM aim at integrating the professionals in the field of traditional and modern sleep medicine together and to prompt the development of sleep medicine in China.

Academic Works of Sleep Medicine in TCM

Through 5 years' hard work, the first academic book of sleep medicine in TCM, *Sleep Medicine in Traditional Chinese Medicine,* edited by Professor Liu Yanjiao and Professor Gao Ronglin from Guang'anmen Hospital, China Academy of Chinese Medical Sciences, was published in AD 2003. This book systematically presents the basic theories and clinical treatment of sleep medicine in TCM. It promoted the establishment of the discipline of sleep medicine of TCM and won the third prize for academic works of Chinese Association of Chinese Medicine.

In AD 2012, Professor Wang Weidong, Professor Liu Yanjiao, and Professor Ci Shuping wrote *Experimental and Clinical Diagnosis and Treatment for Sleep Disorders by Combination of TCM and Western Medicine,* which provided the basic theories and direction for clinical practice of sleep medicine using the combination of TCM and Western medicine.

Professor Wang Qiaochu from Shanghai Traditional Chinese Medicine Hospital conducted a series of basic researches along with Professor Huang Zhili from Shanghai Medicinal College of Fudan University on using the leaf of peanut to treat insomnia, which has certain influence in China.

With the support of the World Health Organization, experts from China Academy of Chinese Medical Sciences compiled the Clinical Guideline for Insomnia based on the evidence-based medicine. This guideline first spread the differentiation of TCM abroad and received high praise worldwide.

The Professional Training and Popularization for Sleep Medicine of TCM

The professional training for sleep medicine of TCM is focused on internal medicine, psychology, and otorhinolar-yngology of TCM, etc. Most of the students were awarded a professional degree. China Academy of Chinese Medicine is the first admission unit to enroll students for sleep medicine of TCM. It has cultivated more than 40 graduates and students for advanced study. Twelve training classes have been held and more than 1700 trainees were enrolled in. On World Sleep Day on March 21, doctors from sleep medicine and psychology department of Guang'anmen Hospital go into the local community to publicize knowledge about sleep medicine and conduct epidemiological survey. Through organizing international academic conferences, more and more people from all over the world have begun to pay attention to the development of sleep medicine in TCM.

Reference

1. Liu Y, Gao R. Sleep medicine in traditional Chinese medicine. Beijing: People's Medical Publishing House; 2002.

Sleep in the Biblical Period

Sonia Ancoli-Israel

At the start of the universe, when God was creating the world, it became clear that the rhythm of dark and light was necessary even before the creation of man, creatures, and plants:

> God said, "Let there be light"; and there was light. God saw that the light was good, and God separated the light from the darkness. God called the light Day, and the darkness He called Night. And there was evening and there was morning, a first day. (Genesis, 1:1–5)

Today it is known that light is the strongest zeitgeber (cue) for strong circadian rhythms just as we know that periods of darkness are also necessary. If circadian rhythms are present at the very start of the Bible, it is likely that other information about sleep and sleep disorders may also be found in those pages. This chapter reviews what the Bible and Talmud (a record of rabbinic discussions about Jewish law, ethics, philosophy, customs, and history) say about sleep.

Sleep as a Vulnerable Period and as a Gift from God

Sleep is rarely the focus of any discussion in the Bible but rather occurs as part of a larger discussion of other topics. Sleep can be a gift from God. ("He provides as much for His loved ones while they sleep" Psalms, 127:2). Sleep can be a time of vulnerability as that is a time when enemies would attack. Therefore, many prayers ask God for safety during the night and assurance of waking up in the morning.

Parts of the paper were previously published in: Ancoli-Israel S. Sleep is not tangible or what the Hebrew tradition had to say about sleep. Psychosom Med. 63:778–787, 2001 and in Ancoli-Israel, S. Sleep in the Hebrew Bible. The Jewish Bible Quarterly, 31:143–152, 2003.

S. Ancoli-Israel (✉)
Departments of Psychiatry and Medicine, University of California, 9500 Gilman Drive, # 0733, 92093–0733 La Jolla, CA, USA
e-mail: sancoliisrael@ucsd.edu

Examples of this include the story in Judges when Delilah cut Samson's hair while he was sleeping and thus destroyed his strength. ("And she made him sleep on her knees; and she called for a man, and she caused him to shave off the seven locks of his head: … and his strength went from him" Judges 16:19). Another instance of vulnerability during sleep occurs in Samuel I (I Sam 26:7–12) in the story of David and Saul. David comes upon Saul sleeping and has the opportunity to kill him, but only takes away Saul's water and spear. ("So David…approached the troops by night, and found Saul fast asleep…But David said…" Don't do him violence!… Just take the spear and the water jar at his head and let's be off…all remained asleep; a deep sleep from the Lord had fallen upon them" I Sam 26:7–12) [1]. In yet a third example, also in Judges, Sisera, a cruel Canaanite leader who ruled over the Israelites for 20 years was defeated by the Israelite surprise attack led by the prophetess and Israelite leader Deborah along with Barak. Sisera escaped the battle and sought refuge in the tent of the Jael, wife of Heber the Kenite. Jael invites Sisera into her tent, "…and she covered him with a blanket… Then Yael wife of Heber took a tent pin and grasped the mallet. When he was fast asleep from exhaustion, she approached him stealthily and drove the pin through his temple till it went down to the ground. Thus he died" (Judges 4:17–21).

Sabbath prayers ask God to protect us from this vulnerable period. On Friday night, the prayer says, "Grant that we lie down in peace, secure in Thy protecting love, and shelter us beneath Thy wings to keep us safe throughout the night. On the morrow raise us up in perfect peace to life, O God" [2]. Each morning the service continues with the prayer thanking God for the gift of waking up: "Blessed art thou, Lord our God, King of the universe, who removes sleep from my eyes and slumber from my eyelids" [3, 4].

In the book of Jeremiah, God says, "I will satisfy the weary soul and…every soul I will replenish" (Jer 31: 25). "Thereupon I [Jeremiah] awoke and looked about and my sleep had been pleasant to me" (Jer 31:26). In addition, almost every prayer service ends with the singing of the prayer,

Adon Olam, part of which states, "To Him I entrust my spirit when I sleep and when I wake…" [3].

Sleep Stages

Today we understand that sleep is composed of different levels. There is the state of rapid eye movement (R) sleep (where most dreams take place) and non-rapid eye movement (N) sleep which is further divided into three stages: N1 (the very lightest level), N2, and N3 (deep or slow-wave sleep). These levels of sleep were first identified in the modern world in the 1950s [5, 6]. However, the rabbis believed that sleep is not one continuous state. There is a rather accurate description of stage 1 sleep in the Talmud when Rabbi Yosi discusses when on Passover it is permissible to eat: "If they fell into a light sleep, they may eat; if they fell fast asleep, they must not eat. What is meant by 'a light sleep'?—Said R. Ashi: A sleep which is not sleep, a wakefulness which is not wakefulness, e.g., if he answers when called, cannot make a reasoned statement, yet recollect when reminded" (Talmud Pesahim 120b).

There are different Hebrew words used to describe sleep in different parts of the Bible, and these correspond to what are labeled as stages of sleep today [7, 8, 9]. The word *tenumah* is often used to mean drowsy or what is now called N1 sleep (e.g., Isa 5:27, Ps 76:6). *Yashen* and *shenah* are used to refer to conscious thought which becomes unconscious and involuntary, a good description of N2 (e.g., Gen 28:16). *Radum* implies a heavy or deep sleep or N3. ("Jonah's sleep was so deep, though a storm howled, the Captain had to awaken him" Jonah 1:5–6). R sleep is also represented by the word *tardemah,* which refers to a period where the flow of thoughts continue in dreams or in revelation (e.g., Gen 15:12).

Function of Sleep

The true function of sleep is not yet known, although there are many theories including that it is physiologically restorative and provides for energy conservation [10]. The Bible and Talmud also suggest that the purpose of sleep is to replenish and heal the body. "What did the Holy One, blessed be He, do? He created the sleep of life, so that man lies down and sleeps whilst He sustains him and heals him and [gives] him life and repose" (Pirqe D'Rabbi Eliezer 12:7–8).

Sleep is also part of the two-process model composed of the homeostatic process and the circadian rhythm component [11, 12]. The Talmud also suggests a homeostatic process when it is explained that a wise person finds the balance between sleep and wakefulness (activity) [1]. "Rabbi Simeon ben Eleazar said: 'And, behold, it was very good' means, and, behold, sleep was good. Is there any sleep which is very good! Did we not learn thus:…a man sometimes sleeps a little and arises and toils much in the study of Torah" (Gen. R. 9:6). In this quote, the rabbis implied that sleep at night is very good because it allows the student to be alert enough to study throughout the day [8], i.e., like the homoeostatic theory which suggests that the drive for sleep builds up during the waking state and is alleviated by sleep, or in other words, the more we sleep, the more alert we are the next day [12, 13].

A second function of sleep, healing, is also found in the teachings of the rabbis. "Sleep is like food and medicine to the sick" (Pirkei de Rabbi Eliezer) [14]. "Sleep is the best medicine. It strengthens the natural forces and diminishes the injurious fluids" (Sefer Shaashu'im 9) [14]. The Talmud lists six actions which can heal, including sleep. When a sick person sleeps, he gets well (Talmud Berachot 57b) [15]. "I should have slept; then had I been at rest" (Job 3:13). Sleep is so important when one is ill, that, although usually it is a sin to turn off a light on the Sabbath, it is not a sin when the light is turned off to help the sick person sleep. In addition, a sleeping patient should never be disturbed (Rosh al Hatorah, Vayeira), reinforcing that nothing else is as important as sleep for the healing process [16].

The relationship between sleeping and healing has been endorsed by the studies of endocrine function [17, 18, 19, 20]. Glucose tolerance and thyrotropin concentrations are lower, evening cortisol concentrations higher, and sympathetic nervous system activity is increased in a sleep debt condition compared to a fully rested condition.

Sleep Deprivation

In addition to the relationship with health, sleep deprivation, whether caused by difficulty sleeping or by insufficient time in bed, has also been shown to result in impaired concentration, memory, and performance as well as problems with social, business, and personal relationships, and overall decreased quality of life [19]. Although they likely did not understand why, the rabbis were aware that there were negative effects of sleep deprivation. The absolute importance of sleep was emphasized and abstaining from sleep was considered a sin. "He that stays awake at night imperils his own life" (Talmud Avot 3:4–5), "because sleep is enforced by nature" (Talmud Tamid 28a) (17). The discussion continues with Rabbi Judah explaining that the "night was only created for sleep" and Rabbi Nachman bar Isaac stating that "humans were meant to work during the day" (Talmud Eruvin 65a). For this reason, "If someone swears not to sleep for three days, he is flogged…." (Proverbs, 6:10–11). This verse is interpreted to mean that not only is sleep absolutely necessary but also the person must be lying as the rabbis believed it would be impossible to remain awake for 3 days [16]. Scientific data support this belief that it is impossible to stay awake for too long. A study of rats sleep-deprived for 2 weeks resulted in temperature changes, heat-seeking behavior, and increased food intake but weight loss, increased metabolic rate, and increased plasma norepinephrine. The sleep-deprived rats also showed stereotypic ulcerative and hyperkeratotic lesions localized to the tail and plantar surfaces of the paws, and all died within a matter of weeks [21].

Insomnia

Not only was excessive sleepiness discussed but also insomnia was described. Being awakened too early in the morning, particularly by noise, was seen as a problem, such as in Proverbs, "He who greets his fellow loudly early in the morning shall have it reckoned to him as a curse" (Proverbs 27:14), and "If a man desires to open a shop in a courtyard, his neighbour may prevent him on the ground that he will not be able to sleep through the noise of people coming and going" (Talmud Baba Bathra 21a). Samuel said, "Sleep at the break of dawn is as important as tempering is for iron" (Berachot 62b) [14].

Insomnia, or sleeplessness as it is called, was used in the Bible to stress the severity of whatever was wrong with the person. Loneliness is a common experience for insomniacs as they are alone and awake while everyone else is asleep. "I lie awake, I am like a lonely bird" (Psalms 102.8). In the book of Esther, a guilty conscience led to insomnia. "Sleep deserted the king [Ahasuerus]" when he realized he had not rewarded his wife's uncle, Mordecai, after Mordecai had saved his (the king's) life (Esther 6:1), while in the book of Daniel, King Darius' "sleep fled from him" after he threw Daniel into the den of lions (Daniel 6:19) [15].

Anxiety and stress are also associated with insomnia in the Bible (e.g., Ps 127.2, Proverbs 4.16, 5:11, 8:16–17). "At night I yearn for You with all my being, I seek You with all the spirit within me" (Isaiah 26:9), "I am weary with groaning; every night I drench my bed, I melt my couch in tears" (Ps 6:7–8), "I call on God to mind, I moan, I complain, my spirit fails, You have held my eyelids open; I am overwrought, I cannot speak" (Ps 77:4–7), "Anxiety on his part, he cannot sleep at night" (Talmud Sanhedrin 100b), "All his days his thoughts are grief and heartache, and even at night his mind has no respite" (Ecclesiastes 2:23), "For I have set my mind to learn wisdom and to observe the business that goes on in the world—even to the extent of going without sleep day and night…" (Ecclesiastes 8:16). Job (7:3–4) complained of "nights of misery" where "when I lie down, I think, when shall I rise? Night drags on and I am sated with tossings till morning twilight." Many patients with insomnia have the same complaint of worry at night keeping them awake.

Job has other references to difficulty sleeping, including pain causing insomnia (30:17), "By night my bones feel gnawed; my sinews never rest." Another translation is, "… my arteries pulsate so strongly that I cannot sleep" [15]. There are other references to illness and sleeplessness in other books of the Bible. "Only from daybreak to nightfall was I kept whole, then it was as though a lion were breaking all my bones; I cried out until morning. I piped like a swift or a swallow, I moaned like a dove, as my eyes, all worn, looked to heaven: 'My Lord, I am in straits; Be my surety!' What can I say? He promised me and He it is who has wrought it. All my sleep had fled because of the bitterness of my soul" (Isa 38:12–15). "For my days have vanished like smoke and my bones are charred like a hearth. My body is stricken and withered like grass; too wasted to eat my food; on account of my vehement groaning my bones show through my skin. I am like a great owl in the wilderness, an owl among the ruins. I lie awake; I am like a lone bird upon a roof" (Ps 102:4–8).

Treatment of Insomnia

There are also treatments for insomnia mentioned, although a bit different from treatments used today. One of the first "steps towards sleep" is placing a hand on the forehead (Talmud Pesachim 112a) [15]. Perhaps this lifts the ribs to make it easier to breath, or perhaps it is an attempt to raise peripheral body temperature. Sleep is induced by a drop in core body temperature which results in peripheral body temperature rising [22]. Placing a hand on the forehead may dissipate the heat more swiftly thus accelerating core body temperature drop, thus inducing sleep.

In Talmud Sabbath (67a–67b), it suggests, "One may go out with…a fox's tooth, which is worn on account of sleep; a living [fox's] for one who sleeps [too much], a dead [fox's] for him who cannot sleep." Physical activity is also suggested as a cure. In Ecclesiastes, we are told, "Sweet is the sleep of a labouring man, whether he eats little or much…but the rich man's abundance doesn't let him sleep" (Eccl 5:11). Interpretations of this passage include that the rich man worries about losing his riches, and thus also loses sleep [16], or that sleep is a blessing set upon the laborer by God, thus to soften his difficult life [23, 24]. A more current interpretation may be that the laboring man who is physically active will likely sleep better than the rich man who spends his time counting his money, as exercise is known to help sleep [25].

There are also other suggestions for the treatment of insomnia. The Talmud suggests turning out the light (Talmud Sabbath 2:5) [15]. Today this would be understood as providing the darkness needed to stimulate the secretion of melatonin which induces sleep [26]. There is also a detailed description of how to create the soft sound of dripping water by raising water into the air from a container with a spout which had a double siphon, and allowing the water to slowly trickle out from the other siphon (Talmud Eruvin 104a; Tosefta Sabbath 2:8) [15]. This would be equivalent to white noise generators. Even hypnotics were not unknown as a sleeping potion was given to Rabbi Eleazar for abdominal surgery (for obesity; Talmud Baba Metzia 83b–84a) [15].

Sleep Hygiene

In 2005, the National Institute of Health convened a state of the science conference on insomnia and concluded that the most effective treatment for insomnia was behavior change [11]. A part of the behavioral treatment is teaching good sleep habits, or good sleep hygiene, including information on sleep duration and optimizing sleep [27]. Our forefathers and foremothers also refer to some of the same sleep hygiene rules that sleep medicine health professionals recommend. These include not spending too much time in bed, getting up at the same time every day, keeping the environment comfortable (not too hot and cold) and dark, avoiding alcohol and limiting, if not avoiding, naps [28].

Sleep duration: One of the greatest Jewish philosophers as well as a physician, and considered by some to be the greatest Talmudic authority of the Middle Ages, Maimonides, said,

> A day and night are twenty-four hours. It is sufficient if you sleep one-third of that, i.e., eight hours…You should not sleep face down or face up, only on your side. The first part of the night you should lie on your left side, the latter part of the night on your right side. Don't sleep immediately after eating; wait about three or four hours before going to sleep. And don't sleep in the daytime. (Hilchot De'ot 4:4–5) [15–16]

Post-Talmudic writers determined that although 8 h of sleep were needed, there could be individual differences [15]. In modern times, the recommended amount of sleep is 7–8 h. *Timing of sleep*: Writings in the Talmud advise on the best timing of sleep and wake. "Eight hours of sleep, terminating at dawn…" (Maimonides, Hilchot De'ot, 4:4–5). In several verses of the Psalms, it says: "Awake, O my soul! Awake, O harp and lyre! I will wake the dawn" (Ps 57:9 and 108:3), suggesting that the right time to arise is with the dawn. "Rab Judah observed: night was created for naught but sleep" (Talmud Eruvin 65a). Time to sleep was governed by the timing of prayer, specifically, for the reciting of the Shema (one of the oldest and most important of the Hebrew prayers which affirms Israel's faith), first thing in the morning and last thing at the end of the day. "Rabbi Dosa ben Harkinas says: Morning sleep, and midday wine…drive a man out of the world" (Avot 3:14) [29]. Another source had a rabbi commenting, "Sleeping away the morning hours and indulg-

ing in strong drink dull the mind" (Talmud Aboth 3:10) [15, 16]. The interpretation of this advice was that "man should not wilfully sleep late" so that the time of reciting the Shema passes. Perhaps, as we know today, they understood that it is important to get up at the same time each day in order to keep the circadian clock synchronized. *Environment*: The Bible refers to the need for a comfortable temperature in order to have proper sleep at several different points. Jacob, during his travels through the desert, complains of extreme temperatures robbing him of sleep: "Often scorching heat ravaged me by day and frost by night; and sleep fled from my eyes" (Gen 31:30), and again in similar words in Deuteronomy (24:12–13), God commands that "If you take your neighbor's garment in pledge, you must return it to him before the sun sets, it is his only clothing, the sole covering for his skin. In what else shall he sleep?" (Ex 22:25–26). Yet another reference to keeping warm and comfortable during sleep is found when, as part of an analogy, the rabbis use an example of a physician telling a patient not to drink anything cold and not to sleep in a damp place [15] or to "rub his temples with oil and sleep in the sun" (Talmud Sabbath 129a).

Alcohol and food: While people with insomnia often use alcohol to fall asleep faster, it is known that later in the night, the alcohol results in insomnia [30]. In the Bible, there are also references to wine and difficulty sleeping: "Rami b. Abba stated: A mile's walk or a little sleep removes the effects of wine." The Rabbi replied: "This applies only to one who has drunk one quarter of a log [a Hebrew measure], but if one has drunk more than a quarter, a walk would only cause him more fatigue and sleep would produce more intoxication" (Talmud Eruvin 64b, Talmud Ta'anith 17b, Talmud Sanhedrin 22b).

The effect of specific foods on sleep is also noted, in particular, among other foods, milk, fishbrine, and wine should be avoided [15]. This advice is repeated in Talmud Moed Katan, where it is advised that "after eating fish, cress and milk, occupy your body [i.e., go for a walk] and not your bed" (Talmud Moed Katan 11a) [15].

Earlier in this chapter, under the discussion of vulnerability during sleep, we discussed the story of Yael and Sisera. As described, Sisera escaped the battle and sought refuge in the tent of the Jael, wife of Heber the Kenite. Jael invites Sisera into her tent, and after she covers him with a blanket he says, "Please let me have some water for I am thirsty." But Yael instead "opened a skin of milk and gave him some to drink… When he was fast asleep from exhaustion, she approached him stealthily and drove a pin through his temple till it went down to the ground. Thus he died" (Judges 4:17–21). Yael must have known that milk would make him sleepy; as we know today, milk and fish contain tryptophan, an amino acid known to have sleep-promoting properties [31].

Napping: Sleep is controlled by core body temperature which takes a dip in the afternoon, explaining why people get sleepy after lunch. This is their normal time to want to nap. However, sleeping too long in the afternoon can interfere with nighttime sleep. In the Talmud, napping is not recommended. Maimonides wrote, "don't sleep in the daytime" (Hilchot Dei'ot 4:4, 5) [16]. Studies have shown that blood pressure declines during afternoon naps and this is an independent predictor of mortality [32, 33]. The Talmud, in general, is against naps on all days but the Sabbath, since daytime is a time for study, not sleep. In the Talmud, Rabbi Eliezer and Rabbi Yochanan ben Zakkai are both praised for only dozing off in the house of study on the Sabbath, but never on any other day (Talmud Sukkah 28a) [15]. Sleeping on the Sabbath, the day of rest, is considered a joy.

There are also situations in the Bible where people are found to nap, particularly when it is warm. For example, Abraham, David, and Ishboseth all sleep in the afternoon. "He [Abraham] was sitting at the entrance of the tent [sleeping] as the day grew hot" (Gen 18:1). [Although we are not told that Abraham was sleeping, we are told that it was hot and it was afternoon, and Abraham continues on to tell the visitors, "bathe your feet and recline under tree" (Gen 18:4). One interpretation therefore, is that since Abraham invites his visitors to recline, he too has been taking a nap.] "Late one afternoon, David rose from his couch and strolled on the roof of the royal palaces..." (II Sam 11:2). "And they reached the home of Ishboseth at the heat of the day, when he was taking his midday rest" (II Sam 4:5). Even animals rest at noon, "Tell me, you whom I love so well; where do you pasture your sheep: Where do you rest them at noon?" (Songs of Songs, 1:7).

There is also a discussion about how long the nap should last if one does nap. "A man may indulge in casual sleep while wearing his tefillin, but not in regular sleep" (Talmud Sukkah 26a–26b). The discussion continues, "What constitutes casual sleep? [Sleeping during the time] it takes to walk one hundred cubits" They continue, "It is forbidden for a man to sleep by day [when it is one's duty to study the Torah] more than the sleep of a horse. And what is the sleep of a horse? Sixty respirations."

In one commentary, 60 respirations take about one-half hour [15]. Good sleep hygiene rules today advise trying to avoid naps, but if you do nap, limit the length of naps to half an hour, since longer naps adversely affect the ability to sleep at night.

Excessive Daytime Sleepiness

The Talmud also discusses excessive sleepiness. Eight things were listed as being harmful in excess, but beneficial in small amounts including wine, work, sleep, wealth, business affairs, hot water, cohabitation, and bloodletting (Midrash Lev. Rabbah 4:3) [16, 15]. In fact, it actually says: "Too much sleep is inadvisable" (Talmud, Gittin 70) [14]. Although the rabbis could not have known it, excessive sleepiness is often a sign of insufficient sleep at night, whether due to self-enforced sleep deprivation or sleep deprivation secondary to specific sleep disorders.

The Talmud also suggests that excessive sleepiness is caused in part by food. Being tired after a meal was well known (Talmud Yoma 18a): "The stomach when full induces sleep" (Talmud Berachot 61b) [15]. On holidays when the high priest was not allowed to sleep, he was not allowed to eat a large meal either, so that he would not get tired and be tempted to sleep.

In the Bible and Talmud, excessive sleep often is described as being synonymous with laziness and sloth. "How long will you lie there, lazybones; When will you wake from your sleep? A bit more sleep, a bit more slumber, a bit more hugging yourself in bed, and poverty will come calling upon you..." (Proverbs 6:9–11) and, "laziness induces sleep" (Proverbs 19:15). And if one becomes obligated to another, "Give your eyes no sleep, your pupils no slumber" (Proverbs 6:4) until your obligation is fulfilled (Proverbs 6:9–11, 10:5, 19:15, 20:13, 24:33–34, 26:14).

The ability to work is affected when a person is drowsy [34]. In Proverbs it says, "Drowsiness shall clothe a man with rags" (Proverbs 23:21).

Treatment of Excessive Sleepiness

The rabbis not only described the problems associated with excessive sleepiness but they suggested how to treat the problem. "If he sought to slumber, young priests would snap their middle finger before him and say: Sir High Priest, arise and drive the sleep away. Thus once on the pavement, they would keep him amused until the time for the slaughtering [of the daily morning offering] would approach" (Talmud Yoma 20a).

It is explained that "some of the worthiest of Jerusalem did not go to sleep all the night in order that the high priest might hear the reverberating noise [of the people awake around him, singing and amusing him] and so that sleep should not overcome him suddenly." Priests used to prick themselves with a thorn to stay awake (Talmud Gittin 84a) or walk about on the cold marble floor (Talmud Yoma 1:7) [15]. This explanation is similar to masking which occurs when the environment is stimulating enough to fool (mask) people into thinking they are alert, i.e., keeping them awake even when they are excessively sleepy. When the situation is unmasked and the environment is no longer stimulating, then the person is overcome by sleep.

Sleep Apnea

The Bible and Talmud do not refer specifically to snoring, sleep apnea, or breathing during sleep; however, there are some statements that suggest that perhaps they were aware of this phenomenon. In Talmud Berakhot, it says,

> …the maw [stomach] brings sleep and the nose awakens. If the awakener sleeps or the sleeper rouses (i.e.., if the nose induces sleep or the maw awakens), a man pines away. A Tanna taught: If both induce sleep or both awaken, a man dies forthwith. (Talmud Berakhot 61b)

The rabbis are suggesting that there is some enzyme in the stomach that helps one fall asleep. One group of rabbis considers the work of the stomach to be mechanical, just grating and grinding. Another group believes that the action of the stomach is a chemical one, such that vapors from the stomach ascend and accumulate in the head and thus induce sleep [15]. However, there is no interpretation of the "nose awakening" in the commentaries. Are they suggesting that the "nose awakens" because when a person cannot breathe, they wake up, such as in the case of sleep apnea? "If the nose does not awaken, then one dies." This might also refer to sleep apnea since patients with sleep apnea who are untreated have a higher mortality rate and more often die during sleep [35, 36].

The closest reference to snoring is: "But did not Rabbi Joshua ben Levi curse anyone who slept lying on his back? In reply it was said: To sleeping thus, if he turns over a little on his side, there is no objection, but to read the Shema [prayer] thus is forbidden even if he turns over somewhat" (Talmud Berakhot 13b). Why does he object to having one sleep on his back? Perhaps because the person will be too noisy because he snores loudly on his back and the noise interferes with the sacred prayer.

Nightmares

Nightmares are very prevalent in the Bible. Job not only has difficulty sleeping because of pain but also suffers from nightmares: "When I think, 'My bed will comfort me, my couch will share my sorrow,' you frighten me with dreams and terrify me with visions" (Job 7:13–14).

Treatment of nightmares can also be found in the Talmud, which states that dreams can cause distress (Berachot 55b), which will only subside if the dream is interpreted immediately [37]. As explained by Askenasy and Hackett [37], these anxiety dreams, or nightmares, are divided in the Talmud into three levels of severity, each of which is treated differently. For the lightest level of nightmare, a special prayer is recited in front of the priests in the synagogue. For the middle level of nightmare, i.e., one where the dreamer becomes depressed, verses from the Bible are recited in front of three

people, including, "You turned my lament into dancing, you undid my sackcloth and girded me with joy…" (Ps 30:12). For the most severe of nightmares, one must fast on the day following nightmare, since the dream may be a warning and fasting, which is a form of repentance, allows one to reflect and make amends for whatever he is being warned about.

Circadian Rhythms

One of the morning prayers includes, "Blessed art thou, Lord our God, King of the universe, who hast given the cock intelligence to distinguish between day and night" (Talmud Berakhot 60b). Sleep in the Bible is governed by the rising and the setting of the sun as well as by temperature. People rise when it is light and go to sleep when it is dark and when it is hot:

> He made the moon to mark the seasons; the sun knows when to set. You bring on darkness and it is night, when all the beasts of the forests stir…When the sun rises, they come home and couch in their dens. Man then goes out to his work, to his labor until the evening. (Ps 104:19–23)

This confirms that man is diurnal, rising with the light and going to sleep with the dark, while some animals are nocturnal, rising at night and going to sleep with the light. This also points out that there is a rhythm to life and that sleep is part of the rhythm, i.e., circadian rhythms.

As mentioned above, sleep is controlled in part by our core body temperature rhythm, which as it drops at night causes us to fall asleep and as it rises in the morning causes us to wake up [38]. In Talmud Sabbath, we are told, "Lend me your robe and I will sleep in it. He singed it, wrapped himself therein and slept. As he became heated through and got up, it fell away from him bit by bit" (Talmud Sabbath 110b). Temperature, particularly keeping warm during sleep, is also seen having healing properties. The Talmud suggests that an ill person "wraps himself in his cloak and sleep, and he must not be disturbed till he wakes himself. When he wakes he must remove his cloak otherwise the illness will return" (Talmud Gittin 70a). In both examples, a person needs to wrap himself up at night to keep warm as his body temperature drops, but needs to unwrap to stay cool as body temperature rises.

Sections of the commentaries also refer to circadian rhythm shifts. Research and clinical work in the area of circadian rhythms has shown that it is easier to delay ones circadian rhythm than to advance it and thus it is easier to travel west than east [39]. Talmud Yoma clearly says, "…it is easier to postpone the hour of sleep than to rise from sleep early in the morning" (Talmud Yoma 22a). These statements are in total agreement with what we know today about phase shifts.

Aging

The Hebrew Bible often refers to reduced sleep quality with old age [8]. Old age is described as a time "when one rises up at the voice of the bird" (Ecclesiastes 12:4). With age comes lighter sleep such that even the song of the birds can awaken an older person (Talmud Sabbath 152a) [15, 16]. This is consistent with what we know about changes in sleep architecture that occur with age, particularly decreases in deep sleep which results in most of the night being spent in lighter levels of sleep [40]. Another aspect of the statement is that older people wake up early, even as the early bird begins to sing. This would suggest advanced sleep phase, a situation where the biological clock is out of synchrony with the environmental clock and the older person gets sleepy earlier in the evening and wakes earlier in the morning, a condition that is very common in older adults [41].

But not all older people have difficulty sleeping in the Bible or Talmud. When asked to what they attribute their longevity, the rabbis reply, "nor did I ever sleep in the *Beth Hamidrash* [house of learning] in which one spends the day and night…" (Megillah 28a) [15]. Here is an old man who does not need to nap, implying that he is sleeping sufficiently at night. This is confirmed by data from Foley et al. which suggested that elderly individuals who are healthy have no complaints of sleep and no difficulty sleeping [42].

Conclusion

Scientists today consider their discoveries to be landmarks. Yet thousands of years ago, there was already a tremendous amount of knowledge about sleep. In the Bible, sleep is generally viewed as both pleasant and necessary [1]. There are references to sleep that can be directly interpreted by what we know today about sleep disorders. Our forefathers and foremothers were aware that sleep was not one continuous stage. They refer to the function of sleep as being restorative. They deplored sleep deprivation, believing that it impairs life. They felt that excessive sleepiness is harmful. They understood that insomnia could be caused by stress and anxiety and by excessive alcohol, and that physical activity (exercise) and drinking milk could improve sleep. They suggested cures for insomnia, including some of the ideas included in today's sleep hygiene rules. They understood that there is a rhythm or timing to sleep. They often took naps in the afternoon, but suggested just how long that nap should last—about one-half hour. And they knew that with age, sleep is advanced, but that healthy elderly do not have difficulty sleeping.

Although we think we have discovered many new features about sleep disorders, most of what we have done is match scientific data to ideas documented in the Bible and Talmud. Our modern scientific knowledge about sleep is not new and existed even in biblical times. This wisdom is also mentioned in the Bible: "…what has been is what will be, and what has been done is what will be done; and there is nothing new under the sun" (Eccle 1:9).

References

1. Bromiley GW, editor. The international standard bible encyclopedia. Grand Rapids: William B. Eerdmans; 1988.
2. Universal Jewish Encyclopedia. New York: University of Jewish Encyclopedia Co.;1943.
3. Birnbaum P, editor. Daily prayer book. New York: Hebrew; 1995.
4. Silverman M, editor. Sabbath and festival prayer book. New York: Joint Prayer Book Commission of the Rabbinical Assembly of America and the United Synagogue of America; 1973.
5. Aserinsky E, Kleitman N. Regularly occurring periods of eye motility and concomitant phenomena during sleep. Science. 1953;118:273–4.
6. Dement WC. The occurrence of low voltage fast electroencephalogram patterns during behavioral sleep in the cat. Electroencephalogr Clin Neurophysiol. 1958;10:291–6.
7. Kennedy J. Studies in Hebrew synonyms. London: Williams and Norgate; 1898.
8. McAlpine TH. Sleep, divine & human in the old testament. Sheffield: Sheffield Academic Press; 1987.
9. Thomson JGSS. Sleep: an aspect of Jewish anthropology. Vetus Testam. 1955;4:421–33.
10. Zepelin H, Rechtschaffen A. Mammalian sleep, longevity, and energy metabolism. Brain, Behav Evol. 1974;10:425–470.
11. Borbely AA. A two process model of sleep regulation. Hum Neurobiol. 1982;1:195–204.
12. Naegele B, Thouvard V, Pepin JL, Levy P, Bonnet C, Perret JE, et al. Deficits of cognitive executive functions in patients with sleep apnea syndrome. Sleep. 1995;18:43–52.
13. Borbely AA, Achermann P, Trachsel L, Tobler I. Sleep initiation and initial sleep intensity: interactions of homeostatic and circadian mechanisms. J Biol Rhythms. 1989;4:149–60.
14. Isaacs RH. Judaism, medicine and healing. Jerusalem: Jason Aronson; 1998.
15. Preuss J. Biblical and Talmudic medicine. Northvale: Jason Aronson; 1993.
16. Finkel AY. In my flesh I see god: a treasury of rabbinic insights about the human anatomy. Northvale: Jason Aronson; 1995.
17. Krueger JM, Walter J, Dinarello CA, Wolff SM, Chedid L. Sleep-promoting effects of endogenous pyrogen (interleukin-1). Am J Physiol. 1984;246:R994–9.
18. Moldofsky H, Lue FA, Eisen J, Keystone E, Gorczynski RM. The relationship of interleukiin-1 and immune functions to sleep in humans. Psychosom Med. 1986;48:309–18.
19. Roth T, Ancoli-Israel S. Daytime consequences and correlates of insomnia in the United States: results of the 1991 National Sleep Foundation Survey II. Sleep. 1999;22:S354–8.
20. Spiegel K, Leproult R, Van Cauter E. Impact of sleep debt on metabolic and endocrine function. Lancet. 1999;354:1435–9.
21. Rechtschaffen A, Bergmann BM, Everson CA, Kushida CA, Gilliland MA. Sleep deprivation in the rat. X. Integration and discussion of the findings. Sleep. 1989;121:68–87.
22. Krauchi K, Cajochen C, Werth E, Wirz-Justice A. A functional link between distal vasodilation and sleep onset latency? Am J Physiol. 2000;278:R741–8.
23. Landman I, editor. Universal Jewish encyclopedia. vol. 9.New York: University of Jewish Encyclopedia; 1943.

24. Freedman H, Simon M, (Tanslators). Midrash Rabbah. London: The Sincino Press; 1997.

25. O'Connor PJ, Youngstedt SD. Influence of exercise on human sleep. In Holloszy JO, editor. Exerc Sport Sci Rev. 23 ed. Baltimore: Williams & Wilkins; 1995;23:105–34.

26. Arendt J, Broadway J, Folkard S, Marks M. The effects of light on mood and melatonin in normal subjects. In Thompson C, Silverstone T, editors. Seasonal affective disorder. London: CNS; 1989. pp. 133–143.

27. Ancoli-Israel S. All I want is a good night's sleep. Chicago: Mosby-Year Book; 1996.

28. Zarcone VP. Sleep hygiene. In Kryger MH, Roth T, Dement WC, editors. Principles and practice of sleep medicine. 2 ed. Philadelphia: W.B. Saunders; 1994.pp. 542–547.

29. Cohen A. (Translator). Aboth D'Rabbi Nathan: the minor tractates of the Talmud. London: The Soncino Press; 1965.

30. Roth T, Roehrs T, Zorick F, Conway W. Pharmacological effects of sedative-hypnotics, narcotic analgesics, and alcohol during sleep. Med Clin N Am. 1985;69:1281–8.

31. Spinweber CL, Ursin R, Hilbert RP, Hilderbrand RL. L-tryptophan: effects on daytime sleep latency and the waking EEG. Electroencephalogr Clin Neurophysiol. 1983;55:652–61.

32. Bursztyn M, Mekler J, Ben-Ishay D. The siesta and ambulatory blood pressure: is waking up the same in the morning and the afternoon? J Hum Hypertens. 1996;10:287–92.

33. Bursztyn M, Ginsberg G, Hammerman-Rozenberg R, Stressman J. The siesta in the elderly: risk factor for mortality? Arch Intern Med. 1999;159:1582–6.

34. Zammit GK, Weiner J, Damato N, Sillup GP, McMillan CA. Quality of life in people with insomnia. Sleep. 1999;22:S379–85.

35. Ancoli-Israel S, Kripke DF, Klauber MR, Fell R, Stepnowsky C, Estline E, et al. Morbidity, mortality and sleep disordered breathing in community dwelling elderly. Sleep. 1996;19:277–82.

36. He J, Kryger MH, Zorick FJ, Conway W, Roth T. Mortality and apnea index in obstructive sleep apnea: experience in 385 male patients. Chest. 1988;94:9–14.

37. Askenazy JJ, Hackett PR. Sleep and dreams in the Hebrew tradition. In Shiyi L, Inoue S, editors. Sleep: ancient and modern. Shanghai: Shanghai Scientific and Technological Literature Publishing House; 1995. pp. 34–54.

38. Czeisler CA, Weitzman ED, Moore-Ede MC, Zimmerman JC, Knauer RS. Human sleep: its duration and organization depend on its circadian phase. Science. 1980;210:1264–7.

39. Campbell SS, Murphy PJ, van den Heuvel CJ, Roberts ML, Stauble TN. Etiology and treatment of intrinsic circadian rhythm sleep disorders. Sleep Med Rev. 1999;3:179–200.

40. Bliwise DL. Review: sleep in normal aging and dementia. Sleep. 1993;16:40–81.

41. Campbell SS, Terman M, Lewy AJ, Dijk DJ, Eastman CI, Boulos Z. Light treatment for sleep disorders: consensus report. V. Age-related disturbances. J Biol Rhythms. 1995;10:151–4.

42. Foley DJ, Monjan AA, Brown SL, Simonsick EM, Wallace RB, Blazer DG. Sleep complaints among elderly persons: an epidemiologic study of three communities. Sleep. 1995;18:425–32.

Sleep in the New Testament

Michel Billiard

Abbreviations of Books of the New Testament

Mt	Matthew
Mk	Mark
Lk	Luke
Jn	John
Acts	Acts of the Apostles
1 Thes	1 Thessalonians
2 Thes	2 Thessalonians
1 Tm	1 Timothy
2 Tm	2 Timothy
Rv	Revelation to John

Before being anything else the Hebrew Bible is a story in which people learn about God through the events of their lives, and the Talmud, a record of rabbinic discussions about Jewish law, ethics, philosophy, customs, history, theology, and other topics. The first one is composed of 24 books. It was written from the sixth to fifth century before Christ onward. The second one has two components, the Mishnah written during the second century after Christ and the Gemara written from the fourth to the sixth century after Christ.

In comparison, the New Testament, including the three synoptic gospels by Matthew, Mark, and Luke, the Gospel by John, the Acts of the Apostles, the 20 letters of Paul, James, Peter, John, and the Revelation to John, is the presentation of Jesus's life, teaching, passion, death and resurrection, and of the lives of first Christian communities. The New Testament was written from the 50s to the beginning of the second century after Christ.

Thus, it is no surprise that what the New Testament writes about sleep is different from what the Hebrew Bible and the Talmud write. In particular, although there are references to sleep in the New Testament, there is almost nothing about Sleep Medicine. There is nothing about insomnia, sleep-related breathing disorders, hypersomnias of central origin,

circadian rhythm sleep disorders, parasomnias, and sleep related movement disorders. On the other hand there are allusions to drowsiness and deep sleep, to the homeostatic process of sleep, to the alternation of day and night or night and day, to wakefulness and vigilance, to dreams, and in a single case, to a deadly consequence of excessive daytime sleepiness. Worth noting is that the word sleep often has a double meaning, one that is literal, which we shall consider, and one that is symbolic where sleep may mean lack of commitment, lack of faith, or even death.

Sleep Stages

Sleep stages are not figured out in the New Testament. However, drowsiness and sleep are contrasted [5] *"they all became drowsy and fell asleep"* (Mt 25:5) and there are three reports of deep sleep, one in the synoptic gospels and two in the Acts of the Apostles. The first one is in Mark, Matthew, and Luke: [36] *"Leaving the crowd, they took him* (Jesus) *with them in the boat just as he was. And other boats were with him.* [37]*A violent squall came up and waves were breaking over the boat, so that it was already filling up.* [38] *Jesus was in the stern, asleep on a cushion. They woke him and said to him, "Teacher, do you not care that we are perishing?"'"* (Mk 4:36–38). The second one is during Herod's persecution of the Christians: [6]*"On the very night before Herod was to bring him to trial, Peter, secured by double chains, was sleeping between two soldiers"* (Acts 12:6) and the third one shows a young man [9]*"sinking into a deep sleep as Paul talked on and on"* (Acts 20:9)

The Homeostatic Process of Sleep

In Borbely and Achermann's two-process model of sleep, process S is a homeostatic process increasing exponentially during wakefulness and decreasing exponentially during sleep [1].

M. Billiard (✉)
Department of Neurology, Gui de Chauliac Hospital, 80 Avenue Augustin Fliche, 34295 Montpellier Cedex 5, France

This process is exemplified in several sections of the New Testament.

The first one is on the occasion of the transfiguration of Christ, that is a transient change of his physical appearance, to reveal his divine nature, when Peter and his companions are struck by sleep: [29]*"While he was praying his face changed in appearance and his clothing became dazzling white.* [30] *And, behold, two men were conversing with him, Moses and Elijah,* [31] *who appeared in glory and spoke of the exodus that he was going to accomplish in Jerusalem.* [32]*Peter and his companions had been overcome by sleep."* (Lk 9: 29–32). However, the time of the day is not indicated, and this sleep may not reflect natural sleep but a state of sideration related to this divine event.

The second example is found in the discourse on the final age and judgment (Mt 24:1 to 25:46), in the parable of the ten virgins: [5]*"Since the bridegroom was long delayed and they all became drowsy and fell asleep"* (Mt 25:5).

The third and main example appears in Christ's Passion (Mt 26: 38–43, Mk 14, 37–41, Lk 22, 45–46). Following the Institution of the Eucharist in the evening in Jerusalem, Jesus goes with his disciples to the Mount of Olives, in a place called Gethsemane. [38]*Then he said to them, "My soul is sorrowful even to death. Remain and keep watch with me". He advanced a little and fell prostrate in prayer...* [40]*When he returned to his disciples, he found them asleep, and* [42]*withdrawing a second time, he prayed again...*[43]*Then he returned once more and found them asleep, for they could not keep their eyes open"* (Mt 26: 38–43). This shows that, even in a dramatic situation, the evening pressure to sleep is so strong that the disciples cannot resist it.

The Alternation of Day and Night

A reference to night and day or to day and night is found repeatedly in the New Testament, three times in Matthew, twice in Mark, three times in Luke, twice in John, three times in the Acts of the Apostles, nine times in letters of Paul and seven times in the Revelation to John, that is 29 times in total.

In John it is clearly indicated that [4]*"We have to do the works of the one who sent me while it is day. Night is coming when no one can work* (Jn 9, 4) and that [9] *"If one walks during the day, he does not stumble, while if one walks at night he stumbles, because the light is not in him"* (Jn 11, 9). In Luke, during the last days before Passion, [37] *"During the day, Jesus was teaching in the temple area, but at night he would leave and stay at the place called the Mount of Olives."* (Lk 21, 37)

On the other hand, in the Acts of Apostles, in the letter by Paul and in the Revelation to John, the circadian rhythm of sleep and wakefulness seems to be ignored by the authors, when they refer to tribes, widows, elders or Paul himself praying day and night (Acts 26:7; I Thes 3:10; I Tm 5:5; II Tm 1:3; Rv 4:8; 7:15), to Paul working day and night (I Thes 2:9; II Thes 3:8), to Paul admonishing disciples day and night (Acts 20:31) and to "demons" being tormented day and night (Rv 14:11; 20:10).

Wakefulness Versus Vigilance

The three synoptic evangelists, Matthew, Mark, Luke, and Paul use the expressions: stay awake (four times), keep watch or be watchful (15 times), be alert (once), and be vigilant (four times) corresponding to two verbs in the original Greek text, γρηγορέω, watch, and ἀγρυπνέω, be vigilant. Thus, already in the New Testament, a distinction is made between what can be called "active wakefulness or full alertness," a physiological concept, and what can be called "readiness to adopt the appropriate behavior in a given situation" [2], a cognitive concept.

Dreaming

The New Testament quotes far fewer dreams than the Old Testament. All of them appear in Matthew, probably a Greek-speaking Jewish convert to Christianity, speaking to Jews familiar with God speaking through dreams.

Six dreams are reported in the New Testament. Five are around Jesus's birth and one a few hours before his death. Of the first five dreams, four are from Joseph, Mary's husband and the other one from the Magi.

> [18]Mary was betrothed to Joseph, but before they lived together, she was found with child through the holy Spirit. [19]Joseph her husband, since he was a righteous man, yet unwilling to expose her to shame, decided to divorce her quietly. [20] Such was his intention when, behold, the angel of the Lord appeared to Joseph in a dream and said "Joseph, son of David, do not be afraid to take Mary your wife into your home. For it is through the holy Spirit that this child has been conceived. (Mt 1:18–20)

The second dream is a warning made to the Magi who had come from the east to do homage to Jesus: [12]*"And having been warned in a dream not to return to Herod, they departed for their country by another way."* (Mt 2:12; Fig. 7.1)

The three other dreams are warnings made to Joseph:

> [13]When they had departed, behold, the angel of the Lord appeared to Joseph in a dream and said, "Rise, take the child and his mother, flee to Egypt, and stay there until I tell you. Herod is going to search for the child to destroy him" (Mt 2:13),

> [19]When Herod had died, behold, the angel of the Lord appeared in a dream to Joseph in Egypt [20]and said "Rise, take the child and his mother and go to the land of Israel, for those who sought the child's life are dead" (Mt 2:19–20),

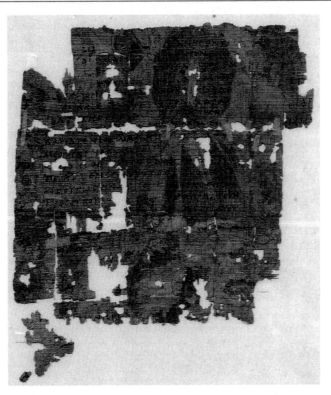

Fig. 7.1 Papyrus 1 (*verso*) designated by β1. This is a papyrus manuscript of the Gospel of Matthew, dating paleographically to the early 3rd century. It was discovered in Oxyrhynchus (Egypt) and is currently housed at the University of Pennsylvania Museum. The surviving text are versus 1:1–9 (recto) and versus 12–13, 14–20 (verso). Parts between square brackets are missing. The words are written continuously without separation. Accents and breathings are absent

²⁰I]δου αγ[γελο]ς KY [κ]α[ο]ναρ [εφανη αυ]τω [λεγων] ἱως[η]φ υἱος] δ[αυίδ] μ[η] φο[βηθη]ς παρ[αλαβ]ει=[μ]αριαν [την] γυναι[κα σου] ²⁰The angel of the lord appeared in a dream and said Joseph son of David do not be afraid to take into your home. Mary your wife

²²But when he heard that Archelaus was ruling over Judea in place of his father Herod, he was afraid to go back there. And because he had been warned in a dream, he departed for the region of Galilee. ²³He went and dwelt in a town called Nazareth. (Mt 2: 22–23)

All these dreams are message dreams and all of them have been fulfilled. On the other hand the last reported dream in Matthew, a dream from Pilate's wife, is a symbolic dream: ¹⁹*"While he was still seated on the bench, his wife sent him a message, have nothing to do with this righteous man. I suffered much in a dream today because of him"* (Mt 27:19), and in this case the advice in the dream is not followed, and Jesus is crucified.

There is a last reference to dreaming in the New Testament, not in Matthew but in the Acts of the Apostles (Acts 2:17), not a dream but a quote of the prophet Joel (Jl 3:1) by the Apostle Peter

¹⁷God says, that I will pour out a portion of my spirit upon all flesh.
   Your sons and your daughters shall prophesy,
   Your young men shall see visions
   Your old men shall dream dreams

simply meaning that all people, whoever they are, will have part in the spirit of God.

A Deadly Example of an Accident Due to Excessive Daytime Sleepiness

The Acts of the Apostles provide us with a clear example of excessive daytime sleepiness facilitated by the young age of a man, the time of the day, midnight, and listening to a man keeping up teaching at night.

⁷"Paul spoke to them because he was going to leave on the next day, and he kept up speaking until midnight. ⁸There were many lamps in the upstairs room where we gathered, ⁹ and a young man named Eutychus who was sitting on the window sill was sinking into a deep sleep as Paul talked on and on. Once overcome by sleep, he fell down from the third story and when he was picked up, he was dead. (Acts 20:7–9)

Conclusion

Although sleep is not considered from a medical point of view in the New Testament, there are many references to it. Sleep can be deep even in inappropriate situations. The drive to sleep builds up during the waking state, to the point that it may be impossible in the evening to stay awake even when it would be appropriate to do so. The alternation of day and night is continuously emphasized in the New Testament. However, Jesus's disciples take some liberty with this rhythm when they do not respect it or even recommend not respecting it. Wakefulness and vigilance, two frequently confounded concepts in the sleep literature are differentiated in the New Testament. Most dreams of the New Testament cannot be considered as true dreams but a way of communication between God and humans, often in critical situations.

Finally, one accident due to excessive daytime sleepiness is alluded to in the New Testament.

References

1. Borbély AA, Achermann P. Sleep homeostasis and models of sleep regulation. J Biol Rhythms. 1999;14:557–68.
2. Koella WP. Vigilance – a concept and its neurophysiological and biochemical implications. Adv Biosci 1978;21:171–78.

The Greco-Roman Period

8

Joseph Barbera

Introduction

To the ancient Greeks and Romans, sleep was a state akin to death, and as such a liminal state between the waking world and the afterlife. Not surprisingly, they attributed great significance to the nocturnal visions that accompanied this state, believing dreams to be communications from the gods (or the dead), and attributing to them the power of prophecy. The belief in the divine and veridical power of dreams is one that the Greeks and Romans shared with the ancient Mesopotamians and Egyptians before them [1, 2]. The Greeks and Romans, however, took this belief in the supernatural etiology of dreams to its ultimate extent. Dreams, in the Greco-Roman world, found a significant place in literary, religious, and historical accounts; and even in the daily life of citizens from slaves to emperors who sought out dream interpreters and dream oracles. At the same time, it is also in this period that we begin to see in Greek and Roman writings the first naturalistic and rationalistic accounts of both sleep and dreaming, paralleling advances in philosophy and natural science. This chapter reviews both the traditional and rationalistic accounts of sleep and dreaming in the classical world, and what "sleep medicine" may have meant in both these perspectives.

Sleep and Dreams in the Greco-Roman World: The Traditional View

In the *Iliad* of Homer [3], Sleep, or Hypnos (Fig. 8.1), is personified in the form of a deity, who is referred to several times as the twin brother of Death (or Thanatos). Various other literary and philosophical references support this ancient view that sleep was a state akin to death. The sig-

nificance of sleep in the ancient mind, however, took a backstage to the significance of the dreams that accompanied this state. Beginning with the *Iliad,* dream narratives were expounded in a number of literary, historical, cultic, and philosophical works spanning the whole of the Greco-Roman era, and such narratives provide us with important insights into how dreams were conceptualized in the ancient world. In such narratives, it is apparent that the ancient Greeks and Romans viewed dreams as an objective phenomenon, independent of the dreamer who experiences the dream as a passive recipient. As Dodds (1951) [4] states, the ancient Greeks never spoke of *having* a dream, but always of *seeing* a dream. Prior to Plato, the word dream is generally used in its nominal form as opposed to a verb [5]. The notion that dreams were a product of the dreamer's mind did not exist in the traditional view of dream in Greco-Roman culture. This objective reality of dreams is most prevalent in archetypal "message dreams" that are frequently described in ancient literary accounts [1]. In such dreams, the dreamer is visited by a dream figure, be they gods, the messengers of the gods, or deceased individuals. In the *Odyssey,* for example, Athene sends Penelope a dream messenger which takes on the form of her sister, Iphthime. The dream messenger is described as slipping past the bolt of Penelope's room and coming to stand by her head to speak to her. Such message dreams find a prominent place in both literary and historical accounts.

Message dreams, as well as "symbolic dreams" [1], which contained more enigmatic imagery, were clearly seen by the ancients as being supernatural in origin. In the *Iliad* [3], dreams are explicitly stated as being sent by Zeus (I.60–64). In the *Odyssey* [6], dreams are said to be the product of two gates located in the underworld: The Gate of Horn, which is responsible for prophetic dreams, and the Gate of Ivory, which is responsible for unfulfilled dreams. This view was reiterated by Plato (*Charmides* 173) [7] and also finds a place in the *Aeneid* (6.890–900) [8]. The godsent dream, or *oneiros,* was sometimes even portrayed as a black-winged creature which could take on various forms as needed [4, 5]. Ovid, in his *Metamorphosis* [9], vividly personifies these

J. Barbera (✉)
The Youthdale Child and Adolescent Sleep Centre, 227 Victoria St.,
M5B 1T8 Toronto, ON, Canada
e-mail: joseph.barbera@utoronto.ca

S. Chokroverty, M. Billiard (eds.), *Sleep Medicine,* DOI 10.1007/978-1-4939-2089-1_8,
© Springer Science+Business Media, LLC 2015,

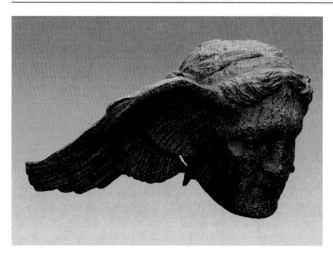

Fig. 8.1 Hypnos, the Greek god of sleep

entities as Morpheus, Icelos, and Phantasos; all of whom were the sons of Hypnos (XI 573–709).

Later accounts view dream visions as the result of the soul being liberated from the body during sleep and undergoing otherworldly journeys [4, 5]. This view was expressed by Plato (427–347 BCE) in *the Republic* (571–572) [10] and the Neoplatonist Synesius of Cyrene (c. 365–414 AD) in his treatise *On Dreams* [11]. In some accounts, these two perspectives—the dream being sent by a god to the dreamer, and the dreamer's soul entering the dream world—may not be mutually exclusive. For example, in the *Odyssey,* the dream figure of Iphthime is portrayed as entering Penelope's bedroom, but Penelope herself is also said to be sound asleep at the "Gate of Dreams" (4.811) [6]. It is as such that sleep, for the ancient Greeks and Romans, may be seen as representing a liminal state between the waking world and the afterlife.

Finally, it is evident in ancient writings that the Greeks and Romans believed in the veridical power of dreams—the ability of dreams to predict the future as well as provide knowledge of the present not immediately available to the dreamer. This is most notable in historical accounts where historical figures, no less than Xerxes [12] and Alexander the Great [13], are said to have been influenced in their actions by dreams they experienced. In practice, the belief in the veridical power of dreams seems to have given rise to the profession of the dream interpreter, or *oneirocritic,* as well as a proliferation of dream interpretation manuals. References to such manuals date back to at least the fifth century BCE with Antiphon the Athenian [11] and reached their zenith with the *Oneirocritica* of Artemidorus [14] in the second century AD. In five books, Artemidorus pours over a variety of dream imagery and indicates their meaning, taking into account the dreamer's personal characteristics in a manner that presages Freud's psychoanalytic perspective.

Paralleling the work of such dream interpreters were the establishment of various dream incubation cults or oracles, wherein supplicants fell asleep in temples or other sacred places in an attempt to induce a divine dream from a deity. Such cults included that of Trophonius in Lebadeia, Amphiaros in Oropos, and Isis and Sarapis from Egypt. The most widespread and influential of such cults, however, was that of the cult of Ascleipius, the God of Medicine [5, 15, 16].

Dreams and the Cult of Asclepius

Asclepius (Fig. 8.2), according to myth, was the son of the god Apollo and the mortal woman Coronos. He was initially revered as a hero and physician of great skill and by the end of the sixth century BC would be elevated to the status of the God of Medicine. His descendents, who carried on the medical arts that he perfected, were known as Asclepiads, a term that would come to refer to all physicians [17]. The Rod of

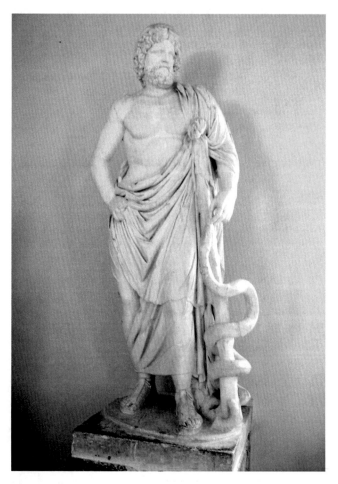

Fig. 8.2 Asclepius, the Greek god of healing. In this statue, he is depicted holding the "Rod of Asclepius," a staff encircled by a single serpent, which continues to be used as a symbol of medicine to this day. (Image courtesy of http://www.HolyLandPhotos.org)

Asclepius, represented by a staff entwined by a single snake, continues to be used as a symbol of medicine to this day1 [18], appearing most notably in the logos of the American Academy of Sleep Medicine (http://www.aasmnet.org/) and the American Board of Sleep Medicine (http://www.absm.org/).

The cult of Asclepius would prove to be one of the most widespread and enduring in the Greco-Roman world. From its origins in Epidaurus, the cult disseminated widely from the fifth century BCE onward, with Asclepieion sanctuaries, or Ascelpieia, being established in an embassy-like fashion throughout the Greco-Roman world [17]. The total number of such sanctuaries has been estimated at up to 513 [18], and it is likely that an Ascleipieoion was a standard institution in any Greco-Roman city or large town. These sanctuaries functioned well into the sixth century AD [17].

The sanctuaries of Asclepius functioned as modern-day spas, if not the precursors to modern-day hospitals. In general, attempts were made to locate Asclepieia in scenic locations, or on sites of religious significance, and almost all of them were built on the site of springs. The Asclepieion of Epidaurus, the center of the cult, boasted an extensive collection of buildings and facilities, including temples to Asclepius, Artemis, Apollo, and Aphrodite; as well as a gymnasium, library, guesthouse, stadium, baths, and a theater. An enigmatic circular building known as the Thalos contained an underground labyrinth and snake pit (an animal considered to be sacred to Asclepius) [17, 18].

The core principle of treatment in the Asclepieion was the practice of dream incubation. Fragments from various literary sources allow us to work out what the process of dream incubation entailed. Prior to undergoing dream incubation, various animal sacrifices were made, the cock being a customary sacrificial animal for Asclepius, with further food offerings of honey cakes, cheese cakes, bakemeats, and figs placed upon a "holy table." Preparatory rituals included prayers in the temple, washings in the sacred well, and the adornment of white robes. Suppliants were then led to the *abaton* where they lay on pallets placed on the floor throughout the sacred room. With the extinguishing of the light, they attempted to fall asleep with the hope of receiving a dream visitation from the god Asclepius [17, 18, 19].

Asclepius, in such dreams, would appear in forms similar to that presented in statues of his likeness, either as a beautiful young man or as an older, bearded man of experience, with a gentle and calm demeanor. He could be accompanied by a retinue of assistants, including his daughters, such as Iaso and Panacea, as well as serpents and dogs. Inscriptions in the Asclepieion of Epidaurus, which date from the fourth century BCE, detail some of the cures carried out by Asclepius:

> Ambrosia of Athens, blind of one eye. She came as a supplicant to the god. As she walked about in the Temple she laughed at some of the cures as incredible and impossible, that the lame and the blind should be healed by merely seeing a dream. In her sleep she had a vision. It seemed to her that the god stood by her and said that he would cure her, but that in payment he would ask her to dedicate to the Temple a silver pig as a memorial of her ignorance. After saying this, he cut the diseased eyeball and poured in some drug. When day came, she walked out sound. (*InscriptionesGraecae*, IV, 1 nos. 121–22, in [17] T. 423)

As alluded to in this passage and others, the early belief was that the dream figure of Asclepius carried out his treatments directly in a miraculous fashion, using both medicinal and surgical means (thus giving the term "sleep medicine" a much more different connotation in the ancient world than we know it today). As suggested by Aristophanes (456–386 BCE) in his play *Platus* [20], the process of dream incubation in the abaton may have involved a certain amount of deceptive theatrics, with temple staff dressing up in the roles of Asclepius and his minions, and appearing at the expected time. Suppliants may even have been given soporific or narcotic substances which may have impaired their judgment and even allowed surgical procedures to be conducted on them [21].

Such miraculous cures, however, are not evident in later accounts of Asclepieion dream incubation. The Greek orator Aelius Aristides (118–180 AD) in his *Sacred Orations* [19] documented the course of an unspecified illness he was suffering from for nearly 17 years, and which brought him into contact with several Asclepieia-seeking treatment. Many of the 130 dreams he described in the work exhibit the discontinuity and bizarreness of content that are reflective of actual dreams. When Asclepius does appear to Aristides in a dream, he acts as more of a consultant, not performing cures directly, but recommending to Aristides various treatments or courses of action. More symbolic dreams seem to have been interpreted by Aristides himself, after discussion with priests, doctors, and friends. Moreover, the medical treatments recommended to Aristides were not out of keeping with rational- or secular-based medicine of the time (Galen noted that such conservative treatments were more likely to be followed by patients when they were recommended by the god Asclepius) [17], T 401). There is evidence to suggest that physicians were at least tangentially associated with the cult of Asclepius [17, 19, 22].

The cult of Asclepius lasted over a millennium, declining only with the decline of paganism itself. Dream incubation would come to be practiced in some early Christian churches, a practice which continued into the Middle Ages. According to Hamilton (1906) [15], remnants of dream-incubation practice could be found in the early twentieth century.

---

1 Not to be confused with the Caduceus, which consists of twin serpents encircling a winged staff, the symbol of Hermes and often erroneously used a symbol of medicine.

Sleep and Dreaming in Greek and Roman Philosophy

While the ancient Greeks and Romans took their belief in the divine nature of dreams to new heights, it is also in this time period that this prevailing view was challenged by philosophers and natural scientists. It is in this time period that we begin to see the first rationalistic accounts of sleep and dreaming in history [23].

Alcmaeon of Croton (early fifth century BCE) provides us with perhaps the first theory of sleep, stating that sleep results from the withdrawal of blood to the "blood-carrying veins," while awakening results from the reverse process [24]. Empedocles (c. 490–430 BCE) described sleep as occurring from a moderate cooling of the blood, with death being the result of total cooling [25]. A similar "cooling" hypothesis was ascribed to Parmenides (early fifth century BCE) [26]. Leucippus (early fifth century BCE) described sleep as something that happened to the body, not the soul, and occurred when "the excretion of fine-textured atoms exceeds the accretion of psychic warmth" (Plutarch *Epitome* V.25.3) [27]. Diogenes of Apollonia (fifth century BCE) believed that sleep resulted from blood filling all the veins and forcing air into the back and belly which warms the breast [28] (Pseudo Plutarch, *PlacitaPhilosophorum*, 5.23).

With respect to dreaming, both Heraclitus (c. 535–475 BCE) and Empedocles alluded to the subjective nature of dreams. Heraclitus further described dreams as the kindling of an "inner light" that occurs when vision is extinguished [29, 30] (Fragment 26 and Fragment 89). However it is Democritus of Abdera (460–370 BCE) who provides us with the first systemic theory of dreams. Democritus, in keeping with the theory of "atomism" he promulgated, described dreams as the result of fast-moving films of atoms or "effluences" (*eidōla*), which are emitted by all objects (including people), penetrating the body during sleep, and impacting directly on the soul [27] (pp. 132–134). This theory, which still sees dreams as a largely externally generated phenomena, would continue to have a long-standing influence [23].

Plato professes several views of dreams throughout his works. In earlier works, he maintains the divine origin of dreams, such as in the *Crito* [31], where he has Socrates divining the timing of his own death based on a dream (44). In a famous passage of the *Republic,* he ascribes to dreams a pseudo-Freudian psychological function, stating that in dreams we express a "lawless wild beast nature" (571c–572b) that we normally repress in wakefulness [10]. Finally, in the *Timaeus* [32], Plato offers a naturalistic account of sleep and dreaming. At night, the "external and kindred fire," responsible for vision, departs with a resultant induction of sleep. With the eyelids closed, the "internal fire" is directed inward. Where such fire equalizes "internal motions," quiet sleep results; where it does not, dreaming occurs (45–46).

Plato is thus perhaps the first individual to distinguish between non-rapid eye movement (NREM) and rapid eye movement (REM) sleep. Despite this naturalistic account, Plato still allows for the possibility of dream divination, even locating the site of dream prophecy to the liver (71).

It is Aristotle (Fig. 8.3) who provides us with the most comprehensive naturalistic account of both sleep and dreaming in the ancient world, writing three full essays on the subject including *On Sleep and Waking* (*De Somno et Vigilia*), *On Dreams* (*De Insomniis*), and *On Divination Through Sleep* (*De Divination per Somnum*) [33]. In *On Sleep and Waking,* Aristotle describes sleep as resulting from the inactivation of the body's primary sense organ, which Aristotle believed to be the heart. Physiologically, he believed, the process of sleep began with the ingestion of food which thickened and heated the blood. This "solid matter" rises to the head where it is cooled by the brain and the subsequent reverse flow back downward causes a "seizure" in the heart which induces sleep. Similar effects were also attributed to soporific agents, states of fatigue, and certain illnesses. Wakefulness followed when digestion was completed with

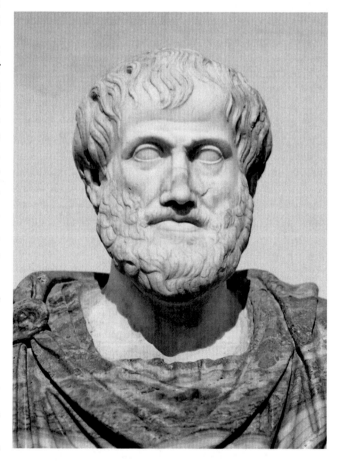

Fig. 8.3 Aristotle. A prolific philosopher and natural scientist, he developed the most comprehensive naturalistic account of sleep and dreaming in the Greco-Roman world. (Image courtesy of Marie-Lan Nguyen/Wikimedia Commons)

a separation between more solid and more pure blood. Aristotle believed that sleep served in the preservation of the organism, in particular, in its exercising of perception and thought.

In *On Dreams,* Aristotle describes dreams in terms of "movements" within the body (presumably the bloodstream) which are created during sensory stimulation in wakefulness. At night, these residual movements impact on the soul/heart to activate perception, but only in its imagining (*phantastikon*) capacity. These residual perceptions produce the appearances (*phantasamata*) of dreams. The turbulence of blood accounts for the variable coherence of such appearances, but, nonetheless, they are taken as real owing to the suspension of judgment during sleep. In *On Divination through Sleep,* Aristotle soundly dismisses the divinatory power of dreams. The foretelling of future events by way of dreams, he contends, is largely a matter of coincidence.

In Hellenistic philosophy, the Stoics, including Chriysipiuus (c. 280–207 BCE) and Posidonius (c. 153–51 BCE) still supported divination in all its forms, including dreaming (Cicero, *On Divination*) [34]. In contrast, Epicurus (341–270 BCE) put forth a theory similar to that of Democritus postulating the existence of effluences or films exuding from the surfaces of bodies and penetrating the sensory organs or going directly into the mind in waking thought and in sleep (*Epicurus to Herodotus*) [35]. This theory was expanded upon by Lucretius (94–49 BCE) in his worth *On the Nature of the Universe s* [36]. Lucretius explained the bizarre nature of dreams as arising from the intermingling of surface films in the air prior to their entering the mind (an image of a centaur, for example, resulting from an amalgamation of surface films from a man and a horse). Lucretius also allowed for the successive images received by the mind to be influenced by what it is "prepared" to see, i.e., by waking preoccupations. Lucretius also conceptualized sleep as the impact of external air and internal respirations on the "vital spirit" or soul atoms diffused throughout the body.

Cicero (106–43 BCE) questioned the divinatory power of dreams in his treatise *On Divination* (*De Divinatione*) [34]. As with Aristotle, he attributed the veridical power of dreams largely to coincidence. He also adds to previous naturalistic accounts of dreaming by suggesting that they result from "an intrinsic internal energy" and even suggests an active cognitive component in the production of dreams as various "reminiscences" and daytime preoccupations come to bear on the mind in a "weak and relaxed state."

Macrobius (c. late third century AD), in his *Commentary on the Dream of Scipio* [37], classifies dreams into five categories: the enigmatic dream, the prophetic vision, the oracular dream, the nightmare, and the apparition. The latter two, he notes, have "no prophetic significance." Nightmares, rather, are caused by "mental and physical distress, or anxiety about the future" with daytime concerns reflecting themselves in nocturnal dreams. His description of "apparitions" amounts to hypnagogic hallucinations, occurring as they do, in "the moment between wakefulness and slumber." It is to this phenomenon that Macrobius ascribes the popular belief of the incubus, a demon said to lie upon sleepers during the night.

Sleep and Dreaming in Secular Greek and Roman Medicine

Traditionally considered to have originated with Hippocrates (c. 460–370 BCE), secular-based medicine in ancient Greece and Rome was characterized by the eschewing of divine causes for disease and the conceptualization of illnesses in terms of environmental influences and humoral imbalances. Dreams continued to find a place in this rationalistic-based medicine. Within the *Hippocratic Corpus,* the treatise *Dreams* [38] maintains that there are dreams that are internally driven and reflective of "bodily states." Dreaming of celestial bodies affected by moisture, for example, indicated an excess of moisture or phlegm within the patient's body. By analyzing the content of a patient's dream, a physician was thus able to diagnose bodily disturbances and direct treatment accordingly [38]. This view was also held by Rufus of Ephesus (c. 100 AD) and Galen (129–216 AD) who authored a treatise on the subject—*Diagnosis in Dreams* [11, 39, 40]. Even Aristotle allowed for the diagnostic use of dreams in medical illness [33], as did Cicero in his own arguments against the divinatory power of dreams (*On Divination*) [34]. On the other hand, there seem to be physicians in ancient Greece and Rome who did not ascribe to the diagnostic value of dreams, including Soranus (*Gynecology*) [41] and those of the Methodist and Asclepiade schools [39].

Disturbances in sleep are frequently noted in the Hippocratic corpus as a symptom to be noted and utilized in prognostication, most notably in the *Epidemics Book I* and *III* and *Prognosis*[42, 43, 44]. The author of *Aphorisms* [45] provides the practical maxim that "both sleep and wakefulness are bad if they exceed their due proportion." In *Prognosis* [44], it is further added that any patient should follow the natural tendency of sleeping at night and being awake during the day and that any alteration from this was problematic. The Hippocratic author of *The Sacred Disease* [46], identifies the brain as the seat of both insomnia and sleepwalking; and notes that excessive blood flow to the brain which heats it is responsible for nightmares. This is in contrast to the traditional view that parasomnic activity was due to "attacks of Hectate and the assaults of the Heroes." In *Regimen II* (Chapter LX) [47] and *Regimen III* (Chapter LXXI) [48], sleep is related to the warming and moistening effects in the body, interacting with the effects of diet and exercise.

Consequently, prescriptions for sleep in relation to diet and exercise occur throughout these texts.

Galen attributed sleep to a cooling of the brain and an increase in its moisture. Insomnia, accordingly, was caused by a brain that was excessively warm and dry. Galen distinguished natural sleep from that of comas and other forms of unconsciousness, as well as from sleep induced from hypnotics which only increases moisture in the body [49, 50]. Galen listed sleep as one of a group of "nonnaturals" that affected the pulse, and, in the ensuing centuries, Galenism would evolve to include sleep as one of the six nonnaturals that on a larger scale affected health and disease [51].

How and to what degree disturbances in sleep were treated by ancient Greek and Roman physicians is unclear. Certainly, the hypnotic properties of various agents were known in antiquity. Aristotle supported his theory of sleep by citing the soporific properties of poppy, mandragora (mandrake), wine, and darnel [33]. Dioscorides (40–90 AD), in his widely influential and long-standing work *De material medica* [52], lists a number of soporific agents including saffron, aloe, rush, opium poppy, henbane, sleepy nightshade, and mandragora. In terms of non-pharmacologic treatments, the Hippocratic treatise, *Regimen in Acute Diseases* [53], offers the advice that "if sleep should not come, a slow prolonged stroll, with no stops, should be taken."

Finally, antiquity provides us with perhaps the first description of sleep apnea, as related by Kryger (1983) [54]. Several sources discuss the case of Dionyisius of Heracleia (360 BCE) who was a man of such morbid obesity that he had difficulties breathing. In addition, he seems to have had significant daytime sleepiness such that his physicians are said to have prescribed him the insertion of long, fine needles into his flesh, in order to awaken him whenever he fell into a deep sleep.

Conclusion

It cannot be said that, in the ancient world, there was anything akin to the field of "sleep medicine" as we know it today. We can, however, see in the Greco-Roman world, a marked preoccupation with sleep and, in particular, dreams. In the Greco-Roman world, the ancient belief in the supernatural origin of dreams was not only held in theory but also in practice, with the proliferation of dream interpreters and dream incubation cults such as that of Asclepius. At the same time, Greek and Roman philosophers began to question the supernatural viewpoint of dreams, and, for the first time in history, offer their own naturalistic accounts of both sleep and dreams. Finally, one can see traces of the importance of sleep and dreams for the earliest practitioners of secular medicine and attempts to translate naturalistic accounts of these phenomena into sound medical practice.

References

1. Oppenheim L. The interpretation of dreams in the Ancient Near East, with a translation of an Assyrian dream-book. Trans Am Philos Soc New Ser. 1956;46(3):179–373.
2. Szpakowska K. Behind closed eyes: dreams and nightmares in ancient Egypt. Swansea: Classical Press of Wales; 2003.
3. Homer. The Iliad (Rieu EV Trans.). Toronto: Penguin Books; 2003.
4. Dodds ER. The Greeks and the irrational. Berkeley: University of California Press; 1951.
5. Flannery-Dailey F. Dreams, scribes and priests: Jewish dreams in the Hellenistic and Roman eras. Leiden: Brill; 2004.
6. Homer. The Odyssey (Rieu EV, Trans.). Markham: Penguin Books; 1991.
7. Plato. Charmides. In: Jowett B, editor. The dialogues of Plato (trans.). 4th ed. Oxford: Clarendon; 1953. pp. 1–37.
8. Virgil. The Aeneid (West D3, Trans.). Toronto: Penguin Books; 1990.
9. Ovid. Metamorphoses (Raeburn D, Trans.). Toronto: Penguin Books; 2004.
10. Plato. The Republic. In: Jowett B, editor. The dialogues of Plato (trans.). 4th ed. Oxford: Clarendon; 1953. p. 1–499.
11. Holowchak. Ancient Science and Dreams. New York: University Press of America; 2002.
12. Herodotus. The histories (De Selincourt A, Trans.). Toronto: Penguin Books; 2003.
13. Hughes DJ. The dreams of Alexander the Great. J Psychohist. 1984;12(2):169–92.
14. Artemidorus D. The interpretation of dreams (Oneirocritica) (White RJ, Trans). 2nd ed. Torrance: Orignian Books; 1990.
15. Hamilton M. Incubation or the cure of disease in pagan temples and Christian churches. St. Andrews: W.C. Henderson & Son; 1906.
16. Ogden D. Greek and Roman necromancy. Princeton: Princeton University Press; 2001.
17. Edelstein EJ, Edelstein L. Asclepius: collection and interpretation of the testimonies. Baltimore: Johns Hopkins University Press; 1945.
18. Hart GD. Asclepius: the god of medicine. London: Royal Society of Medicine Press; 2000.
19. Behr CA. Aelius Aristides and the sacred tales. Amsterdam: Adolf M Hakkert; 1968.
20. Aristophanes. Plutus. In: Oates WJ, O'Neil E, editors. The complete Greek drama. New York: Random House; 1938. pp. 1063–116.
21. Askitopoulou H, Konsolaki E, Ramoutsaki IA, Anastasskai M. Surgical cures under sleep induction in the Asclepieion of Epidauros. Int Congress Ser. 2002;1242:11–7.
22. Nutton V. Ancient medicine. New York: Routledge; 2005.
23. Barbera J. Sleep and dreaming in Greek and Roman philosophy. Sleep Med. 2008;9(8):906–10.
24. Codellas PS. Alcmaeon of Croton: his life, work and fragments. Proc R Soc Med. 1932;25(7):1041–6.
25. Inwood B. The poem of Empedocles. A text and translation with an introduction. Toronto: University of Toronto Press; 2001.
26. Gallop D. Paramenides of Elea. Fragments. A text and translation with an introduction. Toronto: University of Toronto Press, 2000.
27. Taylor CCW. The atomists Leucippus and Democritus. Fragments: a text and translation with a commentary. Toronto: University of Toronto Press; 1999.
28. Pseudo-Plutarch. PlacitaPhilosophorum. (Goodwin WW, editor. Plutarch's Morals. Boston: Little, Brown and Company. Cambridge Press of John Wilson and son; 1874. p. 3.) Perseus Digital Library. http://www.perseus.tufts.edu/hopper/text?doc=Perseus:text:2008.01.0404:book=5:chapter=23&highlight=alcmaeon%2Csleep. Accessed 3 Oct 2012.

29. Freeman K. The pre-socratic philosophers. Oxford: Basil Blackwell; 1959.

30. Robinson TM. Heraclitus. Fragments: a text and translation with commentary. Toronto: Univeristy of Toronto Press; 1987.

31. Plato. Crito. In: Jowett B, editor. The dialogues of Plato (trans.). 4th ed. Oxford: Clarendon; 1953. pp. 367–384.

32. Plato. Timaeus. In: Jowett B, editor. The dialogues of Plato (trans.). 4th ed. Oxford: Clarendon; 1953. pp. 631–780.

33. Gallop D. Aristotle on sleep and dreams. Warminster: Aris and Phillips; 1996.

34. Cicero MT. On divination (Younge CD, Trans.). The nature of the gods and on divination. Amherst: Prometheus Books; 1977. pp. 141–263.

35. Epicurus. Epicurus to Herodotus. In Oates WJ, editor. The stoic and epicurean philosophers. New York: The Modern Library; 1940. pp. 3–18.

36. Lucretius CT. On the nature of the universe (Latham RE, Trans.). London: Penguin Books; 1994.

37. Macrobius. Commentary on the Dream of Scipio. (Stahl WH. Trans.). New York: Columbia University Press; 1952.

38. Hippocrates. Dreams (Regimen IV) (Chadwick J, Mann WN, Trans.). In: Loyd GER, editor. Hippocratic writings. Toronto: Penguin Books; 1983. pp. 252–259.

39. Oberhelman SM. Galen, on diagnosis from dreams. J Hist Med Allied Sci. 1983;38:36–47.

40. Oberhelman SM. Dreams in Graeco-Roman medicine. In: Haase W, editor. Aufstieg, und Niedergang der Romishcen Welt 37.1. Berlin/New York;1993. pp. 121–56.

41. Soranus of Ephesus. Gynecology (Temkin O, Trans.). Baltimore: Johns Hopkins Press; 1956.

42. Hippocrates. Epidemics I (Chadwick J, Mann WN, Trans.). In: Loyd GER, editor. Hippocratic writings. Toronto: Penguin Books; 1983. pp. 87–112.

43. Hippocrates. Epidemics III (Chadwick J, Mann WN, Trans.). In: Loyd GER, editor. Hippocratic writings. Toronto: Penguin Books; 1983. pp. 113–138.

44. Hippocrates. Prognosis (Chadwick J, Mann WN, Trans.). In: Loyd GER, editor. Hippocratic writings. Toronto: Penguin Books; 1983. pp. 170–85.

45. Hippocrates. Aphorisms (Chadwick J, Mann WN, Trans.). In: Loyd GER, editor. Hippocratic writings. Toronto: Penguin Books; 1983. pp. 206–236.

46. Hippocrates. The sacred disease (Chadwick J, Mann WN, Trans.). In Loyd GER, editor. Hippocratic writings. Toronto: Penguin Books; 1983. pp. 237–251.

47. Hippocrates. Regimen II (Jones WHS, Trans.). In: Hippocrates. Loeb classical library. Vol IV. Cambridge: Harvard University Press; 1959. pp. 297–366.

48. Hippocrates. Regimen III (Jones WHS, Trans.). In: Hippocrates. Loeb classical library. Vol IV. Cambridge: Harvard University Press; 1959. pp. 367–420.

49. Galen. On Causes of Symptoms I. In: Johnston I, editor. Galen: on diseases and symptoms. New York: Cambridge University Press; 2006.

50. Siegel RE. Galen on psychology, psychopathology, and function and diseases of the nervous system. New York: S. Karger; 1973.

51. Kroker K. The sleep of others and the transformations of sleep research. Toronto: University of Toronto Press; 2007.

52. Pedanius Dioscorides of Anarzarbus. De materiamedica. (Beck LY, Trans.). New York: Olms-Weidmann; 2005.

53. Hippocrates. Regimen in acute diseases (Chadwick J, Mann WN, Trans.). In Loyd GER, editor. Hippocratic writings. Toronto: Penguin Books; 1983. pp. 186–205.

54. Kryger MH. Sleep apnea: from the needles of Dionysius to continuous positive airway pressure. Arch Intern Med. 1983;143:2301–3.

The Aztec, Maya, and Inca Civilizations

Edgar S. Osuna

The discovery of America placed the European nations in contact with three major civilizations—the Aztecs in the Mexican plateau, the Mayas in the Yucatan peninsula, and the Incas in the Peruvian Andes. The Mayas had been settled for centuries in the same area and developed a civilization with high cultural manifestations, whereas the Aztecs and the Incas, in spite of their political power and strong resistance to the Spanish conquest, were actually cultural parvenues among pre-Columbian people [1].

The Aztecs

The earliest Mexican civilization to leave traces in the central plateau, around 955 BC, was the Olmecs. However, most of the Aztec cultural achievements were inherited from the Toltecs. They were remarkable for city planning, a solid architecture with use of caryatids, and built observatories to plot the movement of the stars and planets.

At the time of the Spanish arrival, the Aztecs capital, Tenochtitlan, was the largest and most beautiful in America, with pyramidal temples, water supply, streets, and gardens [2].

The very name "Aztec" is debated by scholars today. It was first proposed by the explorer naturalist Alexander von Humboldt (AD 1769–1859), and later popularized by William H. Prescott in his remarkable AD 1843 publication: The History of the Conquest of Mexico [3].

Aztec is an eponym of Aztlan, or "Place of the White Heron," a legendary homeland of seven desert tribes called Chichimecs who miraculously emerged from caves located at the heart of a sacred mountain far to the north of the Valley of Mexico, and left the region one by one. The seventh and last tribe, known as the Mexica, decided to move south to Lake Texcoco [3, 4]. They were forced to retreat to an island where they witnessed a miraculous vision of prophecy: An eagle perched on a cactus holding a snake at its mercy. At that moment, the sun rose, and its light caught the eagle's feathers as the bird extended its wings. It was the sign of their sun god, *Huitzilopochtli,* for Tenochtitlan, their final destination, and, in AD 1325, Tenochtitlan was officially founded [1–3].

By the time of the Spanish arrival in AD 1519, the Mexica had formed a strong alliance with their neighbors—the Acolhuacans of Texcoco and the Tepanecas of Tlacopan—and forged a vast empire, the Aztec empire [5]. Eventually, they were to give their name to the nation of Mexico, while their city of Tenochtitlan became what we know as Mexico City.

The diet was based on maize, beans, chili, amaranth, squashes, maguey, and several sources of animal protein were present—turkey, hairless dog, fish, and game. From the maguey plant were produced extensive quantities of an alcoholic drink (*octil or pulque*). Pulque provided relief from gout and was used blended with other substances to heal open wounds.

The Aztecs had an astronomical calendar extending over the solar year of 365 days, divided into 18 months of 20 days each, plus 5 complementary unlucky days *nemontemi.* In addition, there was the astrological or religious calendar *Tonalamatl* of 260 days, divided into 13 months, each under a god. The fate of an individual—health, disease, its prognosis, length of life, besides profession, trade or plain luck—was determined by the *Tonalamatl* calendar [1, 4].

The day started early for Mesoamerican: The people of Tenochtitlan rose before dawn. When the morning star, Venus, appeared in the sky, drums and conch trumpets sounded from the Templo Mayor and the temples that were the focus of religious life in each locality. Many took a steam bath to refresh themselves at the beginning of the day [6].

Explicit cultural codes governed the interpersonal relations and the content of these daily activities. The codes were, in many ways, common to all members of the society,

E. S. Osuna (✉)
Department of Morphology, School of Medicine, National University of Colombia, Bogotá, Colombia
e-mail: edosunas@unal.edu.co

Department of Neurology, University Hospital Fundacion Santa Fe de Bogota, Bogotá, Colombia

S. Chokroverty, M. Billiard (eds.), *Sleep Medicine,* DOI 10.1007/978-1-4939-2089-1_9,
© Springer Science+Business Media, LLC 2015

but varied substantially according to class, gender, age, and special positions. For example, a nobleman advised his son to live in accordance with eight rules:

First: Thou art not to give thyself excessively to sleep... lest thou will be named a heavy sleeper...a dreamer...[5]

The eight rules speak of the ideal attributes of moderation and discretion, only the first was related to sleep.

Other rules were observed during pregnancy. The expectant mother was to eat well and not to be denied anything she desired; she was not to sleep in the daytime, not to look at anything frightening, offending, or red. The Mexica felt that failure to observe these rules could result in a difficult birth, birth defects, stillbirth, or the death of the mother [5].

The home of a common family was a single-room structure arranged in groups of several houses around a common patio. Single-room huts provided little more than a space for sleeping, with the family hearth often situated outside, beneath a canopy. All houses had a shrine to the ancestors. Aztec houses had little or no furniture: People worked, sat, and ate on the floor. They usually slept on woven mats [6, 7].

A most impressive list of works dealing with healing methods and the ideas behind them can be produced, and, practically, all of them are based on the Sahagun Codices—a group of manuscripts, on the Mexicans, written by the Franciscan friar, Bernardino de Sahagun, O.F.M. (AD 1499–1590). Another document, written by Martin de la Cruz, that provides medical information is the *Badianus Codex,* also known as The Codex de la Cruz Badiano, or by its Latin title, *Libellus de Medicinalibus Indorum Herbis.* Visually, the Codex is strikingly similar to a sixteenth-century European herbal [8].

The medical doctrines and practices of the Aztecs were permeated by profound religious elements. The Aztecs believed in the hereafter, with a heaven, *Tonatiuh,* in the sun reserved for the heroes, another heaven, *Tlalocan,* on the earth, and the abode of rest, the underworld *Mictlan.*

The night was a time to be feared. The Aztecs believed that *Tezcatlipoca* was at large in the hours of darkness, sometimes taking the form of the deadliest demon called Night Axe, or sometimes of a wandering demon who approached travelers at the crossroads. It was also the time and realm of the demons called *tzitimime,* malevolent female spirits. Whereas *Tezcatlipoca* was associated with darkness, his eternal rival and counterpart *Quetzalcóatl* was linked to dawn. His rising symbolized resurrection, while the darkness of *Tezcatlipoca* stood for death(Fig. 9.1).

The Aztecs associated owls with *Tezcatlipoca,* with night and sorcery [4, 9].

In the Aztec world, three souls, or animistic entities, inhabited the human body. The *tonalli* (hotness) inhabited the upper part of the head and was responsible for the heat or life force or destiny of an individual. It was associated with the

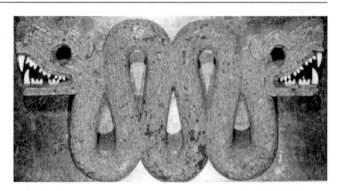

Fig. 9.1 Quetzalcóatl's name has two meanings. Quetzal can mean "green feather" or "precious," and coatl can mean "serpent" or "twin." The elements of the name taken together can mean "Plumed Serpent" or "Precious Twin." Such dual meaning also demonstrates the concept of duality so characteristic of Mesoamerican deities and religion in general. (Taken from ref. [4])

sun, the supreme source of this life force. *Tonalli* could leave the body transiently during sleep [10]. *Tonalli* increased with age, and old people were respected for having strong *tonalli.* When a body lost *tonalli,* death followed, and so corpse was cold. The second entity, the *teyolia,* which resided in the human heart, was the source of thoughts, creative impulses, and human personality [6]. The *ihiyotl,* had its seat in the liver, and was the counterpart of the underworld. Energy, life's breath, passion, and desire were the products of *ihiyotl.* The health of an individual depended on the balance of these three entities, and they were affected by outside forces as well. (Fig. 9.1)

Aztecs knew how to use medicinal plants and roots. A woman or a man could be a *ticitl* (healer), considered to originate from the first wise people. They knew specific methods for how to suture, how to splint, to immobilize a fractured or dislocated bone, and how to bleed a patient [1, 11].

The Aztecs ascribed illnesses of all kinds to three primary causes: supernatural, magical, and natural. They considered sickness the punishment inflicted by their gods for their sins. The power attributed to each deity was in relation with the sickness—the water god sent colds and rheumatism, the love goddess sent venereal diseases etc. [12].

Medical art, *ticiotl,* was believed by the Aztecs to have been developed among the Toltecs by four wise men; *Oxomoc, Cipactonal, Tlatetecui, and Xochicaoaca.* These scholars knew the nature and qualities of herbs, and they developed the astronomical calendar *Tonalamatl.* They were also familiar with the influence of the stars upon the body and were able to interpret dreams [13].

These two elements—one attached to medical botany and the other supernatural—shaped Aztec medicine. Most historians have mentioned that a degree of specialization existed in the Aztec medical profession—the surgeon, phlebotomist, midwife, and the apothecary.

On the eve of the American conquest, Aztec medicine enjoyed considerable prestige among pre-Columbian cultures, and in the eyes of the European arrivals. Many remedies quickly diffused to Europe and became common in the European pharmacopeia of the late sixteenth and subsequent centuries [11].

The Mayas

The ancient Maya created one of the world's most brilliant and successful civilizations. Classic Maya civilization was truly lost until the beginning of the nineteenth century, when brief notices of crumbling jungle cities began to appear in different publications [9].

Maya territory covers roughly the eastern half of Mesoamerica, Yucatan Peninsula, and its broad base. Maya territory covered the western part of Honduras and El Salvador, extended through the lowlands of Petén in Guatemala, Belize, and most of Mexico east of the Isthmus of Tehuantepec—the states of Yucatan, Campeche, and Quintana Roo—and most of Chiapas and part of Tabasco and Veracruz [9, 14].

Maya civilization is divided into three periods: the Preclassic, the Classic, and the Postclassic. The Preclassic includes the origins and apogee of the first Maya kingdoms from about 1000 BC to AD 250. The Classic Maya period started in AD 300, a date which was found carved, as part of the Maya calendar, on a jade plate. The Classic period defines the highest point of Maya civilization in architecture, art, writing, and population size [15].

The highest cultural sophistication of the Maya was hieroglyphic writing going beyond pictographic representation. The finest Mayan hieroglyphs are found in the Maya Codices still extant—one in Dresden, one in Paris, and another in Madrid. As all codices had some religious content, they were destroyed by the Catholic missionaries after the arrival of the Spaniards [9, 14].

The Maya and their ancestors have lived for some 4500 years. The Spanish conquest ended Maya civilization, but the Maya people survived this trauma and 500 years of subsequent oppression. Today, several million Maya people continue to live in their ancient homeland and have retained their culture and languages [15]. Rigoberta Menchu is an indigenous Guatemalan of the Quiche branch of Mayan culture. She received the 1992 Nobel Peace Prize. Over the years, Rigoberta Menchu has become widely known as an advocate of the Indian rights [16].

The Maya believed their world was created by *Hunab,* and his son *Itzammá,* who was the Lord of Heavens, also Lord of Day and of Night. *Ixchel,* his wife, was the goddess of floods, pregnancy, and medical matters [14].

The Maya universe was defined by cosmic trees set at its four cardinal points, together with a fifth, *axis mundi,* placed

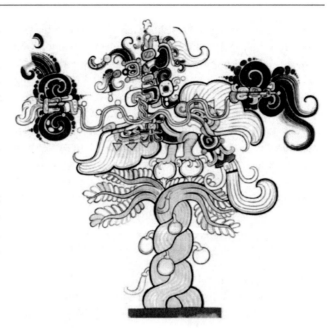

Fig. 9.2 The Maya believed that the center of the world was defined by a cosmic tree. Its upper branches were the heavenly home of the Principal Bird Deity, while its roots sank into the Underworld. This illustration by Heather Hurts (2007) depicts a detail from the West Wall of the murals at San Bartolo

at the center, the ceiba [8]. The ceiba was a sacred tree for the Mayas, and it dominated the center of the cosmos (Fig. 9.2).

There is no other nation in history, where the concept of time produced a stronger impact, nor a people who measured passing time, so accurately, as did the Mayas.

The daily journey formed the basis of the calendar which includes the Sacred Round that was 260 days long, and a second cycle of 365 days long, divided into 18 months *(uinal)* of 20 days with a final period of only 5 days. Each day could be named in terms of both the 260- and 365-day cycles. There was worldwide interest in what might happen on December 21, 2012, as shown by films, books, television specials, and magazines that speak of some kind of universal or cosmic shift in our lives. In fact, the date does mark the completion of a 5125-year Great Cycle. But anyone who understands the Maya timekeeping knows that this date will be followed by a new cosmic cycle that repeats the patterns of the past and reveals new mysteries [13, 17].

In a Maya village, the majority rose before dawn, took a steam bath, ate a maize breakfast, and made their ways to the fields.

Their houses were rectangular, with rounded corners, white walls of stone, mud blocks or adobe, and a special thatch roof. The house contained one or two rooms at most. They slept on mats using cloaks as coverings [6].

They grew corn, beans, squash, groves of fruit, and breadnut trees—a source of food if the corn crops failed. Maize represented more than mere food to the Maya; it was a god—depicted as a young man holding the plant—and the basis of their lives. They believed that man was created by their gods from maize. Protein supplements were obtained from domestic fowls, turkeys, deers, and fishes. Low iodine intake has been mentioned as the cause of pre-Columbian goiter [14].

The physician *ah-men,* was a member of the priestly hierarchy and a product of inherited position and training. The sciences which they taught were the reckoning of the year, the omens of the days, prophecies or events, remedies for sickness, and the art of reading and writing. Physicians imposed the confession upon the patient prior to any treatment as it was customary in the Aztec civilization.

Sweathouses where dry heat with steam was given, perfumed with aromatic plants, were used for the treatment of diseases.

Maya induced cranial deformities during childhood by progressively flattening the frontal and occipital bones between two flat pieces of wood. In this way, Maya obtained the retracted profile which is so characteristic of archeological paintings and bas-reliefs.

The idea of disease of the Mayas was always related to religious and ethical concepts. In the *PopulVuh,* it is asserted that disease is caused by external actions, enemies, or the evil eye.

They identified more clinical syndromes for mental diseases than probably any other culture, for instance, madness, melancholia, delirium, and hallucinations.

A greater part of the treatment was based on the administration of prescriptions made up, in most cases, from medicinal plants. The number of days of treatment was usually 13 for men and 9 for women.

In referring to therapy, it is important to mention that the Mayas used phlebotomy with special lancets, *ta,* as a method of treatment, not only for its physical merit but also as a religious act of penitence.

Tobacco mixed with *cal,* and chewed, was used by them to obtain energy and to quench thirst while at home or traveling or before starting work. Contrary to current sleep hygiene recommendations, the Mayas used tobacco to ease sleep and calm the effects of the daily activities. Tobacco was used also for different diseases such as asthma, fever and convulsions [18].

The Incas

By the early sixteenth century, the Incas built up an empire extending along the Andes, from north Chile and Argentina to south Colombia. The Inca culture was the longest in extension in ancient America.

The Inca empire, called Tawantinsuyu (Four Quarters), was divided into four regions, each supervised by an imperial governor. At the head of the empire was the Inca (lord), who was held to be divine. The Inca ruled from the capital city of Cuzco (currently in Peru), founded by MancoCápac.

The principal crops were corn and potatoes. These were extensively cultivated through a well-planned system of terraces and irrigation canals. A portion of the harvest was kept each year, in storehouses, in case of necessity.

The dwellings of the common people were very primitive. The walls were of beaten earth, and the roof was of thatch. There were no windows. In this dark and smelly hovel, children and guinea pigs were crowded around a little clay hearth. Llama skins, thrown on the ground and folded, served as beds [19].

The Sun was a very useful patron god for the Incas, as he could be perceived, and, therefore, worshipped from anywhere in the empire. It is significant that it is the light not the heat that is emphasized in Inca cosmology.

In the Inca cosmology, the categories of male and female were not ultimately based on biological sex, but rather on cultural ideas. Males were deemed to be dominant, and females subordinate. The fundamental structure of Inca cosmology, the dualities of right (associated with day) and left (associated with night), high and low, male and female, front and back, were in fact, derived from the human body. Although male is usually considered as being superior to female, right superior to left, and so on, in Andean thought, each is essential to the existence of the other. There can be no body without both right and left sides, and no normal adult body is complete without a partner of the opposite sex [20]. The human body, thus, in itself or paired in complementary opposites, is a basic symbol of wholeness and integrity in the Andes.

The duality of sleep and wake could be taken as opposing, and, at the same time, complementary forces, that maintain a constant equilibrium. This has not been described, at least to my knowledge, but it is in accordance with the fundamental structure of Inca cosmology. Sleep is essential to wakefulness, and vice versa, which is similar to the current concept of sleep–wake homeostasis.

The branch of surgery, which seems to have been most practiced in Peru, was trephining (Fig. 9.3).

Medicine consisted of empirical processes and magic practices [21]. The Inca curers, called, in general, *hampiyok,* used various methods for removing a disease from a patient's body; one of the most effective was herbal infusions, of which the *hampiyok* had an extensive knowledge. Other methods included sucking the disease out of a patient, bloodletting, and leaving the patient's clothes by the roadside so that the illness would be carried away by whomever came by and picked the clothes up. According to the Incas, illness was often caused by *hucha* or sin, an element that disrupted the unity of the whole.

According to Garcilaso de la Vega, babies were washed in cold water, exposed to night air, and kept swaddled in cradles

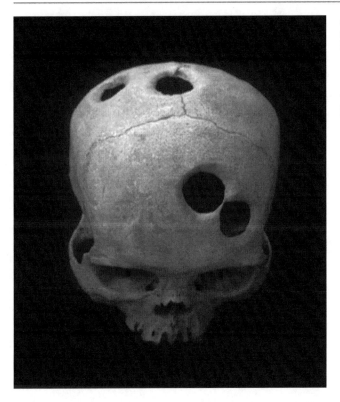

Fig. 9.3 An Inca skull with five healed trepanations (four are visible in this photograph) of similar size and shape. (From the site of Patllacta, near Cuzco, Peru) [21]

until they were three months old. Mothers never held their children in their arms or laps, or even while breast-feeding. The mother placed small planks on the forehead and the back of the head of the baby. To avoid immediate difficulties, the mother tightened these barbarous instruments, a little more each day, until she had obtained the desired shape [23].

The Incas located reason and emotions in the *sonco,* or heart and stomach, and memory in the head or *uma.* Physical sensation was believed to reside in the bones, or *tullu,* and to remain there after death.

Treatment by herbal medicines was, by far, the most important. Available plants that had central effects include maize (which they used to prepare an alcoholic beverage called *chica*). Of course, coca came to head the list [24]. To make it edible, some alkaline material must be added, usually ashes of *quinua*. Coca taken in moderation enables an Indian to show a surprising resistance to fatigue; but taken in excess, it leads to stupidity and laziness [21, 24]. According to the Indians, coca cures sickness and hemorrhages; when infused, it puts a stop to diarrhea and colic, and its juice dries up ulcers. An infusion of *Datura* calmed the nerves and induced sleep, although taken in large doses it could be a poison [25].

Belladona (*Datura ferox*) is well known: It yields atropine and was once widely used as a "twilight sleep" for childbirth [23].

Acknowledgment I thank Jenny Milena Macheta and Diego Prieto for their assistance at the Universidad de los Andes, School of Medicine Library.

References

1. Guerra F. Aztec medicine. Med Hist. 1966;10(4):315–38.
2. Gimeno D. Grandes Civilizaciones de la Historia. Imperio Azteca: Editorial Sol 90; 2008.
3. Pohl J. Aztecs: a new perspective. History Today. 10–17 Dec. 2002.
4. Phillips Ch, Jones D. The mythology of the Aztec and Maya. Southwater: Anness; 2006.
5. Berdan FF. The Aztecs of Central Mexico: an imperial society. 2nd ed. Belmont: Thomson & Wadsworth; 2005.
6. Phillips Ch, Jones D. The Aztec and Maya World. Lorenz Books; 2006.
7. Solis F. The Aztec Empire. Solom R. Guggenheim Museum. Instituto Nacional de Antropologia e Historia/CONACULTA, New York, Oct. 15, 2004.
8. Gimmel M. Reading medicine in the Codex de la Cruz Badiano. J Hist Ideas. 2008 Apr; 69(2):168–92.
9. Stuart G, Stuart G, The mysterious Maya, The National Geographic Society, 1977.
10. Gutierrez MJ, Guierrez CM. Historia de la Medicina: Organización Médica Mexica (Azteca) y sus Tratamientos con Enfasis en la Epilepsia. Revista Mexicana de Neurociencias. Julio-Agosto. 2009;10(4):294–300.
11. Harvey H. Public health in Aztec society. Bull N Y Acad Med. 1981 Mar;57(2):157–65.
12. Aguilar-Moreno Manuel. Handbook to life in the Aztec world. Oxford: Oxford University Press; 2006.
13. Carrasco D. Sessions Scott. Daily life of the Aztecs. 2nd ed. Greenwood; 2011.
14. Guerra F. Maya medicine, lecture Osler Club, at the Wellcome Historical Medical Library, N.W. Feb. 13, 1963.
15. Sharer R. Who Were The Maya? Expedition Spring 2012;54(1):12-16. www.penn.museum.
16. Gimeno D. Cassan F, Contreras J. Grandes Civilizaciones de la Historia. Mayas: Editorial Sol 90; 2008:8.
17. Martin S. Time, Kingship, and the Maya Universe Maya Calendars. Expedition. Spring 2012;54(1):18–24. www.penn.museum.
18. Thompson JE. Historia y religión de los. Mayas: Sigloveintiuno ed.; 2004.
19. Gimeno D. Cassan F, Contreras J. Grandes Civilizaciones de la Historia. Incas y Culturas Andinas. Editorial Sol 90; 2008:2.
20. Classen C. Inca cosmology and the human body. Salt Lake City: The University of Utah Press, 1993.
21. Baudin L, Bradford W. Daily Life in Peru. Allen Unwin; 1St Edn., 1961.
22. Aminoff M, Boller F, Swaab D. Handbook of clinical neurology. 2010;95:3-13.
23. Victor W von Hagen. The ancient Sun Kingdoms of the Americas. Cleveland: The World Publishing; 1961.
24. Golden W. Peru, History of Coca: The Divine plant of the Incas. New York: J.H. Vail & Company. 1901.
25. Fairley HB. La anestesia en el imperioincaico. Rev Esp Anestesiol Reanim. 2007;54:556–62.

Part II

Sleep Medicine from the Medieval Period to the 19th Century

Sleep Medicine in the Middle Ages and the Renaissance

10

A. Roger Ekirch

Early in the Middle Ages, a time of foreign invasions, social upheaval, and feudal warlords, medical texts from the "ancients" found refuge among other prized manuscripts in the cloistered recesses of monasteries. Drawn from Hippocrates, other early Greek writers, and from Galen, the eminent medical theorist of second-century Rome, knowledge of the human body and its care evidenced little advancement until the early twelfth century and the founding of the Salerno medical school in southern Italy. There, ancient texts, formerly preserved in Arabic, became more accessible in Latin. This era witnessed the emergence of a steady succession of universities, commencing with Paris (1110), Bologna (1158), and Oxford (1167), that pursued the study of medicine with newfound enthusiasm. In medieval cities, hospitals and medical guilds also flourished in increasing numbers [1].

For most writers, the ancient Greeks continued to exert immense influence, as did Galen and his emphasis upon a proper regimen in everyday health based upon the management and quality of six "nonnatural things" pertaining to the body (air, exercise and rest, food and drink, sleep and wakefulness, mental activity and emotions, and the retention and discharge of waste). The attraction of classical writings only intensified during the Renaissance with a heightened reliance upon early medical texts in Greek, unadulterated, according to scholarly opinion, by flawed translations into Arabic and Latin. As in poetry and philosophy, so too in medicine, "admiration for all things Greek was in the air," as the historian Roy Porter has written—not, however, to the complete exclusion of other texts, including the influential writings of the eleventh-century Persian scientist Avicenna, whose *Canon of Medicine* became available in Latin in the 1400s. Meanwhile, the advent of printing aided in the rapid dissemination of texts, creating, in turn, new lines of inquiry inspired by Renaissance humanism. Most dramatic, perhaps,

was the advent of diverse drugs and herbs, aided by advances in chemistry, and the discovery of plants and other foreign vegetation in the New World—all of which, by the sixteenth century, popular medical texts, brimming with household advice and no shortage of remedies, made more available to the European public [1].

It is upon these texts that our understanding of early European sleep medicine largely rests, coupled with passing references gleaned from diaries and literary works. Information, as such, is more far plentiful for the Renaissance than for the Middle Ages. Written for the most part by physicians, medical texts typically went through multiple printings. *The Castel of Helthe* (1539), by Thomas Elyot, for example, spawned more than a dozen editions in the 1500s. A number of titles were also translated into English from other tongues, including *The Touchstone of Complexions* by the Dutch doctor Levinus Lemnius and Guglielmo Grataroli's *A Direction for the Health of Magistrates and Students* (1574), originally published in Latin in 1555. Translations, aiding in the cross-pollination of treatments and techniques, only facilitated the congruity of medical opinion during the Renaissance, including discourses about sleep, a topic that most medical texts addressed, however, briefly. With few exceptions, there arose, as a consequence, a broad consensus relating to the physiology of sleep and its role in everyday life [1–3].

As in other medical realms, most physicians depended heavily on the ancients for their understanding of sleep, especially Aristotle and Hippocrates. On the subject of sleep's origins, Aristotle's *De Somnoet Vigilia* was a common source, as it was for Avicenna's "On Sleep and the Waking State" (Hippocrates, by contrast, was notably silent on the subject on what caused sleep). Standard was the Aristotelian notion of "concoction," whereby food, digesting in the stomach, generated warm fumes that ascended to the brain (*somnuscausatur ex vaporecibi, qui vadit ad cerebrum*). There, upon cooling and descending to the chest, they enveloped the heart and precipitated sleep. Later, Galen located the center of sensory perception in the brain rather than the heart, a

A. R. Ekirch (✉)
Department of History, Virginia Tech, Blacksburg, VA 24061, USA
e-mail: arekirch@vt.edu

view that physicians began to adopt by the late Renaissance. Thus, for the English writer Thomas Cogan in *The Haven of Health* (1588), vapors, on reaching the head, became congealed "through coldnesse of the brain" and "do stop the conduits and ways of the senses, and so procure sleep." [2, 4]

Significantly, sleep in the preindustrial age was segmented, consisting of a "first sleep" and a "second sleep" that were bridged by an interval of up to an hour or more of wakefulness during which persons prayed, performed domestic tasks, or, even on occasion, pilfered a neighbor's firewood. "When you do wake of your fyrsteslepe," advised the Tudor physician Andrew Boorde, make water if you feel your bladder charged." [5–7] Other physicians, like Laurent Joubert in France, thought it a prime time for rested couples to conceive children—"after the first sleep" when "they have more enjoyment" and "do it better." Boorde objected to "venerous actes before the fyrsteslepe" lest they "ingendre the crampe, the goute, and other displeasures." [5, 21]

Not all sleepers, of course, followed an identical timetable, though most appear to have awakened not long after midnight [6]. According to Ramón Lull, a medieval Catalan philosopher, *primo somno* extended from midevening to early morning. The English historian William Harrison alluded in his *Description of England* (1557) to "the dull or dead of the night, which is midnight, when men be in their first or dead sleep," whereas Noel Taillepied's *A Treatise of Ghosts* (1588) referred to "about midnight when a man wakes from his first sleep" [9–11].

In the tradition of Aristotle, physicians urged that persons take their first sleep on the right side in order to assist digestion by allowing food to descend "from the mouthe of stomake," near the liver, which operated "as fyre under the pot." Turning, then, to one's left side during second sleep, claimed Cogan, "doth greatly ease the body and helpeth concoction." Doctors also recommended this period of wakefulness for taking medicine, including pills for sores and smallpox [4, 7].

Notwithstanding an early medieval belief that sleep was God's punishment for the fall of man, Renaissance writers celebrated its virtues, all the more, for the importance accorded to sleep in both the holy scriptures and the writings of Aristotle and Hippocrates [2, 7, 12]. Rather than an obligatory hiatus or, worse, a necessary evil, slumber was thought essential to the health of all living creatures. For humans, observed the French doctor André Du Laurens, it was "one of the chief poynts of well ordering and governing one's self." By bringing "all things to rest," it comforted the senses and strengthened the body. Boorde noted approvingly that it not only aided digestion but also made "the body fatter." More than that, it restored spirits and lessened cares, if only by allowing weary souls to forget daily travails. Sleep "taketh away sorrow and asswagethfurie of the minde," wrote William Vaughan [5, 13, 14].

Popular lore echoed medical writings—hence the French proverb, "Quand on estrompu, il fait bon passer le lit." [15] Specially telling was the primacy given to beds and bedding. To judge from surviving wills and estate inventories, beds were the most prized—and the most expensive—articles of household furniture for men and women of property, however modest their means. In the Middle Ages, beds in affluent households consisted of wooden frames generally made of oak or pine. The frame supported a layer of straw topped by a mattress filled with material ranging from straw or woolen wadding to feathers and down. Blankets were commonly lined with fur. For newlyweds a fourteenth-century French writer advised, "For your household you need…mattress, cushions, bed, and straw." [7, 16] And by the mid-1500s, beds had improved in less sumptuous households. Of his youth, Harrison observed, "Our fathers, yea, and we ourselves also, have lien full oft upon straw pallets, on rough mats covered only with a sheet, under coverlets made of dagswain or hapharlots…and a good round log under their heads, instead of a bolster," which was reserved only for women in childbirth. Bedding, praised Harrison, was one of the "things" most "marvelously altered in England," particularly with the growing prevalence of linen sheets and woolen blankets. "Because nothing," wrote Lemnius, "is holesomer than sounde and quiet sleepe," one should "take his full ease and sleepe in a soft bedde." [9, 17] Equally important, the frame needed to be elevated to avoid the cold ground, accompanied, if necessary, by a wooden footstep. In wealthy homes, canopies and curtains enclosed beds in order to block drafts. The poor, however, were fortunate to claim so much as a filthy mattress and tattered bedding, with many indigent families forced to sleep together atop clumps of straw on earthen floors. "Outcasts" slept outdoors "under butchers' stalls," according to the fifteenth-century French poet François Villon [6, 7].

Overwhelmingly, night was the favored time for slumber, according to both God and nature. The shrouded tranquility of evening made it uniquely well suited, as did, in Cogan's view, the value of "its moisture, silence, and darkness" to the progress of concoction [4, 7]. Opinions differed, however, over the proper length of sleep, complicated by allowances for age, health, the seasons (long winter nights required the most), personal temperaments, and diverse tasks and trades. Vaughan, for example, advised extra 2 h for melancholic persons, whereas Lemnius, from his standard prescription of 8 h, excluded porters and sailors among other laborers. In general, a period of 7 or 8 h was advised, except for young children who required more rest [6, 12, 16]. In pointed contrast to Hippocrates, who in "ancient time" had urged a more generous interval, Gratarolo favored 8 h of sleep according to "common custom." Of particular importance, instructed the French surgeon Ambroise Paré, was that food be completely digested in the course of sleep [16, 20].

In spite of its manifold benefits, immoderate rest was deeply discouraged. Not for another century would a heightened sense of time consciousness, fueled, in part, by the growth of puritanism, sharply stigmatize "unnecessary sluggishness." Even so, excessive sleep increasingly became a popular source of ridicule and scorn for its association with indolence, all the more when taken during the day [6, 21]. "A little sleep, a little slumber, a little folding of the hands to rest—and poverty will come on you like a bandit," warned a passage in *Proverbs* (24:33–34).

More alarming, however, were the medical perils that immoderate sleep posed, from indigestion and infertility to palsy and apoplexy. "Much slepingendereth diseases and payne, / It dulles the wyt and hurteth the brayne," declared *The Schoole of Vertue* in 1557 [22]. Then, too, naps allegedly gave rise to fevers and headaches. If unavoidable, they were best kept short and taken in the morning. Vaughan urged the removal of shoes, less thick leather soles prevent dangerous vapors from evaporating. Moreover, napping upright in a chair was thought preferable to lying prone in case the warmth of the bedding proves excessive—"for as too much colde, so too much heate, doth astonish the minde and spirits." [4, 5, 13, 14, 17, 28]

Preparations at bedtime were painstaking. It was not just the quality but also the safety of sleep that stirred concern. Rarely, in Western life, had nighttime appeared so forbidding as during the era from the late Middle Ages to the eighteenth century. Fears, both real and imaginary, fueled anxiety as households readied for bed, and at no point other than sleep were persons more vulnerable, incapable of rational thought, and insensible of their surroundings. Even worse, souls, if death struck during sleep, might not be prepared for salvation. "O Lord," beseeched an Englishman, "now that the darke night is come, which is a signe of horror, death, and woe; and that I am to lie and sleepe on my bedde, which is an image of the grave, protect, direct, and comfort me." [6, 23]

Fire, crime, natural calamities, not to mention satanic spirits, all grew more perilous after dark. "The night is no man's friend," declared a French adage. With dogs and weapons kept close, doors were bolted, shutters closed, and fires banked. The English antiquary John Aubrey recorded that families drew a cross in the ashes of a hearth before assembling to recite evening prayers—or to invoke ancient spells. Affirmed an early Welsh verse, "No ill dreams shall vex his bed, Hell's dark land he ne'er shall tread." [6, 24, 25] Bodies needed to be carefully inspected for lice and fleas. Smoke from burning hay afforded a medieval deterrent to mosquitoes. On cold nights, beds required warming by hot stones wrapped in rags or, in well-to-do homes, by copper pans with coals. Finally, whether one was yet awake or asleep, moral dangers lurked in the dead of night. A twelfth-century theologian warned families "to restrain stirrings of

the flesh and the attacks of the devil which are the most to be feared and avoided in the darkness of this world" [6, 26].

Physicians, for their part, dispensed advice to render sleep both healthy and sound. Common wisdom prescribed that persons not retire immediately after supper. Grataroli and Lemnius advised a minimal period of one and one-half hours, while Du Laurens suggested 3 or 4 h in the event of a heavy meal [13, 17, 19]. "Take heed," warned Cogan, "that wee goe not to bed straightway after supper, but to tarry the time untill the meate be well mingled and gone downe to the bottome of the stomache, which may the better come to passe, [if] we walke softly an houre or two after supper." Boorde also recommended a maximum of two or three dishes [4, 5].

Apart from being encouraged to lie first on their right side, individuals were strongly cautioned against sleeping on their back. "Many thereby, are made starkeded in their sleepe," warned William Bullein [3, 5, 20, 27]. Keeping the head slightly raised was important to keep food in the stomach from reentering the esophagus, and never was the one to sleep with an open mouth [4, 13, 17]. Regardless of social class, sleeping in the nude was customary, with the exception of a nightcap to warm the head. Night garments, consisting chiefly of chemises and smocks, were still a relative novelty by the sixteenth century, even for the propertied classes [2, 6, 16].

Medical knowledge of sleep disorders was at best elementary, confined chiefly to the mysteries of insomnia. An exception was the nightmare, alternately known as the incubus or night hag, which aroused the early interest of classical writers. Symptoms included, in the midst of sleep, a sensation of pressure upon the chest, resulting in breathlessness and an inability to speak. Whereas the Greeks had attributed these frightening sensations to the organic causes, the Church in the Middle Ages blamed the violent attacks of satanic demons seeking sexual intercourse. Renaissance physicians, however, hewed to a wide variety of physiological explanations, from overeating and drinking to fevers [2, 13, 16]. More seriously, Wirsung thought the symptoms might represent an early stage of epilepsy. All the more reason, believed Bullein, not to sleep on one's back. He also ridiculed the writings of "superstitious hypocrites, [and] Infidelles" who touted "charmes, coniurynges, and relickeshangying about the necke, to fraie the Mare." [25, 28]

Occurrences of somnambulism, an affliction that, in time, would figure famously in *Macbeth,* are recorded for the twelfth and thirteenth centuries. In the early 1200s, a work titled *Questions de Maître Laurent* observed, "It happens that many men get up at night while asleep, take up weapons or staffs, or get on horseback." [16] Sensational episodes of sleep violence also drew attention. In the fourteenth century, instances of murder figured in a report by the Council of Vienne in southern France. Even so, physicians appear to have evidenced little interest in such isolated episodes—unlike legal authorities forced to weigh personal culpability. Prevailing opinion exonerated acts, however aggravated, committed during an unconscious state. As early as 1312, the canon *Si Furiosus* observed, "If a madman, a child, or a sleeper mutilates or kills a man, he incurs no penalty for this," a view echoed by the sixteenth-century Spanish scholar Diego de Covarrubias who noted that "such a one lacks understanding and reason and is like a madman." [29, 30]

Far more common was the malady of insomnia, sometimes referred to as "watching" to signify either an inability or a disinclination to sleep. Poor slumber, for many, was commonplace—one of the greatest "miseries in the life of man," thought the Elizabethan poet Nicholas Breton. Illness posed the greatest threat. As in modern life, symptoms associated with cluster headaches, ulcers, gout, and toothaches, among other maladies, all likely intensified at night, as did asthma whose victims were forced to sleep upright. Anxiety contributed to broken sleep, magnified, all the more, by night's perils. "Our thoughts troubled and vexed when they are retired from labour to ease," observed the writer Thomas Nashe [6, 13, 32]. Nor, from a modern perspective, it is easy to appreciate the environmental annoyances of preindustrial life, from timbered homes afflicted by drafty windows, ill-fitted doors, and leaky roofs to infestations of bedbugs, present in England by the 1500s, or the putrid stench of chamber pots. "Some make the chimnie chamber pot to smellyke filthy sinke," complained a sixteenth-century Englishman [6, 33]. Then, as now, some bouts of wakefulness defied explanation during instances of sleep-onset insomnia. In sharp contrast, sleep management insomnia—waking in the middle of the night—was thought utterly normal in the absence of a specific cause such as illness. Rather than a reason for concern or analysis, the interval of "watching" between the first and the second sleep only figured in medical literature as an occasion for engaging in sexual intercourse, ingesting medicine, or for turning from one's right side to assist digestion [6].

In the sentimental view of poets and playwrights, sleep afforded a refuge from the cares and tensions of daily life, particularly for members of the lower ranks, untroubled by the responsibilities of rich and powerful men. In Henry V (ca. 1599), Shakespeare, for example, wrote that none "can sleep so soundly as the wretched slave, / Who with a body fill'd and vacant mind / Gets him to rest." More on the mark was the Bolognese curate who in reference to the poor asked, "Whether due to sleeping on a bed fouler than a rubbish heap, or not being able to cover onseself, who can explain how much harm is done?" [6, 34]

In the absence of safe and effective soporifics, there was no shortage of lotions, potions, and pills purportedly designed to induce sleep—by "inward" as well as "outward means," as Du Laurens wrote [13]. Some remedies, if only by lessening anxiety, may even have afforded a measure of reassurance. Meant to be applied externally were powders, nosegays, ointments, and plasters, with the temples of the forehead and the nostrils often preferred for the most successful application. Du Laurens himself endorsed 11 remedies. Of one, he reported, "There are some which with good successed oeappliehorseleaches behind the eares, and having taken away the horseleaches, they put by little and little a graine of opium upon the hole." [2, 6, 13, 35] Opium figured prominently in medications. In feudal times, "poppy juice" was applied externally. Advised a Neapolitan physician in the late 1200s, "Opium alone, diluted with woman's milk, under the nostrils provokes unlimited sleep." Later, laudanum, a mixture containing alcohol, was employed by the upper ranks despite the danger of being "cast" into "an endlessesleepe." [6, 16] The continental traveler FynesMoryson insisted that Germans, by contrast, refused "to suffer any man to goe to bed" sober [36].

And yet, a significant, if indeterminable, segment of the preindustrial population likely suffered some degree of sleep deprivation. Rather than consisting of two segments of tranquil slumber, their sleep was vulnerable to intermittent disruption—a sequence of "brief arousals" that made daily life all the more arduous in a harsh and punishing age. Medical care remained primitive at best. Despite the earnest advice of physicians, many people may have felt more rested when retiring to bed than rising at dawn [6].

References

1. Porter R. The greatest benefit to mankind: a medical history of humanity. New York: Norton; 1997.
2. Dannenfeldt KH. Sleep: theory and practice in the late Rennaissance. J Hist Med. 1986;41(4):415–41.
3. Elyot T. The castel of helth. London: Thomas Berthelettes; 1541.
4. Cogan T. The Haven of health: chiefly made for the comfort of students, and consequently for all those that have a care of their health. London: Thomas Orwin; 1636.
5. Borde A. A compendious regiment, or dietarie of health. London: 1547.
6. Ekirch AR. At day's close: night in times past. New York: Norton; 2005.
7. Ekirch AR. Sleep we have lost: pre-industrial slumber in the British Isles. Am Hist Rev. 2001 Apr; 105(2):343–87.
8. Joubert L. Popular errors. (De Rocher DG, translator) Tuscaloosa: University of Alabama Press; 1989.
9. Harrison W. The description of England. Edelen G, editor. Ithaca: Cornell University Press; 1968.
10. Lullus R. Liber de regionibus sanitatis et informitatis. 1995. (Unpublished).
11. Taillepied N. A treatise of ghosts. (Summers M, translator) Ann Arbor: University of Michigan Press; 1971.
12. Klug G. Dangerous doze; sleep and vulnerability in medieval German literature. In Brunt L, Steger B, editors. Worlds of Sleep. Berlin: Frank & Timme; 2008. pp. 31–52.
13. Du Laurens A. A discourse of the preservation of the sight; of melancholike diseases; of rheumes, and of old age. ed. Surphlet R, translator. London: Felix Kingston; 1599.
14. Vaughan W. Approved directions for health. London: TS; 1612.

15. Dinges M. Culture matérielle des classes sociales inférieures Ã Bordeaux aux XVIe et XVIIe siècles. Société Archéologique de Bordeaux. 1986;77:85–94.
16. Vernon J. Night in the Middle Ages. (Holch G, translator). Notre Dame: University of Notre Dame Press; 2002.
17. Lemnius L. The touchstone of complexions. (Newton T, translator) London: Thomas Marsh; 1581.
18. Lepper JH. The testaments of François Villon. New York: Boni and Livewright; 1926.
19. Grataroli G. A direction for the health of magistrates and students. (Newton T, translator) London: William How; 1574.
20. Paré A. The workes of that famous chirurgeonAmbroiseParé. (Johnson T, translator) London: T Cotes & R Young; 1634.
21. Innes S. Creating the commonwealth: the economic culture of Puritan New England. New York: Norton; 1995.
22. The schoole of vertue, and booke of good nourture. London: Wyllyam Seares; 1557.
23. F. W. The schoole of good manners. London: W. White; 1609.
24. Burton ES. The home-book of proverbs, maxims, and familiar phrases. New York: Macmillan; 1948.
25. Jones G, compiler. The Oxford book of Welsh verse in English. Oxford: Oxford University Press; 1977.
26. Alanus de Insulis. The art of preaching. (Evans GR, translator) Kalamazoo: Cistercian; 1981.
27. Bullein W. A new ebook eentituled the gouernement of healthe. London: John Day; 1558.
28. Bullein W. Bullein's bulwarke of defence againste all sicknes, sornes, and woundes. London: John Kyngston; 1562.
29. Ekirch AR, Shneerson JM. Nineteenth-Century sleep cases: a historical view. Sleep Med Clin. 2011 Dec; 6(4):483–91.
30. Walker N. Crime and insanity in England: the historical perspective. Edinburgh: Edinburgh University Press; 1968.
31. Grosart AB, editor. The works in verse and prose of Nicholas Breton II, New York: AMS; 1966.
32. McKerrow RB, editor. The works of Thomas Nashe. I. Oxford: Oxford University Press; 1958.
33. Henke JT. Gutter life and language in the early "street" literature of England: a glossary of terms and topics chiefly of the sixteenth and seventeenth centuries. West Cornwall: Locust Hill; 1988.
34. Camporesi P. Bread of dreams: food and fantasy in early Modern Europe. (Gentilcore D, translator) Chicago: University of Chicago Press; 1989.
35. Wirsung C. :Praxis medicinae universalis or a general practise of physicke. (Mosan J, translator) London: George Bishop; 1598.
36. Moryson F. An itinerary containing his ten yeeres travell IV. Glasgow: Macmillan; 1907.

Sleep in the Seventeenth and Eighteenth Centuries

Michael Thorpy

During the seventeenth century, medicine underwent a major change from the doctrines that had influenced it up to that time, such as Aristotelianism, Galenism, and Paracelsianism, to more scientifically directed theories with the underlying teleological desire to accumulate knowledge on the way things work [1]. This time was known as the Age of Scientific Revolution and included the major medical developments of Francis Bacon (1561–1626), William Harvey (1578–1657), and Marcello Malpighi (1628–1694).

Medicine, in general, was then being viewed as advancement in mankind's control over nature and was more soundly based on scientific principles. However, it was still a time to be speculative and philosophical about medicine:

He sleeps well who knows not that he sleeps ill.
(Francis Bacon, Ornamentata Rationalia, IV; quote from Publilius Syrus, Sententiae: Wight Duff and Duff Arnold, 1994) [2]

The scientific revolution began with the theories of Rene Descartes (1596–1650) who rejected Aristotle's doctrines and developed theories based on mechanisms [3]. In this regard, Descartes was similar to Francis Bacon who espoused experimentation and utilitarianism. Descartes developed a hydraulic model of sleep, which considered that the pineal gland maintained fullness of the cerebral ventricles for the maintenance of alertness. The loss of "animal spirits" from the pineal causes the ventricles to collapse, thereby inducing sleep. Descartes also believed that the brain existed in two states; waking, in which its fibers are tense, its spirits strong but rapidly exhausted, and sleep in which its fibers are lax, its spirits gradually replenished (Figs. 11.1 and 11.2).

The beginning of the seventeenth century was the time of William Shakespeare (1564–1616) who made many references to sleep in his writings. Insomnia was a particular topic, as was sleepwalking [4].

...the innocent sleep,
Sleep that knits up the ravell'd sleave of care,
...Chief nourisher of life's feast.
Shakespeare: Macbeth, Act II [4].

The chemical principles of Paracelsus were advanced in the seventeenth century, and medicines, including the use of mercurials, began to take over from treatments such as purging and bloodletting. Illness was then considered to be something that attacked the body in a distinct manner, and the galenic and earlier concepts that disease was a derangement of humors, the essential elements of the body, were starting to fade. The concept of disease was "exogenous" compared to "endogenous" of previous times, so that therapy was aimed at an external cause.

Atomism involved the theory that the natural world consists of two fundamental parts: indivisible atoms and empty void. Atomism, which had been proposed by Democritus, Leucippus, and Epicurus, several centuries before the time of Christ, underwent a revival in the seventeenth century, and was supported by the findings of Jan Baptista van Helmont (1577–1644), who coined the term "gas" and recognized that air was composed of a variety of gases [5]. Van Helmont regarded disease as an internal reaction to some provocation or stimulus from the environment.

Robert Boyle (1627–1691) demonstrated the importance of air for life, and the effect of gases under pressure, which led to the discovery that the reddening of venous blood occurred because of exposure of blood to gases in the air. However, the major discovery of the seventeenth century was that of William Harvey, who was the first to demonstrate that blood was pumped around the body by the heart. It was against this background that the great neurologists, Thomas Willis (1621–1675) and Thomas Sydenham (1624–1689), developed the principles and practice of clinical neurology.

Willis contributed to the knowledge of various disorders in sleep, including restless legs syndrome, nightmares, and insomnia. He recognized that a component contained in coffee could prevent sleep and that sleep was not a disease but primarily a symptom of underlying causes. His book *The Practice of Physick* devoted four chapters to disorders

M. Thorpy (✉)
The Saul R. Korey Department of Neurology, Albert Einstein College of Medicine, Yeshiva University, 111 East 210th Street, 10461 Bronx, NY, USA
e-mail: thorpy@aecom.yu.edu

S. Chokroverty, M. Billiard (eds.), *Sleep Medicine*, DOI 10.1007/978-1-4939-2089-1_11,

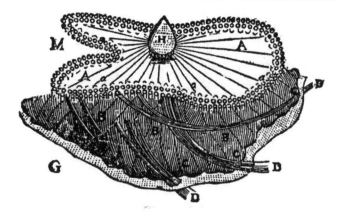

Fig. 11.1 Descartes' (1632) model of the brain awake showing tense fibers and strong spirits. Diagram M. The spirits leave gland **h** (*pineal*), having dilated **a** (*ventricles*) and having partly opened all pores (**a**), and flow to **b** (*fibrous mesh of the brain substance*) and then to **c** (*membrane enveloping this mesh*) and finally into **d** (*origins of the cranial nerves*) [3]

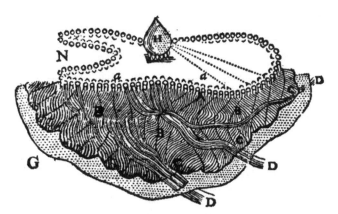

Fig. 11.2 Descartes' (1632) model of the brain asleep, showing lax fibers, and spirits reduced and gradually become replenished. Diagram **n**. The spirits have left gland **h** (*pineal*), the ventricles are mainly reduced and the pores (**a**) become shut down, and flow to **b** (*fibrous mesh of the brain substance*) and **c** (*membrane enveloping this mesh*) is reduced and the nerves **d** (*origins of the cranial nerves*) become relaxed. Parts of the ventricles are still dilated (*dotted lines*) that allows for dreaming during sleep [3]

producing sleepiness and insomnia [6]. As with Descartes, he considered that the animal spirits contained within the body undergo rest during sleep. However, he believed that the animal spirits residing in the cerebellum became active during sleep to maintain a control over physiology. He believed that some of the "animal spirits" became intermittently unrestrained, leading to the development of dreams. He also described restless legs syndrome, which he considered an escape of the animal humors into the nerves supplying the limbs:

> when being abed, they betake themselves to sleep, presently in the arms and legs, leapings and contractions of the tendons, and so great a restlessness and tossings of their members ensue, that

the diseased are no more able to sleep, than if they were in a place of the greatest torture.
(Willis, 1684) [6]

Willis discovered that laudanum, a solution of powdered opium, was effective in treating the restless legs syndrome. Willis also wrote extensively about sleepiness and lethargy. One form of sleepiness that was often reported in the seventeenth and eighteenth centuries and discussed by Willis was "continual sleepiness":

> …the affected as to other things are well enough, they eat and drink well, they walk about,…they now and then nod, and unless they are stirred by others, they are presently overwhelmed with sleep: and after this manner they sleep almost continual sleep, not only for some days or months, but for many years… Thomas Willis 1684 [6]

In 1705, William Oliver described a patient in detail in an article entitled "An account of an extraordinary sleepy person," who was 25 years of age when he developed sleepiness which initially lasted a month, where he could only arouse to eat and drink [7]. Two years later, he had further episodes that lasted 6 weeks and 10 weeks. One year later, after a brief acute illness, he again fell into a deep sleep that lasted 3 months. The nature of these prolonged sleep episodes has never been explained; however, a number of additional reports around the sixteenth, seventeenth, and eighteenth centuries suggest that an infective cause, such as influenza, may have been responsible.

Willis also described, in 1672, a case of "Pickwickian syndrome" [6]:

> …growing aged, being given to idleness and drunkenness, became dull and stupid, and also dropsical, with a great paunch, and his thighs and legs swelled. Yet from these diseases (which he frequently fell into) when he abstained at any time from drinking, and took physick, he oftentimes quickly grew well. But at length, though he was freed from the dropsie, he was oppressed with so heavy a sleepiness, and that he almost perpetually, that in whatever place soever he was, or what ever he was doing he would sleep; then being awakened by his servants or friends, his mind appeared well enough, and for a few minutes he would discourse of any thing well enough, then immediately fall again into sleep. [6]

A few years earlier, in 1614, Felix Platter (1536–1614) had described a man "who tended to fall asleep all the time; in the course of talking, even while eating…. Now this man's body was so enormously fat that he could hardly advance his feet to stride ahead…" [8]. His description predates that of John Fothergill who, in 1781, had described a similar case that suggested the symptoms of Pickwickian syndrome or obstructive sleep apnea [9].

One of the first chronobiological experiments had been that of Sanctorious (1561–1636) who measured the cyclical pattern of change in a number of his own physiological variables [10]. His experimental apparatus has been regarded as the first "laboratory for chronobiology." Subsequently, the intrinsic pattern of circadian activity was demonstrated in the experiment performed by Jacques de Mairan, in 1729, which was reported by M. Marchant [11]. De Mairan placed a heliotrope plant in a dark closet and observed that the leaves continued to open in darkness, at the same time of the day as they had in sunlight. This experiment illustrated the presence of an intrinsic circadian rhythm in the absence of environmental lighting conditions. De Mairan also recognized the importance of this observation for understanding the behavior of patients:

> this seems to be related to the sensitivity of a great number of bed-ridden sick people, who, in their confinement, are aware of the differences of day and night. M. Marchant [11]

Despite some setbacks, a scientific approach to medicine continued with the works of Linnaeus and von Haller. Karl von Linne (1707–1778), called Linnaeus, made important contributions to the classifications of botany, zoology, and medicine [12]. He emphasized the importance of cyclical changes in botany, which was nowhere more clearly presented than in his flower clock. The flower clock was developed upon the principle that different species of flowers open their leaves at various times of the day. Therefore, a garden of flowers, arranged in a circular pattern, could give an estimate of the time of day, by the pattern of flower and leaf openings and closings.

As far back as ancient Greece, there had been some recognition of variation in the behavior of plants and animals, not only on a seasonal basis but also on a daily basis. Linnaeus' finding was an important early milestone in the development of the science of biological rhythms in plants and animals.

During the seventeenth and eighteenth centuries, medical schools had rapidly expanded throughout Europe, with those north of the French–Italian Alps beginning to gain in prominence. The Swiss-born scientist Albrecht von Haller (1708–1777), a pupil of Boerhaave of the University of Leiden, an important medical center in Europe, made major contributions to many scientific topics including medicine. Von Haller performed numerous experiments on the nervous system and demonstrated the sensitivity of nerve and the irritability of muscle; in doing so, he dispelled much of the mysticism of previous eras. Von Haller produced a major work entitled *Elementa Physiologiae* in which he devoted 36 pages to the physiology of sleep and proposed a theory for its cause [13].

The many theories of the cause of sleep can be placed into four main groups: vascular (mechanical, anemic, congestive), chemical (humoral), neural (histological) and a fourth group, which explains the reason for sleep rather than the physiological cause of sleep, the behavioral (psychological, biological) theories [14].

The vascular theories were paramount in the seventeenth and eighteenth centuries. In a vascular concept, similar to that of Alcmaeon in the fifth century BC, von Haller believed that sleep was caused by the flow of blood to the head, which induced pressure on the brain, thereby inducing sleep by cutting off the "animal spirits." Von Haller derived his beliefs from the views of his mentor Hermann Boerhaave (1667–1738). Von Haller's theory was expanded in the nineteenth century into the congestion theory of the cause of sleep, a theory that was still believed into the early part of the twentieth century. Von Haller also considered dreams to be a symptom of disease, "a stimulating cause, by which the perfect tranquility of the sensorium is interrupted."

The vascular theories described the cause of sleep to be related to the blood vessels, either congestion (pressure of blood) or anemia (lack of blood) in the brain. Johann Fredreich Blumenbach (1752–1840), professor at Göttingen, who is regarded as the founder of modern anthropology, was the first to observe the brain of a sleeping subject in 1795 [15]. He noted that the surface of the brain was pale during sleep compared with wakefulness; contrary to earlier theories, he proposed that sleep was caused by the lack of blood in the brain.

The late eighteenth century was also the time of the discovery of oxygen by Karl Scheele (1742–1786) and Joseph Priestley (1733–1804). But it was Antoine-Laurent Lavoisier (1743–1794), who coined the name "oxygen" and recognized its importance in the maintenance of living tissue. Despite the important advances in clinical medicine that occurred in the eighteenth century, there were very few therapeutic advances. Medications still consisted of potions developed from plant and animal tissues, and opium was still the main form of sedation in a common formulation called "Hoffmann's anodyne of opium." The ancient practices of bleeding and purging continued to be widely prescribed throughout the eighteenth century. Infection was a major source of sleep disorders in the seventeenth and eighteenth centuries, both insomnia and excessive sleepiness. An early report of African sleeping sickness was made in 1735 by John Atkins (1685–1757), a naval surgeon, after travels to Guinea and Somalia. [16].

It was not until the late 1700s that the greatest advance of that time was made in the development of sleep medicine. It occurred in Bologna in 1771 with Luigi Galvani's (1737–1798) demonstration of electrical activity of the nervous system in the frog (Fig. 11.3) [17]. Galvani, a professor of anatomy and gynecology, was particularly interested in electricity, and his findings led to the subsequent development of the field of electrophysiology, and the gradual destruction of the humoralist theory of nervous activity.

With the development of the scientific approach to medicine, the discovery of atomism, animal electrophysiology, the advances in respiratory and cardiovascular physiology, as well as treatment advances, such as quinine for malaria and digitalis for heart disease, medicine was about to enter its modern era, the nineteenth century.

Fig. 11.3 Galvani's experiment of the frog with the first demonstration of electrical activity of the nervous tissue [17]

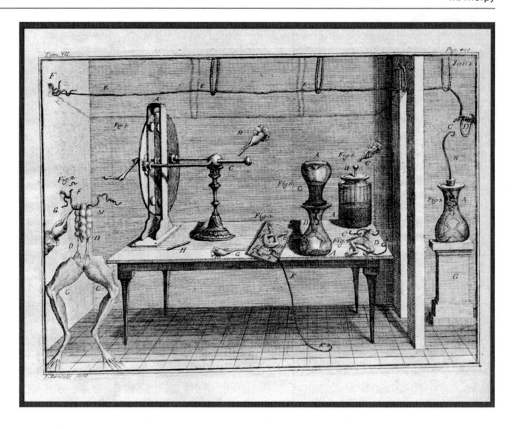

References

1. Thorpy M. History of sleep medicine. Handb Clin Neurol. 2011;98:3–25.
2. Wight DJ, Duff AM. Minor Latin poets. Vol I. Publilius Syrus. Harvard: Harvard University Press; 1994.
3. Descartes R. Treatise of man. Reprinted in 1972. In: Hall TS, editor. Cambridge: Harvard University Press; 1632.
4. Shakespeare W. Macbeth. (Thomas Marc Parrott, editor). New York: American Book; 1904.
5. Van Helmont JB. Ortus medicinæ: id est initia physicæ inaudita. Amsterdam: Apud Ludovicum Elzevirium; 1648.
6. Willis T. Practice of physick. London: Dring T, Harper C, Leigh J; 1684.
7. Oliver O. An account of an extraordinary sleepy person. Philos Trans. 1705;304:2177–82.
8. Platter Felix. Observationum, in hominis affectibus plerisque, corpori et animo, functionum laesione, dolore, aliave molestia et vitio incommodantibus, libri tres, Basel Koenig, 5–6, 1614.
9. Simpson HN. Obesity, heart failure due to (a further note on). New Engl J Med. 1958;259:34.
10. Santorio Santorio. De Statica medicina aphorismorum sectiones septem, accendunt in hoc opus commentarii martini lister, et georgii baglivii. Venice: Novelli; 1759.
11. de Mairan J. Observation Botanique. Paris: Histoire de l'Académie Royale des Sciences; 1729.
12. Linnaeus C. Philosophia Botanica. Stockholm: God of Kiesewetter; 1751.
13. Von Haller A. Elementa Physiologiae Corporis Humani. 8 Vols. Lausannae: Sumptibus; 1766.
14. Wittern R. Sleep theories in the antiquity and in the Renaissance. In: Horne JA, editor. Sleep 88. Stuttgart: Fischer Verlag; 1989. pp. 11–22.
15. Blumenbach J. Anfangs Grande de Physiologie. Göttingen: J.C. Dieterich; 1795.
16. Atkins J. A voyage to Guinea, Brazil, and the West Indies. London: Ward C., Chandler R. 1735. pp. 72–3.
17. Galvani L. De viribus electricitatis in motu musculari commentarius. Bologna: Ex typographia Instituti Scientiarum; 1791.

Part III

The Early Evolution of Modern Sleep Medicine

The Evolution of Sleep Medicine in the Nineteenth and the Early Twentieth Century

Hartmut Schulz and Piero Salzarulo

Introduction

Until the middle of the nineteenth century, knowledge on sleep and its disorders was based exclusively on the information given to the physician by the sleeper himself and the inspection of the sleeper's behavior by an outside observer, interpreted in the frame of the general medical context and philosophical reasoning. This procedure allowed recognition of a wide spectrum of sleep disturbances, characterized by insufficient sleep (insomnia), insufficient wakefulness (somnolence), or strange behaviors during sleep, such as sleepwalking, and some other sleep disturbances.

It was only in the second half of the nineteenth century that sleep was subject to experimental manipulation and measurement. Four main events heralded the transformation of the study of sleep into an experimental science, allowing far reaching consequences for sleep medicine: (1) Kohlschütter's pioneering studies on the depth or "firmness" of sleep by measuring reactions of sleeping subjects to acoustic stimuli [1]; (2) studies on the effect of prolonged sleep deprivation in animals [2] and human subjects [3]; (3) physiological measurements of organic functions, such as body temperature, circulation, respiration, excretion, and others, during sleep or across the sleep–waking cycle; and (4) epidemiological studies using questionnaires and scales to gather information on sleep habits and dreaming [4, 5].

The systematic study of "the sleep of others" [6, 7] became the basis of sleep research as a scientific discipline (Table 12.1). There were two major developments in instrumentation in the early twentieth century, which finally made it feasible to focus on sleep as an object of scientific measurement. One was actimetry which allowed to record rest and activity continuously, and thus sleep–wake cycles in different species, including human beings [8]; and the other was electroencephalography, recording electrical activity of the brain during wakefulness and sleep [9, 10]. Sleep medicine gained from the combination of traditional techniques of medical diagnosis (skilful observation and patient's report) and the availability of technical methods to measure bodily functions in sleep.

Historical Classifications of Sleep Disorders

Early in the nineteenth century, Frank [11, 12] presented a comprehensive classification of sleep disorders, as part of a classification of diseases of the nervous system, updating previous nosological systems [13–15]. Frank described seven classes of sleep disturbances: (1) cataphoria, a more intense and prolonged sleep than normal, which occurs in a symptomatic and an idiopathic form. Cataphoria best corresponds to hypersomnia in actual nosological systems; (2) agrypnia or insomnia, subdivided again into a symptomatic and an idiopathic form. Idiopathic insomnia ("l'agrypnie primitive") occurs in children and adults. In adults, the disorder was classified according to its etiology into (a) inflammatory, (b) gastric, (c) arthritic, and (d) nervous types; (3) a group of disorders characterized by alterations of the appearance of sleep ("par sa manière d'être"), i.e., disorders which are grouped in actual nosological terms as parasomnias. The group includes (a) snoring, (b) jactations, cramps, and episodes of nocturnal heat ("chaleurs nocturnes"), and (c) sleep terrors ("frayeurs nocturnes"); (4) anxiety dreams ("songes effrayants"); (5) nightmare (incubus); (6) somnambulism; and finally (7) somniation, a form of sudden, sometimes periodic episodes of dream-or sleep-like behavior (gesticulation, writhing, speaking, walking, etc.)-during waking, followed by amnesia for the event. For all these disorders, Frank gave a definition, a description of symptoms, causes, diagnosis, and treatment, supplemented by an extensive bibliography, citing all available references from earlier authors.

H. Schulz (✉)
Rankestr. 32, 99096 Erfurt, Germany
e-mail: Hartmut.schulz@gmx.de

P. Salzarulo
Trento, Italy
e-mail: piersal@yahoo.com

S. Chokroverty, M. Billiard (eds.), *Sleep Medicine,* DOI 10.1007/978-1-4939-2089-1_12,
© Springer Science+Business Media, LLC 2015

Table 12.1 Milestones in sleep research and medicine between 1800 and 1953

Year	Event
1862	Ernst Kohlschütter performs laboratory-based measurements of reactivity to stimuli during sleep (depth of sleep curve)
1865	Alfred Maury. *Le sommeil et les rêves*
1867	Hervey de Saint-Denis. *Les rêves et comment les diriger*
1877	Carl Westphal presents a patient with the clinical picture of narcolepsy
1880	Jean Baptiste Gélineau publishes his patient with narcolepsy and coins the term narcolepsy
1890	Ludwig Mauthner. First attempt to localize a "sleep center"
1894	Maria Manaseïna. First study on sleep deprivation in puppies [2]
1896	G. T. W. Patrick and J. A. Gilbert. First study on sleep deprivation in humans
1900	Sigmund Freud. *Die Traumdeutung*
1909	Kuniomi Ishimori. Sleep-inducing substances from sleep-deprived animals
1913	Henri Piéron. *Le problème physiologique du sommeil*
1916	J. S. Szymanski. 24-h rest–activity distribution in different animals, measured by actigraphy
1917	Constantin von Economo. First publications on encephalitis lethargica [16]
1923	I. P. Pavlov. Theory of sleep as "generalized inhibition" [17]
1929	W. R. Hess. Electrical brain stimulation and sleep [18]
1929	Hans Berger. First publications on the electroencephalogram (EEG)
1935	Frédéric Bremer. Cerveau "isolé" and physiology of sleep [19]
1935	A. L. Loomis, E. N. Harvey and G. Hobart. First EEG sleep studies in man
1939	Nathaniel Kleitman. *Sleep and Wakefulness as Alternating Phases in the Cycle of Existence* [20]
1949	G. Moruzzi and H. W. Magoun. Brain stem reticular formation and activation of the EEG [21]
1953	E. Aserinsky and N. Kleitman describe regularly occurring periods of eye motility, and concomitant phenomena, during sleep

About the same time, Hosack [22] published a syllabus containing a synopsis of the main 13 nosological systems of illnesses, published in the second half of the eighteenth and the early nineteenth century. All different sorts of sleep disorders can be found there, with varying terminology and scattered over different diagnostic classes. Table 12.2 summarizes all sleep-related disorders contained in these nosological systems, rearranged according to the categories of the actual International Classification of Sleep Disorders [23]. To get a more complete picture of the historical development, 12 more classifications of sleep disorders were added, which cover the time span from 1838 to 1970. While the selection of these 12 references is fortuitous, the aim was to include diagnostic systems from different countries. These latter entries were not drawn from comprehensive nosological systems of illnesses but from sleep-specific publications. The entries in Table 12.2 show a dominance of three diagnostic categories (insomnias, hypersomnias, and parasomnias) in the considered period; while entries in other American Academy of Sleep Medicine (AASM), diagnostic categories were rare. Abnormal movements in sleep were listed, for the first time, as a separate class of disturbances by Romagna Manoia in 1923 [24]. Most astonishing is the near absence of entries to the category of sleep-related breathing disorders (SRBD), while the lack of circadian sleep rhythm disorders is less surprising for a time when shift work was rare [25], and living conditions of the majority of people were more regular than nowadays.

Publications on Sleep Disorders

Between 1800 and 1880, about 50 publications per decade on sleep disturbances appeared in the medical literature (Fig. 12.1). Publications on sleep and sleep disturbances made up a very small segment of the medical literature. There were very few scientific journals available, mainly in London and Paris. The situation changed clearly in the last third of the nineteenth century with the number of publications on sleep disturbances doubling or tripling at the end of the century. The next steep increase came in the third and fourth decade of the twentieth century, emphasizing the electrophysiological area of sleep research. Figure 12.2 displays publications schematically showing publications in four categories of sleep disorders (insomnia, hypersomnias, parasomnias, and narcolepsy) per decade. Parasomnias dominated the publications in the first six decades; whereas in the seventh decade, insomnia, hypersomnias, and parasomnias had about an equal number of publications. In the eighth decade, narcolepsy appeared as a new diagnosis category. In the past four decades, ending with the year 1950, insomnia was the leading diagnosis, followed by narcolepsy, parasomnias, and hypersomnias.

Insomnia

The definition of insomnia by Macfarlane [35] as "loss of sleep" and "the want of sleep" addresses two different perspectives (one empirical, the other subjective). An important

Table 12.2 Selected nosological systems between 1762 and 1970

Insomnia	Sleep-related breathing disorders	Hypersomnia	Circadian sleep rhythm disorders	Parasomnias	Sleep-related movement disorders	Isolated symptoms	Other sleep disorders	Year of publication
Agrypnia	–	Lethargus,[b] cataphora, carus	–	Ephialte, hallucinations, somnambulism	–	Stertor	–	1762 (1)[a]
Agrypnia	–	Somnolentia, lethargus, cataphora, carus	–	Somnambulism, ephialtes	–	Stertor	–	1763 (2)
	Apnea	Lethargus, torpor, carus, coma, somnolentia	–	Incubus	–	Stertor	Somnium, hypnobatasis	1772 (3)
Agrypnia	–	Lethargus, cataphora, carus	–	Ephialtes, somnambulismus	–	Stertor	–	1776 (4)
–	–	–	–	–	–	–	–	1772 (5)
–	–	–	–	–	–	–	Oneirodynia	1785 (6)
Somnus interruptus, vigilia invita (involuntary watchfulness)	–	Lassitudio (fatigue)	–	Somnambulism, incubus (nightmare)	–	–	Somnium (dreams), somnus periodicus (periods of sleep), Studii inanis periodus (periods of reverie)	1796 (7)
–	–	Lethargus, catalepsis	–	Somnambulans, incubus	–	–	–	1804 (8)
–	–	–	–	Somnambulism, nocturna oppressio	–	–	–	1809 (9)
–	–	–	–	–	–	–	Oneirodynia	1809 (10)
Agrypnia	–	–	–	–	–	–	–	1812 (11)
–	–	–	–	–	–	–	–	1813 (12)
Agrypnia	–	–	–	Ephialtes (nightmare), paroniria (sleepwalking)	–	Rhonchus (snoring, wheezing), paroniria (sleep-talking, night pollution)	–	1817 (13)
Agrypnia	–	Cataphoria	–	Sleep terrors, nightmare, somnambulism	Jactations, cramps	Snoring	Nocturnal heat, anxiety dreams, somniation	1838 (14)
Agrypnia	–	Cataphora	–	Pavor nocturnus, Incubus	–	–	–	1863 (15)
Insomnia	–	Narcolepsy (all forms of hypersomnia)	–	Somnambulism	–	–	–	1896 (16)
Insomnia	–	Narcolepsy,	–	–	–	–	Sleeping sickness (Trypanosomiasis), hysterical sleep (lethargy)	1914 (17)

Table 12.2 (continued)

Insomnia	Sleep-related breathing disorders	Hypersomnia	Circadian sleep rhythm disorders	Parasomnias	Sleep-related movement disorders	Isolated symptoms	Other sleep disorders	Year of publication
Insomnia	–	Hypersomnia, narcolepsy	–	Parasomnia (incubus, sleep terrors, somnambulism)	Abnormal movements in sleep	Confusional awakening	Dreamy states	1923 (18)
Insomnia	Respiratory failure in sleep (remark: not by nasopharyngeal obstruction)	Somnolence, narcolepsy	Reversal of sleep-rhythm	Night terrors, nightmares, Somnambulism, sleep drunkenness, nocturnal enuresis, sleep paralysis	–	Sensory and motor shocks (at sleep onset), states of fear (at awakening), sleep numbness	Nocturnal epilepsy, sleeppains	1929 (19)
Insomnia	–	Narcolepsy	–	Somnambulism, confusional states	–	–	–	1931 (20)
Insomnia	–	Hypersomnias	–	Parasomnias (nightmares, night terrors, somniloquy, somnambulism, teeth grinding, jactations, enuresis, numbness, hypnalgia, personality dissociations)				1932 (21)
Insufficient and restless sleep	–	Excessive sleepiness, drowsiness, narcolepsy	Inversion of the natural order of sleeping and waking	Nightmare, night terrors, sleepwalking				1935 (22)
Insomnia	–	Hypersomnias (encephalitis lethargica), narcolepsy	–	Somnambulism	–	–	Sleep epilepsy, Addison disease	1940 (23)
Insomnia or hyposomnia	–	Narcolepsy; encephalitis lethargica, hypersomnias, and comas		Sleep paralysis			Catalepsy, epilepsy	1963 (24)
Insomnia	Pickwick syndrome	Hypersomnias, Narcolepsy, Kleine–Levin syndrome, encephalitis lethargica		Somnambulism, enuresis	Bruxism		Cranial pain, sleep epilepsy	1970 (25)

[a] Sources: 1. Sauvages, 2. Linnaeus, 3. Vogel, 4. Sagar, 5. Macbride, 6. Cullen, 7. Darwin, 8. Crichton, 9. Pinel, 10. Parr, 11. Swediaur, 12. Young, 13. Good, 14. Frank [12], 15. Dobbert [26], 16. Manacéine [27], 17. Dejerine [28], 18. Romagna Manoia [24], 19. Gillespie [29], 20. Lhermitte [30], 21. Roger [31], 22. Kanner [32], 23. Müller [33], 24. Kleitman [20], 25. Finke and Schulte [34]; For Sources 1 to 13, see Hosack 1821 [22]; sources 14 to 25 see References.

[b] Terminology: Agrypnia insomnia, Lethargus lethargy, Carus deep sleep, Catalepsis suspension of sensation and rigid posture, Cataphora somnolence, Ephialte/Incubus sleep paralysis, Stertor heavy snoring, Paroniria morbid dreaming, Somnium dreaming, Hypnobatasis sleepwalking, Oneirodynia distressing dreams, Somniation dreamlike state during wakefulness

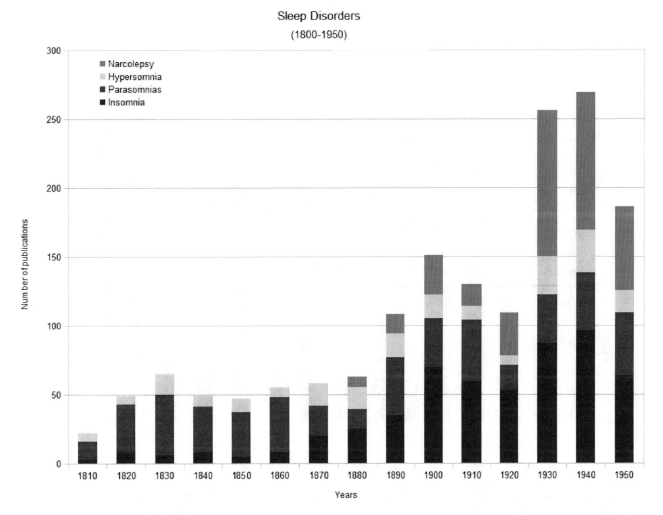

Fig. 12.1 The figure shows the total number of publications on sleep disturbances from 1800 to 1950 in 10-year segments. Data were drawn from the literature data bank of one of us (H.S.) using words from titles, excerpts, summaries, and added key words. If more than one sleep disorder was treated in the same publication, this resulted in double or multiple counting of the same publication. While the rate of publications on sleep disorders was quite stable before 1880, there was a steep rise in the number of publications thereafter. This trend was inverted twice, presumably as a consequence of the First and Second World War. The total number of references was $n = 1616$ which corresponds to 22.3 % of all stored sleep-related references for that period. While the absolute number of publications on sleep disorders increased, the relative proportion of publications on sleep disorders decreased from 31.1 % (1800–1849) to 26.7 % (1850–1899) and finally to 19.5 % (1900–1950)

point, still discussed today, concerns the status of insomnia: Is it a symptom or a disease? The majority of authors at the end of the nineteenth and in the first half of the twentieth century considered insomnia as a symptom, similar to Macfarlane's concept who stated: "It is not a disease, but a symptom of many diseases, differing widely in their nature and complexity, as well as gravity." [35, p. 28]

Kroker, in his book on the history of sleep research, claimed that from 1960 onward "The diagnosis and treatment of insomnia came to rely on laboratory-based studies of sleep." and "sleep…emerged to become a public concern by the end of the twentieth century." [6, p. 349] Kroker further stated that insomnia was a "crucial component of the medical knowledge of sleep" (p. 349) but "if insomnia was a routine concern for clinicians, its status in terms of medi-

cal research was virtually non-existent." "Its experience was personal, as was knowledge and diagnosis of its condition. The physician's role was simply to facilitate the treatment of what the patient already knew to be the problem." (p. 350) Early writers were concerned with the search for an etiology and also for pharmacological treatment (hypnotics) of insomnia.

Classifications of Insomnia

Macfarlane [35, pp. 61–63] gave an overview of the causes of insomnia, based on his own record of patient data and those from two other general practitioners. The combined statistics of 273 cases showed that eight causes accounted for

Sleep Disorders

(1800-1950)

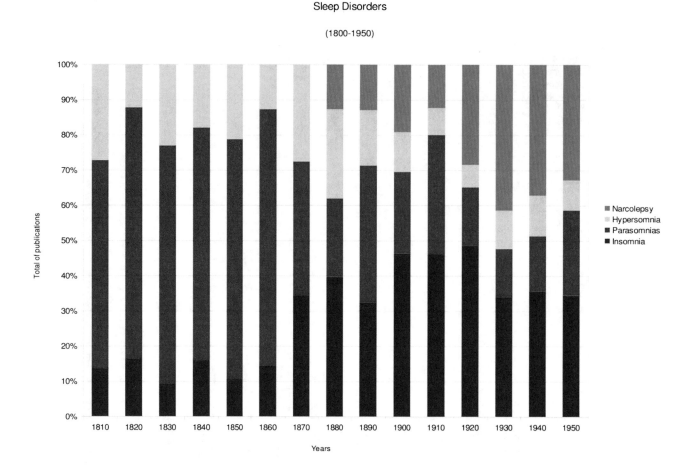

Fig. 12.2 The figure displays the same data as Fig. 12.1, however, referenced to the total number of publications on the four diagnostic groups of sleep disorders. While publications on parasomnias dominated the field before 1870, insomnia became the leading topic of later publications. Reasons for an enhanced interest in insomnia may have

been the rising physiological research on the central nervous system and its pathologies, changes in work, social and environmental conditions [27] and, finally, the development of new hypnotics, which quickly replaced opium as the earlier treatment of choice. Especially psychiatrists, who had to care for sleepless insanes, became interested in new treatment options

67.4 % of all insomnia cases (Table 12.3). Leading causes were neurasthenia (13.6 %) and worry (13.2 %).

A further analysis of the same 273 cases by age and sex showed a wide age distribution of insomnia onset with an earlier onset in females. Apparently, in both genders, it started rarely before the age of 10 or after 70 years, and the distribution reached its maximum at the age 40–50 years (Table 12.4).

Different aspects of these historical data reflect characteristics of insomnia which are also valid today such as the prevalence of psychological factors and higher prevalence and earlier onset of insomnia in females.

Sée [36], cited by Hurd [37, p. 29] and Clarke [38, p. 853], listed nine etiological categories as causes of insomnia: (1) dolorous, (2) digestive, (3) cardiac and dispnoeal, (4) cerebrospinal and neurotic (general paralysis, acute and chronic mania–hysteria–hypochondriasis), (5) psychic insomnia, (6)

insomnia of physical fatigue, (7) genito-urinary, (8) febrile and autotoxic, and (9) toxic. Sée's classification was later mentioned also by the pharmacologist Rudolf who, however, criticized the nine classes as "pigeon-holes in which we may put most cases of insomnia, but beyond that they were not

Table 12.3 Main causes of insomnia for 273 insomnia cases. (Adapted from [35, p. 64])

Cause	Cases	Percent
Neurasthenia	37	13.6
Worry	35	13.2
Gout	26	9.5
Overwork	23	8
Menopause	18	6.6
Dyspepsia	17	6.2
Alcoholism	16	5.9
Senility	12	4.4

Table 12.4 Ages of onset of insomnia. (Adapted from [35, p. 65])

Age	1–10	10–20	20–30	30–40	40–50	50–60	60–70	70–80	80–90	Total
Males	5	7	7	18	31	18	8	7	4	105
Females	5	11	17	40	51	16	16	7	5	168
Total	10	18	24	58	82	34	24	14	9	273

of much value, as these did not follow any rational basis of classification" [39, p. 378]. He classified causes of insomnia into two categories:

I. Nervous system hypersensitivity owing to:
a. Inheritance, bad habit, alteration in habits
b. Fatigue or neurasthenia
c. Circulatory disturbances, especially arteriosclerosis and aortic regurgitation
d. Excitatory toxins produced in the alimentary tract or other body tissues, or introduced from outside.
II. Increase in afferent impulses (e.g., from noise, light, heat, cold, mental and physical discomfort, or pain).

This classification, of causes of insomnia anticipated the present-day concept of "hyperarousal" [40], as a major cause of insomnia.

A further etiological classification proposed in the same period by the neurologist Symonds [41], included three categories: (1) disease of the central nervous system (CNS; e.g., certain cases of encephalitis lethargica), (2) hyperexcitability of the cortical cells due to intoxication, and (3) insomnia caused by unwanted stimuli (e.g., muscular, pain, emotional factor).

Treatment

At the end of the nineteenth and beginning of the twentieth century, several substances to induce sleep were used—in particular, chloral hydrate and bromides. Clarke [38] mentions some "new" hypnotics like paraldehyde and sulphonal. Clarke pointed out that "it is difficult to find any particular drug likely to meet all physiological requirements" (p. 854). Oswald reiterated the same theme much later in 1968 [42]. The pharmacologist Cushny [43, p. 1005] wrote: "the ideal hypnotic should depress CNS (cerebrum) and be devoid of effects on other organs."

Several clinicians drew attention to the danger of routine use of hypnotics [38, 44, p. 854, 45]. Similar warning was given later by Rudolf [39].

It is interesting to compare the role of pharmacological and non-pharmacological treatment options for sleeplessness in the medical literature from 1850 to 1950. Non-pharmacological treatment options included sleep hygiene [46], psychotherapy [47], behavioral procedures [48], relaxation therapy [49], hydrotherapy [50, 51], and electrotherapy [52]. The data in Table 12.5 show a comparable increase of publications for both treatment strategies between 1850 and 1910. In the following years, however, the situation changed dramatically. While the number of papers on treatment of insomnia with hypnotics increased further, those on non-pharmacological treatments fell back to a very low level. It was only much later in the twentieth century that behavior therapy was developed by psychologists, and, even later, specific behavioral and cognitive techniques were introduced into the field of sleep medicine and became a valuable alternative to pharmacotherapy of insomnia.

Sleep-Related Breathing Disorders

It is an enigma that physicians in the nineteenth and early twentieth century rarely reported on SRBD [53–56]. Was the disease infrequent at that time? There were good reasons for such an assumption because the general population was much younger [57, 58], and the distribution of body mass measures was shifted to lower values compared to present-day values [59, 60], probably associated with changes in food supply, meal habits, and physical activity. According to Helmchen and Henderson [59], the percentage of overweight persons among white American men aged 50–59 years increased from 3.4 to 35.0 % between 1890 and 2000. Respiratory difficulties, associated with vascular signs, and somnolence or daytime sleepiness were known mainly in very obese persons, later referred to as Pickwickian syndrome [61], or mistaken for narcolepsy [62, 63]. Recurrent respiratory pauses in sleep were also observed occasionally in stroke patients as described by Broadbent [64] in a stroke patient:

Table 12.5 Comparison of the number of publications[a] on treatment of sleeplessness either with hypnotics or with non-pharmacological treatment options from 1850 to 1950

Treatment	1850–1869	1870–1889	1890–1909	1910–1929	1930–1949
Pharmacological	4	9	25	28	44
Non-pharmacological	5	10	26	21	13

[a] Data were drawn from our data bank of historical sleep references

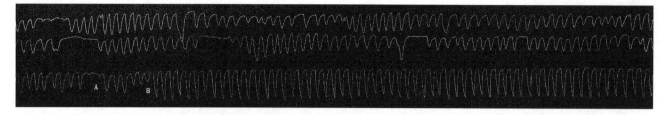

Fig. 12.3 Three continuous tracings which show periodic breathing of a 70-year-old healthy male subject during sleep (pneumographic recording from the thorax). Apneic pauses are most marked in the second tracing. In the third tracing, *A* indicates the restart of respiratory movements and *B* a head movement, followed by normal respiration for the next quarter of an hour. (From [65], plate IV)

The breathing then began in shallow and gentle inspirations and expirations, and gradually rose to a sort of climax, when the movements of the chest were free and forcible and the entry and exit of air at the nostrils or mouth noisy. There was then a gradual subsidence, and a complete arrest in from thirty to thirty-five seconds. This cycle of breathing and pause was maintained with great regularity, the breathing going on for thirty or thirty-five seconds, the cessation lasting fifteen or twenty seconds. It was scarcely disturbed by conversation, but was at times interrupted by yawns. (p. 308)

This case reminded Broadbent what he had observed many years before "something like Cheyne–Stokes' respiration during sleep in a gentleman now more than 80 years of age." He continued:

When a person, especially advanced in years, is lying on his back in heavy sleep and snoring loudly, it very commonly happens that every now and then the inspiration fails to overcome the resistance in the pharynx of which stertor or snoring is the audible sign, and there will be perfect silence through two, three, or four respiratory periods, in which there are ineffectual chest movements; finally air enters with a loud snort, after which there are several compensatory deep inspirations before the breathing settles down to its usual rhythms. In the case to which I allude there was something more than this. The snoring ceased at regular intervals, and the pause was so long as to excite attention, and indeed alarm; I found, on investigation, that there was not simply obstruction by the falling back of the tongue, but actual cessation of all respiratory movements; these then began gradually, but did not at first attain sufficient force to overcome the pharyngeal resistance.

Here, we have, in 1877, the perfect clinical description of what is called today obstructive (case 1) and central (case 2) sleep apnea, both included under the term Cheyne–Stokes respiration almost a century before cardiorespiratory polysomnography came into use as a diagnostic procedure.

Angelo Mosso, an early expert in respiratory physiology, described periodic breathing and luxury respiration [65] as follows: "In sleep a momentary interruption of the respiratory movements is a fairly common phenomenon, and I have to regard it as absolutely physiological, if in sleep, beside the aforementioned fluctuations even complete interruptions occur, just as if a respiratory movement would be absent" (p. 60, our transl). Mosso documented intermittent respiratory pauses with a duration of up to 30 s in a 70-year-old spritely subject who showed no pathological changes in the

heart, lungs, or any other organ (Fig. 12.3). The occurrence of respiratory pauses during sleep, in normal subjects, was later confirmed by Pembrey [66].

It is interesting that George Johnson, a physician at King's College Hospital, London, England, presented the case of a 45-year-old lady who experienced nightly attacks of suffocation. An examination of her throat showed a "very long and slender uvula, which was always in contact with the back of her tongue." Johnson "cut off about two-thirds of the uvula, and from that time she had no more attacks of suffocation." [67, p. 654] This is obviously an early case of surgical treatment for probable obstructive sleep apnea by resection of the soft tissue which blocked the airway passage during sleep. Another English surgeon, Thorne in 1902 [68] removed parts of the soft palate to treat obstructive breathing in sleep. The effect of the operation was to increase the width of margin of the soft palate and to shorten its length from below upward, thus affording a freer passage for nasal respiration, and making it much less likely that the postnasal space will be glued up with tenacious mucus and so obstruct respiration through the nose.

Hypersomnias

In the nineteenth and early twentieth century, three major events strongly influenced the concept of excessive sleepiness, and these included African sleeping sickness (described in Chap. 21), narcolepsy (see also Chap. 26), and encephalitis lethargica (see Chap. 20).

Excessive Sleepiness and Narcolepsy

Impressive case reports on severe sleepiness appeared from time to time in the Western medical literature. Many of them were collected by Heinrich Bruno Schindler and integrated, together with his own extensive case reports, into his book *Idiopathische, chronische Schlafsucht* (idiopathic chronic sleepiness), the first book completely devoted to hypersomnia [69]. He described varieties of sleep attacks, short sleep episodes, periodic sleep episodes, and continuous sleepiness lasting for days, months, even years, combined with a characteristic inability to awaken the person while in a state of pathological sleepiness. In most of the 20 case reports, which he assembled, the etiology was obscure. Physiological knowledge and clinical experience were insufficient, at that time, to explain the observed phenomena of hypersomnia and sort out potential neurological, psychiatric, and other aspects that induced the prolonged and recurrent states of sleepiness. For historical evaluation and general description of idiopathic and recurrent hypersomnia, see Chaps. 27 and 28 in this volume.

A very different type of sleepiness was reported later in the nineteenth century by Westphal ([70] see also [71] and [72]) who had made both careful observations of patients with irresistible sleep attacks and sudden loss of muscle tone, typically evoked by surprise or emotional excitement. Based on these two core symptoms of the disease, Gélineau coined the term narcolepsy from the greek ναρκωσις (somnolent) and λαμβανειν (seize). Earlier case reports with narcolepsy-like symptoms were described by Bright [73, case no. 5], Graves [74], Caffe [75], and Jones [76, case no. 82]; however, in all these cases SRBD could not be ruled out. Narcolepsy quickly gained a special significance for further development of sleep medicine since narcoleptic sleep attacks associated with cataplexy were very different from other forms of protracted sleep or hypersomnia. In the following years, however, confusion arose when some sleep experts included any form of excessive sleepiness under the new diagnostic category [see 27, pp. 106–119]. Brailovsky [77] distinguished the following five etiological groups for individuals complaining of sleepiness: (1) functional narcolepsy, triggered by a special event, (2) narcolepsy associated with morbid physical conditions, (3) narcolepsy in organic disease of the central nervous system (CNS), (4) narcolepsy in toxic–infectious conditions of the CNS, and (5) genuine narcolepsy. This latter group was the most difficult one from an etiological point of view, and Brailovsky wrote: "Finally one can identify a group in which the underlying disease is hard to determine; this problematic group we must treat separately as genuine narcolepsy" (p. 267, our transl.). Brailovsky accepted Pavlov's concept of spread of inhibition as a common mechanism for different forms of sleepiness; however, he emphasized the role of subcortical centers (not considered by Pavlov) in the causation of narcolepsy to explain the rapid onset of sleep and cataplectic attacks. In sharp contrast to the broad concept of narcolepsy, Redlich [78] and others favored a much more strict use of the term narcolepsy to include sleep attacks and cataplexy as the core symptoms. Much later, Yoss and Daly [79], based on the analysis of 241 of their own cases, suggested the narcoleptic tetrad, a symptom complex of daytime sleepiness, cataplexy, sleep paralysis, and hypnagogic hallucinations.

Parasomnias and Sleep-Related Movement Disorders

Parasomnias and sleep-related movement disorders, including restless legs syndrome and rhythmic movement disorder, were known and described in the nineteenth- and twentieth-century sleep medicine. The readers are referred to Chaps. 29, 44, and 45, for evolution and description of some of these entities. Here, we briefly mention about nightmare disorders (REM parasomnias) as well as sleepwalking, sleep terrors, and confusional arousal (all grouped under non-REM parasomnias). The term parasomnia was probably first used by the Swiss psychologist Claparède [80, p. 333] when he spoke about three forms of pathological sleep (insomnia, hypersomnia, and parasomnia). A few years later, Salmon [81] included nightmares, sleep talking, and sleepwalking into the category of parasomnias.

In contrast to motor parasomnias, sleep-related movement disorders "are conditions that are primarily characterized by relatively simple, usually stereotyped, movements that disturb sleep or by other sleep-related monophasic movement disorders such as sleep-related leg cramps" [23, p. 177]. Romagna Manoia [24] was presumably the first who made a distinction between sleep-related movement disorders and parasomnias when he classified sleep disorders (see Table 12.2). Incubus or nightmare, a typical rapid eye movement (REM) sleep parasomnia disorder, which attracted observer's attention all along, is reviewed in the following section.

Nightmare Disorders

The most impressive treatise on nightmare stems from John Waller, a ship doctor of the Royal Navy who himself was severely afflicted by the disorder [82]: "As I have so long been an unfortunate victim to this enemy of repose, and have suffered more from its repeated attacks than any other person I have ever met with, I hope to be able to throw some light on the nature of this affection, and to point out some mode of relief to the unfortunate victims of it." (p. 11) Waller's treatise is a suspense-filled piece of literature, though a few of the dramatic case reports, which he presents, would be rather categorized today as REM sleep behavior disorder (e.g., p. 16 f.). When the nightmare attack occurs, the afflicted person is either just fallen asleep or in deep sleep:

> If the patient be in a profound sleep, he is generally alarmed with some disagreeable dream; he imagines that he is exposed to some danger, or pursued by some enemy which he cannot avoid; frequently he feels as though his legs were tied, or deprived of the power of motion; sometimes he faces himself confined in some very close place, where he is in danger of suffocation, or at the bottom of a cavern or vault from which his return is inter-

cepted. It will not infrequently happen, that this is the whole of the sensation which the disease, for the time, produces, when it goes off without creating any further annoyance: the patient either falls into an oblivious slumber, or the alarming dream is succeeded by one more pleasant. In this case the disease is not fully formed, but only threatens an invasion; it proves however that the pre-disposition to it exists, and that the person is in danger of it. But when the paroxysm does actually take place, the uneasiness of the patient in his dream rapidly increases, till it ends in a kind of consciousness that he is in bed, and asleep; but he feels to be oppressed with some weight which confines him upon his back and prevents his breathing, which is now become extremely laborious, so that the lungs cannot be fully inflated by any effort he can make. The sensation is now the most painful that can be conceived; the person becomes every instant more awake and conscious of his situation: he makes violent efforts to move his limbs, especially his arms, with a view of throwing off the incumbent weight, but not a muscle will obey the impulse of the will: he groans aloud, if he has strength to do it, while every effort he makes seems to exhaust the little remaining vigour. The difficulty of breathing goes on increasing, so that every breath he draws, seems to be almost the last that he is likely to draw; the heart generally moves with increased velocity, sometimes is affected with palpitation; the countenance appears ghastly, and the eyes are half open. The patient, if left to himself, lies in this state generally about a minute or two, when he recovers all at once the power of volition: upon which he either jumps up in bed, or instantly changes his position, so as to wake himself thoroughly. If this be not done, the paroxysm is very apt to recur again immediately, as the propensity to sleep is almost irresistible, and, if yielded to, another paroxysm of Night-Mare is for the most part inevitable. (p. 21)

Finally, it is mentioned that nightmares are frequently accompanied by penile erections, thus completing a set of events (sleeping, dreaming, muscle atonia, and erections) which is typical for a state of sleep which is known as REM sleep today [83]. Waller discusses many occasions of nightmare-associated hallucinations and "visions", produced by a state of consciousness between sleep and wakefulness. More recently hypnagogic mental states were analyzed in detail by Mavromatis [84]. From his own experiences, Waller concluded that neither lying on the back, what most authors gave as primary reason for a nightmare attack, nor late meals and a full stomach, are responsible for nightmares. Waller, who admits his ignorance on the true causes of the disease, recommends to avoid dyspepsia and over-acidification by a careful diet and the use of carbonate of soda in a palatable form.

Nightmare, as described in the nineteenth century medical literature and earlier, differs from the actual classification [23], in that it combined what is now separated into two distinct sleep disorders, (i) recurrent isolated sleep paralysis and (ii) nightmare disorder. In the historical literature, the feeling of oppression in combination with an inability to move and bad dreams was seen as a disease unit. Familial occurrence of the disease has been exemplified with two pedigrees by Ebstein [85].

Somnambulism or Sleepwalking

The nineteenth century became the peak time of publications on somnambulism or sleepwalking (a non-REM parasomnia) with more than 200 publications, well above the number of publications before (eighteenth century: just over 60) or after (1900–1950: about 50). Manacéïne [27] confirmed that somnambulism occurred primarily in adolescents and young persons, i.e., those who required high amounts of muscular activity during daytime, and she raised the question whether somnambulism could result from a lack of physical activity during the day which, in turn, may provoke motor events at night. She referred to cases where somnambulism disappeared after extensive physical work. Somnambulism gained renewed interest for army psychiatrists who had to diagnose soldiers who were sleepwalking. Sandler [86] noted in afflicted subjects "a great number of concomitant neurotic symptoms of other kinds" besides somnambulism, and the treatment of choice was psychotherapy in combination with sodium amytal.

Pavor Nocturnus: Sleep Terrors

"Sleep terrors consist of arousals from slow-wave sleep accompanied by a cry or piercing scream and autonomic nervous system and behavioral manifestations of intensive fear" [23]. Pavor nocturnus was known to the nineteenth-century Saxonian physician, Carl Gustav Hesse, who had written a remarkable monograph of this sleep disorder, which typically affects children [87]. One of the aims of Hesse's treatise was to differentiate pavor nocturnus from nightmare disorders and sleepwalking. The attacks start most frequently 1 or 2 h after sleep onset, the child startles up "as hit by an electrical shock" in full panic, mostly with a shrieking-shrill cry, sometimes jumping out of bed, obviously in avoidance of the horrible scene. Consciousness of the concerned child (or adult) seems to be altered; he or she does not recognize persons and does not understand when someone speaks to them, much in contrast to nightmare sufferers. After the incidence, many children are unable to report what was horrifying them; others are remembering frightening persons, animals, fire, or other phantasms. The event lasts in most cases from 15 to 30 min and it comes only slowly to its end. The frequency of occurrence and the intervals between recurring events vary widely. Hesse, as others, differentiated between symptomatic and idiopathic forms.

The classification into idiopathic and symptomatic forms of pavor nocturnus was later rejected by Braun [88] who regarded the disease as a form of neurasthenia, defined as an increased irritability of the nervous system. He emphasized educational measures for prevention, medication (bromides, chloral, chinin) in severe cases only, and warm or tepid baths.

Confusional Arousal and Its Forensic Aspects

An early and detailed account of a case of violent confusional arousal was presented by the Berlin physician Heim [89, 90]. The person concerned was a longtime friend of Heim who described him as an honest businessman, with lively and jovial temperament, and a powerful body. One night, about an hour after going to bed, his wife became alarmed when she heard him groan, and she tried to awaken him by shaking. The man sat up and opened his eyes without recognizing his wife, and, after a short while, the man jumped out of bed, grabbed her by the hair, and tried to throw her out of the window. About half an hour later, the doctor arrived and saw the wife, covered with blood. The man recognized the doctor, called him by name, and asked him why he and the other persons were there. Heim's report rekindled interest in questions of consciousness in the borderland between sleep and wakefulness, and captured the lawyers' attention regarding questions of responsibility for acts committed during such states of reduced or unclear consciousness. Nearly a century later, the psychiatrist Gudden reviewed 18 published cases of confusional arousal, raising medico-legal questions [91]. He understood confusional arousal, calling it *Schlaftrunkenheit* or *sleep drunkenness* at that time, as a disorder of consciousness out of sleep, associated with hyperesthesia, psychomotor agitation, and a lack of prudence. Schmidt [92] had reviewed the medico-legal literature over a time span of 150 years and was able to locate 15 case reports of homicide and 20 cases of other crimes. Wharton and Stillé [93] emphasized that it is important to distinguish "Somnolentia or Sleep-drunkenness, which is a state which to a greater or less extent is incidental to every individual, from Somnambulism, which is an abnormal condition incident to a very few" (p. 122).

Circadian Rhythm Sleep Disorders

In the period from 1800 to mid-twentieth century, a basis was provided for the later intensive research on circadian rhythms. The Belgian astronomer and social statistician Adolphe Quetelet was one of the first who collected statistical data on the influence of annual and daily rhythms on human life and functioning. He showed that the number of births is higher in the night compared to the daytime hours at a ratio of 5:4. [94]. The influence of the night on diseases was also discussed at that time [95, 96]. Later, in the nineteenth century, an increasing amount of physiological studies was devoted to 24-h alterations of body temperature

[97], metabolism [98], urine secretion and its constituents [99], and the activity of different organs [100]. It was recognized that most of these diurnal changes were independent of sleep and continued even when sleep was prevented or shifted [101]. In the early twentieth century, it was shown in rodents, kept under constant conditions (total darkness), that the daily cycle of activity and rest was self-sustained and not driven by external cues [102]. This finding became the starting point for a search for pacemakers or biological clocks that regulate the timing of behavior, performance, and mood. Curt Richter was one of the early researchers contributing to an understanding of biological clocks in medicine and psychiatry [103]. Early examples of circadian rhythm sleep disturbance were provided by Von Economo's [104] description of encephalitis lethargic and Roasenda's [105] description of inversion of sleep in encephalitis. Another field which gained growing importance in the twentieth century was shift work causing disruption of the alignment of sleep and circadian clock, giving rise to a shift work disorder [106]. However, a more deep understanding of the interaction between sleep and circadian rhythms began only in the second half of the twentieth century, when results from circadian and sleep research were combined [107–109].

Sleep Disturbances and Childhood Development

Most of the papers published in the beginning of the eighteenth century concerned episodic phenomena occurring during sleep, such as sleep terrors and enuresis in children, while much less interest was devoted to insomnia. In addition to some interest in sleep disorders, the relevance of sleep for the development was also pointed out including information for mothers [110, 111]. Capuron [112] dedicated six pages of his handbook "Traité des maladies des enfants" to sleep disturbances and Fonssagrives [113] devoted a section of his book "Leçons d'hygiène infantile" to sleep and insomnia. He underscored the danger of sleep disturbances to general health due to physical causes and use of opioids. However, most books on sleep disturbances did not include diseases of the children and the elderly (Hammond 1869).

It is worth mentioning a publication (probably the first description of obstructive sleep apnea in infants and consequences) by the otolaryngologist Bosworth in 1896 [114] describing upper airway obstructions by enlargement of adenoids causing frequent occurrence of nightmares in children: "While the interference with respiration may not cause any conscious symptoms of dyspnœa, yet it does cause the nightmare so frequently observed in children. It arises from the fact that, the entrance of air to the lungs being slightly impeded during sleep, there follows a slowly but surely increasing lack of proper oxygenation of the blood, resulting in an increase of the *besoin de respirer,* until it culminates in a sense of oppression or suffocation, under the influence of which the child awakens alarmed and terrified" (p. 433).

The term "sleep disorders" became more frequent after 1920 since Goldschmidt's [115] publication of a case of narcolepsy and Pototzky's [116] work on infantile sleep, insomnia, and disturbances of sleep. Pototzky assumed that sleep disturbances were related to four constitutional types, and therapy was different for each type.

The growth of child neuropsychiatry began in the 1920s and 1930s [32, 117–120]. Kanner, a well-known child psychiatrist, emphasized the necessity to consider global aspects of behavior to understand sleep problems in older children. He pointed out the importance of the behavior before sleep proposing a continuity between waking and sleeping behavior. Many of the points raised by Kanner were developed further in the second half of the twentieth century; whereas in the first half of the twentieth century, experimental psychophysiology [121] made important contributions to children's sleep problems.

Before 1950, statistics about frequencies of sleep disturbances in children were extremely rare. There was one remarkable study by Benjamin [122] on the frequency of sleep disturbances in relation to other neurotic symptoms (Table 12.6) presenting data from 205 children (63 % males, 37 % females): "In the course of childhood a *symptom*

change of the neurosis occurs, in such a way that eating disorders decrease from 44 to 11 %, habits from 40 to 8 %, fear from 40 to 19 %, sleep disturbances from 42 to 14 %, vomiting from 28 to 2 %, enuresis from 20 to 8 %, and language impairment decrease from 16 to 4 %. Noteworthy is the temporary increase of enuresis from the 8th to the 11th year of life" (p. 88, our transl.).

Conclusions

In the beginning of the period under consideration, physicians had to rely on reports of patients and occasional observations of the sleeper's behavior as sole sources of information for diagnosis and treatment. Knowledge on the physiology of sleep was extremely limited at that time. The situation changed with the rapid development of physiology and other branches of medicine, organic chemistry, psychology, and availability of instruments for measurement and recording devices [123, pp. 9–26]. In addition, the pharmaceutical industry started to produce new hypnotic agents.

Among the different sleep disorders, insomnia gained its leading position in the second half of the nineteenth century (Figs. 12.1 and 12.2). Since insomnia was seen by the majority of authors as a symptomatic disorder, treatment was primarily aimed at removing or alleviating the assumed

Table 12.6 Frequency of sleep disturbances in relation to demographic data and neurotic symptoms

Sleep disturbances				
Age	4-5 years	6-7 years	8-11 years	12-15 years
Boys	32	37	37	16
Girls	30	35	23	33
Enuresis				
Age	4-5 years	6-7 years	8-11 years	12-15 years
Boys	20	15	27	8
Girls	25	5	11	0
Anxiety				
Age	4-5 years	6-7 years	8-11 years	12-15 years
Boys	40	22	12	19
Girls	30	45	34	40
Tics				
Age	4-5 years	6-7 years	8-11 years	12-15 years
Boys	7	15	10	28
Girls	20	30	15	7

causal factor [35]. While opium was traditionally used for sleeplessness, the situation changed later in the nineteenth century, when a whole series of newly developed hypnotics like bromide salts, chloral hydrate, paraldehyde, and others were marketed, and finally in the twentieth century when barbiturates were introduced. Any new drug met with caution and an ambivalent reaction was seen throughout the history of hypnotic drug use [124]. The most popular non-pharmacological treatment option was sleep hygiene. Only in the first half of the twentieth century, psychotherapy [125] and behavioral therapy (e.g., muscle relaxation therapy) [49] became treatment options for insomnia.

Hypersomnias due to brain diseases, such as tumors or encephalitis, were separated from genuine narcolepsy and recurrent hypersomnia. Narcolepsy was quickly recognized as a potential key for understanding of sleep–wake regulation as confirmed in later studies [126].

The term RLS was introduced by Ekbom [127] giving a full clinical description based on a series of his own cases. Even more surprising is the near-total absence of description of SRBD throughout the nineteenth and the first half of the twentieth century.

References

1. Kohlschütter E. Messung der Festigkeit des Schlafes. Z Ration Med. 1863;17:209–53.
2. Manacéïne M de. Quelques observations expérimentales sur l'influence de l'insomnie absolue. Arch Ital Biol. 1894;21:322–5.
3. Patrick GTW, Gilbert JA. On the effects of loss of sleep. Psychol Rev. 1896;3:469–83.
4. Heerwagen F. Statistische Untersuchungen über Träume und Schlaf. Philosophische Studien. 1889;5:301–20.
5. Weed SC, Hallam FM. A study of dream-consciousness. Am J Psychol. 1896;7:405–11.
6. Kroker K. The sleep of others and the transformations of sleep research. Toronto: University of Toronto Press; 2007.
7. Kronthal P. Der Schlaf des Andern: Eine naturwissenschaftliche Betrachtung über den Schlaf. Halle: C Marhold; 1907.
8. Szymanski JS. Eine Methode zur Untersuchung der Ruhe- und Aktivitätsperioden bei Tieren. Pflügers Arch ges Physiol. 1914;158:343–85.
9. Berger H. Über das Elektrenkephalogramm des Menschen. Arch Psychiat Nervenkr. 1929;87:527–70.
10. Loomis AL, Harvey EN, Hobart GA. Potential rhythms of the cerebral cortex during sleep. Science 1935;81:597–8.
11. Frank J. Praxeos medicae universae praecepta. 2 Vols. (Partis secundae volumen primum, sectio prima, continens Doctrinam de morbis systematis nervosi in genere, et de iis cerebri in specie). Lipsiae: Kuehniani; 1811.
12. Frank J. Maladies du système nerveux. Encyclopédie des Sciences Médicales; III, Pathologie médicale. Paris: Bureau de l'Encyclopédie; 1838, S 27–72.
13. Astruc J. Tractus pathologicus. Paris: P G Cavelier; 1767.
14. Boissier de Sauvages F. Nosologie méthodique. Tome sixième. Lyon: Jean-Marie Bruyset; 1772.
15. Le Camus A. Médecine de l'esprit, où l'on traite des dispositions et des causes physiques qui, en conséquence de l'union de l'âme avec le corps, influent sur les opérations de l'esprit et des moyens de maintenir ces opérations dans un bon état, ou de les corriger lorsqu'elles sont viciées. Paris: Ganeau; 1755.
16. Economo C von. Die Encephalitis lethargica. Monographie. Leipzig: Deuticke; 1917.
17. Pavlov IP. Conditioned reflexes. An investigation of the physiological activity of the cerebral cortex. New York: Oxford University Press; 1927.
18. Hess WR. Hirnreizversuche über den Mechanismus des Schlafes. Arch. Psychiat. Nervenkrankh. 1929;86:287-292.
19. Bremer F. Cerveau "isolé" et physiologie du sommeil. C R Soc Biol. 1935;118:1235–41.
20. Kleitman N. Sleep and wakefulness. (Rev. and enl. ed). Chicago: Univ Chicago Press; 1963.
21. Moruzzi G, Magoun HW. Brain stem reticular formation and activation of the EEG. Electroencephal Clin Neurophysiol. 1949;1:455–73.
22. Hosack D. A system of practical nosology: to which prefixed, a synopsis of the systems of Sauvages, Linnæus, Vogel, Sagar, Macbride, Cullen, Darwin, Crichton, Pinel, Parr, Swediaur, Young, and Good. With references to the best authors on each disease. 2nd ed. New-York: CS Van Winkle; 1821.
23. American Academy of Sleep Medicine. ICSD–2–International classification of sleep disorders, 2nd ed. Diagnostic and coding manual. Westchester: American Academy of Sleep Medicine; 2005.
24. Romagna Manoia A I disturbi del sonno e loro cura. Roma: L Pozzi; 1923.
25. Ramazzini B. De Morbis Artificum Diatriba. Mutinae: Typis Antoni Capponi; 1700.
26. Dobbert G. Der Schlaf und die Schlaflosigkeit in semiotischer Hinsicht. Würzburg: Becker; 1863.
27. Manacéïne M de. Le sommeil. Tiers de notre vie. (French transl. From Russian) Paris: G Masson; 1896 (engl. transl. Sleep: Its Physiology, Hygiene, and Psychology. London: Walter Scott; 1897.
28. Dejerine J. Sémiologie des affections du système nerveux. Paris: Masson; 1914.
29. Gillespie RD. Sleep and the treatment of its disorders. London: Ballière, Tindall & Cox; 1929.
30. Lhermitte J. Le sommeil. Paris: Armand Colin; 1931.
31. Roger H. Les troubles du sommeil : hypersomnies, insomnies, parasomnies. Paris: Masson; 1932.
32. Kanner L. Child psychiatry. Springfield, Ill.: Thomas; 1935.
33. Müller LR. Über den Schlaf. Studien über die Ermüdung, über den Schlaf, über Erholung, über Schlafstörungen und über deren Behandlung. München: Lehmann; 1940.
34. Finke J, Schulte W. Schlafstörungen. Ursachen und Behandlung. Stuttgart: G. Thieme; 1970.
35. Macfarlane AW. Insomnia and its therapeutics. London: HK Lewis; 1890.
36. Sée G. Leçons sur le sommeil, les insomnies et les somnifères. La Médecine moderne, 1890, février 27.
37. Hurd EP. Sleep, insomnia, and hypnotics. Detroit: GS Davis; 1891.
38. Clarke CK. A discussion on the treatment of insomnia. Brit Med J. 1897;2:853–66.
39. Rudolf RD. The treatment of insomnia. Brit Med J. 1922;1:377–9.
40. Riemann D, Spiegelhalder K, Feige B, Voderholzer U, Berger M, Perlis M, Nissen C. The hyperarousal model of insomnia; A review of the concept and its evidence. Sleep Med Rev. 2010;14:19–31.
41. Symonds CP. Sleep and sleeplessness. (An address delivered before the Oxford Medical Society) Brit Med J. 1925;1:869–71.
42. Oswald I. Drugs and sleep. Pharmacol Rev. 1968;20:272–303.
43. Cushny AR. A discussion on the treatment of sleeplessness and pain. Brit Med J. 1905;2:1002–8.
44. Barnes H. A discussion on the treatment of insomnia. Brit Med J. 1897;2:853–66.

45. Sawyer J. Clinical lectures on the causes and cure of insomnia: delivered at the Queen's Hospital, Birmingham. Brit Med J. 1900;2:1551–3, 1627–9.

46. Hall WW. Sleep; or, The hygiene of the night. New York: Hurd and Houghton; 1870.

47. Pötzl O. Der Schlaf als Behandlungsproblem. In Sarason D, editor. Der Schlaf. Mitteilungen und Stellungnahme zum derzeitigen Stande des Schlafproblems. München: JF Lehmanns Verlag; 1929. p. 64–75.

48. Ebaugh FG. Sleep disorders in clinical practice. Calif West Med 1936;45:5-9, 128â€"132.

49. Jacobson E. You can sleep well. The A B C's of restful sleep for the average person. New York: Whittlesey House; 1938.

50. Straßer A. Die hydrotherapeutische Behandlung der Schlaflosigkeit. In D Sarason, editor. Der Schlaf. Mitteilungen und Stellungnahme zum derzeitigen Stande des Schlafproblems. München: JF Lehmanns Verlag; 1929. p. 93–107.

51. Pedersen VC. Insomnia from another point of view. Med Rec NY. 1938;246:434–8.

52. Rockwell AD. Medical and surgical uses of electricity. New edition. New York: William Wood and Co; 1896.

53. Kryger MH. Sleep apnea. From the needles of Dionysius to continuous airway pressure. Arch Intern Med. 1983;143:2301–3.

54. Lavie P. Nothing new under the moon. Historical accounts of sleep apnea syndrome. Arch Intern Med. 1984;144:2025–8.

55. Lavie P. Who was the first to use the term Pickwickian in connection with sleepy patients? History of sleep apnoea syndrome. Sleep Med Rev. 2008;12(1):5–17.

56. Kryger M. Fat, sleep and Charles Dickens. Literary and medical contributions to the understanding of sleep apnea. Clin Chest Med. 1985;6:555–62.

57. Wrigley EA, Schofield RS. The population history of England 1541–1871: a reconstruction. London: Edward Arnold; 1981.

58. The Human Mortality Database. www.mortality.org/.

59. Helmchen LA, Henderson RM. Changes in the distribution of body mass index of white U.S. men 1890–2000. Ann Hum Biol. 2004;31:174–81.

60. Saint Onge JM, Krueger PM, Rogers RG. Historical trends in height, weight, and body mass: Data from U.S. Major League Baseball players, 1869–1983. Econ Hum Biol. 2008;6:482–8.

61. Burwell CS, Robin ED, Whaley RD, Bickelmann AG. Extreme obesity associated with alveolar hypoventilation: a pickwickian syndrome. Am J Med. 1956;21:811–8.

62. Caton R. A case of narcolepsy. Clinical Society of London. Transactions. 1889;22:133–7.

63. Spitz A. Das klinische Syndrom: Narkolepsie mit Fettsucht und Polyglobulie in seinen Beziehungen zum Morbus Cushing. Dtsch Arch Klin Med. 1937;181:286–304.

64. Broadbent WH. On Cheyne-Stokes respiration in cerebral haemorrhage. Lancet. 1877;I:307–309.

65. Mosso A. Periodische Athmung und Luxusathmung. Arch Physiol. 1886;(Suppl):37–116.

66. Pembrey MS. Some observations upon Cheyne-Stokes respiration. Brit Med J. 1899;2:835.

67. Johnson G. On some nervous disorders that result from overwork and mental anxiety. Lancet. 1875; 85–7, 155–7, 651–4.

68. Thorne JM. Notching the soft palate for cure of post-nasal obstruction in adults. Brit Med J. 1902;1:962.

69. Schindler HB. Die idiopathische, chronische Schlafsucht. Beschrieben und durch Krankheitsfälle erläutert. Hirschberg: CWI Krahn; 1829.

70. Westphal C. Zwei Krankheitsfälle, vorgetragen in der Berliner Medicinisch-Psychologischen Gesellschaft. I. Anfälle larvierter Epilepsie, dem Ausbruche paralytischer Geistesstörung Jahre lang vorausgehend. II. Eigenthümliche mit Einschlafen verbundene Anfälle. Arch Psychiat Nervenkr. 1877;7:622–35.

71. Schenck CH, Bassetti CL, Arnulf I, Mignot E. English translation of the first clinical reports on narcolepsy by Westphal and Gélineau in the late 19th century, with commentary. J Clin Sleep Med. 2007;3:301–11.

72. Gélineau JBE. De la narcolepsie. Gaz des Hôp Civ et Milit Empire Ottoman 1880;53:626–28, 635–37.

73. Bright R. Cases illustrative of the effects produced when the arteries and brain are diseased: selected chiefly with a view to the diagnosis in such affections. Guy's Hosp Rep. 1836;1:9–40.

74. Graves RJ. Observations on the nature and treatment of various diseases. Dubl Quart J Med Sci. 1851;11:1–20.

75. Caffe. Maladie du sommeil. Jounal des connaissances médicales pratiques et de le pharmacologie 1862;29ᵉ année, 10 et 20 août, p. 323.

76. Jones CH. Clinical observations on functional nervous disorders. Philadelphia: Henry C. Lea; 1867.

77. Brailovsky V. Über die pathologische Schläfrigkeit und das Schlafzentrum. Z ges Neurol Psychiat. 1926;100:272–88. (in Russian: Sovremennaja pschoneurologija 1925;1(3/4):16–31.)

78. Redlich E. Zur Narkolepsiefrage. Monatsschr Psychiat Neurol. 1915;37:85–94.

79. Yoss RE , Daly D. Criteria for the diagnosis of the narcoleptic syndrome. Proc Staff Meet Mayo Clin. 1957;32:320–8.

80. Claparède E. Esquisse d'une théorie biologique du sommeil. Archives de Psychologie. 1905;4:246–349.

81. Salmon A. La Fonction du Sommeil. Paris: Vigot Frères; 1910.

82. Waller JA Treatise on incubus or night-mare, disturbed sleep, terrific dreams and nocturnal visions with the means of removing these distressing complaints. London: E Cox and Son; 1816.

83. Schulz H, Salzarulo P. Forerunners of REM sleep. Sleep Med Rev. 2012;16:95–108.

84. Mavromatis A. Hypnagogia. The unique state of consciousness between wakefulness and sleep. London: Routledge & Kegan Paul; 1987.

85. Ebstein E. Über den Pavor nocturnus (sog. Alpdrücken) und sein familiäres Auftreten. Z ges Neurol Psychiat. 1920; 62:385–401.

86. Sandler SA. Somnambulism in the armed forces. Ment Hyg. 1945;29:236–47.

87. Hesse CG. Über das nächtliche Aufschrecken der Kinder im Schlafe und die psychisch-gerichtliche Bedeutung des Aufschreckens in den späteren Lebensaltern. Altenburg: HA Pierer; 1845.

88. Braun L. Über das nächtliche Aufschrecken der Kinder. Jahrb Kinderheilk. 1896;43:407–56.

89. Heim EL. Von einer kaum eine Stunde lang gedauerten Tobsucht (Mania furibunda). Horn's Archiv für medizinische Erfahrung. 1817;I:73–84.

90. Schulz H. Die geschichtliche Entwicklung der Schlafforschung in Berlin. Ein historischer Streifzug. Somnologie 2010;14:140-56 and 221–33.

91. Gudden H. Die physiologische und pathologische Schlaftrunkenheit. Arch Psychiat. 1905;40:989–1013.

92. Schmidt G. Die Verbrechen in der Schlaftrunkenheit. Z ges Neurol Psychiat. 1943;176:208–54.

93. Wharton F, Stillé M. Treatise on medical jurisprudence. Second and revised edition. Philadelphia: Kay & Brothers; 1860.

94. Quetelet A. Sur l'homme et le développement de ses facultés, ou essai de physique sociale. Bruxelles: L Hauman; 1836.

95. Busmann K. Ueber nächtliche Krankheiten. Journal der practischen Arzneykunde und Wundarzneykunst 1800;10:120–42.

96. De la Prade R. De l'influence de la nuit sur les malades. Mémoires cour. de l'Acad. de Bruxelles. Bruxelles: Weissenbruch; 1806.

97. Ogle W. On the diurnal variations in the temperature of the human body in health. St George's Hosp Rep. 1866;I:221–45.

98. Johannson JE. Über die Tagesschwankungen des Stoffwechsels und der Körpertemperatur im nüchternen Zustande und vollständiger Muskelruhe. Skand Arch Physiol. 1898;8:85–142.

99. Bert P. Sur les phases horaires d'excrétion de l'urine et de l'urée. C R Soc Biol. 1878;30:255–58.

100. Dastre A. Recherches sur les variations diurnes de la sécrétion biliaire. Arch Physiol Norm Path. 1890;2:800–9.

101. Hoffmann RW. Periodischer Tageswechsel und andere biologische Rhythmen bei den poikilothermen Tieren. In: A Bethe, G v Bergmann, G Embden, A Ellinger, editors. Handbuch der normalen und pathologischen Physiologie mit Berücksichtigung der experimentellen Pharmakologie, vol. 17. Correlationen III. Berlin: Springer: 1926, 644–658.

102. Johnson MS. Activity and distribution of certain wild mice in relation to biotic communities. J Mammal. 1926;7:245–7.

103. Richter CP. Biological clocks in medicine and psychiatry. Springfield, Ill: CC Thomas; 1965.

104. Economo C von Die Pathologie des Schlafes. In: A Bethe, G v Bergmann, G Embden, A Ellinger, editors. Handbuch der Normalen und Pathologischen Physiologie Mit Berücksichtigung der Experimentellen Pharmakologie, 17. Vol., Correlationen III. Berlin, Springer, 1926, S. 591–610.

105. Roasenda G. Inversione del ritmo del sonno, con agitazione psicomotoria notturna (sindrome post-encephalitis). Policlinico (Sez. Prat.). 1921;28:181–6.

106. Menzel W, Bagelmann E, Dassau Hj, Ewert H, Heise U, Schönwald R, Seiferlein K, Wrage H. Zur Physiologie und Pathologie des Nacht- und Schichtarbeiters. Arbeitsphysiol. 1950;14:304–18.

107. Borbély AA. A two process model of sleep regulation. Hum Neurobiol. 1982;1:195–204.

108. Czeisler CA, Zimmerman JC, Ronda JM, Moore-Ede MC, Weitzman ED. Timing of REM sleep is coupled to the circadian rhythm of body temperature in man. Sleep. 1980;2:329–46.

109. Zulley J, Wever R, Aschoff J. The dependence of onset and duration of sleep on the circadian rhythm of rectal temperature. Pflügers Arch. 1981;391:314–8.

110. Anonym. Letters to a mother on the watchful care of her infant. London: Seeley & Burnside; 1831.

111. Menke A. Taschenbuch für Mütter über die physische Erziehung der Kinder in den ersten Lebensjahren und über die Verhütung, Erkenntniß und Behandlung der gewöhnlichen Kinderkrankheiten. vol. 2. Frankfurt a. M.: Friedrich Wilmans Verlagshandlung; 1832.

112. Capuron J. Traité des maladies des enfants, jusqu'à la puberté. Paris: Croullebois; 1820.

113. Fonssagrives J-R. Leçons d'hygiène infantile. Paris: Adrien Delahaye et Émile Lecrosnier; 1882.

114. Bosworth FH. Disease of the nose and throat. New York: William Wood & Co.; 1896.

115. Goldschmidt S. Über die Friedmann'sche Narkolepsie des Kindesalter. Diss Med Univ Würzburg. 1920.

116. Pototzky C. Insomnia and disturbances of sleep. Bull NY Acad Med. 1930;6:330–48.

117. Cameron HC. Sleep and its disorders in childhood. Br Med J. 1930;2:717–9.

118. De Sanctis S. Neuropsichiatria infantile: patologica e diagnostica. Roma: Stock; 1925.

119. Despert LJ. Sleep in pre-school children: a preliminary study. Nerv Child. 1949;8:8–27.

120. Heuyer G. Les troubles du sommeil chez l'enfant. Epinal: Imp Coopérative; 1928.

121. Giddings G. Child's sleep-effect of certain foods and beverages on sleep motility. Am J Public Health. 1934;24:609–14.

122. Benjamin E. Grundlagen und Entwicklungsgeschichte der kindlichen Neurose. Leipzig: Georg Thieme; 1930.

123. Siegel J. The neural control of sleep & waking. New York: Springer; 2002.

124. Renner A. Schlafmitteltherapie. Berlin: Springer; 1925.

125. Crichton-Miller H. Insomnia. An outline for the practioner. London: Edward Arnold & Co; 1930.

126. Fromherz S, Mignot E. Narcolepsy research: past, present, and future perspectives. Arch Ital Biol. 2004;142:479–486.

127. Ekbom KA. Restless legs: clinical study of hitherto overlooked disease in legs characterized by peculiar paresthesia ('Anxietas tibiarum'), pain and weakness and occurring in two main forms, asthenia crurum paraesthetica and asthenia crurum dolorosa. Acta Med Scand. 1945; 121(S 158):7–123.

The History of Polysomnography: Tool of Scientific Discovery

Max Hirshkowitz

EEG and Sleep: The Beginnings

Berger and the String Galvanometer

Hans Berger, considered the father of electroencephalography (EEG), made his first recordings using a device called the string galvanometer in 1924 [1]. It involved suspending a reed between electromagnets using a string so that the oscillations could expose a light-sensitive material (see Fig. 13.1). With this device, he was able to record EEG activity (fluctuating potential differences) and found an 8–13-cycle-per-second waveform when an individual remained relaxed but wakeful. He named this rhythm "alpha" but many referred to it as the "Berger's wave." Another finding, for which he is much less known, was that when a person fell asleep, the alpha rhythm disappeared. As unlikely as it seems, almost a century later we still essentially define sleep onset by determining the point at which alpha EEG activity diminishes. This simple finding conceptually marked the beginning of what decades later would evolve into polysomnography (PSG). Nonetheless, at the time Berger was not highly regarded and considered by many a "crank" until Lord Adrian confirmed his findings [2]. By 1938, EEG gained general recognition. Accounts vary concerning Berger's life after

1938. Whether the Nazi regime forced his retirement or he joined the Schutzstaffel (SS) is unclear; however, he committed suicide in 1941.

Oscillographs, Drum Kymographs, and Strip Chart Recorder

The string galvanometer was not suitable for making recordings over extended time periods. Oscillographs could also be used with bromide paper but long-duration recordings presented a technical problem. However, another device invented decades earlier could be adapted. A German physiologist named Carl Ludwig invented a "wave writer" or kymograph [3] that utilized a cylinder or drum around which a piece of paper could be attached (see Fig. 13.2). A stylus marked the paper as the drum rotated. Early versions used the stylus to scrape off soot from pre-smoked sheet but eventually ink became the preferred writing medium. In this manner, scientists could make recordings over longer time periods, especially when the stylus traversed a worm screw preventing overwriting after the drum completed a full rotation. An alternative approach involved moving a continuous strip of paper (from a roll or fanfolded) under ink pens at a constant speed. The drive mechanism typically incorporated several gear ratios that could move the paper ribbon or strip with rotating sprockets, pinch rollers, or some other mechanism.

Gibbs and Garceau were able to construct a one-channel EEG machine by adapting the Weston Union Morse Code inkwriting undulator while Albert Grass who was working on earthquake seismographs created a three-channel EEG machine. After 1938, EEG rapidly gained popularity as both a research and clinical tool. Polygraphic recording devices (e.g., the grass model 1) became commercially available (see Fig. 13.3). Groups in both Europe and America applied this new approach to psychiatric and neurologic disorders, describing, documenting, and naming various waveforms. Some recordings were made during sleep by sampling EEG and researchers described periods of low-amplitude mixed-

M. Hirshkowitz (✉)
Michael E. DeBakey Veterans Affairs Medical Center, 2002 Holcombe Blvd-Stop Code 111i, Sleep Center, 3426 LinkwoodTX, USA
e-mail: max.hirshkowitz@gmail.com

Department of Medicine and Menninger, Baylor College of Medicine, Houston, USA

Department of Psychiatry, Baylor College of Medicine, Houston, USA

Sleep Disorders & Research Center, Michael E. DeBakey Veterans Affairs Medical Center, Houston, TX 77030, USA

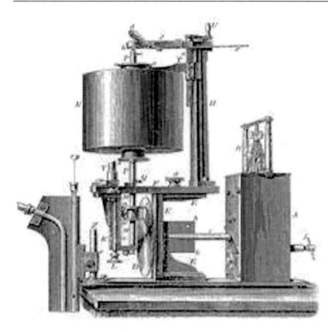

Fig. 13.1 Illustration of a drum kymograph

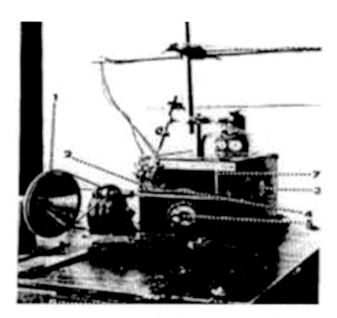

Fig. 13.2 Hans Berger's string galvanometer

frequency activity alternating with high-amplitude slow waves. Gibbs and Gibbs also remarked that EEG was mostly symmetrical during sleep, except during the low-voltage, mixed-frequency episodes [4].

Tuxedo Park

Alfred Loomis was an eccentric, and very wealthy, lawyer-turned Wall Street tycoon who established a research center in Tuxedo Park in the 1930s sometimes called the Loomis Laboratories [5]. Loomis excelled at mathematics and had a

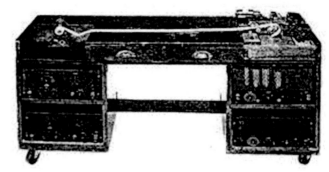

Fig. 13.3 Grass model I polygraph

passion for science. He spent the fortune he made through investments to fund scientific research by the greatest minds in his time (including Heisenberg, Bohr, Fermi, and Einstein). In 1937, Loomis, along with Harvey and Hobart, published the first report from continuous, all-night studies of human sleep [6]. They had constructed an 8-ft.-long, 44-in.-circumference drum recorder (see Fig. 13.4) and monitored up to three channels at a time of signals switched through some sort of selector panel. Recording sites included (midline vertex, midline occiput, behind left and right ears, and just above and to the left of the left eye). They described a fourth channel that could be used to record signal markers, heartbeats, or respiration. They could manage 3.5 h of recording before paper needed changing. They wrote the following "… we have been able to establish very definite *states of sleep* which change suddenly from time to time, and to correlate

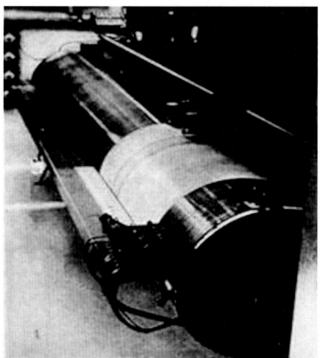

Fig. 13.4 Loomis's drum recorder designed to conduct sleep studies

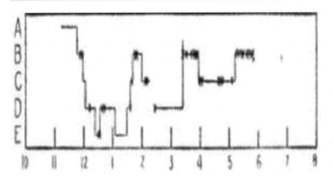

Fig. 13.5 Hypnogram as depicted by Loomis and colleagues**Fig.**

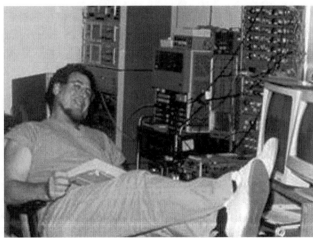

Fig. 13.6 Present author with sleep analyzing hybrid computer

these with movements, with dreams, and with external stimuli applied to the sleeping subject." They described alpha, low voltage, spindles, "random," and spindles plus random sleep state sequences. Interestingly, they recorded and described eye movement activity but did not establish an eye movement dreaming state of sleep. Their graphical depiction of sleep's progression across the night looks remarkably similar to our contemporary hypnograms (see Fig. 13.5). Loomis invited Harvard professor Hallowell Davis and his wife Pauline to TuxedoPark and offered to fund his clinical EEG research. Davis accepted the offer. Loomis had a hopeful but ultimately misguided belief that EEG could be applied to psychological and psychoanalysis and he invited many distinguished psychiatrists to his laboratory. When World War II broke out, the Loomis Laboratories changed direction to help in the war effort. He helped by bankrolling the development of high-powered radio detection and ranging (RADAR) and Loomis radio navigation (LRN), later renamed long range navigation (LORAN); technologies that ultimately helped win the war (Fig. 13.6).

Discover of REM Sleep

In 1953, Aserinsky and Kleitman published data showing dreaming occurred during the sleep stage associated with low-voltage, mixed-frequency activity [7]. Furthermore, rapid eye movement (REM) accompanied these events. In his book *Sleep and Wakefulness,* Kleitman describes the discovery in the following manner: "…we literally stumbled on an objective method of studying dreaming while exploring eye motility in adults…" [8]. He further noted that Ladd (in1892), based only on introspection, posited eye movements during dreaming and Jacobson (in 1937) had written "When a person dreams…most often his eyes are active." Nonetheless, the electrophysiological evidence in their landmark paper officially ushered in a key step toward more fully describing sleep. Meanwhile, Jouvet found his cats lost muscle tone during "paradoxical sleep" episodes which completed our picture of stage REM sleep [9]. These discoveries also marshaled the beginning of multichannel electro-

physiological recording of EEG, electrooculogram (EOG), and sometimes electromyogram (EMG) for studying sleep.

Exploring REM sleep and comparing its mental and physiological correlates to other stages of sleep became a standard paradigm. Dream content, both spontaneous and provoked, during REM represented a very hot topic. After all, Freud had called dreaming the royal road to the unconscious mind [10]. Sleep studies targeting stage REM now provided a laboratory tool to explore the unconscious processes. Concomitant recordings of respiration, heart rhythm, electrodermal activity, paved the way toward what we now call PSG.

The Standardized Manual

As more investigators began researching sleep phenomena, scientists realized that a standardization of techniques could immensely facilitate communication and possibly progress. After REM sleep's discovery, summarizing sleep integrity, continuity, and architecture required more sophistication that the Loomis system offered. Thus, research groups created their own terminology and scoring rules. Dement and Kleitman evolved a system to classify sleep according to EEG criteria [11]. Essentially, a time domain of the set duration was established and the dominant activity within that timeframe-dictated classification. This time domain, called an epoch, could be classified as sleep stage 1, 2, 3, or 4 or awake according to EEG characteristics. When REMs occurred during stage 1 sleep, the stage was designated REM sleep. However, recording technique and terminology differed between sleep laboratories. REM sleep was also called paradoxical sleep, desynchronized sleep, active sleep, D sleep, and even unorthodox sleep.

Ultimately, an ad hoc committee was formed to develop "A Manual of Standardized Terminology, Techniques and Scoring System for Sleep Stages of Human Subjects." [12]

Chaired jointly by Drs. Allan Rechtschaffen and Anthony Kales the committee was a who's who of sleep experts, including William C. Dement, Michel Jouvet, Bedrich Roth, Laverne C. Johnson, Howard P. Roffwarg, Ralph J. Berger, Allan Jacobson, Lawrence J. Monroe, Ian Oswald, and Richard D. Walter. The group standardized procedures, scoring rules, and terminology. More important, they reached consensus and thereafter used the procedures (for the most part) to conduct human sleep research. In essence, this was the real key to R&K (as it was called after the chairmen's initials) successes. My understanding from stories I have been told by various participants indicated there were very strong (verging on violent) disagreements, shouting arguments, and name calling. In the heat of one less than civil debate, reportedly one of the chairmen barred the doors, decreeing that no one could leave until consensus was reached. Ultimately, consensus was reached and this is why R&K succeeded.

PSG, at least for sleep staging was established!

Psychophysiological Study of Normal Sleep

This new field, PSG, was ripe for discovery. In 1961, a research society emerged called the Association for the Psychophysiological Study of Sleep (APSS) and annual meetings were held to discuss research findings. The meeting proceedings were originally published in the *Psychophysiology* (the journal for the Society for Psychophysiological Research) which sported the image of a PSG tracing on its cover. Research laboratories at major universities, at US Naval and Army research centers, in European research institutes, and large medical centers began recording human sleep to describe its biology and to try to understand its underlying process. Whether a particular line of inquiry aimed to elucidate the function of sleep or to derive the intricacies of its process, progress, and some breakthroughs were being made. Sleep deprivation was a popular paradigm in the attempt to infer function. The examination of sleep stage rebound in response to selective stage deprivation provided a model to explore sleep's homeostatic regulation. The military was interested in the adverse effects sleep deprivation had on behavior, attention, cognition, and physical ability.

Many studies focused on REM sleep phenomena. Obviously, dreaming represented a very seductive and intriguing topic; however, no unified theory of dreaming grew out of PSG research. Nonetheless, scientists found the eye movements generally corresponded to direction of gaze in the dream sensorium, middle ear muscle activity concorded with dreamt sounds, and nocturnal erections accompanied REM sleep but did not correspond to sexual dream content. Physiologic events associated with PSG stages other than REM sleep included timing and release of growth hormone during slow-wave sleep, slow-wave activity as a marker for homeostatic drive, other endocrine secretions in sleep, and physiological stability of cardiopulmonary functions during non-REM (NREM) sleep. Note the intuitive appeal of referring to sleep as REM and NREM. However, this terminology highlights how enamored polysomnographers were with REM sleep. REM sleep is the minor partner in sleep, yet we label the majority of sleep as not REM. Perhaps we should refer to wakefulness as non-sleep.

Sleep Latency Tests

Multiple Sleep Latency Test

The sleep studies performed in the Stanford summer sleep camp on children and teenage as well as other studies performed on college students and patients with sleep disorders led to conceptualization of daytime sleep latency as a biomarker for sleepiness. The studies in children were part of Mary A. Carskadon's doctoral dissertation "Determinants of Daytime Sleepiness: Adolescent Development, Extended and Restricted Nocturnal Sleep (1979)." Carskadon and Dement [13] described multiple sleep latency changes across the day during an experimental 90-min sleep–wake schedule in Sleep Research. Sleep Research, at the time, was a major vehicle for sharing information in the sleep community. Their subjects had 16 opportunities to fall asleep (and were instructed to "close your eyes, lie quietly, and try to fall asleep") over each 24-h period as they underwent baseline, sleep deprivation, and recovery periods. PSG recordings from these studies helped form procedures later used in multiple sleep latency test (MSLT). The following year, Richardson et al. [14] published daytime sleep latency findings for patients with narcolepsy and controls. Sleep latency as a biomarker for sleepiness validation came soon after with experimental studies of acute sleep deprivation, chronic sleep restriction, and concordance with other performance measures [15, 16].

The PSG and operational procedures for conducting and analyzing the MSLT were extremely well thought out and effective right from the start. Methods quickly became standardized and a coherent body of literature emerged. A research version (minimizing accumulated sleep) and a clinical version (providing 15 min of sleep to permit REM occurrence) evolved. MSLT's utility for objectively measuring sleepiness and confirming narcolepsy (by REM occurrence) made MSLT an essential part of sleep research and sleep medicine. Guidelines for MSLT were formally adopted in 1986 in the journal *Sleep* [17]. Current clinical guidelines continue to endorse MSLT for diagnosing narcolepsy [18] and research projects still turn to the MSLT when they need an objective measure for sleepiness.

Maintenance of Wakefulness Test

While the ability to fall asleep depends on underlying sleep drive, the ability to remain awake in the face of sleepiness involves additional factors. The inability to volitionally maintain wakefulness in soporific circumstances became the focus of many sleep researchers, clinicians, and regulators. The role of sleepiness in fatigue-related accidents needed definition. The failure of the brain's alertness system in sleep restricted, deprived, or impaired individuals contributes to fatigue in a manner that cannot be engineered away by human factors or ergonomic improvements. Mitler et al. developed maintenance of wakefulness test (MWT) using procedures similar to MSLT but changed the instructions from "try to fall asleep" to "try to remain awake." Criterion group validation in patients suffering from sleepiness succeeded [19, 20]. MWT is a powerful tool (the US Federal Aviation Administration endorsed its use) but methodology varied from study to study, sometimes making it difficult to compare results. A critical variation is test session length which ranges from 20 to 60 min. After a normative data trial [21], test session length settled on 40 min. Current clinical guidelines published in 2005 endorse 40-min sessions, provide standard procedures, and stipulate clinical indications for use [18].

Clinical PSG

Exploration, Biomarkers, and Diagnostics

Just as EEG proved useful in clinical applications, PSG held similar promise. Robert L. Williams was a pioneer and unsung leader in sleep medicine. He explained to me that understanding sleep disorders first required characterizing normal human sleep. Beginning in 1959, his sleep laboratory at the University of Florida, College of Medicine in Gainesville began making continuous all-night sleep recordings in normal, healthy male and female children, adolescents, teenagers, young adults, adults, and seniors. A decade and a half later these "norms" were published in *The EEG of Human Sleep* [22].

It was well known that in adults, REM sleep did not occur until after approximately 70–100 min of NREM sleep. Furthermore, REM sleep seldom, if ever, occurred during daytime naps. PSG evidence verified REM sleep occurring on or near sleep onset both during nocturnal sleep studies and during daytime naps in patients with narcolepsy [23]. *This finding established a PSG diagnostic marker.* The hunt was on! It was noted that patients with major depressive disorders had shorter than normal REM sleep latencies [24]. Sleep-related erection monitoring helped differentiate men suffering from organic versus psychological erectile dysfunction

to aid clinicians in selecting appropriate therapeutic interventions [25].

PSG illuminated sleep pathophysiologies. Obvious ones like cessation of breathing with arousals, oxyhemoglobin desaturations, or both were soon discovered. Driven by technological advances in oximetry, thermistors, thermocouples, and devices/techniques to detect respiratory effort, sleep apnea syndromes were indisputably verified [26]. Commercially available fast-response oximetry systems included the Waters, Hewlett-Packard, and eventually the Biox devices. Airflow detection devices were still largely homemade but ready-to-use commercially available recording sensors quickly followed. Periodic leg movement activity became apparent and its potential for disturbing sleep understood. Abnormal EEG activity or lack thereof, during some sleep-related odd or abnormal behaviors provided differentiation between nocturnal seizure and parasomnias. Also, clinical PSG led to discovery of new sleep disorders; for example, REM sleep behavior disorder [27].

PSG also provided an objective technique to assess insomnia. While this approach ultimately was deemed impractical except under specific circumstances [28], PSG application for investigating drug effects on sleep was a more productive enterprise, especially if waveform changes were analyzed [29]. PSG testing of new drugs for treating insomnia became *de rigueur*. Multi-night, multicenter, randomized controlled trials with PSG primary and/or secondary outcome measures provided the objective evidence to determine whether an investigational new drug will be approved by federal oversight agencies, such as the US Food and Drug Administration. This represents applied clinical science in its ultimate form.

Clinical Guidelines and Professional Society Recommendations

The sudden and rapid expansion of clinical PSG application quickly outdistanced any standardized recommendations. To a large degree, methods for various PSG procedures were scattered in dozens of papers and textbooks, and they all differed. The pivotal publication with respect to PSG methods was Guilleminault's 1982 book *Sleeping and Waking Disorders: Indications and Techniques* [30]. This text immediately became a de facto standard. The methods described by Bornstein's (a.k.a. Sharon Keenan) to record and assess sleep-disordered breathing served as the basic roadmap in many laboratories [31]. It was not until many years after the book was out of print that the *Chicago Group's* sleep apnea recommendations were published [32] (and these were endorsed for research rather than for standard clinical routine). Richard Coleman's chapter [33] served as a primer for PSG evaluation of periodic leg movements. Other chapters detailed MSLT, gastroesophageal (GE) reflux monitoring, and sleep-related erection testing. The book also contained a comprehensive sleep questionnaire.

The original sleep society, APSS, was now trying to serve both scientists and clinicians. Similarly, the annual meetings had basic research, clinical research, and clinical developments on its agenda. Eventually, the Association of Sleep Disorders Centers (ASDC) was formed in 1975 and it ultimately grew an individual member wing called the Clinical Sleep Society (CSS) in 1984. In the meanwhile, the Association of Polysomnographic Technologists (APT) formed in 1978 and a board of polysomnographic technologist registry (BRPT) administered its first examination in 1979. These groups ultimately formed a confederation in 1986 called the Association of Professional Sleep Societies (reusing the initials APSS) and ASDC was renamed the American Sleep Disorders Association (ASDA) the following year (eventually becoming the American Academy of Sleep Medicine (AASM) in 1999). All the while, some progress was being made to have societally endorsed PSG standards. There were task forces to establish procedures for conducting the MSLT [34], recording, and scoring central nervous system (CNS) arousals from sleep [35] and periodic leg movements [36]. The AASM finally formed a standards of practice committee to make recommendations concerning clinical PSG and diagnostics using evidence-based medicine and Rand appropriateness approaches [37, 38]. Additionally, international groups formed to develop standards for recording and scoring clinical PSG information. Notable among these are the group that published an atlas for cyclic alternating pattern scoring [39] and the World Association of Sleep Medicine (WASM) in collaboration with the International Restless Legs Syndrome Study Group (IRLSSG) who updated the guidelines for periodic leg movement assessment (which ultimately was adopted virtually unchanged by AASM) [40].

Finally, in 2007, the AASM published a manual that covered recording and scoring all of the routinely used clinical PSG data [41]. The manual includes terminology, technique, and scoring criteria for sleep staging, CNS arousals, respiratory events, periodic leg movements, other movements, and electrocardiographic abnormalities. The AASM seems committed to updating the manual regularly and providing web-based availability through subscription. The other area of standardization addressed in the manual relates to digital PSG. Sorely needed minimum specifications for computerized PSG systems were developed by a task force I cochaired with Thomas Penzel. These guidelines were long overdue and hopefully will set a standard to assure that our clinical tools remain reliable and valid.

Growth of Sleep Disorders Laboratories and PSG's "Killer App"

As clinical PSG gained ground, sleep disorders center began to open. Some notable early program included the ones in Baptist Memorial (Memphis), Baylor College of Medicine (Houston), Western Psychiatric (Pittsburgh), Presbyterian (Oklahoma City), Ohio State (Columbus), Montefiore (New York), Henry Ford (Detroit), Mount Sinai (Miami), Stanford University (Palo Alto, CA), University of California (Irvine, CA), and Holy Cross (Mission Hills). This core group collaborated on a variety of projects and their leaders were instrumental in developing PSG applications for sleep medicine [42]. These sleep disorders centers created a nucleus from which the ASDC grew. The main focus of these sleep centers was the laboratory designed to conduct clinical PSG procedures. As of 2011, there were nearly 2000 AASM-accredited sleep disorders centers [43].

Sleep apnea was the engine driving this huge expansion of sleep laboratories conducting clinical PSGs. Currently, 80–90 % of all clinical PSG conducted attempt to rule-in or rule-out sleep-disordered breathing. In the parlance of Silicon Valley, this makes sleep apnea PSG's "killer app" (application). Although sleep-disordered breathing was first identified in 1965 by Gastaut et al. [44], it took a decade before clinical and research machinery were adequately mobilized. In 1975, sleep apnea papers still only registered trace amounts in the overall sleep literature. If we inspect journal publication trends, however, by 1995, sleep apnea papers reached approximately 50 % of the overall sleep literature.

Computerization

Signal Processing

One thing about PSG was painfully clear from the beginning to researchers and clinicians. It is an intensively time-consuming process. Even after 6–8 h of recording, analysis could require another 2+ h. From a data processing perspective, each night created a near-Herculean task. As laboratory minicomputers evolved in the 1970s, signal processing techniques held the promise of reducing workload and providing new perspectives to expand scientific horizons by automating sleep analysis.

EEG characterization had already matured and automated spike detection, power analysis, and compressed spectral arrays dazzled onlookers. Signal analysis could characterize ongoing EEG according to frequency, duration, and/or power. These indices could be grouped according to bandwidths relevant to human physiology. The Dement–Kleitman scoring system was particularly amenable to this approach. Fourier transforms, period amplitude analysis, complex demodulation, and coherence analysis were some of the techniques applied. The text *Principles of Neurobiological Signal Analysis* by Glasser and Ruchkin [45] became a standard reference for some developers. Concerns about the details of aliasing, leakage, analog-to-digital conversion, multiplexing, cross talk, digital, and recursive filtering occupied the minds of programmers and engineers involved with PSG applications. Three issues reared up to impede progress of the completely digital analytic approach: artifacts, event detection, and technological limitations.

PSG Artifacts

The first, most important, and even now not fully resolved issue involves artifact recognition. An artifact is an electrical signal arising from activity other than that under study and may masquerade as potentially valid data. PSGs always contain artifact (at least I have never seen an overnight sleep study that was completely artifact free). Artifacts contaminate data and can compromise analysis. Perhaps the earliest adage popularized in computer sciences was "garbage-in, garbage-out" (GIGO). Undetected electrophysiological artifact represents garbage. Artifact can be biological or environmental; it can take many shapes and forms. While humans can (usually) easily detect artifacts, programmers must invent strategies and write code to recognize hundreds of possible scenarios.

Biological artifacts include blinking and eye movements masquerading as EEG waveforms, movement, and EMG activity contaminating EEG signals with high-frequency components, and heartbeat intruding into other bioelectric tracings. Other biological sources of EEG artifact include sweating, twitching, coughing, teeth clinching or grinding, and shivering, to name a few. Environmental artifacts include electrode popping, alternating current (50 or 60 cycles per second) interference, and any other electrical signal in contact with the sleeping subject (for example, a pacemaker). Furthermore, each of these potential artifacts can manifest in dozens of ways, making automated recognition difficult and programming complicated.

Event Detection

Signal processing techniques mostly served to decompose electrophysiological data into its frequency components that could be expressed as duration or power. By contrast, specific event detection requires feature or envelop analysis. Spike detection came early on in clinical EEG but K-complex, sleep spindle, REMs, and slow eye movements lagged far behind. More importantly, some of these waveforms defined sleep stages and have overlapping frequency signatures. Available laboratory computers had far less capacity than today's powerful microprocessors. Thus, some automation attempts approached signal detection using hybrid analog–digital techniques. One of the great pioneers in

PSG computerization, Jack Smith, an engineering professor at the University of Florida developed the sleep-analyzing hybrid computer (SAHC). The SAHC contained specific analog waveform detectors whose output was compiled with a laboratory minicomputer. In later reincarnations, the detectors were interfaced with microcomputer systems.

Technological Limitations

Looking back on laboratory minicomputers, it seems amazing that we were able to accomplish anything. What seemed like the frontiers of high technology now looks like stone knives and axes, in retrospect. Using assembly language (or sometimes compilable languages like FORTRAN II), limited addressable memory space (sometimes only 64 KB), very expensive but quite limited overhead storage devices (Digital Equipment Corporation (DEC) tapes, Diablo or Pertec 15-in. removable disk drives offering maybe 5 MB storage) PSG analysis systems were constructed, programmed, and used in large laboratories. These systems mainly analyzed research data; a particularly popular application involved describing drug effects on sleep in great detail. The promise of automatic sleep stage, sleep apnea, and periodic movement scoring took much longer to reach fruition. Processing speed represented another major hurdle (which is why assembly language was used). Squeezing enough cycle time to process incoming signals was a challenge using OS8 and RT11 operating systems. More complex processing often proceeded offline by playing instrument-analog-recorded PSG data into computers (using Hewlett-Packard, Ampex, Sangamo, Honeywell, and other very expensive tape machines). Eight-bit laboratory minicomputers like the DEC PDP12, 8, Link 8, 8e progressed to 16-bit systems like the Texas Instrument 980, DEC PDP 11/03,/23,/38, and eventually VAX. Each innovation added power, speed, and storage capacity. However, upward migration was sometimes painful because assembly languages were not necessarily compatible which sometimes meant having to jettison software libraries and data as a sacrifice to implementing more capable hardware.

Commercialization

By the mid-1970s, microcomputer began to appear in laboratories. Microcomputers could fit on a desktop (rather than take up the entire end of a room) and cost a fraction of the price. Microcomputers rapidly gained popularity both in the PSG analysis world as well as in all other work environments, becoming smaller and smaller and more and more powerful. By the time I retired my homebrewed original Imsai 8080 and Altair-MITS disk subsystem, IBM had entered the market with their "personal computer," and commercial integrations for PSG applications had appeared. There was a tipping point sometime in the early 1990s where microcomputer systems reach adequate power at a low enough cost to become marketable. Improving software, programming video graphics, and integrating large and larger capability storage devices became imperative.

Oddly enough, the original systems mainly provided a technique for replacing paper. A single PSG was recorded, stored, and could be retrieved, viewed, and annotated on a video display. Automatic scoring was unreliable. The savings in paper cost and paper record storage expense drove the market. Most paper PSGs recorded 30 s of data on one sheet of fanfolded paper. Thus, an 8-h recording required 960 PSG pages. Not accidentally, a box of paper had 1000 fanfolded sheets and usually measured 12.5 × 12.5 × 3.0 in. Thus, each night, our four-bed laboratory produced more than a cubic foot of paper to store. Ten nights would fill a file cabinet. Today, an equivalent number of PSGs would fit in my shirt pocket. The promise of automated scoring and expanding horizons of sleep science were temporarily forgotten.

Scaling data represented the other major advantage when reviewing digital PSGs. With paper, once recorded, the PSG's temporal resolution is set and immutable. Digital PSGs can be viewed as a slow trace (2–5 min per page), at traditional resolution (30 s per page), or expanded (10 s per page). Some systems evolved to allow split screen display with different resolution for selected channels. Initially signal quality eroded but, in time, digital amplifier quality improved. Soon, trade journals, society newsletters, and exposition areas at annual meetings became crowded with digital PSG advertising. Systems like CNS, Telefactor Sassy, Oxford Medilog SAC, Telediagnostic Vista, Melville Diagnostics Sandman, Biologic, Healthdyne NightWatch competed for space with positive airway pressure machines. Traditional pen-and-paper PSG systems were on their way out; eventually even Grass, Nihon Kohden, Nicolet, and TECA developed digital PSG systems.

The Rise of Home Sleep Testing

The most significant change for clinical sleep evaluation is happening right now. For 40 years, attended PSG dominated as the preferred technique for evaluating sleep apnea and/or titrating positive airway pressure therapy. As previously explained, diagnosing sleep apnea is PSG's "killer app." The widespread recognition of sleep apnea as a significant medical condition, paired with PSG's billable current procedural terminology (CPT) code produced the meteoric rise of sleep medicine. However, economics are now driving the market toward finding a less expensive alternative; thus, the new "killer app" for diagnosing sleep apnea is becoming cardiopulmonary recording, also known as home sleep testing (HST) [46]. HST involves making overnight recordings of

airflow, respiratory effort, oxyhemoglobin saturation level, heart rate, and sometimes snoring sounds and EEG. Its only validated use is to verify the presence of sleep apnea.

HST technology is not new. It being recommended for first-line routine clinical use is! As with many new applications, its proper use and limitations are poorly understood. As a tool, it has specific utility but improper use can be dangerous. Our group has used HST for many years and the three most important things we have learned are: (1) HST requires a full-scale clinical sleep program to be effective, (2) HST can rule-in but not rule-out sleep apnea, and (3) careful review to determine technical recording quality is absolutely essential. As HST can rule-in but not rule-out sleep apnea, only those patients with a high pretest probability based on signs, symptoms, and comorbidities should be tested. If individuals for whom there is not a high clinical suspicion are tested, HST becomes an additional, ineffectual test. Follow-up laboratory PSG is needed in two circumstances. (1) Patients with high pretest probability and negative HST require attended laboratory PSG. (2) Patients in whom HST confirms sleep apnea but who continue to have sleep problems after the apnea is treated also require PSG to assess for other sleep pathophysiologies. Thus, PSG still represents the "gold standard" for evaluating sleep disorders.

Conclusion

A significant part of the sleep science and sleep medicine history coincides with the history of PSG. The polysomnogram, born out of EEG, raised by psychophysiology, matured with clinical science, and ultimately became employed by sleep medicine. Amazingly, PSG continues to be our major tool for evaluating sleep and sleep disorders. Originally our analog amplifiers displayed bioelectrical activity by inking tracings on paper. Now, digital amplifiers record similar information on magnetic, silicon, and/or optical media that can be retrieved for display on flat panel screens. Although the recording devices and the display medium have changed dramatically in the past 40 years, how we apply this tool has not. Indeed, the scoring system has evolved somewhat with successive refinements but except for data-tracing scalability (which was not possible with paper recordings), the basic polysomnographer's review process is remarkably similar to what it was 25–35 years ago. Does this mean the field's pioneers had tremendous acumen and incredible insight concerning the immediate and future needs? Does it mean that PSG sufficiently met our needs? Or, does it mean that PSG has reached asymptote and is no longer progressing? This empirical question will be answered as history continues to unfold.

References

1. Berger H. Ueber das Electroenkephalogramm des Menschen. J Psychol Neurol. 1930;40:160–179.
2. Adrian ED, Matthews BHC. Berger rhythm: potential changes from the occipital lobes in man. Brain 1934;57:355–85.
3. Titchener EB. Experimental psychology, a manual of laboratory practice I: quantitative experiments, part II. Instructor's manual. New York: Macmillan; 1918. p. 172–176.
4. Gibbs FA, Gibbs EL. Atlas of electroencephalography. I. Methodology and normal controls. Cambridge: Addison-Wesley; 1950.
5. Conant J. Tuxedo park. New York: Simon and Schuster; 2002.
6. Loomis AL, Harvey N, Hobart GA: Cerebral states during sleep, as studied by human brain potentials. J Exp Psychol. 1937;21:127–144.
7. Aserinsky E, Kleitman N. Regularly occurring periods of eye motility, and concomitant phenomena, during sleep. Science 1953;118:273–4.
8. Kleitman N. Sleep and wakefulness. Chicago: University of Chicago Press; 1967.
9. Jouvet M, Michel F. Sur les voies nerveuses responsables de l'activité rapide au cours du sommeil physiologique chez le chat (phase paradoxale). CR Soc Biol. 1960;154:995–8.
10. Freud S: The interpretation of dreams. New York: Random House; 1950.
11. Dement W, Kleitman N. Cyclic variation in EEG during sleep and their relation to eye movements, body motility, and dreaming. Clin Neurophysiol. 1957;9:673–90.
12. Rechtschaffen A, Kales A. A manual of standardized terminology, techniques and scoring system for sleep stages in human subjects. NIH Publication No. 204. Washington: U.S. Government Printing Office; 1968.
13. Carskadon MA, Dement WC. Sleep tendency: an objective measure of sleep loss. Sleep Res. 1977;6: 200.
14. Richardson GS, Carskadon MA, Flagg W, van den Hoed J, Dement WC, Mitler MM. Excessive daytime sleepiness in man: multiple sleep latency measurement in narcoleptic and control subjects. Electroencephalogr Clin Neurophysiol. 1978;45:621–7.
15. Carskadon MA, Dement WC. Effects of total sleep loss on sleep tendency. Percept Motor Skills. 1979;48:495–506.
16. Carskadon MA, Dement WC. Cumulative effects of sleep restriction on daytime sleepiness. Psychophysiology 1981;18:107–13.
17. Carskadon MA, Dement WC, Mitler MM, Roth T, Westbrook P, Keenan S. Guidelines for the multiple sleep latency test (MSLT): a standard measure of sleepiness. Sleep 1986;9:519–24.
18. Standards of practice committee of the American academy of sleep medicine. Practice parameters for clinical use of the multiple sleep latency test and the maintenance of wakefulness test. Sleep 2005;28:113–121.
19. Mitler MM, Gujavarty KS, Browman CP. Maintenance of wakefulness test: a polysomnographic technique for evaluating treatment efficacy in patients with excessive somnolence. Electroenceph clin Neurophysiol. 1982;53:658–61.
20. Browman CP, Gujavarty KS, Sampson MG, Mitler MM. REM sleep episodes during the maintenance of wakefulness test in patients with sleep apnea syndrome and patients with narcolepsy. Sleep 1983;6(1):23–8.
21. Doghramji K, Mitler MM, Sangal RB, Shapiro C, Taylor S, et al. A normative study of the maintenance of wakefulness test (MWT). Electroencephalogr Clin Neurophysiol. 1997;103(5):554–62.
22. Williams RL, Karacan I, Hursch CJ. EEG of human sleep: clinical applications: New York: Wiley; 1974.
23. Rechtschaffen A, Wolpert EA, Dement WC, Mitchell SA, Fisher C. Nocturnal sleep of narcoleptics. Electroencephalogr Clin Neurophysiol. 1963;15:599–609.
24. Reynolds CF, Kupfer DJ. Sleep research in affective illness: state of the art circa 1987. Sleep 1987;10:199–215.
25. Karacan I, Salis P, Williams RL. The role of the sleep laboratory in diagnosis and treatment of impotence. In: Williams RL, Karacan I, edtors. Sleep disorders: diagnosis and treatment. New York: John Wiley and Son; 1978.
26. Guilleminault C, Dement WC. Sleep apnea syndromes (The Kroc Foundation series: v 11). New York: AR Liss; 1978.
27. Schenck CH, Bundlie SR, Ettinger MG, Mahowald MW chronic behavioral disorders of human REM sleep: a new category of parasomnia. Sleep 1986;9:293–308.
28. Littner M, Hirshkowitz M, Kramer M, Kapen S, Anderson WM, Bailey D, Berry RB, Davila D, Johnson S, Kushida C, Loube DI, Wise M, Woodson BT. Practice parameters for using polysomnography to evaluate insomnia: an update. An American Academy of Sleep Medicine report. Sleep 2003;26(6):754–60.
29. Hirshkowitz M, Thornby JI, Karacan I. Sleep pharmacology and automated EEG analysis. Psychiatr Ann. 1979;9:510–20.
30. Guilleminault C, editor. Sleeping and waking disorders: indications and techniques. Menlo Park: Addison-Wesley; 1982.
31. Bornstein SK. Respiratory monitoring during sleep: polysomnography. In: Guilleminault C, editor. Sleeping and waking disorders: indications and techniques. Menlo Park: Addison-Wesley; 1982. pp. 183–212.
32. The report of an American academy of sleep medicine task force. Sleep-related breathing disorders in adults: recommendations for syndrome definition and measurement techniques in clinical research. Sleep 1999;22(5):667–89.
33. Coleman RM: Periodic movements in sleep (nocturnal myoclonus) and restless legs syndrome. In: Guilleminault C, editor. Sleeping and waking disorders: indications and techniques. Menlo Park: Addison-Wesley; 1982. pp. 267–295.
34. Carskadon MA, Dement WC, Mitler MM, Roth T, Westbrook PR, Keenan S. Guidelines for the multiple sleep latency test (MSLT): A standard measure of sleepiness. Sleep 1986;9:519–24.
35. ASDA Report. Bonnet M, Carley D, Carskadon M, Easton P, Guilleminault C, Harper R, Hayes B, Hirshkowitz M, Ktonas P, Keenan S, Pressman M, Roehrs T, Smith J, Walsh J, Weber S, Westbrook P, Jordan B. EEG arousals: scoring rules and examples. Sleep 1992;15:173–84.
36. ASDA Report. Bonnet M, Carley D, Guilleminault C, Hirshkowitz M, Keenan S, Roehrs T, Weber S. Recording and scoring leg movements. Sleep 1993;16:748–59.
37. ASDA Report. Chesson AL, Ferber RA, Fry JM, et al. Practice parameters for the indications for polysomnography and related procedures. Sleep 1997;20:406–22.
38. Standards of practice committee of the American academy of sleep medicine. Practice parameters for the indications for polysomnography and related procedures: An update for 2005. Sleep 2005;28:499–521.
39. Terzano MG, Parrino L, Smerieri A, Chervin R, Chokroverty S, Guilleminault C, Hirshkowitz M, Mahowald M, Moldofsky H, Rosa A, Thomas R, Walters A. et al. Atlas, rules, and recording technique for scoring of cyclic alternating pattern (CAP) in human sleep. Sleep Med. 2002;3:187–199.
40. Zucconi M, Ferri R, Allen R, Baier PC, Bruni O, Chokroverty S, Ferrini-Strambi L, Fulda S, Garcia-Borreguero D, et al. The official World Association of Sleep Medicine (WASM) standards for recording and scoring periodic leg movements in sleep (PLMS) and wakefulness (PLMW). Developed in collaboration with a task force from the international restless legs syndrome study group (IRLSSG). Sleep Med. 2006;7:175–183.
41. Iber C, Ancoli-Israel S, Chesson A, Quan SF. For the American academy of sleep medicine: The AASM manual for the scoring of sleep and associated events: rules, terminology and technical specifications. Westchester, Ill: American Academy of Sleep Medicine; 2007.

42. Coleman Coleman RM, Roffwarg HP, Kennedy SJ, Guilleminault C, Cinque J, Cohn MA, Karacan I, Kupfer DJ, Lemmi H, Miles LE, Orr WC, Phillips ER, Roth T, Sassin JF, Schmidt HS, Weitzman ED, Dement WC. Sleep-wake disorders based on a polysomnographic diagnosis. A national cooperative study. JAMA. 1982;247:997–1003.

43. Kryger MH, Roth T, Dement WC. Priniciples and practice of sleep medicine, 5th ed. St. Louis: Elsevier Saunders; 2011. p. xxvii.

44. Gastaut H, Tassinari C, Duron B. Etude polygraphique des manifestations episodique (hypniques et respiratoires) du syndrome de Pickwick. Rev Neurol. 1965;112:568–79.

45. Glaser EM, Ruchkin DS. Principles of neurobiological signal analysis. New York: Academic Press; 1976.

46. Hirshkowitz M, Sharafkhaneh A. Comparison of portable monitoring with laboratory polysomnography for diagnosing sleep-related breathing disorders: scoring and interpretation. Sleep Med Clin 2011; 6: 283–292.

Part IV
Sleep Medicine Societies, Professional Societies, and Journals

A History Behind the Development of Sleep Medicine and Sleep Societies

Brendon Richard Peters and Christian Guilleminault

In considering the founding and development of the major sleep societies, it is useful to recall that the entire process is ultimately about people and the exchange of ideas. This "history" is a personal (CG) one and its narrative is inspired by individuals who shared a passion and interest in advancing sleep medicine.

The first sleep society created was the "Association for the Psycho-physiological Study of Sleep" or APSS. It was created by William C. Dement as an informal society where individuals interested in the investigation of sleep could interact. At that time, there were no clear standards to score sleep and wakefulness in laboratory animals or in humans and there was the need to have a forum where ideas could be exchanged between researchers. Its initial members were few but it had an international representation. Individuals integrating sleep and circadian rhythms as well as those interested in sleep and dreams were involved. The early members included many enthusiastic individuals attracted by this new field of research, e.g., Michel Jouvet, Danielle Mounier, Allan Rechtschaffen, Eliot Weitzman, Howard Roffwarg, Michael Chase, Gerald Voegel, Laverne C. Johnson, Rosalind D. Cartwright, Wilse Webb, Truett Allison, Ralph Berger, Frank Snyder, Ismet Karacan, Charles Fisher, Milton Kramer, David Foulkes, Thomas Anders, Allan Hobson, M. Barry Sterman, Peter Hauri, Antony Kales, Walter Baust, Werner Koella, Pier Parmegggiani, Peter Morgane, Olga Petre-Quadens, and Ian Oswald. These participants helped develop structure and purpose for the group.

In addition, there were specific places that quickly became important to the study of sleep and generated increasing interest and membership. In the USA, Chicago, New York, and Stanford became especially influential. Dement, working at Stanford, the University of California, Los Angeles (UCLA) group, and the navy hospital in San Diego brought many individuals into the society. These members included the following: Vincent Zarcone, Georges Gulevitch, Jon Sassin, Ardie Lubin, Denis McGinty, Anna Taylor, and Ronald Harper. In Lyon, France, Marc Jeannerod, and Odile Benoit were brought into the fold. Not everyone was convinced, however, of the utility of binding common interests.

In particular, two individuals were missing from this effort: Nathaniel Kleitman and Eugene Aserinsky. Much later, Nathaniel Kleitman explained his lack of involvement in this way when speaking with one of the authors (CG) of this chapter about rapid eye movement (REM) sleep, "this is the stuff of Dement." The implication was that this was not his primary interest. Greater importance was placed on the understanding of the sleep rhythms in general, with REM sleep being only one of them.

There were clear divisions of interest within sleep. There were a large number of individuals interested in the electrophysiology, pharmacology, and cellular mechanisms of sleep. Still others were more focused on "sleep and dreams." Some people pursued the interactions between seizures and sleep or on other brain disorders and sleep. Finally, there was a small group who was interested in the development of sleep from infancy to childhood. Many times it proved difficult to unite these divergent interests into a common set of purpose and agenda. It became clear early on that it was necessary to develop a common language when considering sleep in humans. Moreover, it was critical to "codify" the electroencephalography (EEG) changes seen when monitoring the brain, in either animals or humans. One of the major early accomplishments of this heterogeneous group, brought together in part by Dement, was the creation of two sleep atlases that are still used today. This was no small feat.

C. Guilleminault (✉)
Sleep Medicine Division, Stanford University Outpatient Medical Center, 450 Broadway, Redwood City, CA 94063, USA
e-mail: cguil@stanford.edu

B. R. Peters
Stanford Sleep Medicine Center, Stanford School of Medicine, Redwood City, CA, USA

S. Chokroverty, M. Billiard (eds.), *Sleep Medicine,* DOI 10.1007/978-1-4939-2089-1_14,
© Springer Science+Business Media, LLC 2015

In order to develop these standards, numerous initial obstacles had to be overcome, including differing techniques and equipment. In North America, the standard equipment used to investigate sleep was the "Grass recorder." In Europe, where sleep was part of the tools used by clinical neurophysiologists in their search for seizure disorders, the most common recorder was the Alvar™ equipment. Even the speed at which the paper moved through the equipment varied. In general, a large amount of recording paper was needed to study sleep, but the goals were often different. EEG specialists wanted to see many EEG leads at a fast speed. However, individuals investigating "sleep and dreams," or the body phenomena associated with sleep onset, were more parsimonious with paper. They wanted to recognize non-REM and REM sleep as well as other phenomena. The basic recording speed was 20 s per epoch in western Europe and 30 s per epoch in the USA. Compromise was eventually reached, but only after individuals committed to their interests were involved (sometimes following heated battles).

One hard-working individual was Dr. Dreyfuss-Brissac in the Port Royal Maternity Hospital in Paris. She was involved in continuous monitoring of premature and newborn infants. She also had an integral role in educating a large number of infant sleep researchers in western Europe. She faced off with Dement who was looking to understand REM sleep in humans and the possible use of sleep recording to investigate psycho-physiology and the role of sleep, and particularly REM sleep deprivation, a research topic far separated from an understanding of the development of sleep in premature infants. These had been quite divergent goals for many years. In Europe, many more EEG leads than in USA were used in monitoring, reflecting very different agendas of the sleep researchers. To their credit, these individuals ultimately knew how to compromise and were able to join efforts to set minimum standards and create a work that is still today the basis of human sleep recording.

The informal gathering of the early APSS became more structured with advancing years. Dement was always a driving force behind this group, pushing the development of the field. He understood that there was the need for a unified front if basic sleep research were to gain a foothold in the National Institute of Health grant funding. Cohesion and growth were central in his view to advance the field of sleep research. The presentation of scientific results in front of peers, as is the standard in many other fundamental research fields, was the only way to have recognition of sleep as a valid, independent, scientific field. Dement had many friends who joined him in these efforts, but two were important at this stage: Allan Rechtschaffen and Michel Jouvet.

Both Dement and Jouvet were fascinated by REM sleep and were dedicated to understanding its mechanisms as well as the development and maintenance of the state of alertness.

Both gave the impression of being "REM or paradoxical sleep scientists." They both had great mutual respect for each other's work. Jouvet would come and visit Dement regularly in the basement of the Stanford anatomy building where cats and mice were continuously monitored. They exchanged data and discussed hypotheses. As funding was still difficult for sleep research in France (even though Jouvet had a much more luxurious university setting compared to Dement), Dement played a critical role in supporting Jouvet on a project submitted to the US Air Force. They also jointly supported the advances presented at the now yearly meetings of the APSS more than any other scientists in the field.

The APSS was still a young society with little formal activity between annual meetings. The organization of the meetings that did occur was thus vitally important. It was coordinated by senior investigators and always located in the USA. The cost of travel was still high for the Europeans and Japanese, who were the two major groups joining the research efforts on sleep. In 1970, the USA was in the middle of an important crisis related to the war in Vietnam. The APSS annual meeting was scheduled to be in Santa Fe, New Mexico in the mid-spring. Snow was still on the surrounding mountains, but the sun was everywhere in the small town. The meeting occurred in a room that could contain about 150 people. Many were young college students taking a year off to do research as pre- and postdoctoral fellows. The APSS had succeeded in attracting young individuals securing its chance to survive over time. The Dement group was the largest with Stephen Henricksen, James Ferguson, Eric Hoddes, as well as young associates from Jack Barchas's biochemistry laboratory and the neurophysiology laboratory of Dr. Chow. There were foreign scientists, not only Jouvet and Olga Petre-Quadens but also Swedish scientists, particularly K. Fuxe and Anita Dahlstrom indicating the extension of their interest in the field of sleep research. It was decided that the next meetings would be held internationally every 5 years opening opportunities for foreign young scientists to come and listen to the senior researchers from other parts of the world.

The first meeting abroad was in 1971, organized by Dr. Olga Petre-Quadens. Though held in Belgium, it was not in Brussels, but in the city of Bruges, a somewhat smaller place and a tourist attraction. For the first time, there was a book published out of the meeting, *The Sleeping Brain*. The organizing committee included Walter Baust, Carmine Clemente, William C. Dement, Laverne Johnson, Michel Jouvet, Anthony Kales, Werner Koella, Toshioko Tokirane, and Jolyon West. Olga Petre-Quadens was the local host and new figures were involved in the program, including Ronald Harper and Barry Jacobs. Frederic Bremer and Nathaniel Kleitman were named the two "honorary presidents." Bremer wrote that this first international meeting of the APSS "marks the date when sleep research became a discipline into itself." Nathaniel Kleitman was less enthusiastic about the accomplishments, writing, "The topic of the ten symposia…are representative of the current concerns of investigators that are interested in the understanding of the processes underlying sleep and wakefulness." He added, "Future sleep research may lead to the elucidation of the mechanism of wakefulness, as well as that of sleep." His remarks reflected his belief that the field was missing the real goals. It was also at this meeting that for the first time the role of computers in sleep research was approached with timidity. These efforts were led by Antoine Remond of France and Jack R. Smith of Florida. In addition, Mary Brazier championed the potentially incredible role that computers could play in EEG analysis, but she was not invited.

It was also at this meeting that two very different groups met for the first time: the European neurologists who had studied disorders of sleep within the context of neurological disorders and the US-based "sleep researchers" who had created the APSS. The scientific symposium was organized under the guidance of Roger Broughton who had been a student of Henri Gastaut (the individual who could have created the field of sleep medicine, but did not believe in it). Elio Lugaresi, Alberto Tassinari, Pierre Passouant, and Bederich Roth represented European neurology. They did not see a new field, but rather a subdiscipline of neurology, an error that pulmonary specialists repeated later on after investigation of the sleep apnea syndrome. Despite their support for the investigation of the brain during sleep, it was clear that it was viewed as only a small part of neurology, the "noble science," and not a new field. Ten years later, Elio Lugaresi was invited to another international sleep meeting where he indicated his strong views on the subject in a conversation involving Dement and Guilleminault, stating, "Do you realize that you are making me a simple sleep researcher, when I am a Neurologist?" Clearly, following Gastaut, most of the famous neurologists did not want the label of "sleep researchers." What was sleep when you were the head of the Neurological Institute? Sleep was viewed as a minor segment of neurology. Two years later, Pierre Passouant expressed the same views when he decided to send Michel Billiard for one year to Stanford; sleep was to be part of a great neurology department. Such philosophy persisted in Montpellier until the second millennium. The term sleep department never emerged, but the sleep laboratory (probably one of the largest in Europe for a long time) was part of the department of neurology of the Montpellier Medical School in France. In some respects, the first international APSS congress demonstrated the isolation of the few individuals who wanted to create a new research discipline, a primary goal of the APSS. In addition, the European neurologists realized that there was a complete absence of the concept of a clinical discipline, and that the APSS was essentially an American-based sleep research society including PhDs with little clinical interest or expertise. And, at that time, none of the senior members of the APSS were interested in clinical sleep medicine.

One individual (CG) had a very different view. He attended the 1970 APSS meeting and had decided that there was a new discipline that he called sleep medicine. CG opened a sleep medicine laboratory in La Salepetriere Hospital, against the desire of his chair and dean. Through contact with his contemporary colleagues who also had just finished or were finishing their residencies, CG monitored adults and children from different departments, including internal medicine, metabolism and endocrinology, and pediatrics. He was effectively alone, having only the help of young individuals he taught such as interns and medical students. The only professional support was from his direct colleagues that he had spent the past 4 years with in that very large hospital in Paris. He was financially supported by a one-year grant from the "Societe Medicale des Hopitaux de Paris." In June 1971, he attended the first international meeting in Bruges and the future did not look promising; the same head of La Salpetriere neurology department was not supportive of his venture, despite the fact that the laboratory had been a success with more than 400 sleep medicine patients monitored in a two-bedroom EEG laboratory. During a lunch break with Vincent Zarcone, who was doing alcohol and sleep research at the Palo Alto VA Hospital and who also worked at the animal sleep laboratory of Dement, CG expressed his views and his belief in a new specialty called sleep medicine. Returning to California, Zarcone learned that Dement wanted to secure a large grant to investigate narcolepsy as a disorder of REM sleep incorporating both animal and human research for a better understanding of REM sleep. Neurologists were not interested as it was mostly a low-paid research position based on a grant. Zarcone suggested that Dement should contact Guilleminault, which he did in August 1971. Guilleminault was initially not very interested, considering the conditions and the focus on only narcolepsy and not on sleep medicine, including adults and children. As his situation deteriorated in France within the following four months, Guilleminault agreed to go to Stanford and arrived on January 4, 1972, to take the position and participate in the write-up of a very large grant on narcolepsy. He succeeded in including 10 pages (out of the 300 of the total grant) on breathing and heart monitoring in adults and children. The grant was funded and most of the next three years were used to perform the work outlined in those 10 pages.

Meanwhile, Anthony Kales at UCLA had opened a human sleep and pharmacology unit and was performing research for the pharmaceutical industry, testing the effects of hypnotics on sleep of normal volunteers and insomniacs. Dement saw a way to support basic research through similar funds from pharmaceutical research. The Dement laboratory had most of its research focused on animal models and on narcolepsy as a disorder of REM sleep. There was a postdoctoral fellow, Terry Pivick, who was doing a research project on sleep in pregnant women, monitoring them in the medical center in a two-bedroom laboratory. Recruitment for pharmacological studies on insomnia was also happening there. It was decided that studies on narcoleptics would also be performed in the same place. The recruitment of patients complaining of insomnia quickly expanded to include various sleep disorders. A young neurologist, Dr. Robert Wilson, doing a year of fellowship was there to help, and CG pushed forward with his idea to develop a sleep disorders clinic. Pursuing his own interest, CG went to the Veterans Administration Hospital to work in collaboration with pulmonary medicine (Dr. Fred Eldridge, the senior researcher) and cardiology (Dr. Ara Tilkian, a fellow in cardiology). He attracted the interest of the head of the pediatric intensive care unit (ICU; Dr Philip Sunshine) whose office was just opposite the two-bedroom sleep laboratory, in referring infants and children for monitoring and evaluation of sleep complaints. Adding the information collected in Paris to that gathered at Stanford, new findings became apparent and CG was able to present these at an international meeting organized by Elio Lugaresi on Pickwickian syndrome and hypersomnia. Guilleminault and Dement had many discussions on the possibility of creating a clinical service where money would be obtained for services and tests. But at the 1972 APSS meeting, the presentation of clinical results fell mostly on deaf ears. The society was much more focused on fundamental research and not interested in any clinical endeavor. William Dement was himself somewhat ambivalent: pharmaceutical research was very different from the creation of a clinical field. For many years, the goal of advancing sleep research would be the primary concern for Dement, and the goal of creating a clinical field of sleep medicine remained primarily with Guilleminault. Nevertheless, these two goals were complementary to ultimately create a specialty of sleep medicine, establish a sleep center at the National Institutes of Health (NIH), and have a medical board recognized by Educational Council for General Medical Education (ECGME). Before any of these achievements, it became quickly apparent that the APSS was not the avenue to create such a clinical field. In fact, many participants were outright opposed to it. The senior members of the APSS were already appointed to faculty positions within well-established departments, and there was no reason to disrupt this well-organized order with a well-established line of advancement and research support. The only individuals who could be interested were young individuals who were not established and thus had nothing to lose, or good friends who wanted to change careers and aim for something different.

In order to secure fee for service, the field needed a well-defined test. Guilleminault proposed to perform nocturnal sleep recording and 24-h sleep recording for individuals with excessive daytime sleepiness. There was the need for a name and Jerome Holland, a retired psychiatrist tapped by Dement to help with administrative issues (particularly with California insurance companies), came up with one. He coined the name "polysomnogram" in 1974. Shortly thereafter at a meeting, Jouvet jokingly indicated that this new field of sleep medicine started with the demonstration of illiteracy, as it should have been either "polyhypnogram" or "multisomnogram." Nevertheless, the name stuck, and it was subsequently recognized and placed in insurance books and thus was not changed in the future.

The resistance to establishing sleep medicine as a field within the APSS body extended to rebutting the suggestion of creating a journal supporting the field. Michael Chase, representing the majority opinion, responded that there was no need for a new journal, as all the good articles were published in neuroscience or physiological journals. Such a move would be detrimental to the recognition of the field of sleep research in neuroscience and in funding research grants. There were many further discussions between Dement and Guilleminault, the latter indicating that there would be no long-term future for sleep research in the medical field if there was not a strong medical service and patient care unit behind it. Things seemed to be at an impasse. Regardless, the Stanford sleep clinic was slowly growing. There was also a unit led by Antony Kales at UCLA. In addition, Ismet Karacan was doing a patient-related service using nocturnal sleep recording to differentiate organic from psychogenic impotence, and this was paid by insurance companies in Texas.

Around this time, Eliott Weitzman, a good friend of Dement, was found to have a hematological cancer and the number one treatment place in the USA for this malady was Stanford. He came on sabbatical to the hospital and became interested in the sleep service. Weitzman also worked with a Stanford medical student Charles Czeisler, who was very much interested in the integration of sleep and circadian rhythms. Further, Weitzman decided to leave Montefiore Hospital and join Cornell University where very large, new sleep research facilities were built. Volunteers could live in isolation from day–night cues and the interaction between circadian rhythms and sleep–wake cycles in normal and pathological conditions could be investigated. Concurrently, there was the beginning of a feud between Dement and Kales about short- and long-acting benzodiazepine hypnotics and support from the pharmaceutical industry. This feud was never resolved and lasted a long time. Ultimately, Kales moved from UCLA to Hershey, Pennsylvania and with his students created a separate society related to sleep and its disorders that ended with his retirement.

The only way to advance the medical arm of sleep research was to create an association of individuals interested in the clinical aspect of sleep. There were many people who would clearly participate, including Howard Roffward and

Eliott Weitzman, Ismet Karacan, Peter Hauri (at Dartmouth who was interested in insomnia), Milton Kramer and a young PhD, Thomas Roth, working in his department. All told, there were about five or six centers that would join, enough to create an official association. There was also a need to cultivate support outside of research, including political influence in the evolving health care system. The efforts at Stanford could raise the standards of clinical service and develop research clinical protocols, but there was also the need to face insurance companies and to gain support from many quarters, including the Congress people in Washington, DC. This latter role was nearly exclusively fulfilled by William Dement. Young medical graduates and specialists were the most enthusiastic about the potential opening of a new clinical field. One of these recruits was Helmut Schmidt, who was trying to set up a sleep disorders unit in the department of psychiatry at Ohio State University. As most sleep disorders at this time included insomnia which was addressed by psychiatrists, David Kupfer was also a choice recruit for the field. As these clinicians sought inclusion in the APSS, there was resistance by members within the USA who were basic science researchers.

In 1975, there were frequent meetings at Stanford and Dement was going regularly to the East Coast. Overall, numbers were still low, but there were more and more places where clinical sleep disorder patients were being seen. It became evident that it would be possible to join these efforts to raise funds and advance the clinical field. There were also discussions on the recruitment of more members. One individual, Roger Broughton, who had trained with Henri Gastaut, became involved. Coming from the Canadian health system, he did not see the problems in the same way. In fact, the only questions and opposition to diverse proposals seemingly came from him. But he also supported the creation of a broader society. Finally, in the winter of 1975 in Chicago, the decision to create a new society called the Association of Sleep Disorder Centers (ASDC) was voted upon. Once passed, there was the need to write bylaws and formalize the society. Initially, there were only five centers that could pay dues, but this was the beginning of clinical sleep medicine.

Early in 1976, the society began to function with William Dement as president, Eliott Weitzman as vice president, Merrill Mitler as secretary (a crucial role as raising funds was a key issue), and two members at large, Peter Hauri and David Kupfer. One of the urgent goals of this society was to gain recognition of sleep specialists who could be reimbursed by insurance companies under a fee-for-service arrangement. Discussions indicated that there was great concern within the business community that anybody could bill for a "sleep work-up." One of the first decisions of this new society was to form an education committee in charge of developing a recognized body of knowledge. This would be outlined in a formal textbook and would include the procedures to be performed by the specialist. In addition, a method was created for practitioners to demonstrate competency. Guilleminault was selected as head of this committee and within a year there was a subcommittee in charge of examination headed by Helmut Schmidt.

There was a need to employ an examination for certification quickly. Materials were gathered, including tests and recordings previously prepared by Mary Carskadon to test graduate students who had training with her to help in a very large project at Stanford, called sleep camp. In addition, recordings performed at Stanford and Cincinnati, Ohio, were used by Thomas Roth to prepare the first examination. This was administered at Stanford by Thomas Roth, Helmut Schmidt, and Christian Guilleminault. Ultimately, the task of developing a professional examination was given to Helmut Schmidt. He engaged the help of developers involved in the board examination for neurology and psychiatry located at Ohio State University. As a result, for the next 12 years the examination would be administered in Columbus, Ohio.

With a long-standing history, sleep medicine also continued its development in Japan. Early contributors included Dr. Kazoo Azumi, who had spent months at Stanford University in late 1960. Dr. Y. Hishikawa was a neurologist from Osaka University and in the late 1960s he traveled via the trans-Siberian train for days to go to Europe and visit Henri Gastaut and Elio Lugaresi who represented clinical neurology and sleep research, particularly related to sleep and epilepsy. In the early 1970s, he studied overweight, Pickwickian-type patients, and reported on the abnormal breathing observed during sleep. He was one of the participants at the Bologna Symposium organized by Elio Lugaresi on hypersomnia in Pickwickian syndrome. Basic researchers in Japan were very much influenced by Michel Jouvet, and many of them went to spend time in his research laboratory. There was not a formal society dedicated to sleep, however, with most individuals belonging to neurophysiological and neurologic societies that had sleep sections. Nevertheless, sleep research was much developed in Japan, and Japanese researchers had gone to the APSS meetings from the very beginning. Armed with a strong interest in fundamental and clinical sleep research combined with contacts in major research centers in Europe and USA, Japan became the place where major advancements occurred. The association between human leukocyte antigen (HLA)-DR2 and narcolepsy–cataplexy was first described by Juji and Honda. What later became known as REM behavior disorder (RBD), was first described by Tachibana et al. and Hishikawa et al. as "stage 1 REM" and "dissociation of REM sleep." In the context of this rich environment, a formal Japanese sleep society was created.

With a typical Japanese twist, the officers of the society were very senior individuals, reflecting the respect of elders integral to the more formal Japanese society. William Dement sought assistance, including financial support, from the

Japanese laboratories and clinical sleep researchers for the new clinical sleep society. He contacted Dr. Azumi to see what the potential involvement of the Japanese specialists could be. The Japanese were surprised by the inquiry, but the individuals involved in the new ASDC were very well known by their Japanese counterparts, and nobody wanted to abruptly reject the offer. The Japanese scientists responded by asking for a visit to Japan by a member of the group. Dement, who traveled extensively within the USA, was uncomfortable traveling abroad and ruled out going to Japan. He suggested that Guilleminault go in his place as an envoy. Considering the age differences and the structure of the Japanese society at that time, this was probably a poor choice. Nevertheless, the Japanese scientists accepted the envoy.

Guilleminault planned to go before the Christmas season in 1975. He intended to meet with the scientists and spend the official Christmas vacation visiting Japan in winter. However, the Japanese scientists were faced with a difficult decision. They wanted to have the presence and involvement of all the senior members working in sleep, independent of their primary specialty. Upon arriving, the envoy was informed that a response to the proposal would not be given as planned. Instead, it would have to wait until after the ceremonies associated with the first of the year in Japan. A formal meeting was organized on January 5. There were about 50 individuals invited to a formal dinner. The response was that the Japanese sleep researchers would not support the new society, but that they would like to organize the 3rd International APSS Meeting or an equivalent international meeting to present Japanese sleep research to the world. This congress would prove to be the last international meeting of the APSS. It was held in Tokyo in July 1979. Yashuo Shimazono was president, Teruo Okuma served as secretary, and Kazoo Azumi was in charge of local accommodations. The Japanese Sleep Society further grew and led to the creation of the regional sleep society called the Asian Sleep Society, keeping for years the presidency of the regional sleep society and supporting it financially.

Although the APSS had been very indifferent to the efforts toward a clinical field, having voted down the idea of having a journal representing the field with clinical articles in 1974, things began to change. Between this vote and the second international meeting of the APSS held in Edinburgh, Scotland, in 1976 with Ian Oswald as the local host, new developments happened in Europe.

A group led by German-Swiss researchers organized a mostly European congress on the "Nature of Sleep" in Wurzburg, Germany in September 1971. Dr. Uros J. Jovanovic was the local host and Professor Werner Koella, who had left his US university position to go back to Switzerland and work in part for Ciba-Geigy and the University of Basel (Switzerland), was the central figure. The majority of the participants were German, but clinical groups not belonging to the APSS, for example, the Italian and French constituen-

cies of the European clinical neurophysiology society were also present, and they were very much involved in the clinical syndromes associated with sleep. Science was presented, but there were also political decisions made, including a large push to organize a European society. This initiative was particularly emphasized by the German group led by Koella and Jovanovic. The society was not created at the meeting, but seeds were planted, including establishing a more clinically oriented focus compared to the APSS. And, within a brief period, a European Sleep Research Society (ESRS) was eventually formed from this initial effort.

These movements in Europe had some consequences, including the creation of a new sleep journal. The Germano-Swiss group that had grants from the pharmaceutical companies decided to create a journal representing the field of sleep called *Sleep and Wakefulness* with Dr. Uros J. Jovanovic from Wurzburg, Germany as editor-in-chief. The first issue was published in 1976 before the international meeting in Scotland. There was a strong opposition to this journal as it was created without any input from the APSS and it had received clear support from the pharmaceutical industry. At the next meeting, this new development was hotly discussed, and the APSS voted to reverse its prior position to support a journal. The membership was not really convinced, refusing to support the journal by having their dues in any way used for it or to publish an abstract of the yearly meeting as there was a prior agreement with Michael Chase and Brain Information Service to do so. Moreover, nobody wanted to be in charge of this new journal.

In this context, there was a reunion of the APSS board members and the executive committee at the international meeting. Some expressed the view that the Europeans were responsible for the existence of the other journal and they should take charge now. Ian Oswald was selected by consensus as the best candidate for the position of editor-in-chief and he absolutely refused. Dement asked Guilleminault, "Would you take the job?" Guilleminault believed that a clinical field needed a journal where advances could be presented. He also believed that it could be used to show outside individuals and organizations that there was a body of knowledge that directly supported the field. He agreed to take the job.

There was then a closed-door meeting of the senior members of the APSS. About one hour later, while Guilleminault was drinking beer in the hotel bar, a small delegation of the APSS council, including Laverne Johnson and Dement, arrived. They conveyed his selection as editor-in-chief of the new journal. The financial issues related to the journal would be handled by Dement. Unfortunately, there was no budget to support the journal and no financial commitment from the society, just the right to indicate "sponsored by the APSS." Soon thereafter there was also an agreement to have the sponsorship of the ASDC, with the same conditions as the APSS. Any formal plan had to be approved by the executive committees of the two societies before going ahead.

Between this nomination and the publication of the first issue, there was a full year of setbacks and continuous efforts. No publishing company wanted to publish a journal that they did not own or where the associated societies did not give some financial support from annual dues or request member subscription, even with reduced fees. Negotiation with all major publishers ended negatively. Elliott Weitzman knew a recently created and aggressive publishing company named Raven Press. The publisher was willing to take the risk and leave ownership to the society, but had a specific request: The journal would be quarterly initially and the first issue would be published only when the content of the first four issues had been received by the publisher. The articles must have been reviewed not only for content but also for grammar by the editorial office, and galley proofing would be done by the editor's office only after receiving back galley proofs from the authors. This required an editorial assistant in the editorial office, with no funding from anywhere. Dement, who remained in charge of finance for the journal, and Guilleminault met several times with the publisher. These meetings were always very difficult with great disagreement between the publisher and Dement. The publisher finally agreed to support a portion of the salary of the assistant, but refused to go any further. After a particularly difficult meeting, with refusal by the publisher to pay for an electric typewriter for the editorial assistant, there was a complete severance of communication between the two individuals, and the two persons never met face to face again leaving Guilleminault as the "go-between" on all financial issues.

In spite of this turmoil, the journal came to life with four issues in the hands of the publisher by the fall of 1977. This was due in large part to the help of the managing editor at Raven Press, Ms. Charlotte Fan. She was the wife of a well-known professor of neurology in New York and she understood the potential of the field and the research behind it. She gave a very helpful and diplomatic hand to the journal with the additional editorial assistance of Ms. Mary Smith who spent many unpaid hours to "translate" into English many valid submissions from foreign researchers. The creation of the journal and the adherence to scientific excellence helped to reinforce the goals of the ASDC. Progressively, members of the APSS gave more attention to this instrument of the field, despite the fact that for many years there remained no official support. In fact, for two years the legal ownership was in the hands of Guilleminault and Dement as "sponsorship" was not even legally approved. With the election of Pierre Passouant as the second president of the European society and Michel Billiard as secretary of the ESRS, the ESRS became one of the three societies sponsoring the journal *Sleep.* This persisted until the creation of the *Journal of Sleep Research,* the official journal of the ESRS, with the first publication in March 1992 with Dr. J. A. Horne as first editor.

The development of the APSS and ASDC and the continued expansion of the field led to the founding of the Southern Sleep Society in 1978. Ed Lucas and Helio Lemmi served as the first officials. Ed Lucas had spent a sabbatical time at Stanford and Helio Lemmi was one of the early members of the ASDC with a sleep disorders center in Memphis, TN. Many of these individuals, while originally from abroad and working in the USA, served as beacons for the development of sleep medicine throughout the world. Dr. Lemmi remembering his origins, often received fellows from Brazil who would spend a year in his center learning about sleep medicine. Similarly, Dr. Ismet Karacan always had numerous Turkish physicians involved in sleep research. His legacy included the founding and development of the first Turkish sleep society, originating from the sleep laboratory created by his students in the Neurological University Department in Istanbul and Dr. Sergio Tufik after his time in Memphis with Dr. Lemmi was quite prolific and he went on to create the department of psychobiology of the Federal University of Sao Paulo, the Sleep Institute (Instituto de Sono) in Sao Paulo, the regional Latin America Sleep Society, and the Brazilian Sleep Society, where he was reelected president for many years.

After his own reelection several times over as president of the ASDC, William Dement saw materialization of his efforts to create a sleep center at the NIH signed into law by President Bill Clinton in 1993. By this time, the two major branches of sleep medicine had moved much closer together and there was a need to unify the efforts. The Association for the Psychophysiology Study of Sleep, representing a large number of fundamental researchers, became the Sleep Research Society. The ASDC became first the American Association of Sleep Medicine and, a short time later, the American Academy of Sleep Medicine.

During this time, national sleep societies burgeoned all over the world. An important one was the Australian sleep society, championed by a charismatic individual who died too soon to see the success of his efforts, Dr. David J. C. Read. He made Australians realize that there was a field in which they could play a major role. His interest was not met without its own resistance.

In 1977, Guilleminault and Dement wanted to organize a meeting on the sleep apnea syndromes. Guilleminault wanted to differentiate these from the Pickwickian syndrome and the obstructive sleep apnea (OSA) associated with this obesity-related syndrome, well reported previously at the 1972 congress in Rimini, Italy. The Krock Foundation, after hesitation and one rejection, agreed to sponsor a "small meeting" with a limited number of participants at its facilities in the Santa Ynez Mountains of California in July 1977. Dr. David Henderson-Smart, involved in pediatric research, was the individual selected to attend from the department of physiology in Sydney. From the same department, and with a great interest in the subject, Dr. Read asked if he could come at his own expense to participate in the meeting. The administrative arm of the foundation initially refused, but under pressure from the organizers finally accepted. Unfriendly provisions were made; however, including the request that Dr. Read come only at the time of the presentations and then promptly leave the premises to go to a motel, miles away and not involving the foundation in any way. Dr. Read agreed to these negative conditions and came on the morning of the first day. However, after the head of the foundation Dr. Robert L. Krock and his head administrator Dr. Peter Amacher met him, they were immediately impressed by his brightness and social skills. By the end of the first day, he had received a personal invitation from Dr. Krock to stay and had the most luxurious room of all the participants. By the end of the conference, when the official photo was taken, in the front row sat Amacher, Krock, and Read indicating the social skills of Dr. Read.

Dr. Read strongly believed that the field was ripe for important advances and he wanted Australia to be very much involved. He had many substantive conversations during the 1977 conference and asked to host the next meeting in Sydney. This assured that Australian sleep researchers would be centrally involved in the organization of the conference. He had sent young researchers, including Drs. Colin Sullivan and Berthon-Jones, to work in Toronto with Professor Eliot A. Phillipson in sleep. He assured leaders in the field that there were many other individuals interested in the field. As a result, in 1980, Dr. Read welcomed researchers from all over the world to Sydney in a brilliant reunion that strongly established the interests of Australia in sleep research. Unfortunately, he died of a rare, untreatable cancer shortly thereafter, but he had started a movement that led to the establishment of a strong society. His superlative social skills were greatly missed in time to come as dissention grew between more senior and very productive researchers.

Another individual responsible for the creation of a strong presence of sleep medicine was Professor Xi Zhen Huang from the department of pulmonary medicine in Peking Union Hospital at Beijing University in China. Dr. Huang came to Stanford's sleep center in 1986 to study sleep medicine and spent both days and nights doing the tasks of physicians and technologists alike. She enchanted the entire clinic with her Chinese cooking and her continual search for novel ideas to bring back to China. In the medical field, exchanges with China were still rare at that time, but Dr. Huang was determined to create a new field. Upon her return to China, she immediately opened a service at her hospital and began training many individuals coming from all over China. She came from a very different province than the capital, and kept her accent when speaking her language, but her enthusiasm was tremendous. Even into her early 80s she was still recently presiding at international meetings bringing sleep researchers to China.

The first society created was the Chinese Sleep Research Society that was established in 1994. But this society's members were doing more fundamental research and the sleep-medicine field was attracting attention from different specialists. Each specialty began pushing the development of the field and created more focused educational programs. One of these very successful and important programs was led by otolaryngologists, most particularly by Professor Denim Han. He was also president of the otolaryngological institute within Tongren Hospital at Capital University in Beijing. These influential individuals were involved in congresses on specialties within sleep medicine, bringing foreign specialists to China and educating young individuals. There was also the creation of clinical sleep societies, including the Sleep Assembly of the Chinese Thoracic Society in 2000 and the Sleep Assembly of the Chinese Neurologic Society in 2010. But realizing the danger of segmenting the field, under the leadership of Dr. Fang Han from Beijing University, the Chinese Sleep Research Society decided to unify all parties. Fundamental and clinical researchers as well as sleep medicine practitioners were brought together under one large roof, with the first newly styled meeting in 2012.

In Europe, several national societies were created early on, largely due to the efforts of one individual in each country. Dr. J. Herman Peters in Germany was one of these individuals. He had done physiological work and public health studies looking at train drivers and their risk of falling asleep during nocturnal duties. He worked in internal medicine and within the subsection of pulmonary medicine. The head of the department of medicine at the University of Marburg was Professor P. von Wichert. He let Dr. Peters develop a research and clinical service oriented toward sleep and pulmonary medicine, with great attention paid to OSA and the associated cardiovascular complications. Given that OSA had first been described in Germany in Pickwickian patients by Jung and Kuhlo, it should not have been unexpected that it attracted the attention of German specialists. Germany also had clinical electrophysiologists that had done sleep research, particularly on narcolepsy. Germany had also had a strong involvement in the creation of the ESRS. Dr. Peters attracted a faithful following of young specialists with interests not only in pulmonology but also in cardiology and surgery. Marburg became the first place where maxillo-mandibular advancement for OSA was performed in Europe as an example. It was also the first place where electrical stimulation of the hypoglossal nerve was done. Individuals including Thomas Podszus, Thomas Penzel, Riccardo Stoohs, and Hartmut Schneider were active in research while completing their specialization in internal medicine by working in the sleep center, headquartered in an old military—style house called "The Barrack." Professor von Wichert was not completely sold on the integration of sleep into his internal medicine department. He came to visit the Stanford Sleep Center and, after his visit, Guilleminault received a Humboldt grant to spend 12 months in Marburg in 1989. Unfortunately, Dr. Peters broke several vertebrae while skiing during the winter, limiting the interaction between these two individuals. However, Dr. Peters always envisioned a strong sleep medicine service and desired to unite the specialists involved into one society. This included not only colleagues in pulmonary medicine but also neuropsychiatry, such as Professor Meier-Ewert, and physiology, such as Professor Marianne E. Schlake. In many ways, Dr. Peters had the same political acumen as William Dement; he understood that support was needed from everywhere, including the state insurance and the federal government. He fought hard to obtain such support. His efforts resulted in a very strong German sleep society. This was the first national society to have a well-read journal, *Somnology*, that became the official journal not only of the German sleep society but also of the Austrian and Swiss sleep societies. Unfortunately, cancer forced Dr. Peters to depart the scene early to fight another battle. Nevertheless, he had created a strong field in his country with a wide-reaching influence. His students including Drs. Riccardo Stoohs, Hartmut Schneider, and Thomas Penzel became internationally well-known sleep medicine specialists working beyond Germany.

Another individual in Europe who was behind the buildup of a national sleep society was Dr. Markku Partinen in Finland. He had trained in part at the Montpellier Medical School in France and had been in the neurology department headed by a well-known French sleep researcher, Professor Pierre Passouant. He also spent over a year at the Stanford Sleep Clinic. After returning to Helsinki, he decided to put sleep medicine on the map of his country. He had Christian Guilleminault visit for some months to provide guidance. He also had the help of Dr. Olli Pollo in Turku, Christian Hublin, and Tina Telakivi in Helsinki. They also had a dedicated group of young specialists interested in the field. One of the first efforts of the Finnish Sleep Society, supported by the Sillampaa foundation, was the organization of a large international symposium on Sleep Disordered Breathing in 1989, showcasing the strength of the Nordic research.

Early in the history of sleep medicine, many societies were created throughout the world under the efforts of only a handful of individuals, some working in isolation and under duress. These efforts persist to this day as sleep medicine gains footing throughout the world. Rene Druker Colin in Mexico had the support of his old colleagues at UCLA in California as well as years of experience organizing national and international meetings and congresses, including the 1975 international congress on the "Neurobiology of Sleep and Memory" in Mexico. This no doubt helped him to create the Mexican Sleep Society. This was not the case for Edgar Osuna, a young neurologist in Bogota, Colombia in the mid-1980s who struggled to convince foreign researchers attending official meetings in Argentina or Chile to take a detour to Bogota to present their latest research results to the few interested members of the sleep section of the Colombian Neurology Association. The same was true, much later in the second millennium, when Dr. Darwin Vizcarra in Lima, Peru had to push hard to bring sleep medicine to his corner of the world.

Far-East Asia was sometimes even more complicated. South Korea at one time had three different sleep societies due to dissention between different types of specialists. As had been seen earlier in history, the more democratic and open society has been the one to grow and survive. Dr. Ning-Hung Chen in Taiwan and Dr. K. Puvanendram in Singapore worked for many years in the field. They were successful in attracting the attention of their colleagues to the world of sleep, leading to the creation of national sleep societies. The work of Dr. J. C. Suri in New Delhi furthered India's sleep society and journal, uniting the efforts with Indian researchers around the world.

The grand history of sleep medicine and its societies unfolded with layered efforts occurring throughout the world. This short history cannot hope to summarize all of these diverse efforts, championed by countless individuals. Hopefully, these gaps will be filled by more in-depth histories written by each individual society as recognition of its founders and contributors.

References

1. Dement, WC, Vaughan C. The promise of sleep Delaporte Press-Random House, New York, NY 1999. pp. 1–521.
2. Chase M, editor. The sleeping brain. BIS/BRI. Los Angeles: University of California; 1972, pp. 1–537.
3. Jovanovic UJ, editor. The nature of sleep. Stuttgart: G. Fisher Verlag; pp. 1–308.
4. Guilleminault C, Dement WC, Passouant P, editors. Narcolepsy, vol. 3, advances in sleep research. New York: Spectrum Publications; 1976. pp. 1–684.
5. Guilleminault C, Dement WC, editors. Sleep apnea syndromes. New York: Alan R. Liss, Inc.; 1978. pp. 1–372.
6. Guilleminault C and Partinen M. Obstructive sleep apnea syndrome: clinical research and treatment. New York: Raven Press; 1990.
7. Sullivan CE, Henderson-Smart DJ, Reid J, editors. The control of breathing during sleep. Sleep 1980;3:221–467.
8. Peters JH, Podszus T, von Wichert P. Sleep related disorders and internal diseases. Berlin: Spinger-Verlag; 1987. pp. 1–393.
9. Drucker-Colin RR, McGaugh JL. Neurobiology of sleep and memory. New York: Academic; 1977. pp. 1–456.

Development of Sleep Medicine in Europe

Michel Billiard

To present a history of sleep medicine in Europe is certainly a great challenge given the number of countries, cultures and political regimes in Europe at the dawn of this new medical era. Moreover there is a great risk in citing the names of historical figures and centres because of inadvertent omission of the names of others for which the author apologizes in advance for any frustration that may be caused. In order to cover the field, this chapter will first consider the European neurophysiological background, and then review the main precursors of sleep medicine and the founding congresses, and finally the first and second periods of sleep medicine centres will be mentioned. In addition a list of the first sleep medicine centres in each single European country is attached. (Table 15.1)

The Neurophysiological Background

Europe is certainly the place where first fundamental neurophysiological studies on sleep were undertaken.

Maria de Manacéine (1843–1903), a physiologist in Saint-Petersburg, carried out in France, in 1894, the first well-documented experiments of prolonged sleep deprivation in puppies, using forced walking and handling. Doing so, she inspired the first sleep deprivation study in human subjects, conducted by Patrick and Gilbert at the Iowa University Psychological Laboratory in USA [1] and the sleep deprivation experiments in dogs by Legendre and Pieron in Paris [2].

Ivan Pavlov (1849–1936), also from Saint-Petersburg, a medical doctor and a physiologist, was not only the inventor of the classical conditioning, a form of learning in which the first conditioned stimulus signals the occurrence of a second

stimulus, the unconditioned stimulus but also was interested in sleep that he defined as "spreading cortical inhibition".

Sigmund Freud (1856–1939) from Vienna, a neurologist and a psychiatrist, developed his psycho-analytic theory of dreaming and attributed three functions to dreams. First, they allow the expression of unconscious wishes. Second, by disguising the wishes and allowing them to be expressed, they provide a safety valve, a means of "discharging" the unconscious and releasing the psychic tension and excitation that result from the unconscious wishes. Third, they serve as a "guardian" for sleep and allow it to continue, the dreamwork transforming the wish so thoroughly, that full arousal and awakening do not occur despite the release of the unconscious excitation [3].

Hans Berger (1873–1941), a neurologist from Jena (Germany), recorded the electrical activity of the brain through the scalp with an original method which he called electroencephalogram [4].

Constantin von Economo (1876–1931) worked in Vienna (Austria). His broad education in physiology, neurology, psychiatry and comparative neuro-anatomy set the ground for outstanding contributions. He was the first to describe encephalitis lethargica in 1917 [5], and then went on to propose his concept of a sleep-regulation centre distinguishing two distinct areas: one rostral, in the diencephalic-mesencephalic region, responsible for sleep and one posterior, in the mesencephalic tegmentum and posterior hypothalamus, responsible for waking [6].

Henri Pieron (1881–1964), a psychologist in Paris (France), studied the effects of sleep deprivation. Together with René Legendre, in the years 1907–1910, they subjected dogs to complete sleep deprivation for several days and then had their serum or cerebrospinal fluid injected to nonsleep-deprived dogs. They observed extremely accentuated sleep phenomena in these dogs, suggesting the existence of a sleep factor that they called "hypnotoxine" [2].

Walter R. Hess (1881–1973), a physiologist in Zurich (Switzerland), received the Nobel Prize for his stimulation

M. Billiard (✉)
Department of Neurology, Gui de Chauliac Hospital
80 Avenue Augustin Fliche, 34295 Montpellier, Cedex 5, France
e-mail :mbilliard@orange.fr

S. Chokroverty, M. Billiard (eds.), *Sleep Medicine,* DOI 10.1007/978-1-4939-2089-1_15,
© Springer Science+Business Media, LLC 2015

Table 15.1 List of the first sleep medicine centres in European countries (up to five per country)

Country	Town	Institution	Chairman or Director	Initial main interest	Approximate date of first clinical polysomnography
Austria	Vienna	Dept. of Psychiatry, Vienna General Hospital	Bernd Saletu	Pharmacopsychiatry	1975
	Vienna	Dept. of Neurology, Vienna General Hospital	Josef Zeitlhofer	Sleep and neurological disorders	1985
	Innsbruck	Dept. of Neurology, Innsbruck University	Gerhard Bauer	Sleep and neurological disorders; Sleep related breathing disorders	1988
	Austrian Society for Sleep Medicine and Sleep Research (ASRA), 1992 Journal: "Somnologie" (Journal of the German Sleep Medicine Society), 2007				
Belgium	Brussels	Dept. Development and Sleep Saint Pierre Hospital	André Kahn	Sudden infant death syndrome; Nutrition and sleep	1978
	Brussels	Dept. Clin Neurophysiol, Cliniques Univ. Saint-Luc	Geneviève Aubert	Sleep related breathing disorders	1979
	Liege	Dept. of Neurology, University Hospital	Georges Frank	Sleep and epilepsy	1979
	Antwerp	Dept. of Psychiatry, University Hospital	Roger Matthys	Insomnia	1979
	Brussels	Dept. of Psychiatry, Erasme Hospital	Julien Mendelwicz	Sleep and psychiatric disorders	1980
	Belgian Association for the Study of Sleep (BASS), 1983 Book: 25 years of Belgian Sleep (2008)				
Bulgaria	Sofia	Dept. of Neurology, Alexandrovska Hospital	Alexander Alexiev	Narcolepsy; Sleep related breathing disorders	1975
	Plovdiv	Dept. of Neurology, Sveti Georgi Hospital	Zacharie Zachariev	Full spectrum of sleep disorders	1984
	Bulgarian Society of Sleep Medicine, 2008				
Croatia	Zagreb	EEG and Clin Psychophysiol, Psychiatric Hospital Vrapce	Vera Dürrigl	Sleep and schizophrenia; Sleep and epilepsy	early 1970s
	Split	Sleep laboratory, University Hospital Split	Zoran Dogas; Goran Racic	Sleep related breathing disorders	2001
	Society for Sleep Medicine of the Croatian Medical Association, 1994				
Czech	Prague	Dept. of Neurology 1st, Faculty of Medicine, Charles University	Bedrich Roth	Hypersomnias of central origin	1965[a]
	Brno	Dept. of Neurology, University Hospital	Miroslav Moran	Sleep and epilepsy; Sleep related breathing disorders	1995
	Prague	Prague Psychiatric Centre	Milos Matousek	Insomnia; Sleep and psychiatric disorders	1998
	Plzen	Dept. of Pulmonology, University Hospital	Jana Vyskocilova	Sleep related breathing disorders	2000
	Czech Sleep Research and Sleep Medicine Society, 2001				
Denmark	Copenhagen	Danish Centre of Sleep Medicine Dept. of Clin Neurophysiol, Glostrup Hospital	Gordon Wildschiödtz	Sleep and mood disorders	1981
	Danish Society for Sleep Medicine, 1996				
Estonia	Tartu	Sleep Disorders Centre, Psychiatry Clinic, Tartu University Hospital	Veiko Vasar; Tuuliki Hion	Full spectrum of sleep disorders	1996
	Tartu	Lung Clinic, Tartu University Hospital	Enn-Jaagup Püttsepp; Erve Sooru	Sleep related breathing disorders	1997
	Estonian Sleep Medicine Association (2005)				

Table 15.1 (continued)

Country	Town	Institution	Chairman or Director	Initial main interest	Approximate date of first clinical polysomnography
Finland	Helsinki	Dept. of Neurology, Meilahti Hospital	Markku Partinen	Hypersomnias Snoring	1978
	Turku	Dept. of Physiology, University of Turku	Jukka Alihanka Joel Hasan	Sleep related breathing disorders Autonomous nervous activity during sleep	1978
	Helsinki	Ullanlinna Sleep Disorders Clinic	Markku Partinen	Narcolepsy Seasonal affective disorders	1986
	Tempere	Dept. of Pulmonary Medicine, Tampere University Hospital	Joel Hasan Jaakko Herrala	Computer aided analysis of sleep Sleep related breathing disorders	1993
	Finnish Sleep Research Society (SUS), 1988 Journal: Sleep News (Uniuutiset), 1999				
France	Montpellier	Dept. Clin Neurophysiol, St Charles Hospital	Pierre Passouant Jean Cadilhac Michel Baldy-Moulinier Marion Delange	Epilepsy Narcolepsy	1960
	Lyon	Sleep Laboratory, Neurology Hospital	Michel Jouvet	Sleep and neurological disorders Narcolepsy and hypersomnia	1962[b]
	Paris	Centre for Neonatal Biological Research, Port-Royal Hospital	Colette Dreyfus-Brisac Nicole Monod	Neonatal medicine (epilepsy, sleep related breathing disorders, sudden infant death syndrome)	1962
	Strasbourg	Dept. Clin Neurophysiol, Hôpitaux Universitaires	Daniel Kurtz	Sleep related breathing disorders	1970
	Paris	Dept. Clin Neurophysiol, Pitié-Salpêtrière Hospital	Jean Scherrer Lucile Garma Françoise Goldenberg	Parasomnias Insomnia	1971
	French Sleep Research and Medicine Society, 1986 Journal: Sleep Medicine, 2004				
Germany	Würzburg	Dept. of Neurology, University Hospital	Uros J. Jovanovic	Sleep and neurologic disorders Sleep and psychiatric disorders Sleep and sexual disturbances	1964
	Munich	Max Plank Institute für Psychiatry	Hartmut Schulz	Sleep structure Sleep and depression Narcolepsy	1972 1976
	Treysa	Neurological Clinic, Hephata	Karl-Heinz Meier-Ewert	Narcolepsy	1978
	Munich	Dept. of Psychiatry, University Hospital	Eckart Rüther	Sleep and psychiatric disorders Insomnia	1979
	Marburg	Dept. of Internal Medicine, Philipps University Hospital	Jörg-Hermann Peter	Sleep related breathing disorders	1981
	German Sleep Society,1992 Journal: Somnologie/Somnology, 1997				

Table 15.1 (continued)

Country	Town	Institution	Chairman or Director	Initial main interest	Approximate date of first clinical polysomnography
Greece	Athens	Dept. of Psychiatry, Eginition Hospital	Constantin Soldatos	Insomnia Sleep and psychiatric disorders	1979
	Thessaloniki	Dept. of Pulmonology, Papanikolaou Hospital	Dimitris Patakas	Sleep related breathing disorders	1983
	Athens	Dept. of Critical Care and Pulmonary Medicine, Evangelismos Hospital	Charalampos Roussos	Sleep related breathing disorders	1990
	Hellenic Sleep Research Society, 1995				
Hungary	Budapest	National Institute of Neurology and Psychiatry	Péter Halasz	Sleep and epilepsy	1991
	Budapest	National Insitute of Neurology and Psychiatry Army Hospital	Péter Köves	Sleep related breathing disorders Movement disorders in sleep	1995
	Budapest	Koranyi National Institute for Tuberculosis and Pulmonology	Nagy György Boszormenyi	Sleep related breathing disorders	1996
	Hungarian Sleep Society, 1997				
Iceland	Reykjavik	Dept. of Respiratory Medicine and Sleep, Landspital Univ. Hospital	Thorarrin Gislasson Helgi Kristbjarnarson	Sleep related breathing disorders	1987
	The Icelandic Sleep Research Society (1991)				
Ireland	Dublin	Sleep Laboratory, St Vincent's Hospital	Walter McNicholas	Sleep related breathing disorders	1984
	Irish Sleep Society, 2004				
Italy	Bologna	Institute of Neurology, University of Bologna	Elio Lugaresi	Sleep related movement disorders Sleep related breathing disorders Parasomnias	1965
	Milan	Dept. of Neurology, Institute San Raffaele	Salvatore Smirne	Insomnia Parasomnias Sleep related breathing disorders	1969
	Pisa	Institute of Neurology, University of Pisa	Alberto Muratorio	Sleep and depression, and neuro-logical diseases	1969
	Parma	Dept. of Neurology, University of Parma	Mario G. Terzano	Sleep and epilepsy	1979
	Udine	Dept. of Neurology, University of Udine	Gian L. Gigli	Sleep and neurological	1981
	Italian Sleep Medicine Society, 1991				
	Journal: AIMS Bulletin, 1995-2007, Somnomed, 2008				
Lithuania	Kaunas	Dept. of Cardiology, University Hospital	Giedrius Varoneckas	Sleep and cardiovascular diseases	1984
	Kaunas	Dept. of Neurology, University Hospital	Vanda Liesiene	Epilepsy	2001
	Kaunas	Dept. of Pulmonology and Immunology, University Hospital	Skaidrius Miliauskas	Sleep related breathing disorders	2003
	Vilnius	Centre of Neurology, Vilnius Univ. Hospital	Raminta Masaitiene	Sleep and neurological disorders	2005
	Lithuanian Sleep Medicine Society, 2000				
Luxembourg	Esch-sur-Alzette	Emile Mayrisch Hospital	Michel Kruger	Full spectrum of sleep disorders	1996
	Luxembourg	Dept. of Neurosciences, Luxembourg Hospital	Nico Diederich	Sleep and neurological disorders	1996
Netherlands	Heeze	Centre for Sleep-Wake Disorders Kempenhaeghe	Guus Declerck	Insomnia & Narcolepsy Sleep related breathing disorders	1994
	The Hague	Dept. of Neurology and Clin Neurophysiol, Westeinde Hospital	Hilbert Kamphuisen	Full spectrum of sleep disorders	1995

Table 15.1 (continued)

Country	Town	Institution	Chairman or Director	Initial main interest	Approximate date of first clinical polysomnography
	Leiden	Dept. of Neurology and Clin Neurophysiol, Leiden Univ. Medical Center	Gert Jan Lammers, Gert Jan Dijk	Narcolepsy and related disorders	1995
	Dutch Society for Sleep-Wake Research (NSWO), 1990				
	Journal: Sleep-Wake Research in the Netherlands, 1990 (one issue per year)				
Norway	Bergen	Bergen Sleep Disorders Centre (private)	Several doctors	Full spectrum of sleep disorders	1998
	Bergen	Norwegian Competence Centre for Sleep Disorders, University of Bergen	Bjorn Bjorvatn	Full spectrum of sleep disorders	2004
	Norwegian Society for Sleep Research and Sleep Medicine (2007)				
	Journal: SOVN, 2009 (two issues per year)				
Poland	Warsaw	Dept. of Psychiatry, Medical University	Andrzej. Jus, Karolina Jus	Sleep and mental disorders / Evaluation of psychotropic drugs	1966
	Torun and Bydgoszcz	Dept. of Pediatric Neurology	Juliusz Narebski	Sleep in children	1972
	Warsaw	Institute of Psychiatry and Neurology	Halina Ekiert	Sleep and mood disorders	1978
	Gdansk	Dept. of Psychiatry and Neurology	Zbigniew Nowicki	Sleep and mood disorders	1983
	Polish Society of Sleep Research, 1991				
	Journal: Sen, 2001				
Portugal	Lisbon	EEG and Sleep Dept., Centro Estudos Egas Moniz, Hospital Santa Maria	Teresa Paiva	Sleep and psychiatry / Biomedical methodologies for sleep	1983
	Oporto	Dept. Clin Neurophysiol, Hospital Santo Antonio	Antonio Martins da Silva	Sleep and epilepsy	1983
	Coimbra	Sleep laboratory, Centro Hospit de Coimbra	José Moutinho dos Santos	Sleep related breathing disorders	1991
	Portuguese Sleep Association, 1991				
Romania	Tirgu-Mures	Department of Neurology, Tirgu-Mures Hospital	Liviu Popoviciu	Hypersomnias of central origin	1971
	Bucharest	Romanian Institute of Pneumology	Florin Mihaltan	Sleep related breathing disorders	1994
	Timisoara	Victor Babes University of Medicine and Pharmacy, Victor Babes Hospital	Stefan Mihaicuta	Sleep and cardiovascular disorders	2005
	Romanian Sleep Society, 2006				
Russian Federation[c]	Moscow	Sechenov 1st Moscow Medical Institute, Dept. of Neurology, Faculty of Advanced Postgraduate training	Alexander M. Vein, Valeriy L. Golubev	Sleep and neurological disorders / Hypersomnias	1992[d]
		Dept. of the Pathology of Autonomic Nervous System	Gennadiy V. Kovrov	Sleep and stress / Insomnia	1994
	Moscow	Centre of Sleep Medicine	Mikhail G Poluektov	Full spectrum of sleep disorders	1994
	Moscow	Clin Sanatorium "Barvikha" Sleep Medicine Division	Roman V. Buzunov	Sleep related breathing disorders	1995
	Moscow	Federal Medical-Biological Centre of Sleep Medicine	Alexander L. Kalinkin	Sleep related breathing disorders	1998
	Russian Sommological Society (section of the Pavlovian Physiological Society of the Russian Academy of Sciences), 2007				
	National Society for Sommology and Sleep Medicine, 2010				
Serbia	Belgrade	Dept. of Epilepsy and Clin Neurophysiol, Institute of Mental Health	Zarko Martinovic	Dreams in chronic alcoholism / Epilepsy	1978
	Serbian Sleep Society, 2011				
Slovakia	Kosice	Dept. of Pathophysiology, University of Kosice	Zoltan Tomori	Sleep related breathing disorders	1996

Table 15.1 (continued)

Country	Town	Institution	Chairman or Director	Initial main interest	Approximate date of first clinical polysomnography
Slovenia	Ljubljana	Institute Clin Neurophysiol, University Medical Centre	Leja Dolenc-Groselj	Full spectrum of sleep disorders	1994
	Golnik	University Clinic of Respiratory and Allergic Diseases	Matjaz Flezar	Sleep related breathing disorders	1994
	Slovene Sleep Society, 2005				
Spain	Madrid	Dept. Clin Neurophysiol, University Hospital San Carlos	Rosa Peraita-Adrados Antonio Vela-Bueno	Sleep and epilepsy Full spectrum of sleep disorders Pharmacology	1971
	Barcelona	Dept. Clin Neurophysiol, Hospital Vall d'Hebron	Teresa Sagales Dolores de la Calzada	Sleep related breathing disorders Sleep and neurological disorders	1972
	Valencia	Dept. Clin Neurophysiol, University Hospital La Fe	Antonio Beneto	Sleep and neurological disorders	1972
	Zaragoza	Dept. Clin Neurophysiol, University Hospital Miguel Servet	José M. Vergara	Pediatric sleep disorders	1980
	Santander	Dept. Clin Neurophysiol, University Hospital Marqués de Valdecilla	Rosario Carpizo	Sleep and neurological disorders	1980
	Iberian Association of Sleep Pathology (AIPS) now Spanish Sleep Society, 1991 Journal : Vigilia-Sueno, 1992				
Sweden	Uppsala	Dept. of Psychiatry, Uppsala University Hospital	Björn-Erik Roos Jerker Hetta	Sleep and psychiatry Pharmacotherapy	1985
	Gothenburg	Dept. Clin Neurophysiol, Sahlgren's Univ. Hospital	Gaby Bader	Hypersomnias Insomnia	early 1980s
	Gothenburg	Centre for Sleep and Wake Disorders, Remströmska Hospital	Jan Hedner	Sleep related breathing disorders	1990s
	Lund	Dept. Clinical Neurophysiol, Lund University Hospital	Sören Berg	Sleep related breathing disorders	1990s
	Swedish Society for Sleep Research and Sleep Medicine, 1989				
Switzerland	Zurich	EEG Laboratory, Neurological Univ. Dept.	Rudolph Max Hess	Sleep and neurological disorders	1960
	Geneva	EEG laboratory, University Hospital, Chêne-Bourg	Jean-Michel Gaillard	Insomnia Pharmacology of sleep Quantitative analysis of sleep	1969
	Berne	EEG Laboratory, Neurogical Univ. Dept., Inselspital	Christian W. Hess	Narcolepsy Sleep related breathing disorders	1982
	Swiss Society for Sleep Research, Sleep Medicine and Chronobiology, 1991				
Turkey	Istanbul	Dept. of Neurology, Cerrahpasa Faculty of Medicine	Erbil Gözükirmizi Hakan Kaynak	Full spectrum of sleep disorders	1985
	Ankara	Dept. of Psychiatry, Gulhane Military Med Acad	Hamdullah Aydin	Full spectrum of sleep disorders	1987
	Ankara	Yildrim Beyazit Training and Research Hospital	Sadik Ardic	Sleep related breathing disorders	1994
	Turkish Sleep Medicine Society, 1992 Journal: Journal of Turkish Sleep Medicine, 2009				

Table 15.1 (continued)

Country	Town	Institution	Chairman or Director	Initial main interest	Approximate date of first clinical polysomnography[e]
United Kingdom	Edinburgh	Dept. Psychol Medicine, Royal Edinburgh Hospital	Ian Oswald	Insomnia Pharmacology of sleep	1959[e]
	London	Academic Department of Psychiatry, Middlesex Hospital	Arthur Crisp Georg Fenton Peter Fenwick	Sleep and mental disorders	1972
	Edinburgh	Department of Medicine, Royal infirmary	Neil Douglas	Sleep related breathing disorders	1979
	Oxford	Chest Clinic, Churchill Hospital	John Stradling	Sleep related breathing disorders	1979*
	Leicester	Sleep Disorders Service, Leicester General Hospital	Christopher Hanning	Sleep related breathing disorders	1986
	British Sleep Society, 1989				

This list has been established thanks to the help of senior sleep disorder specialists in each European country. The names of institutions and chairmen or directors are those of the centres at the origin. The date of first polysomnography is approximate and it does not necessarily match with the date of opening of the sleep medicine centre

[a] Bedrich Roth was interested in patients with hypersomnias of central origin as soon as 1949, performed his first all night EEG recordings in 1951, but due to political situation could not perform polysomnography before 1965

[b] Michel Jouvet's main activity was animal research but he run in parallel a human sleep medicine centre

[c] Russian Federation is a very large country. Only the first sleep medicine centers located in Moscow are presented here

[d] Alexander Vein performed his first polysomnography in 1968, but the sleep medicine centre was opened later in 1992

[e] The main activity of the centre was research, but Ian Oswald would see now and again patients with sleep disorders

studies in freely moving cats with electrodes located at precisely defined anatomical sites in the brain. By stimulating a relatively widespread region extending from the medial thalamus towards the caudate nucleus, at a low frequency of 4–12 c/sec and with stimuli of long duration, typically 12.5–25 ms, with ramp-like, attenuated upward and downward slopes and trains of stimulation lasting from 30 s to 1 min, he obtained what appeared to be physiological sleep [7]. The cat first looked for a suitable sleeping place, then curled up comfortably before falling asleep. Moreover, the cat, like in physiological sleep, could be re-awakened at any time. All these findings were in favour of sleep as an active process.

Frederic Bremer (1897–1982), a brilliant neurologist in Brussels (Belgium), performed his famous "cerveau isolé" and "encéphale isolé" preparations in the cat. In the first experiment the cat was in a state of deep sleep with a regular rhythm of highly synchronous 6–10 Hz waves. Bremer attributed this finding to the deafferentation of the telencephalon, which deprived the brain from the flow of sensory impulses [8]. In the second experiment, the transection of the brainstem above its junction with the spinal cord left intact a majority of sensory pathways, and a normal alternation between sleep and wakefulness was maintained. Bremer interpreted these results, as an evidence that sleep in mammals results from a decrease in cortical tone which is maintained by the flux of sensory information to the brain, a view in favour of sleep as a passive phenomenon [9].

Thereafter, Giuseppe Moruzzi (1910–1986), a neurophysiologist in Pisa (Italy), worked with Horace Magoun (1907–1991) in Chicago. Together they discovered "the presence in the brainstem of a system of ascending reticular relay, whose direct stimulation activates or desynchronizes the EEG", which they called the activating reticular system [10]. This discovery paved the way for a greater understanding of sleep-wakefulness mechanisms.

Michel Jouvet (1925-), the last but not the least on the list, a neurophysiologist in Lyon (France), is famous for having implanted electrodes in or very near the oculomotor nuclei (VI) in the pons, and in the neck of pontine cats, and having observed every 30–40 min a periodic appearance of "spindle-like" activity in the pons, coincident with the total disappearance of the EMG of the neck. These curious episodes lasted about 6 min and occurred periodically every 50 min [11]. Then, performing similar polygraphic recordings in intact cats, he observed a cortical activity similar to that seen during waking, associated with a much increased threshold for arousal. This was a paradoxical finding. Thus, he could state that Dement's rapid eye movement (REM) sleep was a sleep state different from wakefulness and non-REM (NREM) sleep, a kind of rhombencephalic state opposite to the NREM telencephalic type of sleep.

The European Precursors of Sleep Medicine

Rudolph Max Hess (1913–2007), the son of Nobel Laureate Walter R. Hess, studied medicine in Lausanne and Zurich (Switzerland) and in Kiel (Germany), before specializing at the Kantonsspital in Zurich (Switzerland). He then visited the National Hospital for Nervous Diseases, Queen Square in London. In 1948 he was back in Zurich, successively in the EEG, Neurosurgery and Neurology departments. He spent half-a-year in the USA and Canada in 1953–1954. Rudolf Max Hess then came back to Zurich and started to perform clinical polysomnography in 1960.

Pierre Passouant (1913–1983) got his MD in Montpellier (France) in 1943 and created one of the first EEG laboratories in France, at the Saint Charles Hospital in 1947. Beginning in 1953, he assembled a highly talented research group in neurophysiology who worked on the rhinencephalon and the hippocampus, and later on the cerebrum and the bulbar olive. In parallel he was interested in epilepsy. In 1960 he performed polysomnographic studies in epileptic and later in narcoleptic patients. In 1971 he moved to the Gui de Chauliac Hospital and established a fully equipped sleep laboratory starting with two bedrooms. Among his main interests were the effects of sleep on epilepsy and the effects of epilepsy on sleep, the ultradian rhythm of sleep attacks in narcoleptics and the suppression of REM sleep by clomipramine.

Andrzej (1914–1992) and Karolina (1914–2002) Jus are the two researchers who first performed polysomnography in Poland. Andrzej received his MD at the University of Jan Kazimierz in Lwow (Ukraine) in 1939 and Karolina her MD at the University of Wroclaw (Poland) in 1946. They had a very tragic story during Second World War: all the members of Karolina's family were killed in the Holocaust. Andrzej and Karolina married in 1941. In 1947 they participated in a post-doc fellowship at the University Paris Sorbonne. Andrzej worked successively in Wroclaw, Pruszkow and eventually in the Department of Psychiatry at the Medical University of Warsaw in 1950. There, together with his wife, he organized a clinical and scientific laboratory of EEG and sleep research. The first polysomnography was performed in 1966, and the next year they began publishing papers on polysomnography in the international literature [12, 13]. Their main interest was sleep in mental disorders and the influence of psychotropic medications on sleep. In 1970, Andrzej and his wife moved to Canada.

Henri Gastaut (1915–1995) graduated at Marseille University (France) in 1945. He was the scientific director and chief doctor of the Centre Saint-Paul for epileptic children from 1957 to 1968. He devoted his brilliant career in epilepsy with a number of studies on sleep and epilepsy. In 1965, after Richard Jung and Wolfgang Kuhlo in Freiburg (Germany) had published a case report of sleep disordered breathing in a patient with the Pickwickian syndrome [14], technical improvements allowed Gastaut et al. to refine the evaluation performed by the German authors and to clearly identify three different abnormal breathing patterns during sleep in Pickwickian patients, obstructive, mixed and central apneas [15].

Colette Dreyfus-Brisac (1916–2006) graduated in Paris (France) in 1946, after being in the Resistance during the Second World War. She first worked in Fishgolds's EEG laboratory at the Pitié Hospital and in parallel at the Maternity of the Baudeloque Hospital. In 1953, she was joined by Nicole Monod, her closest collaborator during her whole carrier. She headed a team of neurophysiologists working in close contact with neonatologists and paediatric neurologists. She attracted EEG specialists from all over the world. The new Port Royal Hospital was built in the early 1960 and a first paper entitled "Disorders of the organization of sleep in the pathological newborn child" was published by Nicole Monod et al. in 1966 [16].

The very first person interested in sleep medicine in Europe is certainly Bedrich Roth (1919–1989). After a terrible time in Slovakia during Second World War, he fled to Switzerland, studied medicine in Berne from 1943 to 1944, then in Paris from 1945 to 1946, and eventually returned to Prague (Czechoslovakia) where he got his MD in 1947. He specialized in neurology in Hradec Kralové, East of Prague, and came back to the Prague's Neurological Clinic headed by the famous neurologist Kamil Henner in 1949. Not long after his return to Prague he started seeing patients with narcolepsy and hypersomnia. In 1951, he managed to perform his first all night sleep EEG on a Grass machine which was replaced later by a Kaiser EEG machine. Patients were frequently referred to him from Prague and from all over the country. From May 1,1949 to May 1,1955, he saw, in his outpatient clinic, 251 subjects with excessive daytime sleepiness, including 155 with narcolepsy and 96 with hypersomnia [17]. The sleep disorder centre was born. However due to the political situation, the classical polysomnographic recordings did not start before 1965 on a Bioscript apparatus from East Germany.

Uros Jovan Jovanovic was a member of the University Department of Neurology in Würzburg (Germany). He worked in the fields of epilepsy and sleep, psychiatric diseases and sleep and penile erections during sleep. He was famous for organizing an international sleep symposium "the Nature of Sleep", during which a "founding committee" including Drs Baust, Gottesmann, Jovanovic, Koella (Chairman), Oswald and Popoviciu was established, as a preparation for the future first European Congress of Sleep Research which took place one year later in Basel. In addition, he launched the first international journal on sleep, "Waking and Sleeping", in 1976. Unfortunately the journal went out of business in 1980 and a few years later Uros J. Jovanovic quitted the field of sleep.

Elio Lugaresi (1926–) is in every respect a giant in the field of sleep. He graduated from the Bologna University School of Medicine in 1952 and became a post-graduate fellow in the same university. In 1956–1957, he spent one year in the EEG laboratory chaired by Henri Gastaut at the Hospital la Timone in Marseille. Then he returned to Bologna where he set up a research team at the Neurology clinic with the help of Giorgio Coccagna. Elio Lugaresi must be acknowledged for being the first to document the major fluctuations in pulmonary and systemic arterial pressure during obstructive apneas [18], describe restless legs syndrome and periodic leg movements in sleep [19], identify nocturnal paroxysmal dystonia [20] and last but not the least, discover a new prion disease, the "Fatal Familial Insomnia" [21].

Alexander Vein (1928–2003) was the disciple of the distinguished neurologist Nicolay Grashchenkov who died in 1966. He was the founder of sleep medicine and human sleep physiology in Russia. He was interested in insomnia, sleep apneas, movement disorders in sleep, sleep and epilepsy, sleep and stress. His first polysomnographic recordings were performed at the Grashchenkov laboratory in 1968 and he set up the first Russian sleep medicine centre at the Sechenov first Moscow medical Institute in 1992.

Ian Oswald (1929–2012) graduated in both experimental psychology and medicine at Cambridge University and was awarded an MD for research. His first use of EEG was when he did his national service in the Royal Air Force and was involved in checking airmen for possible epileptic propensity. He then, had a fellowship at Oxford University where he did many research studies using EEG equipment. He moved to Edinburgh in 1959 to become a lecturer in Psychological Medicine at Edinburgh University, with clinical duties in the Royal Edinburgh Hospital. He continued his research on sleep using polysomnography and would now and then see patients with sleep disorders.

Key Meetings

A few meetings can be considered as cornerstones in the development of sleep medicine in Europe.

The first one is probably the 1963 meeting of the French Speaking Society of Electroencephalography and Clinical Neurophysiology devoted to night sleep. This meeting was held in Paris under the chairmanship of Henri Fischgold. It gathered speakers from Belgium, France, Germany, Italy and the UK. The primary clinical emphasis in this meeting was the documentation of sleep-related epileptic seizures and a number of related studies on sleep and tumours, sleep-related movement disorders, African sleeping sickness and sleep in patients with mental disorders. This program certainly did not cover all range of sleep disorders, but it served as an incentive to direct the attention to sleep and sleep disorders.

Proceedings of this congress were gathered in a book entitled "Le sommeil de nuit normal et pathologique, Etudes électroencéphalographiques" [22].

The second important meeting is the XVth European meeting on electroencephalography, which was organized in Bologna in 1967 under the chairmanship of Henri Gastaut and Elio Lugaresi. This meeting gathered a large number of speakers and participants. The program covered a more representative range of sleep disorders with sessions on neurophysiological and neurochemical basis of sleep, insomnia, narcolepsy, Pickwickian syndrome and episodic phenomena of sleep. Proceedings of this congress can be found in a book entitled "The abnormalities of sleep in man" [23].

Then came four International congresses within a 16-month period. Ten years after the first meeting of the Association for the Psychophysiological Study of Sleep (APSS), the APSS organized an international congress in Bruges, Belgium (June 19–24, 1971). About three months later another International Symposium, "the Nature of Sleep", was organized by Uros J. Jovanovic in Würzburg (Germany) (September 23–26, 1971) and at the end of this symposium, a preliminary committee headed by Werner P. Koella was formed to organize a European Society of Sleep Research. About eight months later (May 25–27, 1972) a symposium entitled "Hypersomnia with periodic breathing", was organized in Rimini, a small resort on the Adriatic coast". This symposium was organized by Elio Lugaresi and Paul Sadoul, a pulmonologist from Nancy (France). It was mostly devoted to defining the Pickwickian syndrome into different sleep-related breathing disorders. Proceedings were published in 1972, in a special issue of the Bulletin de Physiopathologie Respiratoire (Nancy) under the auspices of the French National Institute of Health and Medical Research [24]. Finally, the first European Congress of Sleep Research was organized by Werner P. Koella in Basel (October 3–6, 1972). It was there that the European Sleep Research Society (ESRS) was founded and it was agreed that the ESRS would organize a scientific Congress every other year. The 40th anniversary of the Society was celebrated during the 21st congress held in Paris in September 2012 and the 22nd Congress of the ESRS was held in Tallin (Estonia) (September 16–20, 2014).

Sleep Medicine Centres

The Beginning of All Night Sleep Recordings (1950–1975)

The use of all night sleep recordings started in the 1960s, mostly in departments of clinical neurophysiology interested in epilepsy and in departments of psychiatry interested in insomnia and the effects of psychotropic drugs on sleep. Apart from insomnia, sleep disorders were neither identified nor recognized by the medical community and recording sleep throughout the night was viewed with scepticism. Medicine occupied itself wholly with diseases and disorders that could be seen and diagnosed in waking patients. Formal outpatient clinics devoted to sleep disorders and sleep medicine centres did not exist, with the notable exception of the Prague sleep medicine centre organized by Bedrich Roth in the early 1950s, which included clinical evaluation and nocturnal EEG recording. At best, patients with sleep disorders could be diagnosed and treated if they were lucky enough to be referred to one of the rare physicians interested in these disorders. Patients benefitted from all night sleep recording on the basis of manifestations occurring during the night, such as epileptic seizures or movement disorders rather than because of insomnia or hypersomnia. There were no established sleep facilities. Patients had their sleep recorded wherever it was possible, often in a nurse's or a physician's office or even in a corridor. There was no technician and patients were hooked up and observed by the doctors themselves at night. To be a sleep doctor was a real challenge as it did not exempt from daily duties and did not match well with family life. In an article entitled "A personal history of sleep disorders medicine", William Dement writes that, during his residency at the Mount Sinai Hospital in New York in 1958–1959, "I worked nearly every night at the Hospital. This finally became intolerable to my wife. However, because federal funds were so loosely administered at that time, I was able to obtain a grant that paid the rent on a large apartment, half of which I converted into my family's living quarters and half into a comfortable two-bedroom sleep laboratory" [25]. At the beginning, only sleep EEG was recorded, and only later EOG and EMG were added. EEG machines consisted of Artex and Alvar in France, Marconi and Ediswan in England, Toenniies and Schwarzer in Germany, and van Gogh in the Netherlands [26]. There were technical problems with fixation of electrodes on the patients' scalp, with electric wires, ink pens, ink pots and blocks of papers. The quality of the tracings often failed to meet expectations. Analysis of tracings still rested on EEG criteria suggested by Loomis et al. [27]. It took time for the definition of sleep stages as proposed by Dement and Kleitman in 1957 [28] and later elaborated by Rechtschaffen and Kales in the "Manual of standardized terminology, techniques and scoring system for sleep stages of human subjects" in 1968 [29], to be introduced in Europe and accepted by EEG specialists. All these limitations explain the time it took to implement real sleep medicine centres.

The Development of Sleep Medicine Centres (1975–2000)

Several factors played in favour of establishing sleep medicine centres.

First of all, the identification of the sleep apnoea syndrome by Christian Guilleminault in 1976 [30], the progressive perception of its high prevalence in the general population and of its health consequences on the short and long terms, and the introduction of continuous positive airway pressure (CPAP) as an effective treatment of this syndrome in 1981 [31]. Second, the publication of the "Diagnostic Classification of Sleep and Arousal Disorders" in 1979, after 3 years of extraordinary efforts by a small group of dedicated individuals who composed the "nosology" committee chaired by Howard Roffwarg [32]. This classification contained four major groupings of sleep disorders, disorders of initiating and maintaining sleep, disorders of excessive somnolence, disorders of the sleep-wake schedule and dysfunctions associated with sleep, sleep stages, or partial arousals. It raised sleep medicine to the rank of other medicine specialties. Third, the publication of epidemiologic surveys showing the high prevalence of different sleep disorders and their cost for the entire society. Fourth, the progressive interest of pulmonologists, neurologists, cardiologists, psychiatrists, paediatricians, ENT surgeons, etc., for the manifestations of their respective diseases during sleep. Fifth, the introduction of new techniques including computerized polysomnography and automatic analysis of sleep.

This is reflected in the rapid development of sleep medicine centres with a primary interest in sleep-related breathing disorders and then of sleep disorders centres interested in the full range of sleep disorders. A good thing or a bad thing? On one hand, sleep disorders medicine was born and accepted, and a crowd of unrecognized patients could now benefit from diagnoses and treatments. On the other hand, untrained and incompetent doctors used automatic analysis of sleep and ended up with incorrect diagnoses and treatments, hence the action plan was initiated by the European Sleep Research Society including the process of accreditation of sleep medicine centers and certification of sleep medicine experts [33–34].

References

1. Patrick GT, Gilbert JA. On the effects of loss of sleep. Psychol Rev. 1896;3:469–83.
2. Legendre R, Piéron H. Des résultats histophysiologiques de l'injection intra-occipito-atlantoïdienne de liquides insomniques. C R Soc Biol. 1910;68:1108–09.
3. Freud S. The interpretation of dreams. New York: Macmillan; 1913.
4. Berger H. Ueber das Elektroencephalogramm des Menschen. J Psychol Neurol. 1930;40:160–79.
5. Von Economo C. Encephalitis lethargica. Wien Klin Wochenschr. 1917;30:581–85.
6. Von Economo C. Sleep as a problem of localization. J Nerv Ment Dis. 1930;71:249–59.
7. Hess WR. Das Schlafsyndrom als Folge dienczephaler Reizung. Helv Physiol Pharmacol Acta. 1944;2:305–44.
8. Bremer F. Cerveau "isolé" et physiologie du sommeil. C R Soc Biol. 1935;118:1235–41.
9. Bremer F. L'activité cérébrale au cours du sommeil et de la narcose. Contribution Ã l'étude du mécanisme du sommeil. Bull Acad R Med Belg. 1937;4:68–86.
10. Moruzzi G, Magoun HW. Brain stem reticular formation and activation of the EEG. Electroencephalogr Clin Neurophysiol. 1949;1:455–73.
11. Jouvet M, Michel F. Corrélations électromyographiques du sommeil chez le chat décortiqué et mésencéphalique chronique. C R Soc Biol. 1959;153:422–25.
12. Jus A, Jus K. Some remarks on the relevance and usefulness of polygraphic sleep studies in psychiatry. Wien Z Nervenheilkd Grenzgeb. 1967;25:250–8.
13. Jus K, Kiljan A, WilczaK H, et al. Polygraphic study of night sleep in schizophrenia before and during treatment with phenothiazine derivatives. Ann Med Psychol (Paris). 1968;126:713–25.
14. Jung R, Kuhlo W. Neurophysiological studies of abnormal night sleep and the Pickwickian syndrome. Prog Brain Res. 1965;18:140–59.
15. Gastaut H, Tassinari CA, Duron B. Etude polygraphique des manifestations épisodiques (hypniques et respiratoires) du syndrome de Pickwick. Rev Neurol (Paris). 1965;112:568–79.
16. Monod N, Dreyfus-Brisac C, Eliet-Flescher J et al. Disorders of the organization of sleep in the pathological newborn child. Rev Neurol (Paris). 1966; 115: 469–72.
17. Roth B. Narcolepsie a Hypersomnie S. Hlediska Fysiologie Spanku. (Narcolepsy and hypersomnia from the aspect of physiology of sleep). Praha: Statni Zdravonické Nakladatelstvi; 1957.
18. Lugaresi E, Cirignotta F, Coccagna G, et al. Some epidemiological data on snoring and cardiocirculatory disturbances. Sleep. 1980;3:221–24.
19. Lugaresi E, Cirignotta F, Coccagna G, et al. Nocturnal myoclonus and restless legs syndrome. Adv Neurol. 1986;43:295–307.
20. Lugaresi E, Cirignotta F. Hypnogenic paroxysmal dystonia: epileptic seizure or a new syndrome? Sleep. 1981;4:129–38.
21. Lugaresi E, Medori R, Montagna P, et al. Fatal familial insomnia and dysautonomia with selective degeneration of thalamic nuclei. N Engl J Med. 1986;315:997–1003.
22. Fischgold H, editor. Le sommeil de nuit normal et pathologique. Paris: Masson & Cie; 1965.
23. Gastaut H, Lugaresi E, Berti-Ceroni C, Coccagna G, editors. The abnormalities of sleep in man. In: Proceedings of the XVth European meeting on electroencephalography. Aulo Gaggi, Bologna, 1968.
24. Gastaut H, Lugaresi E, Berti-Ceroni G, et al., editors. Pathological, clinical and nosographic considerations regarding hypersomnia with periodic breathing. Bull Physiopath Resp. 1972;8:1249–56.
25. Dement WC. A personal history of sleep disorders medicine. J Clin Neurophysiol. 1990;7:17–47.
26. Collura TF. History and evolution of electroencephalographic instruments and techniques. J Clin Neurophysiol. 1993;10:476–504.
27. Loomis AL, Harvey EN, Hobart GA. Cerebral states during sleep, as studied by human brain potentials. J Exp Psychol. 1937;21:127–44.
28. Dement W, Kleitman N. The relation of eye movements during sleep to dream activity: an objective method for the study of dreaming. J Exp Psychol. 1957;53:339–46.
29. Rechtschaffen A, Kales A, editors. A manual of standardized terminology, techniques and scoring system for sleep stages of human subjects. Los Angeles: UCLA Brain Information Service/Brain Research Institute; 1968.
30. Guilleminault C, Tilkian A, Dement WC. The sleep apnea syndromes. Annu Rev Med. 1976;27:465–84.

31. Sullivan CE, Issa FG, Berthon-Jones M, et al. Reversal of obstructive sleep apneas by continuous positive airway pressure applied through the nares. Lancet. 1981;1(8223):862–5.

32. Association of sleep disorders centers. Diagnostic classification of sleep and arousal disorders. First edition, prepared by the Sleep Disorders Classification Committee, HP Roffwarg, Chairman. Sleep. 1979;2:1–137.

33. Pevernagie D, Stanley N, Berg S, et al. European guidelines for the accreditation of Sleep Medicine Centers. J Sleep Res. 2006;15:213–38.

34. Pevernagie D, Stanley N, Berg S, et al. European guidelines for the certification of professionals in sleep medicine: report of the task force of the European Sleep Research Society. J Sleep Res. 2009;18:136–41.

Evolution of Sleep Medicine in Japan

Masako Okawa

Ishimori [1] from Japan in 1909 and Pieron and Legendre in 1913 from France [2] independently performed sleep-deprivation experiments in dogs and then injected the cerebrospinal fluid from the dogs into the cerebral ventricles of nonsleep-deprived dogs. The recipient animals quickly fell asleep, suggesting the accumulation of sleep-inducing factors (called "hypnotoxin" by Pieron) in the brain during waking state. The discovery of sleep substance by Ishimori was considered to be the first milestone of sleep research in Japan. The Japanese researchers continued investigative work on sleep factors and discovered in the 1990s sleep-inducing factors from the brainstems of sleep-deprived rats [3].

Japanese Society of Sleep Research

In 1973, the Japanese Research Committee of Sleep (JRCS) was formed, and in 1977, JRCS was renamed as Japanese Society of Sleep Research (JSSR). Since then, the society had regular annual meetings, and in 1979, it successfully organized the third International Conference of Sleep Research jointly with the 19th APSS meeting in Tokyo. Japanese sleep researchers have made significant contributions in sleep research (e.g., early description of rapid eye movement (REM) sleep behavior disorder in patients with delirium tremens and multiple system atrophy by Hishikawa [4], the discovery of the association of specific human leukocyte antigen (HLA) antigen with narcolepsy–cataplexy by Honda [5], and the discovery of sleep factors, such as uridine, by Inoue [6], oxidized glutathione by Komoda [3], and prostagrandin D_2 by Hayaishi [7]). The research field of sleep later expanded to include biological rhythms. The membership grew rapidly in the past 10 years, and the numbers reached more than 3000 in 2012 (Fig. 16.1).

The history of growth of sleep medicine in Japan is rather recent. It was only in 1994 when all night polysomnography (PSG) was covered by the public health insurance. Prior to that, PSG was performed only for research purposes in a few university hospitals or research institutes, mostly by psychiatrists or basic researchers. No clinical polysomnographer existed at that time. The number of sleep disorder clinics increased rapidly, since PSG was covered by the public health insurance. Pulmonologists and otolaryngologists, who were not sleep specialists, ran most of the newly developed sleep disorder clinics, only caring for patients with sleep-disordered breathing (SDB). The growth of sleep medicine clinics and laboratories accelerated rapidly following the news in 2003 that the bullet train driver dozed off while driving, and he was reported to be suffering from sleep apnea (Fig. 16.2).

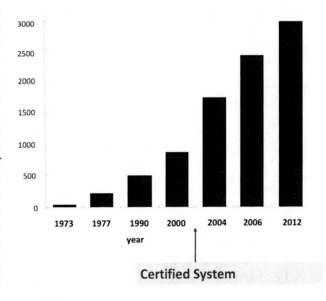

Fig. 16.1 The research field of sleep later expanded to include biological rhythms. The membership grew rapidly in the past 10 years, and the numbers reached more than 3000 in 2012

M. Okawa (✉)
Department of Sleep Medicine, Shiga University of Medical Science, Otsu, Japan
e-mail: Okawa10022@gmail.com

S. Chokroverty, M. Billiard (eds.), *Sleep Medicine*, DOI 10.1007/978-1-4939-2089-1_16,
© Springer Science+Business Media, LLC 2015

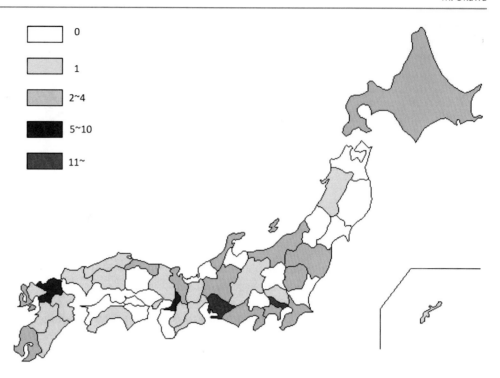

Fig. 16.2 The growth of sleep medicine clinics and laboratories accelerated rapidly following the news in 2003 that the bullet train driver dozed off while driving, and he was reported to be suffering from sleep apnea

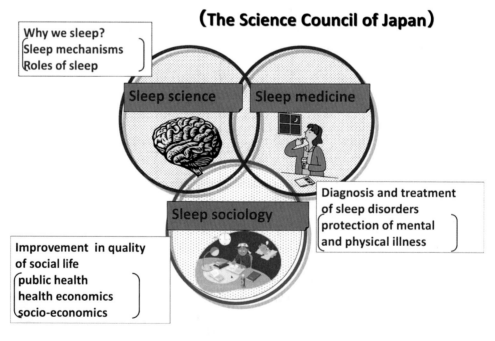

Fig. 16.3 An important contribution to sleep research in Japan was the establishment of "somnology" proposed by the Japanese Society of Sleep Research (JSSR) Commission in 2002

The *Journal of Sleep and Biological Rhythm* (SBR), launched in 2001, became the official journal of JSSR and the Asian Sleep Research Society (ASRS) in 2002.

Establishment of Somnology

An important contribution to sleep research in Japan was the establishment of "somnology" (Fig. 16.3) proposed by the JSSR Commission in 2002.

Somnology consisted of three divisions: (1) sleep science, concerned with basic science aspects of sleep; (2) sleep medicine, dealing with clinical disorders of sleep; (3) sleep sociology, dealing with sleep issues in industry, schools, the community, as well as those related to environmental, public health, and economic situations.

It is our hope that the establishment of this new specialty of somnology will lead to further progress in sleep and biological rhythm research not only in Japan but also throughout the world.

References

1. Ishimori K. Sleep-inducing substance(s) demonstrated in the brain parenchyma of sleep-deprived animals – a true cause of sleep. Tokyo Igakkai Zasshi 1909; 23: 429–57. (Japanese).
2. Legendre R, Pieron H. Recherches sur le besoin de sommeil consécutif à une veille prolongée. A Allgem Physiol. 1913;14:235–62.
3. Komoda Y, Honda K, Inoue S. SPS-B, a physiological sleep regulator, from the brainstems of sleep-deprived rats, identified as oxidized glutathione. Chem Pharm Bull (Tokyo). 1990;38:2057–9.
4. Tachibana M, Tanaka K, Hishikawa Y, et al. A sleep study of acute psychotic states due to alcohol and meprobamate addiction. Advances Sleep Res. 1975; 2:177–205.
5. Honda Y, Juji T, Matsuki K, et al. HLA-DR2 and Dw2 in narcolepsy and in other disorders of excessive somnolence without cataplexy. Sleep. 1986; 9(1 Pt 2):133–42.
6. Inoue S, Schneider-Helmert D, editors. Sleep peptides: basic and clinical approaches. Tokyo: Japan Scientific Societies Press/Springer; 1988.
7. Hayaishi O. Humoral mechanisms of sleep-wake regulation: historical review of prostaglandin D2 and related substances. Sleep Biol Rhythms. 2011;9(Suppl. 1):3–9.

History of Japanese Clinical Sleep Medicine

17

Naoko Tachibana

Introduction

Clinical sleep medicine in Japan is still in developing stage. There is no established consensus about what sleep medicine is, what kind of disorders sleep medicine should deal with, who should be involved in practicing sleep medicine, and how sleep disorders should be investigated and treated. In order to make progress to step into the next stage, establishing an identity of clinical sleep medicine is an urgent matter. People in different countries who are tackling with the practice of sleep medicine should find some information in here.

The Earliest Days

The beginning of Japanese clinical sleep medicine can be dated back to 1990 when polysomnography (PSG) was first covered by the national health insurance. It was achieved by the petitionary activity by Japanese Society of Electroencephalography and Electromyography (currently, Japanese Society of Clinical Neurophysiology), Japanese Society of Sleep Research (JSSR), and The Japan Epilepsy Society. Until that year sleep had been considered one of the subjects of research in psychology, physiology, and psychiatry, and PSG had not been performed routinely for the purpose of clinical diagnosis and treatment. As the Japanese medical care system is virtually controlled by the government, anything without official reimbursement cannot be recognized as clinically necessary; therefore, this was the first step into clinical sleep medicine [1]. However, PSG reimbursement at that time was only 15000 JPY (33000 JPY in 2015), and the manpower resource for PSG remained in the side of physicians who worked without salary in university hospitals as postgraduate students doing clinical sleep research at the same time [2].

The Fragmentary Clinical Sleep Practice in the 1990s

JSSR in the 1990s was composed of mainly psychiatrists, neurophysiologists, and psychologists. Among this group of people, only psychiatrists were allowed to directly deal with patients under the Japanese Medical Service Act. Since these psychiatrists did not compose the major portions of psychiatry community, therefore, sleep was not within psychiatrists' interest except that insomnia widely received psychiatric attention. Although JSSR organized a special symposium about sleep apnea syndrome (SAS) at the 9th Annual Meeting held as early as 1984, they failed to transmit the new knowledge to wider medical community.

On the other hand, some pulmonologists who had been involved in physiological research of sleep apnea started to hold regular meetings organizing Sleep-disordered Breathing Research Group in 1988, which was differently composed from JSSR in that their members are mostly respiratory physicians and otorhinolaryngologists who are more interested in treatment of SAS. In addition, their approach was based on traditional medical methods and they focused on definition of SAS and its epidemiology at the kickoff point. However, the other important aspects of sleep medicine such as sleep health, circadian rhythm, or sleep disorders other than SAS were beyond their scope.

Another important aspect that should be mentioned was that under the Japanese Medical Service Act, the practice of sleep medicine or practice of seeing patients with sleep disorder was not allowed to advertise. This rule applied to the naming of departments of clinics and hospitals, for example, you were allowed to show the name of Sleep Disorders Center inside the clinic or hospital buildings, but not outside. This situation precluded patients seeking for help to their sleep problems from finding proper places to go for a long time until the Internet information had got the status of exception.

N. Tachibana (✉)
Center for Sleep-related Disorders, Kansai Electric Power Hospital, 2-1-7 Fukushima, Fukushima, Osaka 553–0003, Japan
e-mail: NanaOsaka@aol.com

S. Chokroverty, M. Billiard (eds.), *Sleep Medicine*, DOI 10.1007/978-1-4939-2089-1_17,
© Springer Science+Business Media, LLC 2015

In summary, in 1990s, although sleep medicine practice partially started, its existence was hard to be recognized and different places offered different medical services that were fragmentary to the patients [3].

Complicated Reimbursement on Continuous Positive Airway Pressure (CPAP)

The second important milestone in the development of clinical sleep medicine was when continuous positive airway pressure (CPAP) treatment was covered by the national health insurance in 1998. For this coverage, some pulmonologists, acting as a pressure group, had a lot of difficulty to prescribe CPAP. Although CPAP machines themselves had been already available in Japan in the early 1990s, the only way to let obstructive sleep apnea syndrome (OSAS) patients use CPAP machines was first to purchase them by research money at some universities, then prescribe them in the affiliated university hospitals. Direct purchase from CPAP dealers by patients was strictly forbidden by the regulation.

Reimbursement for CPAP treatment in Japan was somewhat unique and complicated, as the insurance covers all the CPAP machines and expendable supplies at the same price on a monthly basis (12100 JPY per month) regardless of the type of machines, attached humidifiers, and how often the patient needs to replace masks. This insurance coverage is only available with the mandatory monthly consultation, which means that the CPAP users should come up to the clinics once per month despite their medically good conditions, until they become free from the CPAP machines or opt out for other treatment.

This reimbursement was a great progress in respect of treatment option, but the definition of OSAS for patients under this CPAP treatment insurance coverage included an apnea–hypopnea index (AHI) of ≥ 20 proven by PSG or AHI ≥ 40 by portable respiratory monitoring with other complications such as hypersomnolence. This definition was not evidence-based or the result of expert opinions, rather influenced by lobbying activity by the industry. It should be especially noted that home monitoring was already included as the method to make a diagnosis in 1998 with the national insurance coverage, which was later regarded as one of the reasons why in-lab full PSG was not widely available in Japan [4].

Accreditation System by JSSR

In 1998, Dr. Meir Kryger, who came to Japan as an invited speaker at various meetings related to OSAS, visited some sleep labs and exchanged information with Japanese sleep researchers and clinicians about the current status of practice of sleep medicine. Summing up his experience, he expressed his view and recommended necessary measures to promote clinical sleep medicine in newsletter of JSSR. He pointed out the importance of organizing a taskforce for standardizing sleep lab and the finalized standard should be approved by not only JSSR but also by other related societies of neurology, psychiatry, and pulmonology [5].

In response to this proposal and in line with the growing interest in OSAS among physicians who do not belong to JSSR, this society started to build an accreditation system that is for sleep physicians, sleep dentists, sleep technologists, and sleep labs. This business was in action in 2001. However, now that there are so many societies and certifications about various subspecialties in Japan where no additional doctors' fee is accepted under the national insurance, the significance of this kind of certification at least for physicians is getting questionable.

Sudden Public Recognition of OSAS

How people began to recognize sleep-related problems in Japan was strongly influenced by a single incident on 26th February, 2003. On this day, a bullet train driver was found to have been sleeping for 8 min while operating a train at 270 km/h and the train was eventually stopped by an emergency device. Several days after this incident, this driver was found to have suffered from unrecognized OSAS, which helped OSAS to be widely recognized under the mass-media coverage. As the public was made to believe that OSAS was the only reason for sleepiness and dozing off, sleepy people were screened by Epworth Sleepiness Scale at the annual checkup organized by their companies, and there was a strong demand for sleep labs and sleep specialists for making a diagnosis of OSAS.

As a result, a lot of possible OSAS patients (or they may suffer from lack of sleep because of poor working condition) have been seen by non-sleep specialists or the value of AHI alone was used for diagnosis and treatment decision without questioning about his/her sleep health. Since there has been no umbrella clinical sleep organization including all the clinicians who actually see patients on the ground, this situation has not been controlled by JSSR or other societies related to OSAS.

Foundation of Clinical Sleep Society

Looking back on this Japanese situation, the dichotomy of academic somnology with little emphasis on sleep apnea and SAS medicine under the compelling circumstance have not yet merged. What is more remarkable is that recently CPAP dealers started marketing CPAP and assisted servo-ventilation to cardiologists for the treatment of patients with heart failure. Because of an unsatisfactory and confusing situation, a group of people established a completely new society, Integrated Sleep Medicine Society Japan (ISMSJ) in 2008. The urgent need is to develop infrastructure of sleep medicine (i.e., modified sleep labs suitable for Japanese medical care system) and to offer basic, but comprehensive, education about sleep and sleep disorders for the younger generation to have practical medical training, because specialists cannot function properly without good collaboration with primary care physicians or other specialists in different fields. People with other careers such as medical technicians who perform PSG, nurses, psychologists, and school teachers should be encouraged to join the field of sleep medicine to set up a team for good medical care. There is further work to be done until clinical sleep medicine is established in Japan.

References

1. Campbell JC, Ikegami N. The art of balance in health policy: maintaining Japan's low-cost, egalitarian system. Cambridge: Cambridge University Press; 2008.
2. Coleman S. Japanese science: from the inside. Abington: Routledge; 1999.
3. Tachibana N. Imbalance between the reality of sleep specialists and the demands of society in Japan. Ind Health. 2005;43:49–52.
4. Tachibana N, Ayas NT, White DP. Japanese versus USA clinical services for sleep medicine. Sleep Biol Rhythm. 2003;1:215–20.
5. Hishikawa Y. The message for Japanese sleep medicine researchers from Dr. M. Kryger. JSSR Newsl. 1999;19:1–3. (In Japanese).

Sleep Medicine Around the World (Beyond North American and European Continents, and Japan)

18

Sudhansu Chokroverty

Introduction

This chapter will briefly summarize the development of sleep medicine beyond North American (See Chap. 14) and European (See Chap. 15) continents and Japan (See Chap. 16 and 17). The major focus will be the current state-of-the-art involving growth and development of sleep medicine in Latin America and Asia (briefly alluded to in Chap. 14) as well as some comments about contemporary sleep medicine in Africa and Australasia. Finally, developmental milestones of international sleep organizations will be briefly mentioned. Tables 18.1, 18.2, 18.3 and 18.4 list the National and Continental, the Latin American, the Asian, and the International Sleep Societies, respectively.

Sleep Medicine in Latin America

As it has been the case in North America and even more in Europe, basic animal and human research has preceded the development of sleep medicine in Latin America. In the 1960s, pioneering research in those fields was conducted by Raul Hernandez Peon (Neurophysiology) in Mexico and Jaime Monti (Pharmacology) in Uruguay. In the 1970s, Rene Drucker Colin (Neurophysiology) in Mexico, Daniel Cardinali (Neuroendocrinology) in Argentina, Sergio Tufik (Psychobiology) in Brazil, and Ricardo Velluti (Neurophysiology) in Uruguay conducted similar research. It was only in the 1980s that many individuals became interested in clinical sleep medicine, and after having training in sleep medicine either in North America or Europe, established sleep disorders centers initially in Brazil, Argentina, Uruguay, Chile, and Colombia, later in Peru, with representatives from Bra-

zil, Argentina, Chile, Uruguay, Colombia, and Peru and later Venezuela, Panama, Ecuador, and Paraguay [1,2].

The major milestone in the development of clinical sleep medicine in Latin America was the foundation of the Federation of Latin American Sleep Societies (FLASS) in 1985. Many exchanges developed between those countries and North America and Europe (mainly Spain) with sleep specialists being invited to participate in FLASS meetings, national sleep societies meetings and sleep training courses, and Latin American sleep specialists presenting their work in the meetings of the Associated Professional Sleep Societies (APSS), the European Sleep Research Society (ESRS), the World Federation of Sleep Research Societies (WFSRS), and the World Association of Sleep Medicine (WASM). From the very beginning, the WASM has been promoting clinical sleep medicine in South America as part of its mission of spreading sleep health worldwide.

In fact, some key members of the FLASS served or are presently serving on the governing councils of the WASM (Sergio Tufik and Dalva Poyares from Brazil) and the World Sleep Day committee (Julia Santin from Chile).

Since the foundation of FLASS and the WFSRS (Ennio Vivaldi from Chile), several Latin American countries established sleep societies (See Table 18.2) to promote research, patient care, and education in sleep medicine.

Except for Brazil, the rest of the Latin American countries do not have facilities for normal training, certification, or guideline assessing minimal competences to practice sleep medicine at present. The field is still young but there is intense interest in advancing the field in Latin America which bodes well for future development of sleep medicine.

Sleep Medicine in India

Great strides have been made in promoting sleep medicine in India in the last two decades [3]. As in the USA and other parts of the world, sleep medicine is a multidisciplinary specialty, but the pulmonary physicians took the lead in

S. Chokroverty (✉)
JFK New Jersey Neuroscience Institute, 65 James Street,
Edison, NJ 08818, USA
e-mail: schok@att.net

S. Chokroverty, M. Billiard (eds.), *Sleep Medicine*, DOI 10.1007/978-1-4939-2089-1_18,
© Springer Science+Business Media, LLC 2015

Table 18.1 Historical milestones for the national and continental sleep societies

Name of society	Year founded
The Association for the Psychophysiological Study of Sleep (APSS)	1964
The European Sleep Research Society (ESRS)	1971
The Japanese Research Committee of Sleep (JRCS)	1973
The Association of Sleep Disorders Centers (ASDC)	1975
The Japanese Society of Sleep Research (JSSR)	1977
The Association of Polysomnographic Technologists (APT)	1978
The APSS is renamed the Sleep Research Society (SRS)	1983
The Clinical Sleep Society (CSS) is founded as a branch of ASDC	1984
The Latin American Sleep Society (LASS)	1985
The Federated Association of Professional Sleep Societies (APSS) composed of ASDC, CSS, APT, and SRS. A few years later the APT withdrew from the Federation following which the name was changed to Associated Professional Sleep Society (The acronym APSS was retained)	1986
The Sleep Society of Canada (SSC)	1986
The ASDC and CSS were reorganized changing the name to The American Sleep Disorders Association (ASDA)	1987
The National Sleep Foundation (NSF) was created	1990
The Academy of Dental Sleep Medicine (ADSM)	1991
The Sleep Society of South Africa (SSSA)	1992
The United States Congress passed a legislation to create The National Centers for Sleep Disorders Research (NCSDR)	1993
The Asian Sleep Research Society (ASRS)	1994
The ASDA was renamed The American Academy of Sleep Medicine (AASM)	1999
The Australasian Sleep Association (ASA)	1999
The Society of Behavioral Sleep Medicine (SBSM)	2010
The Society of Anesthesia and Sleep Medicine (SASM)	2011

Table 18.2 Current Latin American sleep societies

Name	Year founded
The Brazilian Sleep Society (The Associacao Brasileira do Sono (ABS)	1985
The Argentinian Sleep Association (Asociacion Argentina de Medicina del Sueno [AAMS])	1995
The Chilean Sleep Society (Sociedad Chilena de Medicina del Sueno) [SOCHIMES])	2006
The Mexican Sleep Society (Sociedad Mexicana para la Investigacion y Medicina del Sueno [SMIMS])	1997
The Colombian Sleep Society (Asociacion Colombiana de Medicina del Sueno [ACMES])	1999
The Uruguayan Sleep Society (La Sociedad Uruguaya de Investigaciones del Sueno [SUIDES])	2001
The Peruvian Sleep Society (Asociacion Peruana de Medicina del Sueno [APEMES])	2007
The Ecuadorian Sleep Society (La Sociedad Equadoriana de Medicina del Sueno [SEMES])	
The Bolivian Sleep Society (la Asociacion Boliviana de Medicina del Sueno [ABOMES])	

developing and running sleep laboratories, however, neurologists, psychiatrists, otolaryngologists, and dentists had been increasingly interested in practicing sleep medicine. In absence of guidelines with strict enforcement, sleep laboratories had been popping up in a variety of hospitals, nursing homes, and diagnostic centers to diagnose and treat sleep apnea with positive pressure therapy using continuous positive airway pressure (CPAP) equipment. It is hoped that this situation will soon be rectified because the standardization and certification process in sleep medicine are underway. There are some 120 sleep laboratories across India (a trivial number in a country with more than a billion population) with over 20 in Delhi. Most of the sleep-related activities initially happened in New Delhi quickly followed by centers and laboratories in Chennai, Mumbai, Kolkata, Kerala, Ban-

galore, and Hyderabad. The initial push for sleep medicine came from basic scientists led by Dr. V Mohan Kumar at the All India Institute of Medical Sciences (AIIMS) in New Delhi with the founding of the Indian Society for Sleep Research (ISSR) in 1992. It is notable that as early as 1934, when sleep medicine was in its infancy, Dr. Dixshit had provided experimental evidence to show the existence of sleep center in the hypothalamus [4]. The clinicians did not wait too long to spread the mission of promoting clinical sleep medicine. In these efforts Dr. JC Suri, Head of the Department of Pulmonary, Critical Care and Sleep Medicine at Safdarjung Hospital, Delhi where the first sleep laboratory of the country was established, took the lead in founding the Clinical Sleep Medicine Society, the Indian Sleep Disorders Association (ISDA) in 1995. Dr. Suri became the founding

Table 18.3 Asian sleep societies

Name of the organization	Year founded
The Asian Sleep Research Society (ASRS)	1994
The Indian Society for Sleep Research (ISSR)	1992
The Indian Sleep Disorders Association (ISDA)	1995
The Israel Sleep Medicine Association (ISMA)	
The Israel Sleep Research Society (ISRS)	
The Japanese Society of Sleep Research (JSSR)	1977
The Chinese Sleep Research Society (CSRS)	1994
The Korean Society of Sleep Medicine (KSSM)	2010
The Taiwan Sleep Society (TSS)	
The Hong Kong Society of Sleep Medicine (HKSS)	
The Thailand Sleep Medicine Society (TSMS)	
The Singapore Sleep Research Society (SSRS)	
The Palestinian Sleep Medicine Society (PSMS)	

Table 18.4 International sleep societies

Name of organization	Year founded
World Federation of Sleep Research Society (WFSRS)	1987
WFSRS was renamed to World Federation of Sleep Research and Sleep Medicine Societies (WFSRSMS)	2006
WFSRSMS later adopted an abbreviated name, World Sleep Federation (WSF)	2008
World Association of Sleep Medicine (WASM)	2003
World Congress on Sleep Apnea (WCS)	1985
International Pediatric Sleep Association (IPSA)	2005

president. Since 1996, the ISDA has been organizing annual meetings and courses under the heading "Sleepcon" at various cities across the country, and inviting foreign dignitaries from USA, UK, Canada, Israel, China, Europe, Japan, and Australia, including the present writer (Sudhansu Chokroverty), Drs. Christian Guilleminault, Robert Thomas, Claudia Trenkwalder, Patrick Strollo, and Neal Douglas. The other significant activities of the ISDA include introduction of fellowships and conferring diploma in sleep medicine after successfully completing a certification examination, and initiation of a sleep technologists' certification examination.

Drs. Garima Shukla and Manvir Bhatia, two neurologists from the AIIMS in New Delhi quickly joined Dr. Suri and other physicians in the late 1990s in promoting sleep medicine by organizing symposia and courses. Soon, Dr. Anand Kumar at Amrita Institute of Medical Sciences (AIMS) in Cochi, Kerala, Dr. Suresh Kumar, and later Dr. N. Ramakrishnan from Chennai began organizing symposia with participation by sleep specialists from the USA (Drs. Sudhansu Chokroverty, Wayne Hening, Robert Thomas) and other foreign countries. In these endeavors, WASM actively collaborated with the Indian sleep specialists to promote sleep health throughout India and other parts of the world. Currently, most of the major cities including Kolkata (the city where I grew up) are actively practicing and promoting sleep disorders medicine. As in other parts of the world pulmonologists took lead in establishing sleep laboratories and clinics in Kolkata and unfortunately, most of the senior neurolo-

gists there showed a distinct lack of interest in sleep medicine but the junior neurologists are increasingly becoming interested in understanding the basic and clinical science of sleep which is very encouraging. Dr Dhrubajyoti Roy, a pulmonary-sleep specialist at PULSAR clinic in Kolkata, took the lead on behalf of ISDA and Indian Chest Society (ICS) in organizing educational activities. India is on the move and I am very optimistic that sleep medicine will be in the forefront of medical science there in not too distant future.

Sleep Medicine in China

Sleep medicine is still in its infancy in China, but because of increasing interest and awareness amongst physicians and the public, the field has been growing rapidly in the last decade [5]. There are two major sleep medicine organizations in China: One based on the modern Western tradition (Allopathic Medicine) is the Chinese Sleep Research Society (CSRS) and the other based on Traditional Chinese Medicine (TCM) is the TCM Sleep Medicine Society. The CSRS was founded in 1994 and initially was fragmented but later became truly multidisciplinary encompassing members from pulmonary medicine, psychology, ENT, physiology, neuroscience, basic science, and other fields interested in sleep medicine. This society is affiliated with China Association for Science and Technology and has been expanding and promoting the integration and development of clinical and basic sleep science. There are more than 1500 sleep centers in

China (small number considering a population of over a billion), mostly in major cities like Beijing, Shanghai, Guangzhou, Nanjing, Xi'an. CSRS holds its academic meeting every 2 years with participation from many foreign countries including members of the WASM (e.g., Drs. Christian Guilleminault, Sudhansu Chokroverty, Kingman Strohl, and others). There are, however, no standard guidelines, training program, or certification to assess minimal competence to practice sleep medicine. The practice of modern sleep medicine in China actually started with the first recognition of sleep apnea in a patient in 1981 by Dr. Xi-Zhen Huang of Peking Union Hospital [5]. Dr. Huang has rightly been recognized as the founder and the mother of Chinese Sleep Medicine. Dr. Huang's group designed the first polysomnographic system from the existing electroencephalography (EEG) machine in 1983. Dr. Huang also set up the first sleep laboratory in China in 1986 after completing six months of training in sleep medicine at Stanford University in the USA. She is also actively involved in WASM activities being a member of the program committee of the 2nd WASM Congress in 2007. The contemporary physicians contributing significantly toward growth and development of clinical sleep medicine in China include Drs. Yuping Wang, Chairman of Neurology Department at Xuanwu Hospital, Peking University, Beijing; Fang Han at the Department of pulmonary medicine, The People's Hospital, Peking University, Beijing; Han Denim, Chairman of Otolaryngology at Peking University, Beijing; Shen Xiaoming, a pediatrician at Shangai Children's Medical Center affiliated with Shangai Jiao Tong University's School of Medicine; and Yuoming Luo at the department of pulmonary medicine, Guanzhou General Hospital in addition to numerous other multidisciplinary physicians in different universities throughout China. It is interesting to note that the first continuous positive airway pressure (CPAP) machine was used in 1987 in China and in 1995 China began to use its own homemade CPAP machines.

The man spearheading promotion of TCM sleep medicine in China is Professor Weidong Wang of Beijing Guang'anmen Hospital with the founding of the International Sleep Medicine Society of Traditional and Modern Medicine (ISMSTM). Professor Wang had been ably assisted by many doctors including Wang Fang (Jenny) and others at Guang'anmen Hospital. At the second ISMSTM meeting in 2008, several WASM members (e.g., Drs. Sudhansu Chokroverty, Christian Guilleminalt, Wayne Hening, and Arthur Walters) were invited. Three years later, Professor Wang founded the World Sleep Medicine Association holding the first TCM Congress in Beijing. TCM sleep medicine provides a different philosophical perspective to the general population, practitioners, and researchers.

Sleep Medicine in Other Parts of Asia

Sleep medicine (both clinical and basic science) in Israel is at par with that in the USA and Western Europe. It has its own Research and Clinical Sleep Medicine Societies (See Table 18.3). Drs. Peritz Lavie and Jean Askenasy are two prominent sleep scientists and clinicians who have played a significant role in elevating the standard of sleep medicine in Israel.

Sleep medicine is well advanced in South Korea with an established society, Korean Society of Sleep Medicine (KSSM) whose members are derived from multiple disciplines (e.g., neurology, pulmonary, psychiatry, psychology, ENT, etc). The society conducts regular meetings with participation of foreign sleep specialists. In 2010, KSSM established its own journal. KSSM collaborate with WASM in organizing the sixth WASM World Congress in Seoul on March 21 to March 25, 2015. Besides Dr. Seung Bong Hong, several other prominent sleep physicians (e.g., Drs. Seung Chul Hong, Chul Hee Lee, Chol Shin, Jung Hie Lee, and others) took the lead in promoting sleep medicine in South Korea.

Taiwan, Hong Kong, Singapore, Thailand, and Malaysia have made great strides in sleep medicine and have been trying to promote sleep medicine by conducting research, publishing in peer-reviewed journals and trying to practice high-standard patient care. Most of these places, however, lack standard guidelines and certification process in sleep medicine. Thailand is very active in sleep medicine and research and is being spearheaded by Dr. Nick Kotchabhakdi. Thailand Sleep Society (TSS) was the local organizer for the second WASM Congress in Bangkok in 2007. TSS also organized International Sleep Brain and Behavior Symposium with participation by foreign delegates including several active WASM members.

Sleep Medicine in Africa

Sleep medicine has not been a top priority accounting for a lack of growth and development in continental Africa except in South Africa and later in Egypt. Sleep Society of South Africa (SSSA) was established early in 1992 but the speed of growth has been rather sluggish [6]. Dr. Alyson Bentley of Johannesburg (a member of the WASM governing council from 2003–2011) played an important role in pushing for sleep medicine in that region. Later Dr. Tarek Asaad, Professor of Psychiatry at the Institute of Psychiatry in Ain Shams University in Cairo, Egypt, began to organize symposia and courses in sleep medicine in order to stimulate public and professionals' interest in understanding sleep and its disorders which may have serious consequences for individuals and society. Several other individuals in Cairo, Egypt (e.g., Drs. Lamia Afifi, Shahira Loza), had been devoting their time and effort to promote sleep medicine in Africa. In 2011, Dr. Afifi was elected to the WASM governing council to represent Africa which opened an opportunity for her to promote sleep medicine there through WASM activities. In 2013, at the fifth WASM congress in Valencia, Spain, Dr. Loza replaced Dr. Afifi as the WASM Governing Council member to represent Africa. When I visited Ain Shams University in Cairo in 2010 just before the Arab Spring and revolution began to spread, I saw a great deal of interest and enthusiasm for sleep medicine there. Unfortunately, spread of people's unrest subsequently impeded the rapid and progressive growth of sleep medicine. It is hoped that the leaders in South Africa and Egypt realizing the importance of sleep health will be able to overcome the obstacles to stimulate public and the profession to be aware of the importance of a good night's sleep and adverse consequences in its absence.

Sleep Medicine in Australia and New Zealand

Australia and New Zealand have strict training requirements in sleep medicine certification without an exit examination [7]. These two countries have high standard of practice of sleep medicine concentrated mostly in major cities. It is important to remember that the recommended treatment of moderate to severe obstructive sleep apnea syndrome (OSAS) is upper airway pressurization using CPAP equipment which was invented by Dr. Colin Sullivan, a pulmonologist from Sydney, Australia in 1981. Naturally, there is a major emphasis on sleep apnea treatment, research, and education in Australia. The Australasian Sleep Association (ASA) was founded in 1999.

International Sleep Societies

Currently, there are four major organizations dealing with dissemination of knowledge in sleep medicine and research worldwide (Table 18.4).

The World Federation of Sleep Research Society

The World Federation of Sleep Research Society (WFSRS) was founded in 1987 to represent international sleep researchers. Dr. Michel Chase, a noted basic scientist from California, USA making fundamental contributions in understanding rapid eye movement (REM) sleep atonia mechanism, and other basic sleep research took the lead in founding the

Federation. Since founding the organization, the Federation had been conducting quadrennial congress to promote sleep medicine to the international community. In 2006, WFSRS changed its name to World Federation of Sleep Research and Sleep Medicine Societies (WFSRSM) driven by the competitive incentive from other organizations and to reflect its involvement in clinical besides basic science research in sleep medicine. In 2008, however, the governing council decided to use the abbreviated name of World Sleep Federation (WSF) to circumvent the cumbersome and perceived media unfriendly name of WFSRSM. The WSF is composed of the continental and two regional member societies, ESRS, SRS, AASM, ASRS, ASA, LASS, JSRS, and SSC unlike other international organizations catering to individual members rather than sleep societies.

The World Association of Sleep Medicine

The idea for forming a world association for the sleep clinicians came from Dr. Sudhansu Chokroverty (the author of this chapter) who floated the concept in Parma, Italy in November 2001 during the first international EEG cyclic alternating pattern (CAP) meeting organized by Professor Mario Terzano assisted by Dr. Liborio Parrino [8]. The response was sufficiently encouraging to move ahead. We sent an invitation to many sleep clinicians in each continent of the world and organized a planning meeting to found a new WASM on June 11, 2002, in the Hilton Hotel during the APSS annual meeting in Seattle, Washington State, USA. During the planning meeting, Dr. Chokroverty (the present author) gave an introductory statement explaining the rationale and mission. Most spoke in favor of the formation of a new world body, catering to the sleep clinicians. Few, however, had reservation about starting another new world organization.

WASM was chosen as the best name for the new organization by those present at the planning meeting. The founding members (39) at the planning meeting (those who agreed to be members and indicated so by signing the agreement) elected a bylaws committee chaired by Dr. Wayne Hening with members drawn from the USA, Europe, and Asia. Between June 2002 and June 2003, the bylaws committee developed the bylaws, which had been revised several times after receiving comments from the initial founding members.

Next, an organizational meeting was held on June 6, 2003, at the Swissotel, Chicago, Illinois, USA, to officially found the WASM during the APSS meeting. The founding members (39 from the initial planning meeting) and those present at the organizational meeting (an additional 29) for a total of 68 members voted to accept the final version of the WASM bylaws, requiring biennial meetings and incorporating the organization in Kassel, Germany. By a secret ballot, the founding members voted for the officers of the WASM executive committee for a 2-year term as follows: President, Dr. Sudhansu Chokroverty; President Elect, Dr. Markku Partinen; Secretary, Dr. Richard Allen; and Treasurer, Dr. Claudia Trenkwalder.

On a beautiful bright Saturday morning (June 7, 2003), the officers of the executive committee and the chair of the bylaws committee went to the German consular office on Chicago's Michigan Avenue to ratify the bylaws to officially found WASM with the office incorporated in Kassel, Germany.

In course of the next few years, WASM captured the enthusiasm and strong support from many sleep clinicians throughout the globe who embraced WASM as an exciting international organization. WASM had six very successful world congresses: The first one was in Berlin, Europe, in 2005; the second one was in 2007 in Bangkok, Thailand; the third congress was in 2009 in Sao Paulo, Brazil; the fourth one was in 2011 in Quebec City, Quebec, Canada; the fifth one was in 2013 in Valencia (Spain) and the sixth one in Seoul, South Korea, on March 21–25, 2015.

WASM has a noble mission of promoting sleep medicine and sleep health throughout the globe, particularly in those parts of the world where sleep medicine has not sufficiently progressed (our mission and bylaws are available on the Internet at the Web site address: www.WASMonline.org).

WASM has an affiliated journal—*Sleep Medicine*, an international journal—published by Elsevier Publishing Company in Amsterdam, Europe. The journal was founded in 2000 and Dr. Sudhansu Chokroverty is the founding editor in chief. Initially, the journal was published 4 times a year and the frequency of publication was increased to 6, then 8, 10, and currently 12 issues a year. WASM has established two awards for young investigators: The Christian Guilleminault WASM-Elsevier Award for Sleep Research and Elio Lugaresi WASM-Elsevier Award for Sleep Medicine. WASM had sponsored regional workshops and endorsed meetings in different parts of the world. WASM developed WASM—International Restless Legs Syndrome Study Group (IRLSSG) guidelines for periodic limb movements in sleep (PLMS) and periodic limb movements in wakefulness (PLMW) (published in *Sleep Medicine* in 2006).WASM has developed educational guidelines and international certification for practice of sleep medicine in every region of the world, taking into consideration regional concerns and culture. WASM will continually encourage young physicians to develop skills in sleep science. These are the people who are the future of this world and who will be the driving force to fulfill the mission and vision of WASM. The WASM later formed a World Sleep Day (WSD) committee. WSD is an annual event to celebrate sleep around the globe, and it is organized by the WSD Committee of the WASM. It is co-chaired by Dr. Antonio Culebras, Professor of Neurology, Syracuse University, Syracuse, New York, USA, and Dr. Liborio Par-

rino, Associate Professor of Neurology, Parma, Italy, and is assisted by several international committee members.

The idea of a "World Sleep Day (WSD)," to celebrate sleep on a particular day in the year (generally around middle of March), came about during the WASM Governing council meeting at the second WASM Congress in Bangkok, Thailand, February 4th–8th in 2007.

The first WSD was held on March 14, 2008, under the slogan, "Sleep Well, Live Fully Awake." The 2009 WSD was held on March 20 under the slogan, "Drive Alert, Arrive Safe." In 2010, it was held on March 19 and the slogan was "Sleep Well, Stay Healthy." The 2011 WSD was held on March 18 under the slogan, "Sleep Well, Grow Healthy." The WSD in 2012 was celebrated on March 16 under the slogan, "Breathe Easily, Sleep Well." The slogan for 2013 was "Good Sleep, Healthy Aging" and was held on March 15th, and that for 2014 was "Sleep, Easy Breathing, Healthy Body" which was held on March 14, 2014. The slogan for 2015 WSD (held on March 13, 2015) was "When sleep is sound, health and happiness abound."

The WSD events take place primarily online at www.WorldSleepDay.org, featuring educational and historical videos, educational materials, and public service announcements. WSD has grown steadily since its inception and currently has over 120 WSD delegates spreading awareness of sleep issues in over 50 countries around the globe. These delegates contact local media, organize public awareness events, host conferences, translate WSD materials in different languages, and much more.

World Congress on Sleep Apnea (WCS) This international organization was founded in 1985 by a group of sleep specialists interested in increasing awareness of the international community about a common but often undiagnosed or under-diagnosed condition of sleep apnea and its adverse (short-term and long-term) consequences. The WCS has been conducting an international meeting every 3 years in different parts of the world with participation of sleep specialists catering to patients with sleep apnea to highlight important areas of research in sleep apnea. The ninth WCS Congress was held in Seoul, South Korea on March 25–28, 2009, and the tenth Congress was held in Rome on August 27–September 1, 2012. Many WASM members including the present writer and Dr. Christian Guilleminault as well as WSF members had participated in these meetings as invited delegates.

International Pediatric Sleep Association

This international association originated as an offshoot from the European Pediatric Sleep Club (EPSC) and the IPSA was founded in 2005 (See also Chap. 54) following the valiant efforts of Professor Andre Kahn of Belgium assisted by many noted pediatric sleep clinicians from Europe including Dr. Oliviero Bruni of Rome. Sadly, Andre Kahn died prematurely in 2004 before the actual founding of the IPSA on October 13, 2005, following the first congress of the WASM in Berlin. The IPSA decided to affiliate with *Sleep Medicine* journal which has already been an affiliate journal of the WASM. Initially, IPSA met during WASM congress but in 2010 the second IPSA Congress was organized separately by Oliviero Bruni in Rome which was a huge success. IPSA continued its meeting every 2 years in different parts of the world. The third IPSA meeting was held in Manchester, England in 2012, and the fourth meeting was held in 2014 in Porto Alegre in Brazil.

References

1. Averbuch M, Paez S, Meza M, Pedemonte M, Velluti R, Escobar F, et al. Current status of Latin American sleep societies. Sleep Sci. 2011;4(1):34–6.
2. Osuna E. Sleep medicine in South America. In: Sleep health around the world [Internet]. 2006;1(1):15. http//www.friglobalevents.com/wasmonline/PDF/WASM_Newsletter_2_final.pdf   2006:1(1):15. Accessed 12 Jan 2011.
3. Shukla G, Bhatia M. The sleep scenario in India. In: Sleep health around the world [Internet]. 2006;1(1):15. http//www.friglobalevents.com/wasmonline/PDF/WASM_Newsletter_2_final.pdf 2006:1(1):15. Accessed 12 Jan 2011.
4. Dikshit VV. Action of acetylcholine on the "sleep center". J Physiol. 1934;83:42–….
5. Han F. Development of modern sleep medicine in China. In: Sleep health around the world [Internet]. 2006;1(1):15. http//www.friglobalevents.com/wasmonline/PDF/WASM_Newsletter_2_final.pdf 2006:1(1):15. Accessed 12 Jan 2011.
6. Bentley AJ. Sleep medicine in South Africa. In: Sleep health around the world [Internet]. 2006;1(1):15. http//www.friglobalevents.com/wasmonline/PDF/WASM_Newsletter_2_final.pdf 2006:1(1):15. Accessed 12 Jan 2011.
7. Cunnington D. Sleep medicine training in Australia and New Zealand. In: Sleep health around the world [Internet]. 2007;(1):12. http://www.friglobalevents.com/wasmonline/PDF/WASM_Newsletter_2_final.pdf. Accessed 12 Jan 2011.
8. Chokroverty S. Historical milestones. In: Sleep health around the world [Internet]. 2006;1(1):15. http//www.friglobalevents.com/wasmonline/PDF/WASM_Newsletter_2_final.pdf 2006:1(1):15. Accessed 12 Jan 2011.

Cholera

Donatien Moukassa, Obengui and Jean-Rosaire Ibara

Cholera is a highly contagious acute intestinal infection that is specific to humans. It is caused by a Gram-negative bacterium belonging to the 0:1 or 0:139 *Vibrio cholerae* serotypes. The pathogen bears an endotoxin that provokes cataclysmic diarrhea causing severe dehydration that may trigger shock. If untreated, cholera proves to be fatal in 25–30 % of cases. Treatment, especially rehydration, reduces the mortality rate to less than 1 % [1].

Early descriptions date back to the beginning of the sixteenth century, but cholera epidemics only started in the nineteenth century. The disease spread out across all continents, sometimes implying devastating demographic consequences. Since its first occurrence in Sub-Saharan Africa in 1971, cholera has become endemic and epidemic in sub-Saharan Africa. Nowadays, cholera represents a real public health problem in large African cities where refugees concentrate after fleeing away from wars and political unrest.

Although, the current volume is concerned with the impact of diseases in sleep medicine, no scientific reports have been made on cholera and sleep to our knowledge, except anecdotal observations.

Natural History of Cholera

The Growth of Epidemic Waves into Pandemics (Sixteenth Century to Twenty-first Century)

Historically, the first case of cholera was reported in 1503 in one of the Vasco de Gama officers. The outbreak of profuse cataclysmic diarrhea became rapidly fatal to some 20,000 individuals in Calicut, India [2]. For more than three centuries, cholera was confined to Asia (India, China, and Indonesia). From the delta of the Ganges in the nineteenth century, cholera spread out in a pandemic manner to Europe, North Africa, and the Americas (Table 19.1), killing millions of individuals.

The seventh epidemic hit sub-Saharan Africa in 1971. Since initial reports, several epidemic outbreaks were reported. The recent Congo–Brazzaville (2009–2013) epidemic is illustrated in Table 19.2. The epidemic spread widely in the Likouala region—an area where forestry alternates with marshes drained by large rivers (Likouala aux herbes, Sangha, Likouala Mossaka, Oubangui). It affected populations living in scattered villages and campsites. The epidemic was less active in the Cuvette and Plateaux regions. The outbreak concentrated in the large cities of Brazzaville (in 2009 and 2012) and Pointe-Noire (2012–2013). The number of casualties was greater in Brazzaville than in other cities, despite modern hospital facilities. This paradox may be linked to the degraded environment created by poor water supply and sanitation.

Vibrio cholerae and Pathogenicity

Vibrio cholerae was discovered by Filippo Pacini in 1854 [3, 4], but the bacterium microscopic structure was only specified by Robert Koch in 1884 [3] in Calcutta, India. Koch linked his *Bacillus komma* to cholera. In 1885, Ferran proposed the concept of cholera vaccine for humans [5]. In 1894, Pfeiffer initiated the concept of "endotoxin" released

D. Moukassa (✉)
Medical and Morphology Laboratory, Loandjili General Hospital, Pointe-Noire, Congo
e-mail: donatienmoukassa@gmail.com

Obengui
Department of Infectious Disease, University Hospital of Brazzaville, Congo

J.-R. Ibara
Department of Gastroenterology and Medicine, University Hospital of Brazzaville, Congo

S. Chokroverty, M. Billiard (eds.), *Sleep Medicine,* DOI 10.1007/978-1-4939-2089-1_19,
© Springer Science+Business Media, LLC 2015

Table 19.1 The seven cholera epidemics

Dates	Geographical reaches	Public health measures and particular events
1817–1825	Asia and East Africa, spreading to Russia and Europe in 1823	
1826–1841	Spreading from Mecca to Egypt, Europe and Algeria	
1846–1861	Spreading from China to Maghreb, crossed the Atlantic to Latin America	The 1851 International Health Conference edited hygiene measures that allowed to spare the United States and England
1863–1876	Starting from India and China, invading Europe via the French troops coming back from Indochina, and reaching the United States, Latin America, Russia and Poland (1866), and North Africa	Helped by the opening of the Suez Canal (1863), by the Secession War and by population displacements in Eastern Europe
1883–1896	Starting from India	Bouchet observes the bacteria. Koch describes its characteristics. Ferran proposes the first vaccine
1899–1923	Spread from Asia to Russia, and Central and Eastern Europe	
1961 on	Starting from Indonesia, generalized to Asia (1962), India (1964), Middle East (1966) and Eastern Europe (1970), and Latin America (1991). The epidemics reached sub-Saharan Africa (1970), extended to the Great Lakes region (1973) and generalized to the whole continent (1979)	The new extension to Latin America came after almost a century free of the disease. It has been attributed to climatic disasters

Table 19.2 Epidemiological situation during the Congo outbreaks (2009-2013)

Region	Population	Cholera cases	Incidence per 100,000	Casualties	Proportion of casualties (% of cholera cases)
Likouala	154,115	739	479.5	22	3.0
Cuvette	156,044	60	38.5	1	1.7
Plateaux	174,591	87	49.8	4	4.6
Brazzaville	1,373,382	180	13.1	9	5.0
Pointe-Noire	715,334	240	33.6	8	3.3
Total	2,573,466	1306	50.7	44	3.4

by the *Vibrio cholerae* membrane. The choleragen toxin was identified in the 1950s in India and was purified and crystallized by Finkelstein in 1969 [4, 6, 7]. The bactericidal action of the waters of the Ganges River was described in 1896, especially on *Vibrio cholerae* [8]. The El Tor biotype was discovered in 1905 from pilgrim corpses in the Sinai. Between 1907 and 1920 in Indela, Sir Leonard Rogers rehydrated the patients with intravenous hypertonic saline, which significantly changed the death toll of patients from 60–70 % to 3–0 %. In 1911, a cholera epidemic was stopped in Marseille by water chlorination. In 1931, Hérelle and Eliava marketed the first anticholera Tbilisi phages [1, 8, 9].

Descriptive Epidemiology

Incidence (OMS [10])

Nearly all developing countries are dealing with a cholera outbreak or threat of an epidemic. According to the World Health Organization (WHO) [10], in 2003, 45 countries reported a total of 111,575 cases and 1984 deaths (CFR 1.7 %). African cases amounted to 108,067, representing 96 % of the world incidence. In 2004, 56 countries reported 101,389 cases and 2,345 deaths (CFR 2.31 %). Although the number of cases had decreased by 9 % compared to 2003, the number of deaths had increased by 24 %. In contrast, the number

of cases remained low in America (36 cases, with 5 cases in the USA, and 3 cases in Canada), and 7 European countries reported only 21 imported cases (13 in UK).

The number of reported cases increased to 230,000 in 2006 with approximately 6000 deaths [11]. However, the true incidence is probably higher.

Factors Favoring Outbreaks (OMS [24])

Cholera outbreaks are favored by degraded environments. Natural climatic disasters have been followed by epidemics, such as in Haiti after the 2010 earthquake [11], in Central America after Hurricane Mitch (1998), and in Mozambique after large floods in 2000. The El Nino phenomenon may have been at the origin of the Horn of Africa outbreaks in 1997–1998 [11].

Civil war or political unrest may also favor cholera outbreaks. A massive outbreak (58,000 cases and 4200 deaths) hit Rwandan refugee camps in Goma, Democratic Republic of Congo in 1994. Wars favored the appearance of cholera in Darfur, worsened the 1997 and 1998 outbreaks in the Horn of Africa, and caused outbreaks in Kabul (Afghanistan).

Degraded environments, favored by the anarchic development of metropolitan cities, where water supply and treatment are often deficient, contribute to cholera outbreaks.

Analytical Epidemiology [10, 12, 13, 14]

The pathogen is a slightly curved, mobile, 2–3-μm-long, Gram-negative bacterium. It favors a pH 8 milieu at 37 °C and dislikes heat, cold, and acidity. It is sensitive to antiseptics and many antibiotics (including cyclins). It may survive for weeks in shaded fecal matters and 10–15 days in the host. The El Tor biotype of *Vibrio cholerae*, the agent of current outbreaks, has the greatest vitality compared to conventional *cholerae* and *albensis* biotypes.

Serotypes 0:1 and 0:139 of El Tor *Vibrio cholerae* cause outbreaks, the latter having appeared in Bangladesh in 1992. Three 0:1 serotypes combine the A, B, and C antigenic LPS: Ogawa (AB), Inaba (AC), and Hikojima (ABC). Ogawa and Inaba serotypes are mostly responsible for the seventh pandemic, [8] Inaba being responsible for Congo outbreaks.

Factors Leading to Contamination [14, 15]

Genetic Factors

In patients well equipped with intestinal gangliosides (receivers), the incubation period is shorter and the symptoms of cholera are more serious. Alkaline pH multiplies by 40 the risk of severity of cholera (alkalizing consumers, gastrectomized, or vagotomized patients).

Environmental Factors

Vibrio reservoirs are represented by humans and aquatic environments favorable to algal blooms (plankton), such as blackish waters and estuaries. The ongoing climatic warming might create a favorable environment for *Vibrio cholerae*.

Socio–Economic and Demographic Factors

The disease occurs mainly in individuals with poor living conditions, especially in highly populated human concentrations with inadequate water sanitation.

Pathogenic Mechanisms and Tissue Repercussions [14]

The vibrios are ingested through contaminated water and food or through direct contact with patients or carriers. The bacteria multiply in the lumen mucus layer of the small intestine, and adhere intimately to the brush border of enterocytes of type 4 pili. Diarrhea is due to the in situ secretion of the vibrio exotoxin.

Immunity against *Vibrio cholerae* is primarily humoral and short-lasting (2–3 years), being related to the reaction of colonized Peyer's patches that secrete immunoglobulin A (IgA) and immunoglobulin G (IgG)—immunoglobulins in the intestinal lumen. Serum antibodies peak in the second week postinfection and disappear in 4 weeks.

Lungs, liver, and kidney may host *Vibrio cholerae* toxin, provoking specific symptoms. The brain involvement is less documented.

Clinical Symptoms and Time Course [14]

All infected patients do not necessarily develop cholera. When it occurs, the disease is mild in 90 % of cases, typical cholera occurring in less than 10 % of cases.

Silent incubation averages 3 days. Epigastric gurgling precedes a sudden and abundant emission of feces and vomiting. Within 1–2 h, profuse watery colorless rice-water-like diarrhea and vomiting occur repeatedly. They will eventually flow continuously through the anal sphincter and mouth. The odor is bland. The cyanotic and hypothermic (36 °C) patient suffers intense asthenia and muscle cramps. Appreciating the degree of dehydration is crucial, and Table 19.3 lists the criteria for estimating the degree of dehydration.

Untreated, 25–30 % of cholera patients may die from cardiovascular collapse within 1–3 days. Mortality is higher in children, elderly, and malnourished individuals.

The risk of fatal outcome reduces once the patient gets rehydrated quickly (1–5 % of body weight). Healing is completed in 2–3 days without complications or sequels and recovery is rapid. Acute renal failure with anuria complicating acute tubulopathy by hypovolemic shock is rare. Metabolic acidosis due to rapid loss of bicarbonate and hypokalemia

Table 19.3 Criteria for estimating the degree of dehydration in cholera patients

Degree of dehydration	Body weight loss	Skin fold retraction	Eye sockets	Eye balls	Breathing	Voice	Mental state	Radial pulse	Blood pressure	Urine output
Light	6 %	Rapid	Normal	Normal	Normal	Normal	Normal	Normal	Normal	Normal
Medium	6–10 %	Slowed	Hollow	Hollow	Deep	Hoarse	Restlessness	Rapid and weak	Normal or lowered	Decreased
Severe	>10 %	Very slow	Sunken	Dug in	Deep and rapid	Inaudible	Restlessness	Rapid and weak	Low, immeasurable	Oliguria

following vomiting must be corrected rapidly to avoid paralytic ileus.

In children, impaired consciousness or seizures may be observed, along with a rapid development of oliguria or anuria.

Benign forms may appear as acute gastroenteritis with nonfebrile banal vomiting and diarrhea. The abortive form starts as an apparently severe form, but the patient heals spontaneously. Vomiting ceases first allowing rehydration through drinking and feeding. Diarrhea persists for several days, but diuresis recovers and general condition improves. The occurrence of a 38 °C temperature with hot sweats is of good prognosis. However, secondary collapses and cerebral involvement with agitation and delusions are possible.

The dramatic dry cholera is characterized by sudden death occurring in an asymptomatic patient.

Differential Diagnosis [14]

The differential diagnosis includes all causes of bacterial, viral, and parasitic choleriform syndrome. Cholera-like symptoms may be observed in food poisoning due to infection with staphylococcus, salmonella, campylobacter, and anguilules. In children, such symptoms may be observed in rotavirus and enterotoxinogenic *Escherichia coli* infections.

Particular Emphasis on Cholera and Sleep Disorders

The influence of infectious factors on sleep has been stressed for the last 30 years [16]. Pyrogenic bacterial factors are also somnogenic. Muramyl dipeptides and lipopolysaccharide (LPS or endotoxin) trigger the host immune system release of proinflammatory cytokines, such as tumor necrosis factor-α (TNF-α), interferon-β (IFN-β) or interleukin-1 (IL-1), leading to sleep architectural changes. However, as in most other bacterial infections [17], no objective data are available.

Dehydration may also trigger sleep changes, as in military training, impairing performance and mood, promoting fatigue and provoking confusion, depression, and tension [18]. Increased slow-wave sleep after exercise has been related to body temperature elevation [19]. However, such an elevation is lowered by rehydration after exercise [20], agreeing with the fact that rehydration limits exercise-induced hyperthermia [21].

Cholera is accompanied by the release of endotoxin and by dramatic water loss. Sleep–wake disorders may therefore occur in patients with cholera. While we were preparing this chapter, a cholera outbreak struck Pointe-Noire. Sleep disorders were investigated in 36 patients using the sleep diary proposed by Bastuji and Jouvet [22]. Figure 19.1 is a demonstrative example of the major disorganization of the sleep–wake cycle in patients with cholera. They sleep in short bouts that alternate with wakeful bouts during which they can drink and feed. Unfortunately, polysomnography cannot be undertaken in such isolated and highly infectious and toxic patients.

Biological Diagnosis [14]

After confirmation of the first cases at the beginning of the cholera epidemic, the bacteriological diagnosis requires five steps: (I) sampling, (II) transport, (III) direct examination, (IV) culture, and (V) identification.

Sampling is done in several ways, using either swabs, or blotting paper immersed in the feces (Barua's method: The blotting paper is sealed in plastic bags with a cellophane membrane to prevent desiccation) or feces samples.

Samples must be transported directly to the closest laboratory. It can also be transferred at 37°C in liquid (peptone water) or solid Blair's media (taurocholate tellurite peptone).

Direct microscopic examination of a fresh sample reveals suspect mobility. Gram stain will show curved Gram -negative bacilli.

The pathogen may be cultured. After 6 h of incubation at 37 °C, bacteria are seeded in the middle of a Petri's box containing either gelose teepol (bacteria will grow in 2 h) or TCBS buffer (thiosulfate-citrate-bile-sucrose; bacteria will grow in 12 h).

The agglutination technique using polyvalent anti 0:1 and anti 0:139 sera, followed by monovalent anti-Ogawa, anti-Inaba, and anti-Hikojima sera may be employed to identify the pathogen.

In field campaigns and refugee camps, rapid immunochromatography-based strip tests may replace microscopic examination. Simply dipped in a feces sample, the strip will show one or two red lines within 2–5 min (1 line = negative, 2 = positive). Specificity of strip test is 84–100 %, sensitivity 94–100 %.

Treatment [23]

Curative Treatment

Treatment aims at controlling dehydration and its consequences and eliminating *Vibrio cholerae* from the gastrointestinal tract. Rehydration with Ringer lactate can be combined with isotonic saline (SSI) and serum bicarbonate 14 % (2/3 SSI + 1/3 of serum bicarbonate). As an example, in a 60-kg adult who lost 10 % of body weight, 6 l of liquid will be infused during the first 4 h: 1 l during the first 15 min, 1 l during the following 15 min, followed by 1 l in 45 min,

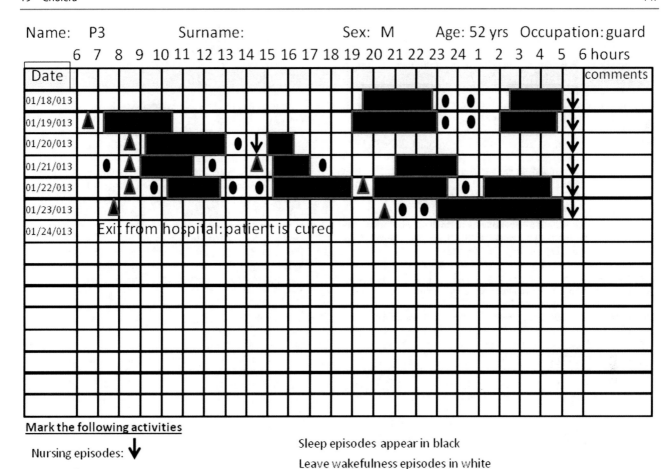

Fig. 19.1 The patient was a 52-year-old guard. He entered the hospital on the 18th of January 2013, in the evening. The diagnosis of cholera was posed, due to profuse uncolored diarrhea and vomiting. Rehydration and antibiotic therapy were immediately prescribed. The patient left the hospital. The sleep–wake cycle was disturbed during 5 days and nights, with a complete insomnia on the fourth night at the hospital. He felt good in the morning of January 23, and only slept at night. He was released the next day in the morning.

and then 1 l hourly. Antibiotic treatment (tetraclyclines, phenicols, sulfonamides) helps breaking *Vibrio cholerae* portage. Antibiotics sometimes develop resistance and in that case fluoroquinolones and third-generation cephalosporins may be used, but their high cost is a limiting factor in countries with limited resources.

Prophylaxis

Strict prophylactic measures will be applied in the context of epidemic risk (war, population displacement, refugee camps, etc.).

When the epidemic has started and after laboratory confirmation of the diagnosis, several steps must be taken: strict isolation of patients; disinfection of vomiting with 5 % bleach during 4 h and disinfection of feces with 4 % cre-

syl sodium or warm milk during 6 h; bleaching or boiling of sanitizing utensils and patient clothes; washing corpses with water and burial disinfectant and enveloping corpses in antiseptic-sprayed shrouds before burial or cremation; disinfection of floors and walls with 5 % cresyl or bleach solutions. Caregivers should be experienced to prevent the spread of germs (wearing coat with long sleeves, boots, and masks; disinfection of hands with soap, alcohol, or bleach before returning home).

Chemoprophylaxis may not be realistic as it requires treating the whole population at risk and may trigger resistance to antibiotics. Furthermore, antibiotic treatment efficacy lasts 3 weeks, after which individuals become again fully susceptible to infection.

Vaccination confers unreliable and incomplete protection, which is only valid for 3–4 months in practice.

References

1. Bourdelais P, Raulot JY. Une peur bleue, histoire du choléra en France, 1832–1854. Paris: Payot; 1987.
2. Metchnikoff E. Sur l'immunité et la réceptivité vis–à–vis du choléra intestinal. In: Recherches sur le choléra et les vibrions. Ann Inst Pasteur. 1894;8:529–89.
3. Ackerknecht EH. Anticontagionism between 1821 and 1867: the Fielding H. Garrison lecture 1948. Int J Epidemiol. 2009;38(1):7–21.
4. Balakrish GN, Narain JP. From endotoxin to exotoxin: De's rich legacy to cholera. Bull World Health Organ. 2010;88(3):237–40.
5. Casanova JM, Ariño Espada MR. Jaime Ferrán and the cholera vaccine. Immunología. 1992;11(1):32–6.
6. Finkelstein R. Cholera enterotoxin (Choleragen): a historical perspective. In: Barua D, Greenough WB III, editors. Cholera. New York: Plenum Medical; 1992. pp.155–218.
7. Sur D, Lopez AL, Kanungo S, et al. Efficacy and safety of a modified killed–whole–cell oral cholera vaccine in India: an interim analysis of a cluster–randomised, double–blind, placebo–controlled trial. Lancet. 2009;74:1694–702.
8. Leca AP. Et le choléra s'abattit sur Paris 1832. Paris: Albin Michel; 1982.
9. Coignerai–Devillers L. La France et le choléra. Revue d'histoire de la pharmacie. 1988;76(276):101–3.
10. WHO. Cholera 2003. Wkly Epidemiol Rec. 2004;79(31):281–8.
11. Piarroux R, Barrais R, Faucher B, Haus R, Piarroux M, Gaudart J, et al. Understanding the cholera epidemic, Haiti. Emerg Infect Dis. 2011;17(7):1161–8.
12. Karki R. Cholera incidence among patients with diarrhea visiting National Public Health Laboratory, Nepal. Jpn J Infect Dis. 2010;63:185–7.
13. Prescott LM, Bhattacharjee NK. Viability of El Tor in common foodstuffs found in an endemic cholera area. Bull World Health Organ. 1969;40(6):980–2.
14. Sack DA, Sack RB, Nair GB, Siddique AK. Cholera. Lancet. 2004;363(9404):223–33.
15. Constantin de Magny G, Colwell RR. Cholera and climate: a demonstrated relationship. TransAm Clin Climatol Assoc. 2009;120:119–28.
16. Krueger JM, Majde JA. Humoral links between sleep and the immune system. Ann NY Acad Sci. 2003;992:9–20.
17. Buguet A, Bouteille B, Cespuglio R, Chapotot F. Maladies infectieuses et sommeil. In: Billiard M, Dauvilliers Y, Editors. Les troubles du sommeil. Paris: Masson; 2005. pp.309–23.
18. Lieberman HR, Bathalon GP, Falco CM, Kramer FM, Morgan CA, Niro P. Severe decrements in cognition function and mood induced by sleep loss, heat, dehydration, and undernutrition during simulated combat. Biol Psychiatry. 2005;57:422–9.
19. Buguet A, Gati R, Soriba M, Melin B, Montmayeur A, Alou S, Wamba B, Bogui P, Lonsdorfer J. Exercise and sleep in a dry tropical climate: preliminary results in 3 subjects. Sports Med Digest. 1991;2:15–7.
20. MontmayeurA, BuguetA, Sollin H, Lacour JR. Exercise and sleep in four African sportsmen living in the Sahel. A pilot study. Int J Sports Med. 1994;15:42–5.
21. Melin B, Curé M, Jimenez C, Savourey G, Bittel J. Déshydratation, réhydratation et exercice musculaire en ambiance chaude. Cah Nutr Diét. 1990;25:383–8.
22. Bastuji H, Jouvet M. Intérêt de l'agenda de sommeil pour l'étude des troubles de la vigilance. Electroencephalogr Clin Neurophysiol.1985;60(4):299–305.
23. Lapeyssonnie L. Chemoprophylaxis of cholera: value, expectations, and limitations. Méd Trop: Rev Corps Santé Col. 1971;31(1): 127–

Encephalitis Lethargica

20

David Parkes

To give even an approximate complete enumeration of the publications relating to encephalitis lethargica since my first communication of 17th April 1917, when I described this new disease, is impossible owing to their immense number. (Constantin von Economo) [1]

It may be stated without reservation that our knowledge of the pathogenesis of epidemic encephalitis leaves much that is obscure…there is no evidence that the disease is contagious, and no light has been thrown on the method of transmission. The therapeutic methods are symptomatic and empirical. (Frederick Tilney and Hubert Shattuck Howe) [2]

Figure 20.1 shows a picture of Constantin von Economo, (1876–1931) in 1910 [3, 4]. From 1906, he worked in the Viennese psychiatric clinic of Wagner von Jauregg, concentrating on mental illness, neurology, neuropathology and later on the care of the war wounded. Following an elder brother's death in the First World War, Constantin, an Austrian soldier and a founder of the Viennese flying club was forbidden to fly by his parents. Medicine was to gain by his monumental studies that included work on the cerebral cortex and on the future evolution of the brain, as well as at least 18 papers on encephalitis lethargica written between 1917 and 1920. Despite a recent review of the subject up to 2011, essential reading for all interested in one of the most unusual of all brain diseases [5, 6], von Economo's 1929 monograph (translated into English by Newman in 1931) remains pre-eminent [7].

Constantin von Economo came to hold the title of professor both of Neurology and Psychiatry in the University of Vienna. Encephalitis lethargica may have affected in total up to a million people worldwide. The disease virtually disappeared in 1927. Vilenski suggests that perhaps only 80 cases with typical clinical features, sometimes also with chorea, dystonia, oromandibular dystonia, myoclonus or other dyskinesia; and in some with magnetic resonance imaging (MRI) scan evidence of inflammatory change in the basal ganglia and midbrain tegmentum [8] were then reported up to 2011.

In 1917, the language of sleep–wake illness was still largely derived from ancient Greek. Rapid eye movement (REM) sleep had not been discovered, and nothing was known of sleep architecture or circadian rhythms. Although the electrical activity of the brain had been studied from the late nineteenth century, electronic amplification of brain signals in man had to await the 1930s development of the valve amplifier. At best, investigation of brain disease was limited to crude examination of the cerebrospinal fluid (CSF) and a test for the then ubiquitous mimic, syphilis, developed by Wassermann and Dean initially using antigen from aborted foetuses from the dustbins of Berlin.[1]

As a medical student in London in the 1950s, encephalitis lethargica as an acute illness had long died out, although assumed 'post-encephalitic' narcolepsy and 'post-encephalitic' Parkinsonism were common topics for presentation at grand rounds in the venerable surroundings of the Saturday morning demonstrations at the lecture theatre of the London Queen Square Hospital for Nervous and Mental diseases. Many of the demonstrators were great demonstrators as well as great physicians. They included the distinguished aphasiologist Macdonald Critchley, author of *The Divine Banquet of the Brain* [9]; a classic precursor of Oliver Sack's *Awakenings*; and the neurologist MacArdle, who may himself have had a delayed sleep phase, being well known for his sometimes late arrivals as well as for his clinical acumen. Several neurologists had first made their reputation in the 1920s by their writings about epidemic encephalitis.

The demonstrations were most valuable for their teaching of clinical examination skills. With hindsight, wrong attribution of several features may not have been uncommon at the time when a formal discipline of sleep medicine did

---

D. Parkes (✉)
Clinical Neurology, The Maudsley Hospital and King's
College Hospital, London, UK
e-mail: dandsparkes@googlemail.com

[1] As frequently recounted by Dean to medical students when professor of pathology at Cambridge in the 1950s. I can find no written evidence however.

S. Chokroverty, M. Billiard (eds.), *Sleep Medicine,* DOI 10.1007/978-1-4939-2089-1_20,
© Springer Science+Business Media, LLC 2015

Fig. 20.1 Constantin von Economo (1876–1931)

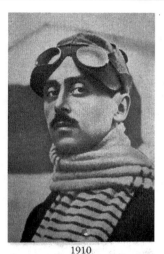

1910

not exist, and the popular name '*sleeping* sickness' for encephalitis lethargica was perhaps not quite correct. However, encephalitis lethargica was one of the most fearful as well as most bizarre afflictions of the brain from 1916–1917 onwards. It breached the previous divide between neurology and psychiatry, sanity and madness, brain and mind. Any potential future epidemic may highlight new areas of molecular biology, epigenetics and protein chemistry in sleep–wake and consciousness research.

Two of these patients remain vividly in my memory. Both, long-term survivors of acute encephalitis, were left with the abnormal postures and involuntary movements of dystonia rather than a sleep–wake disorder. The first made a meagre living as a hymn-writer and the second as a curator in a London art museum. Both men had bizarre postures and gait with torsion, flexion and hyperextension of the trunk, interrupted by functional blindness due to spontaneous oculogyric crises with involuntary upward gaze. Now, such patients are no longer seen. One of the most remarkable memorials to encephalitis lethargica, emphasising movement rather than sleep disorder, can be seen in a Welcome Foundation three-minute film clip from 1924 on You Tube.

As late as 1929, SA Kinnier-Wilson, physician for outpatients at the National Hospital Queen Square thought that sleep disorders could not be alluded to as diseases, and reported that during one 20-year period, he had not seen a case of narcolepsy, 'although it seemed likely that this had a similar physiology to epilepsy' [10]. Wilson, when it suited him, could be a stickler for language, objecting to the term hepatolenticular degeneration when used to describe the condition he had first identified. When this term was used in one occasion in his presence, he is reported to have said, 'Are you referring to my disease?' He argued that 'encephalitis lethargica' was a misnomer since it was the patient, not the

illness that was lethargic.[2] However, by the 1940s, Wilson had come to accept the reality of the narcoleptic syndrome as well as the nomenclature of von Economo.

At the start of the twentieth century, and at the first appearance of epidemic encephalitis lethargica, sleep medicine that existed was largely confined to the study of insomnia rather than to the much less common and unusual cases where apparent sleep could be accompanied by 'numbness', 'powerlessness', 'deadness' or 'apathy' [11]. An odd epidemic of drowsiness or 'trance' known as 'Nona' had been reported to Von Economo by his mother, but this depended largely on folk memory [12]. Excess sleep and lethargy were popularly believed to be the result of low moral fibre, signs of laziness and largely confined to black Africa or the peasantry of Ireland. Thomas Winterbottom (1766–1859) had published his best-known work about sleep, *An account of the Native Africans in the Neighbourhood of Sierra Leone* in 1803, and Gelineau in his monograph of 1881 given his report of 14 patients with the sleep seizures of 'narcolepsy' and so-called *catalepsie* but daytime sleepiness was still largely a medical curiosity [13, 14]. Loose terminology and in particular the term *'narcolepsy'* often led to more confusion than clarity. Also, the literature of psychological medicine in the first half of the twentieth century was influenced by ideas of 'mental' and 'moral' illness, separation of 'mind' and 'brain' and not least by some of the imaginings of Freud, who was an assistant professor (1904) and then full professor (1920) of neurology in Vienna at the first appearance of encephalitis lethargica. Case reports of this illness questioned many previous concepts of clear distinction between disease of the mind and disease of the brain.

Encephalitis Lethargica

With this background, Economo in 1917 described seven patients in a first paper, an additional four in a second, with common features of lethargy and restricted eye movement [15, 16]. The onset was acute, in a matter of hours or days with malaise, fever, headache and neck stiffness, 'subalertness', 'reduced attention', 'mental dazing', 'somnolence', persistent sleep bordering 'stupor' and then 'unrousable' coma. One subject was a somnambulist, another fell asleep 'whenever…standing or walking'. Yet another 'when aroused…(was)…not alert'…with 'attention only possible for short periods'. In contrast, another subject, a boy of 12, 'lay awake in bed day and night'. One patient was deluded, and another hallucinated. There was partial or complete paralysis of eye movement, reduced or absent voluntary

---

[2] . Perhaps it should be pointed out that James Parkinson did not have paralysis agitans, and that the term Parkinson's disease was first used by Charcot.

up-gaze and 'dull, half closed eyes'. The disease was severe, ending in the death of four subjects although three made an initial complete recovery over the next 3–16 weeks. Of the 11 patients, 10 were young, aged from 12 to 38 and one was aged 56.

After Economo's descriptions, many similar cases were reported, and the disease spread worldwide over the next decade, although the presentation was very variable from case to case and from year to year. In addition to lethargy and involvement of the third, fourth, fifth and sixth nerves, Vilenski and Gilman (2011) recorded well over 50 different signs and symptoms that might be present [17]. Both sexes were equally affected. Hall (1924) considered that of each 100 cases, 25 died in the acute phase, 25 recovered practically completely, and 50 went on to develop secondary symptoms after days, weeks or months of apparent recovery. The most serious and frequent of these included motor disorders, change of personality and mental defect, whilst 'lethargy' or sleep disturbances were less pronounced than at initial presentation. The pattern of late disease depended largely on the age of initial infection. Infants went on to develop mental defects, and children personality disorders that were sometimes accompanied by disturbed sleep—nocturnal restless behaviour continuing from the primary illness was more common or possibly more disruptive in children than in adults. The severity of secondary symptoms was largely unrelated to the severity of the initial attack, and with late so-called hypersomnia, narcolepsy and insomnia, it was often difficult or impossible to establish a causal relationship with previous encephalitis. In contrast, Parkinsonism eventually developed in most if not all adults who survived the initial illness, and had a uniformly bad prognosis.

Encephalitis Lethargica and Spanish Flu

Cruchet first reported cases of possible encephalitis lethargica amongst French World War troops in Verdun at the end of 1916 and 1917 [18]. Previous sporadic outbreaks of influenza had occurred in these soldiers from 1915, and it was difficult at first to separate the two illnesses. A great influenza pandemic, later named the Spanish flu, then broke out in Europe between 1918 and 1921. Both diseases went on to spread over all continents. Many physicians, like Cruchet, first saw encephalitis lethargica during or after flu, and it was natural to assume a connection. However, von Economo held from the start that influenza did not cause or lead on to encephalitis lethargica. The name 'Spanish' flu derived from the facts that the Spanish press—Spain not being involved in the Great War—was amongst the first to report extensively on the severity of the pandemic. Three major waves of influenza occurred over the next 10 years, and up to a billion people, quarter to half the world population of 1.86 billion

at that time, were affected. The total loss of life worldwide from Spanish flu was estimated at perhaps 50–100 million, greater than that due to the 1914–1918 war and surpassing even the Black Death of medieval Europe. This compared with the half- to one-million deaths from encephalitis lethargica.

The influenza virus may have predisposed to but did not cause encephalitis lethargica. Influenza, but not encephalitis lethargica, was highly contagious with a high rate of case-to-case, school and family transmission. The peaks of the natural frequency curves of the two conditions did not match, although as with encephalitis lethargica, most cases of influenza occurred in winter. The clinical features of the two conditions were usually quite distinct, and in most cases the tracheitis, upper respiratory infection, malaise, fever, lethargy and muscle aching of influenza recovered within a week following bed rest, although a few subjects died within 24 h of infection. Influenza does sometimes lead to brain inflammation, although this is very uncommon, occurring in perhaps 1 in 100,000 cases who go on to develop headache, vomiting, delirium and coma during influenza outbreaks.

Sleep–Wake Disturbance and Encephalitis Lethargica

Encephalitis lethargica may be more relevant to the study of wakefulness than to that of sleep: in as much as these can be separated. The defining sleep disturbance of encephalitis lethargica was described by von Economo as the inability to maintain wakefulness rather than the occurrence of sleep. His name for the illness was based on the striking lethargy of the initial meningeal and brain involvement of the first phase. Subsequent popular use of the term 'sleeping sickness' in place of 'encephalitis lethargica' may have overstressed the sleep component in a multifaceted disease. In practice, signs and symptoms of extrapyramidal motor disorder and of mental disturbance were more persistent, troublesome, prominent and frequent in the late illness than were lethargy, too much or too little sleep.

Economo suggested that lesions causing *insomnia* were mainly situated in the basal forebrain, those causing *hypersomnia* in the midbrain tegmentum and posterior hypothalamus: but this division may have been more apparent than real and has little value as to the exact localisation of sleep–wake systems in the brain. Encephalitis lethargica was rarely if ever a cause of persistent true hypersomnia as opposed to stupor, of the narcoleptic syndrome, of the complaint of difficulty in falling asleep or in maintaining sleep; although it seems probable that it sometimes might have led to symptomatic central sleep apnoea.

Lethargy, Hypersomnolence, Stupor

What is lethargy? The Greek term 'lethargos' dates from the medical school of Hippocrates, and describes forgetfulness which, when accompanied by *fever*, could lead to rapid death. To drink from Lethe, the river of Hades in mythology, led to forgetfulness of the past. In the middle ages, 'lethargic' came to indicate morbid torpor as well as prolonged unresponsiveness, and in this sense was used by von Economo. 'Lethargy' implies physical 'tiredness' but although we all know what 'tiredness' means, it varies over time and setting, is not quite in the same category as 'fatigue', 'arousal', 'awareness' or 'vigilance', and carries the mental burden of disinclination. Economo did not use the term 'lethargy' in any of his first eleven case descriptions but rather *somnolence, delirium, confusion, stupor, tendency to sleep, mental diminution, continually dazzlement, long reaction time, reduced consciousness, falling asleep standing, walking and sitting; drowsiness, hypersomnolence.*

Lethargy, merging with stupor, may be a disorder of arousal, rather than of sleep. Arousal from stupor demands a stronger stimulus than arousal from sleep. Lethargy, unlike sleep has no definite circadian rhythm, distinction or division into various behavioural stages, and can last days, months or sometimes, years. In lethargy, there is no periodic dream mentation, no regular postural shifts nor intervallic atonia. Muscle tone in patients with post-encephalitic lethargy was sometimes described as increased rather than diminished, with 'catatonic' resistance to the movement and preservation of enforced posture: this observation may, however, have been biased by extrapyramidal damage in patients with encephalitis lethargica.

Hypersomnolence implies definite sleep, and may be misleading if applied retrospectively to encephalitic lethargy. 'Pseudosleep', popular terminology in the pandemic period to describe stupor, does not totally get away with the problem. To further confuse the issue, Economo observed that in three subjects 'somnolence' was independent of the severity of all other conditions, as well as 'not connected with diminished consciousness'. The word 'consciousness' defined as the 'knowledge of what goes on in one's own mind' might today not be used, but the meaning is clear. Subjects with hypersomnolence had an intense desire for sleep, reporting that 'it was impossible... or near-impossible...to stay awake'. The emphasis is on the preservation of vigilance, motor response, and with intact cortical functions of cognition, memory, personality and intellect when aroused despite 'pressure' for sleep or the near inability to remain awake. Several observers stressed that the 'sleep' itself in encephalitis lethargica could be normal, with normal eye closure, meiosis, atonia, and dream report. Any abnormality of sleep lay only in its long duration and considerable depth, a large stimulus being required for arousal. The subject might then be immediately alert.

'Unrousable' sleep was sometimes associated with encephalitis as well as head injury, brain tumours and many other metabolic and cerebral disorders. No clear nomenclature was possible in a pre-encephalographic era, and without careful behavioural studies. This could last days, months, or even in the fabled case of the seven sleepers of Ephesus, for many years. Often likened to hibernation, this is journalistic, not scientific.

One EEG recording in a recent post-encephalitic subject who developed Parkinsonism, during 'stupor' from which the patient could be aroused only by deep painful stimuli, showed diffuse high-voltage delta and theta activity [19]. Perhaps other electroencephalographic parallels to encephalitis lethargica today come from patients with 'idiopathic' hypersomnolence or the Kleine–Levin syndrome, who complain of lethargy and tiredness and go on to develop prolonged sleep episodes lasting up to 20 out of 24 h, usually persisting a few days to several weeks. Here, the EEG between attacks is usually completely normal. During episodes of periodic lethargy or stupor, there may be decrease in stage 3–4 non-rapid eye movement (NREM) and also in REM sleep, interrupted by alpha activity; with occasional early-onset REM sleep and a very short sleep latency.

'Narcolepsy' and Encephalitis Lethargica

The term 'narcolepsy' continues to be one of the most widely misused in journalism if not in medicine. A typical misconception is shown by reports such as that in 2011, when an English burglar was let off from his full sentence when the defence claimed he had 'Attention Deficit Hyperactivity Disorder—which can cause disruption to sleep patterns and narcolepsy, a chronic sleep disorder characterised by an excessive urge to sleep at inappropriate times'. The 20-year-old had stolen DVDs, computer games, sandpaper, toiletries and elastic bands. The court was told that he had a 'sleeping disorder that meant he was awake for up to two weeks at a time and then could be out like a light for one or two days'. As 24-h supervision in the community might prove difficult, health and safety concerns for his attendants combined with powerful medical advocacy and a lenient judge led to a ruling that he could not be sentenced to unpaid work [20].

William Gowers in his *Textbook of the Nervous System* stated in 1904 that most attacks of 'narcolepsy' occurred in hysterical subjects, and that for every case of narcolepsy, 200 cases of epilepsy came under observation. The term 'cataplexy' was first introduced by Henneberg in 1916 [21], the same year as Economo first observed encephalitis. A firm terminology of narcolepsy, the narcoleptic syndrome, and of cataplexy was not established until the second half of the twentieth century although Lowenfeld in 1902 had stated that the association of sleep attacks and 'falls' was necessary for the diagnosis of the syndrome [22]. It is perhaps unfortunate that Lowenfeld's requirement was not always fulfilled; and the term *narcoleptic syndrome* was not always adopted to describe a specific illness, *narcolepsy* for a symptom with many different causes.

Bassetti (2007) reported that by 1924, although the narcoleptic syndrome was known, that a total of only 34 typical cases had been described; in comparison with many thousands of cases of encephalitis lethargica [23]. Although encephalitis could result in profound and continuous sleepiness—or at least, 'pseudosleep'—the concept that it might also have ever been a significant cause of the true sleep and accompanying cataplexy of the narcoleptic syndrome is uncertain. I have seen perhaps a dozen subjects over 50 years with probable or definite post-encephalitic Parkinsonism, and none with a definite post-encephalitis lethargica narcoleptic syndrome as determined by previous acute meningoencephalitis with initial lethargy and ocular palsy. However, there are a few reports of encephalitis lethargica as a probable trigger to the narcoleptic syndrome.

Adie described a boy aged 14 who in 1923 developed sleeplessness, fever, delirium and jerking of the limbs, followed by restlessness during the night and sleepiness during the day; with double vision. He recovered from this state in about three months, but remained apt to drop off to sleep in the daytime, particularly with any monotonous task. He then had attacks in which, if he laughed, his knees gave way and he fell to the ground. He said, 'at the Scout camp the boys used to amuse themselves by making me laugh and then run away, leaving me helpless on the ground. I cannot go to the picture now, because if I am amused my head flops about and people look at me instead of the pictures'. By 1926, the attacks were becoming less frequent [24].

Symonds described a somewhat similar patient who complained of excessive sleepiness, and noticed that whenever he laughed or felt excited, he fell down. An attack was witnessed; 'a little twitching of the facial muscles, short interval of silence, he talked vaguely in Icelandic, then said, "I cannot move my arms"'. As evidence of previous encephalitis, this subject had Parkinsonism [25].

Insomnia and Encephalitis Lethargica

Overall, 'insomnia' was reported in about 10% of cases of acute encephalitis lethargica, almost all in children with hyperkinesis, as opposed to the 50–60% of subjects who developed 'pseudosomnolence' or 'hypersomnolence'. 'Insomnia' was occasionally reported to be atypical, resistant to hypnotics, although Tilney and Howe in 1920 included 'medinol' or barbituric acid dissolved in warm milk in their therapeutic regime. 'Insomnia', when reported in encephalitis lethargica, may not have referred to difficulty in sleeping, staying asleep

or sleep of poor quality but rather was a term used by parents of children affected with night arousal and hyperactivity, often accompanied by restlessness, involuntary movements, dystonia or chorea. The exhausted child would then fall asleep at dawn, and be difficult to arouse until noon. Some reports described this as 'inversion' of the sleep rhythm, and likened this more to sleep patterns in both birds and other animals than to those of normal boys and girls.

Nocturnal excitement in children occurred in both acute and secondary cases of encephalitis; often blamed for 'exhausting the brain' and subsequent lethargy. A typical report of the time, in which observation cannot always be separated from assumption, reads 'After sleep the rested brain is refreshed…and the child is surprisingly normal during the rest of the day. The brain is however soon tired, and with this early fatigue the excitement recurs, once more to go through a familiar train of events. This is emphasised by the fact that other excitomotor phenomena often appear simultaneously—respiratory, spasmodic, etc. It is a matter of common experience that such phenomena are worse when the patient is tired'. Nocturnal excitement sometimes did not begin until 7 or 8 weeks of the onset of illness, often persisted, and could prove one of the most intractable of all symptoms: 'Towards night the parents note a change in the child's behaviour: he becomes restless, excited, and runs about the house prying into things. He will not obey. When put to bed, he does not go to sleep, but jumps up and down, shakes the bed, talks, sings, whistles etc. He spends the whole night in constant activity. Nocturnal enuresis is not uncommon'. In one case of nocturnal wakefulness, the child made continual noises in his throat the whole night through and later was constantly blowing his nose. The syndrome was thought to be so peculiar as to suffice to establish a retrospective diagnosis of encephalitis lethargica.

The more usual nature of insomnia as a self-complaint of difficulty in falling or staying asleep was perhaps no more frequent in encephalitis lethargica than in any other serious physical or mental illness, and related to anxiety, depression, discomfort and pain as well as in particular to the stiffness, tremor and impaired motility of Parkinsonism.

Circadian Rhythms and Encephalitis Lethargica

Although sleep–wake inversion in children such as the above was not uncommon, the effect may have been secondary to environment, motor restlessness, fear, loneliness and the dark rather than to any primary circadian disturbance. The technology to study true circadian rhythm was still half a century distant. However, 'alterations in the sleep cycle' were sometimes described, and Howard and Lees reported in 1987 a post-encephalitic subject with 'sleep inversion'.

Respiration and Encephalitis Lethargica

Respiratory abnormalities, both sleeping and waking, with changes in frequency and rhythm were common in both acute and chronic encephalitis lethargica. Polypnoea was the most usual of these but the opposite, slow breathing, as well as apnoea and periodic respiration were observed in both acute and chronic encephalitis lethargica. Tachypnoea could alternate with periods of apnoea resulting in cyanosis, and paroxysms of hyperpnoea could lead to tetany. Such reports were uncommon and not always clearly separated from the focal dystonias of extrapyramidal disease, as when Schmidt (1921) reported 'tetany' as persisting in the right hand for 2 months in a case 'without respiratory troubles' [26]. Respiratory tics, only briefly controlled by an effort of will, took several forms, with sniffing, blowing, spitting and coughing. A variety of tic-like or myoclonic movements were recorded including jerking of the respiratory muscles, pectorals, and sternomastoids. Cruchet and Rocher described a child with rhythmic 76/min jerking bringing the arms forwards and the shoulders together [27]. Such involuntary movements might be limited, abolished, or confined to sleep although apnoea was almost always most prominent during slumber.

Dreams and Encephalitis Lethargica

Paralysis of eye movements and also gaze palsies would be predicted to interfere with the correlates of REM sleep. That this is the case is suggested by the finding that in progressive supranuclear palsy, comparable to encephalitis lethargica in midbrain damage and with impaired saccadic eye movements and failure of voluntary up-gaze, that it can be difficult to identify REMs during sleep recording. In some but not all subjects there is also loss of dream mentation, with the typical report, 'I have had no dreams for several years'. For von Economo, impaired eye movement at both nuclear and supranuclear levels was a hallmark of acute encephalitis lethargica, although visual perception was retained. This was also the case in the secondary phase Critchley in 1928 reported that 64 of 72 subjects with post-encephalitic Parkinsonism had 'jerky' eye movements [28]. Despite these findings, there are many reports of vivid and frequent dreaming in encephalitis lethargica. Stern (1928) reported that patients might sleep for long periods, days and nights, but continued to have the same 'dreams as normal people': suggesting the preservation of at least one physiologic aspect of REM sleep [29]. A continuum has been suggested between dreams, sleep fragmentation and visual hallucinosis [30] and as with dreaming, visual hallucinosis was not uncommon in encephalitis lethargica. However, the anatomical substrate of dreaming may be different from that of visual hallucinosis; as suggested by the finding that in progressive supranuclear

palsy with ophthalmoplegia, despite a shrunken midbrain with MRI scan showing an axial midbrain diameter less than 17 mm but well preserved cortex, dream mentation or at least dream recall is lost whilst visual hallucinations still occur with the dopaminergic drugs used to treat bradyphrenia and rigidity.

Mental Disorders and Encephalitis Lethargica

The most important message of encephalitis lethargica for sleep medicine may not concern brain waves, the biochemistry or physiology of sleep, but asks a basic question of human freedom: whilst awake, are we slaves or free? In particular, this question was raised by the compulsive behaviour that was especially prominent: as when involuntary upward eye movements could be accompanied by thoughts such as 'kill. kill, kill'. About one third of subjects with acute encephalitis lethargica went on to develop compulsive behaviour, changes in personality, cognition and memory. The typical mental state was of marked slowing of both movement and thought. Depression was common and suicide not infrequent, although some developed hypomania. In the late stages, emotional responses were slow or poor. Many patients were unemployable in the community, impossible in the home and took up numerous places in the mental hospitals of the 1920s and onwards until their death.

Personality changes with hyperactivity and restlessness, both by day and by night, were reported mostly in children; described as having poor control over their behaviour and their instinctual drive, unable to concentrate at school or remain occupied on the same task at home. Both children and adults could steal, take part in inappropriate sexual activity, and previous good behaviour was disturbed by outbursts of anger. Typical reports described previous outgoing and friendly personalities who went on to disturb the peace of their families. Hall (1924) reported a big, powerful girl who had periodic outbursts of violence to her parents if crossed in the mildest of matters, made mischief with the neighbours so that one group took her side, another that of her parents. She eventually was sent to an asylum. Psychosis was frequent and took a bewildering number of forms. Hypochondriasis might be of psychotic severity, paranoid visual and auditory hallucinatory states occurred and there were descriptions of a number of 'schizophrenic-like' illnesses. These states were often accompanied by motor slowing, profound apathy and lethargy as well as by Parkinsonism, overeating and obesity or alternatively and less commonly, by loss of appetite and slenderness.

Criminality was not uncommon. Auden and others reported cases in which the children had fallen into the hands of the police, and amongst these recorded from asylums a certain number who had been unmanageable children [31].

MacPhail recorded a case in a 10-year-old boy who 'took a knife to his mother', 'threatened to cut his brother up', and 'took a hatchet to his sister'. Eventually, it was necessary to send him to an asylum. In the asylum, he was 'quarrelsome and aggressive, but mentally alert and active, and very difficult in consequence [32]'. Amongst other cases reported from the asylums was one of a boy aged 15 who seemed to improve after being there a year. Soon after discharge, however, he was arrested by the police for assaulting a girl of 17 who had laughed at him. He had nearly strangled her. He was bound over on the promise of his brothers to look after him, and a month later committed suicide by hanging himself to the end of his bed by his necktie. Homicide by small children was sometimes reported and encephalitis pleaded in their defence; although any connection may have been tenuous. The medico-legal issues of such cases were difficult, as with the defence of legal 'insanity' raised by the complex concerns of criminality whilst sleep-walking. Fairweather (1947) in the UK described patients in the Rampton State Institution for violent and dangerous offenders admitted following encephalitis with self-mutilation, sexual deviation or perversion and serious aggression of many years duration [33]. One conclusion drawn from cases of encephalitis lethargica like these was that men and women are robotic slaves rather than free agents or that at least any apparent freedom is limited or illusory.

Pathology and Aetiology of Encephalitis Lethargica

In the sleeping sickness called Nona, a probable precursor of encephalitis lethargica, Gayet in 1875 had identified lesions in the midbrain and hypothalamus [34]. Although in patients dying in the acute phase of encephalitis lethargica, the acute disease caused an inflammation of the meninges, supporting tissues and the glia rather than damaging neurones, axons or myelin of the brain, as in Nona, and the changes were usually most severe in brain areas today recognised as associated with cortical activation during wakefulness. These included the central tegmentum (tegmentum—from Latin for 'covering') of the pons and midbrain, the posterior hypothalamus and basal forebrain [35]. Both the gross pathology and its distribution were similar in nature to those of many other forms of encephalitis including other causes of drowsiness such as African sleeping sickness, syphilitic general paralysis of the insane, and Wernicke's encephalopathy. In chronic encephalitis lethargica, in contrast to the acute phase, a 2009 review of 35 epidemic era cases by Anderson, Vilenski and Duvoisin showed that cortical rather than brain-stem damage was the most consistent finding [36].

Physical signs and symptoms in both the acute and chronic stages of encephalitis lethargica had little or no relationship to the exact brain areas showing greatest damage at postmortem. The pathological features pointed to a probable infective cause, perhaps initially via the upper respiratory tract, but no definite virus, bacterium or other organism was identified in the classic era. In later recent somewhat similar examples, Coxsackie, Echo, polio and other viruses have all been isolated: and it seems probable that encephalitis lethargica, despite its 1917–1927 pandemic nature, was not a single disease entity. Specific brain neurotransmitter—protein system attack, metabolic factors, vascular predilection and immune involvement have all been suggested to explain the apparent selectivity of encephalitis lethargica to midbrain amongst other areas, but no theory exactly matches the facts.

In support of neurotransmitter theories, the locus coeruleus, the main brain site of noradrenaline neurones projecting to suprachiasmatic areas as well as to cortex, could be heavily involved—but animal lesions of this nucleus have little effect on sleep or waking, whilst many other neurotransmitter molecules are found in closely adjacent areas. For metabolic theorists, the midbrain tegmental area, one central area of damage in encephalitis lethargica, is also that most targeted in Wernicke's encephalopathy. This causes lethargy, torpor and apathy; and was eventually linked to thiamine deficiency. The metabolic importance of thiamine in glucose metabolism may suggest that brain areas involved in the mechanisms of alertness, attention, vigilance, waking and sleeping are also amongst the most metabolically active regions of the brain: CSF glucose levels were slightly raised in encephalitis lethargica. There is little or no present evidence of an abnormal immune mechanism, despite recent findings of anti-neuronal antibodies and a similar histopathology to that of encephalitis lethargica in immune-mediated Sydenham's chorea.

Finally, many of the symptoms of encephalitis lethargica have a close relation to those of thalamic infarct in vascular disease. The exact presentation here depends on the nuclei involved, but includes early reduced but varying awareness, personality change, apathy and disinhibition as well as psychotic mood changes. Caplan in 1980 reviewed the striking picture that resulted from occlusion of the rostral branches of the basilar artery [37]. This results in infarction of the midbrain, thalamus and portions of the temporal and occipital lobes, producing an array of oculomotor, visual and behavioural abnormalities often with changes in alertness and in the sleep–wake cycle. Perhaps the most remarkable syndrome to appear is that of peduncular hallucinosis, sometimes combined to a half-field, and with or without visual field defects. The hallucinations are recognised as unreal despite their dramatic nature. Caplan's patient saw a parrot in beautiful plumage to the right, and pictures of relatives flashed on the wall to the left.

Terminology of Subalertness

One important lesson for sleep medicine from encephalitis lethargica is the importance of an exact terminology of lethargy, tiredness, fatigue, subalertness, stupor and allied states. However, any 'lethargy' definition and grading, analogous to those of coma, may be impossible to achieve, as dependent on temporal as well as on both 'inside' and 'outside' factors that determine the relationship of self to environment.

It is tempting to speculate that whatever the agent, encephalitis lethargica was localised to a region of the brain with both high blood flow and high metabolic rate, at the centre of a computer-like system that controls wake, rest and sleep switches of the brain. The following terminology of lethargy and associated states is founded not on medicine but on the Oxford Dictionary, where quotation, common usage and habit illustrate the difficult task of matching exact language to brain physiology: of matching brain and mind. Many of these definitions can be questioned, do not fit with medical terminology, involve the idea of 'mind' as independent of 'brain' or depend on philosophy more than physics. Further understanding of these states and the boundaries between brain and behaviour is one important challenge raised by encephalitis lethargica for sleep medicine today.

Alert	Watchful, vigilant, lively
Arousal	Awake from sleep, stir into activity, call into existence
Attention	Turn the mind to, apply oneself, be present
Aware	Conscious, not ignorant, well-informed
Cataplexy	Sudden temporary paralysis
Coma	Unnatural heavy sleep, prolonged unconsciousness
Confusion	Mix up in the mind
Consciousness	Aware, knowing in the mind, totality of a person's thoughts and feelings
Delirium	State of mind with incoherent speech, hallucinations and frenzied excitement
Dementia	Insanity, loss of intellectual power
Dream	Series of pictures or events in mind of sleeping person
Drowsy	Sleepy, half-asleep, dozing, sluggish, slow, languid
Fatigue	Weariness after exertion—weakness
Hallucination	Illusion, apparent perception of external object not actually present
Lethargy	Morbid drowsiness, torpor, inert, apathy, lack of interest, drowsy, trance-like
Narcolepsy	Fits of somnolence
Parkinsonism	Disease of nervous system with tremor, muscular rigidity and emaciation
Sleep	Bodily condition such as that which occurs for several hours each night
Stupor	Dazed state, torpidity
Tire	Grow weary, exhaust patience
Vigilance	Watchfulness, caution, circumspection

References

1. von Economo C. Encephalitis lethargica its sequelae and treatment. Oxford: Oxford University Press; 1931 (Newman K O trans. p. 200. The monograph *EpidemicEncephalitis*, by the Sheffield professor of medicine, Arthur J Hall, 1924, Wright, Bristol, pp. 229, gives 2056 references: Vilensky [2011], suggests over 9000 articles on the topic).
2. Tilney F, Shattuck HL. Epidemic encephalitis. New York: Hoeber; 1920. p. 251.
3. Spillman R. His Wife and Prof J von Wagner- Jauregg. Trans. Spillman R. Baron Constantin von Economo. His life and work. Burlington: Free Press Interstate Printing Corp; 1937. p. 126
4. van Bogaert L, Théodoridès J, von Economo C. The man and scientist. Wien: Verlag der Österreichischen Akademie der Wissenschaften; 1979; p. 138.
5. Vilensky JA. (Ed.) Encephalitis lethargica. Oxford: Oxford University Press; 2011. pp. 316.
6. Vilensky JA, Gilman S. Introduction. In: Vilensky Joel, editor. Encephalitis lethargica. Oxford: Oxford University Press; 2011. p. 3–7.
7. von Economo C. Encephalitis lethargica its sequelae and treatment. Trans. Newman KO. Oxford: Oxford University Press; 1931. pp. 201.
8. Howard RS, Lees AJ. Encephalitis lethargica: a report of four recent cases. Brain. 1987;110:19–33.
9. Critchley M. The divine banquet of the brain. New York: Raven; 1979. pp. 267.
10. Kinnear Wilson SAK. Modern problems in neurology. New York: William Wood and Co; 1929. pp. 364.
11. Macfarlane AW. Insomnia and its therapeutics. London: HK Lewis; 1890. pp. 366.
12. Longuet R. La Nona. Sem Méd. 1892;1:275–8.
13. Winterbottom TM. An account of the native Africans in the neighbourhood of Sierra Leone: to which is added, an account of the present state of medicine among them. London: Hatchard and Morman; 1803. pp. 8.
14. Gélineau JBE. De la Narcolepsie. Tessier et Tessier. Paris: Imprimerie de Sargeres; 1881.
15. von Economo C. Encephalitis lethargica. Wien klin Woch. 1917a;30:581–5.
16. von Economo C. Neue Beitrage zur Encephalitis lethargica. Neurol Cent. 1917b;5:866–78.
17. Vilensky JA, Gilman S. Epidemic encephalitis during the epidemic period. In: Vilenski JA, editor. Encephalitis lethargica. Oxford: Oxford University Press; 2011. p. 8–38.
18. Cruchet R. L'Encephalite épidemique. Paris: Doin and Co; 1929. pp. 135.
19. Rail D, Scholz C, Swash M. Post-encephalitic Parkinsonism: current experience. J Neurol Neurosurg Psychiat. 1981;44:670–6.
20. The Daily Telegraph. Saturday November 19. 2011. p. 17.
21. Henneberg R. Über genuine Narcolepsie. Neurol Zbl. 1916,30:282–90.
22. Lowenfeld L. Über Narcolepsie. Munch Med Wochenschr. 1902;49:1041–5.
23. Bassetti CL. Narcolepsy. In: A Culebras, editor. Sleep disorders and neurological diseases. New York: Informa Healthcare; 2007. pp. 83–116.

24. Adie WJ. Idiopathic narcolepsy: a disease sui generis, with remarks on the mechanisms of sleep. Brain. 1926;49:257–306.

25. Symonds CP. Narcolepsy as a symptom of encephalitis lethargica. Lancet. 1926;ii:1214–5.

26. Schmidt R. Storung des myostatischen Gleichgewichtes der Zunge nach Encephalitis epidemica. Med Klin Berl Wien. 1921;17:210.

27. Cruchet RR. Séquelle du type myorhythmique chez un enfant atteint d'encéphalomyélite epidemique. J Med Bordeaux. 1921;51:230.

28. Critchley AM. Ocular manifestations following encephalitis lethargica. Bristol Med-Chir J. 1928;45:113–24.

29. Stern F. Die Epidemische Encephalitis. Berlin: Julius Springer; 1928. pp. 541.

30. Aarsland D, Larsen JP, et al. Prevalence and clinical correlates of psychotic symptoms in Parkinson disease: a community based study. Arch Neurol. 1999;56:595–601.

31. Auden GA. Behaviour changes supervening upon encephalitis in children. Lancet. 1922;ii:901.

32. Macphail HD. Mental disorder resulting from encephalitis. J Ment Sci. 1922;68:169.

33. Fairweather DS. Psychiatric aspects of the post-encephalitic syndrome. J Ment Sci. 1947;93:201–54.

34. Gayet M. Affection encéphalique localisée aux étages supérieurs des pédoncles cérébraux et aux couches optiques. Arch Physiol. 1875;7:341–51.

35. von Economo C. Sleep as a problem of localization. J Nerv Ment Dis. 1930;71:249–59.

36. Anderson L, Vilenski J, Duvoisin R. Neuropathology of acute phase encephalitis lethargica: a review of cases from the epidemic period. Neuropathol Appl Biol. 2009;35:462–72.

37. Carrera E, Bogousslavsky J. The thalamus and behaviour: effects of anatomically distinct strokes. Neurology. 2006;66:1817–23.

38. Caplan LR. Top of the Basilar syndrome. Neurology. 1980;30:72–9.

African Sleeping Sickness

21

Alain Buguet, Raymond Cespuglio and Bernard Bouteille

Human African trypanosomiasis (HAT) or sleeping sickness is nowadays considered as one of the African "neglected diseases" [1]. Sleeping sickness is a vector-borne parasitic endemic disease in 36 sub-Saharan countries. It ravaged intertropical Africa in at least two epidemic waves in the twentieth century. Sixty million out of 400 million inhabitants are at risk for the lethal disease [2]. Furthermore, HAT represents a tremendous economical burden giving rise to 1.5 million disability-adjusted life years (DALYs), which make it rank just behind malaria [3].This review aims at focusing on the historical development of knowledge in the parasitological, clinical, diagnostic, therapeutic, and epidemiological aspects of HAT.

General History of HAT

Since the initial report of sleeping sickness by Ibn Khaldun [4], sleeping sickness has been studied by physicians who described essentially the clinical signs of the disease, generally focusing on neurological and sleep–wake disturbances. This clinical period ended at the turn of the twentieth century, because of the promotion of research provoked by the first large and devastating epidemic that then spread across colonial Africa. The colonial powers commissioned medical and scientific teams to Africa to develop knowledge on sleeping sickness and improve diagnosis and treatment of the deadly disease. Between 1896 and 1910, trypanosomes were identified as causal agents of the disease, the mode of transmission between sick and healthy persons through the bite of a tsetse fly was discovered, the clinical aspects were specified, diagnostic techniques were elaborated, and therapeutic strategies were proposed. Until then, the disease had been separated into two conditions: *Trypanosoma* fever and sleeping sickness which were integrated into one disease in 1909 as a continuum. The concept of HAT was born. Epidemiological mass screening techniques were developed and the mobile team policy was elaborated, with the goal of eliminating transmission between sick and healthy villagers. At the end of the colonial era, HAT had almost disappeared. However, the integrated control of the disease by the colonial medical services vanished, and, in conjunction with political instability and military unrest, a new epidemic wave emerged in the 1990s. The estimates by the World Health Organization [2] reached up to 500,000 cases. Fortunately, the international community was mobilized and medication manufacturers gave free access to appropriate treatment, with the help of *Médecins sans frontières*. These actions led to resume control of the disease in 2006 [5]. Nevertheless, recently established HAT risk maps demonstrated the persistence of the so-called historical foci [6]. However, as stated by Francis Louis (2012, personal communication), it is hazardous to believe that control has been attained and that HAT is not a public health problem anymore, even though the number of diagnosed new cases continues dropping. One should learn from historical facts.

Parasite and Vector

African Trypanosomes

African Trypanosomes are extracellular unicellular parasites that belong to the Kinetoplastida order, Trypanosomatidae family, Salivaria section. In 1895, Colonel Bruce identified trypanosomes in cattle and horses as the agent of nagana. The parasite was then named *Trypanosoma brucei* (*T. b.*) [7] and Laveran and Mesnil [8] established that humans were

A. Buguet (✉)
Polyclinic Marie-Louise Poto-Djembo, B.P. 49, Pointe-Noire, Congo
e-mail: a.buguet@free.fr

R. Cespuglio
Centre de recherche en neuroscience de Lyon, University of Lyon, Lyon, France

B. Bouteille
Laboratory of Parasitology, Dupuytren University Hospital of Limoges, Limoges, France

S. Chokroverty, M. Billiard (eds.), *Sleep Medicine*, DOI 10.1007/978-1-4939-2089-1_21,
© Springer Science+Business Media, LLC 2015

resistant to *T. b.* Trypanosomes were found in the blood of a feverish British patient in Gambia and were called *T. gambiense* [9]. The same parasite was found in the cerebrospinal fluid (CSF) of Ugandan patients [10]. A few years later, a new species of trypanosomes, *T. rhodesiense* was discovered in East Africa [11].

Trypomastigotes (bloodstream form) can be detected in all body and tissue fluids, particularly in the blood and CSF. They multiply by longitudinal binary fission. The 12–42 μm long and 1.5–3.5 μm wide parasite is animated by the undulations of its flagellum. African trypanosomes cannot be distinguished from one another by conventional microscopic techniques. However, the use of isoenzyme characterization and DNA analysis was able to separate the *T. b.* group into three subspecies, of which two are infective for humans: *T. b. gambiense*, and *T. b. rhodesiense.* The absence of infectivity of *T. b. brucei* to humans has been attributed to a serum haptoglobin-related protein that acts as trypanolytic factor [12]. The *gambiense* group is encountered in West and Central Africa, the *rhodesiense* group in East Africa. Each group is responsible for a different disease, conventional sleeping sickness being due to the *gambiense* group. Today, the genome of trypanosomes has been sequenced [13]. However, the parasite remains aggressive due to its 1000 Variant surface glycoprotein (VSG) genes that allow it to express a continuous variation of glycoprotein shell. Despite the host antibody response, the VSG variation allows some parasites to escape the immune attack, promoting a new parasite population leading to new waves of parasitemia.

The Vector

The vector of trypanosomes is the tsetse fly (*Glossina* sp.). Already in 1857, Livingstone [14] had rendered the "poisonous" tsetse fly responsible for what he called the tsetse fly disease, or nagana. Bruce [15] demonstrated that *Glossina* is the vector of nagana by transmitting the parasite that became *T. b. brucei.* Putting an end to very active scientific controversies, the first report of the British Sleeping sickness commission in Uganda [16] attributed to *Glossina palpalis* the role of vector of African trypanosomes in human sleeping sickness. Entomological studies proved rapidly that the parasite follows a development cycle within the fly [17]. When the tsetse fly bites a vertebrate to take a blood meal, infectious metacyclic trypanosomes that are present in its salivary glands are injected.

Tsetse flies are anchored in Africa and live exclusively in sub-Saharan regions between latitudes 14°N and 20°S. *Glossina (G.) palpalis* (or *G. fuscipes*), that transmits *T. b. gambiense,* lives under hot and humid forest coverage, especially along rivers and lakeshores of West and Central Africa. Man represents the main reservoir of parasites, although both wild and domestic animals (mainly pigs) may also host the trypanosomes. In East Africa, where antelopes are the main reservoir, the *T. b. rhodesiense* vector belongs to the *G. morsitans* group in the savannah or *G. pallipides* at forest edges or *G. fuscipes* in marshlands and river shores.

Clinical Aspects

Historically, clinical presentation of the disease preceded modern biologic diagnostic techniques. Before the turn of the twentieth century, sleeping sickness was a general disease with progressive neuropsychiatric disability and sleep–wake alterations leading to death. The rare pathological analyses revealed meningitis associated with encephalitis. By the end of the first decade of the twentieth century, the clinical characteristics of HAT were well established and the clinical classification of HAT was little modified until today. The French Commission in Congo divided the disease in three successive stages [18]. The hemolymphatic stage 1 marks the invasion of the blood and lymphatic organs by multiplying trypanosomes. It lasts until the appearance of the parasite in the CSF, giving rise to meningoencephalitic stage 2. Preterminal demyelination encephalitis fatally ends the time course of the disease, along with cachexia and doldrums [19].

The Chancre

The first manifestation of the infection is the appearance of a chancre at the bite site. The tender nodule that can reach several centimeters in diameter is hot, edematous and erythematous. It is more frequently observed in *T. b. rhodesiense* HAT and disappears in 2–3 weeks [20]. Trypanosomes can be found after scarification and microscope examination.

Hemolymphatic Stage 1

At stage 1, a general malaise is the rule. Chilliness alternates with irregular feverish bouts that resist to antimalarial drugs. The general malaise is completed by headaches, asthenia, facial edema, prostration, insomnia. Pruritus is discrete, but cutaneous trypanides give rise to large papuloerythematous polycyclic and pruritic plaques over the trunk and/or inferior limbs. Enlarged lymph glands, especially in the lateral cervical area, and splenomegaly result from the invasion of lymphatic organs by trypanosomes. Lumbar and dorsal back pains concomitant to deep muscle and bone pains in response to pressure are common in the still active farmer or fisherman. The conventional Kérandel's key sign was self-described [21]. When the physician tried to turn the key in his door lock, he suffered an acute pain elicited by palmar pressure. Sexual drive drops, and genital frigidity is accompanied by impotence in men and dysmenorrhea in women. Behavioral distemper and mood disorders are frequent with alternation of depressive and manic states. Sleep problems are not uniform and vary in intensity and in course of time, insomnia alternates with excessive daytime sleepiness and normal sleep.

Meningoencephalitic Stage 2

At stage 2, the general symptoms observed at stage 1 are exacerbated, especially headaches and fatigue, and sleep–wake disorders become prominent. Adenopathies and splenomegaly recede. Peaks of fever occur, alternating with hypothermic events. The temperature curve shows periods of hypothermia, especially during the neurological stage in a rat model of HAT [22].

Neuropsychiatric disorders correlate with meningeal inflammation in both forms of HAT. Mental disturbances are dominated by the astonishing disinterest and indifference of the patient towards his own condition and his environment. The apathetic patient with drooping eyelids suffers behavioral disturbances; episodes of agitation and antisocial or aggressive behavior and sudden anger alternate with episodes of confusion, dementia, or delirium. Melancholic and manic episodes may also alternate. Extreme violent behavior has been described with theft, fire lighting, suicide, or homicide.

All types of neurological signs can be observed indicating the involvement of almost all brain structures. Disorders of tone and mobility are constant features of the disease. Extrapyramidal disability is revealed by movement alterations, of which the most characteristic gait disorder (e.g., cerebellar ataxia) was emphasized by nineteenth-century authors. Myoclonic jerks occur during wake and sleep, and restless legs syndrome and periodic limb movements in sleep have been observed during polysomnographic recordings [23, 24]. Movement disorders may also be present in the form of choreic agitation. Tremor is frequently described, starting at the extremities and often generalizing to the whole body. Tongue tremor has been described in nineteenth-century reports. Patients frequently complain of hyperpathia, with bone and muscle pains. Deep tendon reflexes may be hyperactive. Primitive reflexes (palmomental reflex, sucking reflex) may be present, indicating cerebral cortical dysfunction. The Babinski or Hoffman signs indicate pyramidal tract involvement.

Sleep and wake are severely disturbed. In 1890, Mackenzie [25] had observed in a young adult from the Congo Free State "many little sleeps in the daytime, but rarely slept for long together either by night or day, so that the total amount of sleep did not exceed the amount usually taken by healthy people." Lhermitte [26] described the "narcolepsies of sleeping sickness," true sleep attacks starting with brisk

drops in neck muscle tone. Recently, our group confirmed these observations using 24 h polysomnographic recordings, and described the polysomnographic syndrome of HAT that occurs mainly in stage 2 patients. Briefly, the syndrome is made of two features: the loss of circadian alternation of sleep and wakefulness, sleep and wake occurring in bouts of 80–90 min throughout the nychthemeron (24 hours); and sleep structure alterations with the occurrence of sleep-onset rapid eye movement (REM) sleep periods (SOREMP) in several sleep episodes [27]. These alterations have been proposed to be used as a diagnostic tool [28] and have recently been confirmed in a 5-year study on HAT patients in Congo, especially for the diagnosis of relapses during post-treatment follow-up [29].

Diencephalic and hypothalamo–hypophyseal dysfunctions may provoke hunger and thirst contrasting with the state of malnutrition of the patients, as well as hormonal regulation alterations. Multiple endocrine dysfunction including hormonal circadian dysrhythmia may cause loss of libido, impotence, dysmenorrheal, and myxedema. Cortisol and melatonin circadian rhythm is not known to be affected or little influenced by the sleep–wake cycle. The amplitude of cortisol secretion peaks losing its circadian undulation [30], although the overall 24-h mean plasma concentration is unaltered [31]. Melatonin nocturnal peak is delayed by 2 h compared to healthy Africans [32]. Prolactin secretion is linked to sleep and wake alternation, being elevated during sleep. In patients with circadian alterations of the sleep–wake cycle, the prolactin secretion loses its circadian rhythm. Plasma renin activity and growth hormone are tightly linked with slow-wave sleep. Therefore, in HAT patients, the secretion peaks of renin and growth hormone follow the alteration of the circadian distribution of slow-wave sleep, sticking with the hormone–sleep relationship [30, 33].

The Terminal Encephalitis Phase

The terminal encephalitis phase is related to demyelination and atrophy. The degenerative process leads to apathy, dementia, epileptic fits, and incontinence, and death will occur after a chaotic course. Magnetic resonance imaging of the brain has revealed lesions that can also be encountered in other degenerative diseases.

Particular Aspects of Gambian and Rhodesian HAT

Trypanosoma b. gambiense HAT leads to death in several months or years after a complicated and complex neurological and sleep–wake disorder. This form, therefore, deserves the name of sleeping sickness. On the contrary, the acute *T. b. rhodesiense* HAT leads to death in weeks or months after a massive weight loss developing cachexia with cardiovascular failure. The neurological symptoms may not have time to install, although our group found typical sleep–wake alterations in two Caucasians who had caught the disease in Rwanda [34].

Clinical Forms

Healthy carriers have rarely been reported [35]. However, a recent report describes a possible trypanotolerance in man [36].

The observation of symptoms and signs of stage 1 is often persistent during stage 2, and the reverse can be observed concerning the occurrence of neurological signs at stage 1 [29]. In our practice [37], we have encountered discrepancies between clinical symptoms and CSF biology. In Europeans, the time course of the disease has been reported to be rapid [18, 21]. In children, neurological and behavioral symptoms are frequent with an emphasis on sleep disturbances [38, 39]. Neurological and intellectual sequels are often observed [40]. Congenital transmission of the disease has been rarely reported [41].

Diagnosis and Stage Determination

The first biological test to be used in the process of diagnosis was the microscopic search for trypanosomes in the blood, enlarged lymph gland fluid, and CSF, although several other body fluids were investigated in the first half of the twentieth century. The tests followed the already described discovery of trypanosomes in the blood [9] and CSF [10]. The latter author already used centrifugation to concentrate the parasites. Thereafter, the analysis of the CSF was completed by the white blood cell (WBC) count [42]. Several tests were designed in the first half of the twentieth century. However, most developed tests are not easily usable in field conditions. Nowadays, a mixture of "old" techniques (microscopic examination, centrifugation of samples, WBC count) and newer methods (serological tests, modern concentration techniques, CSF lymphocyte count) are in use by mobile teams in their field screening campaigns. An example of field screening for HAT patients by the Congo (Brazzaville) National Program for Control of HAT is detailed in Buguet et al. [37] and Buguet et al. [29].

Several other diagnostic or staging tests have been proposed. However, most of them require a well-equipped laboratory facility and qualified personnel and are not feasible in field conditions. An example is given by the analysis of immunoglobulins M (IgM) that was proposed by Mattern in 1968 [43] for the diagnosis of HAT, as IgM are highly elevated in HAT. A latex technique that can be applied in the field was recently developed [44]. Another example is given by polymerase chain reaction (PCR) that raised hopes after its use in the diagnostic of stage 1 HAT by Truc et al. [45]. The technique is expensive and requires laboratory equipment with uninterrupted cold chain. Furthermore, PCR may remain positive after treatment due to parasite DNA material remaining in body fluids and cannot be used during post-treatment follow-up [46]. The loop mediated isothermal amplification [47] and nucleic acid sequence-based amplification [48] are cheaper and may open a new way for potential field application of DNA amplification techniques.

Treatment

Treatment at Stage 1

The treatment of stage 1 HAT has not changed since the first third of the twentieth century. Since 1936, T. b. gambiense-infected patients are treated with 7–10 intramuscular injections of pentamidine at the dose of 4 mg/kg/day administered daily or every two days to avoid side effects which are rare. These consist of syncope, hypotension, cutaneous eruptions, tachycardia and arrhythmia (cardiac toxicity), hypoglycemia and/or diabetes (pancreatic toxicity), hepatic dysfunction, and hematologic disturbances.

Suramin is used to treat stage 1 T. b. rhodesiense HAT since 1916. Although it is active on T. b. gambiense, it is not used as it may produce a sudden shock in case of co-infection by Onchocerca volvulus. The dosage is 1 g intravenously on days 1, 3, 5, 14, and 21. Side effects are reactive fever, cutaneo-mucous eruptions, nausea, vomiting, polyneuropathy, hematological toxicity, and rarely kidney failure.

Treatment at Stage 2

Melarsoprol is an arsenical released in 1949 that is still used, despite growing resistances and high toxicity, with especially a deadly reactive encephalopathy. It is administered in slow intravenous injections at a maximal dose of 3.6 mg/kg/day, in three 3-day courses at 1 week intervals. A shorter alternative regimen has been proposed, with daily injections of 2.2 mg/kg during 10 consecutive days. However, the risk of complications remains unchanged. Apart from the deadly encephalopathy, other undesirable effects include convulsions, peripheral neuropathies, headaches, tremor, febrile reactions, abdominal pains, chest pains, cutaneous eruptions (potential occurrence of a Lyell's syndrome), peripheral thrombophlebitis, cardiac toxicity, renal or hepatic toxicity, and agranulocytosis. Following the recommendations of the WHO, the proportion of T. b. gambiense patients treated with melarsoprol dropped from 97 % in 2001 to 12 % in 2010 [49].

Eflornithine or difluoromethylornithine has been used to treat stage 2 *T. b. gambiense* HAT since 1986. It is administered during 14 days in 4 daily slow intravenous infusions for a daily dose of 400 mg/kg. The medication is not devoid of adverse effects. Complications concern anemia, leucopenia, diarrhea, convulsions (during the first week), vomiting, thrombopenia, fever, abdominal pains, headaches, alopecia, anorexia, vertigo, sudden deafness.

Nifurtimox is the orally administered medication of Chagas's disease, the American trypanosomiasis. It is active on both stages of *T. b. gambiense* HAT; its activity on *T. b. rhodesiense* remains unknown. Administration of nifurtimox is oral: 5mg/kg twice a day during 10 consecutive days. The adverse effects of nifurtimox consist of convulsions, reversible cerebellar syndrome (ataxia, nystagmus, tremor, and vertigo), psychotic reactions, and anorexia, nausea, vomiting, and weight loss.

Today, the WHO recommends to use nifurtimox in combination with eflornithine for the treatment of *T. b. gambiense* HAT stage 2 [50, 51]. The nifurtimox–eflornithine combination therapy (NECT) has been evaluated recently mainly because of the growing resistance to melarsoprol. The protocol starts with intravenous eflornithine (two 1-h infusions of 200 mg/kg each during 7 consecutive days) followed by by oral nifurtimox as above. The NECT does not, however, meet the expected synergic effects of both molecules regarding trypanocidal activity [52]. Furthermore, resistance phenomena are still under evaluation [53]. Adverse effects are those of eflornithine.

Post-treatment Follow-up

Although a shortening of the follow-up period after treatment has been suggested by certain teams [54, 55], we believe that patients should be reexamined every 6 months during at least 18 months. Considering our own practice [37], relapses at stage 2 were observed 18 months after treatment. It is difficult for the National Programs to follow up patients for such a long time, because of several reasons: the lack of financial and logistic means to launch mobile team campaigns, the poor compliance of the patients to come back for mobile team visits when they occur, certainly for economical reasons and fear of lumbar puncture.

Conclusions on Present Therapeutic Strategies

The available medications are ancient and their efficacy is often imperfect, not accounting for resistance phenomena. However, since the last epidemic, the pharmaceutical industry and WHO have formed a partnership to obtain free treatment for the patients. Nevertheless, research for new therapeutic molecules and strategies should be emphasized. Two molecules are under evaluation: fexinidazole [56] and molecule derived from benzoxaboroles, SCYX-7158 [57].

Conclusion

HAT hits rural populations in remote bush villages that lack adequate healthcare facilities. During the first half of the twentieth century, efforts to control HAT almost led to its elimination. Nowadays, the number of mobile teams remains limited and they still use diagnostic techniques developed 35 years ago. Progress in therapeutic strategies is limited [58]. Medications such as suramine are almost 100 years old. Molecules used at stage 2 are toxic. Nevertheless, because of international and national efforts, the prevalence of HAT is decreasing. This may, however, represent a paradoxical danger as public health authorities may become inattentive and public funds may vanish. The patients themselves often avoid mobile team meetings. They fear lumbar punctures and prefer not to interrupt farming or fishing. Organizing post-treatment follow-up every 6 months during 18–24 months may be difficult or impossible. However, we should have learned from past experience not to alleviate surveillance. New diagnostic tests, especially noninvasive, and nontoxic molecules to treat stage 2 HAT are urgently needed to improve staging and treatment strategies.

Acknowledgments Part of the work received support from the Technical Services Agreement # T7/83/2 of the World Health Organization (2005–2006), from the "Action de recherche en réseau: Le syndrome du cycle veille-sommeil dans la trypanosomiase humaine africaine: méthode noninvasive de diagnostic du stade de la maladie, de validation de tests biologiques et de suivi de traitement" of the Agence universitaire de la Francophonie (2005–2006), and mainly from the UNICEF/UNDP/World Bank/WHO Special Programme for Research and Training in Tropical Diseases (TDR) N° A50468 "Polysomnography, electrochemistry, immunology & neuroanatomy to the diagnosis of Human African Trypanosomiasis" (2006–2009).

References

1. Jannin J, Simarro PP, Louis FJ. Le concept de maladie négligée. Med Trop. 2003;63:219–21.
2. WHO. Control and surveillance of African trypanosomiasis. Report of a WHO Expert Committee. Technical Report Series no.°881. Geneva; 1998.
3. Hotez PJ, Fenwick A, Savioli L, Molyneux DH. Rescuing the bottom billion through control of neglected tropical diseases. Lancet. 2009;373:1570–5.
4. Buguet A, Cespuglio R, Louis F, Bouteille B. Diagnostic de la trypanosomose humaine africaine (maladie du sommeil). Sarrebruck: Editions Universitaires Européennes; 2011.
5. WHO. Human African trypanosomiasis (sleeping sickness): epidemiological update. Wkly Epidemiol Rec. 2006;81:71–80.

6. Simarro PP, Cecchi G, Franco JR et al. Risk for human African trypanosomiasis, Central Africa, 2000–2009. Emerg Infect Dis. 2011;17:2322–4.

7. Plimmer, Bradford. Vorkäufige Notiz über die Morphologie und Verbreitung in der Tsetsekranheit (Fly disease oder Nagana) des gefundenen Parasiten. Centr f Bakter. 1899;26:440.

8. Laveran A, Mesnil F. Recherches morphologiques et expérimentales sur le trypanosome du nagana ou maladie de la mouche tsétsé. Ann Inst Pasteur. 1902;16:1–55.

9. Dutton JE. Note on *Trypanosoma* occurring in the blood of man. Br Med J. 1902;123:881–4.

10. Castellani A. On the discovery of a species of trypanosome in the cerebrospinal fluid of cases of sleeping sickness. Lancet. 1903;161:1735–6.

11. Fantham HB, Thomson JG. Enumerative studies on *Trypanosoma gambiense* and *T. rhodesiense* in rats, guinea-pigs, and rabbits: periodic variations disclosed (preliminary note). Roy Soc Proc B. 1910;83:206–11.

12. Vanhamme L, Pays E. The trypanosome lytic factor of human serum and the molecular basis of sleeping sickness. Int J Parasitol. 2004;34:887–98.

13. Berriman M, Ghedin E, Hertz-Fowler C, et al. The genome of the African trypanosome *Trypanosoma brucei*. Science. 2005;309:416–22.

14. Livingstone D. Missionary Travels and Researches in South Africa: including a sketch of 16 years' residence in the interior of Africa. London: John Murray; 1857.

15. Bruce D. Preliminary report on the tsetse fly disease or nagana in Zululand. Durban: Bennett and Davis; 1895 (Ubombo, Dec 1895).

16. Anonymous. Reports of the sleeping sickness commission. Nr.1. London: Harrison and Sons; 1903 (Reprinted in 2005 by Elibron Classics series, Adamant Media Corporation).

17. Kleine FK. Weitere Beobachtung über Tsetse-fliege und Trypanosomen. Dtsch Med Wochenschr. 1909;35:1956–8.

18. Martin G, Leboeuf, Roubaud. Rapport de la mission d'études de la maladie du sommeil au Congo français 1906–1908. Paris: Masson et Cie Editeurs; 1909.

19. Blum J, Schmid C, Burri C. Clinical aspects of 2541 patients with second stage human African trypanosomiasis. Acta Trop. 2006;97:55–64.

20. Malvy D, Djossou F, Weill Fx, Chapuis P, Longy-Boursier M, Le Bras M. Guess what! Human West African trypanosomiasis with chancre presentation. Eur J Dermatol. 2000;10:561–2.

21. Kérandel J. Un cas de trypanosomiase chez un médecin (auto-observation). Bull Soc Pathol Exot. 1910;3:642–62.

22. Chevrier C, Canini F, Darsaud A, Cespuglio R, Buguet A, Bourdon L. Clinical assessment of the entry into neurological state in rat experimental African trypanosomiasis. Acta Trop. 2005;95:33–9.

23. Bedat-Millet AL, Charpentier S, Monge SMF, Woimant F. Psychiatric presentation of human African trypanosomiasis: overview of diagnostic pitfalls, interest of difluoromethylornithine treatment and contribution of magnetic resonance imaging. Rev Neurol. 2000;156:505–9.

24. Sanner BM, Büchner N, Kotterba S, Zidek W. Polysomnography in acute African trypanosomiasis. J Neurol. 2000;247:878–9.

25. Mackenzie S. Negro lethargy. Lancet. 1890;136: 1100–1.

26. Lhermitte J. La maladie du sommeil et les narcolepsies. Brussels: Etablissements d'imprimerie L. Severeyns; 1910.

27. Buguet A, Bourdon L, Bouteille B, Chapotot F, Radomski MW, Dumas M. The duality of sleeping sickness: focusing on sleep. Sleep Med Rev. 2001;5:139–53.

28. Buguet A, Bisser S, Josenando T, Chapotot F, Cespuglio R. Sleep structure: a new diagnostic tool for stage determination in sleeping sickness. Acta Trop. 2005;93:107–17.

29. Buguet A, Chapotot F, Ngampo S, Bouteille B, Cespuglio R. Management of African trypanosomiasis of the CNS: polysomnography as non-invasive staging tool. Future Neurol. 2012;7:453–72.

30. Brandenberger G, Buguet A, Spiegel K, et al. Disruption of endocrine rhythms in sleeping sickness with preserved relationship between hormone pulses and sleep structure. J Biol Rhythms. 1996;11:258–67.

31. Radomski MW, Buguet A, Montmayeur A Bogui P et al. 24-hour plasma cortisol and prolactin in human African trypanosomiasis patients and healthy African controls. Am J Trop Med Hyg. 1995;52:281–6.

32. Claustrat B, Buguet A, Geoffriau M et al. Plasma melatonin rhythm is maintained in human African trypanosomiasis. Neuroendocrinology. 1998;68:64–70.

33. Radomski MW, Buguet A, Doua F, Bogui P, Tapie P. Relationship of plasma growth hormone to slow-wave sleep in African sleeping sickness. Neuroendocrinology. 1996;63:393–6.

34. Montmayeur A, Brosset C, Imbert P, Buguet A. Cycle veille-sommeil au décours d'une trypanosomose humaine africaine à *Trypanosoma brucei rhodesienne* chez deux parachutistes français. Bull Soc Patholol Exot. 1994;87:368–71.

35. Lapeyssonnie L. Deuxième note concernant un cas exceptionnel de trypanosomiase. Parasitémie observée depuis 21 ans sans signes cliniques appréciables chez une malade traitée inefficacement pendant les 10 premières années. Bull Soc Pathol Exot. 1960;53:28–32.

36. Jamonneau V, Ilboudo H, Kaboré J et al. Untreated human infections by *Trypanosoma brucei gambiense* are not 100 % fatal. PLoS Negl Trop Dis. 2012;6:e1691.

37. Buguet A, Bouteille B, Mpandzou G, et al. La recherche sur la maladie du sommeil (trypanosomose humaine africaine) en République du Congo de 2004 à 2009. Brazzaville: Editions Les Manguiers; 2009.

38. Millogo A, Nacro B, Bonkoungou P et al. La maladie du sommeil chez l'enfant au Centre hospitalier de Bobo-Dioulasso: à propos de 3 observations. Bull Soc Pathol Exot. 1999;92:320–22.

39. Mpandzou G, Ngampo S, Bandzouzi B, Bouteille B, Vincendeau P, Cespuglio R,: Buguet A. Polysomnographic diagnosis of meningoencephalitic *gambiense* African trypanosomiasis in an infant. Sci Med Afr. 2009;1:105–9.

40. Triolo N, Trova P, Fusco C, Le Bras J. Bilan de 17 années d'étude de la trypanosomiase humaine Africaine à " *Trypanosoma gambiense* „ chez les enfants de 0 Ã 6 ans. A propos de 227 cas. Med Trop. 1985;45:251–7.

41. Rocha G, Martins A, Gama G, Brandao F, Atouguia J. Possible cases of sexual and congenital transmission of sleeping sickness. Lancet. 2004;363:247.

42. Broden A, Rhodain J. Le liquide cérébro-spinal dans la trypanosomiase humaine. Bull Soc Pathol Exot. 1908;1: 496–9.

43. Mattern P. Etat actuel et résultats des techniques immunologiques utilisées à l'Institut Pasteur de Dakar pour le diagnostic et l'étude de la trypanosomiase humaine africaine. Bull World Health Organ. 1968;38:1–8.

44. Lejon V, Legros D, Richer M et al. IgM quantification in the cerebrospinal fluid of sleeping sickness patients by latex card agglutination test. Trop Med Int Health. 2002;7:685–92.

45. Truc P, Jamonneau V, Cuny G, Frézil JL. Use of polymerase chain reaction in human African trypanosomiasis stage determination and follow-up. Bull World Health Organ. 1999;77:745–8.

46. Deborggraeve S, Lejon V, Ekangu RA et al. Diagnostic accuracy of PCR in *gambiense* sleeping sickness diagnosis, staging and post-treatment follow-up: a 2-year longitudinal study. PLoS Negl Trop Dis. 2011;5:e972.

47. Kuboki N, Inoue N, Sakurai T et al. Loop-mediated isothermal amplification for detection of African trypanosomes. J Clin Microbiol. 2003;41:5517–24.

48. Mugasa CM, Laurent T, Schoone GJ, Kager PA, Lubega GW, Schallig HD. Nucleic acid sequence-based amplification with oligochromatography for detection of *Trypanosoma brucei* in clinical samples. J Clin Microbiol. 2009;47:630–5.

49. Simarro PP, Franco JR, Diarra A, Ruiz Postigo JA, Jannin J. Update on field use of the available drugs for the chemotherapy of human African trypanosomiasis. Parasitology. 2012;139:842–6.

50. Franco JR, Simarro PP, Diarra A, Ruiz-Postigo JA, Samo M, Jannin JG. Monitoring the use of nifurtimox-eflornithine combination therapy (NECT) in the treatment of second stage *gambiense* human African trypanosomiasis. Res Rep Trop Med. 2012;3:93–101.

51. Priotto G, Kasparian S, Mutombo W et al. Nifurtimox-eflornithine combination therapy for second-stage African *Trypanosoma brucei gambiense* trypanosomiasis: a multicentre, randomised, phase III, non-inferiority trial. Lancet. 2009;374:56–64.

52. Vincent IM, Creek DJ, Burgess K, Woods DJ, Burchmore RJS, Barrett MP. Untargeted metabolomics reveals a lack of synergy between nifurtimox and eflornithine against *Trypanosoma brucei*. PLoS Negl Trop Dis. 2012;6:e1618.

53. Barrett MP, Vincent IM, Burchmore RJ, Kazibwe AJ, Matovu E. Drug resistance in human African trypanosomiasis. Future Microbiol. 2011;6:1037–47.

54. Mumba Ngoyi D, Lejon V, Pyana P et al. How to shorten patient follow-up after treatment for *Trypanosoma brucei gambiense* sleeping sickness. J Infect Dis. 2010;201:453–63.

55. Priotto G, Chappuis F, Bastard M, Flevaud L, Etard JF. Early prediction of treatment efficacy in second-stage *gambiense* human African trypanosomiasis. PLoS Negl Trop Dis. 2012;6:e1662.

56. Torreele E, Bourdin Trunz B, Tweats D et al. Fexinidazole—a new oral nitroimidazole drug candidate entering clinical development for the treatment of sleeping sickness. PLoS Negl Trop Dis. 2011;4:e923.

57. Jacobs RT, Nare B, Wring SA et al. SCYX-7158, an orally-active benzoxaborole for the treatment of stage 2 human African trypanosomiasis. PLoS Negl Trop Dis. 2011;5:e1151.

58. Molyneux D, Ndung'u J, Maudlin I. Controlling sleeping sickness-"when will they ever learn?". PLoS Negl Trop Dis. 2010;4:e609.

Sleep and HIV Disease

Kenneth D. Phillips and Mary E. Gunther

22

Sleep and HIV Disease

Although not the fatal illness it once was, HIV/AIDS remains a life-threatening illness. The worldwide prevalence of HIV/AIDS at the end of 2010 was estimated to be 34 million, which includes 3.4 million children who are less than 15 years of age. The incidence of HIV infection decreased from 3.1 million in 2001 to 2.7 million in 2010. The annual number of deaths worldwide is steadily declining since peaking in 2005 at 2.2 million [1].

With earlier diagnosis, more highly sophisticated monitoring of immune parameters, better antiretroviral therapy, improved recognition of viral mutations and drug resistance, and effective prophylaxis and treatments for opportunistic infections and malignancies, persons with HIV/AIDS (PWHA) are living longer and healthier lives, often many decades beyond their initial infection [2]. While immune status and longevity have improved, PWHA experience many persistent and burdensome symptoms. Insomnia and fatigue are often reported as the most frequent and distressful symptoms associated with HIV/AIDS [3–5]. Even so, insomnia is often underreported, underdiagnosed, and undertreated [6].

Normal Sleep Architecture

Sleep occurs in two distinct stages, rapid eye movement (REM) and non-rapid eye movement (NREM) sleep that are revealed by polysomnography recurrent. Recurrent cycles of REM and NREM sleep occur throughout a 24-h circadian day. In adults, approximately 25 % (90–120 min) of the sleep period is spent in REM sleep, which occurs in early morning.

K. D. Phillips (✉) · M. E. Gunther
The University of Tennessee, College of Nursing, 1200 Volunteer Boulevard, 37996-4180 Knoxville, TN, USA
e-mail: kphill22@utk.edu

M. E. Gunther
e-mail: mgunther@utk.edu

The remaining 75 % of the sleep period is spent in NREM sleep. Adults have four to five bouts of REM sleep per night; the first cycle of REM sleep is shorter in duration with cycles later during the night becoming longer. During REM sleep, rapid movements of the eyes are observed. REM sleep is accompanied by decreased muscle tone and vivid dreams [7].

During wakefulness, the electroencephalogram (EEG) shows two types of brain waves. Beta waves are typical of wakefulness. Beta waves have the highest frequency, the lowest amplitude, and the most desynchronous. As the body becomes more relaxed, just prior to sleep, the brain waves change from beta waves to alpha waves and appear on the EEG as slower frequency, higher amplitude, and more synchronous waveforms. As a person transitions from wakefulness to stage 1 of sleep, the EEG changes from alpha waves to theta waves. Theta waves are even slower in frequency and greater in amplitude. As sleep deepens to stage 2, sleep spindles (sudden increase in frequency) and K complexes (sudden increase in amplitude) appear on the EEG. Stage 3 (delta sleep, slow wave sleep) is the deeper stage characterized by delta waves, which are the slowest waves with the greatest amplitude. Counterintuitively, sleepwalking and sleep talking do not occur during REM, but rather in the deeper stage of sleep (stage 3) [7].

Insomnia in HIV/AIDS

Insomnia is a common complaint in the general population and even higher in PWHA [6, 8–16]. It has been estimated that the prevalence of insomnia in HIV/AIDS ranges from 30 to 100 % [3, 6, 17–21] as compared to 10–35 % in the population at large [22, 23]. The wide variance in the estimated prevalence of insomnia in PWHA may be due to the use of validated and nonvalidated tools for assessing sleep quality, inconsistent inclusion and exclusion criteria, and that objective measures of sleep (e.g., actigraphy and polysomnography) are not often used; therefore, the true rate of sleep disorders is not known. Many studies of the prevalence of insomnia in HIV/AIDS were conducted prior to the advent of combination antiretroviral therapy. These studies need to be repeated giving attention to stage of illness and other potential covariates.

Two 2012 studies looked at the prevalence of sleep quality in cross-sectional samples. Lee and colleagues characterized specific types of sleep difficulty in a sample of 290 adults (men: $n=194.67\%$; women: $n=74.25\%$; and transgendered persons: $n=22.8\%$). Nearly half of the sample (45%) slept less than 6 h per night, 87% slept less than 8 h per night, and 13% sleep 8 h or more per night. Of the 290 participants, 88 (30.4%) reported good sleep; 41 (14%) reported difficulty falling asleep only, 102 (35.2%) reported difficulty staying asleep only, and 59 (20.3%) reported difficulty in falling asleep and staying asleep [24]. Crum-Cianflone and colleagues reported that 46% of 193 HIV-infected military beneficiaries between the ages of 18 and 50 met the criteria for insomnia and 30% reported daytime drowsiness [12].

Insomnia and Stage of HIV Disease

HIV disease has a well-described progression. Stage 1: Acute infection occurs 2–4 weeks after infection with HIV. During the acute infection, the virus is rapidly replicating in the body, the CD4+ cell count drops rapidly, and flu-like symptoms appear. Stage 2: Clinical latency begins at the end of the acute infection when the viral load has dropped to what is termed a "viral set point." During the early period of this stage, the virus replicates slowly and the HIV-infected person is most likely asymptomatic. Toward the end of this period, the rate of viral replication rises and the

CD4+ count declines. Constitutional symptoms such as fever, night sweats, and decreased appetite may appear. This period can last 8 years or longer. Stage 3: AIDS is diagnosed when the CD4+ cell count drops below 200 /mm³. At this point, opportunistic infections and malignancies can occur. Left untreated, life expectancy from the time of the appearance of an opportunistic infection is about 1–3 years. Stage unknown: A person is known to be HIV-infected, but there is no information about the CD4 cell count or AIDS-defining conditions. The Centers for Disease Control and Prevention describes these stages more quantitatively for surveillance. See Table 22.1.

Insomnia has been reported in all stages of HIV/AIDS [25] and has been consistently significantly associated with depression and fatigue [26]. Phillips and colleagues examined the relationships among sleep quality: Pittsburgh Sleep Quality Index (PSQI) and the dimensions of health-related quality of life (SF-36) in a sample of HIV-infected women ($n=144$). Controlling for stage of illness and whether a woman had a paying job or not, global sleep quality explained significant levels of variance in bodily pain, mental health, physical functioning, role physical, social functioning, and vitality. Sleep quality accounted for 20% of the variance in the mental component score, but for none of the variance in the physical component score [27].

Sleep and Immunity

Besedovsky, Lange, and Born provide a thorough synthesis of the evidence supporting the relationships between sleep, circadian rhythm, and immunity [28]. The following section summarizes key conclusion drawn in their article

Table 22.1 Stage of disease. (Source: Centers for Disease Control (2012))

In December 2008, *CDC published Revised Surveillance Case Definitions for HIV Infection Among Adults, Adolescents, and Children Aged< 18 Months and for HIV Infection and AIDS Among Children Aged 18 Months to< 13 Years—United States, 2008* (www.cdc.gov/mmwr/preview/mmwrhtml/rr5710a1.htm). For adults and adolescents (i.e., persons aged ≥ 13 years), the surveillance case definitions for HIV infection and AIDS were revised into a single case definition for HIV infection that includes AIDS and incorporates the HIV infection staging classification system. In addition, the HIV infection case definition for children aged < 13 years and the AIDS case definition for children aged 18 months to < 13 years were revised. No changes were made to the HIV infection classification system, the 24 AIDS-defining conditions for children aged < 13 years, or the AIDS case definition for children aged < 18 months. These case definitions are intended for public health surveillance only and not as a guide for clinical diagnosis

A confirmed case meets the laboratory criteria for diagnosis of HIV infection and one of the four HIV infection stages (stage 1, stage 2, stage 3, or stage unknown)

HIV infection, stage 1: No AIDS-defining condition and either CD4+ T-lymphocyte count of ≥ 500 cells/μL or CD4+ T-lymphocyte percentage of total lymphocytes of ≥ 29

HIV infection, stage 2: No AIDS-defining condition and either CD4+ T-lymphocyte count of 200–499 cells/μL or CD4+ T-lymphocyte percentage of total lymphocytes of 14–28

HIV infection, stage 3 (AIDS): CD4+ T-lymphocyte count of <200 cells/μL or CD4+ T-lymphocyte percentage of total lymphocytes of <14, or documentation of an AIDS-defining condition. Documentation of an AIDS-defining condition supersedes a CD4+ T-lymphocyte count of ≥ 200 cells/μL and a CD4+ T-lymphocyte percentage of total lymphocytes of ≥ 14

HIV infection, stage unknown: No information available on CD4+ T-lymphocyte count or percentage and no information available on AIDS-defining conditions

that support the relationships between sleep and immunity. The onset of sleep is associated with downregulation of the hypothalamic-pituitary-adrenal axis (HPAA) and the sympathetic nervous system (SNS). During that same period, growth hormone, prolactin, melatonin, and leptin steeply rise. These hormones participate in the regulation of the immune response, by stimulating activation, proliferation, and differentiation of immune cells, which then produce proinflammatory cytokines. Proinflammatory cytokines include interleukin-1 (IL-1), tumor necrosis factor (TNF-alpha) and interferon (IFN-gamma). When the HPPA (increasing production of cortisol) and the SNS (increasing the production of catecholamines) are upregulated, proinflammatory immune functions are suppressed. Therefore, during sleep, particularly during slow-wave sleep (SWS), proinflammatory functions peak and during wakefulness anti-inflammatory activity becomes apparent. It has also been demonstrated that immune cell numbers in early differentiation peak during the early sleep period. Production of IL-12, a proinflammatory cytokine, increases and there is a shift of the Th1/Th2 balance toward the production of proinflammatory cytokines. Downregulation of the stress hormones during early sleep may lead to increased proliferation of T helper cell proliferation and migration of naïve T cells to the lymph nodes. Wakefulness is associated with an increase in cytotoxic T lymphocytes and natural killer cells.

Sleep and Immunity in HIV Disease

An inverse relationship was found between frequency of sleep complaint and CD4+ cells which suggests that sleep disturbances may increase as the disease progresses. Relationships between SWS and certain immune variables (i.e., NKCA, antibody production, T cell proliferation and differentiation, and cytotoxic T cell proliferation and differentiation) have been observed. These findings suggest that insomnia adversely affects immunity. Darko et al. hypothesize that IL-1-β and TNF-α may be responsible for the changes in SWS in PWHA [29].

Cruess and colleagues examined the relationship between psychological distress (Impact of Event Scale), subjective sleep disturbance (PSQI) and immune status (CD3+CD4+ [T helper/inducer cells] and CD3+CD8+ [T suppressor cells]) in 57 PWHA. The sample consisted of both men ($n=41$) and women ($n=16$) with a mean age 38.8 ± 8.5. Neither psychological distress nor sleep quality was significantly related to T helper/inducer cells, but both were significantly associated with T suppressor cell even after controlling for age, T helper/inducer cells, and viral load. They concluded that sleep quality mediated the relationship between psychological distress and T suppressor cells [30].

Insomnia and Quality of Life in HIV Infection

HIV/AIDS-related insomnia is associated with a significant burden for PWHA in that it further adds to functional impairment and reduces quality of life (QOL) [19, 27]. Insomnia contributes to fatigue, disability, eventual unemployment, and decreased QOL in PWHIV [8]. Insomnia occurs frequently in PWHIV prior to diagnosis and continues throughout the course of the disease. In fact, excessive daytime sleepiness may be one of the presenting symptoms of HIV disease, [31] and insomnia may even serve as an early marker of HIV disease [13].

Sleep Architecture and HIV/AIDS

Changes in sleep architecture in HIV/AIDS have been studied in small samples. Most of these studies did not include seronegative case controls. Little attention was given to the HIV stage of illness in these small studies. Therefore, the changes in sleep architecture have not been clearly characterized.

Early studies demonstrated an increase in SWS, particularly during the latter half of the sleep period. Norman and colleagues [32] examined sleep architecture in a sample of eight asymptomatic HIV-positive men and compared their sleep to three HIV-negative men. They reported an increase in total percentage of SWS, with most of the SWS occurring in the latter half of the sleep period. This finding has not been replicated in any other study.

A subsequent study by Norman and colleagues compared the sleep architecture of ten HIV-positive men to that of five HIV-negative men. They reported a significant difference (8% more) in the amount of delta (slow wave) sleep in the HIV-positive men [31]. In another study of six asymptomatic HIV-positive men, they reported that alpha-delta patterns were consistently observed throughout the sleep period [33].

Kubicki and colleagues examined sleep architecture in five men with AIDS. They reported a greater number of awakenings and arousals, reduced REM sleep, and a decrease in sleep efficiency in persons who have progressed to AIDS [34].

Wiegand and colleagues [14, 35] on the other hand, found no SWS disruptions in PWHA. Using nocturnal sleep encephalography, they found more frequent shifts to stage 1 sleep equated to a reduction in stage 2 sleep. Sleep-onset latency increased, but total sleep time and sleep efficiency decreased. The number of REM periods increased, but the average duration of a REM episode decreased.

Ferini-Strambi et al. examined sleep architecture in nine HIV-positive men and eight age matched controls. Their study showed a significant reduction in SWS and higher cyclic alternating patterns (CAP), representing the stability st`+ʻ``|$_**`

of sleep in PWHA compared to controls [36]. A significant relationship was found between a higher CAP rate and poor subjective sleep quality. Unlike Norman and colleagues, this group of researchers did not find a higher percentage of SWS in the second half of the night [36].

Wheatley and Smith found that HIV+ patients reported greater delay in sleep onset, earlier morning awakening, more frequent nocturnal awakenings, and poorer well-being on waking. A higher degree of insomnia was observed in individuals who were not taking antiretroviral therapy. They suggested that the observed sleep architecture changes might be related to depression.

Pharmacological Factors Related to Insomnia in HIV/AIDS

Many medications used to treat HIV/AIDS and its complications have insomnia as a side effect.

Adherence to Medications

A high degree of adherence to antiretroviral therapy in HIV/AIDS is necessary to decrease viral replication and to achieve viral suppression (HIV-1 RNA<50 copies per milliliter) [37, 38]. With monitoring and adjustment of combinations of antiretroviral agents, it is possible to decrease the rate of viral mutation and the evolution of drug resistance [39]. Further benefits of viral suppression include: slowing disease progression [40], prolonging life [41], and possibly decreasing the risk of transmitting HIV to others [42]. Viral suppression is also important in reducing overall health care costs.

Many improvements to drug regimens have been made. The number of medications and frequency of medications through the day have decreased by several agents into fewer pills. There are not as many food restrictions as before and it is easier to store medications. However, many barriers to adherence persist. These barriers include stigma, limited access to qualified providers, travel distances to receive care, and limited access to mental health and substance-abuse care. Symptom burden, which is the sum of the severity and impact of symptoms, predict nonadherence to antiretroviral drugs. Depression has been identified in various studies as barriers that decrease adherence to antiretroviral therapy [10, 43–45]. A cross-sectional analysis conducted by Phillips and colleagues demonstrated that HIV-infected women who reported more depressive symptoms and poorer sleep quality also reported lower adherence to medications [44]. Associations between sleep quality and adherence have been demonstrated by others since that study [43, 46].

People who have difficulty sleeping report impaired daytime functioning, which includes decreased attention and concentration, greater fatigue, impaired memory, and decreased ability to carry out daily tasks [10, 47, 48].

In a cross-sectional study of HIV-infected women living in the southeastern USA, Phillips and colleagues [44] found that two thirds of the participants endured severe sleep disturbance and that sleep disturbance was significantly related to adherence to antiretroviral therapy due to daytime dysfunction.

Gay and colleagues, in a study of 350 women and men with HIV infection, found that overall symptom burden was related to medication adherence. Troubling sleep was strongly associated with nonadherence to medications in that study. "Forgetting" and "sleeping through the dose time" were the most frequent reasons identified for failing to take a prescribed dose [49].

Saberi and colleagues [10] conducted a large cross-sectional study ($n=2.846$) of HIV-infected men and women to determine the prevalence of sleep disturbance and to identify the relationship between sleep quality and medication nonadherence. Together, these findings support that sleep disturbances are associated with nonadherence, and future studies of interventions for improving sleep quality should include medication adherence outcome measures.

Correlates of Sleep in HIV/AIDS

In studies involving the general population, researchers recognize the major correlates of diminished quality of sleep as (a) fatigue, (b) excessive daytime sleepiness, (c) perceived stress, and (d) depression. All of these exist in PWHA in addition to anxiety and pain [3, 6, 17]. In an integrated literature review examining insomnia in PWHA, Reid and Dwyer noted that all of the associated correlates are entangled due to "overlap at both measurement and conceptual levels" (p. 267) [9]. Similarly, Nokes and Kendrew [17] reported that the intercorrelations between symptom severity, excessive sleepiness, depression, state anxiety, and functional status precluded attempts to statistically "untangle the effects of the variables" (p. 21). The fact that PWHA usually present with multiple symptoms [50] compounds the difficulty. While both physiologic and psychological variables affect quality of sleep in PWHA, the latter (depression, stress, and anxiety) display strongest statistical correlation. For the PWHA, this manifests as marked delays in sleep onset, more awakenings during the night, and less transition into non-REM sleep [3]. In turn, the resultant insomnia exacerbates the psychological distress of the chronically ill [51].

While existing data sources do not allow calculation of incidence [52], fatigue leads as the most prevalent complaint of PWHA with estimates ranging from less than 50% to more than 80%. Whereas Lerdal et al. [53] simply define fatigue as a "sense of exhaustion, lack of energy, tiredness unrelieved by a night of good quality sleep" (p. 2204), other authors capture a more graphic characterization. In what is considered a classic analysis of the phenomenon, Ream and

Richardson, as cited in Barroso and Voss [52], described fatigue as a "subjective, unpleasant symptom that incorporates total feelings ranging from tiredness to exhaustion, creating an unrelenting overall condition that interferes with individuals' ability to function to their normal capacities" (p. S5). Asked to explain it, PWHA attribute their fatigue to either the disease itself or existing physical attributes (e.g., being overweight), overexertion, or medication side effects [54]. Despite instrument scores indicating significant pathology, respondents have been known to rate the quality of their sleep as "fairly good" [3].

Diminished quality of life arises from the awareness of the imbalance of resources, capacity, and performance [52, 55]. Significantly correlated with quality of sleep, fatigue is a constant across all stages of the disease [56] resulting in persistent impaired daytime functioning [10, 47, 48] and, somewhat paradoxically, increased sleep-onset difficulties [20]. In turn, daytime dysfunction has been significantly related to adherence to antiretroviral therapy regimens [27, 55]. Studying fatigue and insomnia in homosexual men (62 HIV+ and 50 HIV−), Darko et al. [8] found that HIV+ subjects were more likely to: be unemployed, feel fatigued throughout the day, sleep more, nap more, and have diminished alertness. Both fatigue and insomnia significantly contributed to morbidity and mortality in the HIV+ subjects. They concluded that the cognitive dysfunction seen in early HIV infection (asymptomatic) is related more to loss of sleep than to actual neurological impairment.

Twenty years later, Harmon et al. documented that the fatigue PWHA experience differs in both quality and severity than that experienced before becoming infected [57]. HIV-Related Fatigue Scale (HRFS) scores from their study sample ($N=128$) indicated that fatigue interfered with cognition (mental clarity and facility), task performance (activities of daily living), and socialization (work and leisure). The researchers determined that those who have lived the longest with the diagnosis have lower self-reported rates of fatigue attributed to learned coping mechanisms. From this study's findings, increased rates of fatigue can be predicted both in the presence of lower monthly income and pharmacologic treatment of depression. In 2009, Lee et al. [5] reported on clinical characteristics of symptom experiences among PWHA ($N=350$ adults) noting that most prevalent were "lack of energy" and "feeling drowsy" due to "trouble sleeping." These states resulted in difficulty concentrating as well as mild symptoms of depression and anxiety.

A more recent study by Lerdal et al. [53] began exploring patterns of fatigue among PWHA. A sample of 318 PWHA completed self-report questionnaires related to symptoms Memorial Symptom Assessment Scale (MSAS), fatigue (Lee Fatigue Scale; Fatigue Severity Scale 7), sleep quality (PSQI), depression (CES-D), anxiety (POMS), and quality of life (Medical Outcome Study Health Related QOL). Participants were asked to complete the assessments 30 min

after awakening and again 30 min before going to sleep for three consecutive days. Overall, evening fatigue level scores were significantly higher than morning fatigue level scores. While 30% reported fatigue either in the morning or in the evening only, it was noted that those who reported high fatigue in the morning were likely also to report high fatigue in the evening. Using those who reported low levels of fatigue both in the morning and evening (35% of respondents) as a reference group, three patterns were identified: (a) high-fatigue levels only in the morning; (b) high-fatigue levels only in the evening; and (c) high-fatigue levels both morning and evening. High-fatigue levels only reported in the morning were associated with higher anxiety and depression scores; while high-fatigue levels reported only in the evening were associated with high-anxiety scores. Labeled the most debilitating and distressing, high-fatigue levels in both the morning and evening were associated with high-anxiety scores, high-depression scores, and significant sleep disturbances. It is important to note that anxiety is an important antecedent of fatigue regardless of diurnal patterns. Acknowledging the cyclical interaction of psychological variables and quality of sleep suggests once again that mental health states are more predictive of fatigue than the HIV/AIDS disease state. And in turn, while psychological correlates affect sleep, only fatigue maintains statistical significance when exploring the association with sleep quality [3].

EDS is an inability to stay awake in quiet, sedentary situations (such as when reading, watching television, or even driving). While drowsiness (a milder form of daytime sleepiness) may be a by-product of lack of sleep or medication, EDS is usually associated with pathological sleep disorders such as obstructive sleep apnea (OSA) [5, 51]. Prevalence of OSA in PWHA has not been explored or documented despite the presence of several risk factors such as ART-associated lipodystrophy and opioid dependence [51]. In the majority of the studies examining sleep correlates, EDS is determined using the Epworth Sleepiness Scale (ESS), an 8-item self-administered questionnaire validated in obstructive sleep apnea, narcolepsy, and idiopathic hypersomnia. Using this instrument, EDS is defined using a standard cut-point of $ESS \geq 10$.

Crum-Cianflone and colleagues examined sleep quality (PSQI) and daytime sleepiness (Epworth Daytime Sleepiness Scale) in 193 HIV-infected participants and compared them with 50 HIV-negative participants. The HIV-infected group did not differ from the HIV-negative group by mean age, gender, race, rank, or duty status, but they did differ in that the HIV-infected group was slightly better educated, more depressed (Beck Depression Inventory), and were more likely to be hypertensive than the HIV-negative group. No differences were found between the HIV-infected group and the HIV-negative group on the total sleep quality score, any of the seven sleep quality component scores, or on daytime sleepiness. The authors concluded that HIV-infected patients who are diagnosed and treated early may have similar rates of sleep disturbances as the general population [12].

In a similar study examining correlates of sleep in 58 PWHA, Nokes and Kendrew noted that the majority of the participants were unemployed and 79 % reported taking daytime naps at varying frequency [17]. Wanting to determine if sleep quality mediated the stress–fatigue relationship, Salahuddin et al. examined levels of fatigue, sleep quality, and daytime sleepiness in 128 PWHA (majority African-American males; median age 44 years) most of whom had lived with the infection for 10 or more years [58]. Using scores from the HIV-Related Fatigue Scale (HRFS), PSQI, ESS, and a checklist of possibly stressful life events, they found weak correlations between EDS and both fatigue and sleep quality despite the fact that PSQI scores indicated pathological problems. While there was a significant relationship between and among sleep quality, fatigue, and daytime functioning, excessive sleepiness did not add to symptom. Furthermore, Salahuddin et al. found that the association between stress and fatigue-related daytime dysfunction was only marginally explained by EDS and sleep quality yet remains significant when examining daytime dysfunction [58].

The relationship between fatigue and depression is well documented in both the general population and PWHA. Indeed, Lerdal et al. [53] observes that "tiredness" is the second most prevalent symptom among depressed adults while Harmon et al. [57] cites depression as the most influential concomitant accompanying fatigue. Reid and Dwyer noted that the most notable finding of their integrated review of research literature is that the prevalence of depression in PWHA is markedly and significantly related to quality of sleep rather than CD4 count or disease stage [9]. Moneyham et al. observe that it is possible that many of the symptoms manifested in PWHA are manifestations of depression [59].

Working with a sample (*N*=278) of predominantly African-American women, Moneyham and colleagues found that depressive symptoms vary significantly with education, income levels, and living arrangements [59]. These findings are similar to those from studies examining the role of fatigue in the lives of PWHA and support the observed interrelationship between and among the correlates of sleep quality. In this case, analysis of data from a longitudinal study supported their hypothesis that social support and coping strategies can intervene in the relationship between stress (symptom burden and daily functioning) and depression. Indeed, the intensity of symptom burden plus its impact on ability to function in performance of daily activities becomes a significant predictor of depression. These findings are supported by Low et al. who reported that, if present, depression is the central companion of fatigue [60].

Noting that depression levels may decrease as years living with the diagnosis increase [57, 58], contemporary researchers advocate studies that include lifestyle, environmental, cultural, and health belief factors in order to identify and implement interventions leading to effective symptom management [9, 55, 59]. Such interventions might serve to break the patterns of anxiety that have been shown to be associated with therapeutic regimen adherence and quality of life [5, 61].

As life expectancy of PWHA increases, more attention is being given to quality of life. In 2009, Lee et al. reported that reported prevalence of pain in PWHA ranged from 30 to 90 %. The wide range was attributed to varying stages of disease among research participants and the use of different measurement instruments by the researchers. In one of the few studies examining the relationship of pain and sleep quality, Aouizerat and colleagues compared differences in fatigue, sleep disturbances, anxiety, and depression in PWHA with and without pain [50]. They reported significantly greater problems across all variables in the group experiencing pain than in participants reporting no pain. The concern is that providers have been underestimating the relationship between pain and sleep, and therefore, not effectively intervening. From findings of their study of the experience of pain in PWHA, Kowal et al. concluded that interventions strengthening effective coping strategies and improving daily functioning will result in decreased vulnerability to depressive symptoms [62].

Nonpharmacological Treatments for Insomnia

Psychological interventions for PWHA with chronic insomnia offer many benefits when compared to sedative hypnotics [63, 64]. Therefore, it is reasonable and prudent that the first line of treatment should be a psychological intervention.

Cognitive Behavioral Therapy (CBT)

CBT is the current standard of care for first-line treatment of insomnia in the general population. The National Institutes of Health State-of-the-Science Conference on insomnia has listed CBT as a safe and effective means of managing chronic insomnia [65]. Cognitive behavioral therapy and cognitive behavioral therapy with relaxation for insomnia are supported by research. Cognitive behavioral therapy may produce moderate to large effect sizes for sleep-onset latency and sleep quality, and it produces small to moderate effects sizes for number of awakenings, duration of awakenings, and total sleep time [66–74].

Cognitive therapy is based on these premises (1) that cognitive activity (e.g., thoughts, attitudes, and beliefs) affects behavior; (2) cognitive activity can be changed; and (3) behavior and emotions can be monitored and changed [75, 76]. Cognitive activity is part of the adaptive process; however, sometimes cognitions become distorted and lead to maladaptation. Examples of cognitive distortions about sleep include: (1) a person's belief that he or she will not be able to sleep without a medication, (2) a person's belief that if he or she is unable to sleep, it is better to just stay in bed and rest, (3) a person's belief that there is nothing he or she can do to improve sleep, and (4) they will have to deal with insomnia forever. Maladaptive cognitions such as these can lead to chronic insomnia. When cognitive distortions are identified, the goal of therapy is to help the person replace cognitive distortions with adaptive cognitions.

Cognitive behavioral therapy combines cognitive therapy and specific behavioral treatments [77]. Research findings support the efficacy of CBT for primary and comorbid insomnia (associated with a physiological or psychological condition) [78–83]. A randomized, placebo-controlled trial was conducted among 63 young and middle-aged adults with chronic insomnia. Participants were randomly assigned to one of three of three groups: CBT alone, pharmacotherapy alone (zolpidem), or combined CBT and pharmacotherapy. Cognitive behavioral therapy produced greater improvements in sleep-onset latency and sleep efficiency, resulted in the greatest number of normal sleepers following treatment, and maintained these beneficial changes longer [84]. In an earlier clinical trial, 78 adults with chronic and primary insomnia completed an intervention of CBT, pharmacotherapy (temazepam), combined CBT and pharmacotherapy, or a placebo. Treatment outcomes were time awake after sleep onset as measured by sleep diaries and polysomnography and clinical ratings from subjects, significant others, and clinicians. All three active intervention arms resulted in improvements in sleep. The researchers concluded that both CBT and pharmacological interventions were effective for the short time, but the beneficial gains were maintained longer following CBT alone or in or in combination with behavioral treatment [81].

A small pilot study of eight female survivors of breast cancer demonstrated efficacy of CBT by a reduction in total wake time and increased sleep efficiency as measured by a sleep diary and by polysomnography [85]. In a subsequent more adequately powered study, this group of researchers provided 8 weekly sessions of CBT to small groups of participants and compared them to participants in a waitlist control group. They found that CBT effectively increased sleep efficiency, decreased total wake time, decreased sleep onset latency, and decreased wake after sleep onset as measured by polysomnography. Significant reductions in the number of hypnotic medicated nights, insomnia severity, anxiety, and depression were also observed [86].

Many questions about CBT for the treatment of insomnia remain unexplored. These include the number and length of sessions needed to obtain beneficial results.

Sleep Hygiene

Sleep hygiene is a self-managed behavioral intervention that is the most commonly recommended intervention to promote good sleep [87]. Sleep hygiene education can be done easily in a clinician's office.

Sleep hygiene refers to sleep-related behaviors and environmental factors that can be altered to improve sleep quality [88, 89]. The principles of sleep hygiene include eating a healthy diet, limiting the amount of caffeine intake, and going to bed and getting out of bed at consistent times, sleeping in a quiet, dark, temperature-controlled room on a comfortable mattress and pillow. Daytime naps and exercise within 4 h of bedtime are avoided. Eating, drinking (both alcoholic and nonalcoholic beverages), and smoking before going to bed should be avoided. The bed should be used only for sleep and sexual intercourse. The use of electronic devices near bedtime should be avoided [90, 91].

Only two studies have examined the effectiveness of sleep hygiene education for improving the sleep of PWHA [92, 93]. Webel and colleagues tested a sleep hygiene intervention in 40 PWHA. Participants were randomly assigned to one of two groups, with the intervention group receiving a sleep hygiene intervention known as System CHANGE-HIV. Participants in the intervention group had increased sleep efficiency and decreased sleep fragmentation when compared to the control group [93]. Dreher examined the effects of caffeine reduction in an international sample of 88 HIV-positive men and women who experienced insomnia or any other sleeping problem on an occasional or frequent basis. All participants had a total score greater than five on the PSQI at baseline [92]. Participants were randomized to one of two groups. The experimental group was instructed to withdraw from caffeine gradually and then to avoid all caffeine sources for 30 days. In that study, participants in the experimental group reduced their caffeine intake by 90 % compared to a 6 % reduction of caffeine intake in the control group. No difference in the change in sleep quality from pretest to posttest between the groups was observed. However, a 35 % improvement in sleep quality was observed in the experimental group when sleep quality was controlled for health status [92].

Even though sleep hygiene is commonly recommended in clinical practice, randomized studies that are sufficiently powered to demonstrate the efficacy of this intervention do not exist. There is little consensus about which sleep hygiene principles should be included in a treatment plan, and no two studies have used the same set of sleep hygiene principles. Small sample sizes, the inclusion of other interventions, and examining only one aspect of sleep hygiene fail to provide sufficient evidence for the efficacy of sleep hygiene in improving sleep quality [74, 94]. However, sleep hygiene is a common sense approach and the principles of sleep hygiene can be easily taught; therefore, it is one of the most frequently used clinical interventions for disrupted sleep quality.

Relaxation Training

Relaxation training exercises have been used successfully to promote sleep. Relaxation techniques include progressive muscle relaxation and autogenic training (used to reduce somatic tension), and guided imagery and meditation (used to reduce intrusive thoughts at bedtime).

Progressive Muscle Relaxation

Progressive muscle relaxation involves alternately tensing (5 s) and relaxing successive muscle groups (25 s). The person is guided to discriminate between how the muscle feels when contracted and when tensed. As the person becomes more experienced with progressive muscle relaxation over time, the difference between tenseness and relaxation can be discerned without actually having to contract the muscles [95]. Progressive muscle relaxation is a recommended intervention for the treatment of chronic insomnia [74, 78, 96]. *Autogenic training* uses autosuggestions, very similar to self-hypnosis. Autogenic training helps a person to experience relaxation, heaviness, and warmth in the limbs, while at the same time recognizing a calm heart beat and slower respirations [97, 98]. Autogenic training is recommended by the American Association of Sleep Medicine [74, 81, 99]. *Guided imagery* refers to a mind–body technique in which a person is guided to imagine a place that is safe and comfortable to them. During that time the person is imaging this safe and comfortable place, they are instructed to visualize muscle relaxation, to breathe in and out of the nose, and to feel how relaxed they are. Guided imagery is recommended by the Association of Sleep Medicine [74, 81, 99]. *Meditation*, as taught by Benson, [100] uses a word, a prayer, or movement to induce the relaxation response. These inductions are repeated continuously over 10–20 min and are often linked mentally with one's breathing pattern. During this relaxation response, other thoughts may occur, but the person is instructed to not judge the thoughts or respond to them. While learning to meditate, a person is instructed to select the induction behavior, to sit still in comfortable place, to close their eyes, to feel their muscles relax, to focus on their breathing patterns, and to meditate for 10–20 min. When the mind wanders during meditation, the person is taught to return to a focus on the induction behavior [74, 81, 99].

Stimulus Control Therapy

Stimulus control therapy is based on the principles of classical conditioning. For some people, going to bed has become associated with difficulty sleeping. For them, going to bed triggers negative emotions, such as fear, anxiety, frustration, and worry about not being able to sleep. The goals of stimulus control therapy are to help insomnia patients associate the bed and the bedroom only with sleep and to establish regular sleep–wake times. Stimulus control therapy incorporates the following: Use the bedroom only for sleep or sexual activity. Establish consistent times for going to bed, waking up, and getting out of bed and adhere to those times. Get into sunlight or another bright light as soon as possible after awakening. Go to bed only when you become sleepy; sleepiness should be distinguished from fatigue and exhaustion. After going to bed, if you do not fall to sleep within 15–20 min, get out of bed and go to another room to do something relaxing, and when you feel sleepy, return to bed and try to fall asleep again. Do not take daytime naps. It may take several weeks of stimulus control to reestablish normal sleeping patterns. Stimulus control therapy is a recommended psychological intervention for chronic insomnia [74, 101–105].

Sleep Restriction

Sleep restriction is based on the homeostatic sleep drive—the longer a person stays awake, the greater the drive to sleep and the deeper the sleep in the next sleep period [106]. At the beginning of therapy, the person restricts time in bed to the amount of time of actual sleep that is recorded in a sleep diary. This continues for 1 week. At the end of the week if the person has slept at least 90 % of the time actually in bed, then another 15 min is added to the sleep period. If wake time increases resulting in sleep time that is less than 80 % of the time in bed, the sleep period is decreased by 15 min. This process continues until the person achieves the desired amount of sleep. For many people, their sleep becomes more robust as the sleep becomes deeper. They experience fewer awakenings, and maintain sleep for longer periods [106–108].

Pharmacological Treatments for Insomnia in HIV/AIDS

The most common treatments for chronic insomnia are over the counter antihistamines, alcohol, and prescription medications [65]. Other treatments include melatonin and valerian. Prescription medications are frequently prescribed as well. The following is a discussion of the use of medications that promote sleep in HIV/AIDS.

Nonprescription Sleep Aids

Diphenhydramine hydrochloride and doxylamine succinate are over-the-counter H1 receptor antagonists which have historical Food and Drug Administration (FDA) approval for the treatment of insomnia. The American Academy of Sleep Medicine, however, does not recommend either diphenhydramine hydrochloride or doxylamine succinate for the treatment of chronic insomnia, because safety and efficacy data are insufficient [99, 109]. Benadryl may aggravate cognitive impairment in HIV disease and should not be used for the treatment of chronic insomnia [110].

Melatonine is a naturally occurring hormone produced by the pineal gland which helps regulate circadian rhythm [111]. People over 55 years of age often experience a reduction in endogenous melatonin, which may lead to insomnia. The greatest benefits of melatonin use for restoring normal sleep has been for people 55 years of age or older [112]. In HIV/AIDS, mean serum melatonin levels are lower in HIV-infected patients and decline with HIV disease progression [113]. The efficacy and the safety of melatonin for treating chronic insomnia in HIV/AIDS have not been studied.

Sedative Hypnotics

Sedative hypnotics fall into two broad categories: benzodiazepines and nonbenzodiazepine receptor agonists. Benefits of these medications for long-term use have not been studied sufficiently in the general population, and there is a notable absence of comparative effective studies of the safety and efficacy of sleep medications in HIV/AIDS. The lack of research in this area is problematic in that these medications may produce additional daytime sleepiness, daytime dysfunction, cognitive impairment, and motor incoordination [65], in PWHA who may already experience these symptoms.

Metabolism of Sedative Hypnotics

Sedative hypnotics may increase or decrease blood levels of antiretroviral medications. Sedative hypnotics that are *CYP3A inhibitors* are generally expected to increase plasma concentrations of antiretroviral medications that are metabolized by the CYP3A hepatic enzyme system. *CYP3A inducers* are expected to decrease plasma concentrations of antiretroviral medications. See Table 22.2.

Table 22.2 Use of sedative/hypnotics in HIV/AIDS

Brand names	Generic names	Mechanism	Metabolism	Half-life
Benzodiazepines				
ProSom®	Estrazolam	Stimulates the GABA-BZ_1 receptors	CYP3A	10–24 h
Dalmane®	Flurazepam	Stimulates the GABA-BZ_1 receptors	Specific CYP450 enzyme has not been identified	2–3 h; 47–100 h active metabolites
Doral®	Quazepam	Stimulates the GABA-BZ_1 receptors	CYP3A4	39–41 h
Restoril®	Temazepam	Stimulates the BZ_1 receptors	CYP isoforms convert temazepam to oxazepam	3.5–24 h
Halcion®	Triazolam	Stimulates the GABA-BZ_1 receptors	CYP3A	1.5–5.5 h
Nonbenzodiazepines				
Sonata	Zaleplon	Stimulates GABA-BZ1 receptors	CYP3A	1 h
Lunesta®	Eszopiclone	Unknown, but is thought to stimulate the GABA-BZ_1 receptors	CYP3A4	5–6 h
Ambien®	Zolpidem	Interacts with the GABA-BZ1 receptors	Converted to hydroxylated metabolites by CYP3A4 isoenzymes	1.4–3.8 h
Melatonin Receptor Agonist				
Rozerim®	Ramelteon	Stimulates melatonin receptors	CYP1A2 (primarily), CYP2C, and CYP3A4	2–5 h
Histamine-1 Antagonists				
Desyrel®	Trazodone	Antagonizes alpha-1, 5-HT_{2A}, and H-1 receptors at low doses	CYP450 2D6	4–9 h
Elavil®	Amitriptyline	Serotonin-norepinephrine reuptake inhibitor Sedative effect is likely due to histamine-1 receptor antagonism		31–46 h
Sinequan®	Doxepin	Sedative effect is likely due to histamine-1 receptor antagonism	CYP450 2C19 CYP450 2D6	
Remeron®	Mirtazapine	Antagonizes 5-HT2A, 5-HT2C, and H-1	CYP450 2D6	20–40 h

Cytochrome P450 (CYP450) is a class of enzymes usually expressed in liver cells but can also be found in the small intestines, lungs, placenta, and kidneys. These enzymes are located in the smooth endoplasmic reticulum, contain a heme molecule, and absorb light at the wavelength of 450 nm. This class of enzymes is essential for cholesterol, steroid, prostacyclin, and thromboxane A_2 production, in addition to medication metabolism and chemical detoxification. There are over 50 enzymes but six of them constitute approximately 90 % of drug metabolism with CYP3A4 and CYP2D6 being the most significant players [114].

CYP450 enzymes can be inhibited or induced by drugs. Inhibitors are known to block metabolic activity of CYP enzymes while inducers increase the enzyme activity and synthesis, both of which can alter medication blood levels. Some drugs have the ability to be metabolized and then inhibit/induce the same or different enzymes. Medications can be intentionally combined by health care professionals to take advantage of CYP450 enzymes. In HIV patients, liponovir serum levels increased when combined with ritonavir, a protease inhibitor and CYP3A4 inhibitor. However, most combinations of these agents lead to significant adverse drug interactions involving increased side effects or decreased drug effectiveness. This is important since many antiretroviral agents used for HIV contain similar metabolic pathways as most commonly used drugs. Information regarding CYP450 metabolism can be found on drug labels or at the FDA website [114].

Histamine-1 Receptor Antagonists

Histamine helps regulate the sleep–wake cycle [109]. Antidepressant medications (trazodone, doxepin, amitriptyline, and mirtazapine) that are H_1 receptor antagonists are used off label for the treatment of insomnia. An exception to this is doxepin, which has received FDA approval for use in sleep maintenance disorders [109].

Trazodone is widely prescribed for its sedating effects and is one of the most commonly prescribed medications for treating insomnia in the USA [65]. Trazodone most likely results from binding of H1 receptors, alpha-1 receptors, and 5-HT_{2A} receptors. Empirical evidence for using trazodone to treat insomnia is limited. Short-term efficacy of trazodone as a hypnotic has been demonstrated for up to 2 weeks, but its long-term effectiveness is unknown [65].

Doxepin has the most empirical support for the treatment of insomnia, especially for sleep maintenance insomnia. The efficacy of doxepin has been studied in healthy adults, adults with primary insomnia, and elderly adults. These trials have demonstrated consistent improvement in subjective sleep quality and objective sleep measures including wake after sleep onset (a reduction of 5–20 min), total sleep time

(an increase of 25–51 min), and sleep efficiency (an increase of 6–10 %) [115–121]. Doxepin improves appetite, promotes weight gain, helps control diarrhea, and reduces the chronic pain of peripheral neuropathy [122].

Amitriptyline is a tricyclic antidepressant that has sedating effects. Amitriptyline is highly effective in treating major depression. However, the small difference between the therapeutic dose and a toxic dose. Amitriptyline overdose can lead to fatal cardiac arrhythmias. Tricyclic antidepressants are antihistamine (sedation), anticholinergic (constipation), and block alpha adrenergic receptors (erectile dysfunction, orthostatic, and hypotension). Amitriptyline may add to drying of the mouth and other secretions, which is one of the most frequent complaints of PWHA. Amitriptyline may increase appetite and thus be beneficial to persons who need to gain weight. Amitriptyline can be beneficial in the treatment of peripheral neuropathy [109, 122]. There are two studies that suggest that tricyclic antidepressants are not effective in HIV-related peripheral neuropathies [123]. Amitriptyline does not appear to affect immune status in HIV/AIDS [124].

Mirtazapine is an FDA-approved tetracyclic antidepressant. The sedative property of mirtazapine is most likely due to the fact that it blocks the H1 receptors. It also blocks $5HT_{2A}$ and $5HT_{2C}$ receptors which may promote sedation. Lower doses of mirtazapine may produce more sedation than higher doses, because at higher doses it may stimulate noradrenergic responses [125]. Clinical evidence for the use of mirtazapine for the treatment of chronic insomnia in HIV/AIDS is inadequate to recommend it for use solely for its sedative properties for PWHA [109].

The American Academy of Sleep Medicine recommends the use of sedating antidepressants when short-acting or intermediate-acting benzodiazepine receptor agonists have failed. They are particularly beneficial for persons with co-morbid depression or anxiety [99].

References

1. WHO. Global HIV/AIDS response: epidemic update and health sector progress towards universal access. Geneva: World Health Organization; 2011.
2. Gamaldo CE, Spira AP, Hock RS, et al. Sleep, function and HIV: a multi-method assessment. AIDS Behav. 2013;17(8):2808–15;17(8):2808–15.
3. Robbins JL, Phillips KD, Dudgeon WD, H and GA. Physiological and psychological correlates of sleep in HIV infection. Clin Nurs Res. 2004;13(1):33–52.
4. Hudson A, Kirksey K, Holzemer W. The influence of symptoms on quality of life among HIV-infected women. West J Nurs Res. 2004;26(1):9–23.
5. Lee KA, Gay C, Portillo CJ, et al. Symptom experience in HIV-infected adults: a function of demographic and clinical characteristics. J Pain Symptom Manage. 2009;38(6):882–93.
6. Rubinstein ML, Selwyn PA. High prevalence of insomnia in an outpatient population with HIV infection. J Acquir Immune Defic Syndr Hum Retrovirol. 1998;19(3):260–5.

7. Keenan S, Hirchowitz M. Monitoring and staging human sleep. In: Kryger MH, Roth T, Dement WC, editors. Principles and practice of sleep medicine. 5th ed. St Louis: Elsevier-Saunders; 2011. pp. 1602–9.

8. Darko DF, McCutchan JA, Kripke DF, Gillin JC, Golshan S. Fatigue, sleep disturbance, disability, and indices of progression of HIV infection. Am J Psychiatry. 1992;149(4):514–20.

9. Reid S, Dwyer J. Insomnia in HIV infection: a systematic review of prevalence, correlates, and management. Psychosom Med. 2005;67(2):260–9.

10. Saberi P, Neilands TB, Johnson MO. Quality of sleep: associations with antiretroviral nonadherence. AIDS Patient Care STDS. 2011;25(9):517–24.

11. Norman SE, Resnick L, Cohn MA, Duara R, Herbst J, Berger JR. Sleep disturbances in HIV-seropositive patients. JAMA. 1988;260(7):922.

12. Crum-Cianflone NF, Roediger MP, Moore DJ, et al. Prevalence and factors associated with sleep disturbances among early-treated HIV-infected persons. Clin Infect Dis. 2012;54(10):1485–94.

13. Norman SE, Chediak AD, Freeman C, et al. Sleep disturbances in men with asymptomatic human immunodeficiency (HIV) infection. Sleep. 1992;15(2):150–5.

14. Wiegand M, Moller AA, Schreiber W, Krieg JC, Holsboer F. Alterations of nocturnal sleep in patients with HIV infection. Acta Neurol Scand. 1991;83(2):141–2.

15. Terstegge K, Henkes H, Scheuler W, Hansen ML, Ruf B, Kubicki S. Spectral power and coherence analysis of sleep EEG in AIDS patients: decrease in interhemispheric coherence. Sleep 1993;16(2):137–45.

16. Kubicki S, Henkes H, Terstegge K, Ruf B. AIDS related sleep disturbances: a preliminary report. HIV and nervous system. New York: Fischer; 1988. pp. 97–105.

17. Nokes KM, Kendrew J. Correlates of sleep quality in persons with HIV disease. J Assoc Nurses AIDS Care. 2001;12(1):17–22.

18. Justice AC, Rabeneck L, Hays RD, Wu AW, Bozzette SA. Sensitivity, specificity, reliability, and clinical validity of provider-reported symptoms: a comparison with self-reported symptoms. Outcomes Committee of the AIDS Clinical Trials Group. J Acquir Immune Defic Syndr. 1999;21(2):126–33.

19. Hudson AL, Portillo CJ, Lee KA. Sleep disturbances in women with HIV or AIDS: efficacy of a tailored sleep promotion intervention. Nurs Res. 2008;57(5):360–6.

20. Lee KA, Portillo CJ, Miramontes H. The influence of sleep and activity patterns on fatigue in women with HIV/AIDS. J Assoc Nurses AIDS Care 2001;12(Suppl):19–27.

21. Vogl D, Rosenfeld B, Breitbart W, et al. Symptom prevalence, characteristics, and distress in AIDS outpatients. J Pain Symptom Manage. 1999;18(4):253–62.

22. Bayon C, Ribera E, Cabrero E, Griffa L, Burgos A. Prevalence of depressive and other central nervous system symptoms in HIV-infected patients treated with HAART in Spain. J Int Assoc Physicians AIDS Care (Chic) 2012;11(5):321–8.

23. Ohayon MM, Sagales T. Prevalence of insomnia and sleep characteristics in the general population of Spain. Sleep Med. 2010;11(10):1010–8.

24. Lee KA, Gay C, Portillo CJ, et al. Types of sleep problems in adults living with HIV/AIDS. J Clin Sleep Med. 2012;8(1):67–75.

25. Moeller AA, Oechsner M, Backmund HC, Popescu M, Emminger C, Holsboer F. Self-reported sleep quality in HIV infection: correlation to the stage of infection and zidovudine therapy. J Acquir Immune Defic Syndr. 1991;4(10):1000–3.

26. Phillips KD, Sowell RL, Rojas M, Tavakoli A, Fulk LJ, H and GA. Physiological and psychological correlates of fatigue in HIV disease. Biol Res Nurs. 2004;6(1):59–74.

27. Phillips KD, Sowell RL, Boyd M, Dudgeon WD, Hand GA. Sleep quality and health-related quality of life in HIV-infected African-American women of childbearing age. Qual Life Res. 2005;14(4):959–70.

28. Besedovsky L, Lange T, Born J. Sleep and immune function. Pflugers Arch. 2012;463(1):121–37.

29. Darko DF, Mitler MM, Henriksen SJ. Lentiviral infection, immune response peptides and sleep. Adv Neuroimmunol. 1995;5(1):57–77.

30. Cruess DG, Antoni MH, Gonzalez J, et al. Sleep disturbance mediates the association between psychological distress and immune status among HIV-positive men and women on combination antiretroviral therapy. J Psychosom Res. 2003;54(3):185–9.

31. Norman SE, Chediak AD, Kiel M, Cohn MA. Sleep disturbances in HIV-infected homosexual men. AIDS. 1990;4(8):775–81.

32. Norman SE, Shaukat M, Nay KN, Cohn M, Resnick L. Alterations in sleep architecture in asymptomatic HIV seropositive patients. Sleep Res. 1987;16:494.

33. Norman SE, Kiel M, Nay KN, Demirozu MC, Dunbar S, Cohn MA. Alpha-delta sleep pattern and circadian rhythmicity in HIV seropositive patients. Sleep Res. 1989;17:353.

34. Kubicki S, Henkes H, Terstegge K, Ruf B. AIDS related sleep disturbances: a preliminary report. In: Kubicki S, Henkes H, Bienzle U, Pohle HD, editors. HIV and the nervous system. New York: Gustav Fischer; 1988. pp. 97–105.

35. Wiegand M, Moller AA, Schreiber W, et al. Nocturnal sleep EEG in patients with HIV infection. Eur Arch Psychiatry Clin Neurosci. 1991;240(3):153–8.

36. Ferini-Strambi L, Oldani A, Tirloni G, et al. Slow wave sleep and cyclic alternating pattern (CAP) in HIV-infected asymptomatic men. Sleep. 1995;18(6):446–50.

37. Bangsberg DR, Hecht FM, Charlebois ED, et al. Adherence to protease inhibitors, HIV –1 viral load, and development of drug resistance in an indigent population. AIDS. 2000;14(4):357–66.

38. Arnsten JH, Demas PA, Farzadegan H, et al. Antiretroviral therapy adherence and viral suppression in HIV-infected drug users: comparison of self-report and electronic monitoring. Clin Infect Dis. 2001;33(8):1417–23.

39. Bangsberg DR. Less than 95 % adherence to nonnucleoside reverse-transcriptase inhibitor therapy can lead to viral suppression. Clin Infect Dis. 2006;43(7):939–41.

40. Crum NF, Riffenburgh RH, Wegner S, et al. Comparisons of causes of death and mortality rates among HIV-infected persons: analysis of the pre-, early, and late HAART (highly active antiretroviral therapy) eras. J Acquir Immune Defic Syndr. 2006;41(2):194–200.

41. Mocroft A, Ledergerber B, Katlama C, et al. Decline in the AIDS and death rates in the EuroSIDA study: an observational study. Lancet. 2003;362(9377):22–9.

42. CDC. Effect of antiretroviral therapy on risk of sexual transmission of HIV infection and superinfection. Centers for Disease Control and Prevention; 2009. http://www.cdc.gov/hiv/topics/treatment/resources/factsheets/pdf/art.pdf. Accessed 1 Feb 2013.

43. Gay C, Portillo CJ, Kelly R, et al. Self-reported medication adherence and symptom experience in adults with HIV. J Assoc Nurses AIDS Care. 2011;22(4):257–68.

44. Phillips KD, Moneyham L, Murdaugh C, et al. Sleep disturbance and depression as barriers to adherence. Clin Nurs Res. 2005;14(3):273–93.

45. Ammassari A, Murri R, Pezzotti P, et al. Self-reported symptoms and medication side effects influence adherence to highly active antiretroviral therapy in persons with HIV infection. J Acquir Immune Defic Syndr. 2001;28(5):445–9.

46. Pedrol E, Tasias M, Clotet B, et al. Study to determine the improvement in neuropsychiatric symptoms after changing the

responsible antiretroviral drug to nevirapine: the RELAX study. J Int AIDS Soc. 2012;15(6):18347.

47. Roth T, Ancoli-Israel S. Daytime consequences and correlates of insomnia in the United States: results of the 1991 National Sleep Foundation Survey. II. Sleep 1999;22(Suppl 2):S354–8.

48. Ustinov Y, Lichstein KL, Wal GS, Taylor DJ, Riedel BW, Bush AJ. Association between report of insomnia and daytime functioning. Sleep Med. 2010;11(1):65–8.

49. Aouizerat BE, Gay CL, Lerdal A, Portillo CJ, Lee KA. Lack of energy: an important and distinct component of HIV-related fatigue and daytime function. J. Pain Symptom Manage. 2013;45(2):191–201.

50. Aouizerat BE, Miaskowski CA, Gay C, et al. Risk factors and symptoms associated with pain in HIV-infected adults. J Assoc Nurses AIDS Care. 2010;21(2):125–33.

51. Taibi DM. Sleep disturbances in persons living with HIV. J Assoc Nurses AIDS Care. 2013;24(Suppl 1):S72–85.

52. Barroso J, Voss JG. Fatigue in HIV and AIDS: an analysis of evidence. J Assoc Nurses AIDS Care. 2013;24(Suppl 1):S5–14.

53. Lerdal A, Gay CL, Aouizerat BE, Portillo CJ, Lee KA. Patterns of morning and evening fatigue among adults with HIV/AIDS. J Clin Nurs. 2011;20(15–16):2204–16.

54. Siegel K, Bradley CJ, Lekas HM. Causal attributions for fatigue among late middle-aged and older adults with HIV infection. J Pain Symptom Manage. 2004;28(3):211–24.

55. Voss JG, Dodd M, Portillo C, Holzemer W. Theories of fatigue: application in HIV/AIDS. J Assoc Nurses AIDS Care. 2006;17(1):37–50.

56. Darko DF, Mitler MM, Miller JC. Growth hormone, fatigue, poor sleep, and disability in HIV infection. Neuroendocrinology. 1998;67(5):317–24.

57. Harmon JL, Barroso J, Pence BW, Leserman J, Salahuddin N. Demographic and illness-related variables associated with HIV-related fatigue. J Assoc Nurses AIDS Care. 2008;19(2):90–7.

58. Salahuddin N, Barroso J, Leserman J, Harmon JL, Pence BW. Daytime sleepiness, nighttime sleep quality, stressful life events, and HIV-related fatigue. J Assoc Nurses AIDS Care. 2009;20(1):6–13.

59. Moneyham L, Murdaugh C, Phillips K, et al. Patterns of risk of depressive symptoms among HIV-positive women in the southeastern United States. J Assoc Nurses AIDS Care. 2005;16(4):25–38.

60. Low Y, Preud'homme X, Goforth HW, Omonuwa T, Krystal AD. The association of fatigue with depression and insomnia in HIV-seropositive patients: a pilot study. Sleep. 2011;34(12):1723–6.

61. Kemppainen JK, Mackain S, Reyes D. Anxiety symptoms in HIV-infected individuals. J Assoc Nurses AIDS Care. 2013;24(Suppl 1):S29–39.

62. Kowal J, Overduin LY, Balfour L, Tasca GA, Corace K, Cameron DW. The role of psychological and behavioral variables in quality of life and the experience of bodily pain among persons living with HIV. J Pain Symptom Manage. 2008;36(3):247–58.

63. National Institutes of Health. NIH releases statement on behavioral and relaxation approaches for chronic pain and insomnia. Am Fam Physician. 1996;53:1877–80.

64. National Institutes of Health. Consensus development conference statement: the treatment of sleep disorders of older people. Sleep. 1991;14:169–77.

65. NIH. State of the science conference statement on manifestations and management of chronic Insomnia in adults. NIH Consens Sci Statments. 2005;22(2):1–39.

66. Smith MT, Perlis ML, Park A, et al. Comparative meta-analysis of pharmacotherapy and behavior therapy for persistent insomnia. Am J Psychiatry. 2002;159(1):5–11.

67. Morin CM, Benca R. Chronic insomnia. Lancet. 2012;379(9821):1129–41.

68. Murtagh DR, Greenwood KM. Identifying effective psychological treatments for insomnia: a meta-analysis. J Consult Clin Psychol. 1995;63(1):79–89.

69. Morin CM, Culbert JP, Schwartz SM. Nonpharmacological interventions for insomnia: a meta-analysis of treatment efficacy. Am J Psychiatry. 1994;151(8):1172–80.

70. Morin CM, Hauri PJ, Espie CA, Spielman AJ, Buysse DJ, Bootzin RR. Nonpharmacologic treatment of chronic insomnia. Sleep. 1999;22(8):1134–56.

71. Irwin MR, Cole JC, Nicassio PM. Comparative meta-analysis of behavioral interventions for insomnia and their efficacy in middle-aged adults and in older adults 55+ years of age. Health Psychol. 2006;25(1):3–14.

72. McCurry SM, Logsdon RG, Teri L, Vitiello MV. Evidence-based psychological treatments for insomnia in older adults. Psychol Aging. 2007;22(1):18–27.

73. Morin CM, Bootzin RR, Buysse DJ, Edinger JD, Espie CA, Lichstein KL. Psychological and behavioral treatment of insomnia:update of the recent evidence (1998–2004). Sleep. 2006;29(11):1398–414.

74. Morgenthaler T, Kramer M, Alessi C, et al. Practice parameters for the psychological and behavioral treatment of insomnia: an update. Sleep. 2006;29(11):1415–9.

75. Reinecke MA. Cognitive therapies of depression: a modularized treatment approach. In: Reinecke MA, Davison MR, editors. Comparative treatments of depression. New York: Springer; 2002. pp. 249–90.

76. Beck AT. Cognitive therapies and emotional disorders. New York: New American Library; 1976.

77. Hofmann SG. An introduction to modern CBT: pyshcological solutions to mental health problems. Chichester, West Sussex, U.K.: Wiley-Blackwell; 2011.

78. Edinger JD, Wohlgemuth WK, Radtke RA, Marsh GR, Quillian RE. Cognitive behavioral therapy for treatment of chronic primary insomnia: a randomized controlled trial. JAMA. 2001;285(14):1856–64.

79. Mimeault V, Morin CM. Self-help treatment for insomnia: bibliotherapy with and without professional guidance. J Consult Clin Psychol. 1999;67(4):511–9.

80. Morin CM, Kowatch RA, Barry T, Walton E. Cognitive-behavior therapy for late-life insomnia. J Consult Clin Psychol. 1993;61(1):137–46.

81. Morin CM, Colecchi C, Stone J, Sood R, Brink D. Behavioral and pharmacological therapies for late-life insomnia: a randomized controlled trial. JAMA. 1999;281(11):991–9.

82. Savard J, Davidson JR, Ivers H, et al. The association between nocturnal hot flashes and sleep in breast cancer survivors. J Pain Symptom Manage. 2004;27(6):513–22.

83. Perlis ML, Smith MT, Orff H, et al. The effects of modafinil and cognitive behavior therapy on sleep continuity in patients with primary insomnia. Sleep. 2004;27(4):715–25.

84. Jacobs GD, Pace-Schott EF, Stickgold R, Otto MW. Cognitive behavior therapy and pharmacotherapy for insomnia: a randomized controlled trial and direct comparison. Arch Intern Med. 2004;164(17):1888–96.

85. Quesnel C, Savard J, Simard S, Ivers H, Morin CM. Efficacy of cognitive-behavioral therapy for insomnia in women treated for nonmetastatic breast cancer. J Consult Clin Psychol. 2003;71(1):189–200.

86. Savard J, Simard S, Ivers H, Morin CM. Randomized study on the efficacy of cognitive-behavioral therapy for insomnia secondary to breast cancer, part I: sleep and psychological effects. J Clin Oncol. 2005;23(25):6083–96.

87. Homsey M, O'Connell K. Use and success of pharmacologic and nonpharmacologic strategies for sleep problems. J Am Acad Nurse Pract. 2012;24(10):612–23.

88. Hauri P. Current concepts: the sleep disorders. Kalamazoo: The Upjohn; 1977.

89. Gigli GL, Valente M. Should the definition of "sleep hygiene" be antedated of a century? a historical note based on an old book by Paolo Mantegazza, rediscovered: to place in a new historical context the development of the concept of sleep hygiene. Neurol Sci. 2013;26(2):85–91.

90. American Academy of Sleep Medicine. Sleep hygiene: behaviors that promote sound sleep. Westchester: American Academy of Sleep Medicine; 2002.

91. AASM. Sleep hygiene: the health habits of good sleep. 2010. http://yoursleep.aasmnet.org/Hygiene.aspx. Accessed: 18 Jan 2013.

92. Dreher HM. The effect of caffeine reduction on sleep quality and well-being in persons with HIV. J Psychosom Res. 2003;54(3):191–8.

93. Webel AR, Moore SM, Hanson JE, Patel SR, Schmotzer B, Salata RA. Improving sleep hygiene behavior in adults living with HIV/AIDS: a randomized control pilot study of the system CHANGE™-HIV intervention. Appl Nurs Res 2013;26(2):85–91.

94. Stepanski EJ, Wyatt JK. Use of sleep hygiene in the treatment of insomnia. Sleep Med Rev. 2003;7(3):215–25.

95. Jacobson E. Progressive relaxation. Chicago: University of Chicago Press; 1938.

96. Means MK, Lichstein KL, Epperson MT, Johnson CT. Relaxation therapy for insomnia: nighttime and day time effects. Behav Res Ther. 2000;38(7):665–78.

97. Schultz J, Luthe W. Autogenic training a psychophysiologic approach in psychotherapy. New York: Grune and Stratton; 1969.

98. Bowden A, Lorenc A, Robinson N. Autogenic training as a behavioural approach to insomnia: a prospective cohort study. Prim Health Care Res Dev. 2012;13(2):175–85.

99. Schutte-Rodin S, Broch L, Buysse D, Dorsey C, Sateia M. Clinical guideline for the evaluation and management of chronic insomnia in adults. J Clin Sleep Med. 2008;4(5):487–504.

100. Benson H. The relaxation response. New York: Morrow; 1975.

101. Riedel B, Lichstein K, Peterson BA, Epperson MT, Means MK, Aguillard RN. A comparison of the efficacy of stimulus control for medicated and nonmedicated insomniacs. Behav Modif. 1998;22(1):3–28.

102. Espie CA, Lindsay WR, Brooks DN, Hood EM, Turvey T. A controlled comparative investigation of psychological treatments for chronic sleep-onset insomnia. Behav Res Ther. 1989;27(1):79–88.

103. Lacks P, Bertelson AD, Sugerman J, Kunkel J. The treatment of sleep-maintenance insomnia with stimulus-control techniques. Behav Res Ther. 1983;21(3):291–5.

104. Morin CM, Azrin NH. Behavioral and cognitive treatments of geriatric insomnia. J Consult Clin Psychol. 1988;56(5):748–53.

105. Morin CM, Azrin NH. Stimulus control and imagery training in treating sleep-maintenance insomnia. J Consult Clin Psychol. 1987;55(2):260–2.

106. Spielman AJ, Saskin P, Thorpy MJ. Treatment of chronic insomnia by restriction of time in bed. Sleep. 1987;10(1):45–56.

107. Friedman L, Bliwise DL, Yesavage JA, Salom SR. A preliminary study comparing sleep restriction and relaxation treatments for insomnia in older adults. J Gerontol. 1991;46(1):1–8.

108. Rubinstein ML, Rothenberg SA, Maheswaran S, Tsai JS, Zozula R, Spielman AJ. Modified sleep restriction therapy in middle-aged and elderly chronic insomniacs. Sleep Res. 1990;19:276.

109. Vande Griend JP, Anderson SL. Histamine − 1 receptor antagonism for treatment of insomnia. J Am Pharm Assoc. (2003) 2012;52(6):e210–9.

110. Santana CA, Fernandez F. Sleep disorders. In: Fernandez F, Ruiz P, editors. Psychiatric aspects of HIV/AIDS. Philadelphia: Lippincott Williams & Wilkins; 2006:137–46.

111. Maestroni GJ. The immunoneuroendocrine role of melatonin. J Pineal Res. 1993;14(1):1–10.

112. Lemoine P, Zisapel N. Prolonged-release formulation of melatonin (Circadin) for the treatment of insomnia. Expert Opin Pharmacother. 2012;13(6):895–905.

113. Nunnari G, Nigro L, Palermo F, Leto D, Pomerantz RJ, Cacopardo B. Reduction of serum melatonin levels in HIV − 1-infected individuals' parallel disease progression: correlation with serum interleukin − 12 levels. Infection 2003;31(6):379–82.

114. Lynch T, Price A. The effect of cytochrome P450 metabolism on drug response, interactions, and adverse effects. Am Fam Physician. 2007;76(3):391–6.

115. Roth T, Rogowski R, Hull S, et al. Efficacy and safety of doxepin 1 mg, 3 mg, and 6 mg in adults with primary insomnia. Sleep. 2007;30(11):1555–61.

116. Scharf M, Rogowski R, Hull S, et al. Efficacy and safety of doxepin 1 mg, 3 mg, and 6 mg in elderly patients with primary insomnia: a randomized, double-blind, placebo-controlled cross-over study. J Clin Psychiatry. 2008;69(10):1557–64.

117. Krystal AD, Durrence HH, Scharf M, et al.: Efficacy and safety of Doxepin 1 mg and 3 mg in a 12-week sleep laboratory and outpatient trial of elderly subjects with chronic primary Insomnia. Sleep. 2010;33(11):1553–61.

118. Roth T, Heith DH, Jochelson P, et al. Efficacy and safety of doxepin 6 mg in a model of transient insomnia. Sleep Med. 2010;11(9):843–7.

119. Krystal AD, Lankford A, Durrence HH, et al. Efficacy and safety of doxepin 3 and 6 mg in a 35-day sleep laboratory trial in adults with chronic primary insomnia. Sleep. 2011;34(10):1433–42.

120. Lankford A, Rogowski R, Essink B, Ludington E, Heith DH, Roth T. Efficacy and safety of doxepin 6 mg in a four-week outpatient trial of elderly adults with chronic primary insomnia. Sleep Med. 2012;13(2):133–8.

121. Hajak G, Rodenbeck A, Voderholzer U, et al. Doxepin in the treatment of primary insomnia: a placebo-controlled, double-blind, polysomnographic study. J Clin Psychiatry. 2001;62(6):453–63.

122. Pieper AA, Treisman GJ. Drug treatment of depression in HIV-positive patients: safety considerations. Drug Saf. 2005;28(9):753–62.

123. Saarto T, Wiffen PJ. Antidepressants for neuropathic pain: a Cochrane review. J Neurol Neurosurg Psychiatry. 2010;81(12):1372–3.

124. Hill L, Lee KC. Pharmacotherapy considerations in patients with HIV and psychiatric disorders: focus on antidepressants and antipsychotics. Ann Pharmacother. 2013;47(1):75–89.

125. Stimmel GL, Dopheide JA, Stahl SM. Mirtazapine: an antidepressant with noradrenergic and specific serotonergic effects. Pharmacotherapy. 1997;17(1):10–21.

Part VI
Historical Milestones of Individual Sleep Disorders

Evolution of the Classification of Sleep Disorders

23

Michael Thorpy

The classification of sleep disorders continues to evolve as we gain more information about different types of sleep disorders and their pathophysiology. The branch of medicine that deals with the classification of diseases is called nosology, and classification systems have varied uses. The *International Classification of Disease (ICD)* is the main international health classification system used to code illness and to track disease for medical, public health, reimbursement, statistical analysis, and medical informatics reasons. Other classification systems not only have a numerical coding system but are also used to classify diseases and disorders, symptoms, and medical signs for clinical decision making. The American Psychiatric Association's *Diagnostic and Statistical Manual (DSM)* and the *International Classification of Sleep Disorders (ICSD)* fall into this latter category.

For most of recorded history, there was a recognition of predominantly three types of sleep abnormalities: insomnia, excessive sleepiness, and nightmares, and it was not until the nineteenth century that specific sleep disorders, such as narcolepsy, began to be recognized. Differentiation between the causes of sleep disorders reached a peak in the past 50 years following the development of technology for the investigation of sleep.

Early Sleep Diagnoses

Most of our current knowledge of ancient Egyptian medicine derives from the Chester Beatty and the Georg Ebers papyri, written around 1350–1600 BC, but they contain little information on sleep disorders other than dreams [1, 2].

One of the first books published on sleep was *The Philosophy of Sleep* by Robert MacNish in 1830 [3]. MacNish listed several sleep disorders including sleeplessness, nightmares, sleepwalking, and sleep talking, and other authors in the nineteenth century mentioned hypnagogic hallucinations, somnambulism, wakefulness, and somnolence including narcolepsy. Dana in 1884 reviewed the topic of excessive sleepiness and discussed 50 patients and classified the disorders into three categories based on the possible underlying cause: (1) epileptoid state, (2) hysteroid sleeping state, and (3) "puzzling nature" cases not due to the prior two causes [4].

In the early twentieth century, two comprehensive books on sleep had a major influence on the development of sleep disorders medicine: Pieron's *Le Problème Physiologique du Sommeil* and *Sleep and Wakefulness* by Nathaniel Kleitman in 1939 (updated in 1963 to contain 4337 references) [5, 6]. These books were the first to mention many different sleep disorders.

Collins in his book *Insomnia: How to Combat It* in 1930 described three classes of "poor sleepers" [7]. The first class had great difficulty falling asleep which was due to many causes but mainly related to anxiety and worry. In this category, he included "night terrors" predominantly occurring in children. The second class were those who had severe drowsiness in the evening and an early-morning awakening which he thought was due predominantly to "autotoxins" or arteriosclerosis in the elderly. His description most equates with the current diagnostic category of "advanced sleep phase syndrome." The third class he described as those who sleep an adequate amount of hours at night but have severe daytime sleepiness. Gillespie had a greater listing of sleep disorders in his book *Sleep,* also published in 1930 [8]. He discussed insomnia, narcolepsy, sleep–wake rhythm disturbance, hypnagogic hallucinations, somnolence, sleep paralysis, night terrors, somnambulism, nocturnal enuresis, nocturnal epilepsy, and "sleep pains."

Interestingly, many authors in the nineteenth century and the first part of the twentieth century described patients who

M. Thorpy (✉)
111 East 210th Street, Bronx, NY 10467, USA
e-mail: thorpy@aecom.yu.edu

The Saul R. Korey Department of Neurology, Albert Einstein College of Medicine, Yeshiva University, Bronx, NY, USA

S. Chokroverty, M. Billiard (eds.), *Sleep Medicine,* DOI 10.1007/978-1-4939-2089-1_23,
© Springer Science+Business Media, LLC 2015

slept for months or even years before returning to full alertness, often called "protracted sleep," a condition still not understood or even included in modern-day sleep classifications. However, in the second half of the twentieth century, sleep classification was established with greater detail and accuracy.

Evolution of Specific Diagnoses

Narcolepsy and Other Hypersomnias

Westphal first described a patient with narcolepsy in 1877, but it was Gelineau in 1880 who described astasia (cataplexy) in detail and coined the term "narcolepsy" [9, 10]. Following Gelineau's description in the late nineteenth century, narcolepsy was brought to general recognition in 1926 by the Australian-born neurologist William John Adie [11]. There were many attempts to distinguish true narcolepsy, or as Adie called it "idiopathic narcolepsy," from secondary causes of narcolepsy. Adie used the term "pyknolepsy" for alternative causes of sleepiness. Wenderowic in 1924 used the terms "genuine narcolepsy," "hypnolepsy" for mainly postencephalitic sleepiness, and a symptomatic "hypnoid state" for other causes [12]. Lhermitte in 1930 called narcolepsy "paroxysmal hypersomnia" to distinguish it from prolonged hypersomnia [13]. Wilson (1928) and Daniels (1934) regarded narcolepsy as "true narcolepsy" if accompanied by cataplexy [14, 15].

Henneberg in 1916 first used the term "cataplectic inhibition" which was subsequently called "cataplexy" by Adie in 1925 [16]. Prior to that, cataplexy had been called "astasia" by Gelineau [10].

Critchley and Hoffman in 1942 created the term Kleine–Levin syndrome to describe adolescents with periodic hypersomnia and megaphagia [17]. Menstrual hypersomnia, another form of recurrent hypersomnia associated with menstruation, was first reported by Lhermitte and Dubois in 1941 [18].

Idiopathic hypersomnia, a disorder of excessive sleepiness that was distinguished from narcolepsy, was recognized by Roth in 1976 [19]. He recognized two forms, one with a long nocturnal sleep period and another with a normal nocturnal sleep duration.

The invention of the EEG led to the creation of polysomnography (PSG) that has greatly aided the development of sleep classifications.

Parasomnias

The term "parasomnias" was coined by Roger in 1932 [20]. Roger classified the sleep disorders into three groups: the hypersomnias, the insomnias, and the parasomnias.

Kleitman (1939) recognized that the parasomnias included: nightmares, night terrors, somniloquy, somnambulism, grinding of the teeth, jactations, enuresis, delirium, nonepileptic convulsions, and personality dissociations [6]. Broughton in 1968 developed the classification of the "arousal disorders" that consisted of confusional arousals, night terrors, and sleepwalking [21].

Insomnia

Throughout the years, it was always recognized that insomnia could be both idiopathic as well as "secondary" to psychological stress or other medical disorders. Primary insomnia was regarded as a form of insomnia that was not secondary to other medical or psychiatric disorders. In the late 1970s, insomnia became recognized as a symptom rather than a diagnosis, and treatment was directed to the underlying physical or psychological causes. A large number of different types of insomnia were recognized. The concept of a conditioned insomnia (psychophysiological insomnia) was first presented in the *Diagnostic Classification of Sleep and Arousal Disorders* (DCSAD), and subsequently became recognized as a common form of primary insomnia [22].

In the 2000s, it became clear that it was difficult to determine whether some disorders were causative of the insomnia or whether they were just coincident with the insomnia. The concept of "comorbid insomnia" was promoted at a National Institutes of Health (NIH) State of the Science conference held in 2005. By 2012, despite the many causes of insomnia, it was recognized that pathophysiologically only one type of insomnia existed and the sole diagnosis "insomnia disorder" was promulgated.

Sleep-Related Breathing Disorders

Following the reports of snoring, sleepiness, and obesity in the nineteenth century, Sir William Osler referred in 1906 to Dickens' description of Joe [23]. Charles Burwell in 1956 brought general recognition to obstructive sleep apnea syndrome, which he called the "Pickwickian syndrome" [24].

Circadian Rhythm Sleep Disorders

Circadian rhythm sleep disorders were recognized in the late 1970s, partly due to recognition of the chronobiological features of "jet lag" and "shift work."

The atypical, sleep-onset insomnia called the "delayed sleep phase syndrome" was discovered by Weitzman and colleagues in 1981 [25]. The converse situation, "advanced sleep phase syndrome," was described in 1979 [26]. The "non-24-h sleep–wake disorder" was first described in a blind person [27].

Modern Sleep Classification Systems

International Classification of Diseases

ICD-9-CM In 1967, the eighth revision of the *International Classification of Diseases* listed very few sleep disorders [28]. The main list of sleep disorders was in the Mental Disorders section 306 "Special symptoms not elsewhere classified" that listed hypersomnia, insomnia, nightmare and sleepwalking in a subsection entitled "Specific disorders of sleep." Section 780 "Symptoms and ill-defined conditions" under the subcategory "Disturbance of sleep" listed only "Inversion of sleep rhythm." Cheyne Stokes respiration was indexed under "Dyspnoea" and Pickwickian syndrome was indexed under "Obesity not specified as of endocrine origin."

The North American version of *the International Classification of Diseases (ICD-9-CM)* in 1980 contained an expanded listing of the disorders included under the major sleep disorder headings in the World Health Organization's ninth revision of the *International Classification of Diseases*, the ICD-9, first published in 1977 [29, 30]. The sleep disorder diagnoses in ICD-9-CM are organized under two major headings: "The specific disorders of sleep of non-organic origin" (ICD #307.4) and "The sleep disturbances" (ICD #780.5). Subdivisions of these two ICD-9-CM categories were partly based upon the headings and disorders of the 1979 Association of Sleep Disorders Centers (ASDC) *DCSAD* [22].

ICD-10-CM The ICD-10 was introduced in Europe in 1993 (Table 23.1). The USA revised version, ICD-10-CM, is expected to be implemented on October 1, 2015, and includes a nearly complete listing of the sleep disorders that are contained in the ICSD-2 (Table 23.2) [31]. The disorders are in two main sections: F51 in the "Mental, Behavioral and Neurodevelopmental disorders," subsection "Behavioral syndromes associated with physiological disturbances and physical factors," and G47 in the "Diseases of the nervous system," subsection "Episodic and paroxysmal disorders." The classification is in development and may reflect changes expected in the ICSD-3.

Table 23.1 ICD-10 (1993)

F51 Nonorganic sleep disorders

F51.0 Nonorganic insomnia
F51.1 Nonorganic hypersomnia
F51.2 Nonorganic disorder of the sleep–wake schedule
F51.3 Sleepwalking (somnambulism)
F51.4 Sleep terrors (night terrors)
F51.5 Nightmares
F51.8 Other nonorganic sleep disorder
F51.9 Nonorganic sleep disorder, unspecified

G47 Sleep disorders

G47.0 Disorders of initiating and maintaining sleep (insomnias)
G47.1 Disorders of excessive somnolence (hypersomnias)
G47.2 Disorders of the sleep–wake schedule
G47.3 Sleep apnea
G47.4 Narcolepsy and cataplexy
G47.8 Other sleep disorder
G47.9 Sleep disorder unspecified

Table 23.2 ICD-10-CM outline (proposed 2015)

F51 Sleep disorders not due to a substance or known physiological condition

F51.0 Insomnia not due to a substance or known physiological condition
F51.01 Primary insomnia (idiopathic insomnia)
F51.1 Hypersomnia not due to a substance or known physiological condition
F51.3 Sleepwalking (somnambulism)
F51.4 Sleep terrors (night terrors)
F51.5 Nightmare disorder (dream anxiety disorder)
F51.8 Other sleep disorders not due to a substance or known physiological condition
F51.9 Sleep disorder not due to a substance or known physiological condition, unspecified (emotional sleep disorder NOS)

G47 Sleep disorders

G47.00 Insomnia, unspecified
G47.01 Insomnia due to medical condition
G47.09 Other insomnia
G47.1 Hypersomnia
G47.19 Other hypersomnia
G47.2 Circadian rhythm sleep disorders
G47.3 Sleep apnea
G47.4 Narcolepsy
G47.5 Parasomnia
G47.6 Sleep-related movement disorders
G47.8 Other sleep disorders
G47.9 Sleep disorder, unspecified (sleep disorder NOS)
Restless legs syndrome (G25.81)
Sleep deprivation (Z72.820)

NOS not otherwise specified

DSM of the American Psychiatric Association

DSM-II In 1968, in the second American Psychiatric Association's *Diagnostic and Statistical Manual (DSM-II)*, the only category for sleep disorders was the entry "Disorder of Sleep" [32].

DSM-III In DSM-III (1980), the only two disorders of sleep included sleepwalking (somnambulism) and sleep terrors (pavor nocturnus) which were classified in the section entitled "Other Disorders with Physical Manifestations." DSM-III-R (1987) included an expanded listing of sleep disorders in a separate section entitled "sleep disorders" [33]. It included disorders of at least 1 month in duration that were classified into two groups: the dyssomnias and the parasomnias. The dyssomnias were defined as disorders where the predominant disturbance is in the amount, quality, or timing of sleep. The parasomnias were defined as an abnormal event occurring during sleep. The categories were determined by interrater reliability using a structured interview. The dyssomnias consisted of three main disorders: insomnia disorder, hypersomnia disorder, and sleep–wake schedule disorder. The parasomnias consisted of: nightmare disorder, sleep terror disorder, and sleepwalking disorder.

The revision of the American Psychiatric Association's *DSM-III* was under way when the *ICSD* was in development in the late 1980s. DSM-III-R contained an abbreviated list of sleep disorders that served the purposes of the overall DSM-III-R classification but was not compatible with the *ICSD*.

DSM-IV The DSM-IV, published in 1994, included additional sleep disorders in part based on the ICSD (Table 23.3) [34]. A major section entitled "Primary Disorders" included in the dyssomnia category: primary insomnia, primary hypersomnia, narcolepsy, breathing-related sleep disorders, and circadian rhythm sleep disorder. Another category under parasomnias lists: nightmare disorder, sleep terror disorder, and sleepwalking disorder, as in DSM-III-R. A second major section listed "sleep disorders related to another mental disorder," and there was an "other sleep disorders" category.

The process of revising the DSM-IV to produce DSM-V was initiated in 2010 and was implemented in 2010.

Diagnostic Classification of Sleep and Arousal Disorders

The Association of Sleep Disorder Centers (ASDC) classification committee, chaired by Howard Roffwarg, produced the *DCSAD* in 1979. It ushered in the modern era of sleep diagnoses and became the first classification to be widely used internationally (Table 23.4) [22]. The classification was produced by both the ASDC and the Association for the Psychophysiological Study of Sleep (APSS) and was published in the journal *Sleep*. The development of DCSAD began with a workshop on "Nosology and nomenclature of the sleep disorders" in 1972 at the APSS annual meeting.

The DCSAD classification consisted of four major categories: (A) the Disorders of Initiating and Maintaining Sleep (DIMS), (B) the Disorders of Excessive Somnolence (DOES), (C) the Disorders of the Sleep-Wake Schedule (DSWS), and (D) the Parasomnias. The first two categories were more of a differential diagnosis listing. However, some disorders, such as the sleep-related breathing disorders, could produce symptoms of both insomnia and excessive sleepiness, and the circadian rhythm sleep disorders could produce both symptoms. Many disorders were listed twice, once in each symptom category. The parasomnia listing was long and did not have subcategory organization. By the mid 1980s, a revised classification system was needed.

Table 23.3 DSM-IV (1994)

Primary sleep disorders
Dyssomnias
Primary insomnia
Primary hypersomnia
Narcolepsy
Breathing-related sleep disorder
Circadian rhythm sleep disorder
Dyssomnias NOS
Parasomnias
Nightmare disorder
Sleep terror disorder
Sleepwalking disorder
Parasomnia NOS
Sleep disorders related to another mental disorder
Secondary sleep disorders due to an axis III condition
Substance-induced sleep disorders

DSM diagnostic and statistical manual, *NOS* not otherwise specified

Table 23.4 DCSAD outline (1979)

(A) Disorders of initiating and maintaining sleep
(B) Disorders of excessive somnolence
(C) Disorders of the sleep–wake schedule
(D) Parasomnias

DCSAD diagnostic classification of sleep and arousal disorders

The International Classification of Sleep Disorders

ICSD-1 The *ICSD,* produced by the American Sleep Disorders Association in association with the European Sleep Research Society, the Japanese Society of Sleep Research, and the Latin American Sleep Society, was developed as a revision and update of the DCSAD (Table 23.5) [35]. This revision was necessitated by the description of many new disorders and the further development of information on many of the originally described disorders. Classifying the disorders by pathophysiological mechanism was preferred.

The ASDC initiated the process of revising the DCSAD classification in 1985 by establishing an 18-member Diagnostic Classification Steering Committee under the chairmanship of Michael Thorpy. The first meeting of this group was convened in July 1985 at the Annual Meeting of the ASDC in Seattle. A detailed questionnaire was developed and distributed to members of the Clinical Sleep Society (CSS) in the USA and to sleep specialists around the world to determine the usefulness of the first edition of the classification and to assess the potential usefulness of a number of proposed changes. Members representing the European Sleep Research Society, the Japanese Society of Sleep Research, and the Latin American Sleep Society and the Clinical Sleep Society were involved in the ICSD development of the individual disorders.

Every entry in the *DCSAD* was assessed for content and relevance in the practice of sleep disorders medicine. The questionnaire respondents regarded the original classification highly and the majority of the individual diagnostic entities were considered appropriate and relevant to clinical practice. However, opinions differed on both the overall classification structure and some of the individual diagnostic entries.

Table 23.5 ICSD-1 outline (1990)

(1) Dyssomnias
Intrinsic sleep disorders
Extrinsic sleep disorders
Circadian rhythm sleep disorders
(2) Parasomnias
Arousal disorders
Sleep–wake transition disorders
Parasomnias usually associated with REM sleep
Other parasomnias
(3) Medical/psychiatric sleep disorders
Associated with mental disorders
Associated with neurological disorders
Associated with other medical disorders
(4) Proposed sleep disorders

ICSD international classification of sleep disorders, *REM* rapid eye movement

Of the four main DCSAD diagnostic categories, section (C), "the Disorders of the Sleep–Wake Schedule," now called the "Circadian Rhythm Sleep Disorders," was the most favored grouping, probably because of its pathophysiological consistency due to the underlying chronophysiological basis.

The survey indicated that clinicians required more diagnostic information about respiratory and neurological disorders, so those sections were expanded. In addition, integration of childhood sleep disorders into the overall classification system was recommended. A separate childhood sleep disorders classification was considered, but this may have produced an artificial distinction between the same disorder in different age groups.

A classification for statistical and epidemiological purposes required that each disorder be listed only once. Organization on the basis of symptomatology was unsatisfactory because many disorders could produce more than one sleep-related symptom. The final structure was organized more pathophysiologically and less symptomatically. However, as the pathology is unknown for the majority of the sleep disorders, the classification was organized, in part, on physiological features: a pathophysiological organization.

The ICSD-I grouped the sleep disorders into four major sections. Section (1), the dyssomnias, included those disorders that produced a complaint of insomnia or excessive sleepiness. The dyssomnias were further subdivided, in part along pathophysiological lines, into the intrinsic, extrinsic, and circadian rhythm sleep disorders. Section (2), the parasomnias, included those disorders that intruded into or occurred during sleep but did not produce a primary complaint of insomnia or excessive sleepiness. Section (3) was the medical/psychiatric sleep disorders. Section (4) comprised the proposed sleep disorders, developed in recognition of the new and rapid advances in sleep disorders medicine. New disorders were being discovered, and some questionable sleep disorders had been more clearly described. The inclusion of these disorders encouraged further research to determine whether they were specific disorders in their own right or whether they were variants of other already classified disorders.

The subdivisions of the dyssomnias, intrinsic and extrinsic sleep disorders, divided the major causes of insomnia and excessive sleepiness into those that were induced primarily by factors within the body (intrinsic) and those produced primarily by factors outside of the body (extrinsic). This grouping of the sleep disorders initially had been proposed by Nathaniel Kleitman in his extensive monologue on the sleep disorders that was published in 1939 [6].

The medical/psychiatric sleep disorders comprised the medical and psychiatric disorders commonly associated with sleep disturbance. The use of the terms medical and psychiatric was not ideal, but was preferred to the ICD-9 use of the terms organic and nonorganic. Most medical and psychiatric disorders can be associated with disturbed sleep or impaired alertness, so only those disorders with major features of disturbed sleep or wakefulness, or those commonly considered in the differential diagnosis of the primary sleep disorders, were included in this section.

The ICSD-I consisted of disorders primarily associated with disturbances of sleep and wakefulness, as well as disorders that intrude into, or occur during, sleep. The classification provided a unique code number for each sleep disorder so that disorders could be efficiently tabulated for diagnostic, statistical, and research purposes. The primary aim of the text was to provide useful diagnostic information. Diagnostic, severity, and duration criteria were presented, as well as an axial system where clinicians could standardize presentation of relevant information regarding a patient's disorder.

The axial system, similar to the system used in DSM, was developed to assist in reporting appropriate diagnostic information, either in the clinical summaries or for database purposes. The first axis, axis A, contained the primary diagnoses of the ICSD, such as narcolepsy. The second axis, axis B, contained the names of the procedures performed, such as polysomnography, or the names of particular abnormalities present on diagnostic testing, such as the number of sleep-onset rapid eye movement (REM) periods seen on multiple sleep latency testing. The third axis, axis C, contained ICD-9-CM medical diagnoses that were not sleep disorders, such as hypertension.

A brief text revision of the ICSD-I was produced in 1997 and called *The International Classification of Sleep Disorders: Revised* [36]. This revision did not change the overall structure or names of the disorders but mainly involved updating the text.

ICSD-2 In 2005, the American Academy of Sleep Medicine developed a second edition of the ICSD, called ICSD-2 (Table 23.6) [37]. The classification was divided into eight

main sections: (1) insomnia, (2) sleep-related breathing disorders, (3) hypersomnias of central origin not due to a circadian rhythm sleep disorder, sleep-related breathing disorder, or other cause of disturbed nocturnal sleep, (4) circadian rhythm sleep disorders, (5) parasomnias, (6) sleep-related movement disorders, (7) isolated symptoms, apparently normal variants and unresolved issues, and (8) other sleep disorders. There were two appendices: Appendix A: Sleep Disorders Associated with Conditions Classifiable Elsewhere; and Appendix B: Other Psychiatric and Behavioral Disorders frequently encountered in the Differential Diagnosis of Sleep Disorders. The ICSD-2 contained the majority of the diagnoses included in ICSD-I. However, the severity and duration criteria and the axial system of ICSD-I were not included in ICSD-2.

In 2011, the process was initiated to revise the ICSD-2 to produce ICSD-3. Major changes are likely, based on a better understanding of the pathophysiology of sleep disorders, although the major group headings are unlikely to change. There will be change in the individual disorders some of which will be listed as subtypes. The ICSD-3 was published in 2014 [38].

Table 23.6 ICSD-2 outline (2005)

1. Insomnia
2. Sleep-related breathing disorders
3. Hypersomnias of central origin not due to a circadian rhythm sleep disorder, sleep-related breathing disorder or other cause of disturbed nocturnal sleep
4. Circadian rhythm sleep disorders
5. Parasomnias
6. Sleep-related movement disorders
7. Isolated symptoms, apparently normal variants and unresolved issues
8. Other sleep disorders
Appendix A: Sleep disorders associated with conditions classifiable elsewhere
Appendix B: Other psychiatric and behavioral disorders frequently encountered in the differential diagnosis of sleep disorders

ICSD international classification of sleep disorders

References

1. Ebbell B. The Papyrus Ebers. London: Humphrey Milford; 1937.
2. Kenyon FG. Classical texts from Papyri in the British Museum: including the newly discovered poems of Herodas, with autotype facsimiles of MSS. London: British Museum; 1981.
3. MacNish R. The philosophy of sleep. Glasgow: WR M'Phun; 1830.
4. Dana CL. On morbid drowsiness and somnolence. J Nerv Ment Dis. 1884; 9:153–76.
5. Pieron H. Le Problème Physiologique du Sommeil. Paris: Masson; 1913.
6. Kleitman N. Sleep and wakefulness. Chicago: University of Chicago Press; 1939.
7. Collins J. Insomnia: how to combat it. New York: Appeleton and Company; 1930.
8. Gillespie RD. Sleep. New York: William Wood and Company; 1930.
9. Westphal C. Eigentümliche mit Einschlafen verbundene Anfälle. Arch Psychiatr Nervenkr. 1877;7:631–5.
10. Gelineau J. De la narcolepsie. Gaz des Hôp (Paris). 1880;53:626–8, 635–7.
11. Adie WJ. Idiopathic narcolepsy, a disease sui generis, with remarks on the mechanism of sleep. Brain. 1926;49:257–306.
12. Wenderowic E. Hypnolepsie (Narcolepsia Gélineau) und ihre Behandlung. Arch Psychiat. 1924;72:459–72.
13. Lhermitte J. Le sommeil et les narcolepsies. Progr Med. 1930;1:962–75.
14. Wilson SR. The narcolepsies. Brain. 1928;51:63–77.
15. Daniels LE. Narcolepsy. Medicine. 1934;13:1–122.
16. Henneberg R. Über genuine Narkolepsie. Neuro Zbl. 1916;35:282–90.
17. Critchley M, Hoffman HL. The syndrome of periodic somnolence and morbid hunger (Kleine-Levin syndrome). Br Med J. 1942;1:137–9.
18. Lhermitte J, Dubois E. Crises d'hypersomnie prolongée rythmées par les règles chez une jeune-fille. Rev Neurol. 1941;73:608–9.

19. Roth B. Narcolepsy and hypersomnia: review and classification of 642 personally observed cases. Schweiz Arch Neurol Neurochir Psychiat. 1976;119:31–41.
20. Roger H. Les troubles du sommeil—hypersomnies, insomnies et parasomnies. Paris: Masson et Cie; 1932:206p.
21. Broughton RJ. Sleep disorders: disorders of arousal? Science. 1968;159:1070–8.
22. Association of Sleep Disorder Centers, Sleep Disorders Classification Committee. Diagnostic classification of sleep and arousal disorders. Sleep. 1979;2:1–137.
23. Osler W. The principle and practice of medicine: designed for the use of practitioners and students of medicine. 6. New York: Apple; 1906.
24. Burwell CS, Robin ED, Whaley RJ et al. Extreme obesity associated with alveolar hypoventilation—a Pickwickian syndrome. Am J Med. 1956;21:811–8.
25. Weitzman ED, Czeisler CA, Coleman RM et al. Delayed sleep phase syndrome. Arch Gen Psychiatry. 1981;38:737–46.
26. Kamei R, Hughes L, Miles L, et al. Advanced-sleep phase syndrome studies in time isolation facility. Chronobiologia. 1979;6:115.
27. Miles LE, Raynal DM, Wilson MA. Blind man living in normal society has circadian rhythms of 24.9 hours. Science. 1973;198:421–3.
28. ICD. Manual of the international classification of diseases, injuries, and causes of death, eighth revision. Geneva: World Health Organization; 1967.
29. ICD –9. Manual of the international classification of diseases, injuries, and causes of death. Geneva: World Health Organization; 1977.
30. ICD –9-CM. Manual of the international classification of diseases, 9th revision, clinical modification. Washington DC: U.S. Governmental Printing office; 1980.
31. ICD –10-CM. Manual of the international classification of diseases, 10th revision, clinical modification. Washington DC: U.S. Governmental Printing office; 2012.
32. DSM-II. Diagnostic and statistical manual of the mental disorders. 2nd ed. Washington DC: American Psychiatric Association; 1968.
33. DSM-III-R. Diagnostic and statistical manual of the mental disorders. 3rd ed. Washington DC: American Psychiatric Association; 1987.
34. DSM-IV. Diagnostic and statistical manual of the mental disorders. 4th ed. Washington DC: American Psychiatric Association; 1994.
35. American Sleep Disorders Association, Diagnostic Classification Steering Committee. International classification of sleep disorders: diagnostic and coding manual. Rochester: American Sleep Disorder Association; 1990.
36. American Sleep Disorders Association, Diagnostic Classification Steering Committee. International classification of sleep disorders: diagnostic and coding manual (revised). Rochester: American Sleep Disorders Association; 1997.
37. American Academy of Sleep Medicine. International classification of sleep disorders. Diagnostic and coding manual. 2nd ed. Westchester: American Academy of Sleep Medicine; 2005.
38. American Academy of Sleep Medicine. International classification of sleep disorders, 3rd ed. Davien: IL: American Academy of Sleep Medicine, 2014.

History of Epidemiological Research in Sleep Medicine

24

Markku Partinen

Epidemiological studies on sleeping habits and sleep disorders date back to the beginning of the last century. The earliest studies included clinical case series or simple descriptive surveys about the occurrence of different sleep-related phenomena. Recent epidemiological research includes modern epidemiological methods. Sleep epidemiology, as we can understand it now, is defined as a discipline of how to study the occurrence of phenomena of interest in the field of sleep.

The word "epidemiology" is derived from *epi* (upon), *demos* (people), and *logos* (discourse or study). Originally, epidemiologists studied mainly infections and diseases of epidemic proportion. Modern applications of epidemiology include the study of chronic diseases, evaluation of the health status of populations, and effect of different determinants (genetic and environmental) on different outcomes. Increase of computational power enables complicated methods that a researcher could just dream about some 30 years ago. In the beginning of the 1980s, a time-sharing system was used in huge mainframe computers (at that time, IBM dominated the computer manufacturing companies). Sometimes, it took a week or more to have results of a set of tables with chi-square values. Instructions were given by punched cards, which were invented by Herman Hollerith in 1884 at the Massachusetts Institute of Technology (MIT), Boston.

Early Studies

The oldest epidemiological sleep studies are from the end of the eighteenth century. Clement Dukes from England studied sleep need in young children [1]. Other early studies are those by Claparède [2] from France and Camp from Michigan [3]. Approximately 80–100 years ago, young children slept 10.5–13.5 h, 15-year-olds 9–10 h, and adults between 7 h 25 min and 8 h 23 min. These figures do not differ significantly from those in the present day. Women slept a little longer than men. In 1931, Laird published a large study of 509 men of distinction. Sleep disturbances increased with age, as they do at present. At the age of 25 years, about 90% of men slept well, but by the age of 95 everybody had some sleeping problems. On an average, more than 70% of men of distinction reported some difficulty in going to sleep, and more than 40% reported awakening during the night [4].

The number of epidemiological studies increased in the 1960s. In these studies, the average length of sleep varied between 7 and 8 h. In Scotland, 2446 subjects aged over 15 were studied. Of the older subjects in the age group 65–74 years, 18% complained of awakening before 5 a.m. This decreased to 12% after the age of 75. Less than 10% of men aged 15–64 years complained of disturbed sleep. In the age group 65–74 years, disturbed sleep was a complaint in 25% of men. In women, the respective percentage was 43% [5].

Increase of Epidemiological Studies During Recent Years

In the beginning of 1970, less than 50 publications could be found in PubMed using the following Mesh terms: ("Epidemiology"[Mesh] OR prevalence OR incidence) AND ("Sleep Disorders"[Mesh] OR "Sleep Disorders, Circadian Rhythm"[Mesh] OR "Snoring" OR "Sleep Apnea Syndromes"[Mesh] OR "Sleep Apnea, Obstructive"[Mesh] OR "Sleep Apnea, Central"[Mesh] OR "insomnia" OR "parasomnia") and limiting the publications to original human studies. The number of epidemiological publications started to grow faster at the end of the 1980s. In 1990, already 110 studies were published and the figure increased to more than 300 in 2001. Starting from 2008, more than 1000 epidemiological original articles on sleep have been published each year.

M. Partinen (✉)
Department of Clinical Neurosciences, University of Helsinki, Helsinki, Finland
e-mail: markpart@me.com

Helsinki Sleep Clinic, VitalMed Research Centre, Helsinki, Finland

S. Chokroverty, M. Billiard (eds.), *Sleep Medicine,* DOI 10.1007/978-1-4939-2089-1_24,
© Springer Science+Business Media, LLC 2015

Pioneers of Sleep Epidemiology in the USA

Excellent articles on individual differences of sleep length were published by Wilse B Webb in *Science* [6, 7] and also in the classical book *Sleep and Dreaming* (edited by Ernest Hartmann) in 1970 [8]. Webb as well as Hartmann belong to the pioneers of sleep research. Webb can be considered a pioneer in sleep epidemiology. He has always emphasized the need for using proper methods and criteria. Among many other things, he also investigated short and long sleepers. "Short sleepers" slept less than 5.5 h per night and "long sleepers" slept more than 9.5 h per night [6, 7]. Webb was the first to correlate sleep recording findings with sleep length and stated that short sleepers had reduced amount of stage 2 and rapid eye movement (REM) sleep than average sleepers or long sleepers [6, 7]. Webb studied sleep in the elderly as well as effects of shift work, and he always had strong opinions. A case in point is his letter to the editor of *Sleep* "Opinion Polls and Science" where he questioned the opinion polls as scientific evidence (something that I fully agree with). In general, opinion polls have very little to do with scientific epidemiology. All sleep researchers doing or planning to do epidemiological studies should read Webb's works and verify what he had written about a certain topic.

Edward Bixler started sleep epidemiological studies in the 1970s and he continues to carry on excellent studies [9, 11–13]. He started to work in collaboration with Anthony Kales who is best known for the classic Rechtschaffen and Kales (R&K) scoring system published in 1968 [10]. One of the early classic studies on the prevalence of insomnia is the Los Angeles metropolitan study in 1979 [9]. It was a well-done population-based survey on 1006 individuals that was designed as a sleep epidemiological study. The prevalence of insomnia was 42.5%. Nightmares were reported by 11.2%, 7.1% complained of excessive sleepiness, 5.3% reported sleep talking, and 2.5% had sleepwalking. Insomnia was a major complaint amongst older women and those with lower educational and socioeconomic status [9]. Edward Bixler published several landmark studies on the epidemiology of insomnia, parasomnias and sleep apnea. Already in the beginning of 1980s, he emphasized that the criteria of clinically significant sleep apnea differ by age. His studies also showed a strong correlation between obesity and sleep apnea, and that sleep apnea in postmenopausal women is as common as in men [11–13].

Epidemiology of Snoring and Sleep Apnea

In 1980, Elio Lugaresi and his collaborators published the first results of the San Marino epidemiological population-based survey in the journal *Sleep* [14]. It was the first large population-based study on snoring and about the association of snoring with cardiovascular disease. Also, other sleep disorders were surveyed. The Neurological Clinic of Bologna, Italy, is one of the great schools in clinical and clinical–epidemiological sleep research. Prof. Lugaresi and Giorgio Coccagna were among the first persons together with Henri Gastaut to describe obstructive sleep apnea, which they called hypersomnia with periodic breathing. Also, Lugaresi organized the first international symposium "The Rimini Symposium on Hypersomnia and Periodic Breathing" in 1972. Christian Guilleminault introduced the term "sleep apnea" later, in 1975, soon after he had moved from France to work with William Dement at Stanford, USA.

Shortly after the San Marino studies, the first population-based epidemiological studies on the prevalence of snoring and sleep apnea were published from USA (Sonia Ancoli-Israel, Daniel Kripke, Edward Bixler), Finland (Markku Partinen, Tiina Telakivi), Germany (Jörg Hermann Peter, Thomas Podszus), Israel (Peretz Lavie), Sweden (Thorarinn Gislason), and Denmark (Poul Jennum). Thorarinn Gislason is working presently in his hometown of Reykjavik in Iceland, and he is leading genetic and epidemiological studies in collaborations with Allan Pack at the University of Pennsylvania in Philadelphia, USA. Investigators from Iceland are in a unique position for genetic studies because the genetic roots can be traced back to the AD 800s. Unfortunately, the Icelandic population is isolated, and replication studies in other populations have been often negative. Poul Jennum leads the Danish group of sleep researchers. Using the registries that are unique in all Nordic countries, he recently published excellent papers on economical issues of different sleep disorders.

Prevalence of Sleep Apnea

The prevalence of sleep apnea figures varied, depending on the gender and age, between 1 and 6% which agreed with the results of the Wisconsin population-based study that was published in 1993 by Terry Young and collaborators [15]. The first Wisconsin Sleep Cohort study of 602 employed men and women was published in the *New England Journal of Medicine*. Four per cent of men and 2% of women met the minimal diagnostic criteria of obstructive sleep apnea syndrome. These are the most commonly cited prevalence figures of sleep apnea although they are valid only for an employed population. As has been shown later by Bixler, sleep apnea is about as common in postmenopausal women as in men of the same age [13]. Sleep apnea is very common in elderly people, but the effect on mortality is lower in elderly than in middle-aged people [16, 17]. New studies are warranted. The occurrence of sleep apnea increases with body weight, and with increasing prevalence of obesity sleep apnea has been increasing more and more. This means that the Young figures from 1993 are probably outdated [18].

Sleep and Cardiovascular Disease

Markku Partinen and Michel Billiard were students of Pierre Passouant from Montpellier, France. Partinen studied medicine in France and he became interested in sleep when he was preparing for a special certificate of neurophysiology with Passouant. In 1976, after his return to Finland, he started preparing his doctoral thesis [19] on sleep epidemiology. A few years later, he started to collaborate with Markku Koskenvuo and Jaakko Kaprio who had been working at the University of Helsinki with the Finnish twin cohort. Questions of snoring and more questions on sleep were added to the surveys. A U-type association was found, for the first time between sleep length and occurrence of coronary heart disease [20]. This finding has since been replicated in several other studies. The association of habitual snoring with arterial hypertension as well as the association between snoring, sleep apnea and myocardial infarction were reported for the first time by Partinen and collaborators in 1983 [21, 22]. Since that time, the Finnish group continued reporting on genetic and different environmental effects on sleep [23, 24] and publishing further studies on snoring, sleep apnea, and cardio- and cerebrovascular disease [25–27]. These early results have been confirmed later by several other groups.

Type 2 Diabetes and Sleep Apnea

An association between sleep apnea and type 2 diabetes was reported for the first time by Japanese investigators in 1991 [28]. Soon, Finnish researchers found that the severity of sleep apnea was related to the degree of insulin resistance [29]. The association of sleep apnea with type 2 diabetes was recognized widely including the diabetes research community [30, 31].

Mortality and Morbidity in Patients Diagnosed with Sleep Apnea

The first convincing studies showing that mortality is increased in untreated sleep apnea were published by two groups in 1988 [32–34]. Since then, many other studies have shown an association between sudden death, [35] myocardial infarction, stroke, and sleep apnea. The best studies have been prospective studies [36–45].

Narcolepsy

Narcolepsy studies were initiated in Montpellier, France, and at Stanford University, USA. The prevalence of narcolepsy has been studied in many countries. The prevalence of nar-

colepsy is about 30 per 100,000 people [46–50]. The highest figures are from Japan and the lowest are from Israel. In France, the early epidemiological studies were conducted mainly in Montpellier. Pierre Passouant, teacher of Michel Billiard, organized the First International Symposium on Narcolepsy in La Grande Motte in 1975 together with William Dement and Christian Guilleminault. Passouant was one of the pioneers of clinical sleep medicine, including epidemiological understanding, together with William Dement, Christian Guilleminault, Yasuo Hishikawa, and Yutaka Honda.

Insomnia

Insomnia is the most common sleep disorder. It is very important and more difficult to treat than sleep apnea. Socioeconomically, insomnia poses more economic burden than sleep apnea. Several USA groups dominated this field but Europeans have also published many important epidemiological studies on insomnia. The Swedish (Jerker Hetta, Gunnar Boman, and many others), British (Kevin Morgan and others), and Norwegians (Reidun Ursin, Björn Bjorvatn, and others) have been active together with Finnish, French and German researchers. Sleepiness is an important issue in occupational medicine and in traffic. In these areas, the most important studies were conducted by Pierre Philip from France and Torbjörn Åkerstedt from Sweden. As for epidemiological studies on narcolepsy, many Europeans have been involved in pioneering studies, including Yves Dauvilliers from Montpellier, Christer Hublin from Finland, and the Swiss colleagues.

The first international meeting on epidemiology of sleep/wake disorders was organized in Milano Marittima, Italy, in May 1982 (Fig. 24.1). The proceedings of the excellent meeting were published in the book *Sleep/Wake Disorders: Natural History, Epidemiology, and Long-Term Evolution*, edited by Christian Guilleminault and Elio Lugaresi.

History of Other Epidemiological Studies

Other European names in the early history of epidemiology of sleeping habits, insomnia, and sleep apnea include Heikki Palomäki (stroke), John Stradling (neck circumference, risk factors, hypertension), Neil Douglas (RCTs, cognition, etc.), Erkki Kronholm (sleep length, insomnia), and Claudio Bassetti (stroke) among many others. Talking about history of cardiovascular studies on sleep apnea in Europe, one cannot forget Marburg (Germany). Jörg Hermann Peter was a pioneer in that field, and he organized several important meetings on the topic before he passed away in January 2010. Some of the studies that originated in Marburg are now being

Fig. 24.1 The first international meeting on epidemiology of sleep/wake disorders was organized in Milano Marittima, Italy, in May 1982. Milano Marittima 1982. Bill Dement and Elio Lugaresi are in the middle

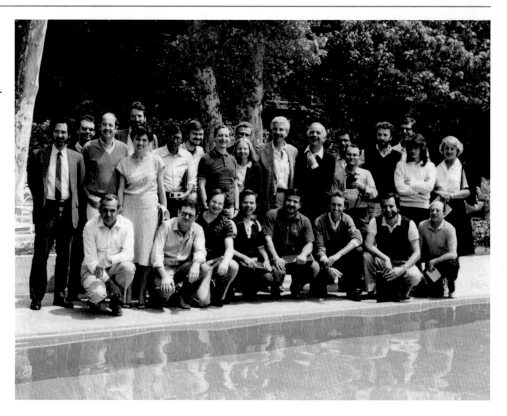

continued in Gothenburg, Sweden, by Ludger Grote and Jan Hedner. One of the pioneers in the area of narcolepsy and hypersomnias had been Prof. Bedrich Roth from Prague (Czech Republic). He was born in 1919 and he passed away in 1989. He published his first monograph on narcolepsy in 1957. His blue book on hypersomnias with epidemiological data remains a classic. Sonia Nevsimalova and Karel Sonka are continuing his pioneering work.

Several US groups, in addition to Bixler and Young, have conducted excellent epidemiological studies. One important researcher is Maurice Ohayon who is a psychiatrist. He became more and more interested in sleep epidemiology after moving from France to Canada. The first epidemiological study using the so-called Sleep-EVAL system was published in 1996 [51]. Since that time, he has published several cross-sectional studies on the occurrence of different sleep disorders.

There are many other Asian, European, and US colleagues who have conducted epidemiological studies in different areas. The list of researchers would be too long, and I have listed only some people who have been important in the history of sleep medicine during its development mainly in the 1980s to the 1990s. I apologize to all of those whose names are missing. Happily, more and more people are interested in sleep epidemiology. With the advent of efficient computers and good registries, studies changed from simple descriptive ones to well-planned case–control, prospective, and multivariate analytic studies of different associations and risk factors.

References

1 Dukes C. Sleep in relation to education. J Roy Sanit Inst. 1905;26:41–4.
2. Claparède E. Théorie biologique du sommeil. Arch de Psychologie. 1905;4:245–349.
3. Camp C. Disturbance of sleep. J Michigan Med Soc. 1923;22:133–8.
4. Laird D. The sleep habits of 509 men of distinction. Am Med. 1931;37:271–5.
5. McGhie A, Russell S. The subjective assessment of normal sleep patterns. J Ment Sci. 1962;108:642–54.
6. Webb WB, Agnew HW, Jr. Sleep stage characteristics of long and short sleepers. Science. 1970;168:146–7.
7. Webb WB, Friel J. Sleep stage and personality characteristics of "natural" long and short sleepers. Science. 1971;171:587–8.
8. Webb W. Individual differences in sleep length. In: Hartmann E, ed. Sleep and dreaming. Boston: Little & Brown; 1970. p. 44–7.
9. Bixler EO, Kales A, Soldatos CR, Kales JD, Healey S. Prevalence of sleep disorders in the Los Angeles metropolitan area. Am J Psychiatry. 1979;136:1257–62.
10. Rechtschaffen A, Kales A. A manual of standardized terminology, techniques, and scoring system for sleep stages of human subjects. Bethesda: National Institute of Neurological Diseases and Blindness, Neurological Information Network; 1968.
11. Bixler EO, Kales A, Soldatos CR, Vela-Bueno A, Jacoby JA, Scarone S. Sleep apneic activity in a normal population. Res Commun Chem Pathol Pharmacol. 1982;36:141–52.
12. Bixler EO, Vgontzas AN, Ten Have T, Tyson K, Kales A. Effects of age on sleep apnea in men: I. Prevalence and severity. Am J Respir Crit Care Med. 1998;157:144–8.
13. Bixler EO, Vgontzas AN, Lin HM, Ten Have T, Rein J, Vela-Bueno A, et al. Prevalence of sleep-disordered breathing in women: effects of gender. Am J Respir Crit Care Med. 2001;163:608–13.

14. Lugaresi E, Cirignotta F, Coccagna G, Piana C. Some epidemiological data on snoring and cardiocirculatory disturbances. Sleep. 1980;3:221–4.

15. Young T, Palta M, Dempsey J, Skatrud J, Weber S, Badar S. The occurrence of sleep-disordered breathing among middle-aged adults. N Engl J Med. 1993;328:1230–5.

16. Ancoli-Israel S, Klauber MR, Stepnowsky C, Estline E, Chinn A, Fell R. Sleep-disordered breathing in African-American elderly. Am J Resp Crit Care Med. 2000;152:1946–9.

17. Bliwise DL, Foley DJ, Vitiello MV, Ansari FP, Ancoli-Israel S, Walsh JK. Nocturia and disturbed sleep in the elderly. Sleep Med. 2008;10:540–8

18. Partinen M, Hublin C. Epidemiology of sleep disorders. In: Meir Kryger TR, Dement WC, editors. Principles and practice of sleep medicine. 5 edn. St. Louis: Elsevier Saunders; 2011. p. 694–715.

19. Partinen M. Sleeping habits and sleep disorders on Finnish men before, during and after military service. Ann Med Milit Fenn. 1982;57:1–96.

20. Partinen M, Putkonen PT, Kaprio J, Koskenvuo M, Hilakivi I. Sleep disorders in relation to coronary heart disease. Acta Med Scand. 1982;660:69–83.

21. Partinen M, Kaprio J, Koskenvuo M, Langinvainio H. Snoring and hypertension: a cross-sectional study on 12808 Finns aged 24–65 years. Sleep Res. 1983;12:273.

22. Partinen M, Alihanka J, Lang H, Kaliomaki L. Myocardial infarction in relation to sleep apneas. Sleep Res. 1983;12:272.

23. Partinen M, Eskelinen L, Tuomi K. Complaints of insomnia in different occupations. Scand J Work Environ Health. 1984;10:467–9.

24. Partinen M, Kaprio J, Koskenvuo M, Putkonen P, Langinvainio H. Genetic and environmental determination of human sleep. Sleep. 1983;6:179–85.

25. Partinen M, Palomäki H. Snoring and cerebral infarction. Lancet. 1985;ii:1325–6.

26. Koskenvuo M, Kaprio J, Partinen M, Langinvainio H, Sarna S, Heikkilä K. Snoring as a risk factor for hypertension and angina pectoris. Lancet. 1985;1:893–6.

27. Koskenvuo M, Kaprio J, Telakivi T, Partinen M, Heikkilä K, Sarna S. Snoring as a risk factor for ischaemic heart disease and stroke in men. Br Med J. 1987;294:16–9.

28. Katsumata K, Okada T, Miyao M, Katsumata Y. High incidence of sleep apnea syndrome in a male diabetic population. Diabetes Res Clin Pract. 1991;13:45–51.

29. Tiihonen M, Partinen M, Närvänen S. The severity of obstructive sleep apnoea is associated with insulin resistance. J Sleep Res. 1993;2:56–61.

30. Tuomilehto H, Peltonen M, Partinen M, Seppa J, Saaristo T, Korpi-Hyovalti E, et al. Sleep-disordered breathing is related to an increased risk for type 2 diabetes in middle-aged men, but not in women—the FIN-D2D survey. Diabetes Obes Metab. 2008;10:468–75.

31. Foster GD, Sanders MH, Millman R, Zammit G, Borradaile KE, Newman AB, et al. Obstructive sleep apnea among obese patients with type 2 diabetes. Diabetes Care. 2009;32:1017–9.

32. He J, Kryger M, Zorick F, Conway W, Roth T. Mortality and apnea index in obstructive sleep apnea. Chest. 1988;94:9–14.

33. Partinen M, Jamieson A, Guilleminault C. Long-term outcome for obstructive sleep apnea syndrome patients. Mortality. Chest. 1988;94:1200–4.

34. Partinen M, Guilleminault C. Daytime sleepiness and vascular morbidity at seven-year follow-up in obstructive sleep apnea patients. Chest. 1990;97:27–32.

35. Seppala T, Partinen M, Penttila A, Aspholm R, Tiainen E, Kaukianen A. Sudden death and sleeping history among Finnish men. J Intern Med. 1991;229:23–8.

36. Ancoli-Israel S, Kripke DF, Klauber MR, Fell R, Stepnowsky C, Estline E, et al. Morbidity, mortality and sleep-disordered breathing in community dwelling elderly. Sleep. 1996;19:277–82.

37. Javaheri S, Parker TJ, Liming JD, Corbett WS, Nishiyama H, Wexler L, et al. Sleep apnea in 81 ambulatory male patients with stable heart failure. Types and their prevalences, consequences, and presentations. Circulation. 1998;97:2154–9.

38. Peppard PE, Young T, Palta M, Skatrud J. Prospective study of the association between sleep-disordered breathing and hypertension. New Engl J Med. 2000;342:1378–84.

39. Kaneko Y, Floras JS, Usui K, Plante J, Tkacova R, Kubo T, et al. Cardiovascular effects of continuous positive airway pressure in patients with heart failure and obstructive sleep apnea. New Engl J Med. 2003;348:1233–41.

40. Campos-Rodriguez F, Pena-Grinan N, Reyes-Nunez N, De la Cruz-Moron I, Perez-Ronchel J, De la Vega-Gallardo F, et al. Mortality in obstructive sleep apnea-hypopnea patients treated with positive airway pressure. Chest. 2005;128:624–33.

41. Lavie P, Lavie L, Herer P. All-cause mortality in males with sleep apnoea syndrome: declining mortality rates with age. Eur Respirat J. 2005;25:514–20.

42. Marin JM, Carrizo SJ, Vicente E, Agusti AG. Long-term cardiovascular outcomes in men with obstructive sleep apnoea-hypopnoea with or without treatment with continuous positive airway pressure: an observational study. Lancet. 2005;365:1046–53.

43. Young T, Finn L, Peppard PE, Szklo-Coxe M, Austin D, Nieto FJ, et al. Sleep disordered breathing and mortality: eighteen-year follow-up of the Wisconsin sleep cohort. Sleep. 2008;31:1071–8.

44. Punjabi NM, Caffo BS, Goodwin JL, Gottlieb DJ, Newman AB, O'Connor GT, et al. Sleep-disordered breathing and mortality: a prospective cohort study. PLoS Med. 2009;6:e1000132.

45. Hudgel DW, Lamerato LE, Jacobsen GR, Drake CL. Assessment of multiple health risks in a single obstructive sleep apnea population. J Clin Sleep Med. 2012;8:9–18.

46. Hublin C, Kaprio J, Partinen M, Koskenvuo M, Heikkilä K, Koskimies S, et al. The prevalence of narcolepsy: an epidemiological study of the Finnish Twin Cohort. Ann Neurol. 1994;35:709–16.

47. Wing YK, Li RH, Ho CK, Fong SY, Chow LY, Leung T. A validity study of Ullanlinna Narcolepsy Scale in Hong Kong Chinese. J Psychosom Res. 2000;49:355–61.

48. Shin YK, Yoon IY, Han EK, No YM, Hong MC, Yun YD, et al. Prevalence of narcolepsy-cataplexy in Korean adolescents. Acta Neurol Scand. 2008;117:273–8.

49. Heier MS, Evsiukova T, Wilson J, Abdelnoor M, Hublin C, Ervik S. Prevalence of narcolepsy with cataplexy in Norway. Acta Neurol Scand. 2009;120:276–80.

50. Partinen M. Epidemiology of sleep disorders. Handb Clin Neurol. 2011;98:275–314.

51. Ohayon M. Epidemiological study on insomnia in the general population. Sleep. 1996;19:S7–15.

The Insomnias: Historical Evolution

Suresh Kumar and Sudhansu Chokroverty

Introduction

To paraphrase David Parkes [1], insomnia can be called by different names just like Wordsworth's [2] cuckoo ("O Cuckoo! Shall I call thee Bird, or but a wandering Voice?") because insomnia is thought to be a symptom of many diseases (medical, psychiatric, and others). For an understanding of insomnia, one should begin by studying the inhabitants of the ancient world and the civilization of the Indus (India), Yangtze (China), the Euphrates (Middle East) [1], and Egypt gradually progressing through to modern industrialized and contemporary culture. The term *insomnia* is derived from Latin meaning literally a total lack of sleep. But from a practical standpoint it is the relative lack of sleep, non-restorative, or inadequate quality of sleep which is relevant. Insomnia is really "hyposomnia" meaning a decrease in duration or depth. Henry Cockeram while working on the dictionary of "hard English words" in the early 1620s [3] used the term *insomnia* synonymous with the word "watching" meaning want of power to sleep.

Developmental Milestones of Insomnia in the Ancient Time

Insomnia

Since ancient times sleep and sleep disorders have been mentioned time and again with particular relevance to sleeplessness and various therapies available for it. Ancient treatises on medicine and surgery have existed as early as 400 BC ca. and have been the forerunners to the present-day modern texts. One such ancient treatise is *Charaka Samhita*. The *Advaita Vedanta* written in Sanskrit (ca. 5000 BC) talks about sleep and wakefulness and the different states were termed *avasthas*; avasthatraya—the three states, namely waking state (*jagrat*), dream sleep (*swapna*), and dreamless sleep (*sushupti*; see also Chap. 4). The *Vedanta* further describes that all human beings without any exception experience all these three states on a daily basis [4]. The vedas, furthermore, elaborate the presence of a fourth state which is described as a state of true awakening. This is defined as a state where there is no interruption by the waking state and is termed "turiyam" or the fourth state. Any disruption of the three states would lead to unsatisfactory sleep and awakening. The vedas also point out that disruption of the peace of mind by stressors can disrupt the natural process of these three states and lead to sleeplessness. The vedas at that time had pointed out the basis of sleep and in fact went on to describe dreamless, and dreaming, motionless sleep which is similar to features of rapid eye movement (REM) sleep. They also described the probable psychophysiological concept of insomnia without directly mentioning it as insomnia.

Ayurvedic medicine existed several thousands of years before Christ. Ayurveda considers sleep to be one of three pillars of health. Ayurveda, a Sanskrit word means the knowledge for a long life (*Ayu* means longevity and *Veda* means knowledge or science). Ayurvedic medicine is a system of traditional Indian medicine (a form of complementary or alternative medicine) practiced from mid- to second millennium BC to contemporary time. During the Buddhist period (ca. 300 BC to AD 1000), the knowledge of Ayurvedic medicine spread to far West and East. This ancient system of medicine is being taught along with the allopathic medicine in many universities and colleges throughout India now.

Traditional Chinese medicine (TCM), existing also since many thousands of years before Christ, approaches insomnia in a different way than Western medicine (see also Chap. 5). TCM using the concept of "root and branch" views insom-

S. Chokroverty (✉)
JFK New Jersey Neuroscience Institute, 65 James Street, Edison, NJ 08818, USA
e-mail: schok@att.net

S. Kumar
Department of Neurology, Sree Balajee Medical College and Hospital, Chrompet, Chennai, India

Chennai Sleep Disorders Centre, Chennai, India

S. Chokroverty, M. Billiard (eds.), *Sleep Medicine,* DOI 10.1007/978-1-4939-2089-1_25,

nia symptoms as the "branches" and the root of the disease as an imbalance of the fundamental substances (e.g., Chi, Yin, Yang, blood, Jing, Shen) or major organ systems (e.g., heart or liver). According to the TCM concept originating from Shamanism and later Taoism, a wandering spirit or Shen disturbance can manifest most commonly as insomnia symptoms. TCM practitioners often combine acupuncture and Chinese herbal medications (e.g., Suan Zao Ren or sour date seed) for treating insomnia. A popular herb, Yi-Gen San has been approved for the treatment of insomnia in Japan. It is interesting to note that this same herb has been reported to be effective in the treatment of three cases of REM sleep behavior disorder [5].

In Western culture, one finds reference to insomnia, probably for the first time in ancient Greeks in the pre-Hippocratic Epidaurian tablets. According to the Greco-Roman concept, the people's lives were controlled by gods and goddesses [6]. The goddess of the night (Nyx) had two sons, namely, Hypnos (the god of sleep) and Thanatos (the god of death). The Greek god Hypnos is often symbolized to hold a poppy flower in the hand with a field of poppies in front of his house [3]. It is described that in ancient Greece, if a person had issues regarding sleeplessness, he would need to visit the sanatorium of Asclepios (the Greek god of medicine) where he would receive the treatment with soothing music, rest, and meditation. This is reminiscent of the cognitive behavioral and relaxation therapies of modern time [7]. The present-day therapy like valerian root was already used in the ancient Greek period for the treatment of sleeplessness. For example, the ancient Greek physician Dioscorides prescribed valerian root as a sedative. Hippocrates (400 BC) mentioned about sleep and sleep-related issues in his writings (Corpus Hippocraticum) [8]. In the Egyptian civilization, medical papyri from the Edwin Smith papyrus, the Ebers papyrus, and Kahun papyrus described the use of opium as a treatment for insomnia [9]. It is stated that the first-century BC Greek physician Heraclides of Taras, who lived in Alexandria, Egypt, recommended opium as the treatment of choice for insomnia [10]. The Indian philosophy describes Nidra Devi as a goddess of sleep and chanting her verses mentioned in the religious book (Chandi path or reading) induces sleep [11].

Aristotle offered the first scientific approach in his writings around 350 BC enumerating the most comprehensive theories of sleep. Three essays in the collection known as Parva Naturalia (on sleep and waking, on dreams, and on divination through sleep) analyzed the genesis of sleep as well as the concept of dreams [12–14]. Quoting Beare's translation "Likewise it is clear that [of those either asleep or awake] there is no animal which is always awake or always asleep, but that both these affections belong [alternately] to the same animal. For if there be an animal not endowed with sense-perception, it is impossible that this animal should ei-

ther sleep or wake; since both these are affections of the activity of the primary faculty of sense-perception." Aristotle stated that no being can remain always awake or asleep permanently. Again quoting Beare's translation "Finally, if such affection is sleep, and this is a state of powerlessness arising from excess of waking, and excess of waking is in its origin sometimes morbid, sometimes not, so that the powerlessness or dissolution of activity will be so or not; it is inevitable that every creature which wakes must also be capable of sleeping, since it is impossible that it should continue actualizing its powers perpetually." Aristotle mentioned that excess of waking would make you powerless and tried to explain the intricate balance between sleep and wakefulness.

Insomnia is mentioned in several places in the Bible (see also Chap. 6) to emphasize the severity, associated loneliness, anxiety, and guilty conscience as well as illnesses causing sleeplessness [15]. An example in the Psalms is: "I lie awake, I am like a lonely bird upon a roof" (102:8). The Bible also mentions physical activity as a treatment for insomnia. The importance of getting enough sleep at night has also been emphasized in Qur'an and the Islamic literature (see also Chap. 3) [16].

Evolution of the Concept of Insomnia from the Nineteenth to Twenty-first Century

Frank in 1811 mentioned agrypnia (meaning insomnia) as one of the seven classes of sleep disturbance [17]. A search of the literature clearly shows that publications on the topic of insomnia dominated the field of sleep research since 1870. For a description of historical evolution of insomnia and its treatment in the nineteenth and early twentieth centuries, the readers are referred to Chap. 12 by Schulz and Salzarulo. Macfarlane [18] in 1890 wrote the definitive text of the nineteenth century defining insomnia as "loss of sleep." It is interesting to note that Macfarlane considered insomnia as a symptom and not a disease, a view still hotly debated in this century.

Contemporary sleep medicine defines insomnia as an inability to fall asleep or maintain sleep associated with an impairment of daytime functioning. International classification of sleep disorders (ICSD-3) [19] classified insomnia into three categories. It can be associated with medical, psychiatric or psychological factors, environmental causes, or ingestion of medication. The term secondary insomnia used in the first National Institute of Health (NIH) consensus development conference in 1983 has been replaced by the term comorbid insomnia in the later NIH consensus conference in 2005 [20] as the cause-and-effect relationship has not been determined. The Diagnostic and Statistical Manual of the American Psychiatric Association (1994; DSM-IV) classified insomnia into primary insomnia and that related to medical or mental disease or to substance abuse or dependency. DSM-V (published in 2013) recommends the term "insomnia disorders" replacing "primary insomnia" and "insomnia associated with medical or mental diseases" [21]. According to the Center for Disease Control (CDC) of the USA, 70 million Americans suffer from chronic insomnia. The lack of a standard definition of insomnia hampered epidemiological studies and limited research on sleep quality. Depending on the definition, up to 30 % of the population in the Western countries may experience insomnia symptoms and insomnia may be persistent in 10 % [22]. Insomnia diagnosis is based on subjective reports (sleep questionnaires and sleep diaries) rather than objective data derived from polysomnographic (PSG) findings. In any case, there appears to be a remarkable discrepancy between PSG and subjective measures. Edinger et al. published research diagnostic criteria for insomnia [23]. Longitudinal studies of the general population in the Western countries suggested high prevalence with varying degrees of persistence with rates varying from 40 to 69 % and the incidence rates of 3.9 to 28.8 % [22]. In a longitudinal study (mean follow-up of 5.2 years) of Chinese adults, the researchers in Hong Kong led by Y. K. Wing found an incidence rate for insomnia symptoms and insomnia syndrome (additional daytime symptoms) of 5.9 %, whereas the persistence rate of insomnia syndrome was 42.7 and 28.2 % for insomnia symptoms [24].

Some major advances in insomnia research occurred in the last half of the twentieth and twenty-first century. Some examples of these include long-term consequences of chronic insomnia, relationship between insomniac and psychiatric disorders, new understanding about pathophysiology of insomnia, and advances in the treatment. First, one must understand that insomnia is a 24-h disease and is not just sleep deprivation. Sleep deprivation is endemic in our modern industrialized society. Average sleep duration in human has decreased by 1.5–2 h in the course of the last 55 years, which may be partly responsible for adverse metabolic and hormonal effects, and increasing incidence of obesity and type 2 diabetes mellitus in the society [25]. Function of sleep, however, remains a mystery but we have enough evidence to show that sleep plays an important role in homeostatic mechanism with restitution of sleep, thermoregulation, immune control, and tissue repair, as well as memory consolidation [26]. Even one night of sleep deprivation impairs hippocampal function resulting in inadequate memory processing [27]. Jenkins and Dallenbach's experiment in 1924 [28] proved that memory retention was better after a night of sleep and this was later supported by behavioral and functional magnetic resonance imaging (fMRI) studies by Stickgold and Walker [29]. An early observation by Kripke et al. [30] in 1979 of increased risk of death from coronary arterial disease, cancer, and stroke in those who sleep less than 4 h

(also those who sleep more than 10 h) was later confirmed [31], but remains controversial without resolving cause and effect and because of the confounding factor of medication ingestion. However, short-term consequences, such as excessive daytime sleepiness, mood disorder, irritability, impaired work efficiency and absenteeism, accidents at work and home, and falls in the elderly, and long-term (remains debatable) consequences, such as increased mortality and morbidity (e.g., obesity, type 2 diabetes mellitus, hypertension, and other adverse cardiovascular consequences, psychiatric disorders, and memory impairment, have been reported in patients with chronic insomnia [32]. Obstructive sleep apnea (OSA) is an additional comorbidity and up to 50 % of OSA patients may suffer from moderate to severe insomnia [33]. There is a clear bidirectional relationship between insomnia and depression [34]. In 1969, Winokur et al. [35] reported that 100 % of their sample of 1257 patients with depression had comorbid insomnia and these observations have been subsequently confirmed in many reports [34].

Significant advances have been made in the last decade of the twentieth and current century in our understanding of the pathophysiology of chronic insomnia. There are many models and theories proposed. Various models focused on primary insomnia rather than comorbid insomnias as the latter represent heterogeneous conditions. Richardson [36] proposed four physiological models: (1) disruption of the sleep homeostat; (2) disruption of the circadian clock; (3) disruption of intrinsic sleep–wake state mechanisms; and (4) disruption (hyperactivity) of extrinsic "override" systems (e.g., stress response mechanisms). A detailed discussion of these models is beyond the scope of this chapter but available data favor the involvement of dysfunctional extrinsic stress response systems. Physiological hyperarousal remains the contemporary theory inspired by studies undertaken earlier by Monroe [37], Kales [38], Adam [39], and coinvestigators, Bonnet and Arand [40], and continuing with Perlis [41], Vgontzas et al. [42], and other investigators [36]. Perlis [41, 43] and coinvestigators have provided a comprehensive review of the hyperarousal theory. The sustained hyperarousal throughout 24 h explains the persistence of chronic primary insomnia. The hyperarousal theory is based on the evidence of physiologic arousal with increased autonomic activity (e.g., elevated heart rate and body temperature), sympathetic arousal (measured by heart rate variability), activation of neuroendocrine (e.g., hypothalamo–pituitary–adrenal [HPA] and neuroimmunological axes), and heightened cortical arousal (e.g., increased beta and gamma frequency electroencephalography (EEG) activity at sleep onset and during non-REM (NREM) sleep with the higher high-to-low frequency ratio in the fast Fourier transformation (FFT) of the EEG signals, and altered brain metabolism as evidenced by the positron emission tomographic (PET) scan findings of heightened neural activation in brain areas subserving arousal and emotion during sleep in insomnias) [41, 43–46]. The increased production of cortisol and interleukin-6 in patients with chronic insomnia support the activation of the HPA and neuroimmunological axes [42]. The finding of a reduction in hippocampal volume [47] in insomnias and the experimental observations of impaired neurogenesis in the hippocampus following sleep loss in rats [48] support cognitive deficits and impaired memory consolidation in patients with chronic insomnia. Finally, using a sophisticated immunohistochemical method (Fos activation indicating neuronal activation), Cano et al. [49] produced a stress-induced insomnia model in rats to show simultaneous activation of both sleep-promoting and arousal-related brain regions similar to the observations in human insomniacs of simultaneous fatigue throughout the day and an inability to "de-arouse" on attempting to sleep.

Evolution of Insomnia Treatment from the Ancient Time to Twenty-First Century

Natural remedies to promote sleep and as a treatment for sleeplessness were popular in the ancient time with the use of chamomile (medicinal herb in the form of tea). St John's Wort and mandragora (mandrake tree) as sleeping aid have a history of use over 2400 years for various disorders including sleeplessness. Ayurvedic medicine, the oldest comprehensive medicinal system of India, describes the use of yoga and "ashwagandha" to cure insomnia [49a]. Ashwagandha, also known as *Withania somnifera* in Latin or "Indian winter cherry" or "Indian ginseng," contains steroidal lactones, anaferine, and heterogonous alkaloids, which reduce the production of cortisol. Ashwagandha promotes a calm state of mind by its restorative action in the nervous system, which counteracts tension and high blood pressure. This brings the body to a state of equilibrium, making the body to relax during stress and fatigue thus restoring sleep to insomnia patient. Likewise, "brahmi," also known as *Bacopa Monnieri* in Latin, was also used in the ancient times to promote sleep. The current concept is that "brahmi" increases the levels of serotonin and bacosides.

Insomnia treatment includes pharmacological therapy using hypnotic medications and non-pharmacologic treatment using lifestyle and behavior modifications. In the nineteenth and twentieth centuries, hypnotic medications had been used frequently for insomnia (see also Chap. 12). As mentioned earlier, opium was first used as a hypnotic in Egypt (ca. 1000 BC). From the ancient time until the nineteenth century, alcohol, opium, or a dilute solution of the active ingredient in the opium poppy seed, morphine, was the ingredient for sleeping medications. Morphine may have

been named after Morpheus (the god of dream and the son of Greek god of sleep Hypnos and the equivalent Italian god of sleep Somnus). In the nineteenth century, bromides, chloral hydrate, and paraldehyde were used as hypnotics, which were later superseded by barbiturates in the beginning of the twentieth century. Benzodiazepines replaced barbiturates in the second half of the twentieth century followed later in the past decade of the twentieth century by imidazopyridines, the non-benzodiazepine $GABA_A$ receptor agonists (popularly known as Z drugs: zolpidem, zopiclone, including eszopiclone, and zaleplon). Over-the-counter (OTC) medications (all containing antihistamines) and alcohol are frequently used by the public presently as nonprescription aids for insomnia. Other prescription drugs currently used as hypnotics include antidepressants (Trazodone and Mellaril (Elavil) in particular); however, at the 2005 NIH state-of-the science consensus conference [20], these medications were discouraged to be used as hypnotics.

The role of non-pharmacological treatment for insomnia was clearly evident even in the nineteenth century in the form of sleep hygiene, and the other measures (e.g., behavioral therapy) were mentioned in the twentieth century (see also Chap. 12). As early as 1880s, hydrotherapy (e.g., baths, showers, wraps, warm douching) was used for sleeplessness [50, 51].

Spielman's 3P (predisposing, precipitating, and perpetuating factors) model of insomnia [52] paved the way for modern cognitive behavioral therapy for insomnia (CBT-I; see also Chaps. 58 and 60). CBT-I basically consists of five components [53–58]: (1) sleep hygiene measures [56]; (2) stimulus control therapy (SCT) of Bootzin [57]; (3) sleep restriction therapy (SRT) of Spielman [58]; (4) progressive muscle relaxation (PMR); and (5) cognitive therapy (CT). Later a web-based (internet-based intervention) CBT treatment was introduced in a 2012 publication [59]. The two main goals of the treatment for chronic insomnia advocated by the American Academy of Sleep Medicine (AASM) are to improve the quality of sleep and to improve the next-day impairment of function [60]. AASM guidelines recommend CBT for chronic primary as well as comorbid insomnias. Non-pharmacological intervention is shown to be superior to hypnotic treatment alone in a head-to-head comparison [61] and CBT is considered the treatment of choice for chronic insomnia [62]. Combined behavioral and pharmacological treatment may be needed in some patients but many unresolved issues remain in this approach [63, 64]. Comorbid insomnia including comorbid depression and insomnia requires a treatment for both the primary condition and insomnia itself. It is generally agreed that acute insomnia should be treated with short-term hypnotic medications during the stressful situation triggering acute insomnia to prevent the development of chronic insomnia.

References

1. Parkes JD. The culture of insomnia: book review. Brain. 2009;132:3488–93.
2. Wordsworth W. To the Cuckoo. In: William Wordsworth, selected poetry. Penguin; 1992.
3. Sullivan E. Insomnia. The Lancet. 2008;371:1497.
4. Sharma A. Sleep as a state of consciousness in Advaita Vedanta. State University of New York Press; 2004.
5. Shinno H, Kamei M, Nakamura Y, Inami Y, Horiguchi J. Successful treatment with Yi-Gan San for rapid eye movement sleep behavior disorder. Prog Neuropsychopharmacol Biol Psychiatry. 2008;32:1749–51.
6. Leadbetter R. Nyx. In: Encyclopedia mythica. Rome: Pantheon; 1999.
7. Poortvliet R, Huygun W. What is sleep? The book of the sandman and the alphabet of sleep. New York: Harry N Abrams; 1989.
8. Jones WHS Trans. Hippocrates on dreams, Loeb Classical Library Vol IV. Cambridge: Harvard University Press; 1923.
9. Silverburg R. The dawn of medicine. New York: Putnam Publishing; 1975.
10. Attarian HA. Defining insomnia. In: Attarian HA, ed. Insomnia. Totowa: Humana; 2004. p. 3.
11. Dash VB, Kashyap VL. Diagnosis and treatment of diseases in Ayurveda. New Delhi: Concept; 1981.
12. Gallop D. Aristotle on sleep and dreams. Warminster; 1996.
13. Gallop D. Aristotle on sleep, dreams, and final causes. In: Cleary JJ, Shartin DC, eds. Boston area colloquium in ancient philosophy. 1988; 4:pp. 257–90.
14. On sleep and sleeplessness, by Aristotle translated by J. I. Beare (year and publisher are missing).
15. Ancoli-Israel S. Sleep is not tangible or what the Hebrew tradition has to say about sleep. Psychosom Med 2001;63:778–87.
16. BaHammam AS, Gozal D. Qur'anic insights into sleep. Nat Sci Sleep. 2012;4:81–87.
17. Frank J. Praxeos medicae universae praecepta. 2 vols. (partis secundae volumen primum, sectio prima, continens Doctrinam de morbis systematis nervosa in genere, et de iis cerebri in specie). Lipsiae: Kuehniani; 1811.
18. Mcfarlane AW. Insomnia and its therapeutics. HK Lewis; 1890. p. 366.
19. American Academy of Sleep Medicine. International Classification of Sleep Disorders. Diagnostic and coding manual. 3rd ed. Westchester: American Academy of Sleep Medicine; 2014.
20. National Institutes of Health State of the Science conference statement. Manifestations and management of chronic insomnia in adults; 13–15 June 2005. Sleep. 2005;28:1049–57.
21. The American Psychiatric Association. Diagnostic and Statistical Manual of Mental Disorders (DSM), the DSM –5. 5th ed. Arlington: The American Psychiatric Association; 13 May 2013.
22. Ohayon M. Epidemiology of insomnia: what we know and what we still need to learn. Sleep Med Rev. 2002;6:97–111.
23. Edinger JD, Bonnet MH, Bootzin RR, Doghramji K, Dorsey CM, Espie CA, et al. Derivation of research diagnostic criteria for insomnia report of an American Academy of Sleep Medicine Work Group. Sleep. 2004;27:1567–96.
24. Zhang J, Lam SP, Li Sx, Yu MWM, Li AM, Ma RCW, et al. Long-term outcomes and predictors of chronic insomnia: a prospective study in Hong Kong Chinese adults. Sleep Med. 2012;13:455–62.
25. Van Cauter E, Spiegel K, Tasali E, Leproutt R. Metabolic consequences of sleep and sleep loss. Sleep Med. 2008;9(suppl. 1):S23–8.
26. Siegel JM. Clues to the functions of mammalian sleep. Nature. 2005;437:1264.
27. Yoo SS, Hu PT, Gujar N, Jolesz FA, Walker MP. A deficit in the ability to form new human memories without sleep. Nat Neurosci. 2007;10:385–92.
28. Jenkins JG, Dallenbach KM. Oblivescence during sleep and waking. Am J Psychol. 1924;35:605–12.
29. Stickgold R, Walker MP. Sleep-dependent memory consolidation and reconsolidation. Sleep Med. 2007;8:331–43.
30. Kripke DF, Simons RN, Garfinkel L. Short and long sleep and sleeping pills: is increased mortality associated? Arch Gen Psychiatry. 1979;36:103–16
31. Hublin C, Partinen M, Koshenvuo M, Kaprio J. Sleep and mortality: a population-based 22 year follow-up study. Sleep. 2007;30:1245–53
32. Grandner MA, Jackson NJ, Pak VM, Gehman PR. Sleep disturbance is associated with cardiovascular and metabolic disorders. J Sleep Res. 2012;21:427–33.
33. Beneto A, Gomez-Siurana E, Rubio-Sanchez P. Comorbidity between sleep apnea and insomnia. Sleep Med Rev. 2009;13:287–293.
34. Reimann D. Insomnia and comorbid psychiatric disorders. Sleep Med. 2007;8 (suppl. 4):S15–20.
35. Winokur G, Clayton PJ, Reich T. Manic depressive illness. St. Louis: Mosby; 1969.
36. Richardson GS. Human physiological models of insomnia. Sleep Med. 2007;8:S9–14.
37. Monroe LJ. Psychological and physiological differences between good and poor sleepers. J of Abnorm Psychol. 1967;72:255–64.
38. Kales A, Kales JD. Sleep disorders: recent findings in the diagnosis and treatment of disturbed sleep. N Engl J Med. 1974;290:487–99.
39. Adam K, Tomeny M, Oswald L. Physiological and psychological differences between good and poor sleepers. J Psychiatr Res. 1986;20:301–16.
40. Bonnet M, Arnad D. Hyperarousal and insomnia. Sleep Med Rev. 1997;1:97–108.
41. Perlis ML, Giles DE, Mendelson WB, Bootzin RR, Wyatt JK. Psychophysiological insomnia: the behavioral model and a neurocognitive perspective. J Sleep Res. 1997;6:179–88.
42. Vgontzas AN, Bixler EO, Lin HM, Prolo P, Mastorakos G, Vela-Bueno A, et al. Chronic insomnia is associated with nyctohemeral activation of the hypothalamo-pituitary-adrenal axis: clinical implications. J Clin Endocrinol Metabol 2001;86:3787–94.
43. Perlis ML, Pigeon WR, Drummond SP. The neurobiology of insomnia. In: Gilman S, ed. Neurobiology of disease. Burlington: Elsevier; 2006. pp. 735–44.
44. Reimann D, Kloefer C, Berger M. Functional and structural brain alteration in insomnia: implications for pathophysiology. Eur J Neurosci. 2009;29:1754–60.
45. Krystal AD, Edinger JD, Wohlgemuth WK, Marsh GR. NREM sleep frequency spectral correlates of sleep complaints in primary insomnia subtypes. Sleep. 2002;25:630–40.
46. Nofzinger EA, Buysse DJ, German A, Price JC, Miewald JM, Kupfer DJ. Functional neuroimaging evidence for hyperarousal in insomnia. Am J Psychiatry. 2004;161:2126–9.
47. Reimann D, Voderholzer U, Spiegelhalder K, Homyak M, Buysse DJ, Nissen C, et al. Chronic insomnia and MRI-measured hippocampal volume: a pilot study. Sleep. 2007;30:955–8.
48. Meerlo P, Mistlberger RE, Jacobs BI, Heller HC, McGinty D. New neurons in the adult brain: the role of sleep and consequences of sleep loss. Sleep Med Rev. 2009; 13:187–94.
49. Cano G, Mochizuki T, Saper CB. Neural circuitry of stress-induced insomnia in rats. J Neurosci. 2008;28:10167–84.
49a. Kulkarni SK, Dhir A. Withania somnifera: an Indian ginseng. Prog Neuropsychopharmacol Biol Psychiatry. 2008 Jul 1;32(5):1093–105.
50. Campbell AJ. Warm douching of the head and neck in the insomnia of continued or eruptive fevers. Br Med J. 1885;1(1256):176–7.
51. Hance IH. Hydrotherapy in the treatment of insomnia. Trans Am Climatol Assoc. 1899;15:137–43.

52. Spielman AJ. Assessment of insomnia. Clin Psychol Rev. 1986;6:11–25.
53. Morin CM, Bootzin RR, Buysee DJ, et al. Psychological and behavioral treatment of insomnia: update of the recent evidence (1998–2004). Sleep. 2006; 29:1393-414.
54. Espie CA, Inglis SJ, Tessier S, Harvey L. The clinical effectiveness of cognitive behavior therapy for chronic insomnia: implementation and evaluation of a sleep clinic in general medical practice. Behav Res Ther. 2001;39:45–60.
55. Edinger JD, Wohlgemuth WK, Radtke RA, Marsh GR, Quillian RE. Cognitive behavioral therapy for treatment of chronic primary insomnia: a randomized controlled trial. JAMA. 2001;285:1856–64.
56. Hauri P. The sleep disorders. In: Current concepts. Kalamazoo: Scope/The Upjohn Co; 1977.
57. Bootzin RR. Stimulus control treatment for insomnia. Proc Am Psychol Assoc. 1972;7:395–6.
58. Spielman A, Yang CM, Glovinsky PB. Sleep restriction therapy. In: Sateia MJ, Buysee DJ, eds. Diagnosis and treatment. Informa; UK 2010. pp. 277–89.

59. Manber R, Carney C, Edinger J, Epstein D, Friedman L, Haynes PL, et al. Dissemination of CBTI to the non-sleep specialist: protocol development and training issues. J Clin Sleep Med. 2012;8(2):209–18.
60. Schutte-Rodin S, Broch L, Buysee D, Dorsey C, Sateia M. Clinical guidelines for the evaluation and management of chronic insomnia in adults. J Clin Sleep Med. 2008;4:487–504.
61. Jacobs GD, Pace-Schott EF, Stickgold R, Otto MW. Cognitive behavioral therapy and pharmacotherapy for insomnia: a randomized control trial and direct comparison. Arch Int Med. 2004;164:1888–96.
62. Morgenthaler T, Kramer M, Alessi C, et al. Practice parameters for the psychological and behavioral treatment of insomnia: an update. An American Academy of sleep medicine report. Sleep. 2006;29(11):1415–19.
63. Morin CM. Combined therapeutics for insomnia: should our first approach be behavioral or pharmacological? Sleep Med. 2006;7(suppl. 1): S15–19.
64. Reimann D, Perlis MI. The treatment of chronic insomnia: a review of benzodiazepine receptor agonists and psychological and behavioral therapies. Sleep Med Rev. 2009;13:205–14.

Narcolepsy–Cataplexy Syndrome and Symptomatic Hypersomnia

Seiji Nishino, Masatoshi Sato, Mari Matsumura
and Takashi Kanbayashi

Introduction

In this chapter, the clinical and pathophysiological aspects of idiopathic and symptomatic narcolepsy–cataplexy syndromes and hypersomnia (or excessive daytime sleepiness, EDS) are discussed. Although no systematic epidemiological study has been conducted, available data suggest that hypersomnia (both idiopathic and symptomatic) is common but under-diagnosed; both types of hypersomnia significantly reduce the quality of life (QOL) of the subjects. Narcolepsy–cataplexy type 1, narcolepsy without cataplexy (a prototypical hypersomnia) type 2, and idiopathic hypersomnia (a primary hypersomnia not associated with rapid eye movement [REM] sleep abnormalities) are three major idiopathic hypersomnias [1], but substantial clinical overlap among these disorders has been noted, as each disorder is currently diagnosed by mostly sleep phenotypes and not by biologically/pathophysiologically based tests. Similarly, symptomatic hypersomnia is a heterogeneous disease entity and the biological/pathophysiological mechanisms underlying symptomatic hypersomnia are mostly unknown.

Recent progress for understanding the pathophysiology of EDS particularly owes to the discovery of narcolepsy genes (i.e., hypocretin receptor and peptide genes) in animals in 1999 and the subsequent discovery in 2000, of hypocretin ligand deficiency (i.e., loss of hypocretin neurons in the brain) in idiopathic cases of human narcolepsy–cataplexy. The hypocretin deficiency can be clinically detected by cerebrospinal fluid (CSF) hypocretin-1 measures; low CSF hypocretin-1 levels are seen in over 90% of narcolepsy–cataplexy patients. Since the specificity of the CSF finding is also high (no hypocretin deficiency was seen in patients with idiopathic hypersomnia), low CSF hypocretin-1 levels have been included in the third revision of the international classifications of sleep disorder as a positive diagnosis for narcolepsy–cataplexy [1].

Narcolepsy–cataplexy is tightly associated with human leukocyte antigen (HLA) DQB1*0602. Hypocretin deficiency in narcolepsy–cataplexy is also tightly associated with HLA positivity, suggesting an involvement of immune-mediated mechanisms for the loss of hypocretin neurons. However, the specificity of HLA positivity for narcolepsy–cataplexy is much lower than that of low CSF hypocretin-1 levels, as up to 30% of the general population shares this HLA haplotype.

The prevalence of primary hypersomnia, such as narcolepsy and idiopathic hypersomnia, is not high at 0.05 and 0.005%, respectively, but the prevalence of symptomatic (secondary) hypersomnia may be much higher. For example, about several million subjects in the USA suffer from chronic brain injury, and 75% of those people have sleep problems, and about half of them claim sleepiness [2]. Symptomatic narcolepsy has also been reported, but the prevalence of symptomatic narcolepsy is much smaller, and only about 120 cases have been reported in the literature in the past 30 years [3]. The meta-analysis of these symptomatic cases indicates that hypocretin deficiency may also partially explain the neurobiological mechanisms of EDS associated with symptomatic cases of narcolepsy and hypersomnia [3].

Anatomical and functional studies demonstrate that the hypocretin systems integrate and coordinate the multiple wake-promoting systems, such as monoamine and acetylcholine systems to keep subjects fully alert [4], suggesting that understanding of the roles of hypocretin peptidergic systems in sleep regulation in normal and pathological conditions is important, as alternations of these systems may also be responsible not only for narcolepsy but also for other less well-defined hypersomnias.

S. Nishino (✉) · M. Sato · M. Matsumura
Stanford University Sleep and Circadian Neurobiology Laboratory, Department of Psychiatry and Behavioral Sciences, Stanford University School of Medicine, 3165 Porter Drive, RM1195, Palo Alto, CA 94304, USA
e-mail: nishino@stanford.edu

T. Kanbayashi
Department of Neuropsychiatry, Akita University, Akita, Japan

S. Chokroverty, M. Billiard (eds.), *Sleep Medicine*, DOI 10.1007/978-1-4939-2089-1_26,
© Springer Science+Business Media, LLC 2015

Since a large majority of patients with EDS are currently treated with pharmacological agents, new knowledge about the neurobiology of EDS will likely lead to the development of new diagnostic tests as well as new treatments and managements of patients with hypersomnia with various etiologies.

This chapter focuses on pathophysiological mechanisms and nosological aspects of idiopathic and symptomatic hypersomnia. For the treatments of these conditions, refer to more specific publications available [5–8].

Symptoms of Narcolepsy

Excessive Daytime Sleepiness

EDS and cataplexy are considered to be the two primary symptoms of narcolepsy, with EDS often being the most disabling symptom. The EDS most typically mimics the feeling that people experience when they are severely sleep-deprived but may also manifest itself as a chronic tiredness or fatigue. Narcoleptic subjects generally experience a permanent background of baseline sleepiness that easily leads to actual sleep episodes in monotonous sedentary situations. This feeling is most often relieved by short naps (15–30 min), but in most cases the refreshed sensation only lasts a short time after awaking. The refreshing value of short naps is of considerable diagnostic value. Sleepiness also occurs in irresistible waves in these patients, a phenomenon best described as "sleep attacks." Sleep attacks may occur in very unusual circumstances, such as in the middle of a meal, a conversation, or riding a bicycle. These attacks are often accompanied by microsleep episodes [9], where the patient "blanks out." The patient may then continue his or her activity in a semiconscious manner (writing incoherent phrases in a letter, speaking incoherently on the phone, etc.), a phenomenon called automatic behavior [9–11]. Learning problems and impaired concentration are frequently associated [9–13], but psychophysiological testing is generally normal.

Sleepiness is usually the first symptom to appear, followed by cataplexy, sleep paralysis, and hypnagogic hallucinations [14–18]. Cataplexy onset occurs within 5 years after the occurrence of daytime somnolence in approximately two-thirds of the cases [15, 17]. Less frequently, cataplexy appears many years after the onset of sleepiness. The mean age of onset of sleep paralysis and hypnagogic hallucinations is also 2–7 years later than that of sleepiness [14, 19].

In most cases, EDS and irresistible sleep episodes persist throughout the lifetime although they often improve after retirement (possibly due to better management of activities), daytime napping, and adjustment of nighttime sleep.

Cataplexy

Cataplexy is distinct from EDS and pathognomonic of the disease [20]. The importance of cataplexy for the diagnosis of narcolepsy has been recognized since its description [21, 22] and in subsequent reviews on narcolepsy [23, 24]. Most authors now recognize patients with recurring sleepiness and cataplectic attacks as a homogeneous clinical entity, and this is now shown to be tightly associated with hypocretin deficiency (see the section on the pathophysiology of the disease). Cataplexy is defined as a sudden episode of muscle weakness triggered by emotional factors, most often in the context of positive emotions (such as laughter, having good cards at card games, the pull of the fishing rod with a biting fish, and the perfect hit at baseball), and less frequently by negative emotions (most typically anger or frustration). All antigravity muscles can be affected leading to a progressive collapse of the subject, but respiratory and eye muscles are not affected. The patient is typically awake at the onset of the attack but may experience blurred vision or ptosis. The attack is almost always bilateral and usually lasts a few seconds. Neurological examination performed at the time of an attack shows a suppression of the patellar reflex and sometimes presence of a Babinski's sign.

Cataplexy is an extremely variable clinical symptom [25]. Most often, it is mild and occurs as a simple buckling of the knees, head dropping, facial muscle flickering, sagging of the jaw, or weakness in the arms. Slurred speech or mutism is also frequently associated. It is often imperceptible to the observer and may even be only a subjective feeling difficult to describe, such as a feeling of warmth or that somehow time is suspended [24, 25]. In other cases, it escalates to actual episodes of muscle paralysis that may last up to a few minutes. Falls and injury are rare and most often the patient will have time to find support or will sit down while the attack is occurring. Long episodes occasionally blend into sleep and may be associated with hypnagogic hallucinations.

Patients may also experience "status cataplecticus." This rare manifestation of narcolepsy is characterized by subintrant cataplexy that lasts several hours per day and confines the subject to bed. It can occur spontaneously or more often upon withdrawal from anticataplectic drugs [16, 26, 27].

Cataplexy often improves with advancing age. In rare cases, it disappears completely but in most patients it is better controlled (probably after the patient has learned to control their emotions) [14, 28].

Sleep Paralysis

Sleep paralysis is present in 20–50 % of all narcoleptic subjects [17, 29–31]. It is often associated with hypnagogic hallucinations. Sleep paralysis is best described as a brief inability to perform voluntary movements at the onset of sleep, upon awakening during the night, or in the morning. Contrary to simple fatigue or locomotion inhibition, the patient is unable to perform even a small movement, such as lifting a finger. Sleep paralysis may last a few minutes and is often finally interrupted by noise or other external stimuli. The symptom is occasionally bothersome in narcoleptic subjects, especially when associated with frightening hallucinations [32].

Whereas EDS and cataplexy are the cardinal symptoms of narcolepsy, sleep paralysis occurs frequently as an isolated phenomenon, affecting 5–40% of the general population [33–35]. Occasional episodes of sleep paralysis are often seen in adolescence and after sleep deprivation, thus prevalence is high for single episodes.

Hypnagogic and Hypnopompic Hallucinations

Abnormal visual (most often) or auditory perceptions that occur while falling asleep (hypnagogic) or upon waking up (hypnopompic) are frequently observed in narcoleptic subjects [36]. These hallucinations are often unpleasant and are typically associated with a feeling of fear or threat [29, 32]. Polygraphic studies indicate that these hallucinations occur most often during REM sleep [29, 37]. These episodes are often difficult to distinguish from nightmares or unpleasant dreams, which also occur frequently in narcolepsy.

Hypnagogic hallucinations are most often associated with sleep attacks and their content is well criticized by the patient. The hallucinations are most often complex, vivid, dream-like experiences ("half sleep" hallucinations) and may follow episodes of cataplexy or sleep paralysis, a feature that is not uncommon in severely affected patients. These hallucinations are usually easy to distinguish from hallucinations observed in schizophrenia or related psychotic conditions.

Other Important Symptoms

One of the most frequently associated symptoms is insomnia, best characterized as a difficulty to maintain nighttime sleep. Typically, narcoleptic patients fall asleep easily, only to wake up after a short nap and are unable to fall back asleep again for before an hour or so. Narcoleptic patients do not usually sleep more than normal individuals over the 24-h cycle [38–40], but frequently have a very disrupted nighttime sleep [38–40]. This symptom often develops later in life and can be very disabling.

Frequently associated problems are periodic leg movements [41, 42], REM behavior disorder, other parasomnias [43, 44], and obstructive sleep apnea [42, 45, 46].

Narcolepsy was reported to be associated with changes in energy homeostasis several decades ago. Narcolepsy patients are frequently (1) obese [47, 48], (2) more often have insulin-resistant diabetes mellitus [47], (3) exhibit reduced food intake [49], and (4) have lower blood pressure and temperature [50, 51]. These findings, however, had not received much attention since they were believed to be secondary to sleepiness or inactivity during the daytime. More recently, however, it was shown that these metabolic changes may be found more specifically in hypocretin-deficient patients [52, 53], suggesting a direct pathophysiological link. Additional research in this area is warranted to clarify this association.

Narcolepsy is a very incapacitating disease. It interferes with every aspect of life. The negative social impact of narcolepsy has been extensively studied. Patients experience impairments in driving and a high prevalence of either car- or machine-related accidents. Narcolepsy also interferes with professional performance, leading to unemployment, frequent changes of employment, working disability, or early retirement [54–56]. Several subjects also develop symptoms of depression, although these symptoms are often masked by anticataplectic medications [10, 54, 57].

Neurobiology of Wakefulness

In order to help in the understanding of the neurobiology of hypersomnia, we will discuss current understandings of the neurobiology of wakefulness. Sleep/wake is a complex physiology regulated by brain activity, and multiple neurotransmitter systems such as monoamines, acetylcholine, excitatory and inhibitory amino acids, peptides, purines, and neuronal and nonneuronal humoral modulators (i.e., cytokines and prostaglandins) [58] are likely to be involved. Monoamines are perhaps the first neurotransmitters recognized to be involved in wakefulness [59], and the monoaminergic systems have been the most common pharmacological targets for wake-promoting compounds in the past years. On the other hand, most hypnotics target the γ-aminobutyric acid (GABA) ergic system, a main inhibitory neurotransmitter system in the brain [60].

Cholinergic neurons also play critical roles in cortical activation during wakefulness (and during REM sleep) [58]. Brainstem cholinergic neurons originating from the laterodorsal and pedunculopontine tegmental nuclei activate thalamocortical signaling, and cortex activation is further reinforced by direct cholinergic projections from the basal forebrain. However, currently no cholinergic compounds are used in sleep medicine, perhaps due to the complex nature of the systems and prominent peripheral side effects.

Monoamine neurons, such as norepinephrine (NE)-containing locus coeruleus (LC) neurons, serotonin (5-HT)-containing raphe neurons, and histamine-containing tuberomammillary neurons (TMN), are wake active and act directly on cortical and subcortical regions to promote wakefulness [58]. In contrast to the focus on these wake-active monoaminergic systems, researchers have often underestimated the importance of dopamine (DA) in promoting wakefulness. Most likely, this is because the firing rates of midbrain DA-producing neurons (ventral tegmental area [VTA] and substantia nigra) do not have an obvious variation according to behavioral states [61]. In addition, DA is produced by many different cell groups [62], and which of these promote wakefulness remains undetermined. Nevertheless, DA release is greatest during wakefulness [63], and DA neurons increase discharge and tend to fire bursts of action potentials in association with significant sensory stimulation, purposive movement, or behavioral arousal [64]. Lesions that include the dopaminergic neurons of the VTA reduce behavioral arousal [65]. Recent work has also identified a small wake-active population of DA-producing neurons in the ventral periaqueductal gray that project to other arousal regions [66]. People with DA deficiency from Parkinson's disease are often sleepy [67], and DA antagonists are frequently sedating. These physiologic and clinical evidences clearly demonstrate that DA also plays a role in wakefulness.

Wakefulness (and various physiologies associated with wakefulness) is essential for the survival of creatures and thus is likely to be regulated by multiple systems, each having a distinct role. Some arousal systems may have essential roles for cortical activation, attention, cognition, or neuroplasticity during wakefulness while others may only be active during specific times to promote particular aspects of wakefulness. Some of the examples may be motivated—behavioral wakefulness or wakefulness in emergency states. Wakefulness may thus likely be maintained by many systems with differential roles coordinating in line. Similarly, the wake-promoting mechanism of some drugs may not be able to be explained by a single neurotransmitter system.

Basic Sleep Physiology and Symptoms of Narcolepsy

Since narcolepsy is a prototypical EDS disorder and since the major pathophysiology of narcolepsy (i.e., deficient in hypocretin neurotransmission) has recently been revealed, the discussion of neurophysiological aspects of narcolepsy will help for a general understanding of neurobiology in EDS.

Narcolepsy patients manifest symptoms specifically related to the dysregulation of REM sleep [68]. In the structured, cyclic process of normal sleep, two distinct states—REM and three stages (S1, S2, S3) of non-REM (NREM) sleep—alternate sequentially every 90 min in a cycle repeating four

to five times per night [69]. As electroencephalography (EEG) signals in humans indicate, NREM sleep, characterized by slow oscillation of thalamocortical neurons (detected as cortical slow waves) and muscle tonus reduction, precedes REM sleep when complete muscle atonia occurs. Slow-wave NREM predominates during the early phase of normal sleep, followed by a predominance of REM during the later phase [69].

Notably, sleep and wake are highly fragmented in narcolepsy, and affected subjects could not maintain long bouts of wake and sleep. Normal sleep physiology is currently understood as dependent upon coordination of the interactions of facilitating sleep centers and inhibiting arousal centers in the brain, such that stable sleep and wake states are maintained for specific durations [69]. An ascending arousal pathway, running from the rostral pons and through the midbrain reticular formation, promotes wakefulness [69, 70]. As discussed earlier, this arousal pathway may be composed of neurotransmitters (acetylcholine, NE, DA, excitatory amino acids), produced by brainstem and hypothalamic neurons (hypocretin/orexin and histamine) and also linked to muscle tonus control during sleep [69, 70]. Whereas full alertness and cortical activation require coordination of these arousal networks, effective sleep requires suppression of arousal by the hypothalamus [70]. Narcolepsy patients may experience major neurological malfunction of this control system.

Narcoleptics exhibit a phenomenon termed short REM sleep latency or sleep-onset REM period (SOREMP), in which they enter REM sleep more immediately upon falling asleep than normal [68]. In some cases, NREM sleep is completely bypassed and the transition to REM sleep occurs instantly [68]. SOREMS are not observed in idiopathic hypersomnia.

Moreover, intrusion of REM sleep into wakefulness may explain the cataplexy, sleep paralysis, and hypnagogic hallucinations, which are symptoms of narcolepsy. Significantly, whereas paralysis and hallucinations manifest in other sleep disorders (sleep apnea syndromes and disturbed sleep patterns in normal population) [71], cataplexy is pathognomonic for narcolepsy [68]. As such, identifying cataplexy's unique pathophysiological mechanism emerged to be potentially crucial to describing the pathology underlying narcolepsy overall.

Discovery of Hypocretin Deficiency and Postnatal Cell Death of Hypocretin Neurons

The significant roles, first of hypocretin deficiency and subsequently of postnatal cell death of hypocretin neurons as the major pathophysiological process underlying narcolepsy with cataplexy, were established from a decade of investigation in both animal and human models. In 1998, the simultaneous discovery of a novel hypothalamic peptide neurotransmitter by two independent research groups proved pivotal [72, 73]. One group called the peptides "hypocretin" because of their primary hypothalamic localization and similarities with the hormone "secretin" [73]. The other group called it "orexin" after observing that central administration of these peptides increased appetite in rats [72]. These neurotransmitters are produced exclusively by thousands of neurons, which are localized in the lateral hypothalamus, and project broadly to specific cerebral regions and more densely to others [74].

Within a year, Stanford researchers identified an autosomal recessive mutation of hypocretin receptor 2 (Hcrtr 2) responsible for canine narcolepsy characterized by cataplexy, reduced sleep latency, and SOREMPs, using positional cloning of a naturally occurring familial canine narcolepsy model [75]. This finding coincided with the observation of the narcolepsy phenotype, characterized by cataplectic behavior and sleep fragmentation in hypocretin-ligand-deficient mice (prepro-orexin gene knockout mice) [76]. Together, these findings confirmed hypocretins as principal sleep/wake-modulating neurotransmitters and prompted investigation of the hypocretin system's involvement in human narcolepsy.

Although screening of patients with cataplexy failed to implicate hypocretin-related gene mutation as a major cause of human narcolepsy, narcoleptic patients did exhibit low CSF hypocretin-1 levels [77] (Fig. 26.1). Postmortem brain tissue of narcoleptic patients assessed with immuno-chemistry, radioimmunological peptide assays, and in situ hybridization revealed hypocretin peptide-loss and undetectable levels of hypocretin peptides or prepro-hypocretin RNA (Fig. 26.1). Further, melanin-concentrating hormone (MCH) neurons, located in the same brain region [78], were observed intact, thus indicating that damage to hypocretin neurons and its production is selective in narcolepsy, rather than due to general neuronal degeneration.

As a result of these findings, a diagnostic test for narcolepsy based on clinical measurement of CSF hypocretin-1 levels for detecting hypocretin ligand deficiency is now available [1]. Whereas CSF hypocretin-1 concentrations above 200 pg/ml almost always occur in controls and patients with other sleep and neurological disorders, concentrations below 110 pg/ml are 94% predictive of narcolepsy with cataplexy [79] (Fig. 26.2). As this represents a more specific assessment than the multiple sleep latency test (MSLT), CFS hypocretin-1 levels below 110 pg/ml are indicated in the International Classification of Sleep Disorders (ICSD)-3 as diagnostic of narcolepsy with cataplexy [1].

Moreover, separate coding of "narcolepsy with cataplexy" (type 1) and "narcolepsy without cataplexy" (type 2) in the ICSD-3 underscores how discovery of specific diagnostic

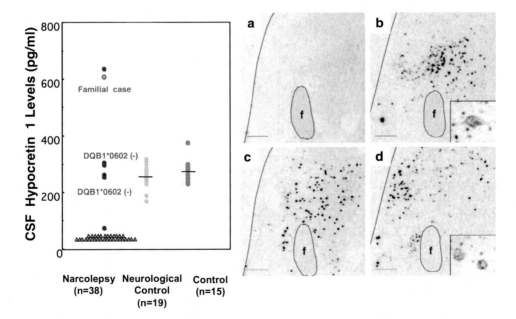

Fig. 26.1 Hypocretin deficiency in narcoleptic subjects. **a** CSF hypocretin-1 levels are undetectably low in most narcoleptic subjects (84.2%). Note that two HLA DQB1*0602-negative and one *familial case* have normal or high CSF hypocretin levels. **b** Prepro-hypocretin transcripts are detected in the hypothalamus of control (**b**) but not in narcoleptic subjects (**a**). Melanin-concentrating hormone (*MCH*) transcripts are detected in the same region in both control (**d**) and narcoleptic (**c**) sections. **c** Colocalization of IGFBP3 in HCRT cells in control and narcolepsy human brain. *Upper panel*: **e** Distribution of hypocretin cells and fibers in the perifornical area of human hypothalamus. **f** In control brains, HCRT cells and fibers were densely stained by an anti-HCRT monoclonal antibody (red fluorescence: VectorRed), while in narcolepsy brains, staining was markedly reduced. *Lower panel*: HCRT immunoreactivity (**g**: *red fluorescence*) and IGFBP3 immunoreactivity (**h**: *green fluorescence*; Q-dot525) and a composite picture (**i**) arrows indicate HCRT cells colocalized with IGFBP3). Note: nonneuronal autofluorescent elements. f and fx, fornix. Scale bar represents 10 mm (**a–d**), 500 mm in (**e** and **f**), 100 mm in g, h, and i (from [78] and [81]). *CSF* cerebrospinal fluid, *HLA* human leukocyte antigen, *HCRT* hypocretin, *IGFBP3* insulin-like growth factor-binding protein 3

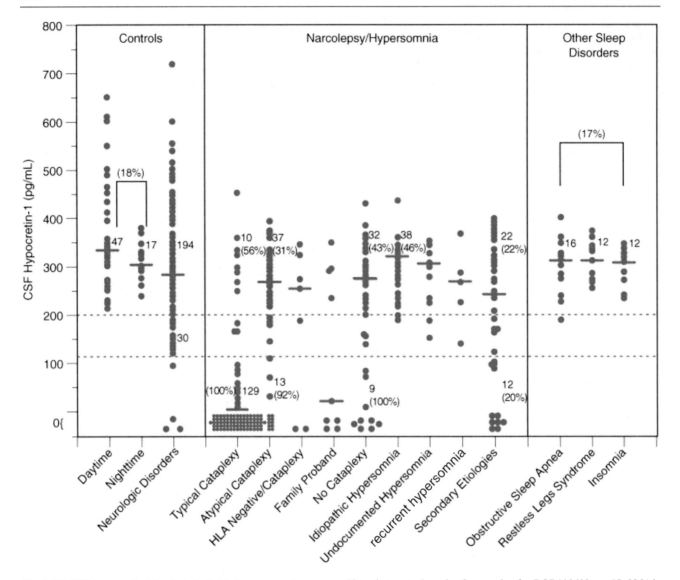

Fig. 26.2 CSF hypocretin-1 levels in individuals across various control and sleep disorders. Each point represents the crude concentration of hypocretin-1 in a single person. The cutoffs for normal (>200 pg/mL) and low (<110 pg/mL) hypocretin-1 concentrations are shown. Also noted is the total number of subjects in each range, and the percentage human leukocyte antigen (HLA)-DQB1*0602 positivity for a given group in a given range is parenthetically noted for certain disorders.

Note that control carrier frequencies for DQB1*0602 are 17–22% in healthy control subjects and secondary narcolepsy, consistent with control values reported in whites (see Table 64.3). In other patient groups, values are higher, with almost all hypocretin-deficient narcolepsy being HLA DQB1*0602 positive. The median value in each group is shown as a horizontal bar. (Updated from previously published data [79])

criteria now informs our understanding of narcolepsy's nosology; narcolepsy with cataplexy, as indicated by low CSF hypocretin-1, appears etiologically homogeneous and distinct from most patients with narcolepsy without cataplexy, exhibiting normal hypocretin-1 levels [79]. Further, the potential of hypocretin receptor agonists (or cell transplantation) in narcolepsy treatment is currently being explored, and CSF hypocretin-1 measures may be useful in identifying appropriate patients as candidates for a novel therapeutic option, namely hypocretin replacement therapy.

Soon after the discovery of human hypocretin deficiency, researchers identified specific substances and genes, such as dynorphin and neuronal activity-regulated pentraxin (NARP)

[80] and most recently, insulin-like growth factor-binding protein 3 (IGFBP3) [81], which colocalizes in neurons containing hypocretin. These findings underscored selective hypocretin cell death as the cause of hypocretin deficiency (as opposed to transcription/biosynthesis or hypocretin peptide processing problems), because these substances are also deficient in postmortem brain HLA of hypocretin-deficient narcoleptic patients [80, 81]. Further, these findings, in view of the generally late onsets of sporadic narcolepsy compared with those of familial cases, suggest that postnatal cell death of hypocretin neurons constitutes the major pathophysiological process in human narcolepsy with cataplexy.

A large kindred with familial narcolepsy (12 affected members) has been reported in Spain [82]. Affected members do not exhibit any symptoms suggesting symptomatic cases of narcolepsy and were diagnosed as familial idiopathic narcolepsy–cataplexy. The family includes a pair of dizygotic twins concordant for narcolepsy–cataplexy in the third generation; the distribution of the disorder indicates an autosomal-dominant transmission of the disease-causing gene. Hor et al. recently performed linkage analysis and sequenced coding regions of the genome (exome sequencing) of three affected members with narcolepsy and cataplexy and had identified a missense mutation in the second exon of myelin oligodendrocyte glycoprotein (MOG) [82]. A c.398 C>G mutation was present in all affected family members but absent in unaffected members and 775 unrelated control subjects [82]. Affected members were hypocretin deficient, but association with HLA DQB1*0602 was not observed [82]. The mutation may secondarily induce hypocretin deficiency with or without immune-mediated mechanisms. MOG has recently been linked to various neuropsychiatric disorders and is considered as a key autoantigen in multiple sclerosis (MS) and in its animal model, experimental autoimmune encephalitis [83]; thus autoimmune mechanisms may also be involved in these cases. However, even if autoimmune mechanisms are involved in these cases, it is possible that the primary target for the immune attack is not the hypocretin system. These results also suggest the heterogeneity of etiology of idiopathic narcolepsy–cataplexy.

How Does Hypocretin Ligand Deficiency Cause the Narcolepsy Phenotype?

Since hypocretin deficiency is a major pathophysiological mechanism for narcolepsy–cataplexy, how the hypocretin ligand deficiency can cause the narcolepsy phenotype is discussed.

Hypocretin/Orexin System and Sleep Regulation

Hypocretins/orexins (hypocretin-1 and hypocretin-2/orexin A and orexin B) are cleaved from a precursor prepro-hypocretin (prepro-orexin) peptide [72, 73, 84]) (Fig. 26.3). Hypocretin-1 with 33 residues contains four cysteine residues forming two disulfide bonds. Hypocretin-2 consists of 28 amino acids and shares similar sequence homology especially at the C-terminal side but has no disulfide bonds

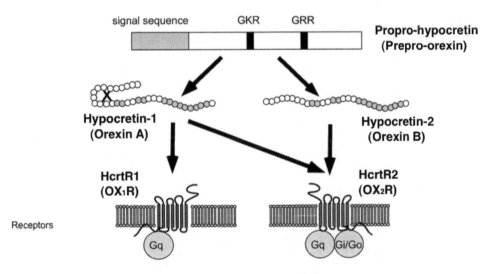

Fig. 26.3 a Structures of mature *hypocretin-1 (orexin A)* and *hypocretin-2 (orexin B)* peptides. **b** Schematic representation of the hypocretin (orexin) system. **c** Projections of hypocretin neurons in the rat brain and relative abundance of hypocretin receptor 1 and 2. **a** The topology of the two intrachain disulfide bonds in orexin A is indicated in the above sequence. Amino acid identities are indicated by shaded areas. **b** The actions of hypocretins are mediated via two G-protein-coupled receptors named hypocretin receptor 1 (*Hcrtr 1*) and hypocretin receptor 2 (*Hcrtr 2*), also known as orexin-1 (OX_1R) and orexin-2 (OX_2R) receptors, respectively. Hcrtr 1 is selective for hypocretin-1, whereas *Hcrtr 2* is nonselective for both hypocretin-1 and hypocretin-2. *Hcrtr 1* is coupled exclusively to the G_q subclass of heterotrimeric G proteins, whereas in vitro experiments suggest that *Hcrtr 2* couples with $G_{i/o}$, and/or G_q. (adapted from Sakurai (2002). **c** Hypocretin-containing neurons project to these previously identified monoaminergic and cholinergic and cholinoceptive regions where hypocretin receptors are enriched. The relative abundance of *Hcrtr 1* versus *Hcrtr 2* in each brain structure was indicated in parenthesis (data from Marcus et al. 2001). Impairments of hypocretin input may thus result in cholinergic and monoaminergic imbalance and generation of narcoleptic symptoms. Most drugs currently used for the treatment of narcolepsy enhance monoaminergic neurotransmission and adjust these symptoms. *VTA* ventral tegmental area, *SN* substantia nigra, *LC* locus coeruleus, *LDT* laterodorsal tegmental nucleus, *PPT* pedunculopontine tegmental nucleus, *RF* reticular formation, *BF* basal forebrain, *VLPO* ventrolateral preoptic nucleus, *LHA* lateral hypothalamic area, *TMN* tuberomammillary nucleus, *DR* dorsal raphe, *Ach* acetylcholine, *Glu* glutamate, *GABA* γ-aminobutyric acid, *HI* histamine, *DA* dopamine, *NA* noradrenalin, *5-HT* serotonin

(a linear peptide) [72]. There are two G-protein-coupled hypocretin receptors, Hcrtr 1 and Hcrtr 2, also called orexin receptor 1 and 2 (OX_1R and OX_2R), and distinct distribution of these receptors in the brain is known. Hcrtr 1 is abundant in the LC while Hcrtr 2 is found in the TMN and basal forebrain (Fig. 26.3). Both receptor types are found in the midbrain raphe nuclei and mesopontine reticular formation [4].

Hypocretins-1 and -2 are produced exclusively by a well-defined group of neurons localized in the lateral hypothalamus. The neurons project to the olfactory bulb, cerebral cortex, thalamus, hypothalamus, and brainstem, particularly the LC, raphe nucleus, and to the cholinergic nuclei (the laterodorsal tegmental and pedunculopontine tegmental nuclei) and cholinoceptive sites (such as pontine reticular formation) [74, 84]. All of these projection sites are thought to be important for sleep regulation.

A series of recent studies have now shown that the hypocretin system is a major excitatory system that affects the activity of monoaminergic (DA, NE, 5-HT, and histamine) and cholinergic systems with major effects on vigilance states [84, 85]. It is thus likely that a deficiency in hypocretin neurotransmission induces an imbalance between these classical neurotransmitter systems, with primary effects on sleep-state organization and vigilance.

Many measurable activities (brain and body) and compounds manifest rhythmic fluctuations over a 24-h period. Whether or not hypocretin tone changes with zeitgeber time was assessed by measuring extracellular hypocretin-1 levels in the rat brain CSF across 24-h periods, using in vivo dialysis [86]. The results demonstrate the involvement of a slow diurnal pattern of hypocretin neurotransmission regulation (as in the homeostatic and/or circadian regulation of sleep). Hypocretin levels increase during the active periods and are highest at the end of the active period, and the levels decline with the onset of sleep. Furthermore, sleep deprivation increases hypocretin levels [86].

Recent electrophysiological studies have shown that hypocretin neurons are active during wakefulness and reduce the activity during slow-wave sleep [87]. The neuronal activity during REM sleep is the lowest, but intermittent increases in the activity associated with body movements or phasic REM activity are observed [87]. In addition to this short-term change, the results of microdialysis experiments also suggest that basic hypocretin neurotransmission fluctuates across the 24-h period and slowly builds up toward the end of the active period. Adrenergic LC neurons are typical wake-active neurons involved in vigilance control, and it has been recently demonstrated that basic firing activity of wake-active LC neurons also significantly fluctuates across various circadian times [88].

Several acute manipulations such as exercise, low glucose utilization in the brain, and forced wakefulness increase hypocretin levels [85, 86]. It is therefore hypothesized that a build up/acute increase of hypocretin levels may counteract homeostatic sleep propensity that typically increases during the daytime and during forced wakefulness [89].

Hypocretin/Orexin Deficiency and Narcoleptic Phenotype

Human studies have demonstrated that the occurrence of cataplexy is closely associated with hypocretin deficiency [79]. Furthermore, the hypocretin deficiency was already observed at very early stages of the disease (just after the onset of EDS), even before the occurrences of clear cataplexy. Occurrences of cataplexy are rare in acute symptomatic cases of EDS associated with a significant hypocretin deficiency (see [3]); therefore, it appears that a chronic and selective deficit of hypocretin neurotransmission may be required for the occurrence of cataplexy. The possibility of involvement of a secondary neurochemical change for the occurrence of cataplexy still cannot be ruled out. If some of these changes are irreversible, hypocretin supplement therapy may only have limited effects on cataplexy.

Sleepiness in narcolepsy is most likely due to the difficulty in maintaining wakefulness as normal subjects do. The sleep pattern of narcoleptic subjects is also fragmented; they exhibit insomnia (frequent wakening) at night. This fragmentation occurs across 24 h, thus, the loss of hypocretin signaling is likely to play a role in this vigilance stage stability (see [90]), but other mechanism may also be involved in EDS in narcoleptic subjects. One of the most important characteristics of EDS in narcolepsy is that sleepiness is reduced and patients feel refreshed after a short nap, but this does not last long as they become sleepy within a short period of time. Hypocretin-1 levels in the extracellular space and in the CSF of rats significantly fluctuate across 24 h and build up toward the end of the active periods [89]. Several manipulations (such as sleep deprivation, exercise, and long-term food deprivation) are also known to increase the hypocretin tonus [86, 89]. Thus, the lack of this hypocretin build up (or increase) caused by circadian time and by various alerting stimulations may also play a role for EDS associated with hypocretin-deficient narcolepsy.

Mechanisms for cataplexy and REM sleep abnormalities associated with impaired hypocretin neurotransmission have been studied. Hypocretin strongly inhibits REM sleep and activates brainstem REM-off LC and raphe neurons and REM-on cholinergic neurons as well as local GABAergic neurons. Therefore, disfacilitation of REM-off monoaminergic neurons and stimulation of REM-on cholinergic neurons mediated through disfacilitation of inhibitory GABAergic inert neurons associated with impaired hypocretin neurotransmission are proposed for abnormal manifestations of REM sleep.

Considerations for the Pathophysiology of Narcolepsy with Normal Hypocretin Levels

There are debates about the pathophysiology of narcolepsy with normal hypocretin levels. Over 90% patients with narcolepsy without cataplexy show normal CSF hypocretin levels, yet they show apparent REM sleep abnormalities (i.e., SOREMS). Furthermore, even if the strict criteria for narcolepsy–cataplexy are applied, up to 10% of patients with narcolepsy–cataplexy show normal CSF hypocretin levels. Considering the fact that occurrence of cataplexy is tightly associated with hypocretin deficiency, impaired hypocretin neurotransmission is still likely involved in narcolepsy–cataplexy with normal CSF hypocretin levels. Conceptually, there are two possibilities to explain these mechanisms: (1) specific impairment of hypocretin receptor and their downstream pathway and (2) partial/localized loss of hypocretin ligand (yet exhibit normal CSF levels). A good example for (1) is Hcrtr-2-mutated narcoleptic dogs; they exhibit normal CSF hypocretin-1 levels [91] while having a full-blown narcolepsy. Thannickal et al. recently reported one narcolepsy without cataplexy patient (HLA typing was unknown) who had an overall loss of 33% of hypocretin cells compared to normal, with maximal cell loss in the posterior hypothalamus [92]. This result favors the second hypothesis, but studies with more cases are needed.

Idiopathic Hypersomnia: A Hypocretin Nondeficient Primary Hypersomnia

With the clear definition of narcolepsy (cataplexy and dissociated manifestations of REM sleep), it became apparent that some patients with hypersomnia suffer from a different disorder. Bedrich Roth was the first in the late 1950s and early 1960s to describe a syndrome characterized by EDS, prolonged sleep, and sleep drunkenness, and by the absence of "sleep attacks," cataplexy, sleep paralysis, and hallucinations. The terms "independent sleep drunkenness" and "hypersomnia with sleep drunkenness" were initially suggested [93], but now this syndrome is categorized as idiopathic hypersomnia (1). Idiopathic hypersomnia should therefore not be considered synonymous with hypersomnia of unknown origin.

In the absence of systematic studies, the prevalence of idiopathic hypersomnia is unknown. Nosologic uncertainty causes difficulty in determining the epidemiology of the disorder. Recent reports from large sleep centers reported the ratio of idiopathic hypersomnia to narcolepsy to be 1:10. [94]. The age of onset of symptoms varies, but it is frequently between 10 and 30 years. The condition usually develops progressively over several weeks or months. Once established, symptoms are generally stable and long lasting, but spontaneous improvement in EDS may be observed in up to one quarter of patients [94].

The pathogenesis of idiopathic hypersomnia is unknown. Hypersomnia usually starts insidiously. Occasionally, EDS is first experienced after transient insomnia, abrupt changes in sleep–wake habits, overexertion, general anesthesia, viral illness, or mild head trauma [94]. Despite reports of an increase in HLA DQ1,11 DR5 and Cw2, and DQ3, and decrease in Cw3, no consistent findings have emerged [94].

The most recent attempts to understand the pathophysiology of idiopathic hypersomnia relate to the investigation of potential role of the hypocretins. However, most studies suggest normal CSF levels of hypocretin-1 in idiopathic hypersomnia [79, 95].

Nosological and Diagnostic Considerations of Major Primary Hypersomnias

Narcolepsy–cataplexy, narcolepsy without cataplexy, and idiopathic hypersomnia are diagnosed mostly by sleep phenotypes, especially by the occurrences of cataplexy and SOREMPS (Fig. 26.4; ICSD-3). Discovery of hypocretin deficiency in narcolepsy–cataplexy was not only a breakthrough but also brought a new nosological and diagnostic uncertainty of the primary hypersomnias. Up to 10% of patients with narcolepsy–cataplexy show normal CSF hypocretin-1 levels (Fig. 26.4). As discussed above, altered hypocretin neurotransmissions may still be involved in some of these cases. However, up to 10% of patients with narcolepsy without cataplexy instead show low CSF hypocretin-1 levels, suggesting a substantial pathophysiological overlap between narcolepsy–cataplexy and narcolepsy without cataplexy, and the hypocretin-deficient status (measured in CSF) does not completely separate these two disease conditions (Fig. 26.4). Similarly, concerns about the nosology of narcolepsy without cataplexy and idiopathic hypersomnia should also be addressed. Since patients with typical cases of idiopathic hypersomnia exhibit unique symptomatology, such as long hours of sleep, no refreshment from naps, and generally resistance to stimulant medications, the pathophysiology of idiopathic hypersomnia may be distinct from that of narcolepsy without cataplexy. However, current diagnostic criteria are not specific enough to diagnose these disorders, especially since the test–retest reliability of numbers of SOREMS during MSLT has not been systematically evaluated.

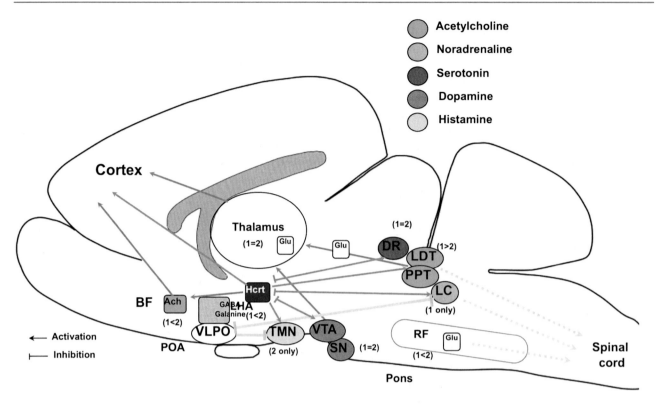

Fig. 26.4 Nosological and diagnostic considerations of major primary hypersomnias. Narcolepsy–cataplexy, narcolepsy without cataplexy, and idiopathic hypersomnia are diagnosed by the occurrences of cataplexy and SOREMPS. Pathophysiology-based marker and low CSF hypocretin levels are included in the ICSD-3 for the positive diagnosis for narcolepsy–cataplexy. However, up to 10 % of patients with narcolepsy–cataplexy show normal CSF hypocretin levels. In contrast, up to 10 % of patients with narcolepsy without cataplexy show low CSF hypocretin-1 levels. These results suggest a substantial pathophysiological overlap between narcolepsy–cataplexy and narcolepsy without cataplexy. Similarly, a substantial overlap likely exists between narcolepsy without cataplexy and idiopathic hypersomnia, as these disorders are diagnosed by the occurrences of SOREMS (two or more). However, the test–retest reliability of detecting number of SOREMS in these conditions has not been systematically evaluated

CSF Histamine and GABAA Receptor Modulator in Narcolepsy and Hypersomnia

Although pathophysiology of hypocretin nondeficient hypersomnia is largely unknown, neurochemical changes in these disease conditions, namely reduced CSF histamine contents and increased activity of GABAA receptor modulator in the CSF, have been reported recently by two groups [96–98].

Histamine is one of these wake-active monoamines [99], and low CSF histamine levels are also found in narcolepsy with hypocretin deficiency [96, 97]. Since hypocretin neurons project and excite histamine neurons in the posterior hypothalamus, it is conceivable that impaired histamine neurotransmission may mediate sleep abnormalities in hypocretin-deficient narcolepsy. However, low CSF histamine levels were also observed in narcolepsy with normal hypocretin levels, and in idiopathic hypersomnia, decreased histamine neurotransmission may be involved in a broader category of EDS than in hypocretin-deficient narcolepsy [97]. Since CSF histamine levels are normalized in EDS patients treated with wake-promoting compounds, low CSF histamine levels may be a new state marker for the hypersomnia of central origin, and functional significances of this finding should further be studied further [97].

Ryer et al. recently reported that activities of substance in CSF that augments inhibitory GABA signaling are enhanced in hypersomnia [98]. The authors demonstrated that in the presence of GABA (10 µM), CSF can stimulate GABAA receptor function in vitro (measures of GABAAR-mediated chloride currents in recombinant pentameric human GABAAR-expressed cultured cells). Interestingly, stimulations of GABAA receptor function by CSF from hypersomnolent patients (idiopathic hypersomnia with and without long sleep, long sleepers and narcolepsy without cataplexy) are significantly enhanced compared to those by CSF from control subjects (84.0 vs. 35.8 %) [98]. This bioactive CSF component had a mass of 500–3000 Da and was neutralized by trypsin. Flumazenil, a benzodiazepine receptor antagonist, reversed the enhancement of GABAA signaling by hypersomnolent CSF in vitro, and flumazenil normalized vigilance in all seven hypersomnolent patients who underwent the drug challenge [98]. The authors conclude that a naturally occurring substance in CSF augments inhibitory GABA signaling, revealing a new pathophysiology associated with

EDS. These results are especially interesting, as GABAAR has never been targeted for the treatment of hypersomnia. It is still unknown if these changes are primary or secondary to the changes in other neurotransmitter systems. It is also critical to test whether the same change is observed in hypocretin-deficient narcolepsy–cataplexy.

Although these new findings are interesting as they are some of the first biomarkers for idiopathic hypersomnia, and these finding may lead to the development of new treatments for somewhat treatment-resistant hypersomnia. However, these markers do not discriminate the types of hypersomnia, and similar changes were observed in various types of hypersomnia.

Symptomatic Narcolepsy and Hypersomnia

Symptoms of narcolepsy can sometimes be seen during the course of a neurological disease process. In such instances, the term "symptomatic narcolepsy" is used, implying that the narcolepsy is a symptom of the underlying process rather than idiopathic. For these cases, the signs and symptoms of narcolepsy must be temporally associated with the underlying neurological process.

In the ICSD-3, narcolepsy with or without cataplexy associated with neurological disorders is classified under "narcolepsy due to medical condition." The criteria for "narcolepsy due to medical condition" is similar to those for "narcolepsy with cataplexy" and "narcolepsy without cataplexy," and the diagnostic criteria include (A) the patient must have a complaint of EDS occurring almost daily for at least 3 months. (B) One of the following must be observed: (i) A definite history of cataplexy. (ii) If cataplexy is not present or is very atypical, polysomnographic monitoring performed over the patient's habitual sleep period followed by an MSLT must demonstrate a mean sleep latency on the MSLT of less than 8 min with two or more SOREMPs. (iii) Hypocretin-1 levels in the CSF are less than 110 pg/mL (or 30 % of normal control values). In addition, (D) a significant underlying medical or neurological disorder must be accountable for the EDS and/or cataplexy, and (E) the hypersomnia is not better explained by another sleep disorder, mental disorder, medication use, or substance use disorder [1]. As mentioned earlier, EDS without cataplexy nor other REM sleep abnormalities is also often associated with these neurological conditions, and is defined as symptomatic cases of EDS (ICSD-3: hypersomnia due to medical condition).

We therefore define "symptomatic narcolepsy" as cases that meet these criteria (if MSLT data were not available, equivalent polygraphic REM sleep abnormalities were also taken into consideration). In addition, an association with a significant underlying neurological disorder that accounts for the EDS and a temporal association (narcolepsy onset

should be within 3 years if the causative diseases are "acute" neurologic conditions) are required [100].

Hypocretin Involvements in Symptomatic Narcolepsy and EDS

Discovery of hypocretin ligand deficiency in idiopathic narcolepsy has also led to new insights into the pathophysiology of symptomatic (or secondary) narcolepsy and EDS. In a recent meta-analysis, 116 symptomatic narcolepsy cases reported in the literature were analyzed [3]. As several authors have previously reported, inherited disorder ($n=38$), tumors ($n=33$), and head trauma ($n=19$) are the three most frequent causes for symptomatic narcolepsy. Of the 116 cases, ten cases are associated with multiple sclerosis (MS), one with acute dissemi- nated encephalomyelitis, and relatively few (n=6) with vascular disorders, 4 with ($n = 4$ encephalitis, one with degeneration ($n = 1$), and three cases in one family with heterodegenerative disorder (autosomal-dominant cerebellar ataxia w/ deafness, (ADCA-DN)., Although it is difficult to rule out the comorbidity of idiopathic narcolepsy in some cases, literature review reveals numerous unquestionable cases of symptomatic narcolepsy [3]. These include cases that are HLA negative and/or late onset and cases where the occurrence of narcoleptic symptoms parallels the rise and fall of the causative disease.

It is important to figure out what mechanisms and which brain sites are involved in the occurrence of symptomatic narcolepsy, especially in relation to the hypocretin system. Although it is not simple to discuss the mechanisms uniformly for symptomatic narcolepsy associated with various genetic disorders, analysis of symptomatic narcolepsy with tumor cases clearly showed that the lesions most often (about 70 % of cases) involved the hypothalamus and adjacent structures (the pituitary, suprasellar, or optic chiasm; Fig. 26.5). The fact that impairments in the hypothalamus are noted in most symptomatic cases of narcolepsy also suggests a possible involvement of impaired hypocretin neurotransmission in this condition.

CSF hypocretin-1 measurement was also conducted in these symptomatic narcolepsy and EDS cases, and reduced CSF hypocretin-1 levels were noted in most cases with various etiologies [3]. EDS in these cases is sometimes reversible with an improvement of the causative neurological disorder or hypocretin status, thus suggesting a functional link between hypocretin deficiency and sleep symptoms in these patients.

Low CSF hypocretin-1 concentrations were also found in some immune-mediated neurological conditions, namely subsets of Guillain-Barré syndrome [101], Ma2-positive paraneoplastic syndrome [102], and MS/neuromyelitis optica (NMO) [3], (see below) and EDS are often associated with the patients with low CSF hypocretin-1 levels.

It should be addressed that Winkelmann et al. recently identified three additional ADCA-DN kindreds [103]. With

Fig. 26.5 Hypothalamic involvement in symptomatic narcolepsy. **a** Category of neurologic diseases associated with symptomatic narcolepsy; **b** Brain lesions involved in symptomatic cases with narcolepsy associated with brain tumor. One hundred and thirteen symptomatic cases of narcolepsy are included. The percentage of each neurologic category (with cataplexy [CA]/with sleep-onset rapid eye movement periods [SOREMP]) is displayed. **a** Tumors, inherited disorders, and head trauma are the three most frequent causes. **b** Analysis of cases of symptomatic narcolepsy with tumor clearly shows that the lesions most often were in the hypothalamus and adjacent structures (the pituitary, suprasellar, or optic chiasm)

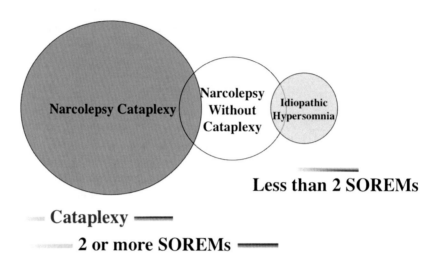

MAJOR HYPERSOMNIAS OF CENTRAL ORIGIN
Cataplexy and MSLT findings

exome sequencing in five individuals from three ADCA-DN kindreds, DNA (cytosine-5)-methyltransferase1 (DNMT1) was identified as the only gene with a mutation found in all five affected individuals [103]. DNMT1 is a widely expressed DNA methyltransferase maintaining methylation patterns in the development and mediating transcriptional repression by direct binding to histone deacetylase 2 (HDAC2) [104].

Based on the available information of crystallographic structures of the DNMT1 [101], the authors speculate that the identified mutations likely affect DNA binding, recognition, or the interaction with other proteins in the DNMT1–HDAC2 complex, causing insufficient CpG methylation and gene silencing in some cases, resulting in the occurrences of ADCA-DN. As the penetrance of the disease is high in the kindred and affected subjects exhibit clear-cut narcolepsy, it is important to further explore the mechanisms of occurrences of narcolepsy–cataplexy in these kindreds.

EDS Associated with MS/NMO: A New Clinical Entity for Autoimmune-Mediated Hypocretin-Deficient Hypersomnia

Of note, Kanbayashi et al. recently encountered seven cases of EDS occurring in the course of MS patients initially diagnosed with symmetrical hypothalamic inflammatory lesions with hypocretin ligand deficiency [106] that contrasts with the characteristics of classic MS cases (Fig. 26.6) (Fig. 26.7).

Symptomatic narcolepsy in MS patients has been reported from several decades ago. Since both MS and narcolepsy are associated with the HLA-DR2 positivity, an autoimmune target on the same brain structures has been proposed to be a common etiology for both diseases [107]. However, the discovery of the selective loss of hypothalamic hypocretin neurons in narcolepsy rather indicates that narcolepsy coincidently occurs in MS patients when MS plaques appear in the hypothalamic area and secondarily damage the hypocretin/orexin neurons. In favor of this interpretation, the hypocretin system is not impaired in MS subjects who do not exhibit narcolepsy [108]. Nevertheless, it is also the case that a subset of MS patients predominantly shows EDS and REM sleep abnormalities, and it is likely that specific immune-mediated mechanisms may be involved in these cases.

CSF hypocretin measures revealed that marked ($\leq$110 pg/ml, $n=3$) or moderate (110–200 pg/ml, $n=4$) hypocretin deficiency was observed in all seven cases [102]. Therefore, four cases met with ICSD-3 criteria [1] for narcolepsy due to medical condition, and three cases met with the hypersomnia due to medical condition. Interestingly, four of them had either or both optic neuritis and spinal cord lesions, sharing the clinical characteristics of NMO. HLA was evaluated in only two cases (case 2 and case 4) and was negative for DQB1*0602. Repeated evaluations of the hypocretin status were carried out in six cases, and CSF hypocretin-1 levels returned to the normal levels or significantly increased with marked improvements of EDS and hypothalamic lesions in all six cases. Since four of them exhibited clinical charac-

Causative Diseases of Symptomatic Narcolepsy (n=116)

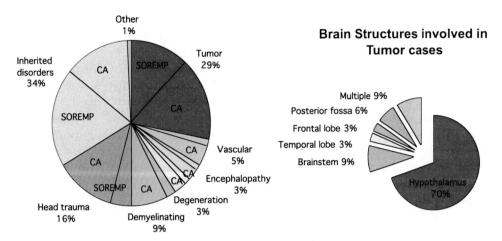

Fig. 26.6 MRI findings (FLAIR or T2) of MS/NMO patients with hypocretin deficiency and EDS. A typical horizontal slice including the hypothalamic periventricular area from each case is presented. All cases were female (*f*) and age (*y*) listed in the parenthesis. * met with ICSD-3 criteria for narcolepsy due to medical condition, and ** met with ICSD-3 criteria for hypersomnia due to medical condition. All cases were initially diagnosed as MS. Cases 3–7 exhibited optic neuritis and/or spinal cord lesions and cases 4, 5, 7 are seropositive for anti-AQP4 antibody and thus being diagnosed as NMO. CSF hypocretin levels are listed below the MRI image. Modified from [102]. *MRI* magnetic resonance imaging, *FLAIR* fluid attenuation inversion recovery, *MS* multiple sclerosis, *NMO* neuromyelitis optica, *EDS* excessive daytime sleepiness, *CSF* cerebrospinal fluid

terization of NMO, anti-AQP4 antibody was evaluated and it was found that three out of seven cases were anti-AQP4 antibody positive, thus being diagnosed as NMO-related disorder [106].

AQP4, a member of the aquaporin (AQP) super family, is an integral membrane protein that forms pores in the membrane of biological cells [109]. Aquaporins selectively conduct water molecules in and out of the cell, while preventing the passage of ions and other solutes and are known as water channels. AQP4 is expressed throughout the central nervous system, especially in periaqueductal and periventricular regions [109, 110] and is found in nonneuronal structures such

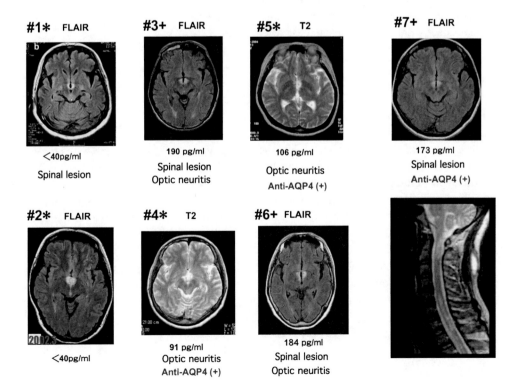

as astrocytes and ependymocytes, but is absent from neurons. Recently, the NMO-IgG (Immunoglobulin G), which can be detected in the serum of patients with NMO, has been shown to selectively bind to AQP4 [111].

Since AQP4 is enriched in periventricular regions in the hypothalamus where hypocretin-containing neurons are primarily located, symmetrical hypothalamic lesions associated with reduced CSF hypocretin-1 levels in our three NMO cases with anti-AQP4 antibody might be caused by the immuno-attack to the AQP4, and this may secondarily affect the hypocretin neurons.

However, the other four MS cases with EDS and hypocretin deficiency were anti-AQP4 antibody negative at the time of blood testing. This leaves a possibility that other antibody-mediated mechanisms are additionally responsible for the bilateral symmetric hypothalamic damage causing EDS in the MS/NMO subjects. There is also a possibility that the four MS cases whose anti-AQP4 antibody was negative could be NMO, since anti-AQP4 antibody was tested only once for each subject during the course of the disease, and the assay was not standardized among the institutes [106]. It is thus essential to further determine the immunological mechanisms that cause the bilateral hypothalamic lesions with hypocretin deficiency and EDS, and their association with NMO and AQP4. This effort may lead to establishment of a new clinical entity, and the knowledge is essential to prevent and treat EDS associated with MS and its related disorders. It should also be noted that none of these cases exhibited cataplexy, contrary to the nine out of ten symptomatic narcoleptic MS cases reported in the past [3]. Early therapeutic intervention with steroids and other immunosuppressants may thus prevent irreversible damage of hypocretin neurons and prevent chronic sleep-related symptoms in these recent cases.

Conclusion

The chapter described the current understanding of pathophysiology of EDS with various etiologies.

The recent progress for understanding the pathophysiology of EDS particularly owes itself to the discovery of hypocretin ligand deficiency in human narcolepsy. Hypocretin deficiency can be clinically detected as low CSF hypocretin-1 level, and low CSF hypocretin-1 levels have been included in the ICSD-3 as a positive diagnosis for narcolepsy–cataplexy.

Symptomatic narcolepsy has also been reported, but the prevalence of symptomatic narcolepsy is much smaller. The meta-analysis of these symptomatic cases indicates that hypocretin deficiency may also partially explain the neurobiological mechanisms of EDS associated with symptomatic cases of narcolepsy.

Although the prevalence of primary hypersomnia such as narcolepsy and idiopathic hypersomnia is not high, that of symptomatic EDS is considerably high, and the pathophysiology of symptomatic EDS likely overlaps with that of primary hypersomnia.

The pathophysiology of hypocretin nondeficient narcolepsy is debated, and the pathophysiology of idiopathic hypersomnia is largely unknown, but hypocretin deficiency is not likely to be involved in this condition. Of interest, decreased histaminergic neurotransmission is observed in narcolepsy and idiopathic hypersomnia, regardless of hypocretin status. Another study reported that activities of substances in CSF that augment inhibitory GABA signaling are enhanced in hypersomnias with various etiologies. Functional significances of these new findings (if this mediates sleepiness or passively reflects sleepiness) need to be evaluated further.

Although much progress was made regarding the pathophysiology of EDS, these new knowledges are not yet incorporated into the development of new treatments, and further research is critical.

References

1. ICSD-3-International classification of sleep disorders: diagnostic and coding manual. 3rd ed. Darien, IL: American Academy of Sleep Medicine; 2014.
2. Verma A, Anand V, Verma NP. Sleep disorders in chronic traumatic brain injury. J Clin Sleep Med. 2007;3(4):357–62.
3. Nishino S, Kanbayashi T. Symptomatic narcolepsy, cataplexy and hypersomnia, and their implications in the hypothalamic hypocretin/orexin system. Sleep Med Rev. 2005;9(4):269–310.
4. Marcus JN, Aschkenasi CJ, Lee CE, Chemelli RM, Saper CB, Yanagisawa M, et al. Differential expression of orexin receptors 1 and 2 in the rat brain. J Comp Neurol. 2001;435(1):6–25.
5. Hirai N, Nishino S. Recent advances in the treatment of narcolepsy. Curr Treat Options Neurol. 2011;13(5):437–57.
6. Nishino S, Mignot E. Narcolepsy and cataplexy. Handb Clin Neurol. 2011;99:783–814.
7. Nishino S, Kotorii N. Overview of management of narcolepsy. In: Goswami M, Pandi-Perumal SR, Thorpy MJ, editors. Narcolepsy. Totowa: Humana; 2009. pp. 251–65.
8. Nishino S. Modes of action of drugs related to narcolepsy: pharmacology of wake-promoting compounds and anticataplectics. In: Goswami M, Pandi-Perumal SR, Thorpy MJ, editors. Narcolepsy. Totowa: Humana; 2009. pp. 267–86.
9. Guilleminault C. Narcolepsy and its differential diagnosis. In: Guilleminault C, editor. Sleep and it disorders in children. New York: Raven Press; 1987. pp. 181–94.
10. Broughton R, Ghanem Q. The impact of compound narcolepsy on the life of the patient. In: Guilleminault C, Dement WC, Passouant P, editors. Narcolepsy. New York: Spectrum; 1976. pp. 201–20.
11. Dement WC. Daytime sleepiness and sleep †attacks". In: Guilleminault C, Dement WC, Passouant P, editors. Narcolepsy. New York: Spectrum; 1976. pp. 17–42.
12. Cohen FL, Smith KM. Learning and memory in narcoleptic patients and controls. Sleep Res. 1989;18:117.
13. Rogers AE, Rosenberg RS. Test of memory in narcoleptics. Sleep. 1990;13:42–52.

14. Billiard M, Besset A, Cadilhac J. The clinical and polygraphic development of narcolepsy. In: Guilleminault C, Lugaresi E, editors. Sleep/wake disorders: natural history, epidemiology and longterm evolution. New York: Raven; 1983. pp. 171–85.

15. Honda Y. Clinical features of narcolepsy. In: Honda Y, Juji T, editors. HLA in narcolepsy. Berlin: Springer; 1988. pp. 24–57.

16. Parkes JD, Baraitser M, Marsden CD, Asselman P. Natural history, symptoms and treatment of the narcoleptic syndrome. Acta Neurol Scand. 1975;52:337–53.

17. Roth B. Narcolepsy and hypersomnia. In: Roth B, Broughton W, editors. Basel: Karger; 1980.

18. Yoss RE, Daly DD. Criteria for the diagnosis of the narcoleptic syndrome. Proc Staff Meet Mayo. 1957;32:320–8.

19. Kales A, Soldatos CR, Bixler EO. Narcolepsy–cataplexy II Psychosocial consequences and associated psychopathology. Arch Neurol. 1982;39:169–71.

20. Guilleminault C, Wilson RA, Dement WC. A study on cataplexy. Arch Neurol. 1974;31:255–61.

21. Henneberg R. Uber genuine Narkolepsie. Neurol Zbl. 1916;30:282–90.

22. Löwenfeld L. Uber Narkolepsie. Munch Med Wochenschr. 1902;49:1041–5.

23. Daniels LE. Narcolepsy. Medicine. 1934;13(1):1–122.

24. Wilson SAK. The narcolepsies. Annu Congress Assoc Phys. 1927;June 3:63–109.

25. Gelb M, Guilleminault C, Kraemer H, Lin S, Moon S, Dement WC, et al. Stability of cataplexy over several months-information for the design of therapeutic trials. Sleep. 1994;17:265–73.

26. Passouant P, Baldy-Moulinier M, Aussilloux C. Etat de mal cataplectique au cours d'ume maladie de Gelineau, influence de la clomipramine. Rev Neurol. 1970;123:56–60.

27. Hishikawa Y, Shimizu T. Physiology of REM sleep, cataplexy, and sleep paralysis. In: Fahn S, Hallet M, Lüders HO, Marsden CDü, editors. Negative motor phenomena. Philadelphia: Lippincot-Raven; 1995. pp. 245–71.

28. Rosenthal L, Merlotti L, Young D, Zorick F, Wittig R, Roehrs T, et al. Subjective and polysomnographic characteristics of patients diagnosed with narcolepsy. Gen Hosp Psychiatry. 1990;12:191–7.

29. Hishikawa Y. Sleep paralysis. In Guilleminault C, Dement W.C., Passouant P, editors. Narcolepsy. New York: Spectrum; 1976. pp. 97–124.

30. Parkes JD, Fenton G, Struthers G, Curzon G, Kantamaneni BD, Buxton BH, et al. Narcolepsy and cataplexy. Clinical features, treatment and cerebrospinal fluid findings. Q J Med. 1974;172:525–36.

31. Yoss RE, Daly DD. Narcolepsy. Med Clin North Am. 1960;44(4):953–67.

32. Rosenthal C. Uber das aufreten von halluzinatorisch-kataplektischem Angstsyndrom, wachanfallen und ahnlichen storungen bei Schizophrenen. Mschr Psychiatry. 1939;102:11.

33. Dahlitz M, Parkes JD. Sleep paralysis. Lancet. 1993;341:406–7.

34. Fukuda K, Miyasita A, Inugami M, Ishihara K. High prevalence of isolated sleep paralysis: Kanashibari phenomenon in Japan. Sleep. 1987;10(3):279–86.

35. Goode B. Sleep paralysis. Arch Neurol. 1962;6(3):228–34.

36. Ribstein M. Hypnagogic hallucinations. In Guilleminault C, Dement WC, Passouant P, editors. Narcolepsy. New York: Spectrum; 1976. pp. 145–60.

37. Chetrit M, Besset A, Damci D, Lelarge C, Billiard M. Hypnogogic hallucinations associated with sleep onset REM period in narcolepsy–cataplexy. J Sleep Res. 1994;3(Suppl 1):43.

38. Hishikawa Y, Wakamatsu H, Furuya E, Sugita Y, Masaoka S, Kaneda H, et al. Sleep satiation in narcoleptic patients. Electroencephalogr Clin Neurophysiol. 1976;41:1–18.

39. Broughton R, Dunham W, Newman J, Lutley K, Dushesne P, Rivers M. Ambulatory 24 hour sleep-wake monitoring in narcolepsy–cataplexy compared to matched control. Electroenceph Clin Neurophysiol. 1988;70:473–81.

40. Montplaisir J, Billiard M, Takahashi S, Bell IR, Guilleminault C, Dement WC. Twenty-four-hour recording in REM-narcoleptics with special reference to nocturnal sleep disruption. Biol Psych. 1978;13(1):78–89.

41. Godbout R, Montplaisir J. Comparison of sleep parameters in narcoleptics with and without periodic movements of sleep. In: Koella WP, Ruther E, Schulz H, editors. Sleep '84. Gustav: Fischer Verlag; 1985. pp. 380–2.

42. Mosko SS, Shampain DS, Sassin JF. Nocturnal REM latency and sleep disturbance in narcolepsy. Sleep. 1984;7:115–25.

43. Mayer G, Pollmächer T, Meier-Ewert K, Schulz H. Zur Einschätzung des Behinderungsgrades bei Narkolepsie. Gesundh-Wes. 1993;55:337–42.

44. Schenck CH, Mahowald MW. Motor dyscontrol in narcolepsy: Rapid-Eye-Movement (REM) sleep without atonia and REM Sleep Behavior Disorder. Ann Neurol. 1992;32(1):3–10.

45. Chokroverty S. Sleep apnea in narcolepsy. Sleep. 1986;9(1):250–3.

46. Lugaresi E, Coccagna G, Mantovani M, Cirignotta F. In: Guilleminault C, Dement WC, Passouant P, editors. Narcolepsy. New York: Spectrum; 1976. pp. 351–66

47. Honda Y, Doi Y, Ninomiya R, Ninomiya C. Increased frequency of non-insulin-dependent diabetes mellitus among narcoleptic patients. Sleep. 1986;9(1):254–9.

48. Schuld A, Hebebrand J, Geller F, Pollmächer T. Increased body-mass index in patients with narcolepsy. Lancet. 2000;355(9211):1274–5.

49. Lammers GJ, Pijl H, Iestra J, Langius JAE, Buunk G, Meinders AE. Spontaneous food choice in narcolepsy. Sleep. 1996;19(1):75–6.

50. Mayer G, Hellmann F, Leonhard E, Meier-Ewert K. Circadian temperature and activity rhythms in unmedicated narcoleptic patients. Pharmacol Biochem Behav. 1997;58(2):395–402.

51. Sachs C, Kaisjer L. Autonomic control of cardiovascular reflexes in Narcolepsy. J Neurol Neurosurg Psychiatry. 1980;43:535–9.

52. Nishino S, Ripley B, Overeem S, Nevsimalova S, Lammers GJ, Vankova J, et al. Low CSF hypocretin (orexin) and altered energy homeostasis in human narcolepsy. Ann Neurol. 2001;50:381–8.

53. Kok SW, Overeem S, Visscher TL, Lammers GJ, Seidell JC, Pijl H, et al. Hypocretin deficiency in narcoleptic humans is associated with abdominal obesity. Obes Res. 2003 Sep;11(9):1147–54.

54. Broughton R, Ghanem Q, Hishikawa Y, Sugita Y, Nevsimalova S, Roth B. Life effects of narcolepsy in 180 patients from North America, Asia and Europe compared to matched controls. Can J Neurol Sci 1981;8(4):299–304.

55. Aldrich MS. Automobile accidents in patients with sleep disorders. Sleep. 1989;12:487–94.

56. Alaila SL. Life effects of narcolepsy: measures of negative impact, social support and psychological well-being. In: Goswanmi M, Pollak CP, Cohen FL, Thorpy MJ, Kavey NB, editors. Loss, grief and care: psychosocial aspects of narcolepsy. New York: Haworth; 1992. pp. 1–22.

57. Roth B, Nevsimalova S. Depression in narcolepsy and hypersomnia. Schweitz Arch Neurol Neurochir Psychiat. 1975;116:291–300.

58. Jones BE. Basic mechanism of sleep-wake states. In: Kryger MH, Roth T, Dement WC, editors. Principles and practice of sleep medicine. 4th ed. Philadelphia: Elsevier Saunders; 2005. pp. 136–53.

59. Jouvet M. The role of monoamines and acetylcholine-containing neurons in the regulation of the sleep-waking cycle. Ergebn Physiol. 1972;64:166–307.

60. Nishino S, Mignot E, Dement WC. Sedative-hypnotics. In: Schatzberg AF, Nemeroff CB, editors. Textbook of psychopharmacology. 2nd ed. Washington, DC: American Psychiatric; 2004. pp. 651–84.

61. Steinfels GF, Heym J, Streckjer RE, Jacobs BJ. Behavioral correlates of dopaminergic activity in freely moving cats. Brain Res. 1983;258:217–28.

62. Björklund A, Lindvall O. Dopamine-containing systems in the CNS. In Björklund A, Hökfelt T, editors. Handbook of chemical

neuroanatomy, vol. 2, Classical Transmitter in the CNS, Part I. Amsterdam: Elsevier; 1984. pp. 55–121.

63. Trulson ME. Simultaneous recording of substantia nigra neurons and voltametric release of dopamine in the caudate of behaving cats. Brain Res Bull. 1985;15:221–3.

64. Ljungberg T, Apicella P, Schultz W. Responses of monkey dopamine neurons during learning of behavioral reactions. J Neurophysiol. 1992;67(1):145–63.

65. Jones BE, Bobillier P, Pin C, Jouvet M. The effect of lesions of catecholamine-containing neurons upon monoamine content of the brain and EEG and behavioral waking in the cat. Brain Res. 1973;58:157–77.

66. Lu J, Jhou TC, Saper CB. Identification of wake-active dopaminergic neurons in the ventral periaqueductal gray matter. J Neurosci. 2006;26(1):193–202.

67. Moller JC, Stiasny K, Cassel W, Peter JH, Kruger HP, Oertel WH. Sleep attacks in Parkinson patients. A side effect of nonergoline dopamine agonists or a class effect of dopamine agonists? Nervenarzt. 2000;71(8):670–6.

68. Nishino S, Mignot E. Pharmacological aspects of human and canine narcolepsy. Prog Neurobiol. 1997;52(1):27–78.

69. Nishino S, Taheri S, Black J, Nofzinger E, Mignot E. The neurobiology of sleep in relation to mental illness. In: Charney DS Nestler, EJ, editor. Neurobiology of mental illness. New York: Oxford University Press; 2004. pp. 1160–79.

70. Saper CB, Scammell TE, Lu J. Hypothalamic regulation of sleep and circadian rhythms. Nature. 2005;437(7063):1257–63.

71. Aldrich MS, Chervin RD, Malow BA. Value of the multiple sleep latency test (MSLT) for the diagnosis of narcolepsy. Sleep. 1997;20(8):620–9.

72. Sakurai T, Amemiya A, Ishii M, Matsuzaki I, Chemelli RM, Tanaka H, et al. Orexins and orexin receptors: a family of hypothalamic neuropeptides and G protein-coupled receptors that regulate feeding behavior. Cell. 1998;92:573–85.

73. De Lecea L, Kilduff TS, Peyron C, Gao X-B, Foye PE, Danielson PE, et al. The hypocretins: hypothalamus-specific peptides with neuroexcitatory activity. Proc Natl Acad Sci U S A. 1998;95:322–7.

74. Peyron C, Tighe DK, van den Pol AN, de Lecea L, Heller HC, Sutcliffe JG, et al. Neurons containing hypocretin (orexin) project to multiple neuronal systems. J Neurosci. 1998;18(23):9996–10015.

75. Lin L, Faraco J, Li R, Kadotani H, Rogers W, Lin X, et al. The sleep disorder canine narcolepsy is caused by a mutation in the hypocretin (orexin) receptor 2 gene. Cell. 1999;98(3):365–76.

76. Chemelli RM, Willie JT, Sinton CM, Elmquist JK, Scammell T, Lee C, et al. Narcolepsy in orexin knockout mice: molecular genetics of sleep regulation. Cell. 1999;98:437–51.

77. Nishino S, Ripley B, Overeem S, Lammers GJ, Mignot E. Hypocretin (orexin) deficiency in human narcolepsy. Lancet. 2000;355(9197):39–40.

78. Peyron C, Faraco J, Rogers W, Ripley B, Overeem S, Charnay Y, et al. A mutation in a case of early onset narcolepsy and a generalized absence of hypocretin peptides in human narcoleptic brains. Nat Med. 2000;6(9):991–7.

79. Mignot E, Lammers GJ, Ripley B, Okun M, Nevsimalova S, Overeem S, et al. The role of cerebrospinal fluid hypocretin measurement in the diagnosis of narcolepsy and other hypersomnias. Arch Neurol. 2002;59(10):1553–62.

80. Crocker A, Espana RA, Papadopoulou M, Saper CB, Faraco J, Sakurai T, et al. Concomitant loss of dynorphin, NARP, and orexin in narcolepsy. Neurology. 2005;65(8):1184–8.

81. Honda M, Eriksson KS, Zhang S, Tanaka S, Lin L, Salehi A, et al. IGFBP3 colocalizes with and regulates hypocretin (orexin). PLoS ONE. 2009;4(1):e4254.

82. Hor H, Bartesaghi L, Kutalik Z, Vicario JL, de Andres C, Pfister C, et al. A missense mutation in myelin oligodendrocyte glycoprotein as a cause of familial narcolepsy with cataplexy. Am J Hum Genet. 2011;89(3):474–9.

83. Clements CS, Reid HH, Beddoe T, Tynan FE, Perugini MA, Johns TG, et al. The crystal structure of myelin oligodendrocyte glycoprotein, a key autoantigen in multiple sclerosis. Proc Natl Acad Sci U S A. 2003;100(19):11059–64.

84. Sakurai T. Roles of orexins in regulation of feeding and wakefulness. Neuroreport. 2002;13(8):987–95.

85. Willie JT, Chemelli RM, Sinton CM, Yanagisawa M. To eat or to sleep? Orexin in the regulation of feeding and wakefulness. Annu Rev Neurosci. 2001;24:429–58.

86. Fujiki N, Yoshida Y, Ripley B, Honda K, Mignot E, Nishino S. Changes in CSF hypocretin-1 (orexin A) levels in rats across 24 hours and in response to food deprivation. NeuroReport. 2001;12(5):993–7.

87. Lee MG, Hassani OK, Jones BE. Discharge of identified orexin/hypocretin neurons across the sleep-waking cycle. J Neurosci. 2005;25(28):6716–20.

88. Aston-Jones G, Chen S, Zhu Y, Oshinsky ML. A neural circuit for circadian regulation of arousal. Nature Neurosci. 2001;4(7):732–8.

89. Yoshida Y, Fujiki N, Nakajima T, Ripley B, Matsumura H, Yoneda H, et al. Fluctuation of extracellular hypocretin-1 (orexin A) levels in the rat in relation to the light-dark cycle and sleep-wake activities. Eur J Neurosci. 2001;14(7):1075–81.

90. Saper CB, Chou TC, Scammell TE. The sleep switch: hypothalamic control of sleep and wakefulness. Trends Neurosci. 2001;24(12):726–31.

91. Ripley B, Fujiki N, Okura M, Mignot E, Nishino S. Hypocretin levels in sporadic and familial cases of canine narcolepsy. Neurobiol Dis. 2001;8(3):525–34.

92. Thannickal TC, Nienhuis R, Siegel JM. Localized loss of hypocretin (orexin) cells in narcolepsy without cataplexy. Sleep. 2009;32(8):993–8.

93. Roth B. Narkolepsie und Hypersomnie. Berlin: VEB Verlag Volk und Gesundheit; 1962.

94. Bassetti C, Aldrich MS. Idiopathic hypersomnia: a series of 42 patients. Brain. 1997;120(Pt 8):1423–35.

95. Bassetti C, Gugger M, Bischof M, Mathis J, Sturzenegger C, Werth E, et al. The narcoleptic borderland: a multimodal diagnostic approach including cerebrospinal fluid levels of hypocretin-1 (orexin A). Sleep Med. 2003;4(1):7–12.

96. Nishino S, Sakurai E, Nevsimalova S, Yoshida Y, Watanabe T, Yanai K, et al. Decreased CSF histamine in narcolepsy with and without low CSF hypocretin-1 in comparison to healthy controls. Sleep. 2009;32(2):175–80.

97. Kanbayashi T, Kodama T, Kondo H, Satoh S, Inoue Y, Chiba S, et al. CSF histamine contents in narcolepsy, idiopathic hypersomnia and obstructive sleep apnea syndrome. Sleep. 2009;32(2):181–7.

98. Ryer EJ, Kalra M, Oderich GS, Duncan AA, Gloviczki P, Cha S, et al. Revascularization for acute mesenteric ischemia. J Vasc Surg. 2012;55(6):1682–9.

99. Brown RE, Stevens DR, Haas HL. The physiology of brain histamine. Prog Neurobiol. 2001;63(6):637–72.

100. Lankford DA, Wellman JJ, O'Hara C. Posttraumatic narcolepsy in mild to moderate closed head injury. Sleep. 1994;17:S25–S8.

101. Nishino S, Kanbayashi T, Fujiki N, Uchino M, Ripley B, Watanabe M, et al. CSF hypocretin levels in Guillain-Barre syndrome and other inflammatory neuropathies. Neurology. 2003;61(6):823–5.

102. Overeem S, Dalmau J, Bataller L, Nishino S, Mignot E, Vershuuren J, et al. Secondary narcolepsy in patients with praneoplastic anti-Ma2 antibodies is associated with hypocretin deficiency. J Sleep Res. 2001;11(suppl. 1):166–7.

103. Winkelmann J, Lin L, Schormair B, Kornum BR, Faraco J, Plazzi G, et al. Mutations in DNMT1 cause autosomal dominant cerebellar ataxia, deafness and narcolepsy. Hum Mol Genet. 2012;21(10):2205–10.

104. Svedruzic ZM. Dnmt1 structure and function. Prog Mol Biol Transl Sci. 2011;101:221–54.

105. Klein CJ, Botuyan MV, Wu Y, Ward CJ, Nicholson GA, Hammans S, et al. Mutations in DNMT1 cause hereditary sensory neuropathy with dementia and hearing loss. Nat Genet. 2011;43(6):595–600.

106. Kanbayashi T, Shimohata T, Nakashima I, Yaguchi H, Yabe I, Shimizu T, et al. Symptomatic narcolepsy in MS and NMO patients; new neurochemical and immunological implications. Arch Neurol. 2009;66:1563–6.

107. Poirier G, Montplaisir J, Dumont M, Duquette P, Decary F, Pleines J, et al. Clinical and sleep laboratory study of narcoleptic symptoms in multiple sclerosis. Neurology. 1987;37(4):693–5.

108. Ripley B, Overeem S, Fujiki N, Nevsimalova S, Uchino M, Yesavage J, et al. CSF hypocretin/orexin levels in narcolepsy and other neurological conditions. Neurology. 2001;57(12):2253–8.

109. Amiry-Moghaddam M, Ottersen OP. The molecular basis of water transport in the brain. Nat Rev Neurosci. 2003;4(12):991–1001.

110. Pittock SJ, Weinshenker BG, Lucchinetti CF, Wingerchuk DM, Corboy JR, Lennon VA. Neuromyelitis optica brain lesions localized at sites of high aquaporin 4 expression. Arch Neurol. 2006;63(7):964–8.

111. Lennon VA, Kryzer TJ, Pittock SJ, Verkman AS, Hinson SR. IgG marker of optic-spinal multiple sclerosis binds to the aquaporin-4 water channel. J Exp Med. 2005;202(4):473–7.

Idiopathic Hypersomnia

Sona Nevsimalova

The history of idiopathic hypersomnia which is distinct from narcolepsy is much shorter, and its biological background is less known than that of narcolepsy–cataplexy. The term idiopathic hypersomnia (*die idiopathische chronische Schlafsucht*) was first used in 1829 by Henrich Bruno Schindler for excessive daytime sleepiness of undetermined origin [1]; however, the description was more suggestive of narcolepsy.

The first author to identify the clinical differences between narcolepsy and other types of hypersomnia was Bedrich Roth, a Czech neurologist, neurophysiologist, and sleep researcher (Fig. 27.1). In 1956, he published a detailed description of difficulties in awakening—sleep drunkenness, recognized later as a leading clinical symptom of idiopathic hypersomnia [2]. He identified sleep drunkenness as a *symptom* (inertia connected with prolonged nocturnal sleep), as *a syndrome* (characterized by patients suffering from prolonged nocturnal sleep, marked difficulty awakening, and daytime sleepiness), and as *an independent nosological* entity. In that paper, he described 20 patients with sleep drunkenness mostly of the independent form (11 patients). The disease usually began in younger age (between 15 and 33 years); the patients often had positive family history (5 out 11 families) and showed features of depression. The most characteristic symptom consisted of prolonged deep nocturnal sleep accompanied by sleep drunkenness during awakening, and prolonged daytime naps generally lasting for 1–3 h or more, but occasionally less. Roth found a secondary cause in two cases (ischemic changes along the borderline between the mesencephalon and diencephalon in one case, and posttraumatic etiology in the other). Sleep drunkenness was also noted in 6 out of 127 narcoleptic patients. This made him suspect the existence of a gradual successive transition from narcolepsy to independent hypersomnia with sleep drunkenness. He found a combination of these entities even in different members of the same family. Only one of his cohort of 20 patients suffered from nocturnal epilepsy in combination with sleep drunkenness during awakening and sleep paralysis while falling asleep. The paper also included the first electroencephalography (EEG) description of sleep drunkenness—sleep activity alternating with alpha rhythm.

Beginning in the early 1950s, Prof. Roth systematically extended his clinical studies of patients with daytime somnolence, and in 1957, he clinically analyzed a cohort of 248 cases [3]. These were divided into two groups: 155 cases of narcolepsy and 93 cases of different types of hypersomnia. The latter cases were classified as: (1) *functional type* (50 cases), in which pathological sleep was not induced by any known disease, (2) cases of *organic origin* (29 patients) determined by some known underlying disease, and (3) *sleepiness with post-dormital drunkenness* (14 cases), specified later as the idiopathic form of hypersomnia with sleep drunkenness.

The discovery of rapid eye movement (REM) sleep [4–6] gave impetus to polysomnographical (PSG) studies of patients with daytime somnolence, previously regarded as narcolepsy. Dement et al. [7] were the first to suggest that patients affected by excessive diurnal somnolence, but not accompanied by signs of REM sleep, and symptoms of cataplexy, hypnagogic hallucinations, or sleep paralysis, should be considered to be suffering from hypersomnolence other than narcolepsy.

At that time, Bedrich Roth had no opportunity to study nocturnal sleep recordings in Prague. That was why he decided to accept an invitation from Allan Rechtschaffen to visit his sleep laboratory in Chicago and examine patients with sleep drunkenness in the USA. The birth of a new clinical entity supported by PSG findings seemed rather amusing there. When Bedrich Roth arrived, everybody in the USA believed that this disease existed only in Prague. However, Roth arranged a short interview in the local television explaining the clinical symptoms of the disease (long nocturnal sleep with difficulty awakening and long-lasting daytime naps) and asked TV viewers for cooperation. Everybody in

S. Nevsimalova (✉)
Department of Neurology, 1st Faculty of Medicine, Charles University, Katerinska 30, 128 00 Prague 2, Czech Republic
e-mail: snevsi@LF1.cuni.cz; sona.nevsimalova@lf1.cuni.cz

S. Chokroverty, M. Billiard (eds.), *Sleep Medicine,* DOI 10.1007/978-1-4939-2089-1_27,
© Springer Science+Business Media, LLC 2015

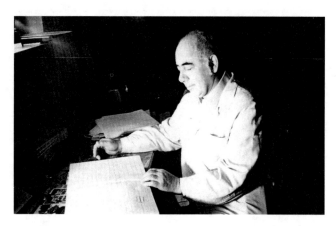

Fig. 27.1 Prof. Bedrich Roth reading polysomnographic recording. He was born on March 23, 1919, and died on November 4, 1989, a few days before the Czech Velvet revolution

the Chicago team was really surprised to see, exactly then and there, the TV show lineup of people waiting to be examined by Bedrich Roth. After a clinical interview, he chose ten patients and the first PSG findings of this ailment were published [8] in patients with idiopathic hypersomnia who underwent PSG recording for two nonconsecutive nights. The organization of sleep was completely normal except for its long duration (12 h or more). The percentage of REM and nonrapid eye movement (NREM) sleep was normal, as was the periodicity of the sleep cycles, the number of which was simply increased. These findings were later published [8].

Three years later, a complete clinical description of hypersomnia with sleep drunkenness (58 cases), enriched by long-term nocturnal monitoring (9 cases), appeared in the literature [9] giving a clear picture of this clinical entity. Sleep drunkenness was characterized by difficulty awakening accompanied by confusion, disorientation, poor motor coordination, slowness, and repeated dosing off. Patients reported that these symptoms occurred almost every morning, and nearly all reported abnormally prolonged sleep. Of 58 cases of hypersomnia with sleep drunkenness, 52 were apparently idiopathic and 6 were possibly symptomatic of organic brain disturbance. A familial history of the disorder was found in 36% of the idiopathic cases. No specific EEG or PSG abnormalities were noted except for relatively increased heart and respiratory rates and extended sleep.

In the late 1960s, the Prague school focused on the pathophysiology of narcolepsy and different types of hypersomnia [10]. Narcolepsy seemed to be associated with REM sleep disturbances and in most instances also with disturbances in NREM sleep, whereas hypersomnia was regarded as involving exclusively the NREM system. The authors assumed that most of the independent narcolepsy cases (without cataplexy) had a mechanism similar to that in hypersomnia patients. This hypothesis was supported also by study of dreams [11].

According to clinical data analyzing 451 patients, 200 were diagnosed with idiopathic narcolepsy, 78 with symptomatic narcolepsy, 47 with hypersomnia with organic basis, and 114 with hypersomnia without organic basis (31 of whom with sleep drunkenness), 2 with independent cataplexy, and 10 with independent sleep paralysis. Hypnagogic hallucinations and vivid, terrifying dreams were frequent in narcolepsy, especially in those suffering also from cataplexy and/or sleep paralysis. In hypersomniac patients, these symptoms were rare. Polygraphic examination of 75 daytime recordings with 215 awakenings showed that 97.4% of patients awakened during paradoxical sleep reporting dreams; 80% of them had experienced vivid dreams with a strong affective component and visual and acoustic perceptions. During synchronous sleep, dreams were reported in 34% of awakenings, usually with vague content. Vivid dreams occurred in only 10% of awakening during synchronous sleep, and these came mostly from within 10 min before or after paradoxical sleep.

Although the first description of a familial occurrence of hypersomnia was reported in Roth's monograph [3], it was only rarely mentioned in later publications. In 1968, Bonkalo [12] described two siblings with a pure form of hypersomnia. A larger material was published in the early 1970s again by the Czech authors [13–14]. They wrote a genealogical study of the families of 30 patients with hypersomnia and 100 patients with narcolepsy. Idiopathic hypersomnia was found to run in the families of more than one third of the cases. The existence of transition from hypersomnia to isolated narcolepsy in patients with heredofamilial occurrence showed a pathogenetic relationship of these disturbances. According to the authors, transfer of the hereditary predisposition towards hypersomnia and isolated narcolepsy is most probably of an autosomal dominant type, while in narcolepsy with cataplexy and other symptoms of sleep dissociation, a multifactorial type of heredity was supposed.

In 1976, Prof. Roth published a review of 642 personally observed cases including 368 cases of narcolepsy and 274 cases of hypersomnia [15]. The largest group of hypersomniac patients consisted of so-called *functional hypersomnias* (213 cases). These were divided into a group with *short sleep cycle* (191 cases) and another with *long sleep cycle* (22 cases). The author distinguished two main forms of short-sleep-cycle hypersomnia: (a) *idiopathic monosymptomatic form* (71 cases), marked solely by excessive daytime sleepiness with long naps, and (b) *idiopathic polysymptomatic form* (103 cases), in which daytime sleepiness was accompanied by prolonged nocturnal sleep and usually also by awakening difficulties (sleep drunkenness or sleep inertia). The rest of functional short-cycle hypersomnias were patients with neurotic hypersomnia (5 cases) and hypersomnia with disorders of breathing during sleep (12 cases). However, nocturnal polygraphic recordings were made only in a minority of these cases, which is why the last mentioned group may have been underdiagnosed.

In the first diagnostic classification of sleep disorders [16], idiopathic hypersomnia was referred to as idiopathic central nervous system (CNS) hypersomnia as one of the disorders of excessive somnolence. The distinction between the two forms proposed by Roth was left out.

In a monograph *Narcolepsy and hypersomnia,* published one year later [17], Roth described a carefully selected group ($n=167$) of idiopathic hypersomnia patients. He characterized this disease as a short-cycle "functional" hypersomnia, not caused by known organic brain disease or by metabolic or toxic condition or of psychogenic origin. Its clinical picture included a short sleep onset and frequently prolonged nocturnal sleep with difficulty awakening in the morning, and accompanied by psychological and autonomic dysfunction including sexual disturbances. Two forms of short-cycle functional hypersomnia—monosymptomatic and polysymptomatic—have a chronic course and severe socioeconomic impact. He drew attention to its relationship to idiopathic narcolepsy, especially the monosymptomatic form, without cataplexy and other disassociated sleep dysfunction. For the treatment, he recommended central stimulants similar to those for narcolepsy. This excellent book served as the most important textbook for physicians and sleep researchers for a long time, as well as for the patients suffering from daytime sleepiness.

In 1981, Roth et al. [18] published a detailed study of neurological, psychological, and polygraphic findings in sleep drunkenness. Eight patients with idiopathic hypersomnia and eight controls were tested after normal sleep duration (patients 12 h, controls 8 h), and after sleep deprivation (patients after 8 and 6 h, controls after 4 and 0 h of nocturnal sleep). A state of sleep drunkenness, characterized by "microsleep" in polygraphic recording, was found in 19 of the patients, but only once in the controls. Clinically prominent features included cerebellar signs, hyporeflexia or areflexia, signs of vestibular involvement, and fine and gross motor dysfunction. The authors presumed that sleep drunkenness develops as a result of chronic relative sleep deprivation in those patients, whose sleep requirements are greater than in normal individuals.

Figure 27.2 illustrates a group of sleep researchers organizing a Symposium on Narcolepsy and Hypersomnia in Prague in honor of Prof. Roth.

A detailed description of nocturnal sleep as well as Multiple Sleep Latency Test (MSLT) results comparing different disorders of excessive daytime somnolence (EDS) came from the Stanford group in the early 1980s [19]. The largest group in a 100-patient cohort consisted of narcoleptic patients (41 with cataplexy, 5 without cataplexy). The rest of the EDS patients formed a rather heterogeneous group: idiopathic CNS hypersomnia (17), EDS associated with psychological and/or psychiatric problem (18), irregular sleep pattern (5), insufficient (disturbed) nocturnal sleep (4), abuse of stimulant drugs (3), neurological conditions (2). In five patients, EDS was associated with no objective abnormality. The authors found a clear intergroup difference in the nocturnal as well as daytime polygraphic examinations. Narcoleptics showed more severe EDS with a shorter MSLT latency and presence of sleep-onset rapid eye movements (SOREMs) (at least two, although their number varied even in the same patient) as compared with others. REM latency during the night was shorter; they had fewer REM segments and more awaken-

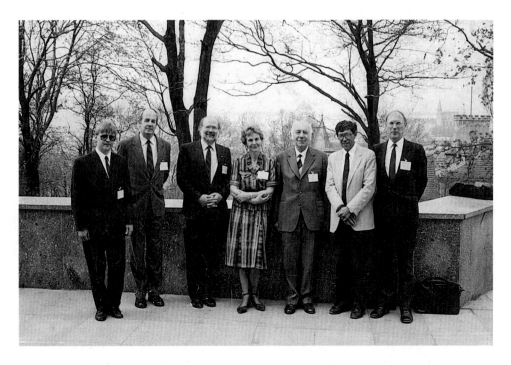

Fig. 27.2 A group of sleep researchers organizing the Symposium on Narcolepsy and Hypersomnia in honor of Prof. Roth in 1988. From the left side: Peter Geisler, Michel Billiard, Roger Broughton, Sona Nevsimalova, Bedrich Roth, Christian Guilleminault, and David Parkes

ings and myoclonic jerks during sleep. In the MSLT, narcoleptics had a mean sleep latency of 3.3 min (standard deviation (SD)±3.3), patients with idiopathic CNS hypersomnia 6.5 min (SD±3.2), and patients with psychological disturbances and those with no objective abnormalities 10.6 min (SD±5.2) and 10.9 min (SD±3.9), respectively. Based on these data, the authors concluded that a mean sleep latency of 5.5 min and less indicates pathological sleepiness which was found in the majority of narcoleptic patients. A value between 6 and 10 min is a "gray area," typical of idiopathic CNS hypersomnia, and mean sleep latency of 10 min and more indicates that pathological sleepiness is unlikely.

Later data [20–21] supported the hypothesis that narcolepsy and *idiopathic CNS hypersomnia* are distinct syndromes with characteristic sleep/wake patterns, EDS symptoms, REM sleep abnormalities, and associated pathophysiological events. Idiopathic CNS hypersomnia patients sleep longer than narcoleptics, enter REM sleep later at night, have more NREM stages 3 and 4, experience fewer and briefer awakenings at night, and are not as sleepy during the day. Sleep apnea and periodic leg movements are less frequent in idiopathic CNS hypersomnia than in narcolepsy. The duality of the two conditions was verified also in human leukocyte antigen (HLA) studies [22]. While narcoleptic patients were invariably associated with HLA-DR2 positivity, idiopathic hypersomnia patients showed an increase of HLA-Cw2, DR5, and B27 antigens. However, Honda et al. [23] found that nearly half the patients suffering from *essential hypersomnia* (34 patients) had a higher frequency of HLA-DR2. Essential hypersomnia was defined by the following criteria: (a) at least a 6-month history of recurrent daytime napping occurring almost daily, (b) absence of cataplexy, and (c) absence of other disorders with daytime somnolence such as sleep apnea.

During the past 30 years, the term idiopathic hypersomnia has been given a variety of clinical labels including idiopathic central nervous hypersomnia or hypersomnolence, functional hypersomnia, mixed or harmonious hypersomnia, and hypersomnia with automatic behavior, and rarely the term was mistaken for NREM narcolepsy. In contrast to narcolepsy, much less interest was shown to this clinical entity over the years (Fig. 27.3).

The 1990 *International Classification of Sleep Disorders* (ICSD-1) [24] defined idiopathic hypersomnia as a presumably CNS-based disorder associated with a normal or prolonged major sleep episode and excessive sleepiness consisting of prolonged (1–2 h) episodes of NREM sleep. The difficulty waking up in the morning and the distinction between the two forms, as proposed by Roth, were not part of the definition. Narcolepsy and hypersomnia were included in a subgroup of dyssomnias—disorders which give rise to insomnia, excessive sleepiness, and eventually both—and referred to as intrinsic sleep disorders, induced primarily by factors within the body.

The clinical significance of idiopathic hypersomnia as an independent clinical entity was questioned. In 1993, Guilleminault et al. [25] suggested that a nonnegligible proportion of subjects previously diagnosed with idiopathic hypersomnia have upper airway resistance syndrome. The clinical features of narcolepsy and idiopathic hypersomnia were seen as substantially overlapping [26]. The same center [27] reviewed clinical and laboratory information on 42 subjects with idiopathic hypersomnia and obtained detailed follow-up evaluation on 28 of them. Only less than one third of the

Fig. 27.3 Differences in the number of quotations listed by PubMed in the last decades. Narcolepsy and idiopathic hypersomnia are correlated

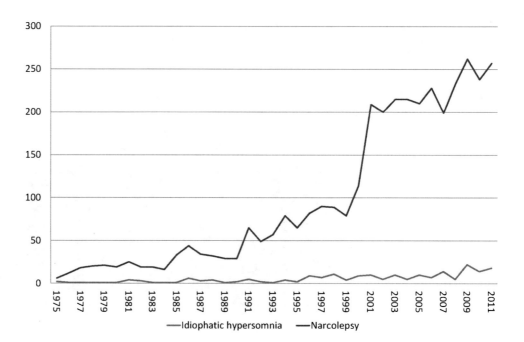

subjects had "classic" idiopathic hypersomnia with nonimperative sleepiness, long unrefreshing naps, prolonged nighttime sleep, difficulty awakening with sleep drunkenness, and prominent mood disturbances. More than one third of the subjects under study had clinical features similar to those of narcolepsy without cataplexy or some other symptoms of abnormal REM sleep. They had short refreshing naps and no problems on awakening. The remaining one third exhibited intermediate clinical characteristics. The authors concluded that idiopathic hypersomnia is a rare syndrome, in which clinical heterogeneity suggests a variable or multifactorial pathogenesis. In ten patients, they were able to identify possible etiological factors—such as viral illness, head trauma, and primary mood disorder. Association with viral illness at the onset of the disease has been reported by other authors as well [28].

In the past two decades, a great deal of progress in the field of research into idiopathic hypersomnia has been made, thanks to Prof. Billiard. He was the first to resurrect Roth's idea of polysymptomatic and monosymptomatic forms of idiopathic hypersomnia [29]; he recommended continuous ad lib recordings of abnormally long major sleep episode as well as long nonrefreshing naps. According to PSG data, idiopathic hypersomnia could also be clearly distinguished from other types of hypersomnia, particularly those associated with mood disorder [30]. A few years later, examining a cohort of 23 subjects, he introduced the terms *complete and incomplete forms of idiopathic hypersomnia*. Detailed clinical, PSG, and immunogenetic data were reported. A strong familial predisposition was found; however, no association with HLAs was observed [31]. Billiard et al. [32] suggested in an excellent review that idiopathic hypersomnia is not a pathological entity in itself, but rather a consequence of chronic sleep deprivation in very long sleepers. The reasons that its pathophysiology is poorly known lie in: (1) the absence of clear clinical and PSG criteria, as well as (2) the absence of a natural animal model comparable with the canine model of narcolepsy.

In 2002, a revision of ICSD-1 was initiated, and Emmanuel Mignot was appointed chairman of the Task Force on "Hypersomnia of Central Origin, not due to a circadian rhythm sleep disorder, sleep related breathing disorders or other cause of disturbed nocturnal sleep" [33]. In the final version of ICSD-2 [34], two distinct entities appeared: (1) *idiopathic hypersomnia with long sleep time* and (2) *idiopathic hypersomnia without long sleep time*. Idiopathic hypersomnia with long sleep time was characterized by EDS lasting at least 3 months, prolonged nocturnal sleep (more than 10 h), documented by interview, actigraphy or sleep logs, and difficulty waking up in the morning or at the end of naps. Nocturnal polysomnography can help exclude other types of EDS and demonstrate a short sleep latency and prolonged sleep period (>10 h). MSLT following overnight polysomnography

shows the mean sleep latency of less than 8 min and fewer than 2 SOREMs. Idiopathic hypersomnia without long sleep time differs from the previous clinical entity by the length of the major sleep episode (longer than 6 h but less than 10 h) and by the absence of difficulty waking up in the morning.

Although this classification responds much better to the clinical description of idiopathic hypersomnia, many questions remain unanswered [33]: Are idiopathic hypersomnia with long sleep time and idiopathic hypersomnia without long sleep time two forms of the same condition or two different conditions? Is there a pathophysiological relationship between narcolepsy without cataplexy and idiopathic hypersomnia?

In their study of 160 narcoleptics, Vernet and Arnulf [35] found 29 (18 %) long sleepers (more than 11 h) with symptoms combining the disabilities of both narcolepsy (severe sleepiness) and idiopathic hypersomnia (long sleep time and unrefreshing naps). In the authors' view, this group may represent a transitional clinical entity with multiple arousal system dysfunctions. The same authors [36] compared 40 hypersomniacs with and 35 without long sleep with 30 healthy matched controls. Hypersomnia patients had greater fatigability and higher anxiety and depression scores, 24 % suffered from hypnagogic hallucinations, and 28 % had sleep paralysis. Sleep drunkenness was present in 36 % and unrefreshing naps in 46 %. They were more frequently evening types as shown also in previous data [37]. MSLT latencies were normal (>8 min) in 71 % hypersomniacs with long sleep time and even longer than 10 min in half of the patients. The authors concluded that MSLT is an inadequate method for the diagnosis of hypersomnia with long sleep time. They recommended at least 24-h monitoring for the verification of idiopathic hypersomnia similar to the suggestion by Billiard and Dauvilliers previously [38]. The patients also showed some subjective symptoms besides excessive sleepiness, particularly attention and memory deficit [39].

Possible common features of narcolepsy, especially the type without cataplexy, and idiopathic hypersomnia are hotly debated currently [40–41]. In contrast to narcolepsy, which is characterized by an abnormal propensity to fall asleep, idiopathic hypersomnia with long sleep time is noteworthy for the patients' inability to terminate sleep. On the other hand, idiopathic hypersomnia without long sleep time seems to be more like narcolepsy without cataplexy with the exception of REM sleep propensity in MSLT, a feature typical for narcolepsy [42]. However, using repeated MSLT tests in the same subject, we can obtain quite different results. Consequently, more research into the pathophysiology and into the predisposing factors of idiopathic hypersomnia is desirable. Genetic studies using genome-wide analysis and other modern methods of molecular genetics can clarify the differences and similarities between these clinical entities.

References

1. Furukawa T. Heinrich Bruno Schindler's description of narcolepsy in 1829. Neurology. 1987;37:146.
2. Roth B. Sleep drunkenness and sleep paralysis [in Czech]. Ceskoslovenska Neurol. 1956;19:48–58.
3. Roth B. Narcolepsy and hypersomnia: from the aspect of sleep physiology [in Czech]. Praha: Stat. Zdrav. Naklad; 1957.
4. Aserinsky E, Kleitman N. Regularly occurring periods of eye motility and concomitant phenomena during sleep. Science. 1953;118:273–74.
5. Aserinsky E, Kleitman N. Two types of ocular motility occurring in sleep. J Appl Physiol. 1955;8:1–10.
6. Dement WC, Kleitman N. Cyclic variation in EEG during sleep and their relation to eye movement, body motility, and dreaming. Electroencephalogr Clin Neurophysiol. 1957;9:673–90.
7. Dement WC, Rechtschaffen A, Gulevich G. The nature of the narcoleptic sleep attack. Neurology. 1966;16:18–33.
8. Rechtschaffen A, Roth B. Nocturnal sleep of hypersomniacs. Activ Nerv Sup.1969;11:229–33.
9. Roth B, Nevsimalova S, Rechtschaffen A. Hypersomnia with sleep drunkenness. Arch Gen Psych. 1972;26:456–62.
10. Roth B., Bruhova S, Lehovsky M. REM sleep and NREM sleep in narcolepsy and hypersomnia. Electroenceph Clin Neurophysiol. 1969;26:176–82.
11. Roth B, Bruhova S. Dreams in narcolepsy, hypersomnia and dissociated sleep disorders. Exp Med Surg. 1969;27:187–209.
12. Bonkalo J. Hypersomnia. A discussion of psychiatric implications based on three cases. Brit J Psychiat. 1968;114:69–73.
13. Nevsimalova-Bruhova S, Roth B. Heredofamilial aspects of narcolepsy and hypersomnia. Schweiz Arch Neurol Psychiat. 1972;110:45–54.
14. Nevsimalova-Bruhova S. On the problem of heredity in hypersomnia, narcolepsy and dissociated sleep disturbances. Acta Univ Carol Med. 1973;18:109–60.
15. Roth B. Narcolepsy and hypersomnia. Review and classification of 642 personally observed patients. Schweiz Arch Neurol Neurochir Psychiat. 1976;119:31–41.
16. Association of Sleep Disorders Centers. Diagnostic classification of sleep and arousal disorders, first edition, prepared by the Sleep Disorders Classification Committee, HP. Roffwarg, Chairman. Sleep. 1979;2:1–137.
17. Roth B. Narcolepsy and hypersomnia. Basel: S. Karger; 1980.
18. Roth B, Nevsimalova S, Sagova V, Paroubkova D, Horakova A. Neurological, psychological and polygraphic findings in sleep drunkenness. Schweiz Arch Neurol Neurochir Psychiatr. 1981;129:209–22.
19. van den Hoed J, Kraemer H, Guilleminault C, Zarcone VP Jr., Miles LE, Dement WC et al. Disorders of excessive daytime somnolence: polygraphic and clinical data for 100 patients. Sleep. 1981;4:23–37.
20. Baker TL, Guilleminault C, Nino-Murcia G, Dement WC. Comparative polysomnographic study of narcolepsy and idiopathic central nervous system hypersomnia. Sleep. 1986;9:232–42.
21. Montplaisir J, Godbout R. Nocturnal sleep of narcoleptic patients: revisited. Sleep. 1986;9:159–61.
22. Poirier G, Montplaisir J, Decary F, Momege D, Lebrun A. HLA antigens in narcolepsy and idiopathic central nervous system hypersomnolence. Sleep. 1986;9:153–8.
23. Honda Y, Juji T, Matsuki K, Naohara T, Satake M, Inko H et al. HLA-DR2 and Dw2 in narcolepsy and in other disorders of excessive somnolence without cataplexy. Sleep. 1986;9:133–42.
24. , Thorpy MJ (Chairman), Diagnostic Classification Steering Committee. International classification of sleep disorders: diagnostic and coding manual. Rochester: American Sleep Disorders Association; 1990.
25. Guilleminault C, Stoohs R, Clerk A, Cetel M, Maistros P. A cause of excessive daytime sleepiness. The upper airway resistance syndrome. Chest. 1993;104:781–7.
26. Aldrich MS. The clinical spectrum of narcolepsy and idiopathic hypersomnia. Neurology. 1996;46:393–401.
27. Bassetti C, Aldrich MS. Idiopathic hypersomnia. A series of 42 patients. Brain. 1997;120:1423–35.
28. Bruck D, Parkes JD. A comparison of idiopathic hypersomnia and narcolepsy-cataplexy using self report measures and sleep diary data. J Neurol Neurosurg Psychiat. 1996;60:576–8.
29. Billiard M. Idiopathic hypersomnia. Neurol Clin. 1996;14:573–2.
30. Billiard M, Dolenc L, Aldaz C, Ondze B, Besset A. Hypersomnia associated with mood disorders: a new perspective. J Psychosom Res. 1994;38 (Suppl.1):41–7.
31. Billiard M, Merle C, Carlander B, Ondze B, Alvarez D, Besset A. Idiopathic hypersomnia. Psychiatr Clin Neurosci. 1998;52:125–9.
32. Billiard M, Rondouin G, Espa F, Dauvilliers Y, Besset A. Physiopathologie de l'hypersomnie idiopathique. Données actuelles et nouvelles orientations. Rev Neurol (Paris). 2001;157:S101–6.
33. Billiard M. Diagnosis of narcolepsy and idiopathic hypersomnia. An update based on the International classification of sleep disorders. 2. Sleep Med Rev. 2007;11:378–88.
34. American Academy of Sleep Medicine. International classification of sleep disorders, 2nd ed.: Diagnostic and coding manual. Westchester, Illinois, American Academy of Sleep Medicine; 2005.
35. Vernet C, Arnulf I. Narcolepsy with long sleep time: a specific entity? Sleep. 2009;32:1229–35.
36. Vernet C, Arnulf I. Idiopathic hypersomnia with and without long sleep time: a controlled series of 75 patients. Sleep. 2009;32:753–9.
37. Nevsimalova S., Blazejova K, Illnerova H, Hajek I, Vankova J, Pretl M. et al. A contribution to pathophysiology of idiopathic hypersomnia. In: Ambler Z, Nevsimalova S, Kadanka Z, Rossini PM, editors. Clinical neurophysiology at the beginning of the 21st century; Suppl Clin Neurophysiol. 2000;53:366–70.
38. Billiard M, Dauvilliers Y. Idiopathic hypersomnia. Sleep Med Rev. 2001;5:349–58.
39. Vernet C, Leu-Semenescu S, Buzare MA, Arnulf I. Subjective symptoms in idiopathic hypersomnia: beyond excessive sleepiness. J Sleep Res. 2010;19:525–34.
40. Sasai T, Inoue Y, Komada Y, Sugiura T, Matsushima E. Comparison of clinical characteristics among narcolepsy with and without cataplexy and idiopathic hypersomnia without long sleep time, focusing on HLA-DRB1(*)1501/DQB1(*)0602 finding. Sleep Med. 2009;10:961–6.
41. Billiard M. From narcolepsy with cataplexy to idiopathic hypersomnia without long sleep time. Sleep Med. 2009;10:943–4.
42. Billiard M. Idiopathic hypersomnia. In: Thorpy MJ, Billiard M, eds. Sleepiness: causes, consequences and treatment. Cambridge: Cambridge University Press; 2011, pp.126–35.

Kleine–Levin Syndrome

Michel Billiard

The term KLS was coined in 1942 by Critchley and Hoffman, surgeon captain and surgeon commander, respectively, at a naval hospital [1]. However, the development of the concept took its roots almost 250 years earlier with the contribution by William Oliver in 1705 [2]. In this chapter, I will refer successively, Section "Scattered Reports of Recurrent Periods of Hypersomnia (1705–1924)" to scattered reports of recurrent episodes of hypersomnia, plus or minus other symptoms from 1705 to 1924, Section "Kleine, Lewis, and Levin's Period (1925–1939)" to a period centered by the first descriptions of recurrent periods of somnolence and morbid hunger by Kleine [3], Lewis [4] and Levin [5, 6], Section "Critchley's Period (1940–2004)" to the Critchley's period introduced by the word KLS coined by Critchley and Hoffman in 1942, and centered on Critchley's milestone publication of 26 cases of "periodic hypersomnia and megaphagia in adolescent males" in 1962 [7], Section "ICSD-2 Period" to the ICSD-2 period starting from 2005 with the description of diagnostic criteria for recurrent hypersomnia [8], and finally Section ICSD-3 Period starting from 2014, with the setting of diagnostic criteria for KLS.

Scattered Reports of Recurrent Periods of Hypersomnia (1705–1924)

Although one may consider Kumbhakarna, the younger brother of the demon king Ravana in the Indian mythological epic Ramayana[1], as a possible case of KLS:

---

[1] The Ramanaya is one of the two great epics of India (third century BC–AD third century), the other being the Mahabharata. Some cultural evidence suggests that the Ramayana predates the Mahabharata.

M. Billiard (✉)
Department of Neurology, Gui de Chauliac Hospital, 80, avenue Augustin Fliche 34295 Montpellier cedex 5, France
e-mail: mbilliard@orange.fr

M. Billiard
School of Medicine, University Montpellier I, Montpellier, France

S. Chokroverty, M. Billiard (eds.), *Sleep Medicine,* DOI 10.1007/978-1-4939-2089-1_28,

"He would sleep for months at a time and, when he wakes up, would eat anything and everything in his path" [9],

(Fig. 28.1a, b), the first account of patients with episodic sleep dates back to the eighteenth century. The first one is by William Oliver in 1705 [2]. (Fig. 28.2)

May the 13th, Anno 1694, one Samuel Chilton, of Tinsburg near Bath, a Labourer, about 25 years of age, of a robust habit of Body, not fat, but fleshy, and a dark brown Hair, happen'd, without any visible cause, or evident sign, to fall into a very profound Sleep, out of which no Art used by those that were near him, cou'd rouze him, till after a month time; then rose of himself, put on his Cloaths, and went about his business of Husbandry as usual; slept, cou'd eat and drink as before, but spoke not one word till about a month after. All the time he slept Victuals stood by him; his Mother fearing he would be starv'd, in that sullen humour, as she thought it, put Bread and Cheese and Small Beer before him, which was spent every day, and supposed by him, tho no one ever saw him eat or drink all that time.

From this time he remained free of any drowsiness or sleepiness till about the 9th of April 1696, and then fell into his Sleeping sit again just as he did before. After some days they were prevail'd with to try what effect Medicines might have on him and accordingly one Mr Gibs, a very able Apothecary of Bath, went to him, Bled, Blister'd, Capp'd and Scarrified him, and used all the external irritating Medicines he could think on, but all to no purpose, nothing of all these making any manner of impression on him; and after the first fortnight he was never observed to open his Eyes. Victuals stood by him.

The second one is by a French physician who studied and graduated in Montpellier, France, Edmé Pierre Chauvot de Beauchêne (1786) [10].

„A girl, in her fourteenth year, was overcome with a lethargic sleep which lasted several days. From that point forward, the affection of sleep recurred at irregular intervals; it usually lasted eight to ten days, continuing at times for fifteen; and upon one sole occasion, it persisted into the seventeenth day.“

There was no typical overeating but "during the first four years of her disease this poor girl had appetite as bizarre as they were dangerous, causing her to eat lime, plaster, soil and vinegar. Thereafter, these appetites subsided, and she nourished herself indiscriminate with all sorts of aliment. This food always occasioned vomiting" (Fig. 28.3).

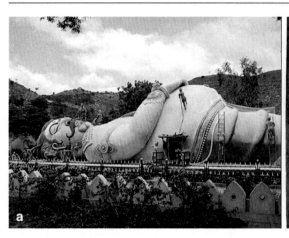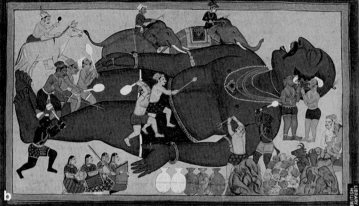

Figs. 28.1 a. Kumbhakarna asleep. **b.** The awakening of Kumbhakarna : the demons try to rouse the giant by hitting him with weapons and clubs and shouting in his ear. A miniature painting by the artist Sahib Din, from an illustrated manuscript of the Sanskrit epic Ramayana, prepared between 1649 and 1653 for Maharana Jagat Singh of Udaipur (Western India), AD 1652. 1977, The British Library Board

During the nineteenth century more cases were published. In a report read at the Royal College of Physicians of London in April 1815, and published later the same year in Medical Transitions,

> "Richard Patrick Satterly described the case of a 16 year old boy who on his return from school was observed to be pale and unwell. He felt cold and complained of a frontal headache. During the following three days, his symptoms appeared to be abating; then the headache worsened, he became flushed, restless and agitated, and his pulse rate was raised. About the seventh day, the patient developed a voracious appetite…he would eat a pound-and-a-half of beef steaks, a large fowl, or a couple of rabbits, at one meal without apparently satisfying his appetite"….."The craving for food came on regularly with the paroxysms of fever, and continued unabated until that subsided, when he usually fell into a sound sleep. The period of the recurrence of the paroxysm was very uncertain, but it was marked by a distinct circumscribed redness of one or both cheeks; the moment this spot became visible, the boy would rouse himself (for he was at other times either sleeping, or dull and torpid)" [11].

Later on, in 1862, Brière de Boismont reported the case of

> a child who, in a recurrent manner, slept a lot, was difficult to arouse, and as soon as he was awakened extemporaneously sang, recited, and acted with great ardor and aplomb. When he was not asleep, he ate ravenously. As soon as he got out of his bed, he would go close to another patient's bed, and overtly seize without any scruple all the food he could find. Apart from this intriguing disease, he was intelligent and skilful [12].

From 1862 onwards, reports became more frequent. Mendel described the case of a soldier, aged 25, who had attacks of 3–5 days' duration at a frequency of 1–2 years. There was no mention whether the patient showed excessive appetite [13]. The same applies to an adolescent girl who had her first attack while sitting in church, went home, and did not wake up for 3 days [14]. Anfimoff, a Russian physician, reported

a youth of 19 years who slept deeply during the first 2 or 3 days of his attacks and then woke up frequently and went to sleep again [15]. His appetite was excellent. In dream, he saw a horse and was scared and afraid of everything. These attacks reappeared every few months.

Later on, case reports concentrated in Germany. Stöcker reported on a 21-year-old man who had experienced headache and frequent epistaxis since childhood, and who, from the ages 19 to 22 years, had recurrent attacks of sleepiness and indifference [16]. Schröder commented on a 17-year-old adolescent who periodically, at intervals of 3 months' duration, had prolonged sleep episodes associated with transient psychological changes and indecent behavior [17]. Such episodes stopped after 3 years. Krüger reported two cases [18]. The first one was in a 44-year-old single woman with recurrent episodes of abnormal sleep at the ages 16, 19, 34, 43, and 44. She did not take any food during the second one and ate normally during the following ones. The second case was a 20-year-old man who had his first attack of sleep during his military service after a grueling day followed by three more attacks lasting for 2–5 days each time at 6–18-month intervals.

Finally, a last case report was by a Russian physician, J.W. Kanabich [19]. The patient was a 19-year-old man who had two attacks of sleepiness accompanied by restlessness, nervousness, and apathy at the age of 14 and 14.5 years.

Thus, from 1786 to 1924, 12 cases of recurrent hypersomnia were published, with an acceleration of the publications in the second half of the nineteenth century. There were nine male and three female cases. The median age of onset was 17 with a range of 12–25. Circumstances at onset included overwork in three cases [16, 18], struggle with a comrade [13], strong emotion [15], sitting in church [14], cold and fever [11], and seasickness [16] in one case each. The duration of the episodes was from 2 days to 12

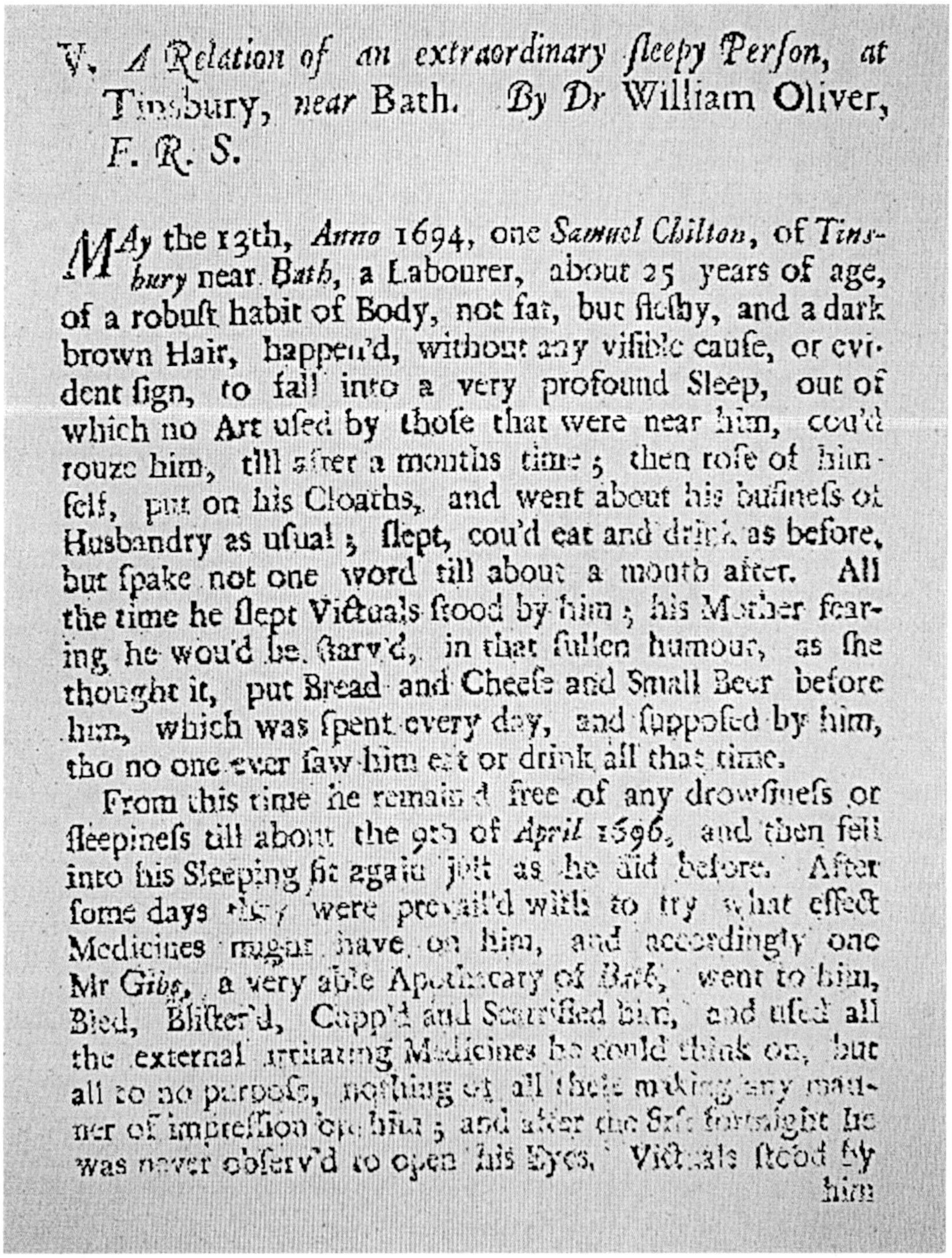

Fig. 28.2 A relation of an extraordinary sleepy person, at Tinsburg, near Bath (UK) by Dr William Oliver, F.R.S. Philosophical Transactions, 1704–1705, vol 24.

V. *A Relation of an extraordinary sleepy Person, at Tinsbury, near* Bath. *By Dr* William Oliver, *F. R. S.*

May the 13th, *Anno* 1694, one *Samuel Chilton,* of *Tinsbury* near *Bath,* a Labourer, about 25 years of age, of a robust habit of Body, not fat, but flabby, and a dark brown Hair, happen'd, without any visible cause, or evident sign, to fall into a very profound Sleep, out of which no Art used by those that were near him, cou'd rouze him, till after a months time ; then rose of himself, put on his Cloaths, and went about his business of Husbandry as usual ; slept, cou'd eat and drink as before, but spake not one word till about a month after. All the time he slept Victuals stood by him ; his Mother fearing he wou'd be starv'd, in that sullen humour, as she thought it, put Bread and Cheese and Small Beer before him, which was spent every day, and supposed by him, tho no one ever saw him eat or drink all that time.

From this time he remain'd free of any drowsiness or sleepiness till about the 9th of *April* 1696, and then fell into his Sleeping fit again just as he did before. After some days they were prevail'd with to try what effect Medicines might have on him, and accordingly one Mr *Gibs,* a very able Apothecary of *Bath,* went to him, Bled, Blister'd, Cupp'd and Scarrified him, and used all the external irritating Medicines he could think on, but all to no purpose, nothing of all these making any manner of impression on him ; and after the first fortnight he was never observ'd to open his Eyes. Victuals stood by him

weeks and the interval between episodes varied from 1 to 2 months to 15 years in one case [18]. Hypersomnia was present in all cases, overeating in four [10–12,15], disinhibited sexuality in one [17], odd behavior, childish, singing, and incoherent utterance in one [10], singing, recitation, and acting with great ardor and aplomb in one [12], agitation in one [11], psychological changes (dull, indifferent, inertia of thought, visual and auditory hallucinations, apathy) in five [15–19], mental symptom (anxiety) in one [15], dysautonomic signs in two [11, 18], and poor sleep for several nights on recovery in three [16–18]. In total, almost all the symptoms and signs later described in KLS were present in a dissociated way.

Kleine, Lewis, and Levin's Period (1925–1939)

In 1925, Willi Kleine, then a young psychiatrist working at Kleist's clinic in Frankfurt, reported on five examples of episodic somnolence, two of which being remarkable for a wealth of symptoms: Hypersomnia, overeating, disinhibited sexuality, odd behavior (in one case), irritability, cognitive disorder, and mental symptom (in one case) [3].

In 1926, Nolan Lewis, a psychiatrist in Washington, introduced a psychoanalytic approach to the problem of four children under 12 years of age, one of whom, aged 10, presenting with attacks of sleepiness, gluttony, odd behavior, irritability, and cognitive symptoms in the form of visual hallucinations [4].

OBSERVATION

S U R

UNE MALADIE NERVEUSE

AVEC complication d'un fommeil, tantôt léthargique, tantôt convulfif.

PAR M. DE BEAUCHÊNE

Médecin de MONSIEUR, Frère du Roi.

À AMSTERDAM;

Et fe trouve à PARIS,

Chez MÉQUIGNON l'aîné, Libraire, rue des Cordeliers, près des Écoles de Chirurgie.

1 7 8 6.

Fig. 28.3 Flyleaf of the article by Edmé Pierre Chauvot de Beauchêne

Next, in 1929, Max Levin, a psychiatrist in Baltimore, described a young man of 19 years with recurrent episodes of hypersomnia, polyphagia, odd behavior, restlessness, irritability, and cognitive symptoms (dull, taciturn) since the age of 16 [5].

Thus, within 4 years, three different authors, all psychiatrists, one from Germany and two from the USA, described patients, all boys or young male adults, presenting with recurrent episodes of severe sleepiness lasting some days associated with hyperphagia, odd behavior, cognitive symptoms, and in one patient disinhibited sexuality.

After a further report by Daniels of a young man aged 18, with four episodes [20] and two reports by Kaplinsky and Schulmann, one in a 14-year-old boy who had attacks lasting for 14–20 days and one in a youth aged 20 years who had two attacks [21], Levin, in 1936, called attention to "a syndrome characterized by recurring periods of somnolence and morbid hunger" and starting from seven "good cases" of this syndrome previously reported in literature [3–5,19, 20], gave the very first comprehensive description of the syndrome:

There are attacks of sleepiness lasting from several days to several weeks with the longest recorded being three months. During the attack the patient sleeps excessively day and night, in extreme instances waking only to eat and go to the toilet. He can always be roused. When roused he usually is irritable and wants to be alone so that he can go back to sleep. He is abnormally hungry and eats excessively. These attacks are separated by intervals of normal health. Besides the two main symptoms, somnolence and hunger, there are incidental symptoms…. (excitement, irritability, difficulty in thinking, forgetfulness, incoherent speech and hallucinations), insomnia at the close of an attack, male sex with a single exception, age of onset in the second decade, onset soon after an acute illness and spontaneous cure in some cases. [6]

Critchley's Period (1940–2004)

Hylkema reported a boy aged 15 who, 2 months after a severe bout of influenza, began to develop recurrent episodes of sleepiness three to twelve times yearly, associated with excessive hunger and drinking, profuse sweating, whistling, and singing to himself [22]. This was followed by the reports of periodic somnolence and morbid hunger in two men, ages 20 and 25, by Critchley and Hoffman (1942) who coined the term KLS, ignoring Lewis's name [1].

In December 1962, Critchley published his milestone article "Periodic hypersomnia and megaphagia in adolescent males" in which he collected 15 "genuine" instances from the literature and 11 cases of his own, gave a comprehensive description of each and defined—

> "a syndrome composed of recurrent episodes of undue sleepiness, lasting some days, associated with an inordinate intake of food, and often with abnormal behaviour" [7].

In addition he emphasized four hallmark features:

1. Males are preponderantly if not wholly affected.
2. Onset in adolescence.
3. Spontaneous eventual disappearance of the syndrome.
4. The possibility that the megaphagia is in the nature of compulsive eating, rather than bulimia.

From this time on, a lot of cases and reviews have been published leading to some remarks about Critchley's hallmarks: Males are preponderantly affected, but the men/women ratio, about four in most series, is not negligible; onset is generally in adolescence, but onset until the age of 80 years has been reported [23]; spontaneous eventual disappearance may take up to more than 30 years [24].

Moreover, further knowledge on the topic covering predisposing and precipitating factors, clinical features, laboratory tests, course, pathophysiology, and treatment has been added. Factors precipitating the first episode of KLS may include upper airway infection, flulike illness, febrile illness, and, in a few cases, emotional stress, alcohol intake, overwork, sunstroke, seasickness. They have been mentioned in

50–70 % of patients. In a multicenter study based on the analysis of gene polymorphism of HLA-DQB1 in 30 unselected patients with KLS, a HLA-DQB1*0201 allele frequency of 28.3 % in patients and 12.5 % in controls ($X^2 = 4.82, p < 0.03$) has been found [25].

In addition to hypersomnia, compulsive eating, disinhibited sexuality, odd behavior, cognitive, and mental symptoms, physical signs such as weight increase and dysautonomic features have been described in quite a number of cases.

Laboratory tests including routine blood tests and anterior pituitary hormonal levels, baseline, or after stimulation have been found normal in almost all cases. Electroencephalography often showed a general slowing of the background activity and polysomnography documented a poor sleep efficiency and frequent sleep-onset rapid eye movement (REM) periods during symptomatic periods. Computed tomography and magnetic resonance imaging of the brain were normal, except case of comorbidity. Neuropathological examinations have been carried out in three cases of typical KLS [26–28] and in one case of KLS, secondary to a presumptive brain tumor [29]: There were intense signs of inflammatory responses within the hypothalamus in two patients [26, 28], mild inflammation in one patient [29], and none in the last patient [27]. More recently, single-photon emission computed tomography (SPECT) studies performed during symptomatic periods and asymptomatic intervals have shown decreased tracer perfusion in several regions, such as basal ganglia, thalamus, hypothalamus, and frontal, parietal, temporal, or occipital lobes [30–35]. A decrease of cerebrospinal fluid (CSF) hypocretin-1 from a normal level during an asymptomatic interval to a low normal level during a symptomatic period has been demonstrated in one case [36]. Based on the generally young age at onset, recurrence of symptoms, frequent infectious trigger, and a significant increased frequency of HLA-DQB1* allele in the above-referred study [25], an autoimmune etiology for KLS has been suggested.

Finally, it has been proposed that in most cases, notably when episodes are not too frequent, the best approach is to do no harm and let the patients sleep through the episodes undisturbed, asking for accommodation at school or at work. In some cases, in which the episodes are prolonged and frequent the only therapy to be efficacious in some cases is lithium.

ICSD-2 Period

A new step in the history of KLS has been the preparation and publication of the second edition of the ICSD, with a sleep disorder referred to as "Recurrent Hypersomnia," including KLS and menstrual related hypersomnia, within the category of hypersomnias of central origin [8].

Diagnostic criteria, that is minimal criteria necessary for a diagnosis of recurrent hypersomnia, include the following:

a. The patient experiences recurrent episodes of excessive sleepiness ranging from 2 days to 4 weeks.
b. Episodes recur at least once a year.
c. The patient has normal alertness, cognitive functioning and behavior between attacks.
d. The hypersomnia is not better explained by another sleep disorder, medical or neurological disorder, mental disorder, medication use, or substance use disorder.

On the other hand, no diagnostic criteria have been settled for KLS and menstrual related hypersomnia. For the former, it is simply indicated that "a diagnosis of KLS should be reserved for cases in which recurrent episodes of hypersomnia are clearly associated with behavioral abnormalities. These may include binge eating, hypersexuality, abnormal behavior such as irritability, aggression, and odd behavior and cognitive abnormalities, such as feeling of unreality, confusion, and hallucinations." For the latter, it is mentioned that "recurrent episodes of sleepiness that occur in association with the menstrual cycle may be indicative of the menstrual related hypersomnia. The condition occurs within the first months after menarche. Episodes generally last one week, with rapid resolution at the time of menses. Hormone imbalance is a likely explanation, since oral contraceptives will usually lead to prolonged remission."

Although it does not look much, making binge eating a facultative symptom modified the definition of KLS as proposed by Levin [21] and Critchley [4] in which "morbid hunger" or "megaphagia" is the second symptom of the syndrome under consideration. It sets the path for considering all recurrent hypersomnias, except menstrual-related hypersomnia, as cases of KLS. As for menstrual related hypersomnia, the definition is somewhat questionable as the first episode may occur several months or years after menarche [37]. Finally, the frequent association of menstrual-related hypersomnia with other symptoms of KLS is not indicated.

Since the publication of ICSD-2, three reviews have been published in 2005, 2008, and 2010 [37–39]. The first one is a very-well-documented review of 186 cases available on Medline (1962–2004), in keeping with the ICSD-2 definition including patients with and without binge eating [38]. This review aimed at reporting on various KLS symptoms, identifying risk factors, and analyzing treatment responses. Median age at onset was 15 (range 4–82 years) and median value of asymptomatic periods 3.5 months. Common symptoms were hypersomnia (100 % of patients), cognitive changes (96 %), eating disturbances (80 %), hypersexuality (43 %), compulsions (29 %), and depressed mood (18 %). Risk factors included sex, women had a longer disease course than men, and the number of episodes during the first year, as patients with a high number of episodes during the first year of KLS had a somewhat shorter KLS duration. Finally, only lithium (but not carbamazepine or other antiepileptics) had a high reported response rate (41%) for stopping relapse, when compared to medical abstention.

The second review is a cross-sectional, systematic evaluation of 108 new cases, and comparison with matched control subjects by the same group [39]. New predisposing factors e.g., increased birth and developmental problem were identified, Jewish heritage was overrepresented, suggesting a founder effect in this population, and five multiplex families were identified. The disease course was longer in men, in patients with hypersexuality and when onset was after age 20. During episodes all patients had hypersomnia, cognitive impairment, and altered perception, 95% had eating behavior disorder (hyperphagia in 66% and increase food intake in 56%); 53%, predominantly men, reported disinhibition, hypersexuality; and 53%, predominantly women, reported a depressed mood. A marginal efficacy for amantadine and mood stabilizers was found.

The last review included 339 cases of recurrent hypersomnia [37] covering a longer period from Kleine (1925) [3] to 2009. It included 239 cases of full-blown KLS according to Levin and Critchley's definitions (192 men and 47 women), 54 cases of KLS without compulsive eating (40 men and 14 women), 18 cases of menstrual-related hypersomnia and 28 cases of recurrent hypersomnia with comorbidity (tumor, encephalitis, head trauma, stroke, and psychiatric disorders) (20 men and 8 women). The main interests of this review were the distinction of several types of recurrent hypersomnia, the largest number of patients of each type ever reported and a statistical analysis taking into account, for each symptom and sign, the yes answers, the no answers and the missing data, allowing valid comparisons between men and women. In the 239 patients with full blown KLS, median age of onset was 15 in both men and women, median duration of episodes 9 days (range 1–180) in men and 8 days (range 1–60) in women, median cycle length (time from onset of one episode to the onset of the next episode) 106.5 days (range 14–1095) in men and 60 days (range 15–1460) in women. All men and women had hypersomnia and compulsive eating, 48.4% of men and 27.6% of women had sexual disinhibition ($p<0.003$), and 29.7% of men and 36.1% of women odd behavior. In the same patients, confusion was present in 47.6% of men and 25.5% of women, feeling of unreality in 37.5% of men and 36.1% of women, delusions/hallucinations in 17.1% of men and 21.2% of women, signs of depression in 19.8% of men and 40.4% of women, and signs of anxiety in 12% of men and 12.8% of women, dysautonomic signs in 18.2% of men and 19.1% of women, and weight gain in 9.9% of men and 44.6% of women ($p<0.0001$).

Besides these reviews, progress has been made in the fields of genetics and functional imaging.

Another study of HLA typing alleles has detected an immunoresponsive HLA DQB1*0602 in significant quantities in patients with KLS (3 of 12, $p=0.046$) [40]. Of 297 patients with KLS, 239 with compulsive eating and 58 without, 9 cases (3%) were familial, suggesting that the familial risk for KLS is extremely high [41]. Three of these families had more than two affected relatives [24, 42, 43] in favor of an autosomal Mendelian inheritance. Two cases of monozygotic twins have been published suggesting a strong genetic basis for the condition [44, 45].

Further SPECT studies [46–48] and imaging subtraction studies by SPECT [49, 50), functional magnetic resonance imaging (fMRI) [51], and positron emission tomography (PET) [52, 53] have confirmed decreased thalamic activity (possibly mediating increase sleep), decreased diencephalic/hypothalamic activity (possibly deregulating instinctual behaviors), and widespread and variable cortical changes (possibly mediating abnormal perception and cognition) [54].

Although it is generally considered that CSF concentrations of hypocretin-1 are most frequently in the normal range, a recent study, in a large population of 42 Chinese KLS patients, has shown that CSF hypocretin-1 levels were lower in KLS patients during episodes, as compared with controls, and in KLS patients during episodes as compared with KLS patients during remissions [55].

On the other hand, not much progress has been made in the management of the condition and multicenter placebo-controlled drug trials are warranted.

ICSD-3 Period

The last step in the history of KLS has been the publication of the third edition of the ICSD [9], remarkable for the replacement of the sleep disorder « recurrent hypersomnia » with its two subtypes, Kleine-Levin syndrome and Menstrual-Related-Hypersomnia, by the sleep disorder « Kleine-Levin syndrome » with one subtype, menstrual-related Kleine-Levin syndrome, and the setting-up of specific diagnostic criteria for KLS :

A. The patient experiences at least two recurrent episodes of excessive sleepiness and sleep duration, each persisting for two days to five weeks

B. Episodes recur usually more than once a year and at least once every 18 months

C. The patient has normal alertness, cognitive function, behavior, and mood between episodes

D. The patient must demonstrate at least *one* of the following during episodes :
   1. Cognitive dysfunction
   2. Altered perception
   3. Eating disorder (anorexia or hyperphagia)
   4. Disinhibited behavior (such as hypersexuality)

E. The hypersomnolence and related symptoms are not better explained by another sleep disorder, other medical, neurologic, or psychiatric disorder (especially bipolar disorder), or use of drugs or medications.

Conclusion

The knowledge of KLS has considerably evolved since the first report by William Oliver. The first definition of the syndrome goes back to Levin in 1936. The quality of the clinical reports has reached its peak with Critchley in 1962. Since that time the quality of clinical reports has diminished to the benefit of laboratory tests, especially various imaging techniques, which have helped approaching the pathophysiology of the syndrome. Yet, several questions remain open: Why do symptoms such as compulsive eating, disinhibited sexuality, odd behavior, and cognitive impairments may be present in one episode and not in the others? Is there any link between KLS and mood disorders? How do infectious diseases act in triggering KLS episodes? Which are the anatomical pathways involved in the different categories of symptoms? Is there a causative mutation involved in both sporadic and familial KLS cases? Is there any opening for future treatments? There is definitely much to discover in KLS.

References

1. Critchley M, Hoffman HL. The syndrome of periodic somnolence and morbid hunger (Kleine-Levin syndrome). Brit Med J. 1942;1:137–9.
2. Oliver W. An account of an extraordinary sleepy person. Philos Trans. 1705;304:2177–82.
3. Kleine W. Periodische Schlafsuch. Mschr Psychiat Neurol. 1925;57:285–20.
4. Lewis NDC. The psychoanalytic approach to the problems of children under twelve years of age. Psychoanal Rev. 1926;13:424–43.
5. Levin M. Narcolepsy (Gélineau syndrome) and other varieties of morbid somnolence. Arch Neurol Psychiat. 1929;22:1172–200.
6. Levin M. Periodic somnolence and morbid hunger. A new syndrome. Brain. 1936;59:494–4.
7. Critchley M. Periodic hypersomnia and megaphagia in adolescent males. Brain. 1962;85:627–57.
8. American Academy of Sleep Medicine. International classification of sleep disorders, 2. Diagnostic and coding manual. Westchester: American Academy of Sleep Medicine; 2005.
9. American Academy of Sleep Medicine. International classification of sleep disorders, 3rd ed. Darien IL: American Academy of Sleep Medicine; 2014.
10. Chauvot de Beauchêne EP. Observation sur une maladie nerveuse, avec complication d'un sommeil, tantôt léthargique, tantôt convulsif. A Amsterdam et à Paris ; chez Méquignon l'aîné. 1786. 22p.
11. Satterley RP. A case of fever, attended with inordinate appetite. Medical Trans. 1815: 350–7.
12. Brière de Boismont A. Des hallucination ou histoire raisonnée des apparitions, des visions, des songes, de l'extase, des rêves, du magnétisme et du somnambulisme. Paris ; Germer Baillière ; 1862.
13. Lyon Med, Mendel M., Oct. 27, 1872, quoted by Dana CL. On morbid drowsiness and somnolence: a contribution to the pathology of sleep. J Nerv Ment Dis. 1884;11:153–76.
14. Laségue. Gaz Hôp (Paris) 1882, quoted by Dana CL. On morbid drowsiness and somnolence: A contribution to the pathology of sleep. J Nerv Ment Dis. 1884;11:153–76.
15. Anfimoff JA (1898). Quoted by Kaplinsky MS and Schulmann ED. Über die periodische Schlafsucht. Acta Med Scand. 1935;85:107–28.
16. Stöcker W. Zur Narkolepsiefrage. Ztschr f d ges Neurol u Psychiat. 1913;18:216–46.
17. Schröder. Ungewöhnliche period. Psychosen. Mtsschr f Psych. 1918;44:S 261.
18. Krüger. Episodisch Schlafzustände (Lethargien). (Inaugural-Dissertation) Greifswald 1920.
19. Kanabich JW. (1923). Quoted by Kaplinsky and Schulmann ED. Über die periodische Schlafsucht. Acta Med Scand. 1935;85:107–28.
20. Daniels LE. Medicine, Baltimore. 1934;13:1.
21. Kaplinsky MS, Schulmann ED. Über die periodische Schlafsucht. Acta Med Scand. 1935;85:107–28.
22. Hylkema EA. Een bijdrage tot de kennis van de narcolepsie. Thesis, Groningen. 1940.
23. Badino R, Caja A, Del Conte I et al. Kleine-Levin syndrome in an 82 year old man. Ital J Neurol Sci. 1992;13:355–6.
24. Ba Hamman AS, GadElRab MO, Owais SM et al. Clinical characteristics and HLA typing of a family with Kleine-Levin syndrome. Sleep Med. 2008;9:575–8.
25. Dauvilliers Y, Mayer G, Lecendreux M, et al. Kleine-Levin syndrome. An autoimmune hypothesis based on clinical and genetic analyses. Neurology. 2002;59:1739–45.
26. Carpenter S, Yassa R, Ochs R. A pathologic basis for Kleine-Levin syndrome. Arch Neurol. 1982;39:25–8.
27. Koerber RK, Torkelson ER, Haven G et al. Increased cerebrospinal fluid 5-hydroxytryptamine and 5-hydroxyindoleacetic acid in Kleine-Levin syndrome. Neurology. 1984;34:1597–600.
28. Fenzi F, Simonati A, Crozato F, et al. Clinical features of Kleine-Levin syndrome with localized encephalitis. Neuropediatrics. 1993;24:292–5.
29. Takrani LB, Cronin D. Kleine-Levin syndrome in a female patient. Can Psychiatr Assoc J. 1976;21:315–8.
30. Lu ML, Liu HC, Chen CH, et al. Kleine-Levin syndrome and psychosis: Observation from an unusual case. Neuropsychiatry Neuropsychol Behav Neurol. 2000;13:140–2.
31. Landtblom AM, Dige N, Schwerdt K, et al. A case of Kleine-Levin syndrome examined with SPECT and neuropsychological testing. Acta Neurol Scand. 2002;105:318–21.
32. Landtblom AM, Dige N, Schwerdt K, et al. Short-term memory dysfunction in Kleine-Levin syndrome. Acta Neurol Scand. 2003;108:363–7.
33. Arias M, Crespo-Iglesias JM, Pérez J, et al. Syndrome de Kleine-Levin : Aportacion diagnostica de la SPECT cerebral. Rev Neurol. 2002;35:531–3.
34. Nose I, Ookawa T, Tanaka J, et al. Decreased blood flow of the left thalamus during somnolent episodes in a case of recurrent hypersomnia. Psychiatry Clin Neurosci. 2002;56:277–8.
35. Portilla P, Durand E, Chalvon A. et al. Hypoperfusion temporo-mésiale gauche en TEMP dans un syndrome de Kleine-Levin. Rev Neurol (Paris). 2002;158:593–5.
36. Dauvilliers Y, Baumann CR, Carlander B, et al. CSF hypocretin −1 levels in narcolepsy, Kleine-Levin syndrome and other hypersomnias and neurological conditions. J Neurol Neurosurg Psychiatry. 2003;74:1667–73.
37. Billiard M, Jaussent I, Dauvilliers Y, et al. Recurrent hypersomnias : A review of 339 cases. Sleep Med Rev. 2011;15:247–57.
38. Arnulf I, Zeitzer JM, File J, et al. Kleine-Levin syndrome: A systematic review of 186 cases in the literature. Brain. 2005;128:2763–76.

39. Arnulf I, Lin L, Gadoth N, et al. Kleine-Levin syndrome: A systematic study of 108 patients. Ann Neurol. 2008;63:482–92.

40. Huang CJ, Liao HT, Yeh GC, et al. Distribution of HLA-DQB1 alleles in patients with Kleine-Levin syndrome. J Clin Neurosci. 2012;19:628–30.

41. Billiard M, Peraita-Adrados R, Tafti M. Genetics of recurrent hypersomnia. In: Shaw P, Tafti M, Thorpy MJ, editors. The genetic basis of sleep and sleep disorders. Cambridge: Cambridge University Press, 2013. 272–77.

42. Suwa K, Toru M. A case of periodic somnolence whose sleep was induced by glucose. Folia Psychiatr Neurol Jpn. 1969;23:253–62.

43. Popper JSD, Hsia YE, Rogers T, et al. Familial hibernation (Kleine-Levin syndrome). Am J Hum Genet. 1980;32:123A.

44. Peraita-Adrados R, Vicario JL, Tafti M, et al. Monozygotic twins affected with Kleine-Levin syndrome. Sleep. 2012;35:595–6.

45. Ueno T, Fukuhara A, Ikegami A, et al. Monozygotic twins concordant for Kleine-Levin syndrome. BMC Neurol. 30 May 2012 ;12:31. (Epub ahead of print).

46. Huang YS, Guilleminault C, Kao PF, et al. SPECT findings in the Kleine-Levin syndrome. Sleep. 2005;28:955–60.

47. Hsieh CF, Lai CI, Lan SH et al. Modafinil-associated vivid visual hallucination in a patient with Kleine-Levin syndrome: Case report. J Clin Psychopharmacol. 2010;30:347–50.

48. Huang YS, Guilleminault C, Lin K, et al. Relatinship between Kleine-Levin syndrome and upper respiratory infection in Taïwan. Sleep. 2012;35:123–9.

49. Hong SB, Joo EY, Tae WS, et al. Episodic diencephalic hypoperfusion in Kleine-Levin syndrome. Sleep. 2006;29:1091–3.

50. Itokawa K, Fukui M, Ninomiya M, et al. Gabapentine for Kleine-Levin syndrome. Intern Med. 2009;48:1183–5.

51. Billings ME, Watson NF, Keogh BP. Dynamics fMRI changes in Kleine-Levin syndrome. Sleep Med. 2011;12:532.

52. Lo YC, Chou YH, Yu HY. PET finding in Kleine-Levin syndrome. Sleep Med. 2012;13:771–2.

53. Haba-Rubio J, Prior JO, Guedj E, et al. Kleine-Levin syndrome: Functional imaging correlates of hypersomnia and behavioral symptoms. Neurology. 2012;79:1927–9.

54. Hirst J, Mignot E, Stein MT. Episodic hypersomnia and unusual behaviors in a 14-year old adolescent. J Dev Behav Pediatr. 2007;28:475–7.

55. Li Q, Wang J, Dong X et al. CSF hypocretin level in patients with Kleine-Levin syndrome. Sleep Med 2013;14,Suppl 1,e47.

Movement Disorders in Sleep

Sudhansu Chokroverty and Sushanth Bhat

Introduction

Clinical and physiological research in understanding normal and abnormal movements occurring during sleep over the past several decades (almost 50 years) uncovered the complexity of sleep-related movements and dispelled the almost universal belief that diurnal movement disorders (e.g., tremor, chorea, dystonia, tics) are abolished by sleep [1]. It is interesting to note that Josef Frank [2], as early as 1811, mentioned about jactations (*jactatio capitis nocturna*) and cramps under "sleep-related movements" in his comprehensive classification of diseases of the nervous system. Manoia, however, in 1923 listed for the first time abnormal movements in sleep as a separate category of sleep disturbance [3]; (see also Chap. 32 in this volume). The sleep community had to wait over 80 years when the 2nd edition of the *International Classification of Sleep Disorders* (ICSD-2) [4] in 2005 published sleep-related movement disorders as a separate and distinct category in the classification of sleep disorders.

Abnormal movements, postures, and behaviors causing "jerks, shakes, and screams" at night have always been challenging to the clinicians posing diagnostic dilemmas. These nocturnal movements and behaviors form a heterogeneous collection of events including both physiological (normal) and pathological (abnormal) types resulting from motor control during sleep (Table 29.1). Some of these movements result from an urge to move with or without uncomfortable feelings in the legs before sleep while lying quietly in bed trying to get to sleep (e.g., restless legs syndrome (RLS)/Willis–Ekbom disease described further on in the next section), some are especially triggered by sleep or occur pref-

erentially during sleep, whereas others are overlapping (i.e., some diurnal movements may be persisting during sleep at night). Physiological motor activity during sleep includes postural shifts, body and limb movements, physiologic fragmentary hypnic myoclonus consisting of transient muscle bursts seen typically in rapid eye movement (REM) sleep but also seen in stage N1, particularly in small babies and children, hypnic jerks, hypnagogic foot tremor (HFT), and rhythmic leg movements.

Abnormal movements that may occur during sleep include motor parasomnias (nonrapid eye movement [non-REM], rapid eye movement [REM], and other parasomnias), sleep-related movement disorders (a separate category was included in the ICSD-2) [4], isolated sleep-related motor symptoms (apparently normal variants), miscellaneous nocturnal motor activities, and traditional diurnal involuntary movements persisting during sleep. Many of these nocturnal motor events may be mistaken for nocturnal seizures (traditionally not classified with movement disorders), especially myoclonic seizures and nocturnal frontal lobe epilepsy (NFLE) or what was originally termed nocturnal paroxysmal dystonia (NPD). Figure 29.1 schematically shows the most common sleep-related movements which need to be considered and differentiated from each other. In this chapter, we describe the evolution and historical milestones of some of those sleep-related movements including the ICSD-3 [4] category of sleep-related movement disorders as well as some diurnal movements persisting during sleep. For a historical account of RLS/WillisEkbom disease, non-REM parasomnias, REM behavior disorder (RBD), and nightmare disorders (REM parasomnias), see other chapters of this book.

Szymanski [5] first attempted to study body motility during sleep using rudimentary actigraphs ("sensitive bed" principle of movement registration) in 1914. It was revealed for the first time that sleep is not just a period of rest and repose but there are interruptions due to body movements. Later, polysomnography (PSG) and particularly video-PSG studies clearly documented physiological body movements and postural shifts during sleep. Gastaut and collaborators

S. Chokroverty (✉) · S. Bhat
JFK New Jersey Neuroscience Institute, 65 James Street, 08818 Edison, NJ, USA
e-mail: schok@att.net

S. Bhat
Seton Hall University, South Orange, NJ, USA

S. Chokroverty, M. Billiard (eds.), *Sleep Medicine,* DOI 10.1007/978-1-4939-2089-1_29,
© Springer Science+Business Media, LLC 2015

Table 29.1 Disorders due to failure of motor control during sleep

A. Failure of motor control at NREM sleep onset
1. Physiological
a. Physiological body movements and postural shifts
b. Physiological hypnic myoclonus
c. Hypnic jerks
d. Hypnagogic foot tremor
e. Rhythmic limb movements
2. Pathological
a. Intensified hypnic jerks
b. Rhythmic movement disorder
c. Propriospinal myoclonus at sleep onset
B. Failure of motor control during NREM sleep
1. Partial arousal disorders
a. Confusional arousals
b. Sleep walking
c. Sleep terror
2. Others
a. Alternating leg muscle activity
b. Periodic limb movements in sleep
C. Failure of motor control during REM sleep
1. Physiological
a. Phasic muscle bursts includingfragmentary hypnic myoclonus
b. Phasic tongue movements
c. Sleep paralysis
2. Pathological
a. RBD
b. Sleep paralysis with narcolepsy
c. Familial sleep paralysis
d. Cataplexy
D. Failure of motor control in both NREM and REM sleep
a. Rhythmic movement disorder
b. Catathrenia
c. Excessive fragmentary myoclonus
d. Sleep bruxism
e. Upper airway obstructive sleep apnea syndrome
E. Failure of motor controlat sleep offset
a. Sleep paralysis
b. Hypnopompic hallucination
c. Sleep inertia ("sleep drunkenness")
F. Diurnal movement disorders persisting in sleep
1. Usually persisting during sleep
a. Symptomatic palatal tremor
2. Frequently persisting during sleep
a. Spinal and propriospinal myoclonus
b. Tics in Tourette's syndrome
c. Hemifacial spasm
d. Hyperekplexia
3. Sometimes persisting during sleep
a. Tremor
b. Chorea
c. Dystonia
d. Hemiballismus

NREM nonrapid eye movement, *RBD* rapid eye movement behavior disorder, *REM* rapid eye movement

from France [6, 7] were the first to study sleep-related normal and abnormal movements using polygraphic technique with multiple surface electromyography (EMG) recordings. Shortly thereafter, Lugaresi and coinvestigators from Italy [8, 9] made important polysomnographic contributions on the evolution of abnormal movements during sleep. Arousals (periods of interruptions from sleep to brief awakenings lasting up to 14 s or less) are often associated with body movements, and these may precede or follow postural shifts. Arousals may be both physiological (e.g., associated with

Fig. 29.1 Most common paroxysmal motor disorders in sleep

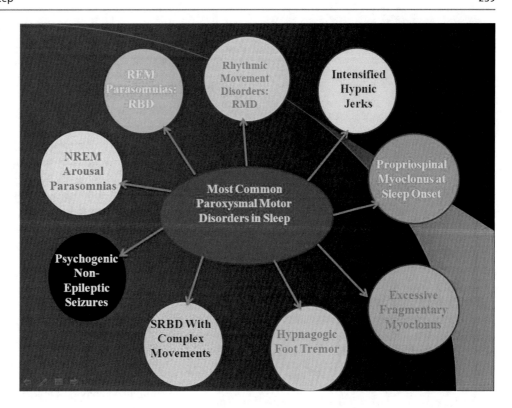

body shifts in normal individuals) and pathological (e.g., on termination of sleep apneic–hypopnic episodes or associated with periodic limb movements in sleep, PLMS). Body movements and postural shifts are frequent at sleep onset and fairly common in stage N1, occur less frequently in stage N2, and are rarely seen in stage N3 but again may be frequent in stage REM [10]. Movements vary not only with sleep stages but also with age. In one study [11], postural shifts during sleep decreased from 4.7/h in 8–12–year-olds to 2.1/h in the elderly (65–80 years). Body motility was among the earliest physiological characteristics of sleep studied [12]. All night polygraphic recordings showed a significant temporal relationship between preceding K-complexes and body movements in the early physiological studies of Gastaut and Broughton [13], and Sassin and Johnson [14].

Disorders of Failure of Motor Control at Non-REM Sleep Onset

Physiological

Physiological Hypnic Myoclonus The term physiological hypnic myoclonus (PHM) was first coined by De Lisi in 1932 to describe brief asynchronous, asymmetric, and aperiodic muscle twitches during sleep in all body muscles of humans and domestic animals resembling fasciculations seen prominently in face and distal body parts (e.g., face, lips, fingers, and toes) [15]. PHM is also known as physiologi-

cal fragmentary hypnic myoclonus and is seen prominently in babies and infants. Quantitative study by Dagnino et al. in 1969 [16] and Montagna and collaborators [17] in 1988 showed the maximum occurrence of these twitches in stage N1 and REM sleep, decreasing progressively in stages N2 and N3. Presence of PHM also during relaxed wakefulness challenges the term hypnic myoclonus [17, 18]; however, it should be noted that propriospinal myoclonus (PSM) at sleep onset and intensified hypnic jerks in many patients [19] are present in relaxed wakefulness before sleep onset. The origin of PHM remains controversial. Facilitatory reticulospinal tract [20], pontine tegmentum [21], and corticospinal tract [16] have all been suggested as the generator of PHM. These movements are physiological without disrupting sleep architecture and these require no treatment.

Hypnic Jerks Including Intensified Hypnic Jerks Hypnic jerks are sudden, brief contractions of the body that occur at sleep onset and are due to excitation of motor centers. They are physiological and occur in up to 70 % of the population at some point in their adult lives. They are often accompanied by a sensation of falling. The earliest mention of this phenomenon is credited to Weir Mitchell [22] (Fig. 29.2), who in 1890 described insomnia occurring as a result of hypnic jerks. Oswald [23] first described the electroencephalography (EEG) correlates of hypnic jerks. In 1965, Gastaut and Broughton performed the first polygraphic study of hypnic jerks [6, 13]. It was not until 1988 that Broughton [24] coined the term "intensified hypnic jerks" to describe the clinical phenomenon of sleep-onset insomnia caused by accentu-

Fig. 29.2 Silas Weird Mitchell (1829–1914)

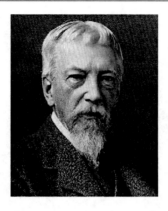

ated and disruptive hypnic jerks occurring at sleep onset. More recently, Chokroverty et al. [19] performed a polysomnographic and polymyographic analysis of ten patients with intensified hypnic jerks and identified four patterns of propagation: synchronous and symmetrical patterned muscle bursts between the two sides and agonist–antagonist muscles similar to those noted in audiogenic startle reflex, reticular reflex myoclonus, dystonic myoclonus, and pyramidal myoclonus with rostrocaudal propagation of muscle bursts.

Hypnagogic Foot Tremor HFT is defined as rhythmic contractions of foot and leg occurring during sleep onset generally bilaterally but asynchronously at a frequency of 0.3–4 Hz, and was first described by Broughton in 1986 [24]. Wichniak and colleagues [25] later performed PSG on 375 consecutive subjects and found HFT (which they called "rhythmic feet movements while falling asleep" and described as rhythmic, oscillating movements of the whole foot or toes) in 7.5 %. The clinical significance of HFT remains undetermined requiring no treatment.

Rhythmic Limb Movements in Sleep and Wakefulness Rhythmic leg movements in non-REM (NREM) sleep, REM sleep, and wakefulness are frequently noted during PSG recordings in the sleep laboratory [26]. Yang and Winkelman [27] recently reported "high-frequency leg movements" in a retrospective study to describe similar phenomena seen in both wakefulness (two-thirds) and sleep (one-third). The significance of these leg movements remains undetermined. There have been brief recent reports of limb and body movements, both rhythmic and complex, on termination of apneas/hypopneas, eliminated by positive pressure therapy [28, 29, 30].

Pathological

Rhythmic Movement Disorder RMD is characterized by repetitive, often dramatic and stereotyped, rhythmic movements involving large muscle groups, occurring predominantly during sleep onset or during sleep–wake transitions,

at a frequency of 0.5–2 Hz [4, 31]. In 1905, Zappert [32] described nocturnal rhythmic head banging in six children and coined the term *jactatio capitis nocturna.* Between 1905 and 1928, Cruchet [33, 34], who used the term *rhythmie du sommeil,* published several observations in French, among which was acknowledgment that credit for the earliest description of this phenomenon should most likely go to Wepfer, who reported a case of rhythmic head movement activity that occurred at night as far back as 1727. There was a report, as early as 1880, by Mary Putnam-Jacobi [35], of a case of nocturnal rotary movement in an 18-month-old boy which appears to be the first clear description of what can be considered to be a case of RMD published in a popular journal of the nineteenth century. RMD generally presents before 18 months of age with head banging, head and body rolling, and body rocking occurring immediately before sleep during relaxed wakefulness continuing into stage N1 and sometimes into stage N2. Leg rolling and leg banging have also been described. RMD is generally benign and the child usually outgrows the movements by the second or third year of life but sometimes may persist into adolescence and adulthood when treatment may be needed. The first line of treatment should be behavioral therapy and in severe cases with potential for inflicting injury clonazepam (0.5–1 mg nightly) or imipramine (10 mg at night) may be helpful [36]. Protective measures should be used in cases with violent movements.

PSM at Sleep Onset PSM, representing myoclonic activity arising in the relaxation period preceding sleep onset, was first described in three patients in 1997 by Montagna et al. [37] They performed polygraphic studies that showed that the myoclonic activity began in spinally innervated muscles, propagating at low speed to rostral and caudal muscular segments, and hypothesized that a spinal generator may be facilitated by changes in supraspinal control related to vigilance levels. They identified it as a potential cause of severe anxiety and insomnia. Subsequently, the same group [38] described another five patients of PSM at wake–sleep transition. Most cases are idiopathic without any structural lesion. PSM has also been described more recently by the same group in three patients with RLS (recently renamed Willi-Ekbom disease) [39]. Manconi et al. [40] described a severe and uncommon case of PSM during wake–sleep transition following a vertebral fracture of T11. The uncommon features of this case include focal myoclonic activity in the axial muscles during stable sleep and later progression into a myoclonic status indicating a very high spinal cord excitability. Recently, a case of PSM at sleep onset was described in an Asian woman from Singapore [41]. The pathophysiological mechanism of PSM at wake–sleep transition stage (predormitum as suggested by Critchley [42]) is hypothesized to be due to the lack of supraspinal inhibitory control at this stage, with resultant spinal cord hyperexcitability propagated through propriospinal pathways [37, 38]. The treatment of this condition is challenging and some cases respond to clonazepam, zonisamide, and other antiepileptic drugs used in the classic PSM [36].

Failure of Motor Control During NREM Sleep

Alternating Limb Muscle Activity During Sleep

Alternating leg muscle activation (ALMA), first described by Chervin and colleagues in 2003, is characterized by brief activation of the anterior tibialis muscle in one leg alternating with similar activation in the other leg, usually lasting up to 20 s and occurring in all sleep stages, but particularly during arousals [43]. In 2006, Consentino and colleagues [44] described a patient with ALMA whose condition responded to pramipexole. Our group [45] documented ALMA in wakefulness, all stages of NREM, and also though less in REM sleep, in patients with a variety of sleep disorders. We observed ALMA also in gastrocnemius and sometimes in quadriceps muscles alternating between two sides. The significance of ALMA remains undetermined but may be a variant of PLMS.

Periodic Limb Movements in Sleep

PLMS is a well-known polysomnographic finding, characterized by repetitive, often stereotyped, and sometimes complex involuntary movements of the limbs, trunk, and occasionally cranially innervated muscles. The first description of this condition was in 1953 by Symonds [46], who used the term "nocturnal myoclonus" to distinguish the phenomenon from hypnic jerking, which he described as "nocturnal jerking." It had been his opinion that both these conditions were associated with an increased risk of epilepsy. A review of his clinical description suggests that Symonds included cases of familial RLS, sleep starts, and myoclonic epilepsy. It was not until 1980 that the term "nocturnal myoclonus" was replaced by "periodic limb movements in sleep" after Coleman et al. [47] clarified that the movements were too prolonged to be classified as myoclonic, and that there was no epileptiform potential associated with them. The association between impaired renal function and PLMS was established in 1985 [48]. The first polygraphic study of PLMS was published by Lugaresi and Coccagna and their collaborators [9, 49, 50] and they demonstrated the common association with RLS as well as the presence of PLMS in normal subjects. An electrophysiological study of PLMS was published later by Wechsler et al. in 1986 [51]. Studying lower limb H-waves,

blink responses, and median nerve somatosensory-evoked responses, they postulated that PLMS was likely secondary to a disorder of the central nervous system producing increased excitability of segmental reflexes at the pontine level or rostral to it. In 2001, Provini et al. [52] studied the motor pattern of PLMS neurophysiologically with EMG/nerve conduction studies, somatosensory-evoked potentials, and transcranial magnetic stimulation, all of which were normal. They found that in PLMS, leg muscles were most frequently involved, often with alternation of sides. Axial muscles were rarely involved and upper limb muscles were involved only sometimes. The tibialis anterior muscle was the most frequent to show the onset of PLMS. There was no constant recruitment pattern from one PLMS episode to another, even in the same patient. There was no orderly caudal or rostral spread of the EMG activity. They speculated about the presence of several generators at various levels of the spinal cord, released by a supraspinal generator. In 2004, de Weerd and colleagues [53] studied activity patterns in patients with PLMS and found that the classic pattern of movement (extensor digitorum brevis, EDB–tibialis anterior, TA–biceps femoris, BF–tensor fascia lata, TFL) or its direct variants was found in only 12 % of the total 469 movements analyzed. The most frequent sequences were characterized by contraction of only the TA, TA–EDB only, or TA–EDB followed by all other combinations (32 %). In 1991, Ali et al. [54] reported the first observation of sympathetic hyperactivity caused by PLMS, noting a mean increase in systolic blood pressure following leg movements of 23 %, comparable to that noted in obstructive sleep apnea. In 1993, Pollmächer and Schulz [55] reviewed PSG characteristics of PLMS and found them most frequent at sleep–wake transition, attenuated during deep NREM sleep and even more during REM sleep. The first description of periodic arm movements in association with periodic leg movements in sleep was made by Chabli et al. in 2000, [56] when they studied 15 cases of patients with RLS who exhibited this phenomenon. That same year, Nofzinger and colleagues [57] described the distinctive characteristic of bupropion of improving rather than worsening PLMS unlike other antidepressants. It is notable that bupropion has some dopaminergic function which may be responsible for this effect. There is currently no scientific evidence that PLMS per se are responsible for insomnia or hypersomnia but they are noted in at least 80 % of cases of RLS. The scoring criteria for PLMS have been updated recently [31].

Failure of Motor Control During REM Sleep

For RBD and narcolepsy–cataplexy, the readers are referred to Chaps. 45 and 26.

Phasic Muscle Movements in REM Sleep (Including Rhythmic Tongue Movements)

REM sleep is associated with a variety of phasic phenomena, such as phasic eye movements, body and limb movements, transient muscle bursts (fragmentary myoclonus), and irregular heart rate and respiration. Less-well-defined and less commonly recognized phasic events in REM sleep include spontaneous middle ear muscle activity (MEMA) in human described by Pessah and Roffwarg in 1972 [58], and phasic movements of the tongue. In 1980, Megirian et al. [59] described rhythmic activity of the tongue in rats during REM sleep. Similar complex tongue movements during REM sleep in human occurring irregularly and lasting for 2–10 s were reported by Chokroverty in 1980 [60]. These complex movements may counteract posterior displacement of the tongue, which may otherwise occur in supine REM sleep because of genioglossal hypotonia, thus functioning as nature's defense against upper airway obstructive sleep apnea during REM sleep.

Failure of Motor Control in both NREM and REM Sleep

Catathrenia

Catathrenia, or nocturnal groaning, is a relatively new isolated symptom characterized by loud expiratory vocalization, whose exact pitch and timber may vary from individual to individual but is fairly stereotyped in a given patient. While far more frequent in REM sleep, it may also occur in NREM sleep and alternate with normal breathing. It was actually first described by Pevernagie et al. [61], but was first named by Vetrugno et al. [62] in 2001. The same group subsequently reported in 2007 [63] that the groaning was accompanied by disproportionately prolonged expiration causing reduced tidal volume and bradypnea without oxygen desaturation, and that patients experienced no additional symptoms after a mean follow-up of 4.9 years. They speculated that catathrenia was due to persistence of a vestigial type of breathing pattern. In 2011, Ott and colleagues [64] performed laryngoscopy under deep sedation in a patient with catathrenia and found that while the glottis was open at inspiration, there was subtotal closure of the glottis at expiration, resulting in the characteristic groaning. The following year, Koo et al. [65] performed acoustic analysis of catathrenia and found that it had morphologic regularity, with two types of sound pitches (either a monotonous sinusoidal pattern or a sawtooth-shaped signal with higher fundamental frequency), as opposed to snoring which was distinct from catathrenia and had an irregular signal. Several authors have reported the efficacy of continuous positive airway pressure (CPAP) in treating this benign but socially awkward condition [66, 67].

Excessive Fragmentary Myoclonus

Excessive fragmentary myoclonus (EFM) is a predominantly PSG finding, currently described as being present if EMG bursts of at least 150 ms occur at a rate of at least 5/min sustained over 20 min of NREM sleep [31]. The first description of EFM was published by Broughton and colleagues in 1985, based on the PSG findings in NREM sleep in 38 consecutive patients [68]. They reported an association with sleep-related respiratory problems, PLMS, narcolepsy, insomnia, and excessive daytime sleepiness. Prior to this, Broughton and Tolentino [69] described what they called fragmentary pathologic myoclonus in a 42-year-old man presenting with excessive daytime sleepiness. In 1993, Lins et al. [70] reported that EFM occurred at high rates in all stages of sleep (including REM) but at a somewhat lower frequency in slow-wave sleep (SWS) explaining, as well, a significantly lower rate in the first hour after onset compared to later hours. More recently, Hoque et al. [71] reported that EFM rates increase with SWS and total REM with the highest EFM rates occurring during phasic REM. The clinical significance and pathophysiology of EFM remain undetermined. A neurophysiologic analysis by Vetrugno et al. failed to disclose any cortical prepotential on EEG–EMG backaveraging suggesting a subcortical origin [72].

Sleep Bruxism

While nocturnal bruxism may occur in patients with daytime tooth grinding, it is clearly a distinct entity in its own right, and can lead to excessive dental wear, autonomic arousals, and sleep fragmentation. One of the earliest works regarding the phenomenon was in 1964 by Reding [73], who predicted a relationship between sleep bruxism and dreaming based on its occurrence in REM sleep. The close association between bruxism and REM sleep was further commented upon by Clarke and Townsend in 1984 [74]. Shortly thereafter, Wieselmann and colleagues [75] analyzed the duration and amount of pressing and grinding jaw movements in ten patients with bruxism, and found that the highest level of activity was during stage N3 and wakefulness, with no difference seen with regard to percentages of the sleep stages. In 2001, Lavigne and colleagues [76] coined the term "rhythmic masticatory muscle activity" (RMMA) in sleep, and found that while the number of episodes of RMMA was comparable between bruxers and controls, the number of EMG bursts per episode was more frequent in the former group. In 2008, Manconi et al. [77] published an interesting case report of a patient with sleep bruxism and catathrenia occurring in a synchronized fashion. They hypothesized about the presence of a common trigger mechanism for both phenomena.

Failure of Motor Control at Sleep Offset

Metabolically [78], physiologically [79, 80], and behaviorally [42, 81, 82], predormitum and postdormitum are two distinct sleep–wake states. Sleep offset occurs with abrupt changes in the EEG activity, unblocking of the afferent stimuli, and restoration of postural muscle tone accompanied by a reduction of cerebral blood flow [78] with concomitant decrement of cerebral metabolism as compared with that in presleep wakefulness. This is in contrast to sleep onset with gradual changes in the EEG, blockade of the afferent stimuli at the thalamic level (essentially converting an "open" brain into a "close" one), and a reduction of postural muscle tone [83]. Because of these differences between the two states, certain motor or other disorders preferentially occur [83] in either predormitum (e.g., PSM at sleep onset, hypnic jerks, RMDs, hypnagogic imagery, and exploding head syndrome) or postdormitum (e.g., sleep inertia, awakening epilepsy of Jung, sleep benefit in some Parkinson's disease (PD) patients). Sleep paralysis (SP) and hallucinations may occur in both states (hypnagogic and hypnopompic).

Sleep Paralysis

SP has been known throughout the history of mankind invoking various interpretations in different cultures and folklore. This physiological phenomenon causing transient immobility is related to REM sleep muscle atonia (body sleep) persisting during wake on (sleep offset) period [4]. This is often associated with intense anxiety and panic. There are three forms of SP: isolated or recurrent sleep paralysis (physiological occurring mostly in adults up to 30–50 % of the population), familial sleep paralysis, and SP as part of narcolepsy tetrad [ICSD 2]. SP may occur at sleep onset (hypnagogic) which is often noted in narcolepsy–cataplexy syndrome but more frequently (physiological type) occurs at sleep offset when it is called hypnopompic. Mitchell [22] is given credit for an early description of SP in 1876 and he termed it "night palsy." Adie [84] in the 1920s observed occurrence of SP in narcolepsy patients and Wilson in 1928 [85] introduced the term "sleep paralysis." There are earlier descriptions in the Chinese, Indian, Persian, and Greek cultures.

The physiologic SP is generally brief, lasting for seconds to a few minutes, but sometimes may last longer, particularly the recurrent isolated SP. On occasions, the episodes are accompanied by hypnagogic or hypnopompic hallucinations. The episodes may be triggered by sleep deprivation, stress, physical exertion, or supine position. Isolated or recurrent SP does not require any specific treatment other than reassurance, lifestyle changes, and regularizing sleep–wake schedule, but in severe cases causing anxiety and panic short-term treatment with selective serotonin reuptake inhibitors (SSRIs) or tricylic antidepressants may be beneficial.

Sleep Inertia

Sleep inertia, also known as sleep drunkenness, is a transient physiologic state of hypovigilance, confusion, impaired cognitive and behavioral performance, and grogginess that immediately follows awakening from sleep [86]. The subject is physiologically awake (body awake) but cognitively asleep (brain asleep). EEG of sleep inertia is characterized by a generalized decrease of high-frequency beta-1 and beta-2 EEG power but an increase of delta power of the posterior scalp region concomitant with decreased frontal delta power [87]. This state can last from minutes up to 4 h, most commonly about 5 min, and rarely may exceed 30 min. Prior sleep deprivation, awakening from SWS and short naps may aggravate sleep inertia. It is also more intense when awakening from near the trough rather than the peak of the circadian core body temperature rhythm [86]. Sleep disorders, particularly idiopathic hypersomnia, as well as narcolepsy–cataplexy syndrome and obstructive sleep apnea syndrome may be associated with prolonged sleep inertia. Bedrich Roth and collaborators were probably the first to describe idiopathic hypersomnia with sleep drunkenness in the 1950s [88]. One suggestion for the pathogenesis of sleep inertia is buildup of adenosine and this state can be reversed by caffeine acting through adenosine A2a receptors.

Diurnal Movement Disorders Persisting in Sleep

Most abnormal movements seen during the daytime persist with decreasing frequency, amplitude, and duration, particularly in stages N1 and N2 [89, 90]. Only tardive dyskinesias (TD) and primary palatal tremor may show complete cessation of movements during sleep. Furthermore, the daytime and nighttime abnormal movements are modulated by sleep–wake states. It is important to understand this interaction so that the clinicians can differentiate between de novo abnormal movements in sleep and those representing reemergence or persistence of those abnormal movements that the patients may have during the daytime [91].

There are various degrees of persistence during sleep of different diurnal movement disorders. In general, the diurnal movements decrease but there are remnants of motor activities that persist during sleep or occur during transitions (stage changes) to lighter sleep. Fish and colleagues [92] using surface EMG and video recordings, and accelerometer studied the relations of a variety of diurnal movements to sleep stages and transitions (monitored both normal and abnormal movements) in PD, Huntington's chorea (HC), Tourette's syndrome (TS), and TD. Forty-one out of 43 patients had persistence of movements during sleep. The movements were seen in descending order during awakenings, stage N1,

REM sleep, and stage N2, and no movements were seen during SWS.

Parkinsonian Tremor

James Parkinson, in his 1817 treatise [93], mentioned about two important observations, long neglected by the contemporary movement disorder specialists until recently: persistence of tremor in the light stage of sleep and sleep dysfunction as an important non-motor symptom. The original quotes from James Parkinson are worthy of note:

> But as the Malady proceeds...." (p. 6)
> "In this stage (stooped posture with "unwillingly a running pace"...most likely stage 3), the sleep becomes much disturbed. The tremulus motion of the limbs occur during sleep and augment until they awaken the patient, and frequently with much agitation and alarm" (p. 7)
> "...and at the last (advanced bedridden stage), constant sleepiness, with slight delirium, and other marks of extreme exhaustion, announce the wished-for release. (p. 9)

Parkinsonian tremor decreases in amplitude and duration in early NREM sleep and may lose its alternating aspects. It is rarely seen in stage N3 and often disappears in REM sleep [94]. In some PD patients, sleep can confer "sleep benefit" to Parkinsonian motor disability [95], perhaps due to the circadian peak of dopamine in the morning or due to altered metabolic state in the postdormitum. Sleep benefit may last from 30 min to 3 h. This is mostly seen in early-onset PD due to recessive Parkin (PARK 2) mutation. Sleep benefit is less consistent in those with the recessive Pink 1 (PARK 6) mutation.

Other Diurnal Movement Disorders

In Huntington's chorea HC, there is variable persistence of chorea during sleep, particularly in stages N1 and N2. Fish and colleagues [92] noted that most of these choreiform movements occurred during awakenings, lightening of sleep stages, or in stage N1 similar to other abnormal daytime movements.

Dystonic movements may persist during sleep at a reduced frequency and amplitude.

In 11 of the 12 patients with *Tourette's syndrome* TS reported by Glaze et al. [96], tic-like movements similar to those noted during wakefulness occurred during NREM and REM sleep. Barabas et al. [97] observed increased frequency of disorders of arousal (e.g., somnambulism and *pavor nocturnus*) in children with TS.

Hemifacial spasm consists of intermittent contraction of one side of the face that can be repetitive and jerk-like or sustained. It is believed to arise from irritation of facial nerve or nucleus. Both central and peripheral (ephaptic transmission between adjacent nerve fibers without synapses) factors are responsible for the spasms. These persist during the lighter stages of sleep [36, 98], decreasing significantly in stage N3 and REM sleep. The best treatment option is botulinum toxin injections into the affected muscles and other options include antiepileptic drugs and muscle relaxants; in refractory cases, vascular decompression of facial nerve may be needed [36].

Palatal Myoclonus (Palatal Tremor)

Palatal myoclonus, described over 100 years ago [99–101], is recently renamed palatal tremor. It is characterized by rhythmic movements of the soft palate and pharynx at a rate of 1–3 Hz [36, 102]. It is sometimes associated with rhythmic ocular, buccal, lingual, laryngeal, and diaphragmatic movements, and occasionally also movements of the upper limbs. Two types have been described: a primary or essential type (no cause found) due to contraction of the tensor veli palatini muscle presenting with a clicking noise in one or both ears, and a secondary type (resulting from a variety of brain stem lesions) due to contraction of the levator veli palatini muscle [36, 102]. The primary type may disappear during sleep but the secondary type persists in sleep although with alteration in amplitude and frequency [99, 100]. Palatal tremor results from an involvement of the Guillain–Mollaret triangle, which is formed by the cerebellar dentate nucleus and its outflow tract in the superior cerebellar peduncle crossing over to the contralateral side in the vicinity of the red nucleus and descending down along the central tegmental tract to the inferior olivary nucleus with a final connection from the inferior olivary nucleus back to the contralateral dentate nucleus [102]. Palatal tremor is mostly refractory to treatment. There are reports of occasional response to anticholinergics, botulinum toxin injections, baclofen, valproic acid, lamotrigine, tetrabenazine, and carbamazepine [36].

References

1. Lugaresi E, Chokroverty S. General introduction and historical review. In: Chokroverty S, et al., editors. Sleep movement disorders, 2 ed. New York: Oxford University Press; 2013. p. 377–81.
2. Frank J. Maladies du système nerveux. In: Bayle M, editor. Encyclopédie des Sciences Médicales Paris: Bureau de l'encyclopedie; 1838.
3. Manoia AR. I disturbi del sonno e loro cura. Roma: L Pozzi; 1923.
4. American Academy of Sleep Medicine. International classification of sleep disorders, 3rd ed. Diagnostic and coding manual. Westchester: American Academy of Sleep Medicine; 2014.

5. Szymanski, JS. Eine Methode zur Untersuchung der Ruhe und Aktivitätsperioden bei Tieren. Pflugers Arch. 1914;158:343–85.

6. Gastaut H, Batini C, Broughton R, et al. Etude électrocéphalographique des phénomènes épisodiques non épileptiques au cours du sommeil. In: Fischgold H, et al., editor. Le Sommeil du nuit normal et pathologique. Paris: Masson & Cie Editeurs; 1965. p. 214.

7. Tassinari CA, Broughton R, Poire R, et al. An electroclinical study of nocturnal sleep in patients presenting abnormal movements. Electroencephalogr Clin Neurophysiol. 1965;18:95.

8. Lugaresi E, Coccagna G, Mantovani M, et al. The evolution of different types of myoclonus during sleep. Eur Neurol. 1970;4:321–31

9. Lugaresi E, Coccagna G, Tassinari CA, et al. Relieve poligrafici sui fenomeni motori nella syndrome delle gambe senza riposo. Riv Neurol. 1965;34:550.

10. Gardner R Jr, Grossman WI. Normal motor patterns in sleep in man. In: Weitzman E, editor. Advances in sleep research (vol 2). New York: Spectrum; 1975. pp. 67–92.

11. De Koninck J, Lorrain D, Gagnon P. Sleep positions and position shifts in five age groups: an ontogenetic picture. Sleep. 1992;15:143–9

12. Kleitman N, Cooperman NR, Mullin FJ. Motility and body temperature during sleep. Am J Physiol. 1933;195:574–84.

13. Gastaut H, Broughton R, A. clinical and polygraphic study of episodic phenomena during sleep. Recent Adv Psychiatry. 1964;7:197–221.

14. Sassin J, Johnson LC. Body motility during sleep and its relation to the K-complex. Exp Neurol. 1968;22:133–44.

15. De Lisi L. Su di un fenomeno motoria constante del sonno normale: le mioclonie ipniche fisiologiche. Riv Pat Ment. 1932;39: 481–96.

16. Dagnino N, Loeb C, Massazza G, et al. Hypnic physiological myoclonias in man: an EEG-EMG study in normals and neurological patients. Eur Neurol. 1969;2:47–58.

17. Montagna P, Liguori R, Zucconi M, et al. Physiological hypnic myoclonus. Electroencephalogr Clin Neurophysiol. 1988;70:172–6.

18. Kunz A, Frauscher B, Brandauer E, et al. Fragmentary myoclonus in sleep revisited: a polysomnographic study in 62 patients. Sleep Med. 2011;12:410–5.

19. Chokroverty S, Bhat S, Gupta D. Intensified hypnic jerks: a polymyographic and polysomnographic analysis. J Clin Neurophysiol. 2013;30:403–10.

20. Gassel MM, Marchiafava PL, Pompeiano O. Phasic changes in muscular activity during desynchronized sleep in unrestrained cats: an analysis of the pattern and organization of myoclonic twitches. Arch Ital Biol. 1964;102:449–70.

21. Gastaut H. Les myoclonies. Semiologie des myoclonies et nosologie analytique des syndromes myocloniques. Rev Neurol. 1968;119:1–30.

22. Mitchell SW. Some disorders of sleep. Int J Med Sci. 1890;100:109–27.

23. Oswald I. Sudden bodily jerks on falling asleep. Brain 1959;82:92–103.

24. Broughton R. Pathological fragmentary myoclonus, intensified hypnic jerks and hypnagogic foot tremor: three unusual sleep-related movement disorders. In: Koella WP, Obal F, Schultz H, Visser P, editors. Sleep '86. Stuttgart: Gustav Fischer Verlag; 1988. pp. 240–42.

25. Wichniak A, Tracik F, Geisler P, et al. Rhythmic feet movements while falling asleep. Mov Disord. 2001;16:1164–70.

26. Chokroverty S, Thomas R, Bhatt M, editors. Atlas of sleep medicine. Philadelphia: Butterworth-Heineman; 2005.

27. Yang C, Winkelman JW. Clinical and polysomnographic characteristics of high frequency leg movements. J Clin Sleep Med. 2010; 6:431–8.

28. Gharagozlou P, Seyffert M, Santos R, et al. Rhythmic movement disorder associated with respiratory arousals and improved by CPAP titration in a patient with restless legs syndrome and sleep apnea. Sleep Med. 2009;10:501–3.

29. Chirakalwasan N, Hassan F, Kaplish N, Fetterolf J, Chervin RD. Near resolution of sleep related rhythmic movement disorder after CPAP for OSA. Sleep Med. 2009;10:497–500.

30. Lysenko L, Bhat S, Patel D, Salim S, Chokroverty S. Complex sleep behavior in a patient with obstructive sleep apnea and nocturnal hypoglycemia: a diagnostic dilemma. Sleep Med. 2012;13:1321–3.

31. Iber C, Ancoli-Israel S, Chesson AL, Quan SF. The AASM Manual for the Scoring of Sleep and Associated Events: Rules, Terminology, and Technical Specifications. Westchester, Ill: American Academy of Sleep Medicine; 2007.

32. Zappert J. Uber nachtliche Kopf bewegungen bei Kindern (jactatio capitis nocturna). Jahrb Kinderheilkd. 1905;62:70–83.

33. Cruchet R. Six nouveaux cas de rythmies du sommeil (les rythmies à la caserne). Gaz Hebd Sci Med. 1912;33:303–8.

34. Cruchet R. Les mauvaises habitudes chez les enfants. Paris: L'Expansion Scientifique Française; 1928

35. Putman-Jacobi M, Case of nocturnal rotator spasm. J Nerv Ment Dis. 1880;7:390–401.

36. Lysenko L, Hanna PA, Chokroverty S. Sleep disruption from movement disorders. In: Barkoukis T, Matheson J, Ferber R, Doghramji K, editors. Movement disorders affecting sleep. Philadelphia: Elsevier; 2011.

37. Montagna P, Provini F, Plazzi G, Liguori R, Lugaresi E. Propriospinal myoclonus upon relaxation and drowsiness: a cause of severe insomnia. Mov Disord. 1997;12:66–72.

38. Vetrugno R, Provini F, Meletti S, Plazzi G, Liguori R, Cortelli P, et al. Propriospinal myoclonus at the sleep-wake transition: a new type of parasomnia. Sleep. 2001;24:835–43.

39. Vetrugno R, Provini F, Plazzi G, Cortelli P, Montagna P. Propriospinal myoclonus: a motor phenomenon found in restless legs syndrome different from periodic limb movements during sleep. Mov Disord. 2005;20:1323–29.

40. Manconi M, Sferrazza B, Iannaccone S, Massimo A, Zucconi M, Ferini-Strambi L. Case of symptomatic propriospinal myoclonus evolving toward acute "myoclonic status". Mov Disord. 2005;20:1646–50.

41. Khoo SM, Tan JH, Shi DX, et al. Propriospinal myoclonus at sleep onset causing severe insomnia: a polysomnographic and electromyographic analysis. Sleep Med. 2009;10:686–8.

42. Critchley M. The pre-dormitum. Rev Neurol (Paris). 1955;93:101–6.

43. Chervin RD, Consens FB, Kutluay E. Alternating leg muscle activation during sleep and arousals: a new sleep-related motor phenomenon? Mov Disord. 2003;18:551–9.

44. Cosentino FI, Iero I, Lanuzza B, Tripodi M, Ferri R. The neurophysiology of the alternating leg muscle activation (ALMA) during sleep: study of one patient before and after treatment with pramipexole. Sleep Med. 2006;7:63–71.

45. Chokroverty S, Thomas R, editors. Atlas of sleep medicine, 2nd ed. Philadelphia Elsevier 2013.

46. Symonds CP. Nocturnal myoclonus. J Neurol Neurosurg Psychiatry. 1953;16:166–71.

47. Coleman RM, Pollak CP, Weitzman ED. Periodic movements in sleep (nocturnal myoclonus): relation to sleep disorders. Ann Neurol. 1980;8:416–21.

48. Bliwise D, Petta D, Seidel W, Dement W. Periodic leg movements during sleep in the elderly. Arch Gerontol Geriatr. 1985;4:273–81.

49. Lugaresi E, Tassinari CA, Coccagna G, Ambrosetto C. Particularités cliniques et polygraphiques du syndrome d'impatiences des membres inférieurs. Rev Neurol (Paris). 1965;113:545–55.

50. Coccagna G, Lugaresi E, Tassinari CA, Amrosetto G. La syndrome delle gambe senza riposo (restless legs). Omnia Med Ther (Nuova Serie). 1966;44:619–84.

51. Wechsler LR, Stakes JW, Shahani BT, Busis NA. Periodic leg movements of sleep (nocturnal myoclonus): an electrophysiological study. Ann Neurol. 1986;19:168–73.

52. Provini F, Vetrugno R, Meletti S, Plazzi G, Solieri L, Lugaresi E, et al. Motor pattern of periodic limb movements during sleep. Neurology. 2001;57:300–4.

53. de Weerd AW, Rijsman RM, Brinkley A. Activity patterns of leg muscles in periodic limb movement disorder. J Neurol Neurosurg Psychiatry. 2004;75:317–9.

54. Ali NJ, Davies RJ, Fleetham JA, Stradling JR. Periodic movements of the legs during sleep associated with rises in systemic blood pressure. Sleep. 1991;14:163–5.

55. Pollmächer T, Schulz H. Periodic leg movements (PLM): their relationship to sleep stages. Sleep. 1993;16:572–7.

56. Chabli A, Michaud M, Montplaisir J. Periodic arm movements in patients with the restless legs syndrome. Eur Neurol. 2000;44:133–8.

57. Nofzinger EA, Fasiczka A, Berman S, Thase ME. Bupropion SR reduces periodic limb movements associated with arousals from sleep in depressed patients with periodic limb movement disorder. J Clin Psychiatry. 2000;61:858–62.

58. Pessah MA, Roffwarg HP. Spontaneous middle ear muscle activity in man: a rapid eye movement sleep phenomenon. Science. 1972;178(4062):773–6.

59. Megirian D, Cespuglio R, Jouvet M. Rhythmical activity of the rat's tongue in sleep and wakefulness. Electroencephalogr Clin Neurophysiol. 1978;44:8–13.

60. Chokroverty S. Phasic tongue movements in rapid eye movements sleep. Neurology 1980;30:665–8.

61. Pevernagie DA, Boon PA, Mariman AN, Verhaeghen DB, Pauwels RA. Vocalization during episodes of prolonged expiration: a parasomnia related to REM sleep. Sleep Med. 2001;2:19–30.

62. Vetrugno R, Provini F, Plazzi G, Vignatelli L, Lugaresi E, Montagna P. Catathrenia (nocturnal groaning): a new type of parasomnia. Neurology. 2001;56:681–3.

63. Vetrugno R, Lugaresi E, Plazzi G, Provini F, D'Angelo R, Montagna P. Catathrenia (nocturnal groaning): an abnormal respiratory pattern during sleep. Eur J Neurol. 2007;14:1236–43.

64. Ott SR, Hamacher J, Seifert E. Bringing light to the sirens of night: laryngoscopy in catathrenia during sleep. Eur Respir J. 2011;37:1288–9.

65. Koo DL, Hong SB, Joo EY. Acoustic characteristic of catathrenia and snoring: different subtypes of catathrenia. Sleep Med. 2012;13:961–4.

66. Songu M, Yilmaz H, Yuceturk AV, Gunhan K, Ince A, Bayturan O. Effect of CPAP therapy on catathrenia and OSA: a case report and review of the literature. Sleep Breath. 2008;12:401–5.

67. Iriarte J, Alegre M, Urrestarazu E, Viteri C, Arcocha J, Artieda J. Continuous positive airway pressure as treatment for catathrenia (nocturnal groaning). Neurology. 2006;66:609–10.

68. Broughton R, Tolentino MA, Krelina M. Excessive fragmentary myoclonus in NREM sleep: a report of 38 cases. Electroencephalogr Clin Neurophysiol. 1985;61:123–33.

69. Tolentino MA. Fragmentary pathological myoclonus in NREM sleep. Electroencephalogr Clin Neurophysiol. 1984;57:303–9.

70. Lins O, Castonguay M, Dunham W, Nevsimalova S, Broughton R. Excessive fragmentary myoclonus: time of night and sleep stage distributions. Can J Neurol Sci. 1993;20:142–6.

71. Hoque R, McCarty DE, Chesson AL Jr. Manual quantitative assessment of amplitude and sleep stage distribution of excessive fragmentary myoclonus. J Clin Sleep Med. 2013;9:39–45.

72. Vetrugno R, Plazzi G, Provini F, Liguori R, Lugaresi E, Montagna P. Excessive fragmentary hypnic myoclonus: clinical and neurophysiological findings. Sleep Med. 2002;3:73–6.

73. Reding GR, Rubright WC, Rechtschaffen A, Daniels RS. Sleep pattern of tooth-greending: its relationship to dreaming. Science. 1964;145(3633):725–6.

74. Clarke NG, Townsend GC. Distribution of nocturnal bruxing patterns in man. J Oral Rehabil. 1984;11:529–34.

75. Wieselmann G, Permann R, Körner E, Flooh E, Reinhart B, Moser F, et al. Distribution of muscle activity during sleep in bruxism. Eur Neurol. 1986;25(S2):111–6.

76. Lavigne GJ, Rompré PH, Poirier G, Huard H, Kato T, Montplaisir JY. Rhythmic masticatory muscle activity during sleep in humans. J Dent Res. 2001;80:443–8.

77. Manconi M, Zucconi M, Carrot B, Ferri R, Oldani A, Ferini-Strambi L. Association between bruxism and nocturnal groaning. Mov Disord. 2008;23:737–39.

78. Braun AR, Balkin TJ., Wesenten NJ, Carson RE, Varga N, Baldwin P, et al. Regional cerebral blood flow throughout the sleep-wake cycle. An H2(15)O PET study. Brain. 1997;120:1173–97.

79. Llinas RR, Steriade M. Bursting of thalamic neurons and states of vigilance. J Neurophysiol. 2006;95(6):3297–308.

80. Horner RL, Sanford LD, Pack AI, Morrison AR. Activation of a distinct arousal state immediately after spontaneous arousal from sleep. Brain Res. 1997;778:127–34.

81. Schacter DL. The hypnagogic state: a clinical review of the literature. Psychol Bull. 1976;83:452–81.

82. Montagna P, Lugaresi E. Sleep benefit in Parkinson's disease. Mov Disord. 1998;13:751–52.

83. Vetrugno R, Montagna P, Sleep-to-wake transition movement disorders. Sleep Med. 2011;12;S11–6.

84. Adie W. Idiopathic narcolepsy: a disease sui generis; with remarks on the mechanism of the brain. Brain. 1926;49:257–306.

85. Wilson S. The narcolepsies. Brain. 1928;51:63–77.

86. Tassi P, Muzet A. Sleep inertia. Sleep Med Rev. 2000;4:341–53.

87. Marzano C, Ferrara M, Moroni F, De Gennaro I. Electroencephalographic sleep inertia of the awakening brain. Neuroscience 2011;176:308–17.

88. Roth B, Nevsimalova S, Rechtschaffen A. Hypersomnia with sleep drunkenness. Arch Gen Psychiatry. 1972;26:456–62.

89. Hening WA, Allen RP, Walters AS, Chokroverty S. Motor functions and dysfunctions of sleep. In: Chokroverty S, editor. Sleep disorders medicine: basic science, technical considerations and clinical aspects, 3rd ed. Philadelphia: Saunders Elsevier; 2009. pp. 397–435.

90. Silvestri RC. Persistence of daytime movement disorders during sleep. In: Chokroverty S, Allen RP, Walters AS, Montagna P, editors. Sleep and movements disorders, 2nd ed. New York: Oxford University Press; 2013. pp. 535–45.

91. Fahn S, Chokroverty S. Movement disorders and sleep: Introduction. In: Chokroverty S, Allen RP, Walters AS, Montagna P, editors. Sleep and movements disorders, 2nd ed. New York: Oxford University Press; 2013. pp 533–34.

92. Fish DR, Sawyers D, Allen PJ, Blackie JD, Lees AJ, Marsden CD. The effect of sleep on the dyskinetic movements of Parkinson's disease, Gilles de la Tourette syndrome, Huntington's disease, and torsion dystonia. Arch Neurol. 1991;48:210–4.

93. Parkinson J. An essay on the Shaking Palsy. London: Whittingham and Rowland; 1817.

94. Askenasy JJ, Yahr MD. Parkinsonian tremor loses its alternating aspects during Non-REM sleep and is inhibited by REM sleep. J Neurol Neursurg Psychiatr. 1990;53:749–53.

95. Merello M, Hughes A, Colosino C, Hoffman M, Starkstein S, Leiguarda R. Sleep benefit in Parkinson's disease. Mov Disor. 1997;12:506–9.

96. Glaze DG, Frost JD Jr, Jankovic J. Sleep in Gilles de la Tourette's syndrome: disorder of arousal. Neurology. 1983;33:586–92.

97. Barabas G, Matthews WS, Ferrari M. Somnambulism in children with Tourette syndrome. Dev Med Child Neurol. 1984;26:457–60.

98. Montagna P, Imbriaco A, Zucconi M, Liguori R, Cirignotta F, Lugaresi E. Hemifacial spasm in sleep. Neurology. 1986;36:270–3.

99. Chokroverty S, Barron KD. Palatal myoclonus and rhythmic ocular movements: a polygraphic study. Neurology. 1969;19:975–82.

100. Deuschl G, Mischke G, Schenck E, Schulte-Mönting J, Lücking CH. Symptomatic and essential rhythmic palatal myoclonus. Brain. 1990;113:1645–72.

101. Lapresle J. Palatal myoclonus. Adv Neurol. 1986;43:265–73.

102. Chokroverty S. Unusual movements disorders. In: Chokroverty S, Allen RP, Walters AS, Montagna P, editors. Sleep and movement disorders, 2nd ed. New York: Oxford University Press; 2013. pp. 710–13.

History of Restless Legs Syndrome, Recently Named Willis–Ekbom Disease

Richard P. Allen

Willis–Ekbom disease (WED) classically known as restless legs syndrome (RLS) has a remarkable history demonstrating interlocking relations between biology and treatment of a medical disorder. WED had little effective treatment or recognition until the later part of the twentieth century when critical advances occurred in understanding the biology of the disorder and treatment options. Prior to these developments, thousands suffered from a tortuous inability to remain at rest in the evening or night. This was well described by Thomas Willis in 1685 [1] as

> leapings and contractions of tendons and so great the restlessness and tossing of their members (arms and legs) ensure, that the diseased are no more able to sleep than if they were in the place of greatest torture.

The actual number with such extreme suffering is somewhat uncertain even today, but the most conservative estimate would be about 0.2–0.8% of the adults in Western Europe and North America (USA and Canada) [2, 3] or more than two million adults. These individuals suffered torturous nights without effective treatment or even recognition of their disorder. The history of WED provides an excellent example of how scientifically based medical developments significantly reduce human suffering.

The history of the WED divides into two phases, i.e., early clinical descriptions of a syndrome and disease conceptualization. Features of the disease conceptualization develop simultaneously along various separate tracks representing developments in diagnosis, patient advocacy, epidemiology, biology, and treatment. This small section can only provide a general overview of this remarkable history and thus focuses on the developments in each area most related to advances in treatment and diagnosis.

Early Reports of WED

Thomas Willis provided the first known medical description of WED in his Latin discourses in 1672 [4] and translated into English in a posthumously published collection of his writings in 1685 [1]. There are scattered limited descriptions of WED after that, mostly from the nineteenth and early twentieth century. The nineteenth-century descriptions were mostly similar to that of Wittmaack who in 1861 referred to WED symptoms as *anxietas tibiarum* [5]. Beard similarly in 1880 refers to WED in relation to "nervous exhaustion" [6]. The nineteenth-century terms used to describe WED at that time indicated a clinical condition without a well-defined biological basis, but these were later read as indicating WED was a psychiatric disorder associated with neuroses and anxiety. This unfortunate linguistic distortion produced a general neglect of WED as a neurological disease.

Diagnosis

It was not until the seminal work by Ekbom in the 1940s [7,8] that WED was restored to consideration as a neurological disease. Others, at about this time, also described the disorder as medical not psychiatric condition, e.g., Mussio-Fournier and Rawak in 1940 refer to inherited familial disease worsening during pregnancy [9], and Allison in 1943 describes "leg jitters" as "a combination of voluntary and involuntary jerks" disturbing sleep [10]. None before Ekbom produced a systematic case series nor a careful description of a large clinical sample. Ekbom's monograph translated into English from Swedish in 1945 [8] provides the first definitive description of the disease and the basis for its current view as neurological disorder. He emphasized both the urge to move and the sensory discomfort with the disorder and named it "restless legs." He clearly identified this as a chronic condition, which he saw as having exclusively or mainly subjective symptoms that "embitter but do not endanger the patient's life."

R. P. Allen (✉)
Department of Neurology, Johns Hopkins University,
Baltimore, MD, USA
e-mail: rallen6@jhmi.edu

S. Chokroverty, M. Billiard (eds.), *Sleep Medicine,* DOI 10.1007/978-1-4939-2089-1_30,
© Springer Science+Business Media, LLC 2015

After Ekbom, the development of attention to physiological recordings of sleep produced a discovery in 1953 of periodic leg movements during sleep (PLMS) [11], which were found to be very common among WED patients [12]. Thus, the sleep field added to the RLS diagnosis the motor signs of PLMS that were found to be fairly specific [13] but not sensitive for diagnosis of WED [14], largely because they occur at high rates in healthy adults over age 45 [15]. Unfortunately, the sleep medicine field when establishing their initial diagnostic criteria for sleep-related disorders distorted the characteristics of WED over emphasizing nighttime symptoms and the sleep disturbance and also PLMS as closely associated with the sleep disruption [16]. This produced considerable confusion about the relation of PLMS to WED that has persisted to some extent. Studies have since clearly demonstrated that the sleep disturbance of WED does not relate to the commonly occurring PLMS but reflects a separate aspect of the disease [13, 17].

At about the same time as the development of sleep medicine interest in WED, three movement disorder experts also "discovered" WED. Arthur Walters and Wayne Hening under the supervision of Sudhansu Chokroverty noted pronounced WED symptoms in a small series of patients and reported for the first time the periodic limb movements during resting wake state [18]. This important work emphasized the need for a diagnostic criteria for WED established not by experts in other fields, but by those working with the disorder. Walters with support from Hening formed the International RLS Study Group (IRLSSG) comprised of 28 WED experts from North American and Europe. Based on their shared clinical experiences, they were able to reach unanimous consensus on a set of four essential diagnostic criteria defining WED [19]. These four criteria emphasize the sensory urge to move (or akathisia) the legs as primary with sensory discomfort common but not always present. The criteria note rest or inactivity engender, and movement relieves the symptoms. Finally, there is a strong circadian component with symptoms exclusive or worse in the evening or night than in the morning. Thus, the patient can remain at rest longer without symptoms in the morning than in the evening.

The initial formulation of the four basic WED diagnostic criteria confounded rest engendering with activity relieving the symptoms, and included a concept of restless feelings that turned out to be confusing. These technical problems were corrected in a 2002 major consensus conference of the IRLSSG held at the National Institute of Health in Washington D.C., USA, chaired by Richard Allen. This led to the definitive four essential diagnostic criteria for WED that have provided the basis for recent major advances in epidemiology, biology, and treatment of WED. This 2002 conference also identified the treatment emergent problem of WED augmentation and noted the special diagnostic considerations for children and cognitively impaired adults [20].

Further clinical experience documented that conditions can "mimic" WED symptoms requiring attention to differential diagnosis to exclude these conditions. The "mimics" produce symptoms that are sometimes hard to discriminate from those defining WED, except the "mimics" are usually closely tied to another condition and the symptoms of the "mimics" almost but not totally match the full extent of the WED symptoms [21]. This pointed out the need for adding a fifth essential diagnostic criterion requiring exclusion of the "mimics." A 4-year process to update the RLS diagnostic criteria started with a 2008 clinical conference sponsored by the IRLSSG at Johns Hopkins in Baltimore, MD, USA. These were approved in 2012 after review at an annual meeting of members followed by a web-based review by all members and are available on www.irlssg.org website [21a]. (See Table 30.1.)

The IRLSSG diagnostic criteria reflect the view that WED is a neurological disease. Two other disciplines have defined WED as either a sleep-related disorder or a psychiatric disorder and in the process have unfortunately distorted the diagnosis to fit their particular discipline ignoring the neurological basis for this disease. So there is one correct set of diagnostic criteria (Table 30.1) and unfortunately two that err particularly in each having a totally arbitrary and different criterion not supported by data for frequency of symptoms required before the diagnosis can be made. RLS diagnosed independently by two neurologists experienced with RLS with 100% agreement included 19% who did not have symptoms at least twice a week (required by the sleep medicine diagnostic criteria) and 33% who did not have symptoms at least three times a week [21b].

Patient Advocacy

Since there had been little professional help available for treatment of WED, the patients themselves organized self-help groups and national organizations around the world to advocate for better recognition, treatment, and eventually a cure for the disease. The experience in the USA started with kitchen table meetings of three RLS patients: Pickett Guthrie, Virginia Wilson, and Robert Balkam. This developed into the current WED foundation with several thousand members and a regular "nightwalkers" publication. Early in this development another WED sufferer, Robert H Yoakum, a well-known humanist and author wrote an article on WED for Modern Maturity. This article produced more reader response as compared to others. More than 40,000 letters were sent to the magazine from older adults reporting relief that someone had identified the cause of their nighttime tortures. Thus, the WED foundation began its continuing campaign for recognition and acceptance of WED in the medical establishment. Today, there are active patient advocacy groups not only in the USA but also in most western European countries. They hold in conjunction with the IRLSSG an annual WED awareness day on Ekbom's birthday.

Severity Assessment

Early in the development of WED evaluations, it became clear that a clinical scale was needed to assess WED severity. A scale called the IRLS, developed and validated in 2002 by the IRLSSG, has since provided a standard unifying clinical WED studies. This ten-item scale has scores ranging from 0 to 40, excellent psychometric properties [22, 23] and two subscales, i.e., symptoms and impact [23]. The scale has been translated into 32 or more languages and is available from Messaging Application Programming Interface (MAPI) Research Trust Patient-Reported Outcome & Quality of Life Instruments Database (Proqolid) at http://www.proqolid.org.

Epidemiology

The initial efforts to determine prevalence of WED used questionnaires asking patients about critical diagnostic symptoms. Efforts before the development of the full diagnostic criteria had a very limited set of questions missing some of the essential features of the diagnosis and produced surprisingly high prevalence, e.g., 15 % of French Canadians [24]. Subsequent better studies relied upon questions covering the four essential diagnostic criteria of IRLSSG and often added some assessment to identify clinically significant RLS. Among the best of these, the RLS epidemiology, symptoms, and treatment (REST) studies have served to define out the understanding of RLS prevalence in Europe and USA. The REST general population study documented a 7 % prevalence for RLS symptoms occurring in the past year and more significantly a 2.7 % prevalence for RLS sufferers, i.e., those with symptoms occurring in the past year usually at least twice a week with moderate to severe distress when occurring [25]. The REST study documents characteristics of the RLS sufferers including the increasing prevalence with

Table 30.1 2013 diagnostic criteria for restless legs syndrome/Willis–Ekbom disease. The preferred diagnostic criteria published by the International Restless Legs Syndrome Study Group). (From Allen, R. P., et al., 2014)

IRLSSG Consensus Diagnostic Criteria for RLS (2012)

Restless legs syndrome (RLS), a neurological sensorimotor disease often profoundly disturbing sleep and quality of life, has variable expression influenced by genetic, environmental, and medical factors. The symptoms vary considerably in frequency from less than once a month or year to daily and the severity varies from mildly annoying to disabling. Symptoms may also remit for various periods of time. RLS is diagnosed by ascertaining symptom patterns that meet the following five essential criteria adding clinical specifiers where appropriate

Essential Diagnostic Criteria (all must be met)

1. An urge to move the legs usually but not always accompanied by or felt to be caused by uncomfortable and unpleasant sensations in the legs[a, b]
2. The urge to move the legs and any accompanying unpleasant sensations begin or worsen during periods of rest or inactivity such as lying down or sitting
3. The urge to move the legs and any accompanying unpleasant sensations are partially or totally relieved by movement, such as walking or stretching, at least as long as the activity continues[c]
4. The urge to move the legs and any accompanying unpleasant sensations during rest or inactivity only occur or are worse in the evening or night than during the day[d]
5. The occurrence of the above features is not solely accounted for as symptoms primary to another medical or a behavioral condition (e.g., myalgia, venous stasis, leg edema, arthritis, leg cramps, positional discomfort, habitual foot tapping.)[e]

Specifiers for Clinical Course of RLS[f]

A. Chronic-persistent RLS: Symptoms when not treated would occur on average at least twice weekly for the past year
B. Intermittent RLS: Symptoms when not treated occured on an average of less than twice per week for the past year, with at least five lifetime events

Specifier for Clinical Significance of RLS

The symptoms of RLS cause significant distress or impairment in social, occupational, educational, or other important areas of functioning by the impact on sleep, energy/vitality, daily activities, behavior, cognition, or mood

[a] Sometimes the urge to move the legs is present without the uncomfortable sensations and sometimes the arms or other parts of the body are involved in addition to the legs
[b] For children, the description of these symptoms should be in the child's own words
[c] When symptoms are very severe, relief by activity may not be noticeable but must have been previously present
[d] When symptoms are very severe, the worsening in the evening or night may not be noticeable but must have been previously present
[e] These conditions, often referred to as "RLS mimics," have been commonly confused with RLS particularly in surveys because they produce symptoms that meet or at least come very close to meeting criteria 1–4. The list here gives some examples that have been noted as particularly significant in epidemiological studies and clinical practice. RLS may also occur with any of these conditions, but the RLS symptoms will then be more in degree, conditions of expression or character than those usually occurring as part of the other condition
[f] The clinical course criteria do not apply for pediatric cases nor for some special cases of provoked RLS such as pregnancy or drug induced RLS where the frequency may be high but limited to duration of the provocative condition

age and a 2:1 female: male ratio. It is often misunderstood that these characteristics were not determined for all RLS but only RLS sufferers.

The developing understanding of WED mimics indicated that the questionnaire approach without any effort to correct for mimics would likely produce a low false positive rate. The 4-item questionnaire diagnosis compared in one large international study with trained physician diagnosis had, indeed, only a 58 % positive predictive value for identification of RLS sufferers [2]. In another study questions asking about the four diagnostic criteria compared to a validated questionnaire excluding mimics had only a 50 % positive predictive value [3]. It takes a very high specificity with reasonable sensitivity to obtain a reasonable positive predictive value for identification of a condition with about a 5 % prevalence. A questionnaire was then developed in a collaborative study involving Cambridge University and Johns Hopkins that included questions designed to exclude common "mimics." The validation compared to a clinical interview found for ascertainment of WED in a population of blood donors a positive predictive value of 86 % [26]. This questionnaire has since been used in other studies and as expected showed that using questions covering only the four-diagnostic criteria has a low positive-predictive value of about 50 % [26]. Moreover, among those determined to have RLS by the Cambridge–Hopkins questionnaire about 8 % had very severe, 38 % severe, and 12 % mild WED as defined by the IRLS.

Thus, the estimated prevalence for WED in Europe and North America is about half that reported in most prior questionnaire survey studies, e.g., about 3–5 % for WED symptoms in the past year, 1–2 % for current clinically significant WED, and about 0.2–0.8 % for very severe WED. The studies conducted in Asia including India have produced conflicting results related to population and methods, but overall indicate lower prevalence than in Europe or the USA.

Biology

There have been two major historic developments in understanding the biology of WED involving iron and genetics. Iron deficiency had long been associated with increased risk of WED and oral iron treatments reversed or reduced WED symptoms [27, 28]. Most RLS patients, however, have normal blood levels of iron and iron-related proteins. This puzzle was resolved by a major breakthrough in understanding WED when magnetic resonance imaging (MRI) studies showed decreased brain iron in the substantia nigra for patients with normal peripheral iron [29] (see Fig. 30.1). This seminal work from Hopkins has since been confirmed by several other studies based on MRI [30], ultrasound [31–34], and autopsy. [35]. The biological basis for the brain iron loss remains to be determined but may reflect a metabolic disorder affecting iron transport to the brain or the distribution and maintenance of

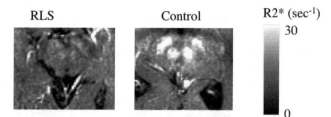

Figure 2. R2* images in a 70 year old RLS patient and a 71 year old control subject. Much lower R2* relaxation rates are apparent in the RLS case in both red nucleus and substantia nigra.
Allen et al , Neurology 56:263-5, 2001

Fig. 30.1 MRI R2* images in a 70-year-old RLS patient and a 71-year-old control subject. Much lower R2* relaxation rates are apparent in the RLS case in both substantia nigra and red nucleus

iron in the brain. An active body of research on iron metabolic disturbances and WED has been produced by Earley and Allen at Johns Hopkins in collaboration with James Conner at Penn State School of medicine. The important historic factor is that these documented a biological basis for WED involving the brain and thus WED is a neurological disease.

The second major biological advance came from genetic studies. The family prevalence of RLS has been known since the early cases reported by Ekbom [8]. Genetic linkage studies from large families failed to produce a genetic basis for any of WED. When genome wide association studies became available and were tried with RLS, they provided clear genetic risk factors for RLS. This was demonstrated in two primary studies published at the same time: Stefansson, Rye, and others working with an Icelandic population found a major allele on the BTBD9 gene that increased risk of RLS and also was associated with peripheral iron status [35a]. Winkelmann and colleagues at the Max Plank found allelic variations increasing the risk of RLS on three genes including BDBT9 [36]. These seminal studies have provided the basis for continuing genetic studies of WED. Presumably, the genetics, environmental factors (iron deficiency, pregnancy, age), and iron biology will coalesce into a better understanding of WED biology. That work is ongoing.

The one major area of disappointment from biological studies remains the failure to date to find any conclusive dopamine abnormalities in RLS, despite the efficacy of dopamine treatment.

Treatment

Success leading to a major disappointment marks the history of WED treatment. The earliest treatments with opioids by among others Willis in the seventeenth century [1] produced good but mixed results [37] and treatment with hypnotics promoted sleep but had limited other benefits for PLMS [38] or other WED symptoms [39]. In contrast, Akpinar reported dramatic benefit from levodopa treatment of WED [40] that was subsequently confirmed in blinded comparator trial between levodopa, propoxyphene, and placebo [41, 42]. At this time, dopamine agonists were being introduced for the treatment of Parkinson's disease. The first of these, pergolide, was shown in initial studies at Johns Hopkins to produce dramatic relief from WED symptoms [43]. This was later also documented for the dopamine agonists pramipexole [44] and ropinirole [45]. Pergolide has since been withdrawn from the market owing to adverse cardiac effects but both ropinirole and pramipexole received wide regulatory approval for treatment of WED and became the drugs of first choice for WED treatment. Patients who had not slept more than 4–6 h a night with these treatments could sleep through most of the night. It seemed a miracle "cure" for WED. But a major disappointment lurked behind the initial success.

Treatment longer than the usual 3-month study revealed disquieting evidence that the dopaminergic medications were making the underlying WED disease worse. This iatrogenic WED augmentation was initially reported and defined by Allen and Earley at Johns Hopkins [46] and later confirmed for other dopaminergic medications [47, 48]. The worsening of WED (augmentation) necessitated increasing the dopaminergic dose. Symptom intensity, amount of the body involved, and amount of the day with symptoms increased for WED. In severe cases patients with initial leg symptoms at night now had leg and arm symptoms 24 h a day, somewhat controlled at night by high doses of dopamine agonists. Adverse effects of compulsiveness and sleepiness became more of a problem. Thus, what started so promising has ended hurting patients. This major problem in WED treatment has led to a reappraisal of treatment approaches.

Fortunately, new studies have documented that the new alpha-2-delta ligand anticonvulsants also provide dramatic benefit for WED that in one study was slightly better than treatment with the dopamine agonists pramipexole. One of these medications, gabapentin enacarbil (Horizant), has been extensively tested [49–51] and is now approved by the Food and Drug Administration (FDA) for WED treatment. There are also indications that high-potency opioid treatment is effective for patients who do not respond to dopaminergic medications [52]. A committee of the IRLSSG met in Madrid in 2012 and under the direction of Diego Garcia Borreguero produced an evidence based and expert consensus on long-term treatment of WED. This emphasizes avoiding dopaminergic augmentation by either keeping the dopaminergic dose low or starting with a very long acting dopamine agonist or an alpha-2-delta ligand as the first medication.

However, perhaps the most interesting treatment development has been the logical development of iron treatment of RLS. The biological studies indicated that increasing peripheral iron to higher levels could produce some increase in brain iron [53] that at least, theoretically, could reduce WED symptoms. IV iron provides one method to produce high peripheral iron status and had been tried with consid-

erable success by Nordlander [54, 55] in the middle of the twentieth century. A recent animal study has indicated that IV iron in mice with experimentally induced decreased iron in the substantia nigra will normalize the iron in that brain area without producing iron overload in other areas [56]. The problem is determining the correct iron formulation and IV dose. The limited data available indicate this may be a promising treatment for 25–50 % of the WED patients producing in one treatment a long lasting relief of more than a year from their symptoms. This treatment development stems from the consideration of the biology of RLS and is supported by preclinical animal studies. More work like that is needed to advance RLS treatments

References

1. Willis T. The London practice of physick. London: Bassett and Crooke; 1685.
2. Allen RP, Stillman P, Myers AJ. Physician-diagnosed restless legs syndrome in a large sample of primary medical care patients in western Europe: prevalence and characteristics. Sleep Med. 2010;11:31–7.
3. Allen RP, Bharmal M, Calloway M. Prevalence and disease burden of primary restless legs syndrome: results of a general population survey in the United States. Mov Disord. 2011;26:114–20.
4. Willis T. De Animae Brutorum. London: Wells and Scott; 1672.
5. Wittmaack T. Pathologie und Therapie der Sensibilitäts neurosen. Liepzig: Schäfer; 1861.
6. Beard G. A practical treatis on nervous exhaustion. New York: William Wood; 1880.
7. Ekbom KA. Asthenia crurum paraesthetica ("irritable legs"). Acta Medica Scandinavica. 1944;118(1–3):197–209.
8. Ekbom KA. Restless legs. Stockholm: Ivar Haeggströms; 1945.
9. Mussio-Fournier JC, Rawak F. Familiäres Auftreten von Pruritus, Utikaria und parästhetischer Hyperkinese der unteren Extremitäten. Confinia Neurol. 1940;3:110–4.
10. Allison FG. Obscure pains in the chest, back or limbs. Can Med Assoc J. 1943;48:36–9.
11. Symonds CP. Nocturnal myoclonus. J Neurol Neurosurg Psychiatr. 1953;16:166.
12. Lugaresi E, Coccagna G, Berti Ceroni G, Ambrosetto C. Restless legs syndrome and nocturnal myoclonus. In: Gastaut H, Lugaresi E, Berti Ceroni G, editors. The abnormalites of sleep in man. Bologna: Aulo Gaggi Editore; 1968. 285–94.
13. Montplaisir J, Boucher S, Poirier G, Lavigne G, Lapierre O, Lesperance P. Clinical, polysomnographic, and genetic characteristics of restless legs syndrome: a study of 133 patients diagnosed with new standard criteria. Mov Disord. 1997;12:61–5.
14. Montplaisir J, Michaud M, Denesle R, Gosselin A. Periodic leg movements are not more prevalent in insomnia or hypersomnia but are specifically associated with sleep disorders involving a dopaminergic impairment. Sleep Med. 2000;1:163–7.
15. Pennestri MH, Whittom S, Adam B, Petit D, Carrier J, Montplaisir J. PLMS and PLMW in healthy subjects as a function of age: prevalence and interval distribution. Sleep. 2006;29:1183–7.
16. ASDA. International classification of sleep disorders, revised: Diagnostic and coding manual. Rochester, Minnesota: American Sleep Disorders Association; 1997.
17. Allen RP, Barker PB, Horska A, Earley CJ. Thalamic glutamate/glutamine in restless legs syndrome: increased and related to disturbed sleep. Neurology. 2013;80:2028–34.

18. Walters AS, Hening WA, Chokroverty S. Frequent occurrence of myoclonus while awake and at rest, body rocking and marching in place in a subpopulation of patients with restless legs syndrome. Acta Neurol Scand. 1988;77:418–21.

19. Walters AS, Aldrich MA, Allen RP, Ancoli-Israel S, Buchholz D, Chockroverty S, et al. Toward a better definition of the restless legs syndrome. Mov Disord. 1995;10:634–42.

20. Allen RP, Picchietti D, Hening WA, Trenkwalder C, Walters AS, Montplaisir J. Restless legs syndrome: diagnostic criteria, special considerations, and epidemiology. A report from the restless legs syndrome diagnosis and epidemiology workshop at the National Institutes of Health. Sleep Med. 2003;4:101–19.

21. Hening WA, Allen RP, Washburn M, Lesage S, Earley C. The four diagnostic criteria for the restless legs syndrome are unable to exclude confounding conditions ("mimics"). Sleep Med. 2009;10:976–81.

21a. Cho, Y.W., et al., *Prevalence and clinical characteristics of restless legs syndrome in diabetic peripheral neuropathy: comparison with chronic osteoarthritis.* Sleep Med, 2013; 14: 1387–92

21b. Allen RP, Picchietti DL, Garcia-Borreguero D, Ondo WG, Walter AS, Winkelman JW, et al. Restless legs syndrome/Willis-Ekbom disease diagnostic criteria: updated International Restless Legs Syndrome Study Group (IRLSSG) consensus criteria history, rationale, description, and signifi cance. Sleep Med, 2014;15:860–73.

22. Walters AS, LeBrocq C, Dhar A, Hening W, Rosen R, Allen RP, et al. Validation of the International Restless Legs Syndrome Study Group rating scale for restless legs syndrome. Sleep Med. 2003;4:121–32.

23. Abetz L, Arbuckle R, Allen RP, Garcia-Borreguero D, Hening W, Walters AS, et al. The reliability, validity and responsiveness of the International Restless Legs Syndrome Study Group rating scale and subscales in a clinical-trial setting. Sleep Med. 2006;7:340–9.

24. Lavigne GJ, Montplaisir JY. Restless legs syndrome and sleep bruxism: prevalence and association among Canadians. Sleep. 1994;17:739–43.

25. Allen RP, Walters AS, Montplaisir J, Hening W, Myers A, Bell TJ, et al. Restless legs syndrome prevalence and impact: REST general population study. Arch Intern Med. 2005;165:1286–92.

26. Allen RP, Burchell BJ, MacDonald B, Hening WA, Earley CJ. Validation of the self-completed Cambridge-Hopkins questionnaire (CH-RLSq) for ascertainment of restless legs syndrome (RLS) in a population survey. Sleep Med. 2009;10:1097–100.

27. O'Keeffe ST, Gavin K, Lavan JN. Iron status and restless legs syndrome in the elderly. Age Ageing. 1994;23:200–3.

28. O'Keeffe ST, Noel J, Lavan JN. Restless legs syndrome in the elderly. Postgrad Med J. 1993;69:701–3.

29. Allen RP, Barker PB, Wehrl F, Song HK, Earley CJ. MRI measurement of brain iron in patients with restless legs syndrome. Neurology. 2001;56:263–5.

30. Earley CJ, Barker PB, Horska A, Allen RP. MRI-determined regional brain iron concentrations in early- and late-onset restless legs syndrome. Sleep Med. 2006;7:459–61.

31. Schmidauer C, Sojer M, Seppi K, Stockner H, Hogl B, Biedermann B, et al. Transcranial ultrasound shows nigral hypoechogenicity in restless legs syndrome. Ann Neurol. 2005;58:630–4.

32. Godau J, Klose U, Di Santo A, Schweitzer K, Berg D. Multiregional brain iron deficiency in restless legs syndrome. Mov Disord. 2008;23:1184–7.

33. Godau J, Manz A, Wevers AK, Gaenslen A, Berg D. Sonographic substantia nigra hypoechogenicity in polyneuropathy and restless legs syndrome. Mov Disord. 2009;24:133–7.

34. Godau J, Schweitzer KJ, Liepelt I, Gerloff C, Berg D. Substantia nigra hypoechogenicity: definition and findings in restless legs syndrome. Mov Disord. 2007;22:187–92.

35. Connor JR, Boyer PJ, Menzies SL, Dellinger B, Allen RP, Earley CJ. Neuropathological examination suggests impaired brain iron acquisition in restless legs syndrome. Neurology. 2003;61:304–9.

35a. Stefansson H1, Rye DB, Hicks A, et al. A genetic risk factor for periodic limb movements in sleep. N Engl J Med. 2007 Aug 16;357(7):639-47.

36. Winkelmann J, Schormair B, Lichtner P, Ripke S, Xiong L, Jalilzadeh S, et al. Genome-wide association study of restless legs syndrome identifies common variants in three genomic regions. Nat Genet. 2007;39:1000–6.

37. Hening WA, Walters A, Kavey N, Gidro-Frank S, Cote L, Fahn S. Dyskinesias while awake and periodic movements in sleep in restless legs syndrome: treatment with opioids. Neurology. 1986;36:1363–6.

38. Mitler MM, Browman CP, Menn SJ, Gujavarty K, Timms RM. Nocturnal myoclonus: Treatment efficacy of clonazepam and temazepam. Sleep. 1986;9:385–92.

39. Boghen D, Lamothe L, Elie R, Godbout R, Montplaisir J. The treatment of the restless legs syndrome with clonazepam: a prospective controlled study. Can J Neurol Sci. 1986;13:245–7.

40. Akpinar S. Treatment of restless legs syndrome with levodopa plus benserazide [letter]. Arch Neurol. 1982;39:739.

41. Kaplan PW, Allen RP, Buchholz DW, Walters JK. A double-blind, placebo-controlled study of the treatment of periodic limb movements in sleep using carbidopa/levodopa and propoxyphene. Sleep. 1993;16:717–23.

42. Allen RP, Kaplan PW, Buchholz DW, Earley CJ, Walters JK. Double-blinded, placebo controlled comparison of high dose propoxyphene and moderate dose carbidopa/levodopa for treatment of periodic limb movements in sleep. Sleep Res. 1992;21:166.

43. Allen R, Early CJ, Hening WA, Walters AS, Wagner MI, Yaffee JB. Double-blind, placebo-controlled, multi-center evaluation of the restless legs syndrome treatment with pergolide (abstract). Sleep. 1998;21:142.

44. Montplaisir J, Nicolas A, Denesle R, Gomez-Mancilla B. Restless legs syndrome improved by pramipexole: a double-blind randomized trial. Neurology. 1999;52:938–43.

45. Freeman A, Rye D, Bliwise DL, Chakravorty S, Krulewicz S, Watts R. Ropinirole fo restless legs syndrome (RLS): an open-label and double-blind placebo-controlled study. Neurology. 2001;56:A5.

46. Allen RP, Early CJ. Augmentation of the restless legs syndrome with carbidopa/levodopa. Sleep. 1996;19:205–13.

47. Silber MH, Girish M, Izurieta R. Pramipexole in the management of restless legs syndrome: an extended study. Sleep. 2003;26:819–21.

48. Winkelman JW, Johnston L. Augmentation and tolerance with long-term pramipexole treatment of restless legs syndrome (RLS). Sleep Med. 2004;5:9–14.

49. Inoue Y, Uchimura N, Kuroda K, Hirata K, Hattori N. Long-term efficacy and safety of gabapentin enacarbil in Japanese restless legs syndrome patients. Prog Neuropsychopharmacol Biol Psychiatry. 2012;36:251–7.

50. Lee DO, Ziman RB, Perkins AT, Poceta JS, Walters AS, Barrett RW, et al. A randomized, double-blind, placebo-controlled study to assess the efficacy and tolerability of gabapentin enacarbil in subjects with restless legs syndrome. J Clin Sleep Med. 2011;7:282–92.

51. Walters AS, Ondo WG, Kushida CA, Becker PM, Ellenbogen AL, Canafax DM, et al. Gabapentin Enacarbil in Restless Legs Syndrome: A Phase 2b, 2-Week, Randomized, Double-Blind, Placebo-Controlled Trial. Clin Neuropharmacol. 2009; 6:311-20.

52. Ondo WG. Methadone for refractory restless legs syndrome. Mov Disord. 2005;20:345–8.

53. Earley CJ, Connors JR, Allen RP. RLS patients have abnormally reduced CSF ferritin compared to normal controls. Neurology. 1999;52 (suppl 2):A111–A2.

54. Nordlander NB. Therapy in restless legs. Acta Med Scand. 1953;145:453–7.

55. Nordlander NB. Restless legs. Brit J Phys Med. 1954;17:160–2.

56. Unger EL, Earley CJ, Thomsen LL, Jones BC, Allen RP. Effects of IV iron isomaltoside-1000 treatment on regional brain iron status in an iron-deficient animal. Neuroscience. 2013;246:179–85.

Sleep and Stroke

Mark Eric Dyken, Kyoung Bin Im and George B. Richerson

Background

Obstructive sleep apnea (OSA) and stroke are common. In the USA, stroke is responsible for half of all acute neurological hospital admissions, while worldwide it is the second major cause of death and the leading cause of long-term disability [1–3]. OSA is also a very frequent and serious problem with a prevalence up to 9% in women and 24% in men in the general adult population [4].

In the past, it was reasonable, given the commonality of stroke and OSA, their association with similar health problems (including hypertension and cardiovascular disease; CVD), and the fact that they share many of the same risk factors (including sex, age, and diabetes), to consider their simultaneous occurrence in any given individual patient as a sheer matter of chance. Nevertheless, over the past few years, research finally allowed for the 2006 guidelines from American Heart Association and American Stroke Association to consider a sleep-related breathing disorder (SRBD) such as OSA among the "less well-documented or potentially modifiable risk factors" for stroke, whereas the literature suggests that a cause-and-effect relationship between OSA and stroke may exist in some cases [5]. In this chapter, we review the history of this literature.

Early Studies: Stroke-Causing Sleep Apnea

Studies from as early as 1962 suggested that sleep apnea could result not only from stroke but also from a variety of degenerative and inflammatory neurological disorders when there was associated injury to the major central nervous system (CNS) respiratory centers [6–11]. Automatic respiration, although subject to modulation by multiple sites in the CNS, is dependent upon the medullary respiratory center (MRC). The MRC is comprised of the dorsal respiratory group (DRG; the nucleus solitarius) and the ventral respiratory group (VRG; which includes the nucleus ambiguous; Figs. 31.1 and 31.2) [8, 12, 13]. Central sleep apnea (CSA) has been documented after stroke involving the nucleus solitarius, presumably due to impairment of inspiratory mechanisms, while OSA has been reported after stroke of the VRG, possibly due to isolated damage of the nucleus ambiguous and consequent dysfunction of the vagal motor innervation to the larynx and pharynx [8]. Nevertheless, individual case reports suggest diffuse injury to the CNS affecting variable areas of respiratory control can also produce apnea [11, 12].

Early Studies: Sleep Apnea and Stroke, an Association

Snoring

Prior to the ready availability of polysomnography (PSG), OSA was often suspected on a clinical basis from the major signs and symptoms of what now constitutes the OSA syndrome, as a continuum has been shown to exist between snoring, obesity, and OSA [14, 15].

In 1989, Palomake et al. suggested that snoring alone was a risk factor for stroke [16]. In their study of 167 men with

M. Eric Dyken (✉)
Sleep Disorders Center, University of Iowa Hospitals and Clinics, 200 Hawkins Drive, Iowa, IA 52242, USA
e-mail: mark-dyken@uiowa.edu

University of Iowa, Roy J and Lucille A Carver College of Medicine, Iowa, IA 52242, USA

K. Bin Im
Department of Neurology, Sleep Disorders Center, University of Iowa, Roy J and Lucille A Carver College of Medicine, Iowa, IA, USA
e-mail: kyoungbin-im@uiowa.edu

G. B. Richerson
The Roy J. Carver Chair in Neuroscience, Roy J and Lucille A Carver College of Medicine, University of Iowa, Iowa, IA, USA
e-mail: George-Richerson@uiowa.edu

S. Chokroverty, M. Billiard (eds.), *Sleep Medicine*, DOI 10.1007/978-1-4939-2089-1_31,
© Springer Science+Business Media, LLC 2015

Fig. 31.1 Afferent and efferent connections of the medullary respiratory center. (From Fig. 19.4, [13], with permission)

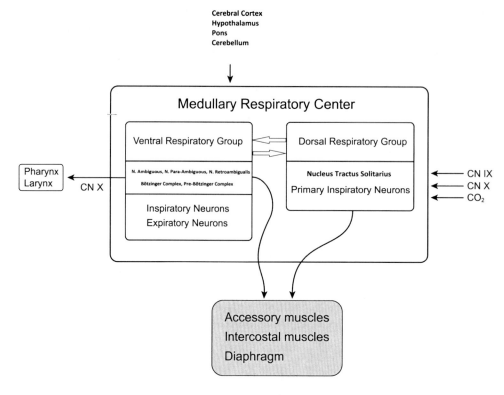

stroke, 36% suffered stroke in sleep. Stepwise multiple logistic regression analysis found snoring to be the only potential risk factor significantly related to stroke in sleep. In 1991, it was reported that the odds ratio (OR) of snoring increased when the combination of obesity and sleepiness (classical signs/symptoms of OSA) was also present [17]. Retrospective analysis of pioneering studies such as these led to the routine use of PSG in similar research, as a significant number of these subjects were suspected to have had OSA.

Early PSG Studies

The foundation of PSG is electroencephalography (EEG). In 1875, Caton performed the first animal studies and in 1929 Berger published recordings from humans [18–21]. By 1936, there were only six EEG laboratories in the USA, including our facility at the University of Iowa, under the direction of my (MED) mentor John Knott [21]. The first continuously recorded all-night EEG sleep studies by Loomis et al. in 1937 were followed by the discovery of rapid eye movement (REM) sleep by Aserinsky and Kleitman in 1953, which showed the utility of the electrooculogram (EOG) [22, 23]. In 1967, Jouvet showed the association of REM sleep with hypotonia justifying the present use of the electromyogram (EMG) [24]. In 1968, the combination of EEG, EOG, and EMG allowed for formal PSG and the first published standardized technique for scoring sleep stages by Rechtschaffen and Kales [25]. In 1978, utilizing the PSG, Guilleminault et al. defined the term apnea index (the average number of

apneas and hypopneas per hour of sleep), to precisely define the presence and severity of OSA [26]. In 2007, the American Academy of Sleep Medicine published the first standard definition for hypopnea in the pediatric population, thus allowing for the routine reporting of the apnea–hypopnea index (AHI; the average number of apneas plus hypopneas per hour of sleep) in children [27]. Today, the AHI is "…the key measure used for case identification, for quantifying disease severity, and for defining disease prevalence in normal and clinical populations" [28] (Table 31.1).

Stroke Case Reports and Case Series

In 1982, Chaudhary et al. published a PSG study of a 46-year-old hypertensive man (performed after a right lateral medullary infarction) that showed an apnea index of 18, with an oxygen saturation (SaO_2) low of 60% [29]. Injury to the nucleus ambiguous was hypothesized to have caused the OSA. Nevertheless, reports of progressive weight gain, snoring, and sleepiness suggested OSA was present prior to stroke.

In 1985, Tikare et al. studied a subject with PSG-documented OSA and recent stroke (the brain computerized tomogram (CT) revealed paraventricular areas of low attenuation) [30]. To our knowledge, this chapter was the first to suggest that OSA-induced hypoxia and cardiac arrhythmia might cause stroke.

In 1991, our group's research interest was piqued by a sleepy, obese 34-year-old man, with a history of snoring, who awoke with left hemiparesis, after which PSG diagnosed severe OSA [31]. A brain CT suggested he had suf-

Fig. 31.2 Neuroanatomy of the medullary respiratory center. The brain stem showing in a parasagittal section **a** the location of the dorsal and ventral respiratory groups (DRG and VRG) and their projection to the spinal cord; in a basal brain view **b** vagus nerve rootlets exiting the lateral surface of the medulla, and in a transverse section of the medulla **c** projections from the DRG to VRG, and the output from both groups to respiratory muscles. (From Fig. 19.5, [13], with permission)

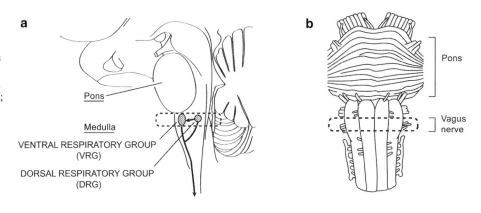

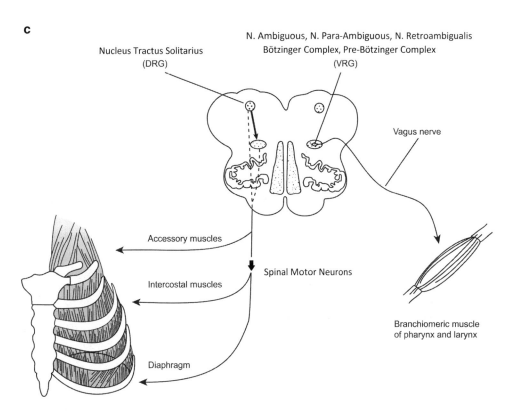

fered a hypertensive hemorrhagic stroke (Fig. 31.3). Our hypothesis, that this stroke could have represented an OSA-precipitated hypertensive bleed, was supported by previous hemodynamic studies which reported elevated blood pressures frequently followed sleep-related obstructive respirations [32–35].

In 1991, Kapen et al. selected 31 subjects with ischemic stroke for PSG [36]. They combined the findings of these studies with those of 16 similar patients who had incomplete sleep studies without respiratory effort or SaO_2 monitoring (S. Kapen, MD, personal communication, 1997). OSA was found in 72 % of these subjects.

Case–Control Stroke Studies

In 1992, our group presented preliminary data from a 4-year follow-up study of 24 consecutively encountered inpatients admitted for stroke, and 27 healthy gender- and age-matched control subjects without stroke [9, 10]. OSA (defined as either an AHI ≥ 10, or any number of obstructive events associated with an SaO_2 value $<86\%$) was found in 71 % of strokes. Closer analysis showed OSA in 10 of the 13 males with stroke (77 %) and in only 3 of the 13 males without stroke (23 %) (P=0.0169). Seven of the 11 females with stroke (64 %) had OSA, whereas only 2 of the 14 females without stroke (14 %) had OSA (P=0.0168).

In 1993, Hudgel et al. selected eight elderly patients, with finger pulse oximetry studies suggesting apnea, and stroke histories ≥ 1 month, for PSG [37]. Stroke subjects were matched to controls in regard to age, gender, weight, and height. Although the type of apnea and the number of individuals with sleep apnea were not defined for either subject group, the respective mean AHI for strokes and con-

Table 31.1 Early reports of stroke patients/populations studied with PSG. (From [68], with permission)

Study type	Number of subjects	% OSA[a]	AHI[b]/RDI[c]	SaO$_2$ (%)[d]	Location	Stroke type (number of patients)
Stroke case reports	–	–	–	–	–	–
Chaudhary et al. [29]	Stroke=1	100.0	18.0	60.0	Brainstem	I
Tilkare et al. [30]	Stroke=1	100.0	78.0	70.0	Hemispheric	I
Rivest/Reiher [41]	Stroke=1	100.0	NG	NG	Brainstem	I
Askenasy/Goldhammer [100]	Stroke=1	100.0	25.0	80.0	Brainstem	I
Dyken et al. [31]	Stroke=1	100.0	36.0	60.0	Subcortical	H
Pressman et al. [42]	Stroke=1	100.0	22.0	<50.0	Hemispheric	I
Selected stroke populations	–	–	–	–	–	–
Kapen et al. [36]	Stroke=47[e](31)	72.0	28.0	NG	Hemispheric	I
Good et al. [101]	Stroke=19	95.0	36.0	NG	Hemispheric (16) Brainstem (3)	I
Case–control studies	–	–	–	–	–	–
Dyken et al. [9]	Stroke=20	70.0	NG	NG	NG	NG
Hudgel et al. [37]	Stroke=8 Control=8	NG NG	44.0 12.0	82.0 90.0	NG NA	I/H NA
Mohsenin/Valor, [38]	Stroke=10 Control=10	70.0 (OSA) 10.0 (CSA) 0	52.0 3.0	70% 80–84%	Hemispheric (7) Subcortical (1)	I (9) H (1)
Dyken et al. [10]	Stroke=24 Control=27	71.0 19.0	26.0 4.0	85.0 91.0	Hemispheric (12) Subcortical (8) Cerebellar (2) Brainstem (2)	I (20) H (4)
Bassetti et al.[f] [43]	Stroke=23 Control=19	70.0 16.0	32.0 6.0	82.0 89.0	Anterior circ. (74%) Posterior circ. (26%)	I
Bassetti et al. [102]	Stroke=39	54.0 (OSA) 10.0 (CSB)	26.0 (NREM) 30.0 (REM)	82.0 (ST) 83.0 (IT)	Hemispheric (28) Brainstem (9) Pontocerebellar (1) Cerebellum (1)	I

OSA obstructive sleep apnea, *SaO$_2$* arterial oxygen saturation, *I* ischemic, *H* hemorrhagic, *circ.* circulation, *ST* supratentorial, *IT* infratentorial, *NG* not given, *NA* not applicable, *CSA* central sleep apnea, *CSB* Cheyne–Stokes-like breathing, *PSG* polysomnography, *REM* rapid eye movement, *NREM* non-REM
[a] Percentage of patients diagnosed polysomnographically with OSA
[b] Apnea/hypopnea index
[c] Respiratory disturbance index
[d] Lowest value during sleep
[e] Only 31 of 47 patients in data pool had full polysomnogram
[f] Data pool was mixed with transient ischemic attack patients

trols was 44.0 and 12.0. The authors suggested that apnea-induced hypoxemia and oscillations of intracranial pressure and blood circulation might increase the risk for ischemic stroke.

In 1995, Mohsenin and Valor selected ten patients from a rehabilitation facility with <1-year histories of hemispheric stroke, for PSG analysis [38]. None had prior apnea, snoring, sleepiness, obesity, or neurological problems. A control group was matched for age, obesity, smoking, and hypertension. The respective mean AHIs for the stroke and control groups was 52.0 and 3.0. The authors hoped to provide new evidence for a cause-and-effect relationship between hemispheric stroke and sleep apnea. Nevertheless, bias was placed against OSA causing stroke as subjects with histories of snoring, obesity, and apnea were selected out.

OSA: A Stroke Risk Factor

Transient Ischemic Attacks

Transient ischemic attacks (TIAs; "ministrokes") are focal neurological deficits resolving within 24 h [3]. Case reports of patients with histories of TIAs during sleep, obesity, and snoring, after the treatment of their PSG-documented OSA led to no further recurrence of TIA, indirectly suggest a cause-and-effect relationship between OSA and stroke, as 15% of strokes are preceded by TIA (90-day risk; up to 17.3%) [3, 39–42]. Nevertheless, case-controlled study reports have been inconsistent and OSA is not considered a TIA risk factor [43, 44].

Fig. 31.3 This brain CT without contrast was performed in a 34-year-old man who awoke with stroke, after which he was diagnosed with obstructive sleep apneas. This study reveals a hemorrhage, with a surrounding area, greater than 1 cm in diameter, of low density, consistent with edema, involving the putamen and posterior limb of the right internal capsule. (From [68], with permission). *CT* computerized tomogram

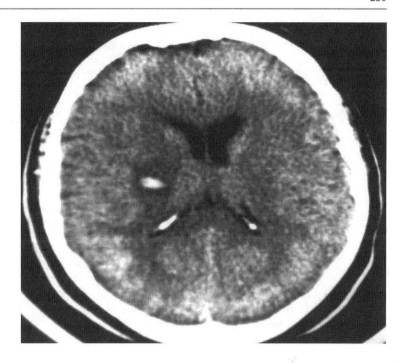

Cohort Studies

Large population and clinically based cohort studies, despite using variable populations, PSG methodologies, OSA definitions, and statistical analyses, and often examining stroke risk in combination with other medical problems, suggest that adults with OSA and an AHI ≥20 are at stroke risks (Table 31.2).

Population-Based Studies

In 2001, Shahar et al. examined the cross-sectional association between sleep-disordered breathing (SDB) and self-reported CVD in 6424 subjects using home (unattended) PSG [45]. Mild-to-moderate SDB was highly prevalent with a median AHI of 4.4; inter-quartile range, 1.3–11.0. At least one element of CVD (stroke, angina, myocardial infarction, heart failure, or coronary revascularization procedure) was reported by 16% ($N=1023$) of subjects. The relative odds ratio (95% confidence interval (CI)) of prevalent stroke (upper vs. lower AHI quartile) was 1.58 (1.02–22.46). This data suggested even mildly elevated AHI values have modest-to-moderate effects on CVD.

In 2005, Arzt et al. addressing 12 years of data from a stratified random sample performed a cross-sectional analysis, utilizing logistic regression, of 1475 subjects (30–60 years) [46]. A baseline AHI ≥20 independently increased the OR for stroke (3.83; 95% CI, 1.17–12.56; $P=0.03$) compared to a reference group with an AHI <5, after adjusting for confounding factors (age, sex, body mass index (BMI; weight in kilograms divided by square of height in meters), alcohol, smoking, diabetes, and hypertension).

From the original population, a longitudinal analysis of 1189 individuals tested whether SDB was associated with increased incident stroke at 4-year intervals throughout the study (at 4, 8, and 12 years). A baseline AHI ≥20 had significantly higher OR for incident stroke compared to the reference group (4.48; 95% CI, 1.31–15.33; $P=0.02$), using a model that controlled for age and sex.

Clinic-Based Studies

In 2005, Yaggi et al. studied an observational cohort of 1022 subjects with suspected SDB [47]. They compared the combined risk of developing composite stroke, TIA, or death from any cause in 697 subjects with OSA (AHI ≥5), to individuals with an AHI <5. Many with SDB received treatment during the study, including diet, positive airway pressure (PAP) therapy, and upper airway surgery.

Follow-up over 3.3–3.4 years of 842 total study subjects showed 22 incident strokes and/or TIAs and 50 deaths in the OSA group, whereas there were only two strokes and/or TIAs and 14 deaths in the comparison group. After adjusting for age, sex, BMI, diabetes, hyperlipidemia, atrial fibrillation, hypertension, race, and smoking, OSA was associated with a significant risk for composite stroke, TIA, or death (hazard ratio (HR), 1.97; 95% CI, 1.12–3.48; $P=0.01$). Trend analysis found an increase in OSA severity associated with increased risk of stroke, TIA, or death from any cause ($P=0.005$).

In 2006, Munoz et al. studied a noninstitutionalized elderly population (range: 70–100 years; median: 77.28), drawn from a random one-stage cluster sampling stratified by age, sex, and census area [48]. After adjusting for sex, a baseline

Table 31.2 OSA and stroke risk: incidence studies. (Modified from Table 1 [8], with permission)

Incidence studies	Subjects studied	Population size	AHI used to define SDB group	SDB prevalence	AHI used to define comparison group	Mean follow-up period (years)	Group outcome Total number of subjects in a given group with outcome	Risk estimate of SDB as risk factor for outcome (95 % CI)
Authors/year								
Arzt et al. [46]	Population based General adult 30 60 years	[a]1475 [b]1189	≥20	7 % (N=99)	<5	Three intervals of 4 years	Stroke SDB=4 Comparison=9	[c]OR=4.48 (1.31–15.33; P=0.02)
Yaggi et al. [47]	Clinic based Referred for suspected SDB ≥50 years	1022	≥5	68 % (N=697)	<5	3.4;SDB 3.3;CG	Stroke, TIA, or death SDB=72 Comparison=16	[d]HR=1.97 (1.12–3.48; P=0.01)
Munoz et al. [48]	Clinic based: Random sample, noninstitutional elderly 70–100 years	394	≥30	25 % (N=98)	<30	4.5	TIA or ischemic stroke SDB=9 Comparison=11	[e]HR=2.52 (1.04–6.1; P=0.04)
Valham et al. [49]	Clinic based Symptomatic angina and CAD	392	≥5	54 %	<5	10.0	Stroke SDB=38 Comparison=9	[f]HR=2.89 (1.37–6.09; P=0.005)
Redline et al. [50]	Community based ≥40 years	5422	≥15	Male 44 % (N=1095) Female 24 % (N=720)	<4.1	8.7	Ischemic stroke Male SDB=54 Female SDB=37	Male: [g]HR=2.86 (1.1–7.4) Female: [h]A 2 % increase in HR (0–5) after threshold OAHI of 25

AHI apnea/hypopnea index=the average number of apneas and hypopneas per hour of sleep, *SDB* sleep-disordered breathing, *CG* comparison group, *CI* confidence interval, *P* probability, *OR* odds ratio, *HR* hazard ratio, *CAD* coronary artery disease, *OAHI* obstructive apnea–hypopnea index, *TIA* transient ischemic attack, *BMI* body mass index

[a] Original population providing original cross-sectional prevalence data

[b] Population used for longitudinal analysis of incident stroke

[c] In a model adjusted for age and sex

[d] In a model adjusted for age, sex, race, smoking, BMI, diabetes mellitus, hyperlipidemia, atrial fibrillation, and hypertension

[e] In a model adjusted for sex

[f] In a model adjusted for age, BMI, left ventricular function, diabetes, sex, intervention, hypertension, atrial fibrillation, previous stroke or TIA

[g] In a model for male subjects comparing the risk for ischemic stroke and the OAHI in the top quartile (quartile IV; OAHI>19) to the lowest quartile (quartile I; OAHI<4.1) of the overall population studied

[h] In a model using nonlinear, covariate-adjusted associations between OAHI and the female sex

AHI ≥30 was a risk factor for incident ischemic stroke or TIA, with a HR of 2.52 (95 % CI=1.04–6.1, P=0.04).

In 2008, Valham et al. studied a population <70-years old, with symptomatic angina and coronary artery disease (verified by angiography and left ventriculography) [49]. The first evaluations of 392 patients randomly selected for modified PSG, without electroencephalography (EEG), using a pressure sensitive bed to monitor respiration, showed sleep apneas (AHI ≥5) in 54 %. All patients were then followed for 10 years (nine receiving OSA therapies), during which 47 (12 %) had strokes. Increased stroke risk was associated with an initial diagnosis of obstructive sleep apneas; HR of 2.89 (95 % CI 1.37–6.09, P=0.005), independent of OSA treatment, previous stroke or TIA, sex, age, BMI, diabetes, hypertension, atrial fibrillation, left ventricular function, or smoking. Independent of confounders, an AHI >5 and <15, and an AHI ≥15, respectively, had 2.44 (59 % CI 1.08–5.52,

P=0.011) and 3.56 (95 % CI 1.56–8.16, P=0.011) times increased risk of stroke compared to those without apnea.

In 2010, Redline et al. followed 5422 subjects, without a history of stroke, for a median of 8.7 years, during which 193 new ischemic strokes occurred [50]. A significantly positive association between initially documented obstructive apnea/hypopnea indices (OAHI) and new ischemic stroke was seen. The greatest risk was for men with an OAHI >19.1 (the top quartile), with an adjusted HR of 2.86 (95 % CI 1.1, 7.4), when compared to men with an OAHI <4.1 (quartile I). In women, stroke risk was not associated with OAHI quartile or oxygen desaturation. Nevertheless, there was, using nonlinear, covariate-adjusted associations with the OSA exposures and interactions with gender, a 2 % increase (95 % C.I. 0, 5) in stroke HR with each unit increment in OAHI after a threshold of 25.

Treatment Versus Non-treatment

Morbidity and Mortality

In 1996, we published a 4-year follow-up on all stroke and sex- and age-matched control subjects from a 1992 prevalence study of OSA in stroke, with the exception of three controls who moved, leaving no contact information [9, 10]. All stroke subjects who died had OSA ($N=5$), of whom only one used continuous PAP (CPAP; death from urosepsis). Only one male control died; without OSA, from prostatic carcinoma. Respectively, stroke subjects dead versus alive had mean AHIs of 41.3 and 22.1, suggesting the diagnosis and severity of OSA in stroke were associated with greater long-term mortality.

A 1990, prospective, treatment versus non-treatment study by Partinen et al. has been used to suggest a cause-and-effect relationship between OSA and stroke [51, 52]. Over 7 years, they followed 198 OSA subjects treated with either weight loss ($N=127$) or tracheostomy ($N=71$); 5.2% of the weight loss group had stroke (17.3% died, 11% from vascular etiologies), whereas only 1.2% with tracheostomy suffered stroke (2.8% died).

CPAP

In 2005, Martinez-Garcia et al. showed, of 51 patients with recent stroke and minimal AHI of 20, only 15 (29.4%) tolerated CPAP after 1 month [53]. In those who could not tolerate CPAP, the probability of a new vascular event increased fivefold (OR 5.09).

In 2006, Palombini et al. studied 32 patients with recent stroke [54]. Only 22% tolerated CPAP for 8 weeks; difficulties with CPAP use as perceived by the patient and family members, facial weakness, motor impairment, and increased difficulties and discomfort using a full-face mask. Brown et al. found stroke patients took longer to put on ($P<0.01$) and remove ($P<0.01$) traditional headgear as compared to a one-piece system [55]. Palombini et al. stated, "Better education and support of patients and families, and special training session in rehabilitation services, will be needed to improve compliance" [54]. Disler et al. showed, in a supportive setting, patients with stroke and OSA, despite moderately severe motor and cognitive functional independence measurement scores, tolerated CPAP with normalization of oxygen saturations [56].

Positional Therapy

Positional sleep apnea (worse supine, due to oropharyngeal gravitational effects) is frequent in acute stroke [57, 58]. In 2008, Dziewas et al. diagnosed OSA in 78% of 55 patients

studied within 72 h of stroke; 65% had positional sleep apnea [58]. Six-month follow-up studies showed OSA in only 49% of the patients, of whom 33% had positional apnea. The authors stated "positional sleep apnea is a predominant feature in acute stroke and its incidence decreases significantly during the following months. These findings may have implications for sleep apnea treatment in patients with acute stroke." They suggest serial PSG studies may permit eventual reductions in OSA treatment.

Other Considerations

The evaluation and treatment in acute stroke must be individually tailored, as a critically ill patient in an intensive care setting may require portable PSG with end-tidal CO_2 monitoring, complemented with an arterial blood gas determination when hypoventilation, CO_2 retention, underlying lung or neuromuscular compromise are suspected. Although positional therapy should be considered, even simple head of bed elevation may be contraindicated due to perfusion pressure issues. PAP therapies (including CPAP, bi-level PAP, and noninvasive positive pressure ventilation) may need to be presented in a supportive educational manner with close follow-up for adherence. Severe cases may require more aggressive therapies, including intubation and tracheostomy.

Potential Mechanisms for OSA-Induced Stroke

The Metabolic Syndrome

OSA increases the odds of having the metabolic syndrome up to ninefold [59, 60]. A cross-sectional case–control study found metabolic syndrome significantly more common in subjects with OSA than controls (49.5 vs. 22.0% for men, $P<0.01$; 32.0 vs. 6.7% for women, $P<0.01$), whereas up to 53% of newly diagnosed apneics have metabolic syndrome [61, 62].

OSA independently associates with obesity, hypertension, and insulin resistance/diabetes, three known stroke risk factors of the metabolic syndrome [3, 63–65]. An elevated BMI by one-standard deviation increases the OR for SDB (AHI ≥ 5) by 4.17 [4]. A prospective, population-based study showed that over a 4-year period, the OR of a subject with an AHI between 5.0 and 14.9 versus ≥ 15.0 for developing hypertension was respectively two versus three times greater, when compared to a non-apneic [66]. A community-based, cross-sectional study of 69 nondiabetics showed mild and moderately severe OSA was associated with significantly reduced insulin sensitivities (38.5 and 51.2%, respectively) compared to non-apneics (AHI <5), independent of percent body fat, sex, age, and race [67].

Autonomic Activity

Microneurographic studies, directly measuring efferent sympathetic neural activity (SNA), have been used to support the hypothesis that OSA-induced hypertensive events can cause stroke through elevations of SNA, from reflex effects of hypoxia, hypercapnia, and decreased input from thoracic stretch receptors (Figs. 31.4 and 31.5) [31, 68, 69]. In 1995, our group studied ten subjects with OSA and found SNA increased by 246% during the last 10 s of apneas, in association with a mean blood pressure increase from 92 mmHg waking to 127 mmHg in REM sleep [70]. Our observations, including finding persistently elevated waking sympathetic tone in apneics, suggested to us that OSA might induce chronic changes that could also predispose to stroke [68, 70].

Autonomic effects could also contribute to the high prevalence of cardiac arrhythmias reported in up to 48% of apneics [71–73]. In 1992, our group showed obstructive apneas (inspiration against a closed glottis with hypoxemia) could cause excessive parasympathetic responses evidenced as recurrent prolonged episodes of sinus arrest with dramatic reductions in blood pressure (180/100 mmHg prior to obstructions to systolic pressures <50 mmHg during obstructions) [74].

Atrial fibrillation provides a 49% risk for OSA [75]. In patients with atrial fibrillation and OSA, CPAP noncompliance is associated with a greater recurrence rate after cardio-version [76]. As a strong stroke risk factor, atrial fibrillation might contribute to stroke in some patients with OSA [3].

Circadian Rhythms

In 1996, our group hypothesized if stroke has an equal probability of occurring at anytime during a 24-h time period, 33% of all strokes should occur during the stereotypical 8-h period of nocturnal sleep [10]. However, stroke has a tendency to occur in the early morning hours and our prospective prevalence study showed a higher-than-expected percentage of patients with OSA who had strokes during sleep (54%; P =0.0304) [77, 10].

Rapid Eye Movement Sleep

Normally, the most prolonged period of REM sleep occurs during the early morning hours, coinciding with the greatest circadian risk for stroke. The hypotonia of REM sleep generally worsens OSA, while OSA negatively accentuates autonomic phenomena associated with REM sleep, including the general elevation of SNA and blood pressures that tend to reach waking levels with surges during the muscle twitches characteristic of phasic REM [78, 79]. Cerebral blood flow normally increases during REM sleep, while obstructive ap-

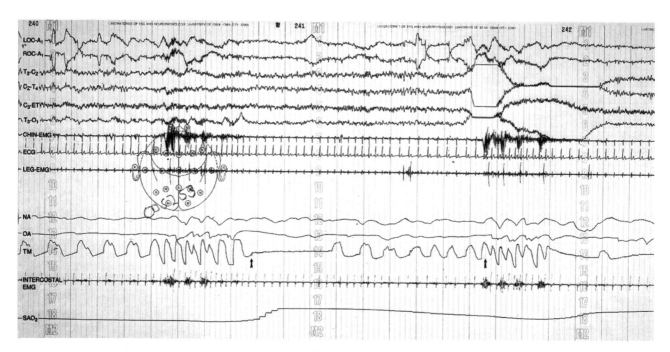

Fig. 31.4 A PSG tracing (paper speed 10 mm/s) has been reduced to correspond to a temporally related microneurographic tracing (Fig. 8.5; paper speed 5 mm/s). *Arrows* indicate a prolonged mixed apnea of approximately 26 s duration occurring during REM sleep, associated with severe oxygen desaturation. *LOC* left outer canthus, *ROC* right outer canthus, *T* temporal, *C* central, *ET* ears tied, *O* occipital, *EMG* electromyogram, *N* nasal airflow, *OA* oral airflow, *TM* thoracic movement, *PSG* polysomnography. (Modified from Fig. 2, [89], with permission)

neas increase intracranial pressure and reduce cerebral perfusion pressure [80, 81].

Early morning normally associates with low fibrinolytic activity and high levels of catecholamines, blood viscosity, and platelet activity and aggregability, during a time when REM-related SNA activation might potentiate platelet aggregation and plaque development [82]. In this otherwise normal hematological milieu, further elevations in catecholamine levels and platelet activation by OSA might increase thrombus and embolus formation and stroke risk [82–84].

Elevated levels of platelet activation proteins, soluble CD40 ligand (sCD40L), and soluble P-selectin (sP-selectin) are linked to silent brain infarctions (SBI) on magnetic resonance imaging (MRI) [85]. Minoguchi et al. showed SBI in 25 % of patients with moderate-to-severe OSA and in only 6.7 % of controls, with significantly higher serum levels of sCD40L and sP-selectin that significantly reduced with CPAP [85].

Arousal

Definition

The phenomena of "arousal" have been variably defined polysomnographically in The American Academy of Sleep Medicine Manual for the Scoring of Sleep and Associated Events [27, 86]. An arousal from any non-REM (NREM) stage of sleep is defined as an abrupt shift of EEG including alpha, theta and/or frequencies > 16 Hz (but not sleep spindles) lasting ≥ 3 s, with ≥ 10 s of stable sleep preceding the change [23, 82]. An arousal from REM sleep also requires a concomitant increase in submental electromyographic activity, lasting ≥ 1 s [27, 86].

Studies suggest upper airway occlusion induces arousal from NREM sleep once inspiratory effort reaches a variable arousal threshold [87]. In one OSA study, it was hypothesized that an impaired arousal response led to prolonged apneas, EEG flattening, and generalized tonic spasms described as "cerebral anoxic attacks" [88].Our group published two PSG

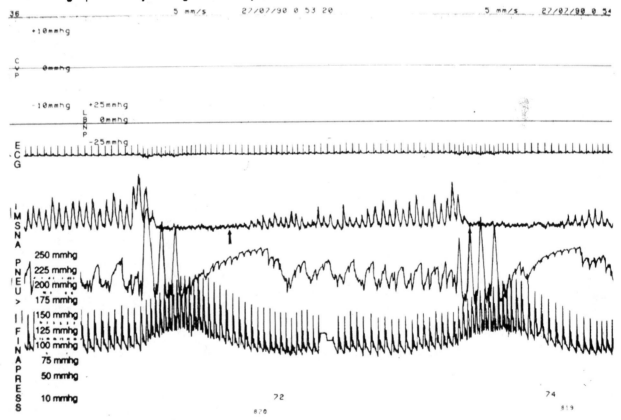

Fig. 31.5 The *arrows* in this microneurographic tracing recorded from the peroneal nerve indicate a gradual elevation of efferent nerve activity during a mixed apnea. The activity peak is immediately followed by cessation of the apnea, with a subsequent marked elevation of arterial blood pressure to 215/130 mmHg from a baseline of 135/80 mmHg. *MSNA* muscle sympathetic nerve activity, *Pneu* chest excursion, *Finapress* fingertip blood pressure. (Modified from Fig. 3, [68], with permission)

cases involving critically ill patients with OSA, where elevated arousal thresholds may also have prolonged obstructions, leading to diffuse cerebral hypoxemic EEGs patterns, followed by transient clinical encephalopathy in one subject and death for the other (Figs. 31.6, 31.7, and 31.8) [89].

White et al. showed the arousal threshold to hypoxia and hypercapnia can be increased by the short-term sleep deprivation. As sleep deprivation is common in acutely ill patients, they could only "speculate—as to the clinical significance of these findings as they apply to the patient with a precarious respiratory status" [90]. Researchers also have shown OSA itself can increase the arousal threshold, possibly due to sleep fragmentation and hypoxemia [87].

Mechanisms of Arousal during OSA

An apnea typically ends with an arousal or "micro-arousal" (of which the patient is usually not aware) [91]. This is an important protective reflex that allows relief of the upper airway obstruction, with an increase in tidal volume and respiratory frequency, without which it is unlikely that the apnea would terminate. There is great interest in the mechanism of arousal in OSA, especially given the associated reports of stroke, cardiovascular catastrophe, and death during sleep. During apnea, there are several stimuli that induce arousal, including hypercapnia, hypoxia, and increased airway resistance.

An increase in partial pressure of carbon dioxide (PCO_2) in arterial blood is a powerful stimulus for arousal. A healthy

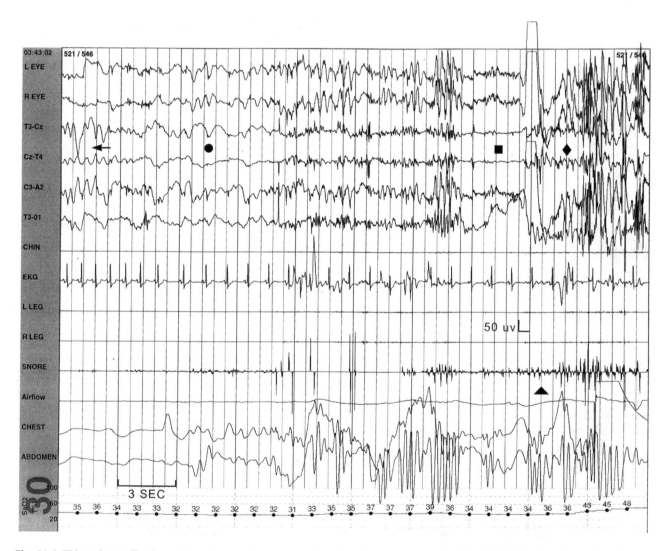

Fig. 31.6 This patient suffered a prolonged obstructive apnea which eventually resulted in a sudden EEG change from a classic REM sawtooth pattern (see *arrows*) to a poorly organized, diffuse delta slow-wave pattern (see *closed circle*), followed by a general flattening of all activity (see *square*) that led to attempts to arouse the patient (as evidenced by diffuse movement artifact; see *diamond*). Nevertheless, persistent obstruction (see *triangle*) necessitated emergency rescue breathing maneuvers. Persistent EEG flattening followed by slowing and eventual recovery of normal waking patterns was appreciated in subsequent epochs. *L* left, *R* right, *T* temporal, *C* central, *O* occipital, *CHIN* mentalis EMG, *L Leg* left anterior tibialis EMG, *R LEG* right anterior tibialis EMG, *SNORE* snoring microphone, *ABDOMEN* abdominal effort, *SaO₂ (%)* oxygen saturation. (Modified from Fig. 1, [89], with permission)

Fig. 31.7 An 80-year-old man with multiple medical problems who was admitted with exacerbation of pulmonary and cardiac disease under a do-not-resuscitate/do-not-intubate status (for whom signed consent had been given for PSG as part of a institutional review board (IRB)-approved study) had a 30 s obstruction that was associated with an SaO_2 low of 12%. At that time, the EEG showed progressive development of a disorganized slow-wave pattern over a 2 ½-min period, followed by ECS (using a recording sensitivity of 1.0 μV/mm). *A1* left ear reference, *A2* right ear reference, *T* temporal, *C* central, *O* occipital, *LL* left leg, *RL* right leg, *NA* nasal airflow, *CE* chest effort, *AD* abdominal effort, *SaO₂* oxygen saturation. (Modified from Fig. 19.10, [13], with permission)

A Hypoxemic Encephalopathic EEG pattern following a prolonged Obstructive Apnea

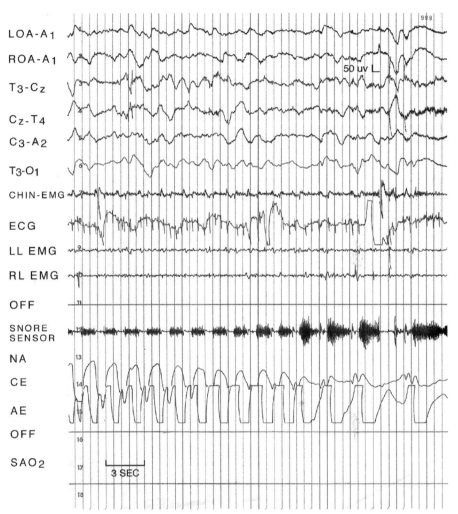

human subject exposed to 8% CO_2 in the ambient air while sleeping will typically wake up within 60 s [92]. Arousal to CO_2 is mediated by serotonin neurons in the raphe nuclei of the brainstem in close association with large branches of the basilar artery [93]. They sense variations in arterial CO_2, responding indirectly to changes in brain pH by increasing their excitatory drive to other neurons that mediate arousal, possibly including those in the thalamus and cortex [94]. Transgenic mice in which all serotonin neurons are deleted from the brain sometimes survive to adulthood and do not wake up from sleep in response to an increase in CO_2 to as high as 10% [95]. There may be differences in hypercapnic arousal due to genetic variations that influence the serotonin system.

Inhalation of hypoxic air alone can induce arousal without hypercapnia [96]. Reductions in arterial PO_2 are sensed by the peripheral arterial chemoreceptors in the carotid and aortic bodies, but central mechanisms are not clear; they do not rely on serotonergic neurons, although they may involve other brainstem neurons of the raphe and solitary tract nuclei [95, 97].

Arousal can be induced by increased work of breathing in response to airway occlusion; an inevitable consequence of upper airway obstruction in OSA [98]. Nevertheless, as arousal does not occur during early airway obstruction (at apnea onset), it is implicit that the development of hypoxia and hypercapnia is critical in the arousal phenomena associated with OSA.

Fig. 31.8 After our patient in Fig. 31.7 (upon whom no heroic therapeutic interventions were allowed) had a final series of apneic events, no discernible EEG activity was captured while utilizing a recording sensitivity or 1.0 μV/mm. A prolonged period of asystole (see arrow) was followed by cardiac arrest, at which time the patient was declared dead (see closed circle). *LOC* left outer canthus, *A1* left ear reference, *A2* right ear reference, *T* temporal, *C* central, *O* occipital, *LL* left leg, *RL* right leg, *NA* nasal airflow, *CE* chest effort, *AD* abdominal effort, *SaO$_2$* oxygen saturation. (Modified from Fig. 2, [89], with permission)

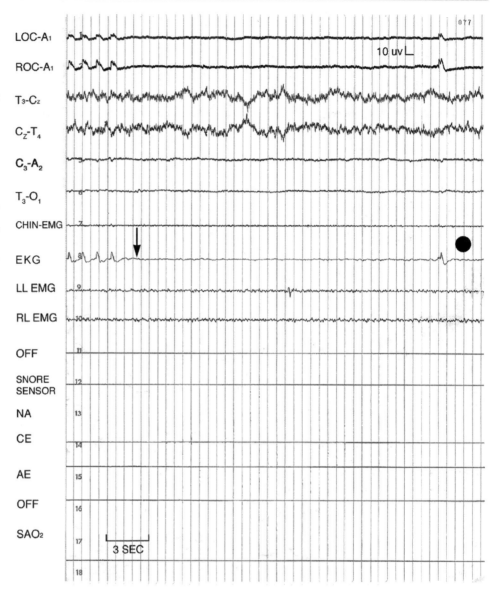

Conclusion

The most important relationship between sleep and cerebrovascular disease is the association of OSA and stroke. Although both are common, multifactorial health problems that share many risk factors, cohort studies show OSA is a risk factor for ischemic stroke. OSA is associated with many stroke risk factors that may independently contribute to stroke risk, suggesting a potential cause-and-effect relationship in some cases (Fig. 31.9). Anecdotal human case reports and laboratory studies suggest depression of arousal, in some

patient populations with OSA could predispose to stroke and death as a result of sustained hypoxemia and hypercapnia.

Although, no double-blind, randomized, controlled, treatment versus non-treatment trial has proven OSA causes stroke, the known pathophysiology mandates therapeutic intervention whenever possible. Once stroke has occurred, Brown et al. suggest if future research can clearly prove that the treatment of OSA significantly reduces morbidity and mortality in a cost-effective manner, then routine screening and more aggressive tailored treatment might become standard of care [99].

Fig. 31.9 This oversimplistic diagram highlights some of the major suspected factors linking OSA, arousal, and stroke. OSA can lead to autonomic instability. Inspiration against a closed airway with hypoxemia can increase parasympathetic activity, potentially leading to bradycardia, sinus arrest, and hypotensive events. Increased sympathetic neural activity (SNA) from the reflex effects of hypoxia, hypercapnia, and decreased input from thoracic stretch receptors can lead to tachycardia, blood pressure surges, and potentially arrhythmias such as atrial fibrillation. While an acute arousal can be protective in preventing untoward effects of a single prolonged apnea, chronic concomitant SNA elevations have been hypothesized to help explain the known associations with a variety of stroke risk factors including the development of thrombus/emboli, diabetes mellitus, and chronic hypertension. (From Fig. 5.6, in Dyken et al., 2013, with permission). *HR* hazard ratio, *BP* blood pressure

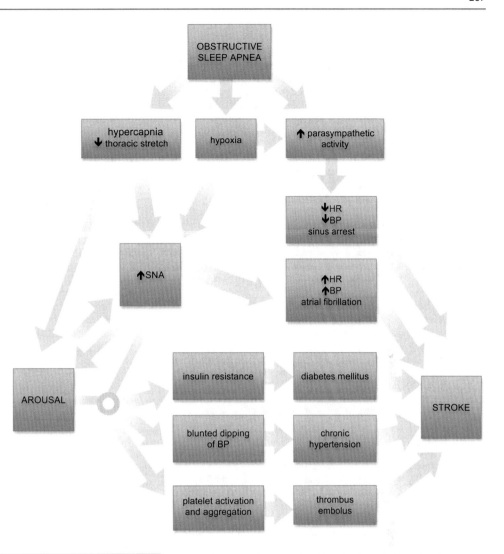

References

1. Murray CJ, Lopez AD. Mortality by cause for eight regions of the world: global burden of disease study. Lancet. 1997;349:1269–76.
2. American Heart Association. Heart and stroke statistics—2004 update. Dallas: American Heart Association; 2003.
3. Lloyd-Jones D, Adams R, Mercedes C, et al. Heart disease and stroke statistics—2009 update. A report from the American Heart Association Statistics Committee and Stroke Statistics Subcommittee. Circulation. 2009;119:e21–181. (Available: circ.ahajournals.org).
4. Young T, Palta M, Dempsey J, et al. The occurrence of sleep-disordered breathing among middle-aged adults. N Engl J Med. 1993;328:1230–5.
5. Goldstein LB, Adams R, Alberts MJ, et al. Primary prevention of ischemic stroke: a guideline from the American Heart Association/American Stroke Association Stroke Council. Stroke. 2006;37:1583–633.
6. Severinghaus JW, Mitchell RA. Ondine's curse-failure of respiratory center automaticity while awake [abstract]. Clin Res. 1962;10:122.
7. Dyken ME, Im KB. Gilman S, eds. Sleep disorders associated with dementia. MedLink Neurology. SanDiego: MedLink Corporation. http://www.medlink.com/. Accessed 11 October 2010.
8. Dyken ME, Im KB. Obstructive sleep apnea and stroke. Chest. 2009;136(6):1668–77.
9. Dyken ME, Somers VK, Yamada T, et al. Investigating the relationship between sleep apnea and stroke [abstract]. Sleep Res. 1992;21:30.
10. Dyken ME, Somers VK, Yamada T, et al. Investigating the relationship between stroke and obstructive sleep apnea. Stroke. 1996;27:401–7.
11. Dyken ME, Yamada T, Berger HA. Transient obstructive sleep apnea and asystole in association with presumed viral encephalopathy. Neurology. 2003;60(10):1692–4.
12. Hugelin A. Forebrain and midbrain influence on respiration. In: Fishman AP, Cherniak NS, Widdecombe JG, Geige SR, editors. Handbook of physiology. Section 3. The Respiratory System Vol 2. Control of Breathing, Part 1. Bethesda: American Physiological Society; 1986. 69–91.
13. Dyken ME, Afifi AK, Im KB. Stroke in sleep. In: Chokroverty S, Sahota P, eds. Acute and emergent events in sleep disorders. New York: Oxford University Press; 2011. 328–48.
14. Berry DT, Webb WB, Block AJ, et al. Sleep-disordered breathing and its concomitants in a subclinical population. Sleep. 1986;4:478–83.
15. Resta O, Foschino-Barbaro MP, Legari G, et al. Sleep-related breathing disorders, loud snoring and excessive daytime sleepiness in obese subjects. Int J Obes Relat Metab Disord. 2001;5:669–75.
16. Palomake H, Partinen M, Juvela S, et al. Snoring as a risk factor for sleep-related brain infarction. Stroke. 1989;10:1311–5.
17. Palomake H. Snoring and the risk of ischemic brain infarction. Stroke. 1991;22:1021–5.

18. Caton R. The electric currents of the brain. Br Med J. 1875;2:278.
19. Berger H. Über das Elektoenkephalogram des Menschen. Arch Psychiat. 1929;87:527–70.
20. Brazier MAB. A history of the electrical activity of the brain: The first half-century. London: Pitman Medical Publishing Co; 1961.
21. Yamada T, Meng E. Chapter 1, Introduction: History and perspective of clinical neurophysiologic diagnostic tests. In: Yamada T, Meng E, editors. Practical guide for clinical neurophysiologic testing—EEG. Philadelphia: Wolters Kluwer/Lippincott Williams & Wilkins. 2010. p. 1–4.
22. Loomis AL, Harvey N, Hobart GA. Cerebral states during sleep, as studied by human brain potentials. J Exp Psychol. 1937;21:127–44.
23. Aserinsky E, Kleitman N. Regularly occurring periods of eye motility, and concomitant phenomena, during sleep. Science. 1953;118:273–4.
24. Jouvet M. Neurophysiology of the states of sleep. Physiol Rev. 1967;47:117–77.
25. Rechtschaffen A, Kales A. A manual of standardized, techniques and scoring system for sleep stages in human subjects. Washington DC: NIH Publication No. 204, US Government Printing Office; 1968.
26. Guilleminault C, van den Hoed J, Mitler M. Clinical overview of the sleep apnea syndromes. In: Guilleminault C, Dement WC, editors. Sleep apnea syndromes. New York: Alan R Liss, Inc; 1978. 1–12.
27. Iber C, Ancoli-Israel S, Chesson A, et al. The AASM manual for the scoring of sleep and associated events: Rules, terminology and technical specifications. 1. Westchester: American Academy of Sleep Medicine; 2007.
28. Ruehland WR, Rochford PD, O'Donoghue FJ, et al. The new AASM criteria for scoring hypopneas: Impact on the apnea hypopnea index. Sleep. 2009;32(2):150–7.
29. Chaudhary BA, Elguindi AS, King DW. Obstructive sleep apnea after lateral medullary syndrome. South Med J. 1982;75:65–7.
30. Tikare SK, Chaudhary BA, Bandisode MS. Hypertension and stroke in a young man with obstructive sleep apnea syndrome. Postgrad Med. 1985;78:59–66.
31. Dyken ME, Somers VK, Yamada T. Hemorrhagic stroke; part of the natural history of severe obstructive sleep apnea? [abstract]. Sleep Research. 1991;20:371.
32. Tilkian AG, Guilleminault C, Schroeder JS, et al. Hemodynamics in sleep-induced apnea: studies during wakefulness and sleep. Ann Intern Med. 1976;85:714–9.
33. Coccagna G, Mantovani M, Brignani F, et al. Continuous recording of the pulmonary and systemic arterial pressure during sleep in syndromes of hypersomnia and periodic breathing. Bull Physiopathol Respir (Nancy). 1972;8(5):1159–72.
34. Lugaresi E, Coccagna G, Mantovani M, et al. Effects of tracheostomy in two cases of hypersomnia with periodic breathing. J Neurol Neurosurg Psychiatry. 1973;36:15–26.
35. Dyken ME, Somers VK, Yamada T. Stroke, sleep apnea and autonomic instability. In: Togawa K, Katayama S, Hishikawa Y, editors. Sleep apnea and rhonchopathy. Basel: Karger; 1993. 166–8.
36. Kapen S, Park A, Goldberg J, et al. The incidence and severity of obstructive sleep apnea in ischemic cerebrovascular disease [abstract]. Neurology. 1991;41(Suppl 1):125.
37. Hudgel DW, Devadatta P, Quadri M, et al. Mechanism of sleep-induced periodic breathing in convalescing stroke patients and healthy elderly subjects. Chest. 1993;104:1503–10.
38. Mohsenin V, Valor R. Sleep apnea in patients with hemispheric stroke. Arch Phys Med Rehabil. 1995;76:71–6.
39. Ovbiagele B, Kidwell CS, Saver JL. Epidemiological impact in the United States of a tissue-based definition of transient ischemic attack. Stroke. 2003;34:919–24.
40. Kleinddorfer D, Panagos P, Pancioli A, et al. Incidence and short-term prognosis of transient ischemic attack in a population based study. Stroke. 2005;36:720–3.

41. Rivest J, Reiher J. Transient ischemic attacks triggered by symptomatic sleep apneas [abstract]. Stroke. 1987;18:293.
42. Pressman MR, Schetman WR, Figueroa WG, et al. Transient ischemic attacks and minor stroke during sleep. Stroke. 1995;26:2361–5.
43. Bassetti C, Aldrich MS, Chervin RD, et al. Sleep apnea in patients with transient ischemic attack and stroke: a prospective study of 59 patients. Neurology. 1996;47:1167–73.
44. McArdle N, Riha RL, Vennelle M, et al. Sleep-disordered breathing as a risk factor for cerebrovascular disease; a case-control study in patients with transient ischemic attacks. Stroke. 2003;34:2916–21.
45. Shahar E, Whitney CW, Redline S, et al. Sleep-disordered breathing and cardiovascular disease. Cross-sectional results of the sleep heart health study. Am J Resp Crit Care Med. 2001;163:19–25.
46. Arzt M, Young T, Finn L, et al. Association of sleep-disordered breathing and the occurrence of stroke. Am J Resp Crit Care Med. 2005;172:1147–51.
47. Yaggi KH, Concato J, Kernan WN, et al. Obstructive sleep apnea as a risk factor for stroke and death. N Engl J Med. 2005;19:2034–41.
48. Munoz R, Duran-Cantolla J, Martinez-Vila E, et al. Severe sleep apnea and risk of ischemic stroke in the elderly. Stroke. 2006;37:2317–21.
49. Valham F, Mooe T, Rabben T, et al. Increased risk of stroke in patients with coronary artery disease and sleep apnea: A 10-year follow-up. Circulation. 2008;118:955–60.
50. Redline S, Yenokyan G, Gottlieb DJ, et al. Obstructive sleep apnea-hypopnea and incident stroke; the sleep heart health study. Am J Respir Crit Care Med. 2010;182:269–77.
51. Partinen M, Jamieson A, Guilleminault C. Long-term outcome for obstructive sleep apnea syndrome patients: mortality. Chest. 1988;94:1200–4.
52. Partinen M, Guilleminault C. Daytime sleepiness and vascular morbidity at seven-year follow-up in obstructive sleep apnea patients. Chest. 1990;97:27–32.
53. Martinez-Garcia MA, Galiano-Blancart R, Roman-Sanches P, et al. Continuous positive airway pressure treatment in sleep apnea prevents new vascular events after ischemic stroke. Chest. 2005;4:2123–9.
54. Palombini L, Guilleminault C. Stroke and treatment with nasal CPAP. Eur J Neurol. 2006;13:198–200.
55. Brown DL, Concannon M, Kare AB, et al. Comparison of two headgear systems for sleep apnea treatment of stroke patients. Cerebrovasc Dis. 2009;27:183–6.
56. Disler P, Hansford A, Skelton J, et al. Diagnosis and treatment of obstructive sleep apnea in a stroke rehabilitation unit: a feasibility study. Am J Phys Med Rehabil. 2002;81:622–5.
57. Wierzbicka A, Rola R, Wichniak A, et al. The incidence of sleep apnea in patients with stroke or transient ischemic attack. J Physiol Pharmacol. 2006;57:385–90.
58. Dziewas R, Hopmann B, Humpert M, et al. Positional sleep apnea in patients with ischemic stroke. Neurol Res. 2008;30:645–8.
59. Coughlin SR, Mawdsley L, Mugarza JA, et al. Obstructive sleep apnoea is independently associated with an increased prevalence of metabolic syndrome. Eur Heart J. 2004;25:735–41.
60. Lam JC, Lam B, Lam CL, et al. Obstructive sleep apnea and the metabolic syndrome in community-based Chinese adults in Hong Kong. Respir Med. 2006;100:980–7.
61. Sasanabe R, Banno K, Otake K, et al. Metabolic syndrome in Japanese patients with obstructive sleep apnea syndrome. Hypertens Res. 2006;29:315–22.
62. Ambrosetti M, Lucioni AM, Conti S, et al. Metabolic syndrome in obstructive sleep apnea and related cardiovascular risk. J Cardiovasc Med. 2006;7:826–9.
63. Roger VL, Go AS, Lloyd-Jones D, et al. Heart Disease and Stroke Statistics—2012 Update: A Report From the American Heart Association (Available: http://circ.ahajournals.org/content/early/2011/12/15/CIR.0b013e31823ac046). Accessed 17 Dec 2010.

64. Rundek T, Gardener H, Xu Q, Goldberg RB, et al. Insulin resistance and risk of ischemic stroke among nondiabetic individuals from the northern Manhattan study. Arch Neurol. 2010;67:1195–200.

65. Tishler PV, Larkin EK, Schluchter MD, Redline S. Incidence of sleep-disordered breathing in an urban adult population. JAMA. 2003;289:2230–7.

66. Peppard PE, Young T, Palta M, et al. Prospective study of the association between sleep-disordered breathing and hypertension. N Engl J Med. 2000;342:1378–84.

67. Aurora RN, Polak J, Punjabi NM, et al. Obstructive sleep apnea is associated with insulin resistance independent of visceral fat. Am J Respir Crit Care Med. 2011;183:A6075.

68. Dyken ME. Cerebrovascular disease and sleep apnea. In: Bradley DT, Floras JS, editors. Sleep disorders and cardiovascular and cerebrovascular disease (Series on Lung Biology and Health in Disease). New York: Marcel Dekker; 2000. 285–306.

69. Somers VK, Mark AL, Abboud FM. Sympathetic activation by hypoxia and hypercapnia. Implications for sleep apnea [abstract]. Clin Exp Hypertens. 1988;A 10:413–22.

70. Somers VK, Dyken ME, Clary MP, et al. Sympathetic neural mechanisms in obstructive sleep apnea. J Clin Invest. 1995;96:1897–904.

71. Guilleminault C, Connolly SJ, Winkle RA. Cardiac arrhythmia and conduction disturbances during sleep in 400 patients with sleep apnea syndrome. Am J Cardiol. 1983;52:490–4.

72. Somers VK, Dyken ME, Skinner JL. Autonomic and hemodynamic responses and interactions during the Mueller maneuver in humans. J Auton Nerv Syst. 1993;44:253–9.

73. Wolk R, Somers VK. Obesity-related cardiovascular disease: Implications of obstructive sleep apnea. Diabetes Obes Metab. 2006;8:250–60.

74. Somers VK, Dyken ME, Mark AL, et al. Parasympathetic hyper-responsiveness and bradyarrhythmias during apnea in hypertension. Clin Auton Res. 1992;2:171–6.

75. Gami AS, Pressman G, Caples SM, et al. Association of atrial fibrillation and obstructive sleep apnea. Circulation. 2004;110:364–7.

76. Kanagala R, Murali NS, Friedman PA, et al. Obstructive sleep apnea and the recurrence of atrial fibrillation. Circulation. 2003;107:2589–94.

77. Marsh E, Biller J, Adams H, et al. Circadian variation in onset of acute ischemic stroke. Arch Neurol. 1990;47:1178–80.

78. Hornyak M, Cejnar M, Elam M, et al. Sympathetic muscle nerve activity during sleep in man. Brain. 1991;114:1281–95.

79. Somers VK, Dyken ME, Mark AL, et al. Sympathetic nerve activity during sleep in normal humans. N Engl J Med. 1993;328:303–7.

80. Klingelhofer J, Hajak G, Sander D, et al. Assessment of intracranial hemodynamics in sleep apnea syndrome. Stroke. 1992;23:1427–33.

81. Jennum P, Borgesen SE. Intracranial pressure and obstructive sleep apnea. Chest. 1989;95:279–83.

82. Tofler GH, Brezinski D, Schafer AI, et al. Concurrent morning increase in platelet aggregability and the risk of myocardial infarction and sudden cardiac death. N Engl J Med. 1987;316:1514–8.

83. Fletcher EC, Miller J, Schaaf JW, et al. Urinary catecholamines before and after tracheostomy in patients with obstructive sleep apnea and hypertension. Sleep. 1987;10:35–44.

84. Geiser T, Buck F, Meyer BJ, et al. In vivo platelet activation is increased during sleep in patients with obstructive sleep apnea syndrome. Respiration. 2002;69:229–34.

85. Minoguchi K, Yokoe T, Tazaki T, et al. Silent brain infarction and platelet activation in obstructive sleep apnea. Am J Respir Crit Care Med. 2007;175:612–7.

86. Berry RB, Brooks R, Gamaldo CE, et al. For the American Academy of Sleep Medicine. The AASM Manual for the Scoring of Sleep and Associated Events: Rules, Terminology and Technical Specifications, Version 2.0. www.aasmnet.org, Darien: American Academy of Sleep Medicine; 2012.

87. Berry RB, Kouchi KG, Der DE, et al. Sleep apnea impairs the arousal response to airway occlusion. Chest. 1996;109:1490–6.

88. Cirignotta F, Zucconi M, Mondini S, et al. Cerebral anoxic attacks in sleep apnea syndrome. Sleep. 1989;12:400–4.

89. Dyken ME, Yamada T, Glenn CL, et al. Obstructive sleep apnea associated with cerebral hypoxemia and death. Neurology. 2004;62:491–3.

90. White DP, Douglas NJ, Pickett CK, et al. Sleep deprivation and the control of ventilation. Am Rev Respir Dis. 1983;198:984–6.

91. Martin SE, Engleman HM, Kingshott RN, et al. Microarousals in patients with sleep apnoea/hypopnoea syndrome. J Sleep Res. 1997;6:276–80.

92. Berthon-Jones M, Sullivan CE. Ventilation and arousal responses to hypercapnia in normal sleeping humans. J Appl Physiol. 1984; 57:59–67.

93. Severson CA, Wang W, Pieribone VA, et al. Midbrain serotonergic neurons are central pH chemoreceptors. Nat Neurosci. 2003;6:1139–40.

94. Richerson, GB. Serotonergin neurons as carbon dioxide sensors that maintain pH homeostasis. Nat Rev Neurosci. 2004;5:449–61.

95. Buchanan GF, Richerson GB. Central serotonin neurons are required for arousal to CO_2. Proc Natl Acad Sci. 2010;107:16354–9.

96. Berthon-Jones M, Sullivan CE. Ventilatory and arousal responses to hypoxia in sleeping humans. Am Rev Respir Dis. 1982;125:632–9.

97. Darnall RA, Schneider RW, Tobia CM, et al. Arousal from sleep in response to intermittent hypoxia in infant rodents is modulated by medullary raphe GABAergic mechanisms. Am J Physiol Regul Integr Comp Physiol. 2012;302:R551–560.

98. Issa FG, Sullivan CE. Arousal and breathing responses to airway occlusion in healthy sleeping adults. J Appl Physiol. 1983;55:1113–9.

99. Brown DL, Chervin RD, Hickenbottom SL, et al. Screening for obstructive sleep apnea in stroke patients: a cost-effectiveness analysis. Stroke. 2005;36:1291–4.

100. Askenasy JJ, Goldhammer I. Sleep apnea as a feature of bulbar stroke. Stroke 1988;19:637–9.

101. Good DC, Henkle JQ, Gelber D, et al. Sleep-disordered breathing in patients with poor functional outcome after stroke. Stroke 1996;27:252–8.

102. Bassetti C, Aldrich MS, Quint D. Sleep-disordered breathing in patients with acute supra- and infratentorial strokes: a prospective study of 39 patients. Stroke 1997;28:1765–72.

Sleep in Neurodegenerative Diseases

32

Alex Iranzo and Joan Santamaria

Introduction

Neurodegenerative diseases are characterized by progressive neuronal loss in the nervous system and abnormal deposition of some proteins such as alpha-synuclein, tau, or amyloid thought to lead to cell dysfunction. The etiology of most of the neurodegenerative diseases is still unknown. Several sleep disorders including insomnia, rapid eye movement (REM) sleep behavior disorder (RBD), periodic leg movements in sleep (PLMS), restless legs syndrome (RLS), excessive daytime sleepiness (EDS), and nocturnal stridor have been described in patients with neurodegenerative diseases. However, the idea that sleep disorders occur commonly in neurodegenerative diseases is relatively new, although one can find descriptions of sleep problems in the classical descriptions of Parkinson disease (PD), multiple system atrophy (MSA), hereditary ataxias, progressive supranuclear palsy (PSP), and Huntington disease (HD). PD can be considered as a representative neurodegenerative disorder where the main sleep symptoms, namely, insomnia, EDS, and parasomnia, commonly occur.

Parkinson Disease

PD is caused by progressive neuronal loss in many regions of the brain leading to dysfunction of several neurotransmitter systems, particularly the nigrostriatal and mesolimbic do-paminergic systems. The structures that regulate the sleep–wake cycle are also damaged by the disease process. PD is clinically characterized by gait and postural abnormalities, resting tremor, rigidity, and bradykinesia. In addition, patients present nonmotor manifestations such as depression, anxiety, dementia, autonomic impairment, and sleep disturbances [20].

In his monograph written in 1817, James Parkinson first recognized that sleep disturbances are an important component of the condition that he originally termed paralysis agitans [96], particularly in patients in the last stage of the disease. For many years, however, neurologists considered insomnia as the only relevant sleep problem. The presence of sleep disruption was considered a risk for developing levodopa psychosis [87, 111] and likely related to chronic levodopa therapy. This attitude changed completely after the publication of two highly relevant papers: one by Schenck et al. in 1996 [108] describing the development of parkinsonism in patients initially diagnosed with idiopathic RBD, and another by Frucht et al. in 1999 [33] describing sleep attacks in patients taking the dopamine agonists pramipexole and ropinirole (Fig. 32.1).

Sleep complaints in patients with PD are more frequently common than in healthy age-matched controls, can be severe, and in some cases are the initial manifestation of the disease [2, 108], and can have a negative impact on quality of life [30, 65, 70, 77, 119]. Insomnia, sleep fragmentation, nocturia, stiffness, difficulties in turning over in bed, akathisia, nocturnal restless legs, cramps, nightmares, vigorous motor and vocal dream-enacting behaviors, visual hallucinations, confusional awakenings, snoring, witnessed apneas, painful early-morning dystonia, and EDS are some of the sleep problems described in PD. Sleep complaints and polysomnography (PSG) abnormalities found in patients with PD are multifactorial. They are related to damage and functional dysregulation of the brain structures and mechanisms involved in sleep origin and maintenance, the effects of antiparkinsonian drugs on sleep, parkinsonism severity,

A. Iranzo (✉) · J. Santamaria
Neurology Service, Hospital Clínic de Barcelona,
C/Villarroel 170, 08036 Barcelona, Spain
e-mail: airanzo@clinic.ub.es

Institut d'Investigació Biomèdiques August Pi i Sunyer
(IDIBAPS), Barcelona, Spain

Centro de Investigación Biomédica en Red sobre Enfermedades
Neurodegenerativas (CIBERNED), Barcelona, Spain

S. Chokroverty, M. Billiard (eds.), *Sleep Medicine,* DOI 10.1007/978-1-4939-2089-1_32,
© Springer Science+Business Media, LLC 2015

Fig. 32.1 Number of articles published between the years 1966 and 2013 dealing with "Parkinson disease" (PD) and with "sleep disorders and PD." The number of publications on the area of PD in 2013 doubled the number of articles published in 1999, whereas for the area of sleep disorders and PD there were six times more articles in 2013 than in 1999. (Source: Pub Med)

SLEEP DISORDERS & PARKINSONS'S DISEASE

n: 1784

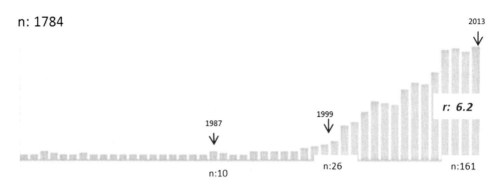

PARKINSONS'S DISEASE

n: 73047

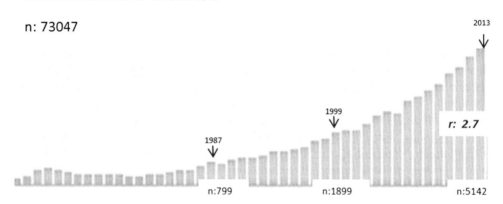

comorbid conditions such as anxiety, depression, and dementia, aging, and genetic individual susceptibility. In general, sleep disturbances gradually worsen with the progression of the disease.

Insufficient and Fragmented Nocturnal sleep

Most patients with PD report insufficient sleep as a result of frequent awakenings, and less commonly, early-onset insomnia and early-morning awakening [65, 70, 77, 119]. In patients with PD, poor and reduced sleep causes severe daytime fatigue and tiredness. Interestingly, as noted in primary insomnia, poor quality and reduced duration of nocturnal sleep in PD are not related to the development of EDS. [6, 103]. Surprisingly, a more robust and continuous sleep architecture has been associated with more severe sleepiness [103]. The main cause of reduced and fragmented sleep in patients with PD is the severity of parkinsonian symptoms. Although muscle tone decreases during sleep, variable degrees of rigidity can be experienced by patients with PD during the different stages of sleep. This rigidity accounts for complaints of stiffness, back pain, and leg cramps. Nocturnal akinesia is responsible, along with

stiffness, for poor nocturnal mobility that manifests as difficulties turning over or getting out of bed. This situation can be extremely distressing to patients who need to go to the toilet several times at night. In patients with advanced PD, chronic treatment with bilateral subthalamic stimulation improves subjective sleep quality, something that is thought to be a consequence of increased nocturnal mobility secondary to a an improvement in rigidity and bradykinesia [5, 54]. Patients with PD who also have dementia may exhibit confusional awakenings and visual hallucinations leading to sleep fragmentation and nonrestorative sleep. The main contributors to early-onset insomnia in patients with PD are anxiety, depression, dyskinesias induced by dopaminergic drugs, and the intrinsic effect of several antiparkinsonian drugs such as selegiline and levodopa. Depression and early-morning trunk and foot dystonia cause early awakening. Circadian sleep–wake cycle disruption is another cause of disturbed nocturnal sleep in patients with PD. These individuals have an exaggerated tendency toward an advancement of phase, thereby developing an irregular sleep–wake pattern characterized by early-morning awakening and evening sleepiness. This situation is frequently associated with an advanced disease state, depression, and dementia.

Excessive Daytime Sleepiness

Most of the studies dealing with EDS in PD have been published after 1999, following the paper by Frucht et al. [33]. It is illustrative, as an example, to review the 1998 [90] and 2001 [92] "Algorithms for the management of PD" in the journal *Neurology* to see how EDS was contemplated before and after the Frucht et al. [33] paper was published. In the twentieth century, EDS in PD was considered rare, and usually related to medications. This perception completely changed after the description of "sleep attacks" in PD patients treated with the dopaminergic agonists pramipexole and ropinirole.

The prevalence of persistent EDS in patients with PD ranges from 15.5 to 74 % [29, 39, 41, 47, 116, 117, 120, 126]. The main factors contributing to persistent EDS are the intrinsic pathology of PD and the sedative effects of the dopaminergic drugs. In patients with PD, the development of persistent EDS may be related to progressive cell loss in the dopaminergic and nondopaminergic brain structures, and circuits that modulate the sleep–wake mechanisms. In general, persistent EDS is associated with advanced parkinsonism and the use of dopaminomimetics. Other possible causes of persistent EDS should be considered before determining whether EDS is caused by the disease itself or by the effects of dopaminomimetics. Circadian dysrhythmia, obstructive sleep apnea, depression, dementia, and the concomitant use of other sedative drugs such as hypnotics are thought to contribute to persistent EDS.

There is a subgroup of sleepy PD patients with short mean sleep latency and the presence of REM sleep periods on the multiple sleep latency test [6, 103]. In PD, cerebrospinal fluid (CSF) hypocretin levels, however, have been reported to be normal [23] and cataplexy does not occur. In unselected PD patients, autopsies show a loss of 23–62 % of hypocretin cells, but CSF hypocretin levels are normal in PD with and without dementia [32, 122] (Table 32.1).

Sudden onset of sleep episodes (SOS), or sleep attacks, are less common than persistent EDS in patients with PD [50]. Among patients with PD treated with dopaminergic drugs, the prevalence of SOS is estimated to range from 0 to 32 % [29, 47, 117, 120]. Episodes of SOS are considered to be the result of a dopaminergic class effect; that is, they have been shown to be associated with the use of virtually all dopaminergic drugs, occur several days or months after the introduction of the dopaminergic drug, and usually resolve or decrease after its withdrawal, reduction, or replacement. The most common variables associated with SOS episodes are therapy with dopamine agonists, duration of parkinsonism, elevated Epworth Sleepiness Scale scores, age, and sex [83, 91, 97]. In PD, modafinil [49] and sodium oxybate [94] may improve EDS.

Sleep-Disordered Breathing

Several studies have shown that sleep-disordered breathing is common in patients with PD, especially in those individuals complaining of sleepiness. However, it is not significantly more prevalent in patients with PD than in age-matched populations [10, 26, 27, 89, 123] (Table 32.2). In PD, the frequency of an apnea–hypopnea index greater than 5 is 27–54 %, and the frequency of greater than 30 is 4–15 %. The number of apneas does not change across consecutive nights and is not modified by the introduction of a dopaminergic agent. The number of apneas per hour in PD is not associated with age, gender, body mass index, the occurrence of RBD, oxyhemoglobin saturation at night, scales that assess sleepiness, and parkinsonism severity. Therefore, it seems that PD itself does not confer an increased risk of obstructive apneas and that the frequent presence of this condition in PD is a reflection of aging or reduction of the upper airway space. Nevertheless, patients with PD who experience EDS should undergo routine PSG to identify the potential for obstructive sleep apneas. In these cases, correct treatment of this condition with continuous positive airway pressure (CPAP) can help them greatly.

Table 32.1 Comparison between Parkinson disease with narcolepsy with cataplexy and with narcolepsy without cataplexy

	Narcolepsy with cataplexy	Narcolepsy without cataplexy	Parkinson disease
Hypersomnia	+	+	+
Sleep attacks	+	+	+
Cataplexy	+	-	-
Hallucinations	+	+	+
Sleep paralysis	+	+	-
REM sleep behavior disorder	+	+	+
HLA DQB1*0602	>90 %	60 %	30 %
Sleep onset REM periods in the multiple sleep latency test	+	+	+/-
Absent hypocretin in cerebrospinal fluid	>90 %	10 %	0 %
Loss of hypocretinergic cells in the hypothalamus	90 %	30 %	23–62 %

Table 32.2 Obstructive sleep apnea in Parkinson disease

Author Year	Country	Patients (n)	Mean age (years)	Mean AHI (n)	AHI >5 (%)	AHI >10 (%)	AHI =5–15 (%)	AHI >15 (%)	AHI =15–30 (%)	AHI >30 (%)
Rye et al. 2000 [103]	USA	27	68	11	–	–	–	–	–	–
Arnulf 2002 [6]	France	54	68	10	47	14	28	20	11	9
Stevens et al. 2004 [116]	USA	19	60	9	–	–	–	–	–	–
Iranzo et al. 2005 [57]	Spain	45	65	16	–	–	–	–	–	–
Diederich 2005 [27]	Luxemburg	49	65	8	43		20	22	8	15
Baumann 2005 [10]	Switzerland	10	69	11	–	–	–	–	–	–
Trotti and Bliwise2010 [123]	USA	55	64	7	44	–	29	15	11	4
Noradina 2010 [89]	Malaysia	46	64	7	54		27	27	18	9
De Cock 2010 [26]	France	100	62	10	27	–	6	21	11	10

AHI apnea–hypopnea index (number of apneas and hypopneas per hour of sleep).

REM Sleep Behavior Disorder

RBD is a parasomnia first described in five patients in 1986 by Schenck et al [106], who expanded the following year [107] the observation to ten new patients, involving predominantly older men (half of whom had a major neurologic disorder including parkinsonism). Since that time, RBD has taken an increasingly important role in understanding sleep in PD. Before the description of RBD, episodes of nocturnal agitation were considered a variant of somnambulism, and thought to appear out of deep nonrapid eye movement (NREM) sleep and probably induced by levodopa (Scharf et al 1978).

RBD is characterized by dream-enacting behaviors, fearful dreams, and REM sleep without atonia. RBD may be idiopathic or associated with neurodegenerative diseases [60]. Studies from three different groups have shown that patients with idiopathic RBD develop the classical motor and cognitive symptoms of PD, dementia with Lewy bodies, and MSA with time [58, 61, 101, 108, 109].

RBD occurs at least in one-third of patients with sporadic PD [34, 105] and is also frequent in patients with PD secondary to mutations in the *parkin* gene [71]. RBD occurs in PD patients untreated or treated with dopaminergic agents. RBD is more common in the rigid-akinetic clinical subtype of the disease than in the tremoric subtype [72]. For reasons not yet known, RBD is more common in male patients with PD than in female patients. Of note, up to 29 % of patients with PD with confirmed RBD by video-PSG are unaware of their abnormal motor and vocal sleep behaviors, and up to 13 % do not recall dreaming [57]. In these cases, history sugges-

tive of RBD can be obtained only from the bed partner. On the other hand, hallucinations, somnambulism, confusional awakenings, and severe obstructive sleep apneas may mimic RBD symptoms in PD [52]. The sensitivity of specialized interviews for identifying RBD in patients with PD varies from 33 to 95 %. There is some evidence that RBD in PD is associated with dementia [128], age, and disease duration [115]. However, the occurrence of RBD in nondemented PD subjects with early stages of the disease is not uncommon. When comparing patients who have PD and RBD with patients who have idiopathic RBD and MSA with RBD, there are few differences in RBD-related clinical and sleep measures [57]. The pathophysiology of RBD in patients with PD is thought to result from the degeneration or dysfunction of the brainstem structures that modulate REM sleep [60]. Such areas include the medial medulla, pedunculopontine, and subcoeruleus mesopontine regions, and their anatomic connections with the substantia nigra pars reticulata, basal ganglia, hypothalamus, and limbic system. Postmortem studies examining the brains of patients with PD have shown that the degenerative process begins in the lower brainstem and advances upward through the pons before reaching the midbrain where the substantia nigra is located [17]. This might account for the observation that RBD precedes the onset of parkinsonism. However, an alternate sequence of neuropathologic events may take place to account for the more common finding of parkinsonism preceding RBD. RBD in PD, and associated with any other condition including the idiopathic form, responds to low doses of clonazepam at bedtime. Melatonin can be a therapeutic alternative in those few cases that do not respond to clonazepam or do not tolerate this drug. In refractory cases, methods of self-protection from injury during episodes of RBD may be necessary. Pramipexole does not improve symptoms of RBD in patients with PD [73], a finding suggesting that dopamine dysfunction does not play a central role in the pathogenesis of RBD.

Restless Legs Syndrome

RLS is a sensorimotor disorder characterized by an urge to move the legs. This impulse is caused by unpleasant sensations that begin during periods of inactivity at night and is relieved by movement. RLS is a condition that affects up to 5–15 % of the general population over 60 years of age and may interfere with sleep initiation and maintenance. Iron and dopaminergic dysfunction in the diencephalo-spinal system are believed to play a critical role in the pathogenesis of RLS because patients with RLS dramatically respond to dopaminergic drugs. Although the description of RLS is several centuries old, the description that levodopa improved their symptoms [3] pointed out the role of the dopaminergic system in RLS and the possible relationship between RLS and PD.

There is no evidence, however, that idiopathic RLS predisposes to develop PD [59] (Table 32.3). On the one hand, patients with idiopathic RLS do not progress to PD [132]. On the other hand, while it had been suggested that there is an association between PD and RLS, the evidence is still limited to few studies with methodological problems that have reported conflicting results [18, 44, 66, 69, 75, 76, 79, 88, 93, 98, 118, 129]. When PD patients are compared with a control group, there is no difference between the rate of RLS between the two groups [2, 19, 42]. It should be noted that RLS must be carefully distinguished by clinical history from other uncomfortable sensations commonly experienced by the PD subjects (stiffness, pain, tingling, heat, cramps) which may be related to parkinsonian features and not to RLS (rigidity, tremor, central pain, off periods, dystonia, and dyskinesias). Like in idiopathic RLS, PD patients with true RLS have low serum ferritin levels. In most of the PD cases with comorbid RLS, parkinsonism precedes the onset of RLS and severity of RLS is mild. This is probably because dopaminergic agents improve both RLS and parkinsonism. However, PD and RLS may be coexistent because they are both prevalent in the elderly. If true RLS is bothersome or prevents the PD patient from sleeping, the evening dose of dopaminergic agents can be increased or a standard formulation can be prescribed. Alternatively, other nondopaminergic drugs that are effective for RLS such as gabapentin and pregabalin can be used.

Periodic Leg Movements During Sleep

PLMS are repetitive, stereotyped leg movements that are 0.5–10 s in duration and are separated by an interval of more than 5 s but less than 90 s. The occurrence of PLMS is thought to be related to the impairment of central dopaminergic function because PLMS decrease in frequency with the use of dopaminergic medications. Moreover, PLMS in PD increase after chronic treatment with bilateral subthalamic stimulation probably because this type of surgery facilitates the reduction or withdrawal of dopaminergic drug treatment [54]. PLMS are more frequent in untreated patients with mild to moderate PD than in healthy individuals [135]. Most patients with PD who experience PLMS are unaware of these leg movements because PLMS are generally not associated with awakenings. Therefore, PLMS in PD may be not considered a main contributing factor for developing insomnia, sleep fragmentation, and EDS.

Table 32.3 Restless legs syndrome in Parkinson disease

Author Year	Country	Patients (n)	Mean age (years)	RLS in PD (%)	RLS in controls (%)
Lang 1987 [75]	Canada	100	62	0	NE
Ondo 2002 [93]	USA	303	67	21	NE
Khan and Sahota 2002 [66]	USA	26	NE	38	NE
Tan et al. 2002 [117]	Singapore	125	65	0	NE
Krishnan et al. 2002 [69]	India	126	57	8	1
Braga-Neto 2004 [18]	Brazil	86	65	52	NE
Nomura 2006 [88]	Japan	165	68	12	2
Gómez-Esteban 2007 [44]	Spain	114	69	22	NE
Loo 2008 [79]	Singapore	200	65	3	0.5
Lee et al. 2009 [76]	Korea	447	64	16	NE
Calzetti 2009 [19]	Italy	118	69	13	6
Peralta et al. 2010 [98]	Austria	113	67	24	NE
Verbaan et al. 2010 [129]	Holland	269	61	11	NE
Angelini 2011 [4]	Italy	109	67	6	4
Gjestard et al. 2011 [42]	Norway	200	65	12	7

NE not evaluated

Multiple System Atrophy

Historically, what is now considered a single disease was first described as three separate entities: striatonigral degeneration, olivopontocerebellar atrophy, and Shy–Drager syndrome [133, 134]. The characteristic pathologic findings, however, are the same and consist of neuronal loss and abnormal intracytoplasmic glial inclusions of alpha-synuclein in widespread areas of the central nervous system most frequently involving the substantia nigra, locus ceruleus, putamen, inferior olives, pontine nuclei, and cerebellar Purkinje cells. There are two main clinical presentations of MSA: the parkinsonian and the cerebellar subtypes, with dysautonomia occurring in both presentations. The disease affects both sexes, usually starts in the sixth decade, and in general progresses invariably with death occurring after an average of 6–9 years [133, 134]. Death during sleep is not infrequent [86, 105, 113].

Multiple central neurotransmitter systems are impaired including dopaminergic, cholinergic, serotonergic, adrenergic, noradrenergic, and glutamatergic. Insufficient and fragmented sleep, stridor, sleep-disordered breathing, and RBD are common among MSA subjects. RBD and stridor are considered red flags of the disease [40].

Insufficient and Fragmented Nocturnal Sleep

MSA patients commonly report sleep onset and maintenance insomnia [36, 130]. Polysomnographic studies in MSA patients frequently demonstrate marked sleep fragmentation and reduced sleep efficiency. Urinary dysfunction related to both urinary incontinence and retention is also a major contributor for reduced and fragmented sleep in subjects with MSA. In some instances, sleep onset insomnia can be associated with anxiety or with agitated depression. Early awakenings may be a sign of depression. Like in PD, the intrinsic pathology in MSA itself is likely to be an important factor for the development of sleep impairment, because early and untreated MSA patients exhibit disturbed and poor sleep. Sleep fragmentation in MSA is more common than in PD, particularly in advanced cases, reflecting the more severe clinical condition and the more diffuse underlying pathological process in MSA. Sleep-related structures such as some brainstem nuclei and basal ganglia are damaged in MSA. The occurrence of sleep complaints in subjects with MSA is related to longer disease, disease severity, and depression. Like in PD, treatment strategies in MSA patients with difficulties in initiating and maintaining sleep need to be highly individualized.

Excessive Daytime Sleepiness

The occurrence of EDS in MSA has not been systematically addressed by either subjective or objective means until recently [84]. It appears to be as frequent as in PD, since approximately a quarter of the patients with moderate disease present this symptom. The underlying cause of hypersomnia may be multifactorial due to obstructive sleep apneas, depression, reduced nighttime sleep, and the effect of some medications such as antidepressants, benzodiazepines, and dopaminergic agents that can even cause sleep attacks [48]. A few patients may show mild reduced mean sleep latency in multiple sleep latency tests and the presence of multiple sleep onset REM periods. Despite the finding that in MSA there is some degree of hypocretinergic cell loss in the posterior hypothalamus [11], the hypocretin-1 levels in the CSF are normal [80].

Sleep-Disordered Breathing and Stridor

There are two different causes of sleep-disordered breathing in MSA. One is central hypoventilation due to degeneration of the pontomedullary autonomic respiratory center. The other is obstructive sleep apnea as a result of upper airway obstruction, mainly at the level of the larynx.

Central Hypoventilation In MSA, many of the areas involved in the automatic control of respiration (nucleus tractus solitarius, pre-Bötzinger complex, medullary raphe, and arcuate nucleus) have severe cell loss [12]. This results in central sleep apneas, Cheyne–Stokes respiration during sleep and during wakefulness in both supine and erect positions, dysrhythmic breathing patterns such as cluster breathing with periods of apneas during wakefulness and sleep, apneustic breathing, periodic inspiratory gasps manifested by a short inspiratory time and prolonged expiratory time, and diminished ventilatory response to both hypercapnia and hypoxemia [21, 22, 78, 124]. These breathing abnormalities occur particularly during sleep and in most of the cases they are subclinical. In a few cases, however, central hypoventilation may manifest as severe dyspnea and respiratory failure. Central sleep apneas are commonly found in later stages of MSA, but in a few cases may be the presenting feature of the disease [24, 43]. In some patients with MSA, failure to increase ventilation in response to hypoxia and hypercapnia may cause sudden death during sleep, particularly in subjects with comorbid untreated obstructive sleep apneas.

Obstructive Sleep Apneas and Stridor In MSA, obstructive sleep apneas are more common than central hypoventilation. It is usually the result of upper airway obstruction at the level of the larynx. PSG with synchronized audiovisual monitoring discloses laryngeal stridor during sleep in up to 36–42% consecutive unselected MSA patients [56, 57, 130]. Detection of stridor in MSA is very important because this condition is associated with life-threatening episodes of respiratory failure, nocturnal choking episodes, sudden death during sleep, and short survival [86, 113, 137]. Nocturnal stridor occurs in all clinical stages of MSA and in few cases it may be the initial symptom of the disease [43]. Between patients with and without stridor, there are no differences in age, sex, body mass index, duration and severity of the disease, and the MSA subtype. Compared to subjects without stridor, patients with stridor have a higher apnea–hypopnea index, oxyhemoglobin desaturations, and vocal cord abnormalities on laryngoscopy [56]. It should be noted that nocturnal stridor and snoring may coexist. The severity of nocturnal stridor increases with the passage of time and invariable worsening of the disease. Stridor during wakefulness follows nocturnal stridor. Daytime stridor reflects marked laryngeal obstruction and potential severe respiratory failure.

In unselected MSA subjects, laryngoscopy may show asymptomatic partial vocal cord abduction restriction. In patients with stridor, laryngoscopy during wakefulness detects normal adduction of the vocal cords in phonation, and partial or complete abduction restriction of the vocal cords during inspiration. This abduction restriction may be unilateral or bilateral. Subjects with complete unilateral vocal cord abduction restriction do not present severe dyspnea because the glottic space is relatively wide during inspiration. Subjects with complete bilateral abduction restriction usually have both diurnal and nocturnal stridor, and are at a high risk of developing episodes of subacute respiratory insufficiency [56]. In some patients with mild stridor, movements of the vocal cords during wakefulness seem to be normal, but flicker-like movements may be seen during inspiration reflecting the possible earliest stage of vocal cord abduction dysfunction that can be detected by direct laryngoscopy. In these subjects, laryngoscopy during anesthesia with propofol or diazepam discloses paradoxical movements of the vocal cords (adduction on inspiration and abduction on expiration) or partial vocal cord abduction [64]. Vocal cord abductor restriction is exacerbated during sleep, and partial abduction limitation during wakefulness may become total during sleep [68]. This is because the vocal cord abductor muscles, like other muscles of respiration, have a reduced tone during sleep.

The origin of laryngeal obstruction in MSA is unclear, but it is thought to be related to a combination of factors including denervation of the vocal cord abductors and abnormal overactivation of the vocal cord adductors [46, 51, 62]. In patients with parkinsonism, the occurrence of vocal cord paralysis indicates underlying MSA and not PD [63]. Management of laryngeal narrowing in MSA is complex.

Laryngeal surgery (vocal cord lateralization, cordectomy) is associated with an increased risk of aspiration. Experience with botulinum toxin is limited to a very few patients [82]. Botulinum toxin therapy may increase the risk of bronchial aspiration, aggravate dysphonia, and dysphagia, and requires electromyographic guidance and repeated injections.

CPAP is an effective noninvasive treatment for eliminating stridor and obstructive sleep apneas in MSA [37, 53, 56]. In patients at early stages of disease, CPAP is an effective long-term therapy for the management of obstructive sleep apneas and nocturnal stridor. Adaptation to the CPAP machine can be difficult in advanced cases. CPAP abolishes stridor because it eliminates the abnormal activity of the vocal cord adductors during inspiration, thereby reducing the laryngeal resistance and increasing the glottic aperture. While untreated stridor is associated with short survival, it has been shown that median survival time is similar between subjects without stridor and those with stridor treated only with CPAP. When CPAP is not tolerated after intensive support, tracheostomy should then be considered. In subjects with daytime stridor, elective tracheostomy should be advised since this condition leads to dramatic subacute episodes of respiratory failure.

Central apneas without important desaturations may appear after tracheostomy and CPAP therapy because of possible unmasking of central apneas after correction of obstructive apneas. Despite the elimination of stridor with tracheostomy some patients have died while sleeping, presumably due to respiratory arrest of central origin or cardiac arrest related to autonomic failure.

REM Sleep Behavior Disorder

The vast majority of patients with MSA have RBD with a prevalence of 90–100% [56, 100]. The finding that in MSA brainstem cell loss is consistently widespread and severe may explain the high prevalence of RBD in this disease. RBD in MSA is unrelated to age, disease severity, disease duration, clinical subtype (parkinsonian or cerebellar), or to any other demographic or clinical feature. In about half of the patients, RBD antedates the onset of parkinsonian, cerebellar, or autonomic symptoms by a mean of 7 years [57].

Huntington Disease

HD is a genetic autosomal dominant neurodegenerative disorder characterized by progressive dementia, chorea, and psychiatric disturbances linked to expanded cytosine–adenine–guanine (CAG) repeats in the Huntington gene. Pathological studies demonstrate severe atrophy of the putamen and caudate, and, to a lesser extent, of the cortex [13].

Sleep disorders are common among patients with HD, particularly in advanced stages. Patients usually report poor sleep quality, sleep fragmentation with frequent awakenings at night, EDS, and the circadian rhythm sleep disorder of the advanced phase type resulting in early-morning awakening [8, 121, 131]. Interestingly, a transgenic model of HD in mice has a disrupted circadian rhythm that worsens as the disease progresses, suggesting a progressive impairment of the suprachiasmatic nucleus in the hypothalamus [85]. In a community survey study with 292 patients, sleep problems were reported by 87% and were rated as important by 62%. Sleep problems, in rank order, were restless limb movements, periodic jerky movements, waking during the night, hypersomnia, and early awakening [121]. In one study involving 25 patients, 64% complained of insomnia, advanced sleep phase occurred in 40%, and hypersomnia in 32% [8].

Overall, PSG studies show reduced sleep efficiency, increased wake time after sleep onset, increased percentage of light sleep, increased REM sleep latency, and reduced percentage of deep sleep and REM sleep [8, 45, 114, 136]. In HD, sleep complaints and PSG abnormalities increase with disease severity and duration. PSG studies have shown a low incidence of sleep apneas in patients with HD [9, 16] and RBD [8]. Multiple sleep latency tests were performed in only one study showing a reduced sleep latency in 4 of 25 patients (16%) and no REM sleep periods [8].

In a pathological study, a mean reduction of hypocretin cells of 27% was observed in five HD brains [99]. However, HD patients do not have a narcoleptic phenotype because cataplexy is absent [8], the multiple sleep latency does not detect sleep onset REM periods [6], and hypocretin-1 level in the cerebrospinal has been found to be normal in 22 alive patients [81] and in samples from ten postmortem patients [35]. Thus, it can be speculated that surviving hypocretinergic neurons in the hypothalamus still provide sufficient hypocretin to prevent the occurrence of hypersomnia and narcoleptic features.

REM Sleep Behavior Disorder

RBD was investigated by clinical history and PSG in one study that involved 25 patients. Three (12%) had video-PSG confirmed RBD. Two were aware of their abnormal behaviors at night, but these behaviors were considered clinically mild. In an additional patient, video-PSG showed RBD but the patient was not aware of displaying dream-enacting behaviors or having unpleasant dreams. Patients were two

women and one man aged 41, 45, and 65 years, respectively. One had mild HD and two moderated HD severity [7]. In another study of 30 HD patients, 7 (23%) patients and bed partners reported symptoms suggestive of RBD but PSG was not performed [131].

Restless Legs Syndrome

In a series of 25 patients, only one (4%) had RLS and a PLMS index greater than 15 was found in six (24%) [6]. PLMS did not fragment sleep. In contrast, one study with six patients found a high mean PLMS index of 123 that fragmented sleep [16]. A 55-year-old man developed RLS 3 years prior the onset of the classical symptoms of HD. PSG demonstrated high indices of periodic leg movements during sleep (index of 58) and wakefulness (index of 79). RLS symptomatology and sleep quality improved dramatically with gabapentin [104]. RLS was described in one family with HD. All five family members affected by RLS were also affected by HD, but some family members with RLS did not have HD suggesting that there may have been the independent occurrence of RLS in this family [28].

Progressive Supranuclear Palsy

PSP is a tauopathy involving the brainstem, basal ganglia, and many other brain areas. It is characterized by dementia, poor levodopa responsive parkinsonism, vertical gaze palsy, and falls. PSG studies show a decreased REM sleep percentage and other features also seen in PD such as decreased total sleep time and reduction in sleep spindles and K complexes. Sleep complaints include insomnia and symptoms suggestive of RBD. The first reported case of RBD linked to PSP was a 70-year-old woman presenting with inhibition of speech during wakefulness and intelligible somniloquy at night due to RBD [95]. Parkinsonism developed one year before the onset of RBD. In a series of 15 patients who underwent PSG, two had clinical RBD, and four exhibited REM sleep with increased tonic electromyographic activity [7]. Clinical manifestations of RBD were severe in one patient, but none of the patients were aware of their abnormal sleep behaviors. The finding that RBD may be found in a tauopathy such as PSP argues against RBD as an exclusive feature of the synucleinopathies (PD, dementia with Lewy bodies, and MSA). Sleep-disordered breathing and RLS are not major complications in PSP.

Hereditary Ataxias

Hereditary ataxias are inherited neurodegenerative disorders that in most cases result from mutations in genes. Modes of inheritance in hereditary ataxias are autosomal dominant (e.g., spinocerebellar ataxias), autosomal recessive (e.g., ataxia telangectasia, Friedreich ataxia), and X-linked (e.g., fragile X tremor ataxia syndrome). These diseases affect the spinocerebellar tracts, cerebellum, brainstem, and many other structures in the brain. They are clinically characterized by progressive ataxia and a wide variety of other neurological symptoms and signs such as polyneuropathy and parkinsonism in addition to nonneurological symptoms including cardiomyopathy and cutaneous telangectasia [67]. Occurrence and clinical relevance of sleep disorders have recently received attention, particularly RBD and RLS.

REM Sleep Behavior Disorder

In one study in spinocerebellar ataxia type 3 (SCA3 or Machado Joseph disease), 53 patients reported more symptoms suggestive of RBD, RLS, obstructive sleep apneas, and insomnia than controls [25]. One study described the presumed presence of RBD in 12 of 22 (56%) SCA3 patients of Portuguese or Azorean origin. Diagnosis was based on a questionnaire, patients were not interviewed by the authors, and PSG was not performed [31]. In a SCA3 patient with clinically suspected RBD video-PSG showed normal REM sleep atonia and non-REM sleep episodes of complex nonrhythmic behaviors lasting more than 10 min [38]. The first reported SCA3 patient with confirmed RBD was a 51-year-old Portuguese man with violent sleep behaviors leading to

injuries. PSG showed increased electromyographic activity in the limbs and chin associated with kicking, thrashing, and yelling [74]. We described the presence of video-PSG confirmed RBD in five of nine (55%) consecutive Spanish SCA3 patients, four men and one woman, with a mean age of 48 years and a mean ataxia duration of 14 years. In two patients, RBD preceded the ataxia onset by 10 and 8 years. Clinical RBD severity was mild or moderate [55].

One study evaluated eight patients with SCA2 from five German families with sleep interviews and video-PSG. All but one reported good quality of sleep. None of the patients and bed partners reported symptoms suggestive of RBD such as nightmares, frequent vocalizations, and aggressive sleep behaviors. Video-PSG, however, showed subclinical RBD (increased submental electromyographic activity not associated with abnormal behaviors) in three patients, normal REM sleep in two, and REM sleep was not observed in three [125]. In another study, four of five SCA2 patients of three different Austrian families had increased electromyographic activity during REM sleep in the video-PSG. These four patients exhibited a mild form of RBD consisting of prominent myoclonic jerks in absence of complex and elaborate behaviors [14]. In one study, RBD was not detected in five patients with SCA type 6 [15].

Restless Legs Syndrome

Several studies have evaluated the occurrence of RLS in subjects with SCAs [1, 14, 15, 55, 102, 110, 127]. Studies found RLS in patients with SCA1, SCA2, SCA3, and SCA6 who were not treated with dopaminergic or antidopaminergic drugs (Table 32.4).The highest frequency of RLS has been

Table 32.4 Studies evaluating the frequency of restless legs syndrome in hereditary ataxias

Author year (Country)	SCA1 patients studied (n)	RLS in SCA1 (%)	SCA2 patients studied (n)	RLS in SCA2 (%)	SCA3 patients studied (n)	RLS in SCA3 (%)	SCA6 patients studied (n)	RLS in SCA6 (%)	RLS in controls (%)
Schöls et al. 1998 (Germany) [110]	6	0	11	18	51	45	21	5	NA
Abele et al. 2001 (Germany) [1]	13	23	22	27	23	30	NA	NA	10
Iranzo et al. 2003 (Spain) [55]	NA	NA	NA	NA	9	55.5	NA	NA	0
Boesch et al. 2006b (Austria) [15]	NA	NA	NA	NA	NA	NA	5	40	NA
Boesch et al. 2006a (Austria) [14]	NA	NA	5	0	NA	NA	NA	NA	NA
Reimold et al 2006 (Germany) [102]	4	25	4	25	2	100	NA	NA	NA
D'Abreu et al. 2008 (Brazil) [25]	NA	NA	NA	NA	53	20.7	NA	NA	4.7

RLS restless legs syndrome, *SCA1* spinocerebellar ataxia type 1, *SCA2* spinocerebellar ataxia type 2, *SCA3* spinocerebellar ataxia type 3, *SCA6* spinocerebellar ataxia type 6, *NA* not available

found in SCA3, ranging from 30 to 55% of the cases [1, 55, 110, 127] a higher figure than what is found in general population based studies. RLS symptoms were mild, moderate, or severe, and RLS was diagnosed only upon specific questioning when the studies were conducted. PSG in SCA1, SCA2, SCA3, and SCA6 showed a high number of PLMS in patients with or without RLS [14, 15, 55, 102, 110]. Most SCA patients were unaware of their leg movements and PLMS were usually not associated with arousals.

Sleep-Disordered-Breathing

PSG studies in patients with autosomal dominant SCAS and ataxia telangiectasia have shown that obstructive sleep apneas are not a common finding, except in one study where an apnea–hypopnea index greater than 5 was detected in four of five patients with SCA6 (range, 6–15) [15]. However, patients with SCA1 [112] and SCA3 [55] may show vocal cord abductor palsy, probably due to neuronopathy of the nucleus ambiguous impairing the recurrent laryngeal nerve fibers that mainly innervate the posterior cricoarytenoid muscle.

References

1. Abele N, Bürk K, Laccone F, et al. Restless legs syndrome in spinocerebellar ataxias types 1, 2 and 3. J Neurol. 2001;248:311–4.
2. Abbott RD, Ross GW, White LR, et al. Excessive daytime sleepiness and subsequent development of Parkinson disease. Neurology. 2005;65:1442–6.
3. Akpinar S. Treatment of restless legs syndrome with levodopa plus benserazide. Arch Neurol. 1982,39:739.
4. Angelini M, Negrotti A, Marchesi E, et al. A study of the prevalence of restless legs syndrome in previously untreated Parkinson's disease patients: absence of co-morbid association. J Neurol Sci. 2011;310:286–8.
5. Arnulf I, Bejjani BP, Garma L, et al. Improvement of sleep architecture in PD with subthalamic stimulation. Neurology. 2000;55:1732–4.
6. Arnulf I, Konofal E, Merino-Andreu M, et al. Parkinson's disease and sleepiness. An integral part of PD. Neurology. 2002;58:1019–24.
7. Arnulf I, Merino-Andreu M, Bloch F. REM sleep behavior disorder and REM sleep without atonia in progressive supranuclear palsy. Sleep. 2005;28:349–54.
8. Arnulf I, Nielsen J, Lehman E, et al. Rapid eye movement sleep disturbances in Huntington disease. Arch Neurol. 2008;68:482–8.
9. Banno K, Hobson DE, Kryger MH. Long-term treatment of sleep breathing disorder in a patient with Huntington disease. Parkinsonism Relat Disord. 2005;11:261–4.
10. Baumann C, Ferini-Strambi L, Waldvogel D, et al. Parkinsonism with excessive daytime sleepiness. J Neurol. 2005;252:139–45.
11. Benarroch EE, Schmeichel AM, Sandroni P, et al. Involvement of hypocretin neurons in multiple system atrophy. Acta Neuropathol. 2007a;113:75–80.
12. Benarroch EE, Schemeichel AM, Low PA, et al. Depletion of putative chemosensitive respiratory neurons in the ventral medullary surface in multiple system atrophy. Brain. 2007b;130:469–75.
13. Biglan KM, Shoulson I. Huntington's disease. In: Jankovic J, Tolosa E, editors. Parkinson's disease and movement disorders. Philadelphia: Lippincott Williams and Wilkins; 2007. pp. 212–227.
14. Bollen EL, Den Heijer JC, Ponsionen C, et al. Respiration during sleep in Huntington's chorea. J Neurol Sci. 1988;84:63–8.
15. Boesch S, Frauscher B, Brandauer E, et al. Disturbance of rapid eye movement sleep in spinocerebellar ataxia type 2. Mov Disord. 2006a;21:1751–4.
16. Boesch SM, Frauscher B, Brandauer E, et al. Restless legs syndrome and motor activity during sleep in spinocerebellar ataxia type 6. Sleep Med. 2006b;7:529–32.
17. Braak H, Del Tredici K, Rüb U, et al. Staging of brain pathology related to sporadic Parkinson's disease. Neurobiol Aging. 2003;24:197–211.
18. Braga-Neto P, Silva-Júnior FP, Monte FS, et al. Snoring and excessive daytime sleepiness in Parkinson's disease. J Neurol Sci. 2004;217:41–5.
19. Calzetti S, Negrotti, Bonavina G, et al. Absence of comorbidity of Parkinson disease and restless legs syndrome: a case-control study in patients attending a movement disorder clinic. Neurol Sci. 2009;30:119–22.
20. Chaudhuri KR, Helay DG, Schapira AHV. Non-motor symptoms of Parkinson's disease: diagnosis and management. Lancet Neurol. 2006;5:235–45.
21. Chokroverty S, Sharp JT, Barron KD. Periodic respiration in erect posture in Shy-Drager syndrome. J Neurol Neurosurg Psychiatry. 1978;41:980–6.
22. Chokroverty S, Sachedo R, Masdeu J. Autonomic dysfunction and sleep apnea in olivopontocerebellar degeneration. Arch Neurol. 1984;41:926–31.
23. Compta Y, Santamaria J, Ratti L, et al. Cerebrospinal hypocretin, daytime sleepiness and sleep architecture in Parkinson's disease dementia. Brain. 2009;132:3308–17.
24. Cormican LJ, Higgins S, Davidson AC, et al. Multiple system atrophy presenting as central sleep apnoea. Eur Respir J. 2004;24:323–5.
25. D'Abreu A, França M, Conz L, et al. Sleep symptoms and their clinical correlates in Machado-Joseph disease. Act Neurol Scand. 2009;119:277–80.
26. De Cock V, Abouda M, Leu S, et al. Is obstructive sleep apnea a problem in Parkinson's disease? Sleep Med. 2010;11:247–52.
27. Diederich NJ, Vaillant M, Leischen M, et al. Sleep apnea syndrome in Parkinson's disease. A case-control study in 49 patients. Mov Disord. 2005;11:1413–8.
28. Evers S, Stögbauer F. Genetic association of Huntington's disease and restless legs syndrome? A family report. Mov Disord. 2003;18:225–7.
29. Fabbrini G, Barbanti P, Aurilia C, et al. Excessive daytime sleepiness in de novo and treated Parkinson's disease. Mov Disord. 2002;17:1026–30.
30. Factor SA, McAlarney T, Sanchez-Ramos JR, et al. Sleep disorders and sleep effect in Parkinson's disease. Mov Disord. 1990;5:280–5.
31. Friedman JH, Fernandez HH, Sudarsky L. REM behavior disorder and excessive daytime somnolence in Machado-Joseph disease (SCA–3). Mov Disord. 2003;18:1520–2.
32. Fronczek R, Overeem S, Lee SY, et al. Hypocretin (orexin) loss in Parkinson's disease. Brain. 2007;130:1577–85.
33. Frucht S, Rogers MD, Greene PE, et al. Falling asleep at the wheel: motor vehicle mishaps in persons taking pramipexole and ropinirole. Neurology. 1999;52:1908–10.
34. Gagnon JF, Bédard MA, Fantini MD, et al. REM sleep behavior disorder and REM sleep without atonia in Parkinson's disease. Neurology. 2002;59:585–9.
35. Gaus SE, Lin L, Mignot E. CSF hypocretin levels are normal in Huntington disease patients. Sleep. 2005;28:1607–8.

36. Ghorayeb I, Yekhlef F, Chrysostome V, et al. Sleep disorders and their determinants in multiple system atrophy. J Neurol Neurosurg Psychiatry. 2002;72:798–800.

37. Ghorayeb I, Yekhlef F, Bioulac B, et al. Continuous positive airway pressure for sleep-related breathing disorders in multiple system atrophy: long-term, acceptance. Sleep Med. 2005a;6:359–62.

38. Ghorayeb I, Provini F, Bioulac B, et al. Unusual nocturnal motor restlessness in a patient with spinocerebellar ataxia 3. Mov Disord. 2005b;20:899–901.

39. Ghorayeb I, Loundou A, Auquier P, et al. A nationwide survey of excessive daytime sleepiness in Parkinson disease in France. Mov Disord. 2007;22:1567–72.

40. Gilman S, Wening GK, Low PA, et al. Second consensus statement on the diagnosis of multiple system atrophy. Neurology. 2008;71:670–6.

41. Gjerstad MD, Aarsland D, Larsen JP. Development of daytime somnolence over time in Parkinson's disease. Neurology. 2002;58:1544–6.

42. Gjerstad MD, Tysnes OB, Larsen JP. Increased risk of leg motor restlessness but not RLS in early Parkinson disease. Neurology. 2011;77:1941–6.

43. Glass GA, Josephs KA, Ahlskog JE. Respiratory insufficiency as the primary presenting symptom of multiple system atrophy. Arch Neurol. 2006;63:978–81.

44. Gómez-Esteban JC, Zarranz JJ, Tijero B, et al. Restless legs syndrome in Parkinson's disease. Mov Disord. 2007;22:1912–6.

45. Hansotia P, Wall R, Berendes J. Sleep disturbances and severity in Huntington's disease. Neurology. 1985;35:1672–4.

46. Hayashi M, Isozaki E, Oda M, et al. Loss of large myelinated nerve fibers of the recurrent laryngeal nerve in patients with multiple system atrophy and vocal cord nerve palsy. J Neurol Neurosurg Psychiatry. 1997;62:234–8.

47. Hobson DE, Lang AE, Martin WWR, Razmy A, et al. Excessive daytime sleepiness and sudden-onset sleep in Parkinson Disease. A survey by the Canadian movement disorder group. JAMA. 2002;287:455–63.

48. Högl B, Seppi K, Brandauer E, et al. Irresistible onset of sleep during acute levodopa challenge in a patient with multiple system atrophy. Mov Disord. 2001:16;1177–9.

49. Högl B, Saletu M, Brandauer E, et al. Modafinil for the treatment of daytime sleepiness in Parkinson's disease: a double-blind, randomized, crossover, placebo-controlled polygraphic trial. Sleep. 2002;25:905–9.

50. Homann CN, Wenzel K, Suppan K, et al. Sleep attacks in patients taking dopamine agonists: review. BMJ. 2002;324:1483–7.

51. Ikeda K, Iwasaki Y, Kuwajima A, et al. Preservation of branchimotor neurons of the nucleus ambiguous in multiple system atrophy (reply letter). Neurology. 2003;61:722–3.

52. Iranzo A, Santamaria J. Severe obstructive sleep apnea-hypopnea mimicking REM sleep behavior disorder. Sleep. 2005;28:203–6.

53. Iranzo A, Santamaría J, Tolosa E, On behalf of the Barcelona Multiple System Atrophy Group. Continuous positive air pressure eliminates nocturnal stridor in multiple system atrophy. Lancet. 2000;356:1329–30.

54. Iranzo A, Valldeoriola F, Santamaría J, et al. Sleep symptoms and polysomnographic architecture in advanced Parkinson's disease after chronic bilateral subthalamic stimulation. J Neurol Neurosurg Psychiatry. 2002;72:661–4.

55. Iranzo A, Muñoz E, Santamaria J, et al. REM sleep behavior disorder and vocal cord paralysis in Machado–Joseph disease. Mov Disord. 2003;18:1179–83.

56. Iranzo A, Santamaría J, Tolosa E, et al. Long-term effect of CPAP in the treatment of nocturnal stridor in multiple system atrophy. Neurology. 2004;63:930–2.

57. Iranzo A, Santamaría J, Rye D, et al. Characteristics of idiopathic REM sleep behavior disorder and that associated with MSA and PD. Neurology. 2005;65:247–52.

58. Iranzo A, Molinuevo JL, Santamaría J, et al. Rapid-eye-movement sleep behaviour disorder as an early marker for a neurodegenerative disorder. Lancet Neurol. 2006;7:572–7.

59. Iranzo A, Comella CL, Santamaria J, et al. Restless legs syndrome in Parkinson's disease and other neurodegenerative diseases of the central nervous system. Mov Disord. 2007;22 (Suppl 18);S424–30.

60. Iranzo A, Santamaria L, Tolosa E. The clinical and pathophysiological relevance of REM sleep behavior disorder in neurodegenerative diseases. Sleep Med Rev. 2009;13:385–401.

61. Iranzo A, Tolosa E, Gelpi E, et al. Neurodegenerative disease status and post-mortem pathology in isolated rapid-eye-movement sleep behavior disorder: and observational cohort study. Lancet Neurol. 2013;12(5):443–53.

62. Isono S, Shiba K, Yamaguchi M, et al. Pathogenesis of laryngeal narrowing in patients with multiple system atrophy. J Physiol. 2001;536:237–49.

63. Isozaki E, Shimizu T, Takamoto K, et al. Vocal cord abductor paralysis in Parkinson's disease: difference from VCAP in multiple system atrophy. J Neurol Sci. 1995;130:197–202.

64. Isozaki E, Naito A, Horiguchi S, et al. Early diagnosis and stage classification of vocal cord abductor paralysis in patients with multiple system atrophy. J Neurol Neurosurg Psychiatry. 1996;60:399–402.

65. Karlsen KH, Larsen JP, Tandberg E, et al. Influence of clinical and demographical variables on quality of life in patients with Parkinson's disease. J Neurol Neurosurg Psychiatry. 1999;66.431–5.

66. Khan SA, Sahota PK. A study look for the incidence of restless legs syndrome in patients with Parkinson's disease. Sleep. 2002;25(Suppl):A378–9.

67. Klockether T. Hereditary ataxias. In Jankovic J, Tolosa E, editors. Parkinson's disease and movement disorders. 5th ed. Philadelphia: Lippincott Williams & Wilkins; 2007. pp. 421–435.

68. Kneisley LW, Rederich GJ. Nocturnal stridor in olivopontocerebellar atrophy. Sleep. 1990;13:362–8.

69. Krishnan PR, Bhatia M, Behari M. Restless legs syndrome in Parkinson's disease: a case-controlled study. Mov Disord. 2003;18:181–5.

70. Kumar S, Bhatia M, Behari M. Sleep disorders in Parkinson's disease. Mov Disord. 2002;17:775–8.

71. Kumru H, Santamaría J, Tolosa E, et al. Rapid eye movement sleep behavior disorder in parkinsonism with PARKIN mutations. Ann Neurol. 2004;56:599–603.

72. Kumru H, Santamaría J, Tolosa E, et al. Relation between subtype of Parkinson's disease and REM sleep behavior disorder. Sleep Med. 2007;8:779–83.

73. Kumru H, Iranzo A, Carrasco E, et al. Lack of effects of pramipexole on REM sleep behavior disorder in Parkinson's disease. Sleep. 2008;31:1418–21.

74. Kushida CA, Clerk AA, Kirsch CM, et al. Prolonged confusion with nocturnal wandering arising from NREM and REM sleep: a case report. Sleep. 1995;18:757–64.

75. Lang AE. Johnson K. Akathisia in idiopathic Parkinson's disease. Neurology. 1987;37:477–81.

76. Lee JE, Shin HW, Kim KS, et al. Factors contributing to the development of restless legs syndrome in patients with Parkinson disease. Mov Disord. 2009;24;579–82.

77. Lees AJ, Blackburn NA, Campbell VL. The nighttime problems of Parkinson's disease. Clin Neuropharmacol. 1988;11:512–9.

78. Lockwood AH. Shy-Drager syndrome with abnormal respirations and antidiuretic hormone release. Arch Neurol. 1976;33:292–5.

79. Loo HV, Tan EK. Case-control study of restless legs syndrome and quality of sleep in Parkinson's disease. J Neurol Sci. 2008;266:145–9.

80. Martinez-Rodriguez J, Seppi K, Cardozo A, et al. Cerebrospinal fluid hypocretin–1 levels in múltiple system atrophy. Mov Disord. 2007;22:1822–4.

81. Meier A, Mollenhauer B, Chores S, et al. Normal hypocretin–1 (orexin A) levels in the cerebrospinal fluid of patients with Huntington's disease. Brain Res. 2005;1063:201–3.

82. Merlo IM, Occhini A, Pacchetti C, et al. Not paralysis, but dystonia causes stridor in multiple system atrophy. Neurology. 2002;58:649–52.

83. Möller JC, Stiasny K, Hargutt V, et al. Evaluation of sleep and driving performance in six patients with Parkinson's disease reporting sudden onset of sleep under dopaminergic medication: a pilot study. Mov Disord. 2002;17:474–81.

84. Moreno-López C, Santamaría J, Salamero M, et al. Excessive daytime sleepiness in multiple system atrophy (SLEEMSA study). Arch Neurol. 2011;68:223–2230.

85. Morton AJ, Wood NI, Hastings MH, et al. Disintegration of the sleep-wake cycle and circadian timing in Huntington disease. J Neurol Sci. 2005;25:157–63.

86. Munsachuer FE, Loh L, Bannister R, et al. Abnormal respiration and sudden death during sleep in multiple system atrophy with autonomic failure. Neurology. 1990;40:677–9.

87. Nausieda PA, Weiner WJ, Kaplan LR. Sleep disruption in the course of chronic levodopa therapy: an early feature of the levodopa psychosis. Clin Neuropharmacol. 1982;5:183–94.

88. Nomura T, Inoue Y, Miyake M, et al. Prevalence and clinical characteristics of restless legs syndrome in Japanese patients with Parkinson's disease. Mov Disord. 2006;21:380–4.

89. Noradina AT, Karim NA, Hamidon BB, et al. Sleep-disordered breathing in patients with Parkinson's disease. Singapore Med J. 2010;51:60–4.

90. Olanow CW, Koller WC. An algorithm (decision tree) for the management of Parkinson's disease: treatment guidelines. Neurology. 1998;58(Suppl 3):S2–57.

91. Olanow CW, Schapira AHV, Roth T. Waking up to sleep episodes in Parkinson's disease. Mov Disord. 2000;15:212–5.

92. Olanow CW, Watts RL, Koller WC. An algorithm (decision tree) for the management of Parkinson's disease: treatment guidelines. Neurology. 2001;56(Suppl 5):S1–88.

93. Ondo WG, Dat Vuong K, Jankovic J. Exploring the relationship between Parkinson disease and restless legs syndrome. Arch Neurol. 2002;59:421–4.

94. Ondo WG, Perkins T, Swick T, et al. Sodium oxybate for excessive daytime sleepiness in Parkinson disease. Arch Neurol. 2008;65:1337–40.

95. Pareja J, Caminiero AB, Masa JF, et al. A first case of progressive supranuclear palsy and pre-clinical REM sleep behavior disorder presenting as inhibition of speech during wakefulness and somniloquiy with phasic muscle twitching during REM sleep. Neurologia. 1996:11:304–6.

96. Parkinson J. An essay on the shaking palsy. London: printed by Whittingham and Rowland for Sherwood, Neely and Jones, 1817.

97. Paus S, Brecht HM, Köster J, et al. Sleep attacks, daytime sleepiness, and dopamine agonists in Parkinson's disease. Mov Disord. 2003;18:659–67.

98. Peralta CM, Frauscher B, Seppi K, et al. Restless legs syndrome in Parkinson's disease. Mov Disord. 2009;24:2076–10.

99. Petersen J, Gil J, Maat-Schieman ML, et al. Orexin loss in Huntington's disease. Hum Mol Genet. 2005;14:39–47.

100. Plazzi G, Corsini R, Provini F. REM sleep behavior disorders in multiple system atrophy. Neurology. 1997;48:1094–7.

101. Postuma RB, Gagnon JF, Vendette M, et al. Quantifying the risk of neurodegenerative disease in idiopathic REM sleep behavior disorder. Neurology. 2009;72:1296–300.

102. Reimold M, Globas C, Gleichmann M, et al. Spinocerebellar ataxia type 1, 2, and 3, and restless legs syndrome: striatal dopamine D2 receptor status investigated by [^{11}C] raclopride positron emission tomography. Mov Disord. 2006;10:1667–73.

103. Rye DB, Bliwise DL, Dihenia B, et al. FAST TRACK. Daytime sleepiness in Parkinson's disease. J Sleep Res. 2000;9:63–9.

104. Savva E, Schnorf H, Burkhard PR. Restless legs syndrome: an early manifestation of Hungtington's disease? Acta Neurol Scand. 2009;119:274–6.

105. Sadaoka T, Kakitsuba N, Fujiwara Y, et al. Sleep related breathing disorders in patients with multiple system atrophy and vocal fold palsy. Sleep. 1996;19:479–84.

106. Schenck CH, Bundlie SR, Ettinger MG, Mahowald MW. Chronic behavioral disorders of human REM sleep: a new category of parasomnia. Sleep. 1986;9:293–308.

107. Schenck CH, Bundlie SR, Patterson AL, Mahowald MW. Rapid eye movement sleep behavior disorder: a treatable parasomnia affecting older adults. JAMA. 1987;257:1786–9.

108. Schenck CH, Bundlie SR, Mahowald MW. Delayed emergence of a parkinsonian disorder in 38 % of 29 older men initially diagnosed with idiopathic rapid eye movement sleep behavior disorder. Neurology. 1996;46:388–93.

109. Schenck CH, Boeve BF, Mahowald MW. Delayed emergence of a parkinsonian disorder or dementia in 81 % of older males initially diagnosed with idiopathic REM sleep behavior disorder (RBD): 16 year update on a previously reported series. Sleep Med. 2013;14(8):744–8.

110. Schöls L, Haan J, Riess O, et al. Sleep disturbances in spinocerebellar ataxias. Is the SCA3 mutation a cause of restless legs syndrome? Neurology. 1998;51:1603–7.

111. Sharf B, Moskovitz C, Lupton MD, Klawans HL. Dream phenomena induced by chornic levodopa therapy. J Neural Transm. 1978;43:143, 151.

112. Shiojori T, Tsunemi T, Matsunaga T, et al. Vocal cord abductor paralysis in spinocerebellar ataxia type 1. J Neurol Neurosurg Psychiatry. 1999;67:695.

113. Silber MH, Levine S. Stridor and death in multiple system atrophy. Mov Disord. 2000;15:699–704.

114. Silvestri R, Raffaele M, De Domenico P, et al. Sleep features in Tourette's syndrome, neuroacanthocytosis and Huntington's chorea. Neurophysiol Clin. 1995;25:66–77.

115. Sixel-Döring F, Trautmann E, Mollenhauer B, et al. Associated factors for REM sleep behavior disorder in Parkinson disease. Neurology. 2011;77:1048–54.

116. Stevens S, Comella CL, Stepanski EJ. Daytime sleepiness and alertness in patients with Parkinson disease. Sleep. 2004;27:967–72.

117. Tan EK, Lum SY, Fook-Chong SMC, et al. Evaluation of somnolence in Parkinson's disease: comparison with age and sex-matched controls. Neurology. 2002a;58:465–8.

118. Tan EK, Lum SY, Wong MC. Restless legs syndrome in Parkinson's disease. J Neurol Sci. 2002b;196:33–6.

119. Tandberg E, Larsen JP, Karlsen K. A community-based study of sleep disorders in patients with Parkinson's disease. Mov Disord. 1998;13:895–9.

120. Tandberg E, Larsen JP, Karlsen K. Excessive daytime sleepiness and sleep benefit in Parkinson's disease: a community-based study. Mov Disord. 1999;14:922–7.

121. Taylor N, Bramble D. Sleep disturbance and Huntingdon's disease. Br J Psychiatry. 1997;171:393.

122. Thannickal TC, Lai YY, Siegel JM. Hypocretin (orexin) cell loss in Parkinson's disease. Brain. 2007;130:1586–95.

123. Trotti LM, Bliwise DL. No increased risk of obstructive sleep apnea in Parkinson's disease. Mov Disord. 2010;25:2246–9.

124. Tsuda T, Onodera H, Okabe S, et al. Impaired chemosensitivity to hypoxia is a marker of multiple system atrophy. Ann Neurol. 2002;52:367–71.

125. Tuin I, Voss U, Kang JS, et al. Stages of sleep pathology in spinocerebellar ataxia type 2 (SCA2). Neurology. 2006;67:1966–72.

126. Valko PO, Waldogavel D, Weller M, et al. Fatigue and excessive daytime sleepiness in idiopathic Parkinson's disease differently correlate with motor symptoms, depression and dopaminergic treatment. Eur J Neurol. 2010;17:1428–36.

127. Van Alfen N, Sinke RJ, Zwarts MJ, et al. Intermediate CAG repeat lengths (53,54) for MJD/SCA3 are associated with an abnormal phenotype. Ann Neurol. 2001;49:805–8.

128. Vendette M, Gagnon JF, Decary A, et al. REM sleep behavior disorder predicts cognitive impairment in Parkinson disease without dementia. Neurology. 2007;69:1843–9.

129. Verbaan D, Rooden SM, van Hilten J, et al. Prevalence and clinical profile of restless legs syndrome in Parkinson's disease. Mov Disord. 2010;25:2142–7.

130. Vertugno R, Provini F, Cortelli P, et al. Sleep disorders in multiple system atrophy: a correlative video-polysomnographic study. Sleep Med. 2004;5:21–30.

131. Videnovic A, Leurgans S, Fan W, et al. Daytime somnolence and nocturnal sleep disturbances in Huntington disease. Parkinsonism Relat Disord. 2009;15:471–4.

132. Walters AS, LeBrocq C, Passi V, et al. A preliminary look at the percentage of patients with restless legs syndrome who also have Parkinson's disease, essential tremor or Tourette syndrome in a single practice. J Sleep Res. 2003;12:343–5.

133. Wenning GK, Colosimo C, Geser F, et al. Multiple system atrophy. Lancet Neurol. 2004;3(2):93–103.

134. Wenning GK, Tison F, Shlomo YB, et al. Multiple system atrophy: a review of 203 pathologically proven cases. Mov Disord. 1997;12(2):133–47.

135. Wetter TC, Collado-Seidel V, Polmächer T, et al. Sleep and periodic leg movement patterns in drug-free patients with Parkinson's disease and multiple system atrophy. Sleep. 2000;23:361–6.

136. Wiegand M, Möller AA, Lauer CJ, et al. Nocturnal sleep in Huntington's disease. J Neurol. 1991;238:203–8.

137. Yamaguchi M, Arai K, Asahina M, et al. Laryngeal stridor in multiple system atrophy. Eur Neurol. 2003;49:154–9.

Sleep, Cognitive Dysfunction, and Dementia

Sleep, Cognitive Dysfunction, and Dementia

33

Stuart J. McCarter, Erik K. St. Louis and Bradley F. Boeve

Disclosures Mr. McCarter has no disclosures.Dr. St. Louis has received grant support from the Mayo Clinic CTSA (Scholarly Opportunity and Small Grants Awards) and from the Mayo Clinic Annenberg and Kinney Career Development Awards.Dr. Boeve has served as an investigator for clinical trials sponsored by Cephalon, Inc., Allon Pharmaceuticals and GE Healthcare. He receives royalties from the publication of a book entitled Behavioral Neurology of Dementia (Cambridge Medicine, 2009). He has received honoraria from the American Academy of Neurology. He serves on the Scientific Advisory Board for the Tau Consortium. He receives research support from the National Institute on Aging (P50 AG16574, U01 AG06786, RO1 AG32306, RO1 AG041797) and the Mangurian Foundation.

Introduction/Background: Sleep, Cognitive Dysfunction, and Dementia

Dementia is an umbrella term which includes several neurodegenerative disorders that cause cognitive decline that interferes with daily life. The decline involves at least one of the following cognitive abilities: (1) learning and memory; (2) speaking or understanding written or spoken language; (3) identifying or recognizing objects; (4) executing motor tasks; and (5) making sound judgments, thinking abstractly, and planning and executing complex tasks [1, 2]. Dementia represents a major health-care burden, affecting an estimated 13.9 % of people aged 71 years and older in the USA [1]. Alzheimer's disease (AD), the most common form of dementia, affects approximately 5.1 million Americans, including 9.73 % of those over age 71 years, the majority being women. As age increases, dementia prevalence increases to 37.4 % in those over age 90 [3]. By the year 2050, 60 % of individuals over age 85 years are projected to have AD, resulting in an immense burden to the health-care system [1].

The restorative properties of sleep have been acknowledged since the time of Hippocrates, while its particular benefits for memory and cognition were recognized much later [4, 5]. Sleep disorders are frequent in dementia. Data suggest that 24.5–88 % of patients with dementia experience sleep disturbances, including insomnia, hypersomnia, sleep-disordered breathing (SDB), rapid eye movement (REM) sleep behavior disorder (RBD), and daytime somnolence, and sleep problems are cited as one of the main factors for the institutionalization of demented persons due to increased caregiver burden [6, 7, 8, 9]. Several studies have highlighted the importance of sleep for normal cognitive function and memory [10, 11, 12, 13, 14, 15, 16, 17, 18]. Therefore, the relationship between sleep disorders and memory impairment, the cardinal and key presenting symptom in most patients with dementia, is vitally important to understand; recognition and timely treatment of sleep disturbances may provide an avenue to improve memory and cognitive functioning and quality of life in patients with dementia.

Sleep, Cognition, and Memory

The importance of REM sleep to memory consolidation was initially postulated in the mid-1960s when subjects undergoing REM sleep deprivation became anxious and developed

B. F. Boeve (✉) · E. K. St. Louis
Mayo Center for Sleep Medicine, Department of Neurology, Mayo Clinic and Foundation, 200 First Street Southwest, 55905 Rochester, MN, USA
e-mail: bboeve@mayo.edu

E. K. St. Louis
e-mail: stlouis.erik@mayo.edu

S. J. McCarter
Mayo Clinic and Foundation, 200 First Street Southwest, 55905 Rochester, MN, USA

S. Chokroverty, M. Billiard (eds.), *Sleep Medicine,* DOI 10.1007/978-1-4939-2089-1_33,
© Springer Science+Business Media, LLC 2015

difficulties with concentration [19, 20]. Hypoxemia and fragmented sleep, the main features of obstructive sleep apnea (OSA), were later shown to be detrimental to cognition [10]. Sleep loss due to insomnia, SDB, or sleep deprivation may also contribute to deficits in cognition. The cognitive functions primarily affected by sleep loss include psychomotor and cognitive speed, attention, working memory, error regulation, complex decision making, and planning [21]. Sleep disturbances along with normal aging cause decreased sleep efficiency, which appears to result in impaired cognition, especially in the domains of vigilance, attention, and executive function, especially when sleep efficiency falls below 70 % [22, 23]. Other measures of sleep quality and structure have also been correlated with cognitive functioning. Individuals with increased wake after sleep onset (WASO) time have poorer attention, visuospatial scanning, and executive functioning [23]. In addition, poor sleep quality due to sleep fragmentation and insomnia has been associated with worsened delayed recall, memory span, naming, and executive functioning. Interestingly, psychomotor skills appear to be less affected by sleep fragmentation than cognitive functions requiring more intense focus [11, 17, 23].

While adequate sleep is necessary for optimal cognitive function, different sleep stages appear to influence different aspects of cognition. Increased amounts of nonrapid eye movement (NREM) sleep appear to improve basic motor skills, while the amount of slow-wave sleep (SWS) and REM sleep correlate with performance on cognitive adaptation, identification, and memory tasks [5, 6, 14]. Higher levels of oxyhemoglobin saturation and fewer respiratory nighttime awakenings are also correlated with improved cognition and motor skills [24]. Very short or very long total sleep duration (as reflected in total sleep time) also appears to be detrimental to cognition [25].

Each stage of sleep contributes differently to the process of memory consolidation and cognition, and sleep has possibly evolved to enable optimally efficient memory encoding and consolidation, while improving executive function, attention skills, motor speed, and accuracy [5]. Subjects who are aroused from SWS have more difficulties with memory recall compared to arousal from light NREM sleep. In addition, more frequent arousals from sleep lead to increased confusion and poorer cognitive abilities [26]. Sleep fragmentation caused by insomnia results in poorer daytime functioning, attention and concentration skills, and overall cognitive flexibility, indicating the necessity of all stages of sleep for optimal cognitive function [11].

While objective sleep data correlate fairly well with cognition, subjective sleep reports are more variable. There appears to be little correlation between subjective reported sleepiness or sleep quality as measured by the Epworth Sleepiness Scale (ESS) or Pittsburgh Sleep Quality Index (PSQI) and objective cognitive measures [23]. However, subjects who believed they slept well performed better cognitively and reported fewer depressive symptoms than if they felt they slept poorly [27, 28]. Interestingly, subjective sleep measures agree better with subjective cognitive measures than objective cognitive measures, indicating that perception of one's sleep plays a large role in cognitive abilities [25]. In addition, poor subjective sleep quality may be an indicator of impending neurodegenerative processes, as older nondemented individuals who took longer to fall asleep performed worse on verbal and long-term memory and visuospatial reasoning tasks, and were more likely to have worse cognition on 3-year follow-up [29, 30].

Sleep and Memory

The importance of sleep and memory has been acknowledged since the beginning of the nineteenth century [4]. For long-term memories to persist, offline encoding and consolidation during sleep is necessary [11, 12, 15, 16, 18]. An early study of the effects of sleep deprivation on declarative memory showed that a night of pre-training sleep deprivation significantly impaired individuals' ability to remember when events occurred [31]. SWS and very slow cortical oscillations of less than 1 Hz appear to be especially important for offline storage and reprocessing of episodic facts, visuomotor learning, declarative memory, memory consolidation, and synaptic reorganization [18, 32, 33, 34, 35, 36]. Recent evidence suggests that cortical slow wave activity is inducible by local neuronal assembly activity, as well as exogenous administration of tumor necrosis factor-alpha (TNF-α) and interleukin (IL)-1, suggesting that bottom-up, localized cortical neurons may participate in homeostatic sleep drive [37]. Memory testing following a full night's sleep compared to acute total sleep deprivation shows a greater resistance to memory interference in word recall tasks, indicating the necessity of sleep for lasting memory [18, 38], and selective interference with NREM sleep slow wave activity impairs visuomotor learning [33]. In addition, while no apparent memory strengthening occurs during the day after learning a new task, continued memory enhancement does occur over the next several nights, forming durable, lasting memories that are more resistant to degradation and interference [5].

Positron emission tomography (PET) scans show activation of hippocampal areas during the learning process, with reactivation of the same areas during the subsequent night of sleep, indicating the necessity of reactivation of hippocampal networks during sleep for the consolidation of new memories. In addition, the amount of reactivation during SWS appears to correlate with next-day improvement in the same task [18, 39, 40]. Ultimately, sleep is necessary for normal hippocampal function during next-day learning. Without adequate sleep, the hippocampus does not possess its full potential for encoding new memories [18].

Sleep spindle density has also been shown to increase after procedural motor and verbal memory tasks. Increased frequency of sleep spindles may assist in synaptic strengthening and memory consolidation. While cortical slow oscillations may be largely responsible for memory consolidation, the faster frequency of sleep spindles is believed to stimulate and facilitate long-term potentiation (LTP), triggering synaptic plasticity. SWS and sleep spindles may work in harmony to regulate brain plasticity and memory [18].

REM sleep, which subsequently activates limbic and paralimbic structures, is integral in emotional processing and may be useful in providing emotional context to new information learned throughout the day. In addition, REM sleep may help with conflict resolution and is especially vital for procedural memory [34, 35]. REM sleep is also important in integrating newly learned information with prior knowledge, and increases problem-solving abilities [34, 41]. Overall, sleep is necessary for optimal next-day learning, problem-solving skills, and for understanding previous day events [34]. Sleep deprivation appears to particularly affect the ability to store and maintain emotionally positive and neutral memories, while the ability to encode negative stimuli remains relatively spared, potentially leading to a greater amount of stored negative memories compared to positive or neutral memories, providing interesting insight into the role of sleep fragmentation and deprivation in depression, since comorbid sleep disorders appear to be of higher frequency in depressed patients [18].

Mechanisms of Sleep-Dependent Memory Processing

There are currently two theories about sleep-dependent encoding and consolidation of declarative memory: the hippocampal–neocortical dialogue and the synaptic homeostasis hypothesis [18, 35]. The hippocampal–neocortical dialogue postulates that during the day as we learn new material, the hippocampus records new information. Then during SWS, the hippocampus is reactivated, replaying the information learned during the day, which is then stored in neocortical structures. With repetitions of this playback in consecutive nights, memories are consolidated and stored, available for long-term retrieval [40, 42]. This theory is supported by functional magnetic resonance imaging (MRI) studies showing decreased hippocampal–medial prefrontal cortex activation during a word recall task following acute sleep deprivation, and chronic studies showing greater medial prefrontal cortex activation 6 months post learning in patients who were not sleep deprived, indicating that sleep following

learning is vital to forming lasting memories [43]. The hippocampal–neocortical dialogue model assumes that information learned during the daytime, followed by full-night sleep, should be more resistant to memory interference than if sleep is restricted [18, 38]. This model further posits that sleep is necessary in order to process ± store new memories in the hippocampus, supported by observations that sleep-deprived individuals have difficulties forming new memories [18, 34, 35].

REM sleep appears to be vital for hippocampal memory consolidation. REM sleep-deprived rats perform significantly worse on a hippocampus-dependent maze than rats allowed full REM sleep. In addition, REM sleep increases in rats previously trained in hippocampus-dependent mazes [44]. During REM sleep, acetylcholine (ACh) levels are increased, suggesting a role for ACh in memory consolidation and LTP in the hippocampus, supported by AD patients having less REM sleep time, poor memory, and decreased ACh production due to cholinergic neuron destruction caused by AD-related pathophysiology [14, 44, 45].

The synaptic homeostasis hypothesis asserts that learning throughout the day increases synaptic connectivity. SWS is then responsible for decreasing synaptic strength to baseline levels to avoid synaptic overpotentiation. This synaptic downscaling or pruning process is necessary for more efficient memory storage and recall. Motor learning triggers a proportional degree of local cortical slow wave activity during SWS, with improvement in the task the next day. Local cortical slow wave activity is believed to prune synaptic connections, erasing unnecessary information, allowing for improved and more efficient memory recall the following day [18, 46].

Most likely, elements of the hippocampal–neocortical and SWS-mediated synaptic plasticity models work in concert with each other for efficient memory encoding and consolidation. The time course of human sleep implies sequential operation of these two memory consolidation processes. Hippocampal–neocortical interaction and information playback resulting in lasting memories would occur early in the night when SWS predominates. Cortico–cortical interactions and neural pruning, which instead occurs most prominently during REM sleep, would occur more during the second half of the night and result in more efficient memory recall, in addition to making room for new memories during the next day [18].

However, the main effect of sleep may not be to facilitate strengthening of individual memories, but to form associations between different memories, allowing for a more efficient memory storage and retrieval, as well as the ability to create generalizable schemas so one can better understand new information learned during the day [18]. Creativity, brought about by the brain's ability to harness previously learned associations and apply these in novel situations requiring unique solutions, has been shown to be heavily REM sleep dependent [18]. REM sleep is not merely a replay of events from the previous day but also a much more active process involving the integration of various associations [47]. However, recent evidence has also linked NREM SWS and slow, sleep-preserving cyclic alternating pattern (CAP) sleep A1 rhythms to aspects of creativity such as originality [48]. In short, a full night of restorative sleep is necessary for assimilation, integration, and storage of memory, so an individual can optimally solve problems and understand new information encountered the following day.

Sleep Architecture in Dementia

Patients with dementia have poorer sleep than nondemented individuals of similar age [49, 50, 51]. Compounding usual age-related changes in sleep architecture, in persons with dementia, degeneration of the nucleus basalis of Meynert (NBM) results in deficient cholinergic input to the cerebral cortex, reflected as diffuse slowing of cerebral activity during both waking electroencephalogram (EEG) and REM sleep [51, 52]. Cerebral slowing and decrease in the frequency of dominant waking alpha EEG activity make the distinction

Table 33.1 Sleep disturbances in dementia subtypes

Dementia type	Sleep disturbances	Causes of sleep disturbances
AD	Insomnia Sundowning Excessive daytime sleepiness Decreased REM sleep time Increased REM latency Increased nocturnal waking Increased daytime napping	Medication side effects Altered sleep/wake cycle SCN degeneration Decreased melatonin production Cholinergic denervation Progression of dementia
DLB	RBD RLS OSA Insomnia Sleep fragmentation Sleep-related leg cramps Excessive daytime sleepiness	RBD Medication side effects Altered sleep/wake cycle α-synuclein-associated degeneration Cholinergic denervation Depression OSA
PD	RBD Insomnia Excessive daytime sleepiness Sleep attacks Sleep fragmentation RLS PLMS OSA Sleepwalking	Muscle rigidity and tremors Dopamine deficiency RBD Medication side effects Depression α-synuclein-associated degeneration Cholinergic denervation Iron deficiency Progression of PD OSA
MCI	Increased WASO Reduced REM sleep time Fragmented SWS RBD OSA Poor sleep quality	ApoE ε4 Genotype RBD Altered sleep/wake cycle Medication side effects
FTD	Decreased TST Fragmented sleep/wake cycle Phase-shifted sleep/wake cycle Nocturnal confusion	Medication side effects Dementia progression Frontal variant FTD
HD	Insomnia Decreased sleep efficiency RBD (infrequent) Decreased SWS Decreased REM time RLS Excessive daytime somnolence	Altered sleep/wake cycle RBD Dopamine deficiency Medication side effects
VaD	OSA	Vascular abnormalities

RBD REM sleep behavior disorder, *REM* rapid eye movement, *RLS* restless legs syndrome, *PLMS* periodic leg movements of sleep, *OSA* obstructive sleep apnea, *WASO* wake after sleep onset, *SWS* slow-wave sleep, *TST* total sleep time, *SCN* suprachiasmatic nucleus, *FTD* frontotemporal dementia, *DLB* dementia with Lewy bodies, *PD* Parkinson's disease, *MCI* mild cognitive impairment, *HD* Huntington's disease, *VaD* vascular dementia

between wake and sleep states difficult to determine in many patients with dementia [49]. Early in the course of AD, there is an increase in mean theta frequency during N3 sleep, but no significant change in theta or delta power, with those having higher mean theta frequency having better memory performance [50]. In general, patients with dementia have more arousals and awakenings from sleep, significantly worse sleep efficiency, and decreased N2 sleep than nondemented individuals. Decrease in N2 is associated with declarative memory dysfunction in dementia [14, 49, 50]. Some dementia subtypes are associated with specific alterations in sleep architecture (Table 33.1). Patients with AD have less REM percentage and increased REM sleep latency when compared to patients with frontotemporal dementia (FTD), which is postulated to be caused by decreased cholinergic inputs from the basal forebrain, leading to deficient initiation and control of REM sleep in AD [14, 45]. In addition, as AD dementia progresses, REM and N3 sleep continually decrease with correspondingly increased sleep fragmentation and reported excessive daytime sleepiness. Unfortunately, naps in AD patients are most often nonrestorative and can further compound nocturnal sleep disturbance and circadian disturbances of sleep–wake cycling due to increased wakefulness at night [52].

Sleep Disturbances in Dementia

Alzheimer's Disease

AD is the most common form of dementia, characterized neuropathologically by neuritic plaques (comprised of beta-amyloid) and neurofibrillary tangles (consisting of abnormal tau protein), and clinically by major disturbances in memory followed by other language, behavioral, and sleep disturbances [1, 52]. Approximately 25–64 % of AD patients report sleep disturbances [9, 53]. Sundowning behaviors occur in 2.4–25 % of patients with AD, and altered circadian rhythm results from progressive degeneration of the suprachiasmatic nucleus (SCN) [8, 54]. Sleep disturbances may be present in the early stages of AD, but usually become worse with progression of dementia [52, 55]. Nocturnal wandering and nighttime confusion are common manifestations of an altered sleep/wake cycle, and lead to insomnia, increased nighttime wakefulness, excessive daytime sleepiness, daytime napping, and altered behavior with worsened cognitive functioning, and increased caregiver burden [7, 56].

There appear to be some genetic underpinnings to sleep disorders in AD. A high-activity four-repeat allele of the monoamine oxidase A variable number of tandem repeats (MAO-A VNTR) promoter polymorphism of the MAO gene has been shown to confer increased susceptibility to sleep

Table 33.2 Treatment options for sleep disorders

Sleep disorder	Treatment options
Insomnia	Discontinue medications known to cause insomnia
	Treat pain-causing medical comorbidities
	Emphasize sleep hygiene and physical activity
	Melatonin 0.5–10 mg
	Rozerem 8–16 mg
	Nonbenzodiazepines (e.g., eszopiclone 2–3 mg, zaleplon 5–10 mg, zolpidem 5–10 mg)
	Bright light therapy
Sundowning	Discontinue medications known to cause insomnia
	Adhere to a strict sleep schedule to help maintain constant sleep/ wake cycle
	Emphasize physical and psychosocial activity
	Melatonin
	Bright light therapy
Excessive daytime sleepiness	Treatment of RBD, OSA, or insomnia
	Discontinuation of dopaminergic agonists
	Stimulants (e.g., Modafinil)
	Discouragement of daytime napping
	Bright light therapy
RBD	Clonazepam 0.25–2 mg
	Melatonin 3–12 mg
RLS	Dopaminergic agonists: Pramipexole, ropinirole, caribidopa–levodopa
	Treatment of iron deficiency
OSA	CPAP
Sleepwalking	Discontinue zolpidem
	Clonazepam 0.25–2 mg

RBD REM sleep behavior disorder, *RLS* restless legs syndrome, *OSA* obstructive sleep apnea, *CPAP* continuous positive airway pressure

disturbance in AD [57]. MAO-A has been implicated in the control of circadian rhythm and sleep regulation [187]. The enzyme MAO-A degrades various neurotransmitters and assists with the conversion of serotonin to melatonin, which is partially responsible for synchronizing the circadian rhythm. In addition, AD patients negative for the ε4 allele of the apolipoprotein E gene also experience greater sleep disruption than those positive for the ε4 allele [57].

Recognition and treatment of common comorbid sleep disorders in patients with dementia may lead to improvements in cognitive and daytime functioning. OSA is particularly common in patients with dementia, with 70–80 % having an apnea–hypopnea index (AHI) of > 5, 48 % with an AHI of > 20, and 24 % having an AHI > 40 [59, 60, 61] (Table 33.2). More severely demented patients appear to have more severe OSA [59]. Whether worsening dementia causes OSA or if severe OSA results in more impaired cognition and dementia remains unclear. Nasal continuous positive airway pressure (CPAP) therapy may benefit cognitive functioning in those with mild/moderate AD, with improvements in attention, vigilance, episodic memory, and executive functioning, as well as daytime sleepiness and mood [60, 61, 62, 64]. In addition, caregiver sleep also reportedly improved when dementia patients with OSA successfully maintained CPAP therapy [61]. Patients with mild dementia who are treated with CPAP may show a slower cognitive decline or even improved cognition [64], although CPAP therapy does not reverse many cognitive deficits [63, 64]. Restless legs syndrome (RLS) may be associated with nocturnal agitation and difficulties initiating or maintaining sleep [65]. Checking ferritin and offering iron replacement therapy for patients having low normal (< 50 µg/L) levels is reasonable, and dopaminergic therapies may be offered for patients with disturbing RLS symptoms or frequent movement-related arousals related to periodic limb movement disorder [66].

Dementia with Lewy Bodies

Dementia with Lewy bodies (DLB) accounts for approximately 15–25 % of dementia cases, and is characterized by diffuse α-synuclein deposits in the neuronal cell bodies (as Lewy bodies) and axons/dendrites (as Lewy neurites) and associated neurodegeneration. The clinical manifestations of DLB include recurrent fully formed visual hallucinations, spontaneous parkinsonism (i.e., unrelated to medications), fluctuations in cognition and/or arousal, and visuospatial and attention deficits, with more variable memory deficits [67, 68, 69, 70]. Sleep disturbances are very common in DLB, impacting up to 88 % of patients [9]. Patients with DLB are twice as likely to report a sleep disorder than those with AD [9, 71].

At least 70 % of neuropathologically confirmed cases of DLB patients have RBD [9, 52, 68, 72]. RBD is so common in patients with DLB that including RBD as diagnostic criteria for DLB increased the likelihood of autopsy-proven DLB diagnosis sixfold [68]. However, RBD is uncommon in tauopathy neurodegenerative diseases such as AD and frontotemporal dementia, suggesting that key neuronal networks involved in REM sleep control are often affected in the synucleinopathies but infrequently affected in the non-synucleinopathy disorders [67, 73, 74, 75].

In a recent analysis of PSG findings in DLB patients with sleep-related complaints [76], RBD was common (83 % of 78 patients had RBD confirmed), yet other findings were observed: reduced sleep efficiency (< 80 % in 72 % of the sample), increased respiratory disturbance index (RDI) despite the relative absence of classic OSA features on history and examination alone (mean RDI = 11.9), and frequent arousals unrelated to disordered breathing or periodic limb movements (> 30 %). The authors interpreted their findings as indicating that multiple sleep disturbances may be present in DLB patients with sleep-related complaints [76].

Patients with DLB are also more likely to report symptoms of daytime somnolence, depression, and anxiety in addition to experiencing significantly more PLMS than other types of dementia [9, 77, 78]. However, when compared to AD, sleep disorders appear to remain constant with DLB progression [71].

Parkinson Disease

Parkinson disease (PD) is another α-synucleinopathy neurodegenerative disorder in which α-synuclein deposits primarily affect the substantia nigra, resulting in a loss of dopaminergic neurons and frequent cognitive and sleep disturbances [52, 54, 75]. RBD is also strongly associated with PD, with about 46 % of patients reporting RBD symptoms that often precede the development of clinically overt motor symptoms [74, 79, 80, 81]. Insomnia, characterized by difficulties initiating and maintaining sleep, affects approximately 60 % of patients with PD, is more severe in patients with longer duration of PD symptoms, and is often comorbid with depression. [56, 82, 83]. Parkinsonian motor features such as muscle rigidity, tremor, and stiffness make sleep initiation and maintenance more difficult and result in more frequent early-morning wakening. RLS affects approximately 20 % of patients with PD and also contributes to an inability to initiate sleep [84, 85]. Sleep apnea symptoms are frequent in PD patients, seen in up to 49.3 % of patients [86]. OSA occurs in 31 % of PD patients, but polysomnographic studies have shown that OSA is no more frequent in PD than in other patients matched for age and gender [87, 88, 89]. Patients with PD may also experience excessive daytime sleepiness and sleep attacks, the sudden onset of sleep in the setting of normal alertness [52, 90]. Dopamine agonists appear to exacerbate excessive daytime sleepiness and may cause sleep attacks, with larger doses causing decreasing daytime alertness, regardless of disease severity or duration [91, 92, 93]. On the other hand, higher doses of levodopa appear to correlate with improved daytime wakefulness [91].

FTD, Vascular Dementia, and Huntington Disease

FTD, characterized by executive and language difficulties as well as personality changes, often involves fragmented sleep/wake rhythms with poorer sleep efficiency and decreased TST, and more pronounced phase advances or delays in the sleep/wake cycle that are accompanied by more prominent nocturnal behaviors when compared to AD [90].

Patients with FTD often have an insidious onset with earlier expression of behavioral changes than other dementias. The temporal variant of FTD has a greater propensity for sleep disorders than the frontal variant of FTD and AD [94]. OSA is a common feature of vascular dementia, and leads to fragmented sleep, increased nocturnal confusion, and excessive daytime sleepiness [90]. Sleep in patients with Huntington disease (HD) is highly variable. Choreiform movements are primarily present in waking and light NREM sleep, and patients often have difficulty falling asleep, resulting in excessive daytime somnolence [95]. In addition, sleep spindle frequency and sleep fragmentation is increased, with decreased sleep efficiency, N3 and REM sleep [52, 90, 96, 97, 98, 99]. RBD has also been described in some HD patients [96]. Case studies have reported a possible relationship between RLS and HD, citing RLS as a possible predictor of HD; however, this connection requires further study [100,101].

Mild Cognitive Impairment

Mild cognitive impairment (MCI) refers to a clinical syndrome with impairment in one or more cognitive domains, with essentially normal performance of activities of daily living. There are two subtypes of MCI: amnestic and nonamnestic MCI [102, 103, 104]. Patients with either subtype of MCI experience sleep disturbances, including reduced REM time, more fragmented SWS, poor sleep quality, and OSA [105]. Patients with amnestic MCI, in which memory is primarily impaired, often develop the neuroimaging and neuropathologic characteristics of AD in terms of hippocampal atrophy on MRI, normal striatonigral uptake on dopamine transmitter scanning (DATscan), and positive uptake on amyloid PET scans [102]. Nonamnestic MCI is more often associated with Lewy body pathology. In a study of the Mayo Clinic aging and dementia databases, all patients with RBD and MCI were shown to have autopsy-proven Lewy body disease [106]. Functional imaging shows normal hippocampal structure, absence of amyloid uptake on PET scan, and reduced striatonigral uptake on DATscan, in addition to more visuospatial disturbances [102]. RBD, increased WASO, and reduced executive functioning are also common in nonamnestic MCI, and can be used to help distinguish between MCI subtypes [102, 107]. In addition, patients with amnestic MCI have a higher 5-year rate of conversion to dementia than nonamnestic MCI patients [108]. MCI patients of the ApoE ε4 genotype, a main risk factor for developing AD, have decreased REM time and are at increased risk for developing OSA, indicating there may be some link between OSA and AD, although this relationship is not well understood [82, 105, 109, 110].

Sundowning and Complex Nocturnal Visual Hallucinations in Dementia Patients

Circadian rhythm disturbances are common in patients with dementia and affect more than 80 % of those over age 65, resulting in insomnia, excessive daytime sleepiness, and day/night reversal [111, 112, 113]. Sundowning, which can be described as the evening or nocturnal exacerbation of behavioral disturbance characterized by agitation, delirium, anxiety, aggression, and other disruptive behaviors, is often cited as the main reason for the institutionalization of patients with dementia. While the exact prevalence of sundowning is difficult to determine, between 2.4 and 25 % of patients with AD, and 13–66 % of elderly individuals living at home exhibit some degree of sundowning behaviors, with higher percentages being reported in patients with more severe dementia [1, 114, 115].

Sundowning may be viewed as a nocturnal expression of delirium, and has been known since the time of Hippocrates [116]. In the modern era, the first experiment to examine sundowning behaviors was performed in 1941, when demented patients were brought into a dark room for an hour during the day, and subsequently developed delirium [117]. The spectrum of sundowning behaviors in dementia patients may also include mood swings, demanding attitude, resistance to caregiver instruction, and visual and auditory hallucinations [114, 115, 118, 119, 120, 121].

Sundowning is reported more often during the fall and winter months, presumably due to decreasing amounts of sunlight available to help synchronize the circadian rhythm [122]. While the function of the SCN decreases through the process of normal aging, the SCN appears to be more damaged in patients with dementia, resulting in a more drastically altered circadian rhythm. Neuropathological studies of the SCN in patients with AD have shown a greater than normal degree of vasopressin and neurotensin loss, resulting in a decreased ability to set the circadian rhythm [123]. Degeneration of the NBM in AD causes the downregulation of choline acetyltransferase activity and deregulated control of acetylcholinesterase, resulting in a significant decrease in ACh, and causing a further altered sleep/wake cycle [119]. Since the NBM is also markedly affected in DLB and PD, sleep/wake cycle disruption in these disorders may have a similar underlying basis. In addition, a rat model of AD has shown increased locomotor activity just prior to the dark phase, with a corresponding increase in acetylcholinesterase expression in the basal forebrain [119]. Melatonin receptors are also substantially reduced in the SCN of patients with AD, resulting in further circadian rhythm dysregulation. Patients with preclinical AD prior to the onset of cognitive symptoms show decreased CSF levels of melatonin, possibly indicating another biomarker for future neurodegeneration, and providing further evidence for potential sources of disturbed circadian regulation in AD [124].

Management of Sundowning

Many predisposing neurobiological alterations underlie circadian rhythm abnormalities in patients with dementia, so it is important to eliminate or control comorbid medical disorders or medication uses that may further disturb the sleep/wake cycle. Beta-blockers, corticosteroids, bronchodilators, and anti-cholinesterase medications may contribute to insomnia in elderly individuals and should be avoided prior to bedtime if possible [52]. Daily physical activity, exposure to light, social interaction, and adherence to a strict sleep schedule may help balance circadian rhythm disturbances and improve nighttime sleep quality. In fact, the best predictor for institutionalized patients with dementia maintaining a normal circadian rhythm is physical and psychosocial activity [113].

The most effective treatment for sundowning behaviors remains controversial. A systematic review showed that melatonin has efficacy in treating sundowning behaviors and agitation, in addition to increasing sleep quality and improving cognition in patients with dementia, although the optimal dose is unclear [114, 124]. Light therapy has also been effective in stabilizing circadian rhythm in institutionalized patients with dementia. Bright light therapy results in decreased nocturnal awakenings, daytime napping, aggression, and sundowning behaviors. In some cases, bright light therapy has resulted in improved cognition, less reported depressive symptoms, and less functional decline [126]. Again, the best "dose" and time frame for administration of bright light therapy is unclear, since studies have used different light sources and intensities for varying durations administered at variable time frames. Bright light therapy of 2500 lx or greater for at least 1 h during the morning or continuous bright light exposure throughout the day (≥ 8 h) appears to be beneficial in regulating the circadian rhythm, improving nighttime sleep, and decreasing sundowning behaviors [126, 127, 128, 129, 130, 131, 132, 133, 134, 135]. Individuals with a phase-advanced circadian rhythm often benefit from bright light therapy in the evening while those who are phase-delayed should have exposure in the morning [136]. The combination of light therapy and melatonin may also be useful for consolidating sleep and improving mood. However, the severity of dementia, as well as the most prominent type of circadian disturbance, most likely determines the optimal timing, dose, and impact of therapy [90, 126].

Complex Nocturnal Visual Hallucinosis

Patients with dementia often experience complex hallucinations, especially in low light or occurring with confusional arousals from sleep. Hallucinations are common throughout the disease course of DLB, with 80 % experiencing visual hallucinations. The hallucinations may contribute to altered thought content, such as beliefs that others are stealing, persecutory delusions, delusions of reference, infidelity, grandiosity, and, occasionally, somatic delusions. Conversely, hallucinations are reported less frequently and later in the course of AD [71, 137, 138]. Approximately 12 % of patients with PD experience hallucinations, and are even more common in DLB and PD dementia, possibly due to defective control of REM sleep causing REM intrusion into wakefulness [139]. Hypnopompic hallucinations often appear as silent, vivid, and brightly colored distortions of people or animals that occur just after sudden arousal from sleep typically lasting a few seconds and disappearing with brighter ambient light. Hypnagogic hallucinations have similar clinical characteristics and instead occur in the state of drowsiness just prior to the onset of sleep [139, 140]. Hypnagogic and hypnopompic hallucinations may represent intrusions of REM sleep into wakefulness and are often difficult to distinguish from dreams. However, as compared with dreams of REM sleep, rarely do sleep–wake transitional hallucinations evolve or contain a plot. Sleepwalking and night terrors can also present with complex nocturnal hallucinations, or as parasomnia behaviors without accompanying hallucinations [140]. Polysomnography (PSG) may be helpful in distinguishing confusional arousals with hallucinations from other parasomnias such as RBD [141].

As dementia progresses, distinguishing between dreams, visual hallucinations, and reality may become more difficult for the patient. Treatment should be reserved for patients who are frightened or bothered by their hallucinations, and other conditions known to precipitate hallucinations such as urinary tract infections or medication side effects must be excluded. Cholinesterase inhibitors and/or atypical neuroleptics may be effective in treating hallucinations in some patients, however, the atypical neuroleptics should be used carefully in patients with dementia [137].

Evidence for Sleep Disturbances that Could Predict Development of Cognitive Impairment ± Dementia

Sleep Deprivation

The first study of sleep deprivation and cognition was performed in 1896 [142]. Numerous studies since have elucidated the deleterious effects of sleep deprivation on cognition, especially demonstrating prominent deficits in alertness, executive function, memory, and learning of novel tasks that usually return to baseline after sufficient recovery sleep [18, 21, 38, 143, 144, 145, 146, 147, 148]. However, more recent evidence indicates that sleep deprivation and disturbance may be associated with permanent neurobiological changes that may accelerate future cognitive decline. Epidemiological studies show that chronic insomnia is an independent predictor for poor cognition in elderly men, but not women [149]. In addition, nondepressed men with chronic insomnia are more likely to develop cognitive impairment than patients reporting normal sleep. Sleep duration less than 6 h or naps greater than 1 h have also been associated with cognitive impairment [150].

One recent study found an increased and earlier expression of amyloid-beta protein deposits in the brains of sleep-restricted mice, indicating that the sleep/wake cycle may be important in regulating amyloid-beta, and a disruption of this cycle may accelerate development of AD [151]. Rats undergoing REM sleep deprivation also have impaired spatial learning and decreased hippocampal excitability and LTP, the major cellular mechanism underlying learning and memory formation, which may be partially responsible for decreased learning and memory abilities resulting from sleep deprivation [143, 145, 152].

Studies using functional imaging have shown patients undergoing sleep deprivation have decreases in alertness and cognitive function, which correspond with a decreased global metabolism of glucose, especially in the thalamus and prefrontal and parietal cortices [148]. In addition, there is a decrease in the activity level of the medial temporal lobe during a verbal learning task with an increase in prefrontal and parietal activation in sleep-restricted individuals compared to controls, indicating a potential compensatory attempt by other brain regions for the decrease in medial temporal function [18, 153]). Neuroimaging has also revealed that frequent and progressively longer cognitive lapses, which are a hallmark of sleep deprivation, involve widely distributed changes in brain regions including frontal and parietal control areas, secondary sensory processing areas, and thalamic areas [21]. Human subjects and rats who have been subjected to sleep fragmentation or deprived of both REM and NREM sleep also show a reduced neuron proliferation and a reduced number of developing neurons, especially in the dentate gyrus of the hippocampus [154, 155, 156]. Growth hormone appears to facilitate neurogenesis in the dentate gyrus, and has even been shown to protect against neuronal loss caused by prolonged sleep deprivation in rats [157]. However, preserved circadian rhythm or melatonin secretion has little effect on neuronal proliferation, indicating the importance of sleep itself in neurogenesis [158]. Longitudinal sleep loss may cause overall decrease in neurogenesis, primarily in the hippocampus, leading to cognitive dysfunction, especially

memory loss, and mood disorders, potentially exacerbating underlying cognitive deficits seen in dementia [155].

Altered Circadian-Activity-Rhythm Architecture

A recent analysis on circadian-activity-rhythm architecture provided insights on whether such rhythms might predict future cognitive decline [159]. The study investigators sought to determine whether circadian activity rhythms as measured by wrist actigraphy in community-dwelling older women are associated with incident dementia or MCI. The subjects were elderly female participants in a longitudinal aging study, in which subjects underwent wrist actigraphy and many other measures during one wave of study (2002–2004), and underwent a comprehensive cognitive assessment in a subsequent wave of the study (2006–2008). This permitted characterization of the subjects ($n = 1282$) as cognitively normal, or meeting criteria for MCI or dementia. Their data showed that older women with decreased activity rhythms had a higher likelihood of developing dementia or MCI when comparing those in the lowest quartiles of amplitude or rhythm robustness to women in the highest quartiles. Furthermore, an increased risk of dementia or MCI was also found for women whose timing of peak activity occurred later in the day (after 3:51 p.m.) when compared to those with average timing (1:34 p.m. to 3:51 p.m.). The authors concluded that women with decreased circadian activity rhythm amplitude and robustness, and delayed rhythms, have increased odds of developing dementia and MCI [159].

The direction of the association could not be surmised from these data. The authors suggested that interventions such as physical activity (which would be reflected on actigraphy as increased amplitude, mesor, and robustness) or bright light exposure in the early morning (which would be reflected on actigraphy as advancing the phase) might reduce the risk of cognitive deterioration in the elderly [159]. Hence, future intervention studies with physical activity and bright light therapy may indicate some readily available and inexpensive therapies that could modify the risk of future cognitive decline.

Sleep-Disordered Breathing

SDB primarily results in impairments in attention/vigilance, executive functioning, and memory in addition to construction and psychomotor skills, with more severe SDB correlating with worse cognition [34, 62, 105, 160, 161, 162, 163]. Whether intermittent hypoxemia, sleep fragmentation, or both cause cognitive dysfunction in SDB is unclear. One study inducing intermittent hypoxia at a simulated altitude of 13,000 ft. for 4 weeks resulted in no deficits in subjective or objective alertness, vigilance, or working memory [164]. However, other studies suggest that hypoxemia associated with sleep apnea may result in greater cognitive impairment. In addition, the degree of sleeping and wakeful hypoxemia appears to correlate with the degree of cognitive impairment [165]. A recent study of nondemented community dwelling women over age 80 found that SDB (measured by an AHI > 15 or greater than 7 % of total sleep time with hypoxemia below the oxyhemoglobin saturation margin of 90 %) were more likely to develop dementia or MCI, while sleep duration and sleep fragmentation did not appear to be risk factors for developing cognitive impairment [166]. However, sleep fragmentation and hypoxemia may result in cognitive impairments through different mechanisms. Sleepiness may result from sleep fragmentation, causing memory and attention deficits, whereas disturbances in executive functioning may be due to brain damage caused by hypoxemia [13].

The prefrontal cortex is particularly susceptible to sleep deprivation and hypoxia. Sleep fragmentation and intermittent hypoxemia have both been shown to lead to neuronal loss in the hippocampus and prefrontal cortex, which are closely associated with memory processes and executive functions. In addition, the prefrontal cortex is believed to be involved in attention control, providing a basis for the attention deficits seen in patients with OSA [64, 167]. Some studies have shown a gray matter reduction in the right middle temporal gyrus, cerebellum, anterior cingulate, hippocampus, and parietal and frontal cortices in OSA patients with cognitive deficits [168, 169, 170, 171, 172]. After 3 months of treatment with CPAP therapy, improvements in cognition were seen with an increase in gray matter density [168]. While white matter changes in OSA have been less extensively studied, patients with OSA do exhibit changes in axonal connections between the limbic system, pons, cerebellum, and the frontal, parietal, and temporal cortices [173]. However, there are currently little data correlating brain morphology changes and cognition in OSA [64].

Recurrent episodes of hypoxia due to OSA may cause structural ischemic lesions in the prefrontal cortex, which could explain the greater cognitive impairment and lack of symptom reversal with therapy in more severe OSA cases [64]. Some individuals possess cognitive reserve marked by a lower resting metabolism and increased neural activation during activity on functional imaging that may allow them to be less susceptible to sleep deprivation caused by frequent arousals in OSA [64].

Recent research suggests that TNF-α may play a role in excessive daytime sleepiness and cognitive dysfunction in mice subjected to recurrent arousals from sleep, such as those seen in OSA. TNF-α induces sleepiness and enhances SWS [174]. However, excessive TNF-α can inhibit LTP and disrupt hippocampus-dependent memory consolidation [175, 176]. Increased TNF has been shown to be a risk fac-

tor for developing AD. Mice subjected to sleep fragmentation showed increased levels of TNF-α around cortical neurons and exhibited cognitive problems and sleepiness, while maintaining baseline amounts of sleep duration and similar sleep architecture. However, double knockout mice without TNF-α receptor, or those treated with a TNF-α antagonist, showed little cognitive dysfunction or daytime sleepiness, indicating that sleepiness and cognitive dysfunction in disorders of frequent arousal may be partially mediated by TNF-α [176].

Whether SDB contributes to the pathophysiologic processes involved in neurodegeneration inherent in the degenerative dementias remains unclear. One recent study suggested that daytime hypersomnia and other sleep disturbances increased the risk of developing vascular dementia [177]. Furthermore, OSA almost certainly exacerbates the cognitive deficits seen in dementia and normal aging, indicating that early treatment may be beneficial if OSA is detected and may prevent faster than normal cognitive decline [64].

REM Sleep Behavior Disorder

RBD, characterized by the loss of skeletal muscle atonia and enactment of dreams, was first described in 1965 in cats with bilateral pontine lesions near the locus coeruleus, and formally identified in humans in 1986 [178, 179]. Traditionally affecting men older than 50, RBD is a hallmark of DLB and other α-synucleinopathy neurodegenerative disorders, including DLB, PD, and multiple system atrophy (MSA) [73, 75, 180]. PSG is required for diagnosis of RBD in order to identify the presence of REM sleep without atonia (RSWA), the neurophysiologic substrate of RBD, in addition to ruling out nocturnal epilepsy or NREM parasomnias [141]. Approximately 80 % of patients with idiopathic RBD (iRBD) develop a synucleinopathy disease given longitudinal follow-up, and RBD symptoms can present up to half a century prior to the onset of neurodegenerative symptoms, providing a potential window of opportunity for delivery of future neuroprotective therapies for individuals who may be predisposed to impending neurodegeneration [73, 74, 75, 79, 181, 182]. The association between RBD and the synucleinopathies has been largely responsible for the growing interest of neurologists in the field of sleep medicine.

Patients with iRBD have shown decreased cerebral glucose metabolism on fluorodeoxyglucose (FDG)-PET scans in the occipital lobe, the area predominantly affected in DLB, while hypometabolism in the left anterior cingulate gyrus, right frontal lobe, and right anterior temporal lobe (areas primarily affected in PD) were the main findings in another subset of patients [69]. These findings support the contention that iRBD is often a very early clinical manifestation of a synucleinopathy neurodegenerative process.

In addition, studies of α-synuclein immunohistochemistry in neurologically normal individuals have shown different regions of α-synuclein deposits in the brain, which may explain the variation in glucose metabolism [69, 183]. Occipital glucose hypometabolism may be related to visuospatial impairments seen in patients with DLB [69. Subjects with iRBD also show decreased striatal dopamine uptake in the substantia nigra on ^{23}I-2β-carbomethoxy-3β-(4-iodophenyl)-N-(3-fluoropropyl)-nortropane (^{123}I-FP-CIT) single-photon emission computed tomography (SPECT) and nigral hyperechogenicity on transcranial sonography (TCS), similar to that seen in PD and DLB [184]. In addition, patients with PD and RBD show neocortical, limbic, and thalamic cholinergic denervation not seen in PD patients without RBD, indicating that RBD may also be associated with cholinergic neuronal degradation [185].

Nondemented iRBD patients followed up for 2 years showed a decline in verbal memory and visuo-constructive functions when compared to nondemented age-matched controls [186]. While none of these patients developed dementia at time of follow-up, impaired visuospatial ability is a hallmark of DLB, indicating that these patients were likely undergoing an alpha-synucleinopathy neurodegenerative process. In a population based study, individuals with iRBD were 2.2 times more likely to develop MCI or PD than those without RBD [187]. RBD is also much more common in PD, with 69 % of those with PD also having probable RBD, while probable RBD was only seen in 20 % of those with RLS and 13 % having essential tremor [188] strengthening the belief that RBD is an early clinical expression of a synucleinopathy neurodegenerative process and suggesting that patients with RLS or essential tremor are not at increased risk for the development of PD [188]. RBD may also be a predictor of dementia in patients with PD. In one study, 48 % of PD patients with RBD developed dementia, while no PD patients without RBD developed dementia [189]. However, all 13 patients who developed dementia had MCI at baseline examination, indicating that they may have already been progressing towards dementia.

Loss of REM muscle atonia (RSWA) during PSG may also be a predictor for future development of dementia. In one recent study of RSWA, patients developing dementia had a 73 % muscle atonia loss, compared to only 40 % in those that did not develop dementia [74, 190]. Finally, RBD is also associated with the development of new hallucinations and cognitive fluctuations in patients with dementia. Patients with DLB or PDD were more likely to have RBD- or NREM-related arousals and hallucinations than nondemented PD patients, with more frequent arousals and dream enactment behaviors (DEB) in more severely cognitively impaired patients [80, 191].

The treatment of RBD focuses on decreasing potentially injurious DEB [72, 75, 192]. Clonazepam and melatonin have been shown to be equally effective in decreasing frequency and severity of DEB and injury occurrence in RBD [192]. However, melatonin was reported to be more effective in RBD patients with a neurodegenerative disorder compared with clonazepam [192]. This finding, coupled with reports of decreased sundowning behaviors in melatonin-treated dementia patients, provide evidence for use of melatonin as a potential first-line treatment for both RBD and sundowning in patients with dementia [192, 193]. Unfortunately, neither melatonin nor clonazepam has been found to slow progression of neurodegeneration in RBD and further research on potentially neuroprotective therapies is needed.

Conclusions

Sleep is vital to normal cognitive functioning, especially for the formation and consolidation of new memories. Altered circadian rhythm and sleep complaints are common in the aging population, especially in those with dementia, and sleep disturbances may further impact cognitive functioning in patients with dementia. While the relationship between sleep disturbances and dementia remain to be fully elucidated, hypoxia related to OSA may result in permanent pathological brain changes that may contribute to the development of dementia. RBD is very likely a very early clinical manifestation of a synucleinopathy neurodegenerative process, primarily PD and DLB. Timely recognition and treatment of sleep disturbances related to medication side effects, altered circadian rhythm, OSA, and RLS may provide an avenue to improve memory and cognitive functioning and quality of life in patients with dementia.

Acknowledgments This work was supported by grants (P50 AG16574, U01 AG06786, RO1 AG32306, RO1 AG041797), the Mangurian Foundation, and by the National Center for Research Resources and the National Center for Advancing Translational Sciences, National Institutes of Health, through Grant Number 1 UL1 RR024150–01. The content is solely the responsibility of the authors and does not necessarily represent the official views of the NIH.

References

1. Alzheimer's Association. Alzheimer's disease facts and figures. Alzheimers Dement. 2012;8:131–68.
2. American Psychiatric Association. Diagnostic and statistical manual of mental disorders. 4th ed. (text rev.). Washington, DC: American Psychiatric Press; 2000.
3. Plassman BL, Langa KM, Fisher GG, et al Prevalence of dementia in the United States: the aging, demographics, and memory study. Neuroepidemiology. 2007;29(1–2):125–32.
4. Hartley, D. (1801). Observations on Man, His frame, his deity, and his expectations (1749/)6691. Gainesville: Scholars Facsimile Reprint.

5. Stickgold R. Sleep-dependent memory consolidation. Nature. 2005;437(7063):1272–8.

6. Ancoli-Israel S. Sleep and its disorders in aging populations. Sleep Med. 2009;Suppl 1:S7–11.

7. McCurry SM, Ancoli-Israel S. Sleep dysfunction in Alzheimer's disease and other dementias. Curr Treat Options Neurol. 2003;5(3):261–72.

8. Moran M, Lynch CA, Walsh C, et al. Sleep disturbance in mild to moderate Alzheimer's disease. Sleep Med. 2005;6(4):347–52.

9. Rongve A, Boeve BF, Aarsland D. Frequency and correlates of caregiver-reported sleep disturbances in a sample of persons with early dementia. J Am Geriatr Soc. 2010;58(3):480–6.

10. Bonnet MH. Effect of sleep disruption on sleep, performance, and mood. Sleep. 1985;8(1):11–9.

11. Haimov I, Hanuka E, Horowitz Y. Chronic insomnia and cognitive functioning among older adults. Behav Sleep Med. 2008;6(1):32–54.

12. Hornung OP, Danker-Hopfe H, Heuser I. Age-related changes in sleep and memory: commonalities and interrelationships. Exp Gerontol. 2005;40(4):279–85.

13. Jones K, Harrison Y. Frontal lobe function, sleep loss and fragmented sleep. Sleep Med Rev. 2001;5(6):463–75.

14. Kundermann B, Thum A, Rocamora R, et al. Comparison of polysomnographic variables and their relationship to cognitive impairment in patients with Alzheimer's disease and frontotemporal dementia. J Psychiatr Res. 2011;45(12):1585–92.

15. Maquet P. The role of sleep in learning and memory. Science. 2001;294:1048–52.

16. Maquet P, Schwartz S, Passingham R, et al. Sleep-related consolidation of a visuo-motor skill: brain mechanisms as assessed by fMRI. J Neurosci. 2003;23:1432–40.

17. Mazzoni G, Gori S, Formicola G, et al. Word recall correlates with sleep cycles in elderly subjects. J Sleep Res. 1999;8(3):185–8.

18. Walker MP. The role of sleep in cognition and emotion. Ann N Y Acad Sci. 2009;1156:168–97.

19. Empson J, Clarke P. Rapid eye movements and remembering. Nature. 1970;227:287–8.

20. Kales A, Hoedemaker F, Jacobson A et al. Dream Deprivation: an Experimental Reappraisal. Nature 1964;204:1337–8.

21. Goel N, Rao H, Durmer JS, et al. Neurocognitive consequences of sleep deprivation. Semin Neurol. 2009;29(4):320–39.

22. Blackwell T, Yaffe K, Ancoli-Israel S, et al. Poor sleep is associated with impaired cognitive function in older women: the study of osteoporotic fractures. J Gerontol A Biol Sci Med Sci 2006;61(4):405–10.

23. Blackwell T, Yaffe K, Ancoli-Israel S, et al. Association of sleep characteristics and cognition in older community-dwelling men: the MrOS sleep study. Sleep. 2011;34(10):1347–56.

24. Cole CS, Richards KC, Beck CC, et al. Relationship among disordered sleep and cognitive and functional status in nursing home residents. Res Gerontol Nurs. 2009;2(3):183–191.

25. Kronholm E, Sallinen M, Suutama T, et al. Self-reported sleep duration and cognitive functioning in the general population. J Sleep Res. 2009;18(4):436–46.

26. Bonnet, MH Cognitive effects of sleep and sleep fragmentation. Sleep 1993 16 Suppl 8:S65–67.

27. Bastien CH, Fortier-Brochu E, Rioux I, et al. Cognitive performance and sleep quality in the elderly suffering from chronic insomnia. Relationship between objective and subjective measures. J Psychosom Res. 2003;54(1):39–49.

28. Nebes RD, Buysse DJ, Halligan EM, et al. Self-reported sleep quality predicts poor cognitive performance in healthy older adults. J Gerontol B Psychol Sci Soc Sci. 2009;64(2):180–7.

29. Jelicic M, Bosma H, Ponds RW, et al. Subjective sleep problems in later life as predictors of cognitive decline. Report from the Maastricht Ageing Study (MAAS). Int J Geriatr Psychiatry. 2002;17(1):73–7.

30. Schmutte T, Harris S, Levin R, et al. The relation between cognitive functioning and self-reported sleep complaints in nondemented older adults: results from the Bronx aging study. Behav Sleep Med.2007;5(1):39–56.

31. Morris GO, Williams HL, Lubin A. Misperception and disorientation during sleep. Arch Gen Psychiatry. 1960;2:247–54.

32. Cantero JL, Atienza M, Salas RM, et al. Effects of prolonged waking-auditory stimulation on electroencephalogram synchronization and cortical coherence during subsequent slow-wave sleep. J Neurosci. 2002;22(11):4702–8.

33. Landsness EC, Crupi D, Hulse BK, et al. Sleep-dependent improvement in visuomotor learning: a causal role for slow waves. Sleep. 2009;32(10):1273–84.

34. Malhotra RK, Desai AK. Healthy brain aging: what has sleep got to do with it? Clin Geriatr Med. 2010;26(1):45–56

35. Marshall L, Born J. The contribution of sleep to hippocampus-dependent memory consolidation. Trends Cogn Sci. 2007;11(10):442–50.

36. Mölle M, Marshall L, Gais S, et al. Learning increases human electroencephalographic coherence during subsequent slow sleep oscillations. Proc Natl Acad Sci U S A. 2004;101(38):13963–8.

37. Krueger JM, Clinton JM, Winters BD, et al. Involvement of cytokines in slow wave sleep. Prog Brain Res. 2011;193:39–47.

38. Ellenbogen JM, Hulbert JC, Stickgold R, et al. Interfering the theories of sleep and memory: sleep, declarative memory, and associative interference. Curr Biol. 2006;16:1290–4.

39. Peigneux P, Laureys S, Fuchs S, et al. Are spatial memories strengthened in the human hippocampus during slow wave sleep? Neuron. 2004;44:535–45.

40. Wilson MA, McNaughton BL. Reactivation of hippocampal ensemble memories during sleep. Science. 1994;265:676–9.

41. Wagner U, Gais S, Haider H, et al. Sleep inspires insight. Nature. 2004;427:352–5.

42. Buzsaki G. The hippocampo-neocortical dialogue. Cereb Cortex. 1996;6:81–92.

43. Gais S, Albouy G, Boly M, et al. Sleep transforms the cerebral trace of declarative memories. Proc Natl Acad Sci U S A. 2007;104:18778–83.

44. Graves L, Pack A, Abel T. Sleep and memory: a molecular perspective. Trends Neurosci. 2001;24(4):237–43.

45. Perry E, Walker M, Grace J, et al. Acetylcholine in mind: a neurotransmitter correlate of consciousness? Trends Neurosci. 1999;22:273–80.

46. Huber R, Ghilardi MF, Massimini M, et al. Local sleep and learning. Nature. 2004;430:78–81.

47. Fosse MJ, Fosse R, Hobson JA, et al. Dreaming and episodic memory: a functional dissociation? J Cogn Neurosci. 2003;15:1–9.

48. Drago V, Foster PS, Heilman KM, Aricò D, Williamson J, Montagna P, Ferri R. Cyclic alternating pattern in sleep and its relationship to creativity. Sleep Med. 2011;12(4):361–6.

49. Bliwise D. Sleep in normal aging and dementia. Sleep 1993 16(1):40–81.

50. Hot P, Rauchs G, Bertran F, et al. Changes in sleep theta rhythm are related to episodic memory impairment in early Alzheimer's disease. Biol Psychol. 2011;87(3):334–9.

51. Prinz P, Vitiello M, Murray R, et al. Sleep disorders and aging N Engl J Med 1990;323:520–6.

52. Chokroverty S. Sleep and neurodegenerative diseases. Semin Neurol. 2009;29(4):446–67.

53. Guarnieri B, Adorni F, Musicco M, et al. Prevalence of sleep disturbances in mild cognitive impairment and dementing disorders: a multicenter Italian clinical cross-sectional study on 431 patients. Dement Geriatr Cogn Disord. 2012;33(1):50–8.

54. Ahlskog JE. Parkinson's disease: is the initial treatment established? Curr Neurol Neurosci Rep. 2003;3(4):289–95.

55. Moe KE, Vitiello MV, Larsen LH, et al. Symposium: cognitive processes and sleep disturbances: sleep/wake patterns in Alzheim-

er's disease: relationships with cognition and function. J Sleep Res. 1995;4(1):15–20.

56. Deschenes CL, McCurry SM. Current treatments for sleep disturbances in individuals with dementia. Curr Psychiatry Rep. 2009;11(1):20–6.

57. Craig D, Hart DJ, Passmore AP. Genetically increased risk of sleep disruption in Alzheimer's disease. Sleep. 2006;29(8):1003–7.

58. Wu YH, Fischer DF, Swaab DF. A promoter polymorphism in the monoamine oxidase A gene is associated with the pineal MAOA activity in Alzheimer's disease patients. Brain Res. 2007;1167:13–9.

59. Ancoli-Israel S, Klauber MR, Butters N, et al. Dementia in institutionalized elderly: relation to sleep apnea. J Am Geriatr Soc 1991;39:258–63.

60. Ancoli-Israel S, Palmer BW, Cooke JR, et al. Cognitive effects of treating obstructive sleep apnea in Alzheimer's disease: a randomized controlled study. J Am Geriatr Soc. 2008;56(11):2076–81.

61. Cooke JR, Ayalon L, Palmer BW, et al. Sustained use of CPAP slows deterioration of cognition, sleep, and mood in patients with Alzheimer's disease and obstructive sleep apnea: a preliminary study. J Clin Sleep Med. 2009;5(4):305–9.

62. Aloia MS, Arnedt JT, Davis JD et al. Neuropsychological sequelae of obstructive sleep apnea-hypopnea syndrome: a critical review. J Int Neuropsychol Soc. 2004;10(5):772–85.

63. Antic NA, Catcheside P, Buchan C, et al. The effect of CPAP in normalizing day-time sleepiness, quality of life, and neurocognitive function in patients with moderate to severe OSA. Sleep. 2011;34:111–9.

64. Sforza E, Roche F. Sleep apnea syndrome and cognition. Front Neurol. 2012;3:87 (Epub 2012).

65. Rose KM, Beck C, Tsai PF, et al. Sleep disturbances and nocturnal agitation behaviors in older adults with dementia. Sleep. 2011;34(6):779–86.

66. Aurora RN, Kristo DA, Bista SR, et al. The treatment of restless legs syndrome and periodic limb movement disorder in adults-an update for 2012: practice parameters with an evidence-based systematic review and meta-analyses: an American academy of sleep medicine clinical practice guideline. Sleep. 2012;35(8):1039–62.

67. Ferman TJ, Boeve BF. Dementia with Lewy bodies. Neurol Clin. 2007;25(3):741–60

68. Ferman TJ, Boeve BF, Smith GE, et al. Inclusion of RBD improves the diagnostic classification of dementia with Lewy bodies. Neurology. 2011;77(9):875–82.

69. Fujishiro H, Iseki E, Murayama N, et al. Diffuse occipital hypometabolism on [18 F]-FDG PET scans inpatients with idiopathic REM sleep behavior disorder: prodromal dementia with Lewy bodies? Psychogeriatrics. 2010;10(3):144–52.

70. McKeith IG, Dickson DW, Lowe J, et al. Diagnosis and management of dementia with Lewy bodies: third report of the DLB Consortium. Neurology. 2005;65:1863–72.

71. Bliwise DL, Mercaldo ND, Avidan AY, et al. Sleep disturbance in dementia with Lewy bodies and Alzheimer's disease: a multicenter analysis. Dement Geriatr Cogn Disord. 2011;31(3):239–46.

72. Boeve BF. Mild cognitive impairment associated with underlying Alzheimer's disease versus Lewy body disease. Parkinsonism Relat Disord. 2012;18 Suppl 1:S41–4.

73. Boeve BF, Silber MH, Ferman TJ. Current management of sleep disturbances in dementia. Curr Neurol Neurosci Rep. 2002;2(2):169–77.

74. Gagnon RB, Vendette JF, Fantini M, et al. Quantifying the risk of neurodegenerative disease in idiopathic REM sleep behavior disorder. Neurology. 2009;72(15):1296–1300.

75. McCarter SJ, St Louis EK, Boeve BF. REM sleep behavior disorder and REM sleep without atonia as an early manifestation of degenerative neurological disease. Curr Neurol Neurosci Rep. 2012;12(2):182–92.

76. Pao WC, Boeve BF, Ferman TJ, et al. Polysomnographic findings in dementia with Lewy bodies. Neurologist. 2013;19(1):1–6.

77. Baumann CR, Dauvilliers Y, Mignot E, et al. Normal CSF hypocretin-1 (orexin A) levels in dementia with Lewy bodies associated with excessive daytime sleepiness. Eur Neurol. 2004;52(2):73–6.

78. Hibi S, Yamaguchi Y, Umeda-Kameyama Y, et al. The high frequency of periodic limb movements in patients with Lewy body dementia. J Psychiatr Res. 2012;46:1590–4.

79. Claassen DO, Josephs KA, Ahlskog JE, et al. REM sleep behavior disorder preceding other aspects of synucleinopathies by up to half a century. Neurology. 2010;75(6):494–9.

80. Postuma RB, Lang AE, Gagnon JF, et al. How does parkinsonism start? Prodromal parkinsonism motor changes in idiopathic REM sleep behaviour disorder. Brain. 2012;135(Pt 6):1860–70.

81. Sixel-Doring F, Trautmann E, Mollenhauer B, et al. Associated factors for REM sleep behavior disorder in Parkinson disease. Neurology. 2011;77(11):1048–54.

82. Dauvilliers Y. Insomnia in patients with neurodegenerative conditions. Sleep Med. 2007;8 Suppl 4:S27–34.

83. Gjerstad MD, Wentzel-Larsen T, Aarsland D, et al. Insomnia in Parkinson's disease: frequency and progression over time. J Neurol Neurosurg Psychiatry. 2007;78(5):476–9.

84. Iranzo A, Comella CL, Santamaria J, et al. Restless legs syndrome in Parkinson's disease and other neurodegenerative diseases of the central nervous system. Mov Disord. 2007;22 Suppl 18:S424–30.

85. Ondo WG, Dat Vuong K, Jankovic J. Exploring the relationship between Parkinson disease and restless legs syndrome. Arch Neurol. 2002;59:421–4.

86. Chotinaiwattarakul W, Dayalu P, Chervin RD, et al. Risk of sleep-disordered breathing in Parkinson's disease. Sleep Breath. 2011;15(3):471–8.

87. Cochen De Cock V, Abouda M, Leu S, et al. Is obstructive sleep apnea a problem in Parkinson's disease? Sleep Med. 2010;11(3):247–52.

88. Trotti LM, Bliwise DL. No increased risk of obstructive sleep apnea in Parkinson's disease. Mov Disord. 2010;25(13):2246–9.

89. Yong MH, Fook-Chong S, Pavanni R, et al. Case control polysomnographic studies of sleep disorders in Parkinson's disease. PLoS ONE. 2011;6(7):e22511.

90. Zhou QP, Jung L, Richards KC. The management of sleep and circadian disturbance in patients with dementia. Curr Neurol Neurosci Rep. 2012;12(2):193–204.

91. Bliwise DL, Trotti LM, Wilson AG, et al. Daytime alertness in Parkinson's disease: potentially dose-dependent, divergent effects by drug class. Mov Disord. 2012;27:1118–24.

92. Ferreira JJ, Galitzky M, Montastruc JL, et al. Sleep attacks and Parkinson's disease treatment. Lancet. 2000;355(9212):1333–4.

93. Gottwald MD, Brainbridge JL, Dowling GA, et al. New pharmacotherapy for Parkinson's disease. Ann Pharmacother. 1997;31:1205–17.

94. Liu W, Miller BL, Kramer JH, et al. Behavioral disorders in the frontal and temporal variants of frontotemporal dementia. Neurology. 2004;62(5):742–8.

95. Videnovic A, Leurgans S, Fan W, et al. Daytime somnolence and nocturnal sleep disturbances in Huntington disease. Parkinsonism Relat Disord. 2009;15(6):471–4.

96. Arnulf I, Nielsen J, Lohmann E, et al. Rapid eye movement sleep disturbances in Huntington disease. Arch Neurol. 2008;65(4):482–8.

97. Fish DR, Sawyers D, Allen PJ, et al. The effect of sleep on the dyskinetic movements of Parkinson's disease, Gilles de la Tourette syndrome, Huntington's disease, and torsion dystonia. Arch Neurol. 1991;48(2):210–4.

98. Goodman AO, Rogers L, Pilsworth S, et al. Asymptomatic sleep abnormalities are a common early feature in patients with Huntington's disease. Curr Neurol Neurosci Rep. 2011;11(2):211–7.

99. Wiegand M, Möller AA, Lauer CJ, et al. Nocturnal sleep in Huntington's disease. J Neurol. 1991;238(4):203–8.

100. Evers S, Stögbauer F. Genetic association of Huntington's disease and restless legs syndrome? A family report. Mov Disord. 2003;18(2):225–7.

101. Savva E, Schnorf H, Burkhard PR. Restless legs syndrome: an early manifestation of Huntington's disease? Acta Neurol Scand. 2009;119(4):274–6.

102. Boeve BF, Silber MH, Parisi JE, et al. Synucleinopathy pathology and REM sleep behavior disorder plus dementia or parkinsonism. Neurology. 2003;61(1):40–5.

103. Petersen RC. Mild cognitive impairment as a diagnostic entity. J Intern Med. 2004;256:183–94

104. Ratcliff R, Van Dongen HP. Sleep deprivation affects multiple distinct cognitive processes. Psychon Bull Rev. 2009;16:742–51.

105. Kim SJ, Lee JH, Lee DY, et al. Neurocognitive dysfunction associated with sleep quality and sleep apnea in patients with mild cognitive impairment. Am J Geriatr Psychiatry. 2011;19(4):374–81.

106. Molano J, Boeve B, Ferman T, et al. Mild cognitive impairment associated with limbic and neocortical Lewy body disease: a clinicopathological study. Brain. 2010;133(Pt 2):540–56.

107. Naismith SL, Rogers NL, Hickie IB, et al. Sleep well, think well: sleep-wake disturbance in mild cognitive impairment. J Geriatr Psychiatry Neurol. 2010;23(2):123–30.

108. Devine ME, Fonseca JA, Walker Z. Do cerebral white matter lesions influence the rate of progression from mild cognitive impairment to dementia? Int Psychogeriatr. 2013;25:120–7.

109. Gottlieb DJ, DeStefano AL, Foley DJ, et al APOE e4 is associated with obstructive sleep apnea/hypopnea: the sleep heart health study. Neurology. 2004;63:664–8.

110. Hita-Yañez E, Atienza M, Gil-Neciga E, et al. Disturbed sleep patterns in elders with mild cognitive impairment: the role of memory decline and ApoE É4 genotype. Curr Alzheimer Res. 2012;9(3):290–7.

111. Desai AK, Schwartz L, Grossberg GT. Behavioral Disturbance in Dementia. Curr Psychiatry Rep. 2012;14:298–309.

112. Foley DJ, Monjan AA, Brown SL, et al. Sleep complaints among elderly persons: an epidemiologic study of three communities. Sleep. 1995;18(6):425–32.

113. Sullivan SC, Richards KC. Predictors of circadian sleep-wake rhythm maintenance in elders with dementia. Aging Ment Health. 2004;8(2):143–52.

114. de Jonghe A, Korevaar JC, van Munster BC, et al. Effectiveness of melatonin treatment on circadian rhythm disturbances in dementia. Are there implications for delirium? A systematic review. Int J Geriatr Psychiatry. 2010;25:1201–8.

115. Gallagher-Thompson D, Brooks JO, et al. The relations among caregiver stress, "sundowning" symptoms, and cognitive decline in Alzheimer's disease. J Am Geriatr Soc. 1992:40:807–10.

116. Lipowski ZJ. Delirium: acute brain failure in man. Springfield: Charles C. Thomas; 1980.

117. Cameron DE. Studies in senile nocturnal delirium. Psychiatr Q 1941;15:47–53.

118. Bedrosian TA, Nelson RJ. Sundowning syndrome in aging and dementia: research in mouse models. Exp Neurol. 2013;243:67–73.

119. Bedrosian TA, Herring KL, Weil ZM, et al. Altered temporal patterns of anxiety in aged and amyloid precursor protein (APP) transgenic mice. Proc Natl Acad Sci U S A. 2011;108(28):11686–91.

120. McCurry SM, Reynolds CF, Ancoli-Israel S, et al. Treatment of sleep disturbance in Alzheimer's disease. Sleep Med Rev. 2000;4(6):603–28.

121. Volicer L, Harper DG, Manning BC, et al. Sundowning and circadian rhythms in Alzheimer's disease. Am J Psychiatry. 2001;158:704–11.

122. Khachiyants N, Trinkle D, Son SJ, et al. Sundown syndrome in persons with dementia: an update. Psychiatry Investig. 2011;8:275–87.

123. Stopa EG, Volicer L, Kuo-Leblanc V, et al. Pathologic evaluation of the human suprachiasmatic nucleus in severe dementia. J Neuropathol Exp Neurol. 1999;58(1):29–39.

124. Cardinali DP, Furio AM, Brusco LI. Clinical aspects of melatonin intervention in Alzheimer's disease progression. Curr Neuropharmacol. 2010;8:218–27.

125. Zhdanova IV, Tucci V. Melatonin, circadian rhythms, and sleep. Curr Treat Options Neurol. 2003;5(3):225–9.

126. Riemersma-van der Lek RF, Swaab DF, Twisk J, et al. Effect of bright light and melatonin on cognitive and noncognitive function in elderly residents of group care facilities: a randomized controlled trial. JAMA. 2008;299(22):2642–55.

127. Dowling GA, Mastick J, Hubbard EM, et al. Effect of timed bright light treatment for rest-activity disruption in institutionalized patients with Alzheimer's disease. Int J Geriatr Psychiatry. 2005;20(8):738–43.

128. Dowling GA, Burr RL, Van Someren EJ, et al. Melatonin and bright-light treatment for rest-activity disruption in institutionalized patients with Alzheimer's disease. J Am Geriatr Soc. 2008;56(2):239–46.

129. Forbes D, Morgan DG, Bangma J, et al. Light therapy for managing sleep, behaviour, and mood disturbances in dementia. Cochrane Database Syst Rev. 2004;(2):CD003946.

130. McCurry SM, Pike KC, Vitiello MV, et al. Increasing walking and bright light exposure to improve sleep in community-dwelling persons with Alzheimer's disease: results of a randomized, controlled trial. J Am Geriatr Soc. 2011;59(8):1393–402.

131. Most EI, Scheltens P, Van Someren EJ. Prevention of depression and sleep disturbances in elderly with memory-problems by activation of the biological clock with light–a randomized clinical trial. Trials. 2010;11:19.

132. Salami O, Lyketsos C, Rao V. Treatment of sleep disturbance in Alzheimer's dementia. Int J Geriatr Psychiatry. 2011;26(8):771–82.

133. Shirani A, St Louis EK. Illuminating rationale and uses for light therapy. J Clin Sleep Med. 2009;5(2):155–63.

134. Skjerve A, Holsten F, Aarsland D, et al. Improvement in behavioral symptoms and advance of activity acrophase after short-term bright light treatment in severe dementia. Psychiatry Clin Neurosci. 2004;58(4):343–7.

135. Sloane PD, Williams CS, Mitchell CM, et al. High-intensity environmental light in dementia: effect on sleep and activity. J Am Geriatr Soc. 2007;55(10):1524–33.

136. Gooley JJ. Treatment of circadian rhythm sleep disorders with light. Ann Acad Med Singapore. 2008;37(8):669–76.

137. Boeve BF. REM sleep behavior disorder: updated review of the core features, the REM sleep behavior disorder-neurodegenerative disease association, evolving concepts, controversies, and future directions. Ann N Y Acad Sci. 2010;1184:15–54.

138. Manford M, Andermann F. Complex visual hallucinations. Clinical and neurobiological insights. Brain. 1998;121(Pt 10):1819–40.

139. Manni R, Terzaghi M, Ratti PL, et al. Hallucinations and REM sleep behaviour disorder in Parkinson's disease: dream imagery intrusions and other hypotheses. Conscious Cogn. 2011;20(4):1021–6.

140. Silber MH, Hansen MR, Girish M. Complex nocturnal visual hallucinations. Sleep Med. 2005;6(4):363–6.

141. American Academy of Sleep Medicine. International classification of sleep disorders, 2nd ed.: diagnostic and coding manual. Westchester, Illinois: American Academy of Sleep Medicine; 2005.

142. Patrick GT, Gilbert JA. On the effects of loss of sleep. Psychol Rev. 1896;3:469–83.

143. Campbell IG, Guinan MJ, Horowitz JM. Sleep deprivation impairs long-term potentiation in rat hippocampal slices. J Neurophysiol. 2002;88:1073–76.

144. Chee MW, Chuah YM. Functional neuroimaging and behavioral correlates of capacity decline in visual short-term memory after sleep deprivation. Proc Natl Acad Sci. 2007;104;9487–92.

145. Davis CJ, Harding JW, Wright JW. REM sleep deprivation-induced deficits in the latency-to-peak induction and maintenance of long-term potentiation within the CA1 region of the hippocampus. Brain Res. 2003;973:293–7.

146. Durmer JS, Dinges DF. Neurocognitive consequences of sleep deprivation. Semin Neurol. 2005;25(1):117–29.

147. Petersen RC. Clinical practice. Mild cognitive impairment. N Engl J Med. 2011;364(23):2227–34.

148. Thomas M, Sing H, Belenky G, et al. Neural basis of alertness and cognitive performance impairments during sleepiness. I. Effects of 24 h of sleep deprivation on waking human regional brain activity. J Sleep Res. 2000;9(4):335–52.

149. Raymann RJ, Swaab DF, Van Someren EJ. Skin temperature and sleep-onset latency: changes with age and insomnia. Physiol Behav. 2007;90(2–3):257–66.

150. Ohayon MM, Vecchierini MF. Normative sleep data, cognitive function and daily living activities in older adults in the community. Sleep. 2005;28(8):981–9.

151. Kang JE, Lim MM, Bateman RJ, et al. Amyloid-beta dynamics are regulated by orexin and the sleep-wake cycle. Science. 2009;326(5955):1005–7.

152. Yang RH, Hu SJ, Wang Y, et al. Paradoxical sleep deprivation impairs spatial learning and affects membrane excitability and mitochondrial protein in the hippocampus. Brain Res. 2008;1230:224–32.

153. Drummond SP, Brown GG, Gillin JC, et al. Altered brain response to verbal learning following sleep deprivation. Nature. 2000 403:655–7.

154. Guzman-Marin R, Bashir T, Suntsova N, et al. Hippocampal neurogenesis is reduced by sleep fragmentation in the adult rat. Neuroscience. 2007;148(1):325–33.

155. Meerlo P, Mistlberger RE, Jacobs BL, et al. New neurons in the adult brain: the role of sleep and consequences of sleep loss. Sleep Med Rev. 2009;13(3):187–94.

156. Sportiche N, Suntsova N, Methippara M, et al. Sustained sleep fragmentation results in delayed changes in hippocampal-dependent cognitive function associated with reduced dentate gyrus neurogenesis. Neuroscience. 2010;170(1):247–58.

157. García-García F, De la Herrán-Arita AK, Juárez-Aguilar E, et al. Growth hormone improves hippocampal adult cell survival and counteracts the inhibitory effect of prolonged sleep deprivation on cell proliferation. Brain Res Bull. 2011;84(3):252–7.

158. Mueller AD, Mear RJ, Mistlberger RE. Inhibition of hippocampal neurogenesis by sleep deprivation is independent of circadian disruption and melatonin suppression. Neuroscience. 2011;193:170–81.

159. Tranah GJ, Blackwell T, Stone KL, et al. Circadian activity rhythms and risk of incident dementia and MCI in older women. Ann Neurol. 2011;70(5):722–32.

160. Antonelli Incalzi R, Marra C, Salvigni BL, et al. Does cognitive dysfunction conform to a distinctive pattern in obstructive sleep apnea syndrome? J Sleep Res. 2004;13(1):79–86.

161. Cohen-Zion M, Stepnowsky C, Marler M, et al. Changes in cognitive function associated with sleep disordered breathing in older people. J Am Geriatr Soc. 2001;49(12):1622–7.

162. Kim HC, Young T, Matthews CG, et al. Sleep-disordered breathing and neuropsychological deficits: a population-based study. Am J Respir Crit Care Med. 1997;156:1813–9.

163. Sforza E, Roche F, Thomas-Anterion C, et al. Cognitive function and sleep related breathing disorders in a healthy elderly population: the SYNAPSE study. Sleep. 2010;33(4):515–21.

164. Weiss MD, Tamisier R, Boucher J, et al. Pilot study of sleep, cognition, and respiration under 4 weeks of intermittent nocturnal hypoxia in adult humans. Sleep Med. 2009;10(7):739–45.

165. Findley LJ, Barth JT, Powers DC, et al. Cognitive impairment in patients with obstructive sleep apnea and associated hypoxemia. Chest. 1986;90(5):686–90.

166. Yaffe K, Laffan AM, Harrison SL, et al. Sleep-disordered breathing, hypoxia, and risk of mild cognitive impairment and dementia in older women. JAMA. 2011;306(6):613–9.

167. Beebe DW, Gozal D. Obstructive sleep apnea and the prefrontal cortex: towards a comprehensive model linking nocturnal upper airway obstruction to daytime cognitive and behavioral deficits. J Sleep Res. 2002;11:1–16.

168. Canessa N, Castronovo V, Cappa, SF, et al. Obstructive sleep apnea: brain structural changes and neurocognitive function before and after treatment. Am J Respir Crit Care Med. 2011;183:1419–26.

169. Joo EY, Tae WS, Lee MJ, et al. Reduced brain gray matter concentration in patients with obstructive sleep apnea syndrome. Sleep. 2010;33(2):235–41.

170. Macey PM, Henderson LA, Macey KE, et al. Brain morphology associated with obstructive sleep apnea. Am J Respir Crit Care Med. 2002;166(10):1382–7.

171. Morrell MJ, Jackson ML, Twigg GL, et al. Changes in brain morphology in patients with obstructive sleep apnoea. Thorax. 2010;65(10):908–14.

172. Yaouhi K, Bertran F, Clochon P, et al. A combined neuropsychological and brain imaging study of obstructive sleep apnea. J Sleep Res. 2009;18(1):36–48.

173. Macey PM;Kumar R;Woo MA;et al. Brain structural changes in obstructive sleep apnea. Sleep 2008;31(7):967–77

174. Krueger JM. The role of cytokines in sleep regulation. Curr Pharm Des. 2008:14:3408–16.

175. Pickering M, Cumiskey D, O'Connor JJ Actions of TNF-alpha on glutamatergic synaptic transmission in the central nervous system. Exp Physiol. 2005;90:663–70.

176. Ramesh V, Nair D, Zhang SX, et al. Disrupted sleep without sleep curtailment induces sleepiness and cognitive dysfunction via the tumor necrosis factor-α pathway. J Neuroinflammation. 2012;9:91.

177. Elwood PC, Bayer AJ, Fish M, et al. Sleep disturbance and daytime sleepiness predict vascular dementia. J Epidemiol Community Health 2010;65(9):820–4

178. Jouvet M, Delorme F. Locus coeruleus et sommeil paradoxal. C R Soc Biol. 1965;159:895–9.

179. Schenck CH, Bundlie SR, Ettinger MG, et al. Chronic behavioral disorders of human REM sleep: a new category of parasomnia. Sleep. 1986;9(2):293–308.

180. Bonakis A, Howard RS, Ebrahim IO, et al. REM sleep behaviour disorder (RBD) and its associations in young patients. Sleep Med. 2009;10(6):641–5.

181. Iranzo A, Tolosa E, Gelpi E, et al. Neurodegenerative disease status and post-mortem pathology in idiopathic rapid-eye-movement sleep behaviour disorder: an observational cohort study. Lancet Neurol. 2013;12(5):443–53.

182. Schenck CH, Boeve BF, Mahowald MW. Delayed emergence of a parkinsonian disorder or dementia in 81% of older men initially diagnosed with idiopathic rapid eye movement sleep behavior disorder: a 16-year update on a previously reported series. Sleep Med. 2013;14(8):744–8.

183. Frigerio R, Fujishiro H, Ahn TB, et al. Incidental Lewy body disease: do some cases represent a preclinical stage of dementia with Lewy bodies? Neurobiol Aging. 2011;32(5):857–63.

184. Iranzo A, Lomeña F, Stockner H, et al. Decreased striatal dopamine zz as risk markers of synucleinopathy in patients with idiopathic rapid-eye-movement sleep behaviour disorder: a prospective study [corrected]. Lancet Neurol. 2010;9(11):1070–7.

185. Kotagal V, Albin RL, Müller ML. Symptoms of rapid eye movement sleep behavior disorder are associated with cholinergic denervation in Parkinson disease. Ann Neurol. 2012;71(4):560–8.

186. Fantini ML, Farini E, Ortelli P, et al. Longitudinal study of cognitive function in idiopathic REM sleep behavior disorder. Sleep. 2011;34(5):619–25.

187. Boot B, Boeve B, Roberts R, et al. Probable REM sleep behavior disorder increases risk for mild cognitive impairment and Parkinson's disease: a population-based study. Ann Neurol. 2012;71(1):49–56.

188. Adler CH, Hentz JG, Shill HA et al. Probable RBD is increased in Parkinson's disease but not in essential tremor or restless legs syndrome. Parkinsonism Relat Disord. 2011;17(6):456–8.

189. Postuma RB, Bertrand JA, Montplaisir J, et al. Rapid eye movement sleep behavior disorder and risk of dementia in Parkinson's disease: a prospective study. Mov Disord. 2012;27(6):720–6.

190. Postuma RB, Gagnon JF, Rompré S, et al. Severity of REM atonia loss in idiopathic REM sleep behavior disorder predicts Parkinson disease. Neurology. 2010;74(3):239–44.

191. Ratti PL, Terzaghi M, Minafra B, et al. REM and NREM sleep enactment behaviors in Parkinson's disease, Parkinson's disease dementia, and dementia with Lewy bodies. Sleep Med. 2012;13(7):926–32.

192. McCarter SJ, Boswell CL, St Louis EK, et al. Treatment outcomes in REM sleep behavior disorder. Sleep Med. 2013;14(3):237–42.

193. Mahlberg R, Kunz D, Sutej I, et al. Melatonin treatment of day-night rhythm disturbances and sundowning in Alzheimer disease: an open-label pilot study using actigraphy. J Clin Psychopharmacol. 2004;24(4):456–9.

Fatal Familial Insomnia and Agrypnia Excitata: Insights into Human Prion Disease Genetics and the Anatomo-Physiology of Wake and Sleep Behaviours

Elio Lugaresi and Federica Provini

Introduction

In May 1984, a young doctor from the Venice region, Dr. R, telephoned one of us (EL) asking for a consultation. For some months, his wife's uncle (Mr. S) had presented the signs and symptoms of a disease that some years earlier had led to the death of his two sisters in the duration of 10–12 months. As Dr. R had already ascertained consulting the parish archives of the villages in the area where Mr. S, his sisters, and their ancestors had lived for centuries, the disease had been in their family at least since the nineteenth century. It probably dated back even further, but this could not be established as the parish records had been destroyed during the Napoleonic Wars.

On behalf of Mr. S and his relatives, Dr. R asked EL to admit Mr. S to the neurology clinic in Bologna for an in-depth investigation into the possible cause of his loss of sleep. Dr. R claimed that for some mysterious reason no one could understand that his family members died because they stopped sleeping. The many doctors, including leading neurologists, who had examined the patients, formulated myriad diagnoses ranging from oneiric-like schizophrenia to hypersomnia-related encephalopathy.

Despite our 20-year experience dealing with sleep and sleep disorders, we had never come across a case of this kind, nor had we read anything of the sort in the literature.

The following day, EL met Dr. R, his wife (Mr. S's niece) and Mr. S. While Dr. R and his wife told me the story of S and his family, S listened in silence, giving short but correct answers to questions he was asked. His face gave nothing

away. Every now and then he would close his eyes or rest his head as if about to drop off to sleep: he was *apathetic* and *somnolent* like all the patients belonging to this and other families we were to examine later.

EL had no doubts that S and his relatives had a hitherto unidentified hereditary disease whose cardinal features were a worsening sleep disorder and apathy. He immediately admitted Mr. S to our clinic and asked his team to undertake an in-depth investigation. Mr. S died 4 months later having completely lost the ability to sleep. An autopsy was performed and S's brain and spinal cord together with histological specimens of the brains of his two sisters were sent to our friend and collaborator P. Gambetti, director of the Neuropathology Division at Case Western University in Cleveland, OH, USA.

We monitored the Italian patients from this and other families while P. Gambetti's group undertook the neuropathological investigations. Some young researchers from Bologna also went to work alongside Gambetti who in turn involved leading US researchers Gajdusek and Prusiner and their groups. This joint collaboration led to the identification of the clinical and neuropathological features of the disease we named fatal familial insomnia (FFI) [1] and its molecular genetic mechanisms [2, 3].

Some 15 years after the discovery of FFI, we realized there existed a syndrome characterized by a permanent daily and nightly state of motor and autonomic activation associated with loss of sleep [4, 5]. This syndrome, which we named agrypnia excitata (AE), was shared by FFI [4–7], Morvan syndrome (MS), a dysimmune encephalopathy caused by autoantibodies binding to subunits of voltage gated K^+ (VGK) channels, prominently expressed by gamma-aminobutyric acid (GABA) neurons of the thalamus [8], and delirium tremens (DT), the acute psychosis following untreated alcohol withdrawal syndrome in chronic alcohol abusers [9]. The most likely cause of AE is a breakage in the circuit running through the limbic portion of the thalamus and connecting the forebrain to the hypothalamus and brainstem [4–7].

F. Provini (✉)
IRCCS Istituto delle Scienze Neurologiche di Bologna
University of Bologna, Ospedale Bellaria,
Via Altura, 3, 40139 Bologna, Italy
e-mail: federica.provini@unibo.it

F. Provini · E. Lugaresi
Department of Biomedical and Neuromotor Sciences,
University of Bologna, Ospedale Bellaria,
Via Altura, 3, 40139 Bologna, Italy

S. Chokroverty, M. Billiard (eds.), *Sleep Medicine,* DOI 10.1007/978-1-4939-2089-1_34,
© Springer Science+Business Media, LLC 2015

Fatal Familial Insomnia: Its Clinical Variants and Sporadic (Nongenetic) Form

FFI is an autosomal dominant hereditary disease with a high penetrance caused by a missense mutation at codon 178 of prion protein gene (PRNP), encoding asparagine for aspartic acid, on one of the alleles of the prion protein gene [2]. Allele-specific sequencing demonstrated that codon 129 of the PRNP, the site of a common methionine/valine polymorphism, is the determinant of the disease phenotypes linked to the 178 mutation. The FFI anatomo-clinical phenotype will become manifest if the mutated allele at codon 129 encodes methionine at the polymorphic methionine–valine codon. Otherwise, the disease shows the anatomo-clinical features of Creutzfeldt–Jakob disease [10, 11].

FFI affects men and women in equal measure. The first symptoms are rapidly progressive worsening insomnia and apathy that gradually turns into obstinate mutism. On average, symptoms arise at around the age of 50 with a broad range spanning two to three decades [12].

From onset, insomnia, somnolence and apathy are flanked by motor activation (focal and diffuse myoclonias mainly in the extremities) and *recurrent stereotyped gestures mimicking daily-life activities* like washing, combing hair, dressing and undressing, handling objects or greeting non-existent persons. We named this stereotype repetition of gestures *oneiric stupor (OS)* as, when questioned, patients would often report an oneiric scene in which they were taking part. *OS* is one of the hallmarks of FFI [7] (Fig. 34.1).

From the early stages of disease, patients also present profuse sweating, abundant salivation and lacrimation and a progressive increase in heart and breathing rates accompanied by a mild but progressive rise in body temperature. Associated disorders include difficulty urinating and impotence in males [1, 12].

As the weeks pass, difficulty standing, a complex gait impairment, distal tremors and tendon hyperreflexia become increasingly evident. Worsening somnolence is transformed into a permanent state of drowsiness ("dormiveglia") or stupor persisting night and day. When stimulated, patients open their eyes and answer correctly but in monosyllables. Death is due to sudden cardiorespiratory arrest or intercurrent febrile illness.

Fig. 34.1 Oneiric stupor. Sequential frames recorded from top to bottom in patients with fatal familial insomnia (*FFI*), Morvan syndrome (*MS*) and delirium tremens (*DT*) showing similar complex semi-purposeful movements during oneiric stupor episodes

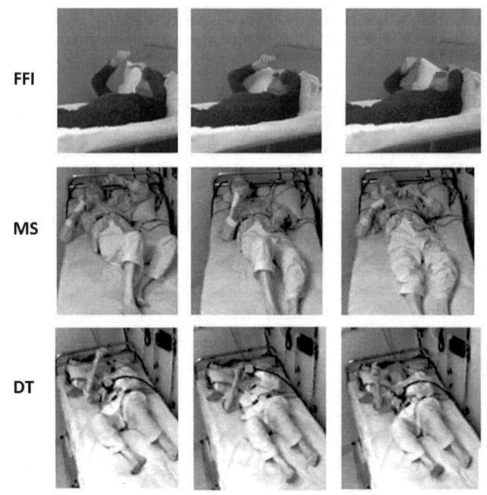

The disease has a rapid course (8–12 months) in around two-thirds of patients. In these cases, both mutated and non-mutated alleles of PRNP at the position 178, and at the polymorphic codon 129 encode methionine [13]. In the remaining cases in which the non-mutated allele in position 129 of the PRNP encodes valine, the clinical course is at least two to three times longer and highly variable.

Serial neuropsychological tests have documented that attention and vigilance progressively decline from the early signs of disease, whereas intellectual functions remain largely spared until the most advanced stages. Given these characteristics, FFI should be considered a chronic confusional state rather than a form of dementia [14, 15].

Serial electroencephalogram (EEG) performed throughout the disease course fail to disclose abnormalities other than those linked to a progressive increase in somnolence. Serial polygraphic recordings for 24 h during disease evolution document a fragmentation and progressive reduction of spindle and delta activities that ultimately disappear completely [16]. Once spindle and delta activities disappear, intravenous injection of benzodiazepines or barbiturates at high doses transform "dormiveglia" or stupor into a deep coma associated with flattening of the EEG, invariably failing to trigger spindle and delta activities [17].

This state of subvigilance persisting day and night is characterized polygraphically by an alternation of stage 1 sleep (EEG theta activity associated with slow eye movement discharges and diminished muscle tone) and very short bursts of rapid eye movement (REM) sleep (lasting 30–40 s) that recur, often in clusters, both day and night. Stage 1 and REM sleep continue to alternate until the preterminal stages of the disease (Fig. 34.2).

Background and stimulated cardiovascular function monitoring documents a state of sympathetic hyperactivity whereas parasympathetic activity is always within normal limits [18]. Serial 24-h recordings disclose a progressive increase in heart and breathing rates, systemic arterial pressure and body core temperature during the clinical course [19]. Circadian cortisol and noradrenaline secretions are two to three time higher than normal, daily and nightly, whereas the nocturnal melatonin peak subsides to almost disappear [20] (Fig. 34.3).

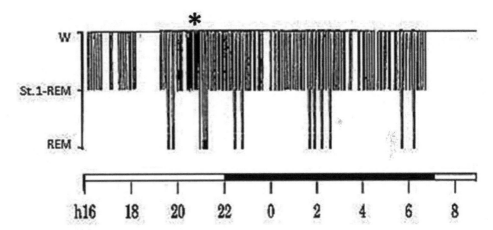

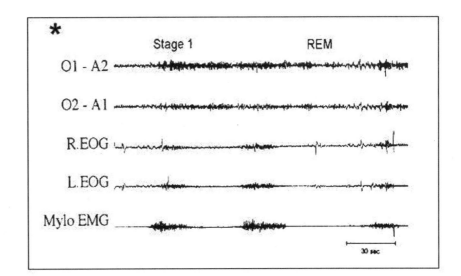

Fig. 34.2 Polysomnographic recording in fatal familial insomnia. *Top*: The 24-h wake–sleep histogram demonstrates reduced total sleep time, absence of synchronized sleep and abnormal cyclic organization of sleep. *Bottom*: Electroencephalographic tracing shows transitions between rapid eye movement (*REM*) and subwakefulness (stage 1) recurring in a quasi-periodic fashion

Fig. 34.3 The 24-h recordings of noradrenaline, cortisol and melatonin concentrations in a patient with FFI and in a control individual. Noradrenaline and cortisol secretions are higher than normal throughout the 24 h. The nocturnal peak of melatonin secretion is lost

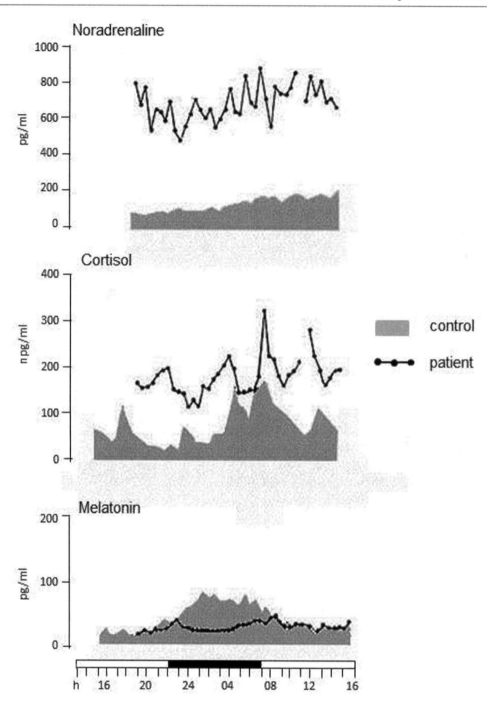

Computed tomography (CT) and magnetic resonance imaging (MRI) scans are unremarkable except for a mild cerebral and cerebellar atrophy in the most advanced disease stages. By contrast, serial positron emission tomography (PET) ([18]fludeoxyglucose(FDG) PET) scans invariably show a bilateral thalamic hypometabolism from the early disease stages [21, 22]. Impaired thalamic metabolism is evident many months before the onset of the early signs of disease in carriers of the FFI mutation [23].

General autopsy fails to disclose findings of significance whereas brain examination reveals bilateral and symmetrical atrophy of the thalami. The thalamic formations invariably

and most severely affected are the anterior and medio-dorsal thalamic nuclei. Neuronal loss in these nuclei exceeds 50%, reaching values of more than 90% in the antero-ventral nuclei and mesial part of medio-dorsal nuclei. The other nuclei, with the exception of the pulvinar, invariably damaged, are inconsistently and scarcely affected.

According to Schulman [24], who observed an ante-litteram FFI case, and Macchi et al. [25] who studied two FFI patients by morphometric analysis, the thalamic reticular nucleus (TRN) was one of the most damaged thalamic formations. However, Gambetti (personal communication) claimed it would be difficult if not impossible to establish whether the entire length of this extremely long and thin layer is involved in the pathological process.

Rapid evolution cases often present areas of spongiform degeneration confined to the *anterior cingulate gyrus* and *mesio-orbital cortical and sub-cortical formations* [26]. In longer evolution cases, cortical spongiform degeneration may extend throughout the frontal lobe to the parieto-temporal regions, but always prevails in the mesio-orbital areas of the frontal lobe. FFI can be defined as a thalamo-limbic or prevalently thalamo-limbic encephalopathy.

Genetic and Molecular Biology of FFI and Other Prion Diseases

As mentioned above, FFI is a prion disease caused by a point mutation at codon 178 of PRNP. The FFI phenotype is seen when the methionine–valine polymorphic codon 129 of the PRNP encodes methionine in the mutated allele. If the mutated allele at codon 178 encodes valine, at position 129, the disease phenotype will be a rapidly evolving dementia associated with diffuse spongiform degeneration of the cortex and subcortical grey matter structures [11].

The most common FFI phenotype (short course and anatomic lesions confined to the thalamus) presents when codon 129 of the prion protein gene encodes methionine in mutated and non-mutated alleles (around two-thirds of patients). When the non-mutated allele encodes valine (methionine–valine heterozygous at codon 129), the disease has a longer more variable course with thalamic atrophy associated with spongiform degeneration of the frontal and parieto-temporal cortices. The prion protein fragment deposited in the brain tissues of FFI patients has a molecular weight and conformation different from that of the fragments found in the brains of patients with the spongiform encephalopathy variant caused by the same mutation at codon 178, co-segregating with valine in the mutated allele. For the first time in human genetics, these molecular and genetic findings showed that the disease generated by a punctiform mutation of the prion protein gene is due to a polymorphism of the same gene [13]. Working with Prusiner and his group, we were able also to demonstrate that transgenic mice infected with FFI brain homogenates develop and transmit a disease characterized by prions that retain the donor prion conformation. Conversely, transgenic mice infected with brain homogenates of patients with Creutzfeldt–Jakob disease develop and transmit a diffuse encephalopathy characterized by prions with a conformation similar to that of the donor [27]. These findings provide convincing evidence of Prusiner's theory that the variable clinical manifestations of prion disease are linked, at least in part, to different prion conformations rather than a hypothetical prion-driven virus.

Clinical and Polygraphic Aspects of Agrypnia Excitata

Some 15 years after the first description of FFI, we realized that at least two other neurological disorders, MS and DT, present features similar to FFI consisting of a confusional state characterized by a polygraphic tracing with intermediate aspects between stage 1 NREM sleep and REM sleep. Stage 1+REM or stage 1 REM were the terms used by Tachibana et al. and Kotorii et al. to define the polygraphic tracing they observed in cases of acute psychosis triggered by untreated sudden alcohol withdrawal in patients with chronic alcoholism [28, 29].

In addition, FFI, MS and DT share the features of a syndrome characterized by a general and permanent state of motor and autonomic activation. We named this condition AE. The hallmark of AE is the stereotyped subcontinuous repetition of gestures mimicking the daily-life activities described above under the name of *OS* (Fig. 34.1).

OS, a sign we invariably observed in cases of FFI, MS and DT, but never encountered in patients with confusional states of different nature and origin, is the most characteristic feature of AE.

Pathophysiology of AE

In FFI, AE is caused by a breakage in the circuit running through the medio-dorsal thalamic nuclei and rostral part of the TRN and interconnecting the basal forebrain formation to hypothalamus and upper brainstem. In MS, autoantibodies binding to subunits of VGK channels, particularly expressed by GABAergic neurons of the thalamus, impair normal thalamic function [8, 30, 31]. This mechanism is responsible for the loss of sleep associated with day and night motor, sympathetic and noradrenergic activation in MS [8, 30, 31]. In DT, the disappearance of sleep combined with a general hyperactivation syndrome ensues from a concomitant downregulation of GABA-A synapses and upregulation of N-methyl-D-aspartate (NMDA) glutamatergic synapses following untreated sudden alcohol withdrawal in chronic alcohol abusers [9].

Clinical and pathophysiological observations in AE suggest that basic wake and sleep behaviours and their orderly succession throughout the 24 h are produced by a neuronal network extending from the neocortex to lower brainstem, and working in an integrated fashion. The most caudal part of the network, contained in the hindbrain, consists of a gatekeeper automatically generating ultradian rhythms of rest periods alternating with shorter periods of activation in man and other mammals. This basic rest activity cycles (of sleep and wakefulness), documented in man and other mammals [32] is probably generated by a single medullary gatekeeper, as demonstrated by the fact that an alternating periodicity of rest and activity with the same duration as the rest–activity cycles of wake and sleep is maintained in medullary and midpontine cats [33]:

- The midbrain, hypothalamus and basal forebrain continuum contain activating and deactivating systems and the ultradian (metabolic) and circadian (physical) mechanisms regulating the transition from wakefulness to sleep and vice versa. The primordial emotional inputs, somnolence (desire for sleep) and sleep satiety, originating at this level, regulate the ultradian and/or circadian alternation of wake and sleep.
- Synchronized sleep originates at thalamo-cortical level. Spindling arises in the rostral portion of the TRN and delta sleep in the neocortex. An intralimbic circuit running through the visceral thalamus controls cerebral and body homeostasis as AE syndrome suggests. This hypothesis seems to be in line with experimental results on the anatomo-physiology of sleep.

Only experimental trials replicating AE in animals will tell us if and to what extent this hypothesis is correct.

Conclusion

The circuit controlling and regulating homeostasis in the brain and the entire organism appears to be interrupted at the thalamic level in FFI, or functionally imbalanced due to a GABA-A neural system block in MS or concomitant downregulation of the GABA system and upregulation of NMDA glutamatergic system in DT. This impaired circuit gives rise to the syndrome we named AE. The resulting homeostatic imbalance leads to an inability to generate synchronized (calm) sleep and hence the inability to stay awake. What remains of sleep and wake is a state of subvigilance in which stage 1 is mixed with fragments of REM sleep. This peculiar electrophysiological condition is accompanied by a permanent state of autonomic and motor activation whose hallmarks are stereotypic repetition of gestures mimicking daily-life activities.

References

1. Lugaresi E, Medori R, Montagna P, et al. Fatal Familial Insomnia and dysautonomia with selective degeneration of thalamic nuclei. N Engl J Med. 1986;315(16):997–1003.
2. Medori R, Tritschler HJ, LeBlanc A, et al. Fatal Familial Insomnia, a prion disease with a mutation at codon 178 of the prion protein gene. N Engl J Med. 1992;326(7):444–9.
3. Monari L, Chen SG, Brown P, et al. Fatal familial insomnia and familial Creutzfeldt-Jakob disease: Different prion proteins determined by a DNA polymorphism. Proc Natl Acad Sci U S A 1994;91(7):2839–42.
4. Lugaresi E, Provini F. Agrypnia Excitata: clinical features and pathophysiological implications. Sleep Med Rev. 2001;5(4):313–22.
5. Montagna P, Lugaresi E. Agrypnia Excitata: A generalized overactivity syndrome and a useful concept in the neurophysiopathology of sleep. Clin Neurophysiol. 2002;113(4):552–60.
6. Provini F, Cortelli P, Montagna P, Gambetti P, Lugaresi E. Fatal insomnia and Agrypnia Excitata: sleep and the limbic system. Rev Neurol (Paris). 2008;164(8–9):692–700.
7. Lugaresi E, Provini F, Cortelli P. Agrypnia Excitata. Sleep Med. 2011;12 Suppl 2:S3–10.
8. Liguori R, Vincent A, Clover L, et al. Morvan's syndrome: peripheral and central nervous system and cardiac involvement with antibodies to voltage-gated potassium channels. Brain. 2001;124(Pt 12):2417–26.
9. Plazzi G, Montagna P, Meletti S, Lugaresi E. Polysomnographic study of sleeplessness and oneiricisms in the alcohol withdrawal syndrome. Sleep Med. 2002;3(3):279–82.
10. Goldfarb LG, Haltia M, Brown P, et al. New mutation in scrapie amyloid precursor gene (at codon 178) in Finnish Creutzfeldt-Jakob kindred. Lancet. 1991;337(8738):425.
11. Goldfarb LG, Petersen RB, Tabaton M, et al. Fatal familial insomnia and familial Creutzfeldt-Jakob disease: disease phenotype determined by a DNA polymorphism. Science. 1992;258(5083):806–8.
12. Montagna P. Fatal familial insomnia and the role of the thalamus in sleep regulation. Handb Clin Neurol. 2011;99:981–96.
13. Montagna P, Cortelli P, Avoni P, et al. Clinical features of fatal familial insomnia: phenotypic variability in relation to a polymorphism at codon 129 of the prion protein gene. Brain Pathol. 1998;8(3):515–20.
14. Gallassi R, Morreale A, Montagna P, Gambetti P, Lugaresi E. "Fatal familial insomnia": neuropsychological study of a disease with thalamic degeneration. Cortex. 1992;28(2):175–87.
15. Gallassi R, Morreale A, Montagna P, et al. Fatal familial insomnia: behavioral and cognitive features. Neurology. 1996;46(4):935–9.
16. Sforza E, Montagna P, Tinuper P, et al. Sleep-wake cycle abnormalities in fatal familial insomnia. Evidence of the role of the thalamus in sleep regulation. Electroencephalogr Clin Neurophysiol. 1995;94(6):398–405.
17. Tinuper P, Montagna P, Medori R, et al. The thalamus participates in the regulation of the sleep-waking cycle. A clinico-pathological study in fatal familial thalamic degeneration. Electroencephalogr Clin Neurophysiol. 1989;73(2):117–23.
18. Cortelli P, Parchi P, Contin M, et al. Cardiovascular dysautonomia in fatal familial insomnia. Clin Auton Res. 1991;1(1):15–21.
19. Portaluppi F, Cortelli P, Avoni A, et al. Diurnal blood pressure variations and hormonal correlates in fatal familial insomnia. Hypertension. 1994;23(5):569–76.
20. Portaluppi F, Cortelli P, Avoni P, et al. Progressive disruption of the circadian rhythm of melatonin in fatal familial insomnia. J Clin Endocrinol Metab. 1994;78(5):1075–8.
21. Perani D, Cortelli P, Lucignani G, et al. [18F]FDG PET in fatal familial insomnia: the functional effects of thalamic lesions. Neurology. 1993;43(12):2565–9.
22. Cortelli P, Perani D, Parchi P, et al. Cerebral metabolism in fatal familial insomnia: relation to duration, neuropathology, and distribution of protease-resistant prion protein. Neurology. 1997;49(1):126–33.
23. Cortelli P, Perani D, Montagna P, et al. Pre-symptomatic diagnosis in fatal familial insomnia: serial neurophysiological and 18FDG-PET studies. Brain. 2006;129(Pt 3):668–75.
24. Schulman S. Bilateral symmetrical degeneration of the thalamus; a clinicopathological study. J Neuropathol Exp Neurol. 1957;16(4):446–70.
25. Macchi G, Rossi G, Abbamondi AL, et al. Diffuse thalamic degeneration in fatal familial insomnia: a morphometric study. Brain Res. 1997;771(1):154–8.
26. Gambetti P, Petersen R, Monari L, et al. Fatal familial insomnia and the widening spectrum of prion diseases. Br Med Bull. 1993;49(4):980–94.

27. Montagna P, Gambetti P, Cortelli P, Lugaresi E. Familial and sporadic fatal insomnia. Lancet Neurol. 2003;2(3):167–76.

28. Tachibana M, Tanaka K, Hishikawa Y, Kaneko Z. A sleep study of acute psychotic states due to alcohol and meprobamate addiction. In: Advances in sleep research, vol. 2. New York: Spectrum; 1975. pp. 177–205.

29. Kotorii T, Nakazawa Y, Yokoyama T, et al. The sleep pattern of chronic alcoholics during the alcohol withdrawal period. Folia Psychiatr Neurol Jpn. 1980;34(2):89–95.

30. Vincent A, Buckely C, Schott JM, et al. Potassium channel antibody-associated encephalopathy: a potentially immunotherapy-responsive form of limbic encephalitis. Brain. 2004;127(Pt 3):701–12.

31. Cornelius JR, Pittock SJ, McKeon A, et al. Sleep manifestations of voltage-gated potassium channel complex autoimmunity. Arch Neurol. 2011;68(6):733–8.

32. Kleitman N. Sleep and wakefulness. Chicago: University of Chicago Press; 1963.

33. Siegel JM, Tomaszewski KS, Nienhuis R. Behavioral states in the chronic medullary and midpontine cat. Electroencephalogr Clin Neurophysiol. 1986;63(2):274–88.

Epilepsy and Sleep

35

Sándor Beniczky and Peter Wolf

Historical Milestones

The close relationship between sleep and epilepsy had been recognised already by the ancient Greeks [1]. In the fourth century BC, Aristotle wrote that "sleep is similar to epilepsy, and in some way sleep is epilepsy". The facilitating effect of sleep deprivation on ictogenesis was described by Galen, in the second century, and the importance of sleep hygiene for the treatment of patients with epilepsy was already emphasised by Hippocrates in the fifth century BC. Aretaeus of Cappadocia (first century) has described that epilepsy could cause sleep disturbance.

In the early nineteenth century, based on clinical observations, Prichard opined that epilepsy, sleepwalking, and nightmares were related [2]. Already at the end of the nineteenth century, distinction between epileptic seizures and parasomnia (sleepwalking) has been made [3].

Analysing the seizure occurrence of hospitalised patients, Féré concluded that two thirds of the seizures occurred during sleep [4]. Based on a large-scale study on hospitalised patients, in 1885, Gowers observed that 1/5 of the seizures only occurred during the night, 2/5 only during the day, and the rest occurred either night or day [5]. Furthermore, he described that falling asleep and awakening were especially vulnerable periods.

The discovery of electroencephalography (EEG) revolutionised both the field of epilepsy and sleep medicine [6]. Based on the EEG changes, sleep stages were established, patterns characteristic for sleep were described [7], and the cyclic alternation of rapid eye movement (REM) sleep and non-REM (NREM) sleep was discovered [8]. In 1968, the still valid consensus on scoring sleep, based on polygraphic recordings including EEG, surface electromyography, and electro-oculography, has been published [9].

In parallel with the development of polygraphic techniques for patients with sleep disorders, sleep-related EEG abnormalities were described in patients with epilepsy. Gibbs and Gibbs observed a significant increase in the amount of epileptiform EEG discharges, during sleep and the occurrence of EEG abnormalities in sleep, even in patients with normal waking recordings [10]. REM sleep was found to inhibit generalised epileptiform discharges [11], whilst epileptic seizures mainly occurred during stage 2 of non-REM sleep [12, 13].

In the late 1950s, electroclinical syndromes of childhood epilepsies with occurrence or strong accentuation in sleep were reported. In 1958, "benign" childhood epilepsy with centro-temporal spikes, focal seizures predominantly during sleep, and a self-limited course has been described [14, 15]. In 1957, Landau and Kleffner published their seminal paper on children with acquired aphasia and seizures [16]. Later, Patry and co-workers reported the electroclinical picture of almost continuous epileptiform EEG activity during sleep (electrical status epilepticus in sleep; ESES), cognitive dysfunctions, and seizures [17].

Janz, in a series of papers in the 1960s, analysed the syndromatic significance of various relations of generalised tonic–clonic ("grand mal") seizures (GTCS) to the sleep–waking cycle particularly distinguishing awakening grand mal and sleep grand mal; the former is related to myoclonic and absence seizures and the latter to complex partial seizures [18]. These also differed in their response to the only available antiepileptic drugs (AEDs) of the time—awakening

S. Beniczky (✉)
Department of Clinical Neurophysiology,
Danish Epilepsy Centre, Dianalund, Denmark
e-mail: sbz@filadelfia.dk

Department of Clinical Neurophysiology,
Aarhus University, Aarhus, Denmark

P. Wolf
Department of Neurology, Danish Epilepsy Centre,
Dianalund, Denmark
e-mail: pwl@filadelfia.dk

S. Chokroverty, M. Billiard (eds.), *Sleep Medicine,* DOI 10.1007/978-1-4939-2089-1_35,
© Springer Science+Business Media, LLC 2015

epilepsies responding best to phenobarbital and sleep epilepsies to phenytoin [19].

In spite of the technological advances, differentiating between parasomnia and nocturnal seizures remained difficult even in the twentieth century. This is probably best illustrated by the history of nocturnal paroxysmal dystonia (bizarre tonic or dystonic movements arising abruptly from non-REM sleep without epileptiform electrographic correlate on scalp recordings) that initially was considered a new form of parasomnia [20]. However, invasive EEG recordings demonstrated that these are epileptic seizures of the frontal lobe, arising from deep foci (supplementary sensorymotor or cingulate cortex) [21, 22].

The first type of human epilepsy, in which the genetic defect was demonstrated, was a sleep-related epilepsy: The autosomal dominant nocturnal frontal lobe epilepsy [23]. This involved mutations in the nicotinic acetylcholine receptor gene [24].

Sleep and Seizure Generation

Sleep-related interictal epileptiform discharges (IEDs) and seizures occur mainly during non-REM sleep and the transition phases between sleep stages or between sleep and wakefulness. In contrast, epileptiform discharges and seizures are almost completely absent during REM-sleep: Only highly localised epileptiform discharges are occasionally recorded during REM-sleep, whilst the inhibition of the motor system prevents ictal manifestations.

As activation with propagation of epileptiform activity is mainly observed during stage 2 of NREM sleep, the neurophysiologic changes during this stage received much attention in an attempt to elucidate the substrates of seizure generation. EEG in non-REM sleep is characterised by a higher level of synchronisation and increase in amplitude. Because epileptic seizures are due to abnormal excessive or synchronised neuronal activity in the brain, it was reasonable to hypothesise that the increased level of neuronal synchronisation during non-REM sleep contributed to seizure generation, whilst the desynchronisation during REM-sleep counteracted seizure generation. As sleep spindles and K-complexes are abundant during stage 2, it was hypothesised that epileptiform discharges could have neural substrates similar to these EEG patterns characteristic for sleep.

Studies on animal models yielded further insights into the intricate interplay between the neural substrates of sleep and epilepsy. Specific stimulation of the thalamic reticular system elicited epileptiform cortical responses during sleep. However, this could not be easily elicited in an alert animal, demonstrating the essential role of sleep in seizure generation [25].

Intracellular recordings (from neurons and glial cells), measurement of extracellular ionic concentrations (K and Ca), and simultaneous recordings of intracortical field potentials in anesthetised cats suggested that sleep slow oscillation was the precursor of the epileptiform activity [26]. Sleep slow oscillation is a cortically generated slow (< 1 Hz) rhythm resulting from the complex interplay within neural and glial networks, modulated by the diffuse action of extracellular ion currents. It is disrupted by wakefulness, as activation of the brainstem elicits a global change in the extracellular space, with profound modifications of glial and cerebral blood flow parameters [26]. It was argued that sleep slow oscillations contributed to the generation of K-complexes (with the exception of occasional sensory-evoked K-complexes). A smooth transition was observed from physiological sleep slow oscillation to paroxysmal, spike-and-slow-wave complexes (2 Hz) and rhythmic fast (15 Hz) ictal activity [27].

Exogenous stimulation (acoustic and photic) evoked K-complexes and sleep spindles, and also precipitated generalised tonic–clonic seizures in amygdala-kindled cats [28]. The most vulnerable periods were those in which the spontaneous seizures occurred most frequently: non-REM sleep and the transition to REM-sleep. It was argued that epileptiform EEG activity was associated with "phasic arousals without awakening" or "aborted arousals" in patients with idiopathic generalised epilepsy (IGE; [29]). Awakening is a particularly seizure-prone phase of the sleep–waking cycle, especially in patients with idiopathic generalised epilepsies. This applies to the end of both night sleep and afternoon naps, whereas the related epileptiform discharge in juvenile myoclonic epilepsy was most prominent in nocturnal intermediate awakenings [30]. The dynamic differences behind this intriguing contrast in behaviour of seizures and interictal discharge, which could reflect differences in inhibitory mechanism, have never been investigated. The relations of cyclic alternating patterns (as part of sleep microstructure), to the epileptiform discharge, in this syndrome, have been described by Gigli et al. [31].

Relationship with sleep phenomena can be found not only at the level of generation of the epileptic seizures but also at propagation and semiological manifestation of the seizures [32]. Based on video-polygraphic recordings, Tassinari and co-workers documented that sleep-related epileptic seizures and non-epileptic events (parasomnias) share similar manifestations/semiological features (oroalimentary automatisms, bruxism, ambulatory behaviours, fear, and violent behaviour). The authors hypothesised that these stereotypical motor sequences resulted from activation of neuronal networks ("central pattern generators") located at the subcortical level (brainstem and spinal cord) that are activated during seizures as well as parasomnia, through a release-like mechanism.

A close relation of the epileptiform discharges of benign Rolandic childhood epilepsy to sleep spindles has been described by Nobili et al. [33]. Avanzini et al. [34] considered this syndrome as a prototypical "system epilepsy".

EEG Recordings and Sleep

The sensitivity of a single EEG recording for detecting IEDs is rather low (50%). However, repeated recordings, including sleep recording, increase the sensitivity to 92% [35]. It was suggested that sleep deprivation had an activating effect on IEDs by modulating cortical excitability [36, 37]. In patients with juvenile myoclonic epilepsy, sleep proved to be one of the major activating factors of the IEDs [38, 39].

Besides the quantitative changes in the IEDs, described above, qualitative changes are also observed. In children with West syndrome, the disorganised delta activity of hypsarrhythmia is enhanced during sleep but often it becomes also more synchronous. In addition, stretches of diffuse flattening appear during sleep. The typical 10-Hz runs-of-rapid spikes in children with Lennox–Gastaut syndrome are only recorded during sleep. In patients with IGEs, the intra-burst frequency of the spike- and slow-wave paroxysms tends to decrease during sleep. In patients with Rolandic epilepsy, the unilateral IEDs become bilateral (synchronous or asynchronous) during non-REM sleep; unilaterality is restored during REM sleep.

Nocturnal Seizures

Seizures occurring during sleep (or mainly during sleep) are not specific for a certain epilepsy type or syndrome. They can occur in focal as well as "generalised" epilepsies, in symptomatic as well as idiopathic epilepsies.

Frontal Lobe Epilepsy

Seizures occur mostly during sleep. Seizures are typically of short duration and occur in clusters, mainly in the first part of the sleep. The patients usually retain consciousness or lose it very briefly, and there is no postictal confusion, unless with evolution to secondarily generalised seizures. The semiology is different, depending on which part of the frontal lobe is involved in the generation of the seizure manifestation: bilateral asymmetric tonic seizures with head version ("fencing posture"), vocalisation, speech arrest, uni- or bilateral somatosensory phenomena (supplementary sensory motor area seizures) [40]; hyperkinetic seizures with large amplitude movements involving the proximal parts of the limbs and/or complex automatisms (mesial or orbitofrontal

cortex); focal tonic, versive, or focal clonic seizures (dorsolateral cortex), mastication, salivation, swallowing (frontal operculum), focal motor seizures according to the involved part of the motor homunculus (motor cortex).

In frontal lobe epilepsies, the risk of secondary generalisation is similar during sleep and wakefulness.

Most of the cases are symptomatic or cryptogenic. The diagnostic workup is often difficult, as many patients have normal EEG recordings and magnetic resonance imaging (MRI).

Autosomal dominant nocturnal frontal lobe epilepsy (ADNFLE) is a genetic epilepsy due to mutation in the gene encoding a subunit of the nicotinic acetylcholine receptor [23, 24]. It begins in childhood (around 10 years). Shortly after falling asleep, clusters of brief (<1 min), stereotyped motor seizures (focal tonic, clonic, hyperkinetic) occur, often preceded by nonspecific aura; up to ten seizures/night. About one quarter of the patients occasionally have seizures also during the day. Half of the patients have occasionally secondarily generalised seizures. The seizure semiology shows a remarkable intra-individual stability, and there is no progression of the symptoms. The neurological examination is unrevealing, and the cognition is normal, except for discrete neuropsychological changes, suggesting affection of the frontal lobe. MRI is normal, but functional neuroimaging can show frontal defects. It is intriguing that the only patient with ADNFLE who was investigated with intracranial electrodes had a seizure onset zone in the insula [41]. Seventy percent of the patients become seizure-free on carbamazepine.

Differentiating nocturnal frontal lobe seizures from parasomnia can be difficult in some cases, and it requires video–EEG and polygraphic recordings in dedicated centres [42]. Sleep seizures occur frequently (>3 seizures/night; >10 seizures/month), occur mainly in stage 2 of non-REM sleep, are short (up to 1–2 min), stereotyped, often with retained consciousness. Family history is usually unrevealing (with the exception of the rare ADNFLE). Parasomnias have less frequent clinical episodes (1–2/night; 1–4/month), occur in non-REM sleep or in REM sleep, later during the sleep (>90 min), have more variable motor manifestation/semiology, and longer duration (up to 30 min). Patients have affected consciousness/responsiveness. Family history is often positive [43].

Temporal Lobe Epilepsy

In the symptomatic/cryptogenic cases, seizures mostly occur in wakefulness. However, sleep modulates these seizures too: Complex partial seizures starting from sleep evolve to secondarily generalised seizures twice as often as the seizures starting from wakefulness.

Familial lateral temporal lobe epilepsy (TLE) is a rare form of genetic (autosomal dominant) epilepsy that starts in late childhood or early adult life. Lateral (neocortical) temporal seizures consist of auditory, vertiginous, visual, or olfactory hallucinations, evolving to complex partial seizures and to mainly nocturnal, secondarily generalised seizures. Seizures have an excellent response to carbamazepine.

Rolandic Epilepsy/Benign Childhood Epilepsy with Centrotemporal Spikes (BECTS)

This syndrome is the most common localisation-related epilepsy in childhood, and it is characterised by "brief, simple, partial, hemifacial motor seizures, frequently having associated somatosensory symptoms which have a tendency to evolve into generalised tonic-clonic seizures. Both seizure types are often related to sleep (70–80% of the seizures occur during sleep). Onset occurs between the ages of 3 and 13 years (peak 9–10 years), and recovery occurs before the age of 15–16 years. Genetic predisposition is frequent, and there is male predominance. The EEG has blunt high-voltage centrotemporal spikes, often followed by slow waves that are activated by sleep and tend to spread or shift from side to side" [44]. In terms of seizures, the prognosis is indeed good: 80–90% of patients who require AED treatment at all become seizure-free on therapy (sulthiame alone or in combination with clobazam; carbamazepine). Seizures usually disappear and EEG normalises before the age of 16 years. However, a significant number of patients have some degree of neuropsychological impairment and educational problems, and the term "benign" has, therefore, been questioned for this syndrome.

Panayiotopoulos Syndrome

This is a form of idiopathic, localisation-related childhood epilepsy, defined as: "a benign age-related focal seizure disorder occurring in early and mid-childhood. It is characterised by seizures, often prolonged, with predominantly autonomic symptoms, and by an EEG that shows shifting and/or multiple foci, often with occipital predominance" [45]. More than two thirds of the seizures are nocturnal, and usually consist of emesis, behavioural changes, and unilateral eye deviation. Consciousness and speech are preserved. The prognosis is excellent. About one quarter of the patients only have a single episode, and half of the patients only have two episodes during their lifetime. Spontaneous remission is often within 1 or 2 years.

Encephalopathy with Electrical Status Epilepticus During Sleep

Several syndromes have been described that have the following common features: (1) epileptic seizures, mostly during sleep, (2) neuropsychological or motor impairment/decline, and (3) significant activation of paroxysmal EEG activity during sleep, leading to a subclinical pattern of almost continuous spike and slow waves (ESES). It has been proposed that the syndromes sharing these features are different manifestations of the same epileptic encephalopathy [46, 47].

Atypical BECTS

Atypical BECTS ("pseudo-Lennox syndrome") is characterised by IEDs similar to the ones recorded in typical BECTS but "generalisation" during sleep, atonic–astatic seizures, atypical absences and myoclonic seizures [48, 49]. In 56% of patients, the accentuation during sleep reached the level of ESES. Besides the above-mentioned seizures, some patients also have focal seizures (mostly originating in the orofacial region), and secondarily generalised tonic–clonic seizures. Notably tonic seizures and 10-Hz run-of-rapid spikes (typical for Lennox–Gastaut syndrome) are absent in atypical BECTS. One quarter of the patients have mental retardation at onset of epilepsy (usually between 2 and 6 years). The course of the epilepsy is self-limited: 84% of patients were in clinical remission at the last follow-up, and all subjects older than age 15 were seizure-free [49]. However, the percentage of patients with cognitive impairment doubled through the course of the disease (56% attended a school for mentally handicapped children).

Landau–Kleffner Syndrome

Landau–Kleffner syndrome (acquired epileptic aphasia) is defined as "a childhood disorder in which an acquired aphasia, multifocal spike, and spike-and-wave discharges are associated. Epileptic seizures and behavioural and psychomotor disturbances occur in two thirds of the patients. There is verbal auditory agnosia and rapid reduction of spontaneous speech. The seizures, usually GTCS or partial motor, are rare, and remit before the age of 15 years, as do the EEG abnormalities" [44]. Before the onset (2–11 years), the children have normal development. The onset is subacute, and starts with gradual development of sensory aphasia. EEG shows focal epileptiform discharges, most often in the temporal lobe on the dominant side (in 67–90% of the patients) or in the frontal lobe. Accentuation during sleep reaches the level of ESES in 40–50% of the patients. Clinical seizures are rare. The main seizure types are: atypical absences, focal motor seizures, atonic seizures, and secondarily generalised tonic–clonic seizures. The seizures are relatively easily controlled with AED (valproate, sulthiam, clobazam), but the prognosis is poor concerning language and cognitive impairment. Less than one fifth of patients achieve complete language recovery, and almost two thirds of the patients develop mental retardation and evolution to CSWS (see below). Steroids and multiple pial transection have been suggested for the treatment of the language impairment.

Epilepsy with Continuous Spike-Waves During Slow Sleep

Epilepsy with continuous spike-waves during slow sleep (CSWS) "results from the association of various seizure types, partial or generalised, occurring during sleep, and atypical absences when awake. Tonic seizures do not occur. The characteristic EEG pattern consists of continuous dif-

fuse spike-waves during slow wave sleep, which is noted after onset of seizures. Duration varies from months to years. Despite the usually benign evolution of seizures, prognosis is guarded because of the appearance of neuropsychologic disorders" [44]. Since then, it has been demonstrated that besides the neuropsychological impairment, motor disturbances can be a part of this encephalopathy: ataxia, dyspraxia, dystonia, and unilateral motor deficit [47]. About one tenth of the patients only have rare nocturnal motor seizures.

CSWS and ESES had been used as synonyms, and this led to some confusion in the literature. It was suggested that the term ESES should be used for the electrographic phenomena, and CSWS for the syndrome.

The hallmark of this epileptic encephalopathy is the strong accentuation of the epileptiform discharges during sleep (Fig. 35.1). Sporadic epileptiform discharges (focal or "generalised") as single discharges or (sometimes) in trains can be seen during wakefulness. During non-REM sleep, the activation of the EEG paroxysms gives the characteristic pattern of almost continuous, diffuse, 1.5–2.5-Hz spike-and-slow-wave discharges that occupy more than 85% of

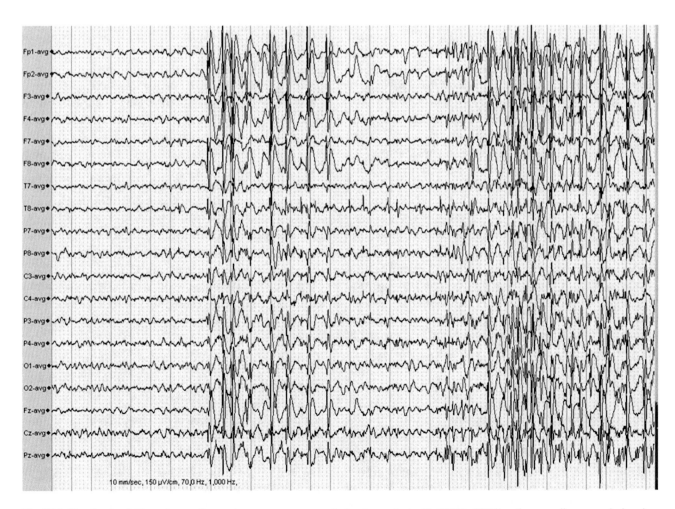

Fig. 35.1 Shortly after falling asleep, spikes-and-wave paroxysm are starting in a patient with CSWS. *CSWS* continuous spike-waves during slow sleep

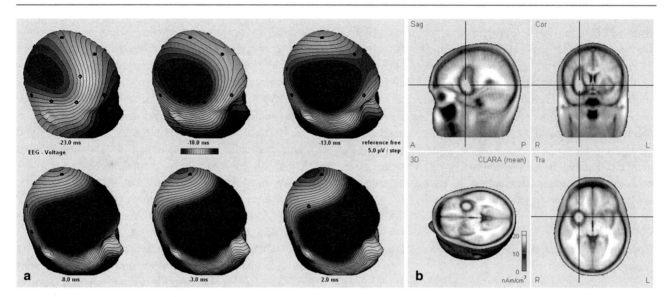

Fig. 35.2 Secondary bilateral synchrony in a patient with CSWS. **a** Sequential 3-dimensional voltage map on the ascending slope of the averages spike. The colour code indicates the polarity and the amplitude; negative potential is in *blue*, positive potentials are in *red*. Notice that at the onset, the negativity is only in the right central region; then it propa- gates bilaterally to the frontal region. **b** Source localisation (distributed source model, using BESA software) at the onset of the spike, suggesting that the initial electric activation is a focal one, localised in the right insula. *CSWS* continuous spike-waves during slow sleep, *BESA* brain electrical source analysis

slow sleep ("spike-wave index"). During REM sleep, the paroxysms are suppressed to below 25 %. Functional neuro-imaging studies, intracranial recordings, and source analysis suggest that the "diffuse" epileptiform discharges are due to secondary bilateral synchrony (Fig. 35.2).

The neuropsychological impairment ranges from language-related impairment, temporo-spatial disorientation to global cognitive decline with marked impairment of IQ, mental retardation, attention deficit and behavioural changes, aggressiveness, and difficulty in contact [47].

As with the other syndromes related to this type of epileptic encephalopathy, the course is favourable concerning seizures and the EEG pattern. Complete control of seizures is usually achieved within one year. Patients respond well to valproate and benzodiazepines. The EEG pattern (ESES) disappears within 3 years. Steroids might help in suppressing the nocturnal paroxysmal EEG activity and improve the neuropsychological functions. In spite of disappearance of seizures and ESES, and the improvement of cognitive functions, the prognosis is guarded: Less than half of the patients manage to live a normal life [47].

Idiopathic Generalised Epilepsies

IGEs represent a group of syndromes, comprising childhood and juvenile absence epilepsies, juvenile myoclonic epilepsy, and epilepsy with generalised tonic–clonic seizures on awakening. They are considered "awakening" type of epilepsies (Fig. 35.3; [19]). However, some patients have rare, nocturnal seizures.

Generalised tonic–clonic seizures, when occurring during sleep, start from stage 2 or during a shift between sleep stages, probably precipitated by a sudden clinical or abortive awakening; they never occur during REM sleep.

Myoclonic seizures can occur during sleep, and this imposes sometimes a differential-diagnostic problem. Periodic paroxysmal leg movements do not have EEG correlate, whilst epileptic myoclonias ictally are associated with polyspike-wave discharges.

Electrographic patterns corresponding to classical, "generalised" spike-and-slow-wave complexes are often recorded during sleep, though with reduction in its frequency. During sleep, it is impossible to assess the major clinical manifestation ("absence"); however, discrete eyelid myoclonia are often noticed time locked to the discharges.

Patients with awakening epilepsies have low-sleep efficiency. Sleep deprivation is an important provocative factor for awakening epilepsies, but it does not seem to affect the sleep epilepsies.

Other Epilepsies

In Lennox–Gastaut syndrome, the 10-Hz run-of-rapid spikes are precipitated during non-REM sleep, and are associated with tonic seizures of variable intensity (from discrete, only detectable by co-registering surface EMG signals, to major, generalised tonic seizures).

Patients with ring chromosome 20 have subtle, nocturnal seizures, often resembling awakening.

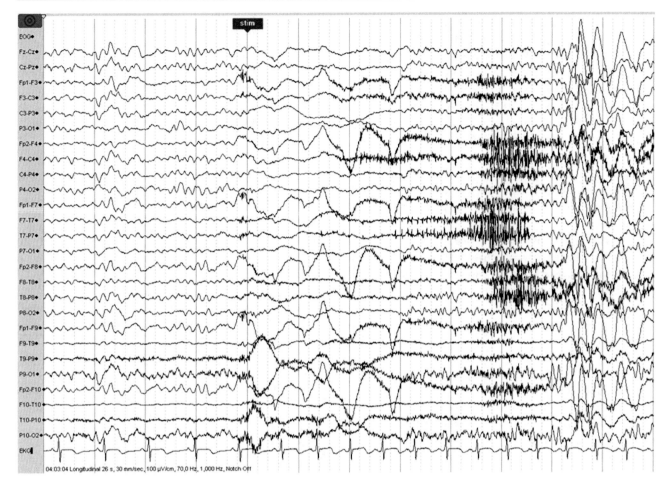

Fig. 35.3 Effect of awakening on the epileptiform activity in a patient with JME: shortly (6 s) after awakening, bilateral, fronto-central paroxysms are triggered. *JME* juvenile myoclonic epilepsy

Several other seizure types occur less often during sleep than in wakefulness: myoclonia in patients with Dravet syndrome, seizures in the late childhood occipital epilepsy (Gastaut-type), and symptomatic parietal and occipital lobe epilepsies.

Effect of Epilepsy and of Antiepileptic Medication on Sleep

Patients with epilepsy often complain about disturbed sleep and excessive daytime drowsiness [50]. This is partly due to the effect of antiepileptic medication, but epilepsy itself affects the sleep structure, especially REM sleep [51].

Nocturnal seizures, especially the temporal seizures cause awakening, and the long postictal period (seen often) interferes with sleep. Nocturnal temporal lobe seizures cause decrease in REM sleep and sleep efficiency [51]. Furthermore, patients with TLE have decreased sleep efficiency also in the seizure-free periods.

As sleep disorders are common in the general population, therefore, these may occur coincidentally in patients with epilepsy [51]. This generates a vicious circle: Sleep disruption worsens epilepsy, which, in turn, worsens the sleep disorder.

A little appreciated aspect of sleep is its being a phase in the circadian rhythm. However, significantly contrasting circadian patterns of sleep and activity in JME versus TLE have been reported by Pung and Schmitz [52].

In a series of investigations with newly diagnosed patients comparing unmedicated baseline sleep with phenobarbital, phenytoin, ethosuximide, and valproate [53], ethosuximide was the only substance that had a major impact on sleep structure producing a marked decrease of depth of sleep with increase of stage 1 sleep. This corresponded well with frequent complaints of patients on this drug about sleep disturbances. Phenobarbital increased stage 2 sleep and decreased REM sleep; in awakening epilepsies, but not in sleep epilepsies, it decreased transitional states around REM phases which correlates with its preferential therapeutic effect in these epilepsies that have their spike maxima here [53]. A longitudinal evaluation of phenytoin as part of this project showed that initial effects largely disappeared over time, and the individual sleep pattern was mostly restored [54].

Likewise, several generally positive initial effects of carbamazepine on sleep have been described but seemed to disappear over time [55]. Whereas vigabatrine seems to have no significant effect on sleep, improvement is noted with gabapentin and clonazepam, the latter though producing an increase in spindle density [55]. Lamotrigine (LTG) was reported to increase REM percentage and decrease slow-wave sleep and the number of stage shifts [56]. This study on 13 patients seems not to have included patients who developed insomnia and delayed sleep onset, otherwise a not infrequent, sometimes rather annoying side effect of LTG. Little is yet known about possible influences of still newer AEDs on sleep.

As a caveat, improvements of sleep with administration of AEDs may be the indirect consequence of the therapeutic effect with reduction or disappearance of sleep-disturbing seizures or epileptiform discharges during sleep.

Conclusions

EEG is the most important investigation for both sleep and epilepsy, and sleep is the most important provocative tool for EEG in the diagnosis and differential diagnosis of epilepsy. Video observation (with and without EEG) may not only be necessary to distinguish epileptic seizures from other sleep-related disorders like parasomnias but also from normal sleep-related motor phenomena. These can be quite similar, especially when they use identical, sometimes complex, phylogenetically old innate motor patterns.

Sleep is a perfectly normal functional state of the brain and the organism, whereas epileptic seizures are characterised by more or less profound deviations from normal brain function. It is, therefore, intriguing that manifold relations seem to exist between both conditions. One probable reason is that the seizure-generating mechanisms are embedded in the complex activities of the central nervous system and subject to many provocative and inhibitory mechanisms. Whereas reflex epileptic seizures are the best-know exogenous modulators of seizure generation [38], the mechanisms regulating sleep are the best-known endogenous modulators. An astonishing number of epilepsy syndromes have clear relations to sleep or, more generally, the circadian rhythm. The relation, however, works both ways and seizures can have an impact on sleep. Syndrome-related peculiarities of circadian rhythms seem to indicate some still only partially revealed common basic mechanisms.

The therapeutic aspects also are twofold. Some therapeutic effects of AEDs may be related to modulations of sleep structures they cause, but sleep can also be negatively influenced by AEDs.

References

1. Grigg-Damberger M, Damberger SJ. Historical aspects of sleep and epilepsy. In: Bazil CW, Malow BA, Sammaritano MR, editors. Sleep and epilepsy: the clinical spectrum. Amsterdam: Elsevier Science; 2002. pp. 3–16.
2. Prichard JCA. Treatise on diseases of the nervous system. London: Thomas and George Underwood; 1822.
3. Echeverria MC. De l'épilepsie nocturne. Ann Méd Psychol. 1879;5:177–97.
4. Féré L. Les epilepsies et les epileptiques, vol. I. Paris: Alcan; 1880.
5. Gowers WR. Epilepsy and other chronic convulsive diseases, vol. I. London: William Wood; 1885.
6. Berger H. Über das Elektroenkephalogramm des Menschen. Arch Psychiatr Nervenkr. 1929;87:527–70.
7. Loomis AL, Harvey EN, Hoban G. Cerebral states during sleep studies by human brain potentials. J Exp Psychol. 1937;21:127–44.
8. Dement WC, Kleitman N. Cyclical variations in EEG during sleep and their relation to eye movements: body motility and dreaming. Clin Neurophysiol. 1957;10:673–90.
9. Rechtschaffen A, Kales A. A manual of standardised technology, techniques and scoring system for sleep stages of human subjects. Los Angeles: UCLA Brain Information Service/ Brain Research Institute; 1968.
10. Gibbs EL, Gibbs FA. Diagnostic and localizing value of electrographic studies in sleep. Res Publ Assoc Res Nerv Ment Dis. 1947;26:366–76.
11. Cadilhac J, Vlahovitch B, Delange-Walter M. Modifications des décharges épileptiques au cours de la période des mouvements oculaires. Sommeil normal et pathologique. Paris: Masson; 1965. pp. 275–82.
12. Passouant P, Besset A, Carriere A, Billiard M. Night sleep and generalised epilepsies. In: Koella WP, Levin P, editors. Sleep 1974. Basel: Karger; 1974. pp. 185–96.
13. Passouant P. Influence des états de vigilance sur les épilepsies. In: Koella WP, Levin P, editors. Sleep 1976. Basel: Karger; 1976. pp. 57–65.
14. Bancaud J, Columb D, Dell MB. Les pointes rolandiques: un symptome EEG propre á l'enfant. Rev Neurol. 1958;99:206–9.
15. Nayrac P, Beaussart M. les pointes-ondes prérolandiques: expression EEG très particulière. Étude electroclinique de 21 cas. Rev Neurol (Paris). 1958;19:25–6.
16. Landau WM, Kleffner FR. Syndrome of acquired aphasia with consvulsive disorder in children. Neurology. 1957;7:523–30.
17. Patry G, Lyagoubi S, Tassinari CA. Subclinical electrical status epilepticus induced by sleep in childresn. Arch Neurol. 1971;24:242–52.
18. Janz D. Epilepsy and the sleeping-waking cycle. In: Vinken PJ, Bruyun GW, editors. Handbook of clinical neurology, vol. XV. North Holland: Amsterdam; 1974. pp. 457–90.
19. Janz D. The grand-mal epilepsies and the sleeping-waking cycle. Epilepsia. 1962;3:69–109.
20. Lugaresi E and Cirignotta F. Hypnogenic paroxysmal dystonia: epileptic seizure or a new syndrome? Sleep. 1981;4:129-38.
21. Rajna P, Kundra O, Halasz P. Vigilance-dependent tonic seizures— epilepsy or sleep. Epilepsia. 1977;24:725–33.
22. Meierkord H. Is nocturnal paroxysmal dystonia a form of frontal lobe epilepsy? Mov Disorder. 1992;7:38–42.
23. Scheffer IE, Bhatia KP, Lopes-Cendes I, Fish DR, Marsden CD, Andermann F, Andermann E, Desbiens R, Cendes F, Manson JI, et al. Autosomal dominant frontal epilepsy misdiagnosed as sleep disorder. Lancet. 1994;343:515–7.

24. Steinlein OK, Mulley JC, Propping P, Wallace RH, Phillips HA, Sutherland GR, Scheffer IE, Berkovic SF. A missense mutation in the neuronal nicotinic acetylcholine receptor alpha 4 subunit is associated with autosomal dominant nocturnal frontal lobe epilepsy. Nat Genet. 1995;11:201–3.

25. Penfield W, Jasper H. Epilepsy and the functional anatomy of the human brain. Boston: Little, Brown and Co.; 1954.

26. Amzica F. Physiology of sleep and wakefulness as it relates to the physiology of epilepsy. J Clin Neurophysiol. 2002;19:488–503.

27. Steriade M, Amzica F, Neckelmann D, Timofeev I. Spike-wave complexes and fast components of cortically generated seizures. II. Extra- and intracellular patterns. J Neurophysiol. 1998;80:1456–79.

28. Shouse MN, Langer J, King A, Alcalde O, Bier M, Szymusiak R, Wada Y. Paroxysmal microarousals in amygdala-kindled kittens: could they be subclinical seizures? Epilepsia. 1995;36:290–300.

29. Halász P, Terzano MG, Parrino L. Spike-wave discharge and the microstructure of sleep-wake continuum in idiopathic generalised epilepsy. Neurophysiol Clin. 2002;32:38–53.

30. Touchon J, Besset A, Billiard M, Baldy-Moulinier M. Effects of spontaneous and provoked awakening on the frequency of polyspike and wave discharges in 'bilateral massive myoclonus'. In: Akimoto S, Kazamatsuri H, Seino M, Ward AA, editors. Advances in epileptology XIII. New York: Raven Press; 1982. pp. 269–72.

31. Gigli GL, Calia E, Marciani MG, Mazza S, Mennuni G, Diomedi M, Terzano MG, Janz D. Sleep microstructure and EEG epileptiform activity in patients with juvenile myoclonic epilepsy. Epilepsia. 1992;33:799–804.

32. Tassinari CA, Cantalupo G, Högl B, Cortelli P, Tassi L, Francione S, Nobili L, Meletti S, Rubboli G, Gardella E. Neuroethological approach to frontolimbic epileptic seizures and parasomnias: the same central pattern generators for the same behaviours. Rev Neurol (Paris). 2009a;165:762–8.

33. Nobili L, Baglietto MG, Boelke M, De Carli F, De Negri E, Rosadini G, De Negri M, Ferrillo F. Modulation of sleep interictal epileptiform discharges in partial epilepsy of childhood. Clin Neurophysiol. 1999;110:839–45.

34. Avanzini G, Manganotti P, Meletti S, Moshé SL, Panzica F, Wolf P, Capovilla G. The system epilepsies: a pathophysiological hypothesis. Epilepsia. 2012;53:771–8.

35. Salinsky M, Kanter R, Dasheiff RM. Effectiveness of multiple EEGs in supporting the diagnosis of epilepsy: an operational curve. Epilepsia. 1987;28:331–4.

36. Terney D, Beniczky S, Varga ET, Kéri S, Nagy HG, Vécsei L. The effect of sleep deprivation on median nerve somatosensory evoked potentials. Neurosci Lett. 2005;383:82–6.

37. Veldhuizen R, Binnie, CD, Beintema DJ. The effect of sleep deprivation on the EEG in epilepsy. Electroencephalogr Clin Neurophysiol. 1983;55:505–12.

38. Beniczky S, Guaranha MS, Conradsen I, Singh MB, Rutar V, Lorber B, Braga P, Fressola AB, Inoue Y, Yacubian EM, Wolf P. Modulation of epileptiform EEG discharges in juvenile myoclonic epilepsy: an investigation of reflex epileptic traits. Epilepsia. 2012;53:832–9.

39. Guaranha MS, da Silva Sousa P, de Araújo-Filho GM, Lin K, Guilhoto LM, Caboclo LO, Yacubian EM. Provocative and inhibitory effects of a video-EEG neuropsychologic protocol in juvenile myoclonic epilepsy. Epilepsia. 2009;50:2446–55.

40. Lüders HO. The supplementary sensorimotor area. An overview. Adv Neurol. 1996;70:1–16.

41. Picard F, Baulac S, Kahane P, Hirsch E, Sebastianelli R, Thomas P, Vigevano F, Genton P, Guerrini R, Gericke CA, An I, Rudolf G, Herman A, Brice A, Marescaux C, LeGuern E. Dominant partial epilepsies. A clinical, electrophysiological and genetic study of 19 European families. Brain. 2000;123:1247–62.

42. Alving J, Beniczky S. Diagnostic usefulness and duration of the inpatient long-term video-EEG monitoring: findings in patients extensively investigated before the monitoring. Seizure. 2009;18:470–3.

43. Husain AM, Sinha SR. Nocturnal epilepsy in adults. J Clin Neurophysiol. 2011;28:141–5.

44. Commission on Classification and Terminology of the International League Against Epilepsy. Proposal for revised classification of epilepsies and epileptic syndromes. Epilepsia. 1989;30:389–99.

45. Ferrie C, Caraballo R, Covanis A, Demirbilek V, Dervent A, Kivity S, Koutroumanidis M, Martinovic Z, Oguni H, Verrotti A, Vigevano F, Watanabe K, Yalcin D, Yoshinaga H. Panayiotopoulos syndrome: a consensus view. Dev Med Child Neurol. 2006;48:236–40.

46. Tassinari CA, Cantalupo G, Rios-Pohl L, Giustina ED, Rubboli G. Encephalopathy with status epilepticus during slow sleep: "the Penelope syndrome". Epilepsia. 2009b;50(Suppl. 7):4–8.

47. Tassinari CA, Rubboli G, Volpi L, Meletti S, Gardella E, d´Orsi G, Zaniboni A, Rondelli F, Cagnetti C, Michelucci R. Encephalopathy with electric status epilepticus during slow sleep. In: Bazil CW, Malow BA, Sammaritano MR, editors. Sleep and epilepsy: the clinical spectrum. Amsterdam: Elsevier; 2002.

48. Aicardi J, Chevrie J. Atypical benign partial epilepsy of childhood. Dev Med Child Neurol. 1982;24:281–92.

49. Hahn A, Pistohl J, Neubauer BA, Stephani U. Atypical "benign" partial epilepsy or pseudo-Lennox syndrome. Part I: symptomatology and long-term prognosis. Neuropediatrics. 2001;32:1–8.

50. Hoeppner JB, Garron DC, Cartwright RD. Self-reported sleep disorder symptoms in epilepsy. Epilepsia. 1984;25:434–7.

51. Bazil CW. Effects of individual seizures on sleep structure. In: Bazil CW, Malow BA, Sammaritano MR, editors. Sleep and epilepsy: the clinical spectrum. Amsterdam: Elsevier; 2002. pp. 181–6.

52. Pung T, Schmitz B. Circadian rhythm and personality profile in juvenile myoclonic epilepsy. Epilepsia. 2006;47(suppl 2):111–4.

53. Wolf P. Relations of epilepsy and the sleep and waking cycle. J Autonomic Nervous System Suppl. 1986; 30: 603–10.

54. Röder-Wanner UU, Noachtar S, Wolf P. Response of polygraphic sleep to phenytoin treatment for epilepsy. A longitudinal study of immediate, short- and long-term effects. Acta Neurol Scand. 1987;76:157–67.

55. Sammaritano MR, Sherwin AL. Effect of anticonvulsants on sleep. In: Bazil CW, Malow BA, Sammaritano MR, editors. Sleep and epilepsy: the clinical spectrum. Amsterdam: Elsevier; 2002: pp. 187–94.

56. Placidi F, Marciani MG, Diomedi M, Scalise A, Pauri F, Giacomini P, Gigli GL. Effects of lamotrigine on nocturnal sleep, daytime somnolence and cognitive functions in focal epilepsy. Acta Neurol Scand. 2000;102:81–6.

Richard J. Castriotta and Mark C. Wilde

Abbreviations

CPAP	Continuous positive airway pressure
CSF	Cerebrospinal fluid
CT	Computerized tomography
DLMO	Dim-light melatonin onset
DSPS	Delayed sleep phase syndrome
EDS	Excessive daytime sleepiness
ESS	Epworth sleepiness scale
GCS	Glasgow coma scale
ICSD 1	International classification of sleep disorders, 1st edition
ICSD 2	International classification of sleep disorders, 2nd edition
MEQ	Morningness eveningness questionnaire
MSLT	Multiple sleep latency test
NPSG	Nocturnal polysomnography
OSA	Obstructive sleep apnea
PLMS	Periodic limb movements in sleep
PSQI	Pittsburgh sleep quality Index
PTH	Posttraumatic hypersomnia
PTSD	Posttraumatic stress disorder
RBD	REM sleep behavior disorder
SOREMP	Sleep-onset REM (rapid eye movement) sleep period
TBI	Traumatic brain injury

R. J. Castriotta (✉)
Division of Pulmonary and Sleep Medicine,
University of Texas Medical School at Houston,
6431 Fannin St., MSB 1.274, Houston, TX 77030, USA
e-mail: Richard.J.Castriotta@uth.tmc.edu

Sleep Disorders Center, Memorial Hermann Hospital—Texas Medical Center, Houston, TX, USA

M. C. Wilde
Department of Physical Medicine and Rehabilitation,
University of Texas Medical School at Houston, Houston, TX, USA
e-mail: Mark.C.Wilde@uth.tmc.edu

Introduction

Traumatic brain injury (TBI) is a growing global problem of increasing importance to both military and civilian populations. Part of the reason is improved survival of both battle-field injuries and motor vehicle and workplace accidents that involve head injury. Severity of a TBI is an important variable as it presages outcome. TBI patients with severe injuries are at increased risk of significant longer-term disabilities, while those with mild injuries almost invariably can expect a complete recovery with no lasting problems past 3 months post injury, and those with moderate injuries fall in the middle [1, 2]. One way that the severity of TBI is graded is based on the best postresuscitation Glasgow Coma Scale (GCS) score considered in consort with computerized tomography (CT) scanning [3–7]. A mild level of injury severity is defined as a GCS of 13–15 with a negative CT of the brain. Moderate and severe TBI are GCS of 9–12 and 3–8, respectively, independent of CT findings or a GCS of 13–15 with a positive CT of the brain [5, 6]. Another method of defining injury severity is based on the length of time from injury onset until the patient follows commands. Specifically, those patients following commands in less than 1 h are considered to have mild injuries, while those following commands in 1–24 h and greater than 24 h have moderate and severe injuries, respectively [4]. Finally, TBI survivors go through a period termed posttraumatic amnesia, which is a trauma-induced confusional syndrome or encephalopathy in which the injured person is unable to form new memories due to the initial effects of the injury. In persons, with concussions, this period is usually brief and circumscribed, lasting seconds to minutes to a few hours. In persons with more serious injuries, this syndrome can last for days to weeks, is a good measure of injury severity and ultimate long-term outcome, and is considered resolved when the person is capable of establishing a consistent pattern of continuous memory [7].

The cumulative number of TBI cases in the US Military from 2000 to 2012 is 266,810 and over 80 % are in the nondeployed setting [8]. It is estimated that there are at least

S. Chokroverty, M. Billiard (eds.), *Sleep Medicine,* DOI 10.1007/978-1-4939-2089-1_36,
© Springer Science+Business Media, LLC 2015

1.7 million cases of TBI each year in the USA [9] and most of these are mild [10] with only a brief change in mental status or consciousness. The annual incidence of hospitalized TBI in Europe is 235/100,000 [11]. We might simply define TBI as "an alteration in brain function or other evidence of brain pathology caused by an external force" [12]. That many TBI patients have sleep disorders should not be surprising, given the fact that some sleep disorders, especially obstructive sleep apnea (OSA) and narcolepsy, are associated with an increased risk of motor vehicle accidents [13–19]. Therefore, there exists a complex relationship between sleep/wake disorders and TBI. The former predisposes to the latter, and yet most sleep problems appear to be chronologic sequelae of the injury.

Early Years

References to changes in sleep/wake status after TBI appear early, but only in recent years have there been the tools (polysomnography, multiple sleep latency tests, actigraphy, etc.) to make accurate diagnoses. With regard to TBI, Hippocrates wrote, "a good prognosis would be the onset of sleep since it means the mind has been healed by sleep," but also "if sleep relieves the delirium, but does not suppress it, this may become extremely dangerous" [20]. Galen noted cases of excessive sleepiness after TBI in Rome in the second century [21]. William Osler wrote about insomnia after TBI in the context of what was called "the traumatic neuroses," and describes the symptoms of "simple traumatic neurasthenia" after an accident in which there has been a shock or concussion: "the patient complains of headache and tired feelings. He is sleepless and finds himself unable to concentrate" [22]. With regard to treatment, he advises: "For the relief of sleeplessness all possible measures should be resorted to before the employment of drugs" [23]. While much of today's TBI is a result of automobile accidents, in the nineteenth century, the terms "railway brain" and "traumatic hysteria" were used to describe the symptoms, so often, associated with trauma induced by train accidents. These symptoms were often attributed to the newly described "neurasthenia" [24]. It is clear that Osler considered most of these cases of "railway brain" were "traumatic hysteria," for which symptoms persisted only as long litigation, but some cases fit the description of TBI-induced insomnia or hypersomnia, and others were what would today be termed posttraumatic stress disorder (PTSD). Large numbers of head injuries during the First World War would lead to more serious attention to TBI and its longer-term consequences with regard to sleep early in the next century.

Twentieth Century

There were quite a few reports of "posttraumatic narcolepsy," which came out of World War I from Germany [25–27] and France [28, 29], at a time when concepts of narcolepsy, cataplexy, and hypersomnia were still in the formative stages. The term narcolepsy had been introduced by Gelineau [30] in 1880, but was still not well understood, and, believed by many, not to be a specific disease. There were cases of head injuries incurred during the war, producing long-lasting sleepiness, with case reports published between 1915 and 1918. Lhermitte reported four cases of "narcolepsy" without cataplexy with onset after cerebral concussion, while Souques [29] may have been the first to use the term "traumatic narcolepsy" (narcolepsie d'origine traumatique) in his report of one case. Both of these French reports were published in 1918, and, today, might be termed posttraumatic hypersomnia (PTH). The term Kataplexie or cataplexy (kataplectische Hemmung) was introduced in 1915 by Henneberg [31]. Adie [32] made a convincing case that the combination of sleep attacks and cataplexy was pathognomonic for narcolepsy as a distinct disease. Haenel [33] reported the first case of posttraumatic narcolepsy with cataplexy in 1929, while Thiele and Bernhardt [34] attributed 3 of their 25 cases of narcolepsy with cataplexy to trauma, reporting in 1931. The first three British cases were reported by Gill [35] in 1941. These were cases of civilian blunt head trauma, which clearly fit our current understanding of mild TBI and narcolepsy. The case reported by Pollock [36], in 1930, of hypersomnolence in a young woman with onset after an automobile accident in the USA makes no mention of cataplexy, but does document sleep attacks which are refreshing. On the other hand, Daniels [37] reported in 1934 a clear case of posttraumatic narcolepsy with cataplexy from the Mayo Clinic. The onset of symptoms for this 22-year-old man was after being knocked unconscious while playing football. The case of posttraumatic narcolepsy reported by Bonduelle, Bouygues, Delahousse, and Faveret [38] from France, in 1959, was one of severe TBI, following which there was narcolepsy with cataplexy and hypnagogic hallucinations. This is the first clear documentation of that symptomatology after TBI. The second can be found in the case reported in 1972 by Amico, Pasquali, and Pittaluga [39] of the sleep-related sequelae of TBI in a non-obese man involved in a motor vehicle accident in Italy. This 58-year-old man was found to have hypersomnia without cataplexy, but with sleep-onset REM sleep periods (SOREMPs), hypnagogic hallucinations, and periodic breathing with periods of apnea. The fact that he also appeared to have heart failure and atrial flutter–fibrillation leads to the possibility that he may have had central apnea as well as OSA. He did have snoring and irregular diaphragmatic contractions and loud breathing with snoring alternating with periods of total quietness. This is the first published report describing sleep-disordered breathing (SDB) associated with TBI.

The first description of the effects of TBI on *dreaming* is a report of three cases by Humphrey and Zangwill in 1951 of cessation of dreaming in three men after TBI sustained in 1944 [40]. These injuries, however, resulted from mortar wounds and were not closed head injuries. The ten cases reported from Italy by Barbano and Bossi [41] in 1964, however, were those of TBI involving young (23–57 years old) civilians from months to years after closed head injury with post-TBI recognizable sleep/wake disorders: insomnia, nightmares, circadian rhythm disorders (*turbi del ritmo veglia-sonno*), and paradoxical restlessness from hypnotics. Eight of the ten had insomnia, two of whom with daytime sleepiness, and two had only tiredness. One of those with insomnia had nightmares. All of these had suffered TBI with loss of consciousness and had objectively normal neurologic exams at the time of report. This is the first mention of circadian rhythm disorders after TBI and also of the *paradoxical effects of hypnotics*. The specifics of the hypnotics are not, however, in this paper. Since most of those available at the time (barbiturates, etc.) are no longer being used, this may be a reason why this phenomenon has not been observed more recently.

In 1966, Meurice [42] studied objective and subjective sleepiness and vigilance in a group of 42 Belgian TBI patients and 42 normal controls isolated in a quiet dark place. He found no correlation between electroencephalographic sleepiness and subjective sleepiness, fatigability, attention, or vigilance in the TBI subjects. This discrepancy between objective and subjective findings would be confirmed over 40 years later [43]. Drowsiness was more intense in the TBI patients. There was no correlation with electroencephalographic (EEG) sleepiness and duration of TBI or length of unconsciousness. There was increased intensity of sleep in the TBI subjects (*le sommeil par ondes lentes et spindles [stade B]*), and a trend toward fewer complaints in the TBI subjects with mild drowsiness and fewer neurologic symptoms. This appears to be the *first detailed polygraphic study of sleep in TBI*, but respiratory parameters were not monitored. The *first polysomnographic study of infants and children after TBI* was done by Lenard and Pennigstorff in Göttingen in 1970, showing a reduction of sleep stages with highly synchronized EEG activity, increased sleep spindles, and increased REM density, but no change in the amount of REM sleep [44]. In 1979, Alexandre et al. [45] reported a proposed *correlation between sleep and cognitive alterations* in a group of 20 patients with severe head injuries in Italy. None of the ten patients with initial severe REM alterations had normal performance 14 months later, while they found REM sleep to be normal in all those without cognitive deficits.

During the 1980s and 1990s, there were case studies reporting mainly posttraumatic narcolepsy. Good et al. [46] described a case of a 37-year-old white man who developed *narcolepsy* (cataplexy, SOREMPs, excessive daytime sleepiness; EDS, hypnagogic hallucinations, and sleep paralysis) 18 months after a presumed mild traumatic injury who also had a positive HLA DR2. They concluded that an interaction between the TBI and a genetic predisposition may have been involved in the development of his disorder. Maccario et al. [47] described a case of *posttraumatic narcolepsy*. However, in this case, the patient did not have cataplexy, and they did not present tissue-typing data. Kapen and Mohan [48] documented three cases of *posttraumatic narcolepsy* after TBI, all of whom had objective evidence of excessive sleepiness on the MSLT, three SOREMPs, and purported symptom onset after TBI. Human leukocyte antigen (HLA) studies were positive in one, negative in another, and not available in a third. One patient also was diagnosed with OSA, and the two patients who accepted treatment reportedly achieved symptomatic benefit. Francisco and Ivanhoe [49] reported a case of a 27-year-old male with posttraumatic narcolepsy who was successfully treated with *methylphenidate*.

Broughton et al. [50] described two cases of significant closed head injury, who presented with complaints of *insomnia* which was confirmed on nocturnal polysomnography (NPSG) as well as *involuntary rhythmic leg movements prior to sleep onset* which stopped during sleep but resumed during nocturnal arousals. In neither case, was there evidence of periodic movements of sleep or restless legs syndrome. One patient had OSA and both had mean MSLT scores less than 10 min, but neither of them had SOREMPs. There were several reports of delayed sleep phase syndrome (DSPS) after TBI during this period [51–54]. One of these studies reported successful treatment of a 15–year-old girl with marked DSPS of almost half a day with 5 mg of melatonin. [51]

The 1980s and 1990s engendered a sea change in the investigation of sleep and TBI. This is clearly when a focus on the individual gave way to more of an emphasis on group-based studies. As the twentieth century began to wind down, the preeminence of the ideographic approach to the study of derangements of sleep after TBI slowly faded away, while the nomothetic (legislative) approach to the examination of the topic took its place. Several different types of group-based studies became popular. They are: (1) studies based on self-report methodologies, (2) studies based on objective laboratory measures, and (3) studies combining both approaches. The findings from these studies are reviewed in the following sections.

Self-report studies have been one of the important components of rehabilitation research [54]. With the increasing interest of the rehabilitation community, on the impact of disordered sleep after TBI, came a wave of studies based on self-report. The strength of this approach is that it affords the economic collection of large amounts of data in a relatively rapid and economic manner. The weakness of self-report data is that they are subject to the multiple distortions of report biases. These biases may flow from distorted perceptions of the reporter due to cognitive deficits or external incentives. This must be kept in mind when reviewing these studies and weighing their relative merits.

Nevertheless, a number of these survey studies have supported the notion that sleep/wake disorders are common after TBI. Parsons and Ver Beek [55] compared self-reported pre- and post-injury sleep/wake patterns in 75 mild head injury patients and found significantly increased sleep complaints following mild TBI and an association between the length of altered consciousness and complaints of altered sleep–wake patterns but no association between length of posttraumatic confusion and sleep wake disturbances. Cohen et al. [56] found that 73 % of a sample of hospitalized TBI patients who were three months post injury reported at least one sleep complaint, usually (80 %) insomnia, while only three patients complained of hypersomnia, and 52 % of the outpatients reported sleep disturbance. Daytime sleepiness was more prevalent (73 %), while insomnia was less prevalent (8 %). Clinchot et al. [57] studied a cohort of TBI patients consecutively admitted to a rehabilitation unit and found that 50 % reported difficulty sleeping; 65 % of whom reported terminal insomnia, 25 % reported oversleeping, and 45 % reported initial insomnia. Eighty-five percent of patients reporting sleep problems also reported daytime fatigue, and the severity of TBI was inversely associated with sleep complaints, while persons with sleep complaints were more likely to be female.

Another new type of nomothetic study that appeared during this period focused *on sleep architecture after TBI*. In one study which compared a single night of sleep recordings in ten mostly severe TBI patients to ten matched controls found that the TBI patients had less stage 1 sleep and a greater number of awakenings [58]. Cohen et al. [59] described the serial NPSG recordings in a series of studies of persons after TBI. Specifics of these studies are not well documented in this abstract. However, the authors reported disorganized sleep patterns in unconscious patients immediately after trauma and decreased REM sleep in confused patients with a gradual increase in REM with the recovery of higher mental function. Other aspects of sleep remained disorganized even after the reestablishment of normal values of REM sleep. Other changes documented included multiple awakenings, decreased sleep efficiency, and reduced slow wave sleep.

One study broke ground, during the 1980s, by applying traditional sleep research methodologies at the group level to a TBI sample. Guilleminault et al. [60] published a review of 20 patients who were referred for sleep studies because of posttraumatic excessive sleepiness. Nine of these patients had a history of coma lasting at least 24 h, five had a history of transient loss of consciousness less than 24-h, and six with no loss of consciousness. All patients underwent NPSG and completed the Stanford Sleepiness Scale and a subgroup underwent cerebrospinal fluid (CSF) investigations. Objective sleepiness was evaluated through various means. Eighteen patients had significant sleeping problems. Eight patients were diagnosed with *sleep apnea*. Nine had significant daytime somnolence. One patient reported episodes of muscle weakness similar to cataplexy and demonstrated two SOREMPs which would be consistent with posttraumatic narcolepsy.

Several group studies were published in the 1990s that focused on specific sleep disorders after TBI. Lankford et al. [61] studied nine cases with complaints of EDS after TBI with NPSG, MSLT, HLA typing (in six cases), and a history and physical examination. The results disclosed a diagnosis of posttraumatic narcolepsy in 8/9 cases, and HLA typing was positive in all six cases. Beetar et al. [62] compared the incidence of self-reported insomnia and pain complaints in a referred cohort of 127 symptomatic (127 mild TBI, 75 moderate to severe) TBI patients to a general neurologic control sample. They found that TBI subjects reported significantly more insomnia than non-TBI subjects, poor sleep maintenance was the most common sleep problem for all patients, TBI patients reported more sleep complaints than non-TBI patients, mild TBI patients reported significantly more insomnia than moderate-to-severe TBI patients, and pain was strongly associated with sleep problems.

Twenty-first Century

The new millennium has seen a burgeoning of studies on sleep and TBI. The types of published projects fall into the familiar categories discussed above, including self-report, laboratory, and combined approaches. The dearth of case studies is rather striking and perhaps suggests that sleep/wake abnormalities are now recognized as a significant comorbidity after TBI, and thus worthy of further rigorous investigation. The following section charts the course of TBI research from the fleeting fears of Y2K and beyond.

The new millennium continued to see studies based on self-report which again reflected an increased incidence of investigations of sleep disorders after TBI in adult and pediatric populations coming mostly from rehabilitation medicine. As in studies from earlier years, investigations based on self-report suggest an increased prevalence of sleep disorders after TBI [63–67]. Unfortunately, because of their nature, this methodology does not lend itself to the diagnosis of specific sleep disorders, and only throws light on the general problem. In addition, there are a number of problems with the use of self-report measures [68]. There are numerous potential biases that exist in mild TBI related to potential malingering, symptom exaggeration, and misattribution of symptom onset [69–72]. We may recall the "railway brain" and "traumatic neurasthenia" described by Osler [22]. However this should be distinguished from the "pseudohypersomnia" seen in 8 of 184 TBI patients reported by Guilleminault et al. [72] who had apathy and subjective sleepiness, but normal MSLT scores. In severe TBI patients, issues with self-awareness and other cognitive deficits could cloud the judgment of the reporter, leading to a distorted or unrealistic self-portrayal [73]. Thus, it is not surprising that one study found that objectively sleepy TBI patients reported the best sleep-related quality of life [43]. This same study also found that the relationship between self-reported daytime sleepiness (Epworth Sleepiness Scale; ESS) and objective sleepiness (MSLT) was close to nil in a TBI cohort. In addition, given the copious evidence suggesting that this clinical population is concerned about their sleep, it would seem that another report further validating what has already been shown would not be necessary. Rather, what would appear to be important would be to determine if there is any objective basis to these concerns and then to characterize the precise clinical problems.

There have been a number of nomothetic studies using NPSG or nocturnal EEG to evaluate sleep architecture of TBI patients without regard to addressing diagnostic issues. The data are mixed on whether there are objective changes in objective sleep parameters after mild TBI [74, 75]. Other reports, including patients with more severe injuries, have found that TBI is associated with increased slow-wave sleep and reduced evening melatonin production, while anxiety and depression may be associated with some of these changes, but not injury severity [76, 77]. In a particularly important series of studies in Switzerland, Baumann et al. [78] collected CSF hypocretin levels in 44 consecutive patients with mild to severe traumatic brain injuries in the acute phase (1–4 days post injury) and found abnormally low levels in 30 of 31 patients with severe TBI, and 7 of 8 patients with moderate TBI. CSF fluid, hypocretin, levels were undetectable in 9 of 39 patients with moderate to severe TBI patients. Lower hypocretin levels were associated with injury severity, a positive CT scan, coma, and having hypothalamic lesions. In a separate study from this group, the number of hypocretin neurons was found to be significantly reduced in a postmortem study of four severe TBI patients relative to controls [79]. While having the advantage of evaluating objective sleep parameters, most of these studies, particularly those that compare nocturnal EEG values and sleep architecture variables to normal controls, simply beg the question as to whether or not underlying disorders of sleep may or may not be driving any of these systematic differences. The exception would be approaches which are similar to those

reported in papers which suggest that hypothalamic abnormalities may underlie some of the posttraumatic sleep disturbances [78, 79]. These findings are particularly important, given the link between the orexins, human narcolepsy, and the maintenance of wakefulness [80].

The new millennium has seen an exponential growth in the number of studies that used both self-report and objective methods to study sleep disorders after TBI. It is in these studies that one begins to see beyond sleeping problems as simply a symptom of acquired brain damage, and thus a clear pattern begins to emerge of an increased prevalence of known sleep disorders in TBI. The first of these studies in the new millennium was undertaken by Guilleminault et al. [72] who comprehensively evaluated 184 victims of head and neck trauma (both TBI and whiplash) with complaints of sleepiness. A significant proportion appeared to have had a verifiable TBI of any severity. Fifty-nine patients (32 %) were diagnosed with sleep disordered breathing (SDB), 51 patients had an MSLT of less than or equal to 5 min, and 101 patients had an MSLT of between 5–10 min. SOREMPs occurred in persons with MSLT scores below 10 min and five patients had two or more of these. Four of these patients, who had two SOREMPs, had DR15, DQ6 (DR6 DQ1) HLA typing, and two were positive for haplotypes. No patients with SOREMPs had cataplexy. Objective sleepiness, in this study, was associated with severity of injury. Castriotta and Lai [81] prospectively studied TBI patients with subjective sleepiness using NPSG and MSLT. A diagnosis of a treatable sleep disorder was made in all subjects and included SDB in 7 of 10 subjects, narcolepsy (2/10), and one case of PTH, defined as hypersomnia with onset after TBI with MSLT score < 10 min and < 2 SOREMPs with a normal NPSG, and no other cause of sleepiness. This was the first paper to use that term as so defined, in contradistinction to "posttraumatic narcolepsy." In the first study of the new millennium to comprehensively study a nonselected TBI sample, Webster et al. [82] evaluated 28 adults with mostly severe TBI who were less than 3 months post injury, and admitted for comprehensive inpatient rehabilitation [82]. This group found sleep apnea in 36 % of the sample. This rate of sleep apnea was found to be significantly higher than would be predicted, based on population norms, and no correlation was found between the occurrence of significant sleep apnea and measures of TBI severity or other demographic variables. There were both cases of central and obstructive apnea in this sample. The second study of a nonselected sample, evaluated 71 subjects enrolled in a residential brain injury program (the majority of which [57] had suffered a TBI), using NPSG and MSLT [83]. Forty-seven percent of the cohort had EDS (defined as mean MSLT score < 10 min). Subjects were classified into three groups: not sleepy, sleepy with abnormal studies, and sleepy with normal studies. They found 53 % of the patients had normal studies and were not sleepy, 17 % were sleepy with abnormal sleep studies, and 30% were sleepy with normal sleep studies. Sleepiness was not associated with TBI severity.

Verma et al. [84] studied 60 adults who presented to a private sleep clinic with sleep complaints months to 2 years following TBI. While they could not present their data in terms of prevalence rates of specific disorders, 30% had an apnea hypopnea index (AHI) of > 10 apneas and hypopneas/h), 35% had a periodic limb movement index (PLMI) > 10 PLMs/h, 9% had a PLM arousal index of > 5 PLM–arousals/h, 53% of the 28 patients receiving MSLT had a mean latency < 5 min, 32% (9/28) of these had two or more SOREMPs, and 13% of the sample had evidence of REM behavior disorder (RBD). Two of the nine patients with abnormal MSLT scores and ≥ 2 SOREMPs tested positive for HLA antigens associated with narcolepsy.

Castriotta et al. [43] consecutively recruited 87 TBI adults without regard to complaints or presenting symptoms and studied them at least 3 months post TBI using NPSG and MSLT and found an *increased prevalence of sleep disorders* in this sample. Specifically, 46% of the sample had abnormal sleep studies: 23% were diagnosed with OSA, 11% with PTH defined as MSLT score < 10 min with < 2 SOREMPs and a normal NPSG, 6% were diagnosed with narcolepsy (MSLT score < 5 min with > 2 SOREMPs), and 7% with PLMS. Twenty-five percent were found to have objective EDS with an MSLT score < 10 min. There was no relationship between injury severity and the presence of EDS or a diagnosed sleep disorder. Baumann et al. [85] comprehensively studied 76 TBI patients and new-onset sleep–wake disturbances following TBI were found in 47 patients (72%). Subjective EDS (defined by an ESS ≤ 10) was found in 28% of the sample, while objective EDS (defined by mean sleep latency < 5 min on MSLT) in 25%, fatigue (daytime tiredness without subjective or objective EDS) in 17%, PTH, here defined as a ≥ 2 h *increased need for sleep per 24-h period* relative to pre-injury baseline), in 22% of patients and insomnia in three patients. Interestingly, low-hypocretin levels were found in 25/27 patients sampled acutely, although this tended to normalize by 6 months. Patients with PTH had lower levels at 6 months. The presence of a sleep disorder was not related to clinical/injury characteristics, outcome, or gender.

Collen et al. [86] retrospectively studied 116 soldiers with combat-related TBIs receiving care at Walter Reed Army Medical Center in the USA and found that 97% reported sleep problems, the majority of which (85%) reported EDS. NPSG was performed in 79% of patients, and OSA was diagnosed in 34.5% of the cohort, while 55% had insomnia based on *Diagnostic and Statistical Manual of Mental Disorders* (DSM) IV criteria. Not surprisingly, given the sample, there was a striking rate of comorbid psychiatric disorder (90.5%) with PTSD, depression, and anxiety being the most commonly diagnosed disorders.

These studies make it clear, whether the samples were selected based on having sleep complaints, or not, that the prevalence of sleep disorders, such as OSA, narcolepsy, PTH and PLMS, are quite high relative to the general population. This has been further highlighted by a recent meta-analysis [87]. One study [88] attempted to address treatment of these patients. This study evaluated the treatment outcome of a cohort of 22 TBI patients with sleep disorders: 13 OSA (23%), 2 PTH (3%), 3 narcolepsy (5%), and 4 PLMS (18%). Twelve who had objective EDS with MSLT score < 10 min were treated. They found that apneas, hypopneas, and snoring were eliminated by CPAP in OSA subjects, but that MSLT scores did not reflect reductions in EDS. PLMs were effectively treated with pramipexole. One of three narcolepsy subjects and one of two PTH subjects had their EDS effectively treated with modafinil. In another treatment study of EDS, the efficacy of modafinil in treating fatigue and EDS was studied in 53 TBI patients who were randomly assigned to receive 400 mg of modafinil or placebo in a crossover design [89]. They found that there were no statistically significant improvements seen with modafinil and placebo on the fatigue severity scale at 4 or 10 weeks of treatment.

Sleep disorders appear to add an additional cognitive burden on top of that produced by the injury itself. For example, TBI patients with EDS have greater difficulties with vigilance than non-sleepy TBI patients, produce slower reaction times and make more lapses than non-sleepy patients on a psychomotor vigilance task [43]. In addition, TBI patients with OSA were found to have greater difficulties with new learning and memory as well as vigilance than TBI patients without OSA [90]. Mahmood et al. [91], in a study of TBI patients with insomnia, found that neuropsychological measures of higher-order cognitive functioning and processing speed were modestly predictive of sleep disturbance independent of gender and injury severity. In another study evaluating cognition in insomnia and TBI, Bloomfield et al. [92] compared TBI patients classified as good or poor sleepers according to self-report and objective sleep measures on a battery of attention measures and found that patients with insomnia had significant deficits on measures of sustained attention.

Studies devoted to specific sleep disorders after TBI are still few in number. However, insomnia appears to be the exception and has been particularly well studied in several well-designed studies. In general, the majority of the studies have shown that insomnia is common after TBI but is most common after mild TBI, and seems to be associated with pain and psychiatric factors. Fichtenberg and associates, at the Rehabilitation Institute of Michigan in Detroit, published a series of careful investigations of insomnia, which along with a group in Quebec, make up the bulwark of the investigations in this area. Fitchtenberg et al. [93] studied 91 consecutive TBI patients with the Pittsburgh sleep quality Index (PSQI), and other self-report sleep measures. Patients were diagnosed with insomnia based on DSM criteria. They found that milder injuries as well as depression and pain were associated with the presence of insomnia but that the presence of financial incentive was not. This same group later found higher rates of insomnia using the PSQI in post-acute spinal cord and musculoskeletal rehabilitation patients relative to TBI survivors with rates 28 % in TBI and 56 % in spinal cord and musculoskeletal groups, respectively [94]. Ouellet et al. [95] found similar associations between severity and comorbidities in a Quebec cohort of 462 participants who sustained minor-to-severe TBI. Specifically, 50.3 % of these subjects reported symptoms of insomnia, whereas 31.1 % met diagnostic criteria for insomnia, 93 % of whom believed that its onset followed their accident. The same group compared objective and subjective measures of insomnia in 14 TBI patients with insomnia syndrome and 14 matched controls and found that 71 % of the TBI patient's sleep problems could be verified with NPSG [96]. Fogelberg et al. [97] assessed 129 moderate-to-severe TBI patients 1 year after injury using the PSQI as a measure of sleep disturbance and self-report measures of depression, anxiety, and pain. Forty-four percent of TBI patients reported significant sleep problems on the PSQI (>5) and depression, pain, and anxiety were associated with poorer sleep. In a multicenter study of 334 TBI survivors studied as two samples, a point prevalence rate for insomnia of 11 and 24 % for the two different samples was found [98]. As in other studies, psychiatric problems were associated with insomnia in both samples. It is likely that insomnia rates are lower in this study than others because the sample was restricted to patients with moderate-to-severe injuries. Similar results and correlates with insomnia have been reported elsewhere as well [99]. There have been few treatment studies of insomnia after TBI. In a single case study, Ouellet and Morin [100] reported the successful treatment of a moderate TBI patient using cognitive behavioral therapy for insomnia.

There have been several investigations of circadian rhythm disorders after TBI. Unfortunately, they have significant weaknesses. One study found an increased prevalence of circadian rhythm disorders in a cohort of individuals with mild TBI recruited from a rehabilitation complaining of insomnia [101]. This study suffers from lack of generalizability due to its use of a highly selected sample of persons with mild TBI with sleep complaints. Another case study was published of a 39-year-old who displayed non-24-h sleep–wake cycles following a motor vehicle accident with a purported mild TBI [102]. There are a number of characteristics of the case that are highly atypical and the link between circadian abnormalities and a mild TBI are not compelling, and, at best, highly speculative. Several studies have been published which, while not formally evaluating circadian rhythm disorders per say, appear to be in the conceptual ballpark. An interesting group study compared the sleeping patterns of 31 TBI patients on an inpatient rehabilitation unit collected by

night nursing staff [103]. Sleep disturbance was defined as at least 1or 2 h wakefulness for more than 50 of the epochs observed. Sixty-eight percent of the sample had sleep–wake disturbances by this methodology. The presence of sleep–wake disturbances was not related to injury severity, age or BMI. The same group, in a later investigation, studied the sleep efficiency of 11 TBI patients on an inpatient rehabilitation unit with a minimum of 7 days of actigraphy [104]. They found that 78 % of subjects had mean week-1 sleep efficiency scores of ≤63 %, that TBI patients without posttraumatic confusion had significantly better week-1 sleep efficiency scores than those with ongoing posttraumatic confusion, and that improving sleep efficiency was associated with resolving posttraumatic confusion. Unfortunately, this study suffers from a small sample size and failure to take full advantage of the data available from actigraphy in diagnosing circadian rhythm disorders in this sample. Another group study was undertaken which attempted to evaluate sleep–wake cycle disturbances in 205 TBI patients using staff ratings and found that 84 % of the patients had a sleep–wake cycle disturbance on admission to a rehabilitation unit with 63 % having moderate-to-severe ratings (at a median 24 days post injury) [105]. A significant percentage showed sleep–wake cycle disturbances throughout rehabilitation stay, although the incidence and severity tended to decrease over time. The presence of moderate-to-severe sleep–wake cycle disturbance at 1 month post injury was predictive of length of posttraumatic confusion and rehabilitation stay.

One potential hypothesis that can be generated from these studies is that the length of posttraumatic confusion, which has also been well established as a measure of brain injury severity and predictor of outcome, is determined, in part, by sleep cycle disturbances [7]. An alternative view is that the latter occur as a consequence of injury to hypothalamic or related brain networks regulating the sleep–wake cycle which are seen in more severe injuries similar to that reported with hypocretin abnormalities [78, 79]. Thus, the sleep–wake disturbance may have an independent mechanism that is related to posttraumatic confusion by way of injury severity and not a direct link to cognitive functioning. While certainly sleep–wake cycle disturbance would exacerbate a host of problems affecting behavioral functioning, cognitive functioning and the ability to participate in rehabilitation, the approach from a scientific and clinical standpoint might be different. Furthermore, carefully designed research will be necessary to address these issues.

Another small study investigated circadian phase changes in post acute TBI patients. Steele et al. [106] compared the responses to the Morningness-Eveningness Questionnaire (MEQ), salivary dim light melatonin onset (DLMO), and sleep diary entries of 10 post-acute (mean days post injury=516) TBI patients to 10 age- and sex-matched controls. The results did not show significant group differences in habitual sleep time, MEQ or DLMO. There was more variability in retrospectively reported pre-injury to current MEQ scores versus initial- and 3-month scores of the controls. They concluded that there was no conclusive evidence of circadian rhythm disorder after TBI but that the MEQ may not be appropriate for TBI patients [106]. This study is an important study because it is the first to use the MEQ in a TBI population and the authors are probably correct that it would be very difficult for cognitively impaired patients to complete. However, this study also suffers from having a small sample size. In addition, the observations reported in the studies discussed above in acute samples would suggest that circadian changes may occur early in the course of relatively severe TBI patients. Therefore, post acute heterogeneous samples may not be the appropriate subject of study. There are many outstanding questions remaining regarding the relationship between circadian phase changes and TBI. Answering these will require carefully designed prospective studies using appropriate techniques and designs.

The most recent sleep disorder to be found associated with TBI is recurrent hypersomnia. Billiard and Podesta [107] reviewed 12 cases of recurrent hypersomnia culled from the world literature and concluded that 2 were directly related to TBI without other associations, 8 were Kleine–Levin syndrome triggered by TBI and 2 could not be verified as TBI-associated recurrent hypersomnia. They defined recurrent hypersomnia by the criteria of the International Classification of Sleep Disorders 2nd Edition [ICSD 2, 108]. These are recurrent episodes of excessive sleepiness of 2 days to 4 weeks' duration; episodes recur at least once yearly, normal cognitive function and behavior between episodes and no other cause of hypersomnia. This paper also raises some questions about our concept of hypersomnia.

Definitions and Diagnostic Criteria for Posttraumatic Hypersomnia

In the 1990 ICSD 1st Edition [1, 109], and also in its revised editions published in 1997 and 2001, the definition of posttraumatic hypersomnia is: *a disorder of excessive sleepiness that occurs as a result of a traumatic event involving the central nervous system.* The ICSD 1 diagnostic criteria for PTH require excessive sleepiness, onset of sleepiness temporally associated with head trauma, no medical disorder that could account for the symptoms, the symptoms do not meet the criteria of other sleep disorders that produce sleepiness (e.g., narcolepsy), and polysomnography demonstrating
1. Normal timing quality and duration of sleep
2. Mean sleep latency of less than 10 min on MSLT
3. Fewer than two SOREMPs on MSLT

These ICSD 1 criteria were used in most of the reports published early during this century, but an alternative definition has been more recently proposed and utilized. Professor Baumann [110, 111] has noted the importance of distinguishing between *EDS* as "increased daytime sleep propensity" and *hypersomnia* as "the increased sleep need per 24 hours." A proposed *alternative definition of PTH* entails *an increased sleep need ≥2 h compared to pre-TBI conditions.* The ICSD 2 mentions PTH under "Hypersomnia Due to Medical Condition" and defines this as *excessive sleepiness due to head trauma* [112]. The *ICSD 2 criteria for the diagnosis of PTH* under this category would include *revised MSLT criteria for hypersomnia: a mean sleep latency <8 min with no more than one SOREMP*, if the MSLT is performed. The other criteria include excessive sleepiness almost daily for at least 3 months, significant medical or neurological disorder (in this case, TBI) accounts for the sleepiness, and no other better explanation exists. Because of the lack of correlation between subjective complaints and objective findings, as well as the possibility of SDB and narcolepsy, it would be reasonable to adhere to the earlier requirement of excluding other sleep disorders and documentation of excessive sleepiness by NPSG and MSLT for the diagnosis of PTH. It also remains possible that two separate forms of what may be called PTH exist: The earlier concept of excessive sleepiness (propensity to fall asleep) incorporated in the more commonly used expressions of hypersomnia, and another group of TBI patients with increased sleep need per 24 h, which could be a circadian rhythm disorder after TBI or some other pathophysiology as yet undetermined. This might be diagnosed with actigraphy rather than with MSLT. The distinction between these two concepts of "hypersomnia" may be important with regard to the possible recognition and treatment of some sleep problems resulting from TBI.

Conclusion

A look at the past milestones in learning about sleep and TBI (Table 36.1) reveals that most of what we know has been learned over a relatively short time span. As more attention is directed toward the sleep/wake problems associated with TBI, and research yields a greater understanding of the associated sleep disorders and their pathophysiological mechanisms, we can anticipate a significant increase in new milestones in discovery. We hope this will also result in more widespread recognition of the importance of employing appropriate diagnostic methods to discover treatable problems ascribed to presumed irreparable brain injury, and use of therapeutic modalities that improve the quality of life and productivity of those with TBI.

Table 36.1 Milestones in sleep disorders with TBI

400 BC	Hippocrates [20]	First mention of sleep and TBI in *Aphorisms*
165 AD	Galen [21]	Excessive sleepiness in head injury
1880	Gelineau [30]	Introduction of term *narcolepsie*
1896	Osler [22]	Insomnia after TBI in "railway brain"
1915	Henneberg [31]	Introduction of term *Kataplexie*
1915	Redlich [25]	*Narkolepsie* associated with TBI
1918	Lhermitte [28]	*Narcolepsie* after cerebral concussion
1918	Souques [29]	Term "Posttraumatic narcolepsy"
1929	Haenel [33]	Posttraumatic narcolepsy with cataplexy
1941	Gill [35]	Narcolepsy after mild TBI
1930	Pollock [36]	Sleep attacks which are refreshing
1951	Humphrey and Zangwell [40]	Cessation of dreaming after TBI
1959	Bonduelle at al [38]	Posttraumatic hypnogogic hallucinations
1964	Barbano and Bossi [41]	Circadian rhythm disorders after TBI
1966	Meurice [42]	First detailed polysomnography in TBI; no subjective–objective correlation
1970	Lenard and Penningtorff [44]	Polysomnography of pediatric TBI
1972	Amico et al. [39]	Sleep-disordered breathing with TBI
1979	Alexandre et al. [45]	Correlation between sleep and cognitive function after TBI
1982	Parsons and VerBeek [55]	Increased sleep complaints after TBI
1983	Guilleminault et al. [60]	Retrospective review of EDS after TBI; freq OSA
1989	Good et al. [46]	Post-TBI narcolepsy with SOREMPs and HLA DR2
1992	Cohen et al. [56]	Increased insomnia in inpatient TBI, EDS in outpatient TBI: temporal changes in complaints
1996	Francisco and Ivanhoe [49]	Satisfactory treatment of posttraumatic narcolepsy with methylphenidate
1997	Nagtegaal et al.	DSPS after TBI, treated with melatonin
1990	American Academy of Sleep Medicine [109]	Definition of posttraumatic hypersomnia with NPSG and MSLT criteria
2000	Guilleminault et al. [72]	"Pseudohypersomnia" after TBI
2001	Castriotta and Lai [81]	Prospective study of EDS in TBI using term PTH by ICSD 1 criteria; predominance of SDB
2005	Baumann et al. [78]	Reduced CSF hypocretin in TBI
2007	Ayalon et al. [101]	Circadian rhythm disorders Dx'd by actigraphy in 36% of TBI with insomnia complaint
2007	Baumann et al. [85]	EDS by MSLT in 25% of TBI subjects
2007	Castriotta et al. [43]	Sleep disorders in 46% of TBI subjects; EDS by MSLT in 25%
2007	Verma et al. [84]	HLA-DQB1*0602 in posttraumatic narcolepsy; REM without atonia in 13% with sleep problems
2009	Baumann [79]	Loss of hypocretin neurons in TBI
2012	Mathias and Alvaro[87]	First meta-analysis of sleep in TBI
2013	Billiard and Podesta [107]	Recurrent hypersomnia after TBI

TBI traumatic brain injury, *SOREMP* Sleep-onset *REM* (rapid eye movement) sleep period, *EDS* Excessive daytime sleepiness, OSA Obstructive sleep apnea, *HLA DR2*, DSPS delayed sleep phase syndrome, *NPSG* nocturnal polysomnography, *MSLT* multiple sleep latency test, *SDB* sleep-disordered breathing, *CSF* cerebrospinal fluid, *REM* rapid eye movement, *ICSD 1* International classification of sleep disorders, 1st edition

References

1. Dikmen SS, Machamer JE, Powell JM, Temkin NR. Outcome 3 to 5 years after moderate to severe traumatic brain injury. Arch Phys Med Rehabil. 2003;84(10):1449–57.
2. Millis SR, Rosenthal M, Novack TA, Sherer M, Nick TG, Kreutzer JS, et al. Long-term neuropsychological outcome after traumatic brain injury. J Head Trauma Rehabil. 2001;16(4):343–55.
3. Levin HS, Benton AL, Grossman RG. Neurobehavioral consequences of closed head injury. New York: Oxford University Press; 1982.
4. Dikmen S, Machamer J, Temkin N. Mild head injury: facts and artifacts. J Clin Exp Neuropsychol. 2001;23(6):729–38.
5. Kashluba S, Hanks RA, Casey JE, Millis SR. Neuropsychologic and functional outcome after complicated mild traumatic brain injury. Arch Phys Med Rehabil. 2008;89(5):904–11.
6. Williams, DH, Levin, HS, Eisenberg, HM. Mild head injury classification. Neurosurgery. 1990;27(3):422–8.
7. Levin HS. Neurobehavioral outcome of closed head injury: Implications for clinical trials. J Neurotrauma. 1995;12(4):601–10.
8. DoD Worldwide Numbers for TBI | DVBIC. Available from: http://www.dvbic.org/dod-worldwide-numbers-tbi.

9. Faul M, Xu L, Wald MM, Coronado VG. Traumatic brain injury in the United States: emergency department visits, hospitalizations, and deaths. Atlanta, GA; 2010.

10. Centers for Disease Control and Prevention (CDC) NC for IP and C. Report to Congress on mild traumatic brain injury in the United States: steps to prevent a serious public health problem. Atlanta, GA; 2003.

11. Tagliaferri F, Compagnone C, Korsic M, Servadei F, Kraus J. A systematic review of brain injury epidemiology in Europe. Acta Neurochir. 2006;148(3):255–68.

12. Menon DK, Schwab K, Wright DW, Maas AI. Position statement: definition of traumatic brain injury. Arch Phys Med Rehabil. 2010;91(11):1637–40.

13. Leger D. The cost of sleep-related accidents: A report for the national commission on sleep disorders research. Sleep. 1994;17(1):84–93.

14. Young T, Blustein J, Finn L, Palta M. Sleep-disordered breathing and motor vehicle accidents in a population-based sample of employed adults. Sleep. 1997;20(8):608–13.

15. Ellen RLB, Marshall SC, Palayew M, Molnar FJ, Wilson KG, Man-Son-Hing M. Systematic review of motor vehicle crash risk in persons with sleep apnea. J Clin Sleep Med. 2006;2(2):193–200.

16. Stradling J. Driving and sleep apnea. Thorax. 2008;63(6):481–3.

17. Stone KL, Ancoli-Israel S, Blackwell T, Ensrud KE, Cauley JA, Redline S, et al. Actigraphy-measured sleep characteristics and risk of falls in older women. Arch Intern Med. 1987;147(16):1768–75.

18. Rodenstein D. Driving in Europe: the need of a common policy for drivers with obstructive sleep apnoea syndrome. J Sleep Res. 2008;17(3):281–4.

19. Daley M, M Morin C, LeBlanc M, P Grégoire J, Savard J, Baillargeon L. Insomnia and its relationship to health-care utilization, work absenteeism, productivity and accidents. Sleep Med. 2009;10(4):427–38.

20. De Gorter J. Medicina hippocratica exponens aphorismos hippocratis, 5th edn. Padova: Typis Seminarii; 1778. p. 71.

21. Jelliffe S. Narcolepsy, hypnolepsy, pyknolepsy. M.J. and Rec. 1929;119:269.

22. Osler W. The principles and practice of medicine, 2nd edn. New York: Appleton & Company; 1896. p. 1035.

23. Osler W. The principles and practice of medicine, 2nd edn. New York: Appleton & Company; 1896. p. 1039.

24. Bouveret L. La Neurasthenie: Epuisement Nerveux. Librairie J-B Baillière et Fils. Paris; 1891.

25. Redlich E. Zur Narkolepsie Frage. Monatsch Psychiat und Neurol. 1915;37:85.

26. Singer K. Echte und pseudo Narkolepsie. Zeitsch. Neurol und Psych. 1917;36:278.

27. Kahler M. Zur Kenntnis der Narkolepsie. Jahrn Psychiat und Neurol. 1921;41:1.

28. Lhermitte J. La forme narcoleptique tardive de la commotion cérébrale. Paris Medical. 1918;8:509.

29. Souques A. Narcolepsie d'origine traumatique: Ses rapports avec une lésion de la region infundibulo-hypophysaire. Revue Neurologique. 1918;1:521.

30. Gelineau J. De la narcolepsie. Gaz des Hôp. 1880;55:626–628; 635–637.

31. Henneberg RH. Über genuine Narkolepsie. Deutsche med Wehnschr. 1915;41:1585.

32. Adie W. Idiopathic narcolepsy: A disease sui generis; with remarks on the mechanism of sleep. Brain. 1926;49:257.

33. Haenel H. Zbl Ges. Neurol Psychiat. 1929;35:282.

34. Thiele R, Bernhardt H. Erfahrungen über Narkolepsie. Zentralnl f d ges Neurol und Psychiat. 1931;61:143–4.

35. Gill A. Idiopathic and traumatic narcolepsy. Lancet Neurol. 1941;1:474–6.

36. Pollock L. Disorders of sleep. Med Clin N Am. 1930;13:1111–20.

37. Daniels L. Narcolepsy. Medicine. 1934;13:1–122.

38. Bonduelle M, Bouygues P, Delahousse J, Faveret C. Narcolepsie post-traumatique. Lille Med. 1959;4 (11):719–721.

39. Amico G, Pasquali F, Pittaluga E. Turbe pickwickiane-narcolettiche post-commotive. Riv Sper Freniatr Med Leg Alien Ment. 1972;96(1):74–85.

40. Humphrey ME, Zangwill OL. Cessation of dreaming after brain injury. J Neurol Neurosurg Psychiatry. 1951;14(4):322–5.

41. Barbano G, Bossi L. Rheography in the subjective syndrome of patients with cranial trauma. Minerva Medica. 1964;55:640–4.

42. Meurice E. Signs of diurnal falling asleep in a group of post-concussion patients compared with a group of normal subjects. Revue Neurologique. 1966;115(3):524–6.

43. Castriotta RJ, Wilde MC, Lai JM, Atanasov S, Masel BE, Kuna ST. Prevalence and consequences of sleep disorders in traumatic brain injury. J Clin Sleep Med. 2007;3(4):349–56.

44. Lenard H, Penningstorff H. Alterations in sleep patterns of infants and young children following acute head injuries. Acta Pediat Scand. 1970;59:565–71.

45. Alexandre A, Rubini L, Nertempi P, Farinello C. Sleep alterations during post-traumatic coma as a possible predictor of cognitive defects. Acta Neurologica. 1979;28 (Suppl):188–92.

46. Good JL, Barry E, Fishman PS. Posttraumatic narcolepsy: the complete syndrome with tissue typing. J Neurosurg. 1989;71:765–7.

47. Maccario M, Ruggles KH, Meriwether MW. Post-traumatic narcolepsy. Mil Med. 1987;152(7):370–1.

48. Kapen S, Mohan K. Post traumatic narcolepsy. A report of three cases. Sleep Res. 1995;24:259.

49. Francisco GE, Ivanhoe CB. Successful treatment of post-traumatic narcolepsy with methylphenidate: a case report. Am J Phys Med Rehabil. 1996;75(1):63–5.

50. Broughton R, Willmer J, Skinner C. Post-traumatic insomnia with rhythmic leg movements. Sleep Res. 1987;16:466.

51. Nagtegaal JE, Kerkhof GA, Smits MG, Swart AC, Van der Meer YG. Traumatic brain injury-associated delayed sleep phase syndrome. Funct Neurol. 1997;12(6):345–8.

52. Patten SB, Lauderdale WM. Delayed sleep phase disorder after traumatic brain injury. J Am Acad Child Adolesc Psychiatry. 1992;31(1):100–2.

53. Quinto C, Gellido C, Chokroverty S, Masdeu J. Posttraumatic delayed sleep phase syndrome. Neurology. 2000;54(1):250–2. [cited 2013 Apr 9]

54. Meyer T, Deck R, Raspe H. Problems completing questionnaires on health status in medical rehabilitation patients. J Rehabil Med. 2007;39(8):633–9.

55. Parsons LC, Ver Beek D. Sleep-awake patterns following cerebral concussion. Nurs Res. 1982;31(5):260–4.

56. Cohen M, Oksenberg A, Snir D, Stern MJ, Groswasser Z. Temporally related changes of sleep complaints in traumatic brain injured patients. J Neurol Neurosurg Psychiatry. 1992;55(4):313–5.

57. Clinchot DM, Bogner J, Mysiw WJ, Fugate L, Corrigan J. Defining sleep disturbance after brain injury. Am J Phys Med Rehabil Assoc Acad Physiat. 1998;77(4):291–5.

58. Prigatano GP, Stahl ML, Orr WC, Zeiner HK. Sleep and dreaming disturbances in closed head injury patients. J Neurol Neurosurg Psychiatry. 1982;45(1):78–80.

59. Cohen M, Groswasser Z, Stern MJ, Costeff H. Sleep disorders following craniocerebral injury. Sleep Res. 1987;16:472.

60. Guilleminault C, Faull KF, Miles L, Van den Hoed J. Posttraumatic excessive daytime sleepiness: a review of 20 patients. Neurology. 1983;33(12):1584–9.

61. Lankford DA, Wellman JJ, O'Hara C. Posttraumatic narcolepsy in mild to moderate closed head injury. Sleep. 1994;17(8 Suppl):S25–8.

62. Beetar JT, Guilmette TJ, Sparadeo FR. Sleep and pain complaints in symptomatic traumatic brain injury and neurologic populations. Arch Phys Med Rehabil. 1996;77(12):1298–302.

63. Beebe DW, Krivitzky L, Wells CT, Wade SL, Taylor HG, Yeates KO. Brief report: parental report of sleep behaviors following moderate or severe pediatric traumatic brain injury. J Pediatr Psychol. 2007;32(7):845–50.

64. Kaufman Y, Tzischinsky O, Epstein R, Etzioni A, Lavie P, Pillar G. Long-term sleep disturbances in adolescents after minor head injury. Pediatr Neurol. 2001;24(2):129–34.

65. Kempf J, Werth E, Kaiser PR, Bassetti CL, Baumann CR. Sleep-wake disturbances 3 years after traumatic brain injury. J Neurol Neurosurg Psychiatry. 2010;81(12):1402–5.

66. Rao V, Spiro J, Vaishnavi S, Rastogi P, Mielke M, Noll K, et al. Prevalence and types of sleep disturbances acutely after traumatic brain injury. Brain Inj. 2008;22(5):381–6.

67. Watson NF, Dikmen S, Machamer J, Doherty M, Temkin N. Hypersomnia following traumatic brain injury. J Clin Sleep Med. 2007;3:363–8.

68. Meyer T, Deck R, Raspe H. Problems completing questionnaires on health status in medical rehabilitation patients. J Rehabil Med. 2007;39(8):633–9.

69. Iverson GL, Lange RT, Brooks BL, Rennison VLA. "Good old days" bias following mild traumatic brain injury. Clin Neuropsychol. 2010;24(1):17–37.

70. Lange RT, Iverson GL, Brooks BL, Rennison VLA. Influence of poor effort on self-reported symptoms and neurocognitive test performance following mild traumatic brain injury. J Clin Exp Neuropsychol. 2010;32(9):961–72.

71. Lange RT, Iverson GL, Rose A. Post-concussion symptom reporting and the "good-old-days" bias following mild traumatic brain injury. Arch Clin Neuropsychol. 2010;25(5):442–50.

72. Guilleminault C, Yuen KM, Gulevich MG, Karadeniz D, Leger D, Philip P. Hypersomnia after head-neck trauma: a medicolegal dilemma. Neurology. 2000;54(3):653–9.

73. Hart T, Seignourel PJ, Sherer M. A longitudinal study of awareness of deficit after moderate to severe traumatic brain injury. Neuropsychol Rehabil. 2009;19(2):161–76.

74. Gosselin N, Lassonde M, Petit D, Leclerc S. Sleep following sport-related concussions. Sleep Med. 2009;10:35–46.

75. Schreiber S, Barkai G, Gur-Hartman T, Peles E, Tov N, Dolberg OT, et al. Long-lasting sleep patterns of adult patients with minor traumatic brain injury (mTBI) and non-mTBI subjects. Sleep Med. 2008;9(5):481–7.

76. Parcell DL, Ponsford JL, Redman JR, Rajaratnam SM. Poor sleep quality and changes in objectively recorded sleep after traumatic brain injury: a preliminary study. Arch Physl Med Rehabil. 2008;89(5):843–50.

77. Shekleton J, Parcell DL, Redman JR, Phipps-Nelson J, Ponsford JL, Rajaratnam SMW. Sleep disturbance and melatonin levels following traumatic brain injury. Neurology. 2010;74(21):1732–8.

78. Baumann CR, Stocker R, Imhof H-G, Trentz O, Hersberger M, Mignot E, et al. Hypocretin-1 (orexin A) deficiency in acute traumatic brain injury. Neurology. 2005;65(1):147–9.

79. Baumann CR, Bassetti CL, Valko PO, Haybaeck J, Keller M, Clark E, et al. Loss of hypocretin (orexin) neurons with traumatic brain injury. Annal Neurol. 2009;66(4):555–9.

80. Siegel JM, Moore R, Thannickal T, Nienhuis R. A brief history of hypocretin/orexin and narcolepsy. Neuropsychopharmacology. 2001;25:S14–20.

81. Castriotta RJ, Lai JM. Sleep disorders associated with traumatic brain injury. Arch Phys Med Rehabil. 2001;82(10):1403–6.

82. Webster JB, Bell KR, Hussey JD, Natale TK, Lakshminarayan S. Sleep apnea in adults with traumatic brain injury: a preliminary investigation. Arch Phys Med Rehabil. 2001;82(3):316–21.

83. Masel BE, Scheibel RS, Kimbark T, Kuna ST. Excessive daytime sleepiness in adults with brain injuries. Arch Phys Med Rehabil. 2001;82(11):1526–32.

84. Verma A, Anand V, Verma NP. Sleep disorders in chronic traumatic brain injury. J Clin Sleep Med. 2007;3(4):357–62.

85. Baumann CR, Werth E, Stocker R, Ludwig S, Bassetti CL. Sleep-wake disturbances 6 months after traumatic brain injury: a prospective study. Brain. 2007;130:1873–83.

86. Collen J, Orr N, Lettieri CJ, Carter K, Holley AB. Sleep disturbances among soldiers with combat-related traumatic brain injury. Chest. 2012;142(3):622–30.

87. Mathias JL, Alvaro PK. Prevalence of sleep disturbances, disorders, and problems following traumatic brain injury: a meta-analysis. Sleep Med. 2012;13(7):898–905.

88. Castriotta RJ, Atanasov S, Wilde MC, Masel BE, Lai JM, Kuna ST. Treatment of sleep disorders after traumatic brain injury. J Clin Sleep Med. 2009;5(2):137–44.

89. Jha A, Weintraub A, Allshouse A, Morey C, Cusick C, Kittelson J, et al. A randomized trial of modafinil for the treatment of fatigue and excessive daytime sleepiness in individuals with chronic traumatic brain injury. J Head Trauma Rehabil. 2008;23(1):52–63.

90. Wilde MC, Castriotta RJ, Lai JM, Atanasov S, Masel BE, Kuna ST. Cognitive impairment in patients with traumatic brain injury and obstructive sleep apnea. Arch Phys Med Rehabil. 2007;88(10):1284–8.

91. Mahmood O, Rapport LJ, Hanks RA, Fichtenberg NL. Neuropsychological performance and sleep disturbance following traumatic brain injury. J Head Trauma Rehabil. 2004;18:378–90.

92. Bloomfield ILM, Espie C, Evans JJ. Do sleep difficulties exacerbate deficits in sustained attention following traumatic brain injury? J Int Neuropsychol Soc. 2010;16(1):17–25.

93. Fichtenberg NL, Millis SR, Mann NR, Zafonte RD, Millard AE. Factors associated with insomnia among post-acute traumatic brain injury survivors. Brain Inj. 2000;14(7):659–67.

94. Fichtenberg NL, Zafonte RD, Putnam S, Mann NR, Millard AE. Insomnia in a post-acute brain injury sample. Brain Inj. 2002;16(3):197–206.

95. Ouellet M-C, Beaulieu-Bonneau S, Morin CM. Insomnia in patients with traumatic brain injury. J Head Trauma Rehabil. 2006;21(3):199–212.

96. Ouellet M-C, Morin CM. Subjective and objective measures of insomnia in the context of traumatic brain injury: a preliminary study. Sleep Med. 2006;7(6):486–97.

97. Fogelberg DJ, Hoffman JM, Dikmen S, Temkin NR, Bell KR. Association of sleep and co-occurring psychological conditions at 1 year after traumatic brain injury. Arch Phys Med Rehabil. 2012;93(8):1313–8.

98. Cantor JB, Bushnik T, Cicerone K, Dijkers MP, Gordon W, Hammond FM, et al. Insomnia, fatigue, and sleepiness in the first 2 years after rraumatic brain injury: an NIDRR TBI model system module study. J Head Trauma Rehabil. 2012; 6:E1–14.

99. Parcell DL, Ponsford JL, Rajaratnam SM, Redman JR. Self-reported changes to nighttime sleep after traumatic brain injury. Arch Phys Med Rehabil. 2006;87:278–85.

100. Ouellet M-C, Morin CM. Cognitive behavioral therapy for insomnia associated with traumatic brain injury: a single-case study. Arch Phys Med Rehabil. 2004;85(8):1298–302.

101. Ayalon L, Borodkin K, Dishon L, Kanety H, Dagan Y. Circadian rhythm sleep disorders following mild traumatic brain injury. Neurology. 2007;68:1136–40.

102. Boivin DB, James FO, Santo JB, Caliyurt O, Chalk C. Non-24-hour sleep-wake syndrome following a car accident. Neurology. 2003;60(11):1841–3.

103. Makley MJ, English JB, Drubach D, Kreuz J, Celnik P, Tarwater PM. Prevalence of sleep disturbance in closed head injury patients in a rehabilitation unit. Neurorehabilitation and Neural Repair. 2008;22(4):341–7.

104. Makley MJ, Johnson-Greene L, Tarwater PM, Kreuz AJ, Spiro J, Rao V, et al. Return of memory and sleep efficiency following moderate to severe closed head injury. Neurorehabilitation and neural repair. 2009;23(4):320–6.

105. Nakase-Richardson R, Sherer M, Barnett SD, Yablon SA, Evans CC, Kretzmer T, et al. Prospective evaluation of the nature, course, and impact of acute sleep abnormality after traumatic brain injury. Arch Phys Med Rehabil. 2013;94(5):875–82.

106. Steele DL, Rajaratnam SMW, Redman JR, Ponsford JL. The effect of traumatic brain injury on the timing of sleep. Chronobiol Int. 2005;22(1):89–105.

107. Billiard M, Podesta C. Recurrent hypersomnia following traumatic brain injury. Sleep Med. 2013;14(5):462–5.

108. American Academy of Sleep Medicine. International classification of sleep disorders, 2nd edn. Diagnostic and coding manual. Westchester, Illinois: Americam Academy of Sleep Medicine; 2005, pp. 95–7.

109. Diagnostic Classification Steering Committee, Thorpy MJ. Chairman. International classification of sleep disorders: Diagnostic and coding manual. Rochester, Minnesota, American Sleep Disorders Association 1990, pp. 49–52.

110. Baumann CR. Traumatic brain injury and disturbed sleep and wakefulness. Neuromolecular Med. 2012;14:205–12

111. Baumann CR. Traumatic brain injury and sleep-wake disorders. Sleep Med Clin. 2012;7:609–17.

112. American Academy of Sleep Medicine. International classification of sleep disorders, 2nd edn. Diagnostic and coding manual. Westchester, Illinois: Americam Academy of Sleep Medicine; 2005, p. 108.

Headache Syndromes and Sleep

37

Munish Goyal, Niranjan Singh and Pradeep Sahota

Introduction

The intimate and complex relationship between sleep and headache has been a concern for many clinicians for ages. In a patient suffering from sleep disorder and headache syndrome, it is difficult and challenging to ascertain whether the sleep disorder leads to headache or the headache syndrome leads to the sleep disorder. It is known that both these disorders are common and occur concurrently, complicating each other.

History

Throughout history there are references about sleep and headaches. For example, Romberg in 1853, writing about migraine, stated that, "the attack is generally closed by a profound and refreshing sleep" [1]; Leiving in 1873 described sleep as a factor terminating headache [2]; Bing in 1945 wrote about headaches occurring on arousal from sleep [3]; Gans described reduction in migraine attacks following selective sleep deprivation, especially deep sleep [4]; Dexter reported an association between morning arousals with headache and increased amount of slow-wave sleep and rapid eye movement (REM) sleep [5]. In 1990, Sahota and Dexter wrote a landmark review article describing the relationship between headache and sleep [4]. Sahota and Dodick then emphasized the relationship between sleep and headache in the second edition of the international classification of sleep disorders

(ICSD), diagnostic and coding manual, in 2005 [5]. Subsequent reports further review this relationship, but the above represent some of the key contributions.

Relationship Between Headache and Sleep

The enigmatic relationship of headache and sleep is bidirectional—sleep affects headache and headache in turn affects sleep. Headaches have been described to occur during sleep [6], following sleep [3, 7, 8], and in relation to different sleep stages [6, 7, 9, 10]. In a review article, Sahota and Dexter [4] proposed a classification about the relationship between sleep and headache. Headache can be broadly classified as primary and secondary headaches. The primary headache is a headache which is not caused by any other medical condition or disorder. The secondary headache is defined as a headache due to other medical disorders. In this chapter, we will focus on primary and secondary headaches related only to sleep disorders.

Primary Headache

Cluster Headache (CH)

Nicolas Tulp has been credited for describing CH in 1641 [11]. CH is classified under the spectrum of disorders called trigeminal autonomic cephalalgias (TACs). CH is characterized by the core features of unilateral, severe excruciating head pain occurring in clusters (1–8 episodes per day), lasting from 15 to 180 min, with accompanying features of autonomic dysfunction (e.g., conjunctival injection, lacrimation, ptosis, miosis, nasal congestion, and rhinorrhea) [5]. Russel et al. found a preponderance of attacks beginning during sleep and the majority of daytime attacks began when patients were physically relaxed [12]. CH attacks have been shown to occur during REM sleep or within 9 min of REM termination [6, 13]. It has been reported in several studies

M. Goyal (✉) · N. Singh · P. Sahota
Department of Neurology, University of Missouri Hospitals & Clinics, 5 Hospital Drive, DC047.00 CE507, Columbia, MO 65212, USA
e-mail: goyalm@missouri.edu

N. Singh
e-mail: singhn@missouri.edu

P. Sahota
e-mail: sahotap@missouri.edu

that the patients with CH have a higher prevalence of obstructive sleep apnea (OSA) [13–17]. Nocturnal hypoxia related to OSA could be a trigger for the CH [14]. A role of hypothalamus in this correlation has also been proposed, as noted by the improvement in sleep architecture in patients treated with deep brain stimulator for chronic CH [18].

Tension-Type Headache (TTH)

Insufficient sleep, oversleeping, and sleep disorders have been implicated as precipitating and aggravating factors for TTH [27–29]. Results from the third Nord-Trøndelag Health Survey indicated that subjects with chronic headache were 17 times more likely to have severe sleep disturbances and the association was somewhat stronger for chronic migraine than for chronic TTH [19].

In a cross-sectional study from Norway, the authors reported that the presence and severity of sleep apnea seem not to influence presence and attack frequency of TTH in the general population [20].

Hypnic Headache (HH)

Raskin in 1988 described a case series of six elderly patients having headaches exclusively in sleep [21]. The criteria for diagnosis of HH were proposed in 1997 by Goadsby et al. [22]. The headache should occur at least 15 times per month for at least 1 month, awaken the patient from sleep, lasting for 5–60 min, the pain being generalized or bilateral and not associated with autonomic features. They proposed that HH should be added to the international headache society classifications under miscellaneous headaches [22]. Later in year 2004, the HH was classified under International Classification of Headache Disorders-II (ICHD II), in the category of "other primary headache." The diagnostic criteria state that the headache is dull, occurs after age of 50 years, develops only during sleep, and awakens the patient.

Migraine

Migraine and sleep disorders can be present in an individual when it is difficult to ascertain if migraine caused the sleep disorder or the sleep disorder is the cause for the migraine. Migraine can emerge during nocturnal sleep or following a brief period of daytime sleep; attacks can be preceded by a lack of sleep; sleep has also been shown to relieve migraine, especially in children [23]. Patients with migraine without aura have a much higher prevalence of sleep abnormalities as compared to controls which may be due to multiple

contributory factors [24]. It has been reported that preferential emergence of attacks during night sleep or upon awakening progressively increases with aging [25].

Migraine and Restless Legs Syndrome (RLS)

The frequency of RLS in migraine patients in pediatric age group was significantly higher than in controls (22 vs. 5 % ($p < 0.001$) [26]. A strong association between migraine and RLS is reported in the women with migraine with and without aura [27]. Rhode et al., in a case-control study of patients with migraine, found a significantly higher lifetime prevalence of RLS than the control group [28]. Similar correlation has been reported by d'Onofrio et al. [29] and by Chen et al. [30]. The underlying pathophysiology has been linked to the dysfunction of dopaminergic metabolism in migraine [28, 31].

Migraine and Parasomnias

A higher incidence of several parasomnias, e.g., bruxism, sleepwalking, sleep talking, and night terrors, has been found in children with migraine [32].

Migraine and Narcolepsy

There has been controversial correlation between migraine and narcolepsy. In two different studies, Dahmen et al. reported two to fourfold increase in the migraine prevalence in patients with narcolepsy [33, 34]. These results were challenged by a multicenter case-control study which concluded that there is no association between migraine and narcolepsy but that patients with narcolepsy show more unspecific headache, probably due to sleep disturbances [35].

Migraine and Insomnia

Sevillano-García et al. reported insomnia in 37.42 % of their patients [36]. In a survey by Lateef et al., adults with migraine reported more frequent difficulty initiating sleep, difficulty staying asleep, early-morning awakening, and daytime fatigue when compared to the individuals without headache [37]. In another survey in Hong Kong Chinese women with different headache diagnoses, the prevalence of insomnia symptoms was reported as problem waking up too early in 29.4 %, difficulty staying asleep in 28.0 %, and difficulty falling asleep in 24.4 % [38].

Migraine and Excessive Daytime Sleepiness (EDS)

EDS has been reported in patients with migraine. The exact mechanism is unknown. Peres et al. reported EDS in patients with migraine. Epworth sleepiness scale(ESS) score ≥ 10 was in 37 % of patients and ESS of ≥ 15 in 10 % of patients [39]. In a case-control study, EDS was more frequent in migraineurs than in controls (14 vs. 5 %) [40].

In summary, there is a broad spectrum of relationships between migraine and sleep. While the above observations are important, a full range of this relationship still needs to be defined. Further research can possibly explain common pathphysiological pathways between these two entities.

Secondary Headaches

Sleep Apnea Headache

According to the ICHD II, sleep apnea headache [10.1.3] has been classified under secondary headaches—headache attributed to disorder of homeostasis. The diagnostic criteria include—a recurrent headache with at least one of the following—headache occurring on more than 15 days per month; headaches being bilateral with pressing quality and not accompanied by nausea, photophobia, or phonophobia; and each headache resolved within 30 min. The headache should be present upon awakening and it ceases within 72 h, and does not recur, after effective treatment of sleep apnea [5]. Aldrich et al. reported a frequency of morning headaches in 18 % of patients with OSA versus 21–38 % in the patients with other sleep disorders versus 6 % in control group. They concluded that the symptom of morning headache is nonspecific in patients with sleep disorders [41]. Morning headaches have been reported to have a 90-day prevalence of around 60 % in habitual snorers as well as in their bed partners [42].

In a recent population-based cross-sectional study from Norway, sleep apnea headache is reported in 11.8 % of the participants with OSA. In a Turkish study, the morning headaches resolved in 90 % of the patients using positive airway pressure [43]. In a large telephone questionnaire study ($n = 18,980$) from the general populations of the UK, Germany, Italy, Portugal, and Spain, prevalence of chronic morning headache was found to be 7.6 %. The headache was most common in patients with depression, insomnia, and sleep-related breathing disorders. The authors concluded that the chronic morning headaches are not specific to sleep-related breathing disorder [44].

Exploding Head Syndrome (EHS)

Described by Armstrong-Jones [45] in 1920, it is a unique and rare syndrome of sudden, loud, painless, explosive sound in the head without actual headache, which can frighten and awaken the subject from sleep. In a study with polysomnographic evaluation in nine patients with EHS, Sachs and Svanborg concluded that EHS occurs during a nocturnal awakening when the subject is relaxed but temporarily awake [46]. In ICSD II, EHS is listed as one of the parasomnias [47]. The treatment options include clomipramine [46, 48] and topiramate [49].

Recent Advances in Treatment of Headache

Given the relationship between sleep and headache, treatment of headache can have implications for sleep. Treatment of headache can be divided into acute and preventive treatment. Acute treatments are required for all patients at some point of time while some patients may need preventive therapy depending upon headache duration, frequency, severity, and response to acute treatment. Migraine being the most common type of headache in practice has gained the most attention.

Historically, acute migraine-specific management was based on the vascular model of headache proposed by Wolff and Graham in 1938 linking migraine to vasoconstriction [50]. As a result, ergot preparations were developed and were efficacious, but with significant side effects. The 1990s saw a major advance with the introduction of sumatriptan. This serotonin receptor hydroxytryptamine 1 (5-HT1) agonist was as effective as ergots but generally produced fewer side effects [51]. Subsequently, several other triptans became available but their exact mode of action is unclear.

In late 2009, calcitonin gene-related peptide (CGRP) came as a hope for new era of treatment for acute migraine. Acute treatment of migraine with triptans presents a clear limitation due to its cardiovascular side effects. Gepants, a CGRP antagonist, might offer a new nonvasoconstrictive approach in the acute treatment of migraine. When compared with triptans, gepants class showed a similar efficacy, moreover corresponding to the best published results for oral triptans. CGRP antagonists are in different phases of their development, and the treatment of migraine could be based on the use of gepants, as class of acute medications.

There are several nonspecific acute treatments including nonsteroidal anti-inflammatory drugs (NSAIDS), antiemetics, antihistaminic agents, opiates, and steroids.

The preventive treatment of migraine began with methysergide in 1960s [52]. Even after half a century, no other medication has been introduced exclusively for migraine prevention. There are a large number of different classes of medication used for preventive therapy that include but are not limited to antiepileptics, antidepressants, beta blockers, calcium channel blockers, NSAIDS, botulinum toxin, and novel peripheral and central neuromodulators. Botulinum toxin was recently approved by Food and Drug Administration (FDA) for use in chronic migraine.

There have been several open label, nonrandomized studies using neuromodulation for chronic migraine, but several questions need to be answered before any further recommendation can be made including cost of therapy.

Several medications used for treatment of migraine have been found successful in CHs including triptans, calcium channel blockers, antiepileptics, steroids, and neurostimulators. Posterior hypothalamic stimulation and occipital nerve stimulation are two procedures used in medically refractory CH [53]

So far no randomized control trial data are available for treatment of HH. All recommendations are based on case reports and smaller case series. Caffeine has been found to be effective for both acute and prophylactic treatment while lithium works best for preventive treatment [54].

In summary, an intimate relationship between sleep and headache is known for centuries. While the initial reports were based on descriptive relationship, addition of polysomnography revealed additional details of relationship between headache, sleep stages, and primary sleep disorders. The purpose of reviewing such a relationship from a historical standpoint is to focus our attention on development of methods for proper treatment which will impact the quality of sleep in such patients.

References

1. Romberg MH. A manual of the nervous diseases of man. (Trans and editor. Sieveking EH.). London: Sydenham Society; 1853.
2. Lieving E. On megrim, sick-headache and some allied disorders. London: Churchill; 1873.
3. Robert B. Lehrbuch der Nervenkrankheiten Bing, R.: Published by Basel, Schwabe; (1947).
4. Sahota PK, Dexter JD. Sleep and headache syndromes: a clinical review. Headache. 1990;30(2):80–4.
5. The international classification of headache disorders: 2nd edition. Cephalalgia. 2004;24(Suppl. 1):9–160.
6. Dexter JD, Weitzman ED. The relationship of nocturnal headaches to sleep stage patterns. Neurology. 1970;20(5):513–8.
7. Dexter JD. The relationship between stage III + IV + REM sleep and arousals with migraine. Headache. 1979;19(7):364–9.
8. Kayed K, Sjaastad O. Nocturnal and early morning headaches. Ann Clin Res. 1985;17(5):243–6.
9. Kayed K, Godtlibsen OB, Sjaastad O. Chronic paroxysmal hemicrania IV: "REM sleep locked" nocturnal headache attacks. Sleep. 1978;1(1):91–5.
10. Pfaffenrath V, Pollmann W, Ruther E, Lund R, Hajak G. Onset of nocturnal attacks of chronic cluster headache in relation to sleep stages. Acta Neurol Scand. 1986;73(4):403–7.
11. Koehler PJ. Prevalence of headache in Tulp's Observationes Medicae (1641) with a description of cluster headache. Cephalalgia. 1993;13(5):318–20.
12. Russell D. Cluster headache: severity and temporal profiles of attacks and patient activity prior to and during attacks. Cephalalgia. 1981;1(4):209–16.
13. Kudrow L, McGinty DJ, Phillips ER, Stevenson M. Sleep apnea in cluster headache. Cephalalgia. 1984;4(1):33–8.
14. Graff-Radford SB, Teruel A. Cluster headache and obstructive sleep apnea: are they related disorders? Curr Pain Headache Rep. 2009;13(2):160–3.
15. Chervin RD, Zallek SN, Lin X, Hall JM, Sharma N, Hedger KM. Sleep disordered breathing in patients with cluster headache. Neurology. 2000;54(12):2302–6.
16. Graff-Radford SB, Newman A. Obstructive sleep apnea and cluster headache. Headache. 2004;44(6):607–10.
17. Nobre ME, Leal AJ, Filho PM. Investigation into sleep disturbance of patients suffering from cluster headache. Cephalalgia. 2005;25(7):488–92.
18. Vetrugno R, Pierangeli G, Leone M, Bussone G, Franzini A, Brogli G, et al. Effect on sleep of posterior hypothalamus stimulation in cluster headache. Headache. 2007;47(7):1085–90.
19. Odegard SS, Engstrom M, Sand T, Stovner LJ, Zwart JA, Hagen K. Associations between sleep disturbance and primary headaches: the third Nord-Trondelag health study. J Headache Pain. 2010;11(3):197–206.
20. Kristiansen HA, Kvaerner KJ, Akre H, Overland B, Russell MB. Tension-type headache and sleep apnea in the general population. J Headache Pain. 2011;12(1):63–9.
21. Raskin NH. The hypnic headache syndrome. Headache. 1988;28(8):534–6.
22. Goadsby PJ, Lipton RB. A review of paroxysmal hemicranias, SUNCT syndrome and other short-lasting headaches with autonomic feature, including new cases. Brain. 1997;120(Pt 1):193–209.
23. Dodick DW, Mosek AC, Campbell JK. The hypnic ("alarm clock") headache syndrome. Cephalalgia. 1998;18(3):152–6.
24. Karthik N, Kulkarni GB, Taly AB, Rao S, Sinha S. Sleep disturbances in 'migraine without aura'—a questionnaire based study. J Neurol Sci. 2012;321:73–6.
25. Gori S, Lucchesi C, Morelli N, Maestri M, Bonanni E, Murri L. Sleep-related migraine occurrence increases with aging. Acta Neurol Belg. 2012;112(2):183–7.
26. Seidel S, Bock A, Schlegel W, Kilic A, Wagner G, Gelbmann G, et al. Increased RLS prevalence in children and adolescents with migraine: a case-control study. Cephalalgia. 2012;32(9):693–9.
27. Schurks M, Winter AC, Berger K, Buring JE, Kurth T. Migraine and restless legs syndrome in women. Cephalalgia. 2012;32(5):382–9.
28. Rhode AM, Hosing VG, Happe S, Biehl K, Young P, Evers S. Comorbidity of migraine and restless legs syndrome—a case-control study. Cephalalgia. 2007;27(11):1255–60.
29. d'Onofrio F, Bussone G, Cologno D, Petretta V, Buzzi MG, Tedeschi G, et al. Restless legs syndrome and primary headaches: a clinical study. Neurol Sci. 2008;29(Suppl. 1):S169–72.
30. Chen PK, Fuh JL, Chen SP, Wang SJ. Association between restless legs syndrome and migraine. J Neurol Neurosurg Psychiatry. 2010;81(5):524–8.
31. Cannon PR, Larner AJ. Migraine and restless legs syndrome: is there an association? J. Headache Pain. 2011;12(4):405–9.
32. Cevoli S, Giannini G, Favoni V, Pierangeli G, Cortelli P. Migraine and sleep disorders. Neurol Sci. 2012;33(Suppl. 1):S43–6.
33. Dahmen N, Kasten M, Wieczorek S, Gencik M, Epplen JT, Ullrich B. Increased frequency of migraine in narcoleptic patients: a confirmatory study. Cephalalgia. 2003;23(1):14–9.
34. Dahmen N, Querings K, Grun B, Bierbrauer J. Increased frequency of migraine in narcoleptic patients. Neurology. 1999;52(6):1291–3.
35. DMKG Study Group. Migraine and idiopathic narcolepsy—a case-control study. Cephalalgia. 2003;23(8):786–9.
36. Sevillano-Garcia MD, Manso-Calderon R, Cacabelos-Perez P. Comorbidity in the migraine: depression, anxiety, stress and insomnia. Rev Neurol. 2007;45(7):400–5. (Comorbilidad en la migrana: depresion, ansiedad, estres y trastornos del sueno).
37. Lateef T, Swanson S, Cui L, Nelson K, Nakamura E, Merikangas K. Headaches and sleep problems among adults in the United

States: findings from the National Comorbidity Survey-Replication study. Cephalalgia. 2011;31(6):648–53.

38. Yeung WF, Chung KF, Wong CY. Relationship between insomnia and headache in community-based middle-aged Hong Kong Chinese women. J Headache Pain. 2010;11(3):187–95.

39. Peres MF, Stiles MA, Siow HC, Silberstein SD. Excessive daytime sleepiness in migraine patients. J Neurol Neurosurg Psychiatry. 2005;76(10):1467–8.

40. Barbanti P, Fabbrini G, Aurilia C, Vanacore N, Cruccu G. A case-control study on excessive daytime sleepiness in episodic migraine. Cephalalgia. 2007;27(10):1115–9.

41. Aldrich MS, Chauncey JB. Are morning headaches part of obstructive sleep apnea syndrome? Arch Intern Med. 1990;150(6):1265–7.

42. Seidel S, Frantal S, Oberhofer P, Bauer T, Scheibel N, Albert F, et al. Morning headaches in snorers and their bed partners: a prospective diary study. Cephalalgia. 2012;32(12):888–95.

43. Goksan B, Gunduz A, Karadeniz D, Agan K, Tascilar FN, Tan F, et al. Morning headache in sleep apnoea: clinical and polysomnographic evaluation and response to nasal continuous positive airway pressure. Cephalalgia. 2009;29(6):635–41.

44. Ohayon MM. Prevalence and risk factors of morning headaches in the general population. Arch Intern Med. 2004;164(1):97–102.

45. Armstrong-Jones R. Snapping of the brain. Lancet. 1920;196(5066):720.

46. Sachs C, Svanborg E. The exploding head syndrome: polysomnographic recordings and therapeutic suggestions. Sleep. 1991;14(3):263–6.

47. American Academy of Sleep Medicine. International classification of sleep disorders: diagnostic and coding manual. 3rd ed. Darien, IL: American Academy of Sleep Medicine; 2014.

48. Chakravarty A. Exploding head syndrome: report of two new cases. Cephalalgia. 2008;28(4):399–400.

49. Palikh GM, Vaughn BV. Topiramate responsive exploding head syndrome. J Clin Sleep Med. 2010;6(4):382–3.

50. Graham JR, Wolff HG. Mechanism of migraine headache and action of Ergotamine Tartrate. Arch Neurpsych. 1938;39(4):737–63.

51. Peroutka SJ. Sumatriptan in acute migraine: pharmacology and review of world experience. Headache. 1990;30(Suppl. 2):554–60.

52. Loder E. Prophylaxis: headaches that never happen. Headache. 2008;48(5):694–6.

53. Goadsby PJ, Cittadini E, Burns B, Cohen AS. Trigeminal autonomic cephalalgias: diagnostic and therapeutic developments. Curr Opin Neurol. 2008;21(3):323–30.

54. Diener HC, Obermann M, Holle D. Hypnic headache: clinical course and treatment. Curr Treat Options Neurol. 2012;14(1):15–26.

Part VIII
Psychiatric and Psychological Sleep Disorders

Depression

38

Michelle M. Primeau, Joshua Z. Tal and Ruth O'Hara

Introduction

Sleep has long been recognized as an associated feature of psychiatric conditions. *The Diagnostic and Statistical Manual of Mental Disorders* [1] (DSM-IV) includes some form of disordered sleep in the diagnostic criteria of a variety of mood, anxiety, and cognitive disorders. Furthermore, on a subclinical level, most people can attest to the subjective mood and cognitive disturbance following even one night of sleep loss. Although conventional now, the connections between psychopathology and sleep were not explored until the 1900s. The first to brave the unchartered intersections of sleep and emotions was Sigmund Freud. He posited that dreaming was a vehicle for the expression of intolerable wishes that waking life could not entertain [2]. Despite its scientific limitations, Freud's interpretation of dreams provided the foundation for both scientific and popular conceptions of sleep.

As a graduate student interested in psychiatry, a young William Dement worked in the lab of physiologist Nathaniel Kleitman, who had pioneered the empiric study of sleep. Dement's hope was to apply the newly established objective measures of sleep to evaluate the speculations of psychoanalysis. With time, Dement's interests became far more extensive, encapsulating many sleep avenues. With the help of Christian Guilleminault, Mary Carskadon, and Vincent Zarcone, Dement went on to found the first Sleep Clinic at Stanford University in the Department of Psychiatry, and he became an outspoken advocate for the recognition and treatment of sleep disorders [3].

Sleep Deprivation and Mood

Early investigations of sleep were descriptive, attempting to outline sleep fundamentals. Guilleminault et al. [4] noted a higher than expected prevalence of depression and anxiety in men presenting with sleep complaints. These symptoms were in part attributed to a "repetitive sleep deprivation syndrome," and the physiologic consequences of sleep-disordered breathing [5]. Early sleep researchers expected that the psychological consequences of sleep loss were restricted to selective deprivation of REM sleep, following Freud's theory [4]. However, patients who were awoken mid-non-REM (NREM) sleep displayed similar effects on mood, so it appeared sleep's impact on mood was not specific to dysfunctional dream sleep [4]. One meta-analysis found that, overall, sleep deprivation appears to have the greatest impact on mood, followed by repercussions on cognitive tasks [5]. Motor performance was shown to be the least affected by sleep deprivation, though the effect size was still large (-0.87) [5]. Furthermore, partial sleep deprivation (<5 h/24 h period), rather than short- or long-term total sleep deprivation, exacted the most acute influences on mood and cognition [5].

The 1970s presented a shift in sleep deprivation research, as sleep deprivation revealed antidepressant effects when applied to people with endogenous depression [6, 7]. One study found significant improvements on multiple objective and subjective mood and cognition ratings in patients with endogenous depression after one night's sleep deprivation, compared to controls [8]. Controls, however, did depict elevated "dysphoria" and "activation" scores under identical procedures [9]. Given the immense effort required to maintain the wakefulness required of sleep deprivation, it was not considered a practical treatment option [9]. Even partial sleep deprivation was found to be too difficult and not potent enough to institute [10]. Regardless, more than 50 % of individuals do achieve an antidepressant response to sleep deprivation [10]. The response is transient as 83 % will relapse after a night of recovery sleep [10], and as such, is little used today.

R. O'Hara (✉) · M. M. Primeau · J. Z. Tal
Department of Psychiatry and Behavioral Sciences, Stanford University, Stanford, CA, USA
e-mail: roh@stanford.edu

VA MIRECC Fellowship Program, VA Palo Alto, Palo Alto, CA, USA

S. Chokroverty, M. Billiard (eds.), *Sleep Medicine,* DOI 10.1007/978-1-4939-2089-1_38,
© Springer Science+Business Media, LLC 2015

Sleep Architecture Changes with Depression

Sixty to ninety percent of individuals with major depressive disorder (MDD) report disrupted sleep [11]. The 1960s introduced clinical recognition of the link between sleep and psychiatric conditions, spurring researchers to investigate the relationship of sleep to the cardinal mood disorder, depression [12]. Initial attempts were unsuccessful in finding a unifying model of the interaction of depression and sleep [13]. Subjective ratings of sleep were not able to explain the cause of depressive symptomatology to a satisfactory degree [13]. Some depressed patients presented chronic insomnia, with increased sleep latency and decreased sleep efficiency. Others presented hypersomnia, sleeping 10–14 h in a 24-h period.

As the field of sleep medicine progressed within the scientific community and the technology became more refined, psychiatrists started to turn to the objective techniques of the burgeoning field in an attempt to understand why so many of their depressed patients complained of difficulties with sleep. Some hoped that sleep in itself would become a biomarker for the disease [14, 15]. With the use of polysomnography (PSG) and electroencephalography (EEG) to characterize sleep stages, shortened REM latency was discovered as a hallmark feature of endogenous depression, with the interval length correlating with the severity of depression [14, 15].

These EEG distinctions presented an opportunity for predicting treatment response. Initially, in studies with patients with depression, it was found that taking tricyclic antidepressants (TCAs) lead to greater suppression of REM, which in turn lead to a greater response to treatment [16]. This finding was confirmed when persistent prolonged REM latency exhibited a sustained response to treatment [17]. Furthermore, the same group found that prolonged sleep latency and shorter REM latency together were best able to predict response to treatment [18].

Over time, further abnormalities of sleep architecture have been substantiated in depression, including decreased slow wave sleep (SWS), increased REM density, prolonged sleep latency, increased fragmentation, and decreased sleep efficiency [19]. For a period, there was an active debate as to which variable was central to depression—REM or SWS changes [18]. However, a groundbreaking meta-analysis by Benca et al. [20] later demonstrated that reduction in REM latency was not specific to depressive disorders. She showed that while no specific sleep finding was pathognomonic for a specific psychiatric condition, there were consistent differences seen, especially when patients with affective disorders are compared with control groups [20].

More recently, researchers have started evaluating sleep microarchitecture utilizing specialized technology. Such techniques allow a finer analysis of the waveforms present in the EEG; shapes that are unable to be appreciated or quantified using the naked eye, but can be distinguished using various computer techniques. Like studies of the sleep macroarchitecture in depression, the results have been mixed [18]. Some studies have found alterations in SWS [21], whereas some found significant SWS patterns are restricted to male depressed sleepers [22]. Others have noted patients with MDD have less beta frequency percentage relative to patients with insomnia or controls [23]. Indeed, distinct microarchitectural patterns were found among patients with insomnia and those with coexisting depression and insomnia [24].

Sleep Disorders and Mood Disorders

Insomnia

Previously, insomnia was considered secondary to either a medical condition or psychiatric condition, and classically it was taught that treatment of the primary condition would; therefore, improve the disordered sleep disturbance [25]. However, with time, research has illustrated a more bidirectional relationship [23], and treatment of disturbed sleep has been recognized as warranting independent clinical attention [10, 26, 27].

Epidemiologic studies have shown that those with insomnia are at an increased risk of developing depression. One prospective epidemiologic study demonstrated that patients with persistent insomnia had three times the risk of developing depression when compared to those whose insomnia resolved [28]. Another epidemiologic study confirmed a sustained, elevated risk for depression lasting 34 years, for those experiencing a bout of insomnia in medical school [29]. In addition, poor sleep quality was related to the development of depressive symptoms with interferon treatment [30], and some studies have suggested an overlap of the genetics of insomnia, depression, and anxiety [31]. Furthermore, sleep disturbance has been shown to be the most common residual symptom following remission of depression [32] and reoccurrence of insomnia may herald recurrence of depression [33].

More recently, a body of literature describing the relationship of sleep disruption to suicidality has emerged. Krakow et al. [34] noted elevated self-reported suicidality in young women with a history of sexual assault, with the greatest incidence in women with symptoms of sleep-disordered breathing or movement disorders. Similarly, in patients with MDD, both insomnia and hypersomnia predict suicide risk [35]. Subjective report of insomnia in particular has been related to increased risk for suicide [36], with one meta-analysis finding a relative risk of having suicidal behavior in the presence of sleep disturbance ranging from 1.95–2.95 [37].

Similar to MDD, sleep disturbance has been implicated in the pathology of bipolar disorder (BD). One of the hallmark features of a manic episode is the "reduced need for sleep" [1], which has been described in 69–99 % of subjects while undergoing a manic episode [38]. Gruber et al. [39] found similar results when they analyzed sleep variables in 468 subjects in the National Institute of Mental Health's Systematic Treatment Enhancement Program for Bipolar Disorder (STEP-BD). They found lower total sleep time (TST) and increased sleep variability were associated with more severe manic symptoms [39]. Research on BD has associated mania's sleep disruption with an instable circadian rhythm due to genetic and social factors [38]. Beyond an emanation of mania, insomnia, and its resulting sleep disruption have been demonstrated to be one of the most robust prodromal symptoms of the onset of a manic episode. Jackson et al. [40] reviewed 73 publications on early signs of mania onset, and identified sleep disruption as the most common symptom of an impending episode. Conversely, just as sleep disruption is associated with the onset and occurrence of mania, improved sleep functioning has been associated with increased BD remission over the course of treatment [39]. One study by Nowlin-Finch et al. [41] used a blinded chart review protocol in an inpatient manic BD group to find that greater TST on the first night of hospitalization was associated with faster response to treatment and earlier discharge. As a result of this association between sleep disturbance and mania, many psychological treatments for BD incorporate components of psychological treatments for insomnia [38].

Beyond BD, there is consistent evidence that the circadian rhythm plays a role in mood disorders. Both depression and BD can manifest variation based on time, whether seasonal differences or diurnal waxing of symptoms [42]. *The Diagnostic and Statistical Manual of Mental Disorders* (DSM-IV) allows for a seasonal pattern specifier on both MDD and BD [1]. For MDD, the seasonal pattern leads to symptoms in the winter season, with full remission during other times of the year [1]. The DSM-IV describes seasonally patterned MDD as usually characterized by hypersomnia [1]. Nevertheless, some studies have documented high reports of combined hypersomnia–insomnia or insomnia alone in subjects with seasonally patterned MDD [43–45] In one of the largest studies on this issue, Øyane, et al.'s [44] group of 8860 subjects found insomnia and fatigue to be the most frequent complaints in participants with high seasonal depressive fluctuations, relative to medium and low seasonal depressive fluctuations. As a result, the authors propose two clinical subgroups of seasonally patterned MDD, one presenting the traditional hypersomnia and one presenting insomnia [44].

Sleep-Disordered Breathing

Clinical studies over the past several decades suggest the existence of a relationship between depression and sleep-disordered breathing, particularly obstructive sleep apnea (OSA). OSA is by far the most common form of sleep-disordered breathing. It is defined by frequent episodes of obstructed breathing during sleep and is characterized by sleep-related decreases (hypopneas) or pauses (apneas) in respiration. The diagnosis of OSA is confirmed when a PSG recording determines an apnea–hypopnea index (AHI) of > 5/h of sleep.

Among the first studies investigating the relation between OSA and depression, Guilleminault et al. [46] reported that 24 % patients with OSA had previously seen a psychiatrist for anxiety or depression. Reynolds et al. [47] also found approximately 40 % of OSA patients met the research diagnostic criteria for an affective disorder. While not all studies have observed a significant association between sleep apnea and depression [48], many investigations of OSA patients have been observed to have higher levels of depressive symptoms [49, 50]. OSA and depression share common risk factors, which may partly explain their high comorbidity in the general population, including obesity, cardiovascular disease, hypertension, and diabetes. Older adults have been observed to have higher rates of both OSA and depression, further underscoring the potential of comorbid medical disorders, so common in the elderly for explaining the association of OSA and depressive symptoms [50]. In a large epidemiological study of 18,980 subjects representative of the general population in their respective countries (UK, Germany, Italy, Portugal, and Spain) and assessed by telephone survey, Ohayon [51] found 17.6 % of subjects with a DSM-IV breathing-related sleep disorder diagnosis also presented with a MDD diagnosis, and vice versa, after controlling for obesity and hypertension.

In one of the most comprehensive investigations of this issue, Peppard et al. [52] conducted a population-based epidemiological study to examine if sleep-disordered breathing was a longitudinal predictor of subsequent depression. This study had a sample of 788 men and 620 women randomly selected and evaluated for sleep apnea with in-laboratory PSG and for depression with the Zung depression scale, assessed at 4-year intervals. The authors found an increase of one sleep-disordered breathing category, e.g., from minimal to mild OSA, to be associated with a 1.8-fold increased adjusted odds for developing depression. Their findings provide evidence for a dose–response association between sleep apnea and depression and suggest a potential causal link between these conditions.

Two factors hypothesized to be responsible for depressive symptoms in OSA are sleep fragmentation and oxygen desaturation during sleep, but systematic studies examining these components in OSA patients with depression are limited. Preliminary imaging data suggest that OSA-associated hypoxemia may result in cerebral white matter hyperintensities (WMH), which in turn have a negative impact on mood. Aloia et al. [53] found more subcortical WMH in the brain magnetic resonance imaging (MRI) of patients with severe OSA, and a tendency for a positive correlation between these subcortical hyperintensities and depression scores on the Hamilton Depression Scale. On the neurotransmitter level, the serotoninergic system has a central role as a neurobiological substrate of mood and sleep regulations, in addition to upper airway muscle tone control during sleep. More recently, in nondepressed subjects, the serotonin transporter polymorphism long allele has been found to be associated with increased levels of OSA, suggesting a potential common biological mechanism for OSA and depressive symptoms [54].

Molecules increasing 5-HT neurotransmission such as the serotonin reuptake inhibitors (SSRI) are widely prescribed and are suggested to improve OSA. However, serotoninergic drugs have already been tested for OSA, with limited success and numerous adverse effects [55]. Several 5-HT receptor ligands and bifunctional molecules are under development, which may in the future be able to target both—the depressive syndrome and OSA.

In sum, the extant literature underscores the existence of a complex relationship between OSA and depression with respect to clinical presentation, treatment, and underlying pathophysiology. Given that up to 20% of all patients presenting with diagnosed OSA may also have depressive syndrome, sleep medicine practitioners should be careful to assess for depression in patients with OSA. Further, the relationship of OSA to depressive symptoms may vary, depending on age, gender, and health characteristics of OSA patients. Future clinical research and basic research studies are required to more fully characterize the relationship between depression and OSA, as well as the potential mechanisms by which both disorders may interact.

Narcolepsy

As a disease, narcolepsy has contributed much to the history of sleep medicine. After it was first described, narcolepsy was proposed to have both a primary and secondary etiology, which could include a psychosomatic component [56]. In 1960, Vogel [57] discovered short REM latencies in patients with narcolepsy, arising from an interest in validating psychoanalytic concepts of sleep and dreams. In fact, when Dement first started the Sleep Clinic at Stanford University, characterizing narcolepsy was one of his primary goals [3].

Narcolepsy remains difficult to recognize by many providers, and it is frequently mistaken for depression [58, 59].

This may partly be due to symptom overlap between the two conditions, such as fatigue, decreased concentration, appetite changes, and sleep disruption, though depressive symptoms are not a prominent component of narcolepsy's presentation [60]. In one study utilizing a semi-structured interview to control for some of the overlapping symptoms, patients with narcolepsy did reveal elevated prevalence of cognitive symptoms of depression, though not reaching the level of major depression [60].

Other similarities have been drawn between narcolepsy and depression using polysomnogram (PSG) measures. Both are characterized by a shortened REM latency and fragmented nocturnal sleep, though certainly to a different extent [59]. Upon meta-analysis, both conditions are associated with significant sleep disruption, with the finding of greater sleep disruption in those with narcolepsy, as would be expected [61].

Interestingly, antidepressants have demonstrated efficacy in treating narcolepsy with cataplexy. TCAs were shown to be successful in decreasing cataplectic attacks, through the REM-suppressing effects of the medication class [62], and newer classes of antidepressants, such as selective serotonin reuptake inhibitors (SSRIs) and serotonin–norepinephrine reuptake inhibitors (SNRIs) are preferred today, due to a more favorable side-effect profile [63]. Unlike the treatment of depression, where antidepressants can take up 4–6 weeks to take effect, antidepressants are immediately helpful in the treatment of cataplexy [61]. Gammhydroxybutyrate (GHB) is another unique treatment for narcolepsy. GHB was initially developed as an anesthetic, but unlike other sedating agents, it was found to increase REM and SWS [61]. Due to the aforementioned debate as to the relative importance of SWS and REM sleep in depression, GHB was hypothesized to remit mood symptoms, but instead induced changes similar to narcolepsy [64]. Based on these findings, some have proposed REM induction as a biological marker for depression [65]. In fact, early in the development of GHB, it was given to psychiatric patients with depression and anxiety, but was abandoned as other medications with a wider therapeutic index, such as TCAs and benzodiazepines, came into wider use [63]. Recent attention has returned to study GHB as a novel treatment for patients with depression [63].

Restless Legs Syndrome

Recent inquiries into comorbid mood and sleep disorders have focused on depressive symptoms in patients with restless legs syndrome (RLS). Elevated rates of depressive symptoms have been described in variety of populations with RLS [66]. One epidemiologic study utilizing the Nurses' Health Study information noted increased risk for depression in those with RLS (RR = 1.6), and higher depression scores at subsequent follow-up in those with RLS [67]. When investigating patients with endogenous depression, research has similarly found an elevated rate of RLS symptoms in these patients [66]. The most striking clinical implication for treatment of depression is research demonstrating that SSRIs and SNRIs increased periodic limb movements and precipitated RLS symptoms [68].

Treatment

Historically, disordered sleep was considered epiphenomena of depression, but with time, the perspective evolved to incorporate a bidirectional relationship between coexisting conditions [69]. This led researchers to target sleep disorders, which have demonstrated antidepressant effects. In one well-designed study of patients meeting DSM-IV criteria for both MDD and insomnia, co-therapy with fluoxetine and eszopiclone versus fluoxetine and placebo led not only to greater improvement in sleep measures but also to a quicker and more sustained antidepressant response, even after discontinuation of the sleep medication [70, 71]. Similarly, cognitive behavioral therapy for insomnia, which has been shown to be effective in the treatment of insomnia, also can enhance treatment of depressive symptoms in patients with comorbid depressive symptoms [72]. With respect to sleep-disordered breathing, a systematic review on the influence of continuous positive airway pressure (CPAP), the gold standard treatment for OSA, on neurobehavioral performance of OSA patients found that depressive symptoms remit along with excessive daytime sleepiness following CPAP treatment [73].

Conclusion

In conclusion, the early history of sleep medicine owes much to the contributions of psychiatrists exploring the fascinating world of sleep; however, time has shown that psychiatrists have much to learn from the field of sleep medicine as well. There is an important, bidirectional relationship between sleep and depression, which has yet to be completely understood. The fields of psychiatry and sleep have expressed a similar pattern of interaction, spurring research in one or the other to parse the components of diagnoses and treatment together. Early interest in sleep biomarkers drove a large amount of PSG data in the past, while recent advances in the study of sleep disorders such as insomnia, sleep apnea, or narcolepsy have uncovered details that inform future research in depression.

References

1. American Psychiatric Association. Diagnostic and statistical manual of mental disorders: DSM-IV-TR. 4th edn. (text revision). Washington, DC: American Psychiatric Association; 2000
2. Freud S. The interpretation of dreams. In: Strachey J, editor. The standard edition of the complete psychological works of Sigmund Freud, vols 4 and 5. London: Hogwarth; 1953.
3. Hobson JA. Sleep medicine and psychiatry: history and significance. In: Winkleman JW, Plante DT, editors. Foundations of psychiatric sleep medicine. New York: Cambridge University Press. 2010.
4. Guilleminault C, Eldrich FL, Tilkian A, et al. Sleep apnea syndrome due to upper airway obstruction. Arch Int Med. 1977;137:296–300.
5. Pilcher JJ, Huffcutt AI. Effects of sleep deprivation on performance: a meta-analysis. Sleep.1996;19:318–26.
6. Pflug B, Tolle R. Therapy for endogenous depression by means of sleep deprivation. Der Nervenarzt. 1971;42:117–24.
7. Svendsen K. Sleep deprivation therapy in depression. Acta Psychiat Scand. 1976;54:184–92.
8. Gerner RH, Post RM, Gillin C, et al. Biological and behavioral effects of one night's sleep deprivation in depressed patients and normals. J Psychiat Res. 1979;15:21–40.
9. Germain A, Buysee DJ, Nofzinger EA. Sleep-specific mechanisms underlying posttraumatic stress disorder: integrative review and neurobiological hypothesis. Sleep Med Rev. 2008;12:185–95.
10. Wu JC, Bunney WE. The biologic basis of an antidepressant response to sleep deprivation and relapse: review and hypothesis. Am J Psychiatry. 1990;147:14–21.
11. Kloss J, Szuba M. Insomnia in psychiatric disorders. In: Szuba MP, Kloss JD, Dinges DF, editors. Insomnia: principles and management. New York: Cambridge University Press; 2003. p. 43–70.
12. Kupfer D, Harrow M, Detre T. Sleep patterns and psychopathology. Acta Psychiat Scan. 1969;45:75–89.
13. Kupfer D, Foster F. Interval between onset of sleep and rapid eye movement sleep as an indicator of depression. Lancet. 1972;2:684–6.
14. Kupfer DJ, Foster FG, Coble P, et al. The application of EEG sleep for the differential diagnosis of affective disorders. Am J Psychiatry. 1978;135:69–74.
15. Kupfer D, Foster F. Interval between onset of sleep and rapid eye movement sleep as an indicator of depression. Lancet. 1972;2:684–86.
16. Kupfer DJ, Foster FG, Reich L, et al. EEG sleep changes as predictors in depression. Am J Psychiatry. 1976;133:622–26.
17. Kupfer DJ. The application of EEG sleep for the differential diagnosis and treatment of affective disorders. Pharmakopsychiatr Neuropsychopharmakol. 1978;11:17–26.
18. Kupfer DJ, Spiker DG, Coble PA, et al. Sleep and treatment prediction in endogenous depression. Am J Psychiatry. 1981;138:429–34.
19. Gerhman PR, Thase ME, Riemann D, et al. Sleep disturbance in psychiatric illness depressive disorders. In: Winkleman JW, Plante DT, editors. Foundations of psychiatric sleep medicine. Cambridge: Cambridge University Press 2011.
20. Benca RM, Obermeyer WH, Thisted RA, et al. Sleep and psychiatric disorders: a meta-analysis. Arch Gen Psychiatry. 1992;4:651–68.
21. Armitage R. Microarchitectural findings in sleep EEG in depression: diagnostic implications. Biol Psychiatry. 1995;35:72–84.
22. Armitage R, Hoffman R, Trivedi M, et al. Slow-wave activity in NREM sleep: sex and age effects in depressed outpatients and healthy control. Psychiatry Res. 2000;95:201–13.
23. Perlis ML, Smith MT, Andrew PJ, et al. Beta/gamma EEG activity in patients with primary and secondary insomnia and good sleeper controls. Sleep. 2001;24:110–7.
24. Staner L, Cornette F, Maurice D, et al. Sleep microstructure around sleep onset differentiates major depressive insomnia from primary insomnia. J Sleep Res. 2003;12:319–30.

25. Benca RM, Peterson MJ. Insomnia and depression. Sleep Med. 2008;9:S3–9.
26. Ancoli-Israel S, Martin J, Jones DW, et al. Sleep disordered breathing and periodic limb movements in sleep in older patients with schizophrenia. Biol Psychiatry. 1999;45:1426–32.
27. Aldrich MS, Brower KJ, Hall JM. Sleep-disordered breathing in alcoholics. Alcohol Clin Exp Res. 1999;23:134–40.
28. Ford D, Kamerow D. Epidemiologic study of sleep disturbances in psychiatric disorders. J Am Med Ass. 1989;262:1479–84.
29. Chang PP, Ford DE, Mead LA, et al. Insomnia in young men and subsequent depression. Am J Epidemiol. 1997;146:105–14.
30. Franzen PL, Buysee DJ, Rabinovich M, et al. Poor sleep quality predicts onset of either major depression or subsyndromal depression with irritability during interferon-alpha treatment. Psychiatry Res. 2010;177:240–5.
31. Gehrman PR, Meltzer LJ, Moore M, et al. Heritability of insomnia symptoms in youth and their relationship to depression and anxiety. Sleep. 2011;34:1641–6.
32. Nierenberg AA, Husain MM, Trivedi MH, et al. Residual symptoms after remission of major depressive disorder with citalopram and risk for relapse: A STAR*D report. Psychol Med. 2010;10:41–50.
33. Perlis ML, Giles DE, Buysse DJ, et al. Self- reported sleep disturbance as a prodromal symptom in recurrent depression. J Affect Disord. 1997;42:209–12.
34. Krakow B, Artar A, Warner TD, et al. Sleep disorder, depression, and suicidality in female sexual assault survivors. Crisis. 2000;21:130–70.
35. Agargun MY, Kara H, Solmaz M. Sleep disturbances and suicidal behavior in patients with major depression. J Clin Psychiatry. 1997;58:249–51.
36. Bernart RA, Joiner TE, Cukrowicz KC, et al. Suicidality and sleep disturbances. Sleep. 2005;28:1135–41.
37. Pigeon WR, Pinquart M, Conner K. Meta-analysis of sleep disturbance and suicidal thoughts and behaviors. J Clin Psychiatry. 2012;73:1160–7.
38. Harvey AG. Sleep and circadian rhythms in bipolar disorder: seeking synchrony, harmony, and regulation. Am J Psychiatry. 2008;165(7):820–9.
39. Gruber J, Miklowitz DJ, Harvey AG, et al. Sleep matters: sleep functioning and course of illness in bipolar disorder. J Affect Disord. 2011;134(1–3):416–20.
40. Jackson A, Cavanagh J, Scott J. A systematic review of manic and depressive prodromes. J Affect Disord. 2003;74(3):209–17.
41. Nowlin-Finch NL, Altshuler LL, Szuba MP, et al. Rapid resolution of first episodes of mania: sleep related? J Clin Psychiatry. 1994;55(1):26–9.
42. Lader M. Limitations of current medical treatments for depression: disturbed circadian rhythms as a possible therapeutic target. Eur Neuropsychopharm. 2007;17(12):743–55.
43. Roecklein KA, Carney CE, Wong PM, et al. The role of beliefs and attitudes about sleep in seasonal and nonseasonal mood disorder, and nondepressed controls. J Affect Disord. 2013;150:466–73.
44. Øyane NM, Ursin R, Pallesen S, et al. Self-reported seasonality is associated with complaints of sleep problems and deficient sleep duration: the Hordaland health study. J Sleep Res. 2008;17(1):63–72.
45. Anderson JL, Rosen LN, Mendelson WB, et al. Sleep in fall/winter seasonal affective disorder: effects of light and changing seasons. J Psychosom Res. 1994;38(4):323–37.
46. Guilleminault C, Eldridge FL, Tilkian A, et al. Sleep apnea syndrome due to upper airway obstruction: a review of 25 cases. Arch Intern Med. 1977;137:296–300.
47. Reynolds CF, Kupfer DJ, McEachran AB, et al. Depressive psychopathology in male sleep apneics. J Clin Psychiatry. 1984;45:287–90.
48. Phillips BA, Berry DT, Lipke-Molby TC. Sleep-disordered breathing in healthy, aged persons. Fifth and final year follow-up. Chest. 1996;110:654–8.
49. Kales A, Caldwell AB, Cadieux RJ, et al. Severe obstructive sleep apnea—II: associated psychopathology and psychosocial consequences. J Chronic Dis. 1985;38:427–34.
50. Schröder CM, O'Hara R. Depression and obstructive sleep apnea. Ann Gen Psychiatry. 2005;27;4:13.
51. Ohayon MM: The effects of breathing-related sleep disorders on mood disturbances in the general population. J Clin Psychiatry. 2003;64:1195–200.
52. Peppard PE, Szklo-Coxe M, Hla KM, et al. Longitudinal association of sleep-related breathing disorder and depression. Arch Intern Med. 2006;18:1709–15.
53. Aloia MS, Arnedt JT, Davis JD, et al. Neuropsychological sequelae of obstructive sleep apnea-hypopnea syndrome: a critical review. J Int Neuropsychol Soc. 2004;10:772–85.
54. Yue W, Liu H, Zhang J, et al. Association study of serotonin transporter gene polymorphisms with obstructive sleep apnea syndrome in Chinese Han population. Sleep. 2008;31:1535–41.
55. Veasey SC. Serotonin agonists and antagonists in obstructive sleep apnea: therapeutic potential. Am J Respir Med. 2003;2:21–9.
56. Foruyn HAD, Mulders PC, Renier WO, et al. Narcolepsy and psychiatry: an evolving association of increasing interest. Sleep Med. 2011;12:714–9.
57. Vogel G. Studies in psychophysiology of dreams III: the dream of narcolepsy. Arch Gen Psychiatry. 1960;3:421–8.
58. Kauta SR, Marcus CL. Cases of pediatric narcolepsy after misdiagnoses. Pediatr Neurol. 2012;47:362–5.
59. Kryger MH, Walid R, Manfreda J. Diagnoses received by narcolepsy patients in the year prior to diagnosis by a sleep specialist. Sleep. 2002;25:36–41.
60. Adda C, Lefevre B, Reimao R. Narcolepsy and depression. Arq Neuropsiquiatr. 1997;55:323–6.
61. Hudson JI, Pope HG, Sullivan LE, et al. Good sleep bad sleep: a meta-analysis of polysomnographic measures of insomnia, depression and narcolepsy. Biol Psychiatry. 1992;32:958–75.
62. Guilleminault C, Caskadon M, Dement W. On the treatment of rapid eye movement narcolepsy. Arch of Neurol. 1974;30:90–3.
63. Mignot E. A practical guide to the therapy of narcolepsy and hypersomnia syndromes. Neurotherapeutics. 2012;9:739–52.
64. Mamelak M. Narcolepsy and depression and the neurobiology of gammahydroxybutyrate. Progress Neurobiol. 2009;89:193–219.
65. Bosch OG, Quednow BB, Seifritz E, et al. Reconsidering GHB: orphan drug or new model antidepressant? J Psychopharmacol. 2012;26:618–28.
66. Picchietti D, Winkelman JW. Restless legs syndrome, periodic limb movements in sleep, and depression. Sleep. 2005;28:891–8.
67. Li Y, Mirzaei F, O'Reilly EJ, et al. Prospective study of restless legs syndrome and depression in women. Am J Epidemiol. 2012;176:279–88.
68. Rottach KG, Schaner BM, Kirch MH, Zivotofsky AZ, Teufel LM, Gallwitz T, et al. Restless legs syndrome as side effect of second generation antidepressants. J Psychiatric Res. 2008 Nov;43(1):70–5.
69. Riemann D. Does effective management of sleep disorders reduce depressive symptoms and the risk of depression? Drugs. 2009;69(S2):43–64.
70. Fava M, McCall WV, Krystal A, et al. Eszopiclone co-administered with fluoxetine in patients with insomnia coexisting with major depressive disorder. Biol Psychiatry. 2006;59:1052–60.
71. Krystal A, Fava M, Rubens R, et al. Evaluation of eszopiclone discontinuation after cotherapy with fluoxetine for insomnia with coexisting depression. J Clin Sleep Med. 2007;3:48–55.
72. Manber R, Edinger JD, Gress JL, et al. Cognitive behavioral therapy for insomnia enhances depression outcome in patients with comorbid major depressive disorder and insomnia. Sleep. 2008;31:489–95.
73. McMahon JP, Foresman BH, Chisholm RC. The influence of CPAP on the neurobehavioral performance of patients with obstructive sleep apnea hypopnea syndrome: a systematic review. WMJ. 2003;102:36–43.

Schizophrenia and Psychosis

Brady A. Riedner, Fabio Ferrarelli and Ruth M. Benca

In a sense, psychosis, loosely defined as "loss of contact with reality," is a state of being that happens to all of us each night when we fall asleep. The association between psychosis and sleep is even further strengthened when one considers that psychosis implies not simply a lack of connection with external reality, but a bizarre transformation of consciousness where the mind sees what is not there, emotional content is intensified, the flow of information or time is disjointed, and the sense of one's self is confused. This is what usually happens when we dream. A link between psychosis and sleep has been hypothesized for a long time. In *De Somniis,* Aristotle stated, "the faculty by which, in waking hours, we are subject to illusion when affected by disease, is identical with that which produces illusory effects in sleep" [1]. More directly, the renowned German philosopher Arthur Schopenhauer, whose writings would significantly influence Sigmund Freud, remarked "a dream is a short-lasting psychosis and psychosis is a long-lasting dream" [2]. The bond between psychosis and sleep seems to have gained even more momentum after the turn of the century as the inquiry into dreams became a central theme in psychiatry. It is noteworthy that almost all of the early papers reporting on sleep in schizophrenia begin with a quote or a reference relating dreams and psychosis. If not from the earlier mentioned philosophers, then from Jung, "Let the dreamer walk about and act like one awakened, and we have the clinical picture of dementia praecox" [3] or noted British neurologist Hughlings Jackson, who quipped, "Find out about dreams and you will find out about insanity." [4]. If so many of the great thinkers recognized it, how could it not be that sleep would tell us all we needed to know about psychosis and schizophrenia?

At about the same time dream research was making an impact in psychiatry, Kraepelin [5] and Bleuler [6] developed the clinical criteria for schizophrenia. Prior to their work, it is likely that most signs of the disease fell under the general rubric of "madness" [7]. Schizophrenia is a complex thought disorder that typically includes several symptoms from the following categories: a psychotic dimension including hallucinations and delusions; a disorganized dimension that includes disorganized speech, bizarre behavior, and inappropriate affect; and a negative dimension including lack of volition and blunted affect [8]. Cognitive impairments, like working memory deficits and attention difficulties, often accompany the disease. Schizophrenia is widely regarded as the most devastating of psychiatric illnesses based on the early age of onset and the socially debilitating nature of the disease for many sufferers. Although treatment has certainly improved outcomes for many sufferers, schizophrenia still places an immense burden on immediate family and society in general and represents a still largely unsolved puzzle for mental health providers. Despite a century of intense research, the origin and pathophysiology of schizophrenia remain elusive.

Psychiatrists were interested in studying the relationship between sleep and schizophrenia even before the discovery of rapid eye movement (REM) sleep and its association with dreaming. Although Kraepelin himself noted, in his seminal work, that "during the whole development of the disease, the sleep of the patients is frequently disturbed even when they are lying quiet," [5] early sleep research focused almost exclusively on the content of dreams in schizophrenic and psychotic patients. The first published work in a scholarly journal studying hallucinations and dreams can be traced back to Trapp in 1937, which included 15 patients diagnosed with dementia praecox, a term initially introduced by Kreepelin to describe schizophrenia [9]. Trapp reported that the content of waking hallucinations often influenced dream content, and

R. M. Benca (✉)
Departments of Psychiatry and Psycology, Center for Sleep Medicine and Sleep Research, University of Wisconsin-Madison, 6001 Research Park Blvd, Madison, WI 53719, USA
e-mail: rmbenca@wisc.edu

B. A. Riedner
Psychiatric Institute, University of Wisconsin-Madison, Madison, WI, USA

F. Ferrarelli
Department of Psychiatry, School of Medicine and Public Health, University of Wisconsin-Madison, Madison, WI, USA

S. Chokroverty, M. Billiard (eds.), *Sleep Medicine,* DOI 10.1007/978-1-4939-2089-1_39,
© Springer Science+Business Media, LLC 2015

that when hallucinations subsided, dream content no longer related to previous hallucinations. Later research, however, found no obvious difference in the amount or content of dreams in schizophrenics relative to normal subjects [10, 11].

After its discovery in 1953, REM sleep quickly became a primary target for the investigation of sleep in schizophrenia [12]. Beginning with Dement's classic work in 1955, researchers looked at how REM sleep might be altered in schizophrenia [13]. Dement was the first to use the electroencephalogram (EEG) and electrooculogram (EOG) to examine alterations in REM sleep in schizophrenic patients. The basic assumption was that if REM sleep represented an electrophysiological correlate of dreaming, and dreaming and psychoses were to share a common neural mechanism, then the study of REM in schizophrenic patients might reveal important insights into this disorder. It was generally postulated that this common mechanism might be overactive in schizophrenics, causing them to have abnormal amounts of REMs during sleep. However, early studies found few consistent differences in the amount of REM sleep between schizophrenics and normal subjects [13, 14], even during periods of the illness when subjects were acutely hallucinating [15, 16].

Influenced heavily by Freud and the psychoanalytic tradition prevalent at the time, some researchers interpreted these early negative results in an alternative light. Instead of schizophrenic patients having too much "dreaming" sleep, perhaps the suppression of dreaming sleep or some modification of dreaming control may lead to waking psychosis in schizophrenics [17]. In other words, was schizophrenia a case of dreaming sleep "bleeding" into wakefulness to cause waking psychoses? Subsequent research would initially diminish support for this hypothesis, as investigators were unable to find consistent evidence during waking of electrophysiological signs of REM sleep in schizophrenics [18]. Nor did it appear that REM sleep-specific deprivation experiments had a unique effect on schizophrenics [19], despite early reports of modified REM rebound [20]. Researchers tended to interpret findings of decreased REM latency, the time it takes to reach the first REM period, as reflecting increased dreaming pressure in schizophrenia [21, 22] but this finding was also not consistently replicated [23]. Attempts to quantify REM density, a measure of the frequency of REMs during REM sleep [23], or other REM phasic events (i.e., middle ear contractions or periorbital integrated potentials, [24] also failed to yield abnormalities specific to schizophrenia.

Although the preponderance of early research efforts examining schizophrenia focused on REM sleep for theoretical reasons, investigators also reported noticeable deficits in the amount of nonrapid eye movement (NREM) sleep in schizophrenic patients. Several studies suggested that there

was a deficit specifically in the amount of deep NREM or slow-wave sleep (SWS) in schizophrenics relative to healthy controls [14, 25, 26]. However, it was clear even at the time that these results lacked specificity for schizophrenia [27]. Still, since it was well known that sleep, especially during periods of acute psychosis, was often severely affected in schizophrenics, including periods of profound insomnia or a complete reversal of the sleep–wake periods, research into the role of sleep in the pathophysiology of the disorder persisted. The late 1970s to early 1990s saw a vast improvement in recording techniques, more consistency in sleep and psychiatric classification, and improved data analysis opportunities as a result of access to computing resources. While the number of studies examining sleep architecture in schizophrenia remained high, subsequent meta-analysis of this work suggested that the most consistent sleep disturbances in schizophrenia were congruent with signs of insomnia (i.e. increased sleep latency and waking after sleep onset), revealing relatively little in terms of diagnostic specificity for schizophrenia [28–30].

Still, scientific interest in the relationship between sleep and schizophrenia has continued. The last two decades have seen a flourishing of sleep research in schizophrenia. This has been propelled by a better understanding of the neural circuitry and the functional significance underlying the two main rhythms that typify NREM sleep-slow waves and spindles. Animal and human studies have demonstrated how sleep slow waves are generated cortically by neuronal intrinsic conductances and are synchronized through cortico–cortical connections [31]. Spindles, instead, originate in a structure called the thalamic reticular nucleus (TRN). They are synchronized and sustained by the TRN connections with the cortex and with the thalamus, long recognized as the sensory gating mechanism for the cortex [31]. Therefore, since the late 1980s, researchers have less often turned to sleep macrostructural elements, such as amounts or timing of a particular sleep stage, in order to explain the pathophysiology of schizophrenia, differentiate schizophrenics from normal controls, and/or characterize various schizophrenic subtypes. Instead, current investigators are using sleep as a unique opportunity to examine the spontaneous activity of brain circuits of schizophrenics, as reflected by sleep-specific EEG rhythms. Exploring those rhythms, particularly during NREM sleep, allows researchers to probe neuronal integrity during a time when other concomitants of the disorder (like hallucinations, diminished attention, and decreased motivation) are relatively diminished.

Feinberg proposed his "synaptic pruning" theory of schizophrenia in 1982, in part based on his observation of sleep slow waves during normal human development. He noted that there were two periods of dramatic change in slow waves, a rapid increase in the first year of life and a precipitous fall during adolescence [32]. As a corollary, cortical synaptic density (the number of neuronal connections within a given area of tissue) appeared to follow a similar pattern, although based on relatively scant postmortem evidence at the time [33]. Feinberg argued that errors in synaptic pruning made during this critical period of neuronal synaptic reorganization could be responsible for schizophrenia [32]. Feinberg and others have focused on the observation that slow waves are homeostatically regulated during sleep. Specifically, larger and more numerous slow waves occur at the beginning of the night proportional to the time spent awake, whereas less frequent and smaller slow waves characterize the end of the night after sleep pressure has been diminished, a finding consistent with the idea that slow waves reflect synaptic plasticity in the cortex [34]. Evidence supporting the idea that changes in synaptic strength are mirrored by changes in slow wave activity (SWA), a measure of EEG power between 0.5 and 4 Hz typically used to capture the amplitude of slow waves, continues to accumulate [35]. While it is not known whether slow waves are actively participating in, or merely reflecting, neuronal change, the observation that the dramatic decline of slow waves during adolescence coincides with the typical age of symptom onset in schizophrenia deserves attention. Intriguingly, longitudinal studies of grey matter volumes in schizophrenia have shown accelerated grey matter losses during adolescence, especially in early onset schizophrenia [36–38], as would be predicted by the Feinberg model. Moreover, recent work has demonstrated that grey matter matures in a regionally and temporally complex pattern which is mirrored by the developmental changes in SWA [39–41]. Still, as was the case with amounts of SWS, the data regarding SWA abnormalities in post-adolescent schizophrenics are not consistent, with some, but not all, showing decreased SWA relative to controls, as would be predicted by the theory [42–45]. Moreover, decreased SWA is not specific for schizophrenia [46]. However, it is clear that inasmuch as they can be used as a proxy for cortical development, when combined with the ease of home monitoring of sleep EEG, as has been used by Feinberg et al. to track adolescent development [47], slow waves may yet provide valuable clues to identify plasticity deficits in schizophrenia, particularly during development. It remains to be seen whether the developmental trajectory of SWA is altered in schizophrenia.

Sleep research in schizophrenia has recently focused on sleep spindles for reasons that are both data driven and hypothesis based. Spindles, recorded from the scalp EEG, are waxing and waning bursts of highly synchronized 12–16 Hz oscillations that are characteristic of NREM sleep. In lighter NREM sleep (stage N2), they are often found in isolation, whereas in SWS, they are often grouped by cortical slow waves [48]. Results from the earliest studies to specifically examine spindles in schizophrenic subjects were inconsistent. Hiatt et al. [44] found an increase in the number of visually detected spindles during the first NREM period, but was only able to record from five unmedicated and recently rehospitalized schizophrenic subjects. Two subsequent studies, instead, found no difference in unmedicated [49] or first-episode, drug-naïve patients [50]. It is notable that all these studies reported on the density (counts/min) of spindles visually identified from only a few channels (usually C3 or C4) in a relatively narrow frequency range, 12–14 Hz, except the Van Cauter study that used a slightly wider range (11.5–15 Hz).

Spindle studies using automated detection methods, a wider frequency range of interest (12–16 Hz), and a larger array of channels, have shown consistent spindle deficits in medicated schizophrenic patients relative to both healthy control subjects as well as nonschizophrenic patients taking antipsychotics [42, 43]. The differences between the earlier studies and the current research are significant because they indicate how quickly the rapid advancement in recording techniques can shape our current understanding of spindles in schizophrenic populations. Although observed even as early as 1950, it is now widely recognized that there are two distinct types of spindles based on their relative frequency and topography: slow (12–14 Hz) frontal spindles and fast (14–16 Hz) centroparietal spindles [51, 52]. As illustrated by these most recent studies and highlighted in a recent review, the traditional electrode placements commonly applied in sleep recordings may miss critical differences in spindle activity between populations based on suboptimal electrode placements [53].

The spindle deficits observed in schizophrenic patients may provide substantial insight into neurobiology of schizophrenia. Spindle activity is initiated in the TRN, and this activity is then amplified by the interplay of reticular neurons with thalamocortical cells [54]. In addition to its role as the spindle generator, the TRN acts as an integrator of multiple functional modalities [55] and plays a role in sensory gating [56] and attention [57]. Deficits in attention and sensory gating [58] have been consistently found in schizophrenics, including first-break and chronic patients, and are thought to represent a core feature of the disorder. Additional evidence from molecular, animal, and human studies indicates a neurobiological dysfunction in the TRN that, intriguingly, may underlie several important features of schizophrenia [53, 59]. While dysfunction in the TRN could potentially explain several of the cardinal features of schizophrenia, it is difficult to neuroimage with other methods, because of its thin, shell-like nature [60]. Therefore, at this time, recording sleep spindles with EEG represents the best opportunity to understand the role of TRN dysfunction in schizophrenia.

The relationship between sleep, cognition, and schizophrenia has also recently garnered significant attention.

Although procedural memory is not typically among the well-known cognitive deficits implicated in schizophrenia, several recent studies have suggested that sleep-dependent improvement in motor sequence learning may be specifically disrupted in schizophrenia. A typical motor sequence learning task involves performing a simple five-element finger-tapping sequence as fast and as accurately as possible for a repeated number of trials. A typical outcome measure is the number of accurate sequences in a 30-s trial, averaged across several trials. Despite performing as well as controls before sleep, schizophrenic subjects have consistently failed to show the same post-sleep improvement as either healthy [61–64] or depressed controls [63] on these types of tasks. Moreover, although it has not been demonstrated in all of the studies [61–63], spindle activity seems to be particularly important for this type of task [65]. The most recent study did show a correlation between spindle reduction and memory impairment in schizophrenics [64]. The same relationship between spindles and overnight improvement was not demonstrated in control subjects; however, it is not clear if the lack of correlation was related to a ceiling effect for post-sleep performance enhancement in healthy individuals. Additionally, all of the studies mentioned above reported decreased spindle activity relative to controls, further solidifying the notion that spindles are defective in schizophrenia. Given the aforementioned role of slow waves in plasticity, it has also been suggested that slow waves may play a part in the cognitive impairments observed in schizophrenia [62, 66–68]. Thus, it may turn out to be the lack of coordination between slow waves and spindles that most dramatically impacts cognition in schizophrenia, as recently suggested by investigators using an animal model of schizophrenia to record sleep intracranially [69].

The route between sleep and the pathophysiology of schizophrenia was not as clearly paved as the famous turn of the century quotes regarding dreams and psychosis would have suggested. Even REM sleep, despite its early promise, did not seem to be uniquely different in schizophrenic patients, at least in terms of its timing, duration, and homeostatic response to deprivation. These early setbacks, however, may have been more related to the analysis tools available to a nascent sleep research field, than to any inherent inability of sleep to provide important insights into the disorder. As the field has developed sophisticated analysis techniques beyond using EEG to measure sleep architecture, several obvious advantages to examining sleep in schizophrenia have emerged. Sleep offers a rare opportunity to directly examine spontaneous neural activity when other confounds associated with schizophrenia (i.e., lack of motivation, attentional deficits, hallucinations) are noticeably diminished. Currently, the findings of consistent deficits in sleep spindle activity represent perhaps the most promising research direction in sleep and schizophrenia, although slow waves may

yet reveal important insights into cortical development, plasticity, or memory dysfunction. The spindle deficit implicates a particular brain structure, the TRN that may be critical to understanding the neurobiology of schizophrenia. Still, whether or not the magnitude or localization of spindle deficits will prove to be a mere correlate of cognitive deficits or whether these spindle abnormalities will further inform our understanding of the disease neuropathology still needs to be assessed. Furthermore, the degree to which pharmacological interventions aimed at reversing spindle deficits will provide novel therapeutic opportunities remains to be tested.

Armed with a new set of techniques and tools for examining sleep, current researchers are also revisiting the relationship between REM sleep, dreaming, and schizophrenia [70]. Instead of trying to find macrostructural differences of REM sleep in schizophrenia, as in the past, investigators are focusing on the similarities between REM and psychosis in order to use this stage of sleep as a model for schizophrenia. For instance, pre-pulse inhibition, the diminished electrophysiological response to the second of a pair of closely timed stimuli, is similarly mitigated in schizophrenia and REM sleep [71]. Neuroimaging results also suggest that a similar area of reduced activation in REM sleep, Finally, the dorsolateral prefrontal cortex [72] is dysfunctional in schizophrenic patients [73]. And although the electrophysiological correlates of dreaming in humans are not yet elucidated as are the main oscillatory rhythms characterizing NREM sleep, it can also be expected that using more sophisticated analyses on the brain activity during sleep will eventually lead to a closer link between dreaming and neuronal activity [74], which may ultimately provide important insights into the pathophysiology of psychosis. Perhaps then, the early prognostications that an understanding of dreaming will allow us to understand psychosis can finally be fulfilled.

References

1. McKeon R. The basic works of Aristotle. New York: Random House; 1941.
2. Kleitman N. Sleep and wakefulness (Midway reprint).Chicago: University of Chicago Press; 1987. (1987-09-15).
3. Jung CG. The psychology of dementia praecox. New York: Nervous and Mental Disease; 1936.
4. Jackson JH. Selected writings. New York: Basic; 1958.
5. Barclay RM, Cranefield PF, Robertson GMb, Kraepelin E. Dementia praecox and paraphrenia. Edinburgh: Livingstone; 1919.
6. Bleuler E. Dementia praecox, or, the group of schizophrenias. New York: International Universities Press; 1950.
7. Heinrichs RW. Historical origins of schizophrenia: two early madmen and their illness. J Hist Behav Sci. 2003;39(4):349–63.
8. Andreasen NC, Black DW. Introductory textbook of psychiatry. Washington, DC: American Psychiatric Pub; 2006.
9. Trapp CE, Lyons RH. Dream studies in hallucinated patients: preliminary study. Psychiatr Q. 1937;11(2):253–66.

10. Kant O. Differential diagnosis of schizophrenia in the light of the concept of personality-stratification. Am J Psychiatry. 1940;97(2):342–57.

11. Noble D. A study of dreams in schizophrenia and allied states. Am J Psychiatry. 1951;107(8):612–6.

12. Aserinsky E, Kleitman N. Regularly occurring periods of eye motility, and concomitant phenomena, during sleep. Science. 1953;118(3062):273–4.

13. Dement W. Dream recall and eye movements during sleep in schizophrenics and normals. J Nerv Ment Dis. 1955;122(3):263–9.

14. Caldwell DF, Domino EF. Electroencephalographic and eye movement patterns during sleep in chronic schizophrenic patients. Electroencephalogr Clin Neurophysiol. 1967;22(5):414–20.

15. Feinberg I, Koresko RL, Gottlieb F, Wender PH. Sleep electroencephalographic and eye-movement patterns in schizophrenic patients. Compr Psychiatry. 1964;5(1):44–53.

16. Koresko RL, Snyder F, Feinberg I. 'Dream time' in hallucinating and nonhallucinating schizophrenic patients. Nature. 1963;199:1118–9.

17. Fisher C, Dement WC. Studies on psychopathology of sleep and dreams. Am J Psychiatry. 1963;119(12):1160–8.

18. Rechtschaffen A, Mednick SA, Schulsin F. Schizophrenia and physiological indices of dreaming. Arch Gen Psychiatry. 1964;10(1):89–93.

19. Vogel GW, Traub AC. REM deprivation I: effect on schizophrenic patients. Arch Gen Psychiatry. 1968;18(3):287–300.

20. Zarcone V, Gulevich G, Pivik T, Dement W. Partial REM phase deprivation and schizophrenia. Arch Gen Psychiatry. 1968;18(2):194–202.

21. Gulevich GD, Dement WC, Zarcone VP. All-night sleep recordings of chronic schizophrenics in remission. Compr Psychiatry. 1967;8(3):141–9.

22. Stern M, Fram DH, Wyatt R, Grinspoo L, Tursky B. All-night sleep studies of acute schizophrenics. Arch Gen Psychiatry. 1969;20(4):470–7.

23. Feinberg I, Koresko RL, Gottlieb F. Further observations on electrophysiological sleep patterns in schizophrenia. Compr Psychiatry. 1965;6(1):21–4.

24. Benson KL, Jr. Zarcone VP. Testing the REM sleep phasic event intrusion hypothesis of schizophrenia. Psychiatry Res. 1985;15(3):163–73.

25. Feinberg I, Braun M, Koresko RL, Gottlieb F. Stage–4 sleep in schizophrenia. Arch Gen Psychiatry. 1969;21(3):262–6.

26. Traub AC. Sleep stage deficits in chronic schizophrenia. Psychol Rep. 1972;31(3):815–20.

27. Gresham SC, Agnew HW, Williams RL. Sleep of depressed patients: an EEG and eye movement study. Arch Gen Psychiatry. 1965;13(6):503–7.

28. Benca RM, Obermeyer WH, Thisted RA, Gillin JC. Sleep and psychiatric disorders: a meta-analysis. Arch Gen Psychiatry. 1992;49(8):651–68.

29. Chouinard S, Poulin J, Stip E, Godbout R. Sleep in untreated patients with schizophrenia: a meta-analysis. Schizophr Bull. 2004;30(4):957–67.

30. Monti JM, Monti D. Sleep disturbance in schizophrenia. Int Rev Psychiatry. 2005;17(4):247–53.

31. Steriade M. Corticothalamic resonance, states of vigilance and mentation. Neuroscience. 2000;101(2):243–76.

32. Feinberg I. Schizophrenia caused by a fault in programmed synaptic elimination during adolescence. J Psychiatric Res. 1982;17(4):319–34.

33. Huttenlocher PR. Synaptic density in human frontal cortex: developmental changes and effects of aging. Brain Res. 1979;163(2):195–205.

34. Tononi G, Cirelli C. Steep function and synaptic homeostasis. Sleep Med Rev. 2006;10(1):49–62.

35. Massimini M, Tononi G, Huber R. Slow waves, synaptic plasticity and information processing: insights from transcranial magnetic stimulation and high-density EEG experiments. Eur J Neurosci. 2009;29(9):1761–70.

36. Gogate N, Giedd J, Janson K, Rapoport JL. Brain imaging in normal and abnormal brain development: new perspectives for child psychiatry. Clin Neurosci Res. 2001;1(4):283–90.

37. Gogtay N. Cortical brain development in schizophrenia: insights from neuroimaging studies in childhood-onset schizophrenia. Schizophr Bull. 2008;34(1):30–6.

38. Thompson PM, Vidal C, Giedd JN, Gochman P, Blumenthal J, Nicolson R, et al. Mapping adolescent brain change reveals dynamic wave of accelerated gray matter loss in very early-onset schizophrenia. Proc Natl Acad Sci U S A. 2001;98(20):11650–5.

39. Buchmann A, Ringli M, Kurth S, Schaerer M, Geiger A, Jenni OG, et al. EEG sleep slow-wave activity as a mirror of cortical maturation. Cereb Cortex. 2011;21(3):607–15.

40. Gogtay N, Giedd JN, Lusk L, Hayashi KM, Greenstein D, Vaituzis AC, et al. Dynamic mapping of human cortical development during childhood through early adulthood. Proc Natl Acad Sci U S A. 2004;101(21):8174–9.

41. Kurth S, Jenni OG, Riedner BA, Tononi G, Carskadon MA, Huber R. Characteristics of sleep slow waves in children and adolescents. Sleep. 2010;33(4):475–80.

42. Ferrarelli F, Huber R, Peterson MJ, Massimini M, Murphy M, Riedner BA, et al. Reduced sleep spindle activity in schizophrenia patients. Am J Psychiatry. 2007;164(3):483–92.

43. Ferrarelli F, Peterson MJ, Sarasso S, Riedner BA, Murphy MJ, Benca RM, et al. Thalamic dysfunction in schizophrenia suggested by whole-night deficits in slow and fast spindles. Am J Psychiatry. 2010;167(11):1339–48.

44. Hiatt JF, Floyd TC, Katz PH, Feinberg I. Further evidence of abnormal non-rapid-eye-movement sleep in schizophrenia. Arch Gen Psychiatry. 1985;42(8):797–802.

45. Keshavan MS, Reynolds CF, Miewald JM, Montrose DM, Sweeney JA, Vasko RC, et al. Delta sleep deficits in schizophrenia—evidence from automated analyses of sleep data. Arch Gen Psychiatry. 1998;55(5):443–8.

46. Ganguli R, Reynolds CF, Kupfer DJ. Electroencephalographic sleep in young, never-medicated schizophrenics: a comparison with delusional and nondelusional depressives and with healthy controls. Arch Gen Psychiatry. 1987;44(1):36–44.

47. Feinberg I, Campbell IG. Sleep EEG changes during adolescence: an index of a fundamental brain reorganization. Brain Cogn. 2010;72(1):56–65.

48. Molle M, Marshall L, Gais S, Born J. Grouping of spindle activity during slow oscillations in human non-rapid eye movement sleep. J Neurosci. 2002;22(24):10941–7.

49. Van Cauter E, Linkowski P, Kerkhofs M, Hubain P, L'Hermite-Baleriaux M, Leclercq R, et al. Circadian and sleep-related endocrine rhythms in schizophrenia. Arch Gen Psychiatry. 1991;48(4):348–56.

50. Poulin J, Daoust AM, Forest G, Stip E, Godbout R. Sleep architecture and its clinical correlates in first episode and neuroleptic-naive patients with schizophrenia. Schizophr Res. 2003;62(1–2):147–53.

51. De Gennaro L, Ferrara M. Sleep spindles: an overview. Sleep Med Rev. 2003;7(5):423–40.

52. Jankel WR, Niedermeyer E. Sleep spindles. J Clin Neurophysiol. 1985;2(1):1–35.

53. Ferrarelli F, Tononi G. The thalamic reticular nucleus and schizophrenia. Schizophr Bull. 2011;37(2):306–15.

54. Fuentealba P, Steriade M. The reticular nucleus revisited: Intrinsic and network properties of a thalamic pacemaker. Prog Neurobiol. 2005;75(2):125–41.

55. Pinault D. The thalamic reticular nucleus: structure, function and concept. Brain Res Rev. 2004;46(1):1–31.

56. Krause M, Hoffmann WE, Hajos M. Auditory sensory gating in hippocampus and reticular thalamic neurons in anesthetized rats. Biol Psychiatry. 2003;53(3):244–53.

57. Guillery RW, Feig SL, Lozsadi DA. Paying attention to the thalamic reticular nucleus. Trends Neurosci. 1998;21(1):28–32.

58. Freedman R, Olincy A, Ross RG, Waldo MC, Stevens KE, Adler LE, et al. The genetics of sensory gating deficits in schizophrenia. Curr Psychiatry Rep. 2003;5(2):155–61.

59. Vukadinovic Z. Sleep abnormalities in schizophrenia may suggest impaired trans-thalamic cortico-cortical communication: towards a dynamic model of the illness. Eur J Neurosci. 2011;34(7):1031–9.

60. Guller Y, Ferrarelli F, Shackman AJ, Sarasso S, Peterson MJ, Langheim FJ, et al. Probing thalamic integrity in schizophrenia using concurrent transcranial magnetic stimulation and functional magnetic resonance imaging. Arch Gen Psychiatry. 2012;69(7):662–71.

61. Manoach DS, Cain MS, Vangel MG, Khurana A, Goff DC, Stickgold R. A failure of sleep-dependent procedural learning in chronic, medicated schizophrenia. Biol Psychiatry. 2004;56(12):951–6.

62. Manoach DS, Tahkkar KN, Stroynowski E, Ely A, McKinley SK, Wamsley E, et al. Reduced overnight consolidation of procedural learning in chronic medicated schizophrenia is related to specific sleep stages. J Psychiatric Res. 2010;44(2):112–20.

63. Seeck-Hirschner M, Baier PC, Sever S, Buschbacher A, Aldenhoff JB, Goeder R. Effects of daytime naps on procedural and declarative memory in patients with schizophrenia. J Psychiatric Res. 2010;44(1):42–7.

64. Wamsley EJ, Tucker MA, Shinn AK, Ono KE, McKinley SK, Ely AV, et al. Reduced sleep spindles and spindle coherence in schizophrenia: mechanisms of impaired memory consolidation? Biol Psychiatry. 2012;71(2):154–61.

65. Fogel SM, Smith CT. The function of the sleep spindle: a physiological index of intelligence and a mechanism for sleep-dependent memory consolidation. Neurosci Biobehav Rev. 2011;35(5):1154–65.

66. Goder R, Boigs M, Braun S, Friege L, Fritzer G, Aldenhoff JB, et al. Impairment of visuospatial memory is associated with decreased slow wave sleep in schizophrenia. J Psychiatric Res. 2004;38(6):591–9.

67. Goder R, Aldenhoff JB, Boigs M, Braun S, Koch J, Fritzer G. Delta power in sleep in relation to neuropsychological performance in healthy subjects and schizophrenia patients. J Neuropsychiatry Clin Neurosci. 2006;18(4):529–35.

68. Goder R, Fritzer G, Gottwald B, Lippmann B, Seeck-Hirschner M, Serafin I, et al. Effects of olanzapine on slow wave sleep, sleep spindles and sleep-related memory consolidation in schizophrenia. Pharmacopsychiatry. 2008;41(3):92–9.

69. Phillips KG, Bartsch U, McCarthy AP, Edgar DM, Tricklebank MD, Wafford KA, et al. Decoupling of sleep-dependent cortical and hippocampal interactions in a neurodevelopmental model of schizophrenia. Neuron. 2012;76(3):526–33.

70. Gottesmann C. The dreaming sleep stage: a new neurobiological model of schizophrenia? Neuroscience. 2006;140(4):1105–15.

71. Kisley MA, Olincy A, Robbins E, Polk SD, Adler LE, Waldo MC, et al. Sensory gating impairment associated with schizophrenia persists into REM sleep. Psychophysiology. 2003;40(1):29–38.

72. Maquet P. Functional neuroimaging of normal human sleep by positron emission tomography. J Sleep Res. 2000;9(3):207–31.

73. Weinberger DR, Berman KF, Zec RF. Physiological dysfunction of dorsolateral prefrontal cortex in schizophrenia 1: regional cerebral blood-flow evidence. Arch Gen Psychiatry. 1986;43(2):114–24.

74. Nir Y, Tononi G. Dreaming and the brain: from phenomenology to neurophysiology. Trends Cogn Sci. 2010;14(2):88–100.

Bipolar Disorder

Sara Dallaspezia and Francesco Benedetti

The clinical observation of sleep alterations in mood disorders is really ancient. In 400 AD, Hippocrates in book II of *Epidemics* in the Hippocratic Corpus described a loss of sleep in a woman of Thasus with a "melancholic turn of mind," showing a concomitant worsening of the woman's clinical condition. Two hundred years later, Aretaeus of Cappadocia not only used term such as "sleepless" to describe depressed patients but also was the first physician who recognized that mania and depression could alternate in the same person, describing for the first time bipolar disorder. Thus, the association of sleep and mood disturbances dates back to the very first descriptive presentation of mood disorders and it has been confirmed in most recent studies showing that sleep changes predict and precede mood swings in bipolar patients [1, 2].

Maintaining stable sleep–wake cycles is of central importance to the maintenance of stability in bipolar disorder. Sleep loss can trigger mania in patients and the reduction of sleep duration is a good predictor of hypomania or mania the next day in rapid-cycling bipolar patients [3]. The causal relationship between sleep loss and mania is bidirectional: the capacity of sleep reduction to cause mania and mania to reduce sleep is a self-reinforcing mechanism that could explain the tendency of mania to escalate out of control and become autonomous through increasing manic symptomatology [4]. This relationship between mania and sleep loss seems to be important mostly in the beginning of a manic episode [5]. Indeed, during depressive episodes, bipolar patients report more hypersomnia than unipolar patients with a prevalence ranging from 35 [6] to 78 % [7] and the symptoms being highly recurrent across separate episodes of bipolar depression as first observed by Leibenluft et al. [8].

With the discovery of rapid eye movement (REM) sleep in the early 1950s, polysomnographic sleep research helped to lead the way to the knowledge of sleep alteration in bipolar disorder. Much of the early sleep research in psychiatry beginning in the mid-1960s was descriptive, laying out what is now a rich picture of polysomnographic features of depression, mania, and other psychiatric diseases [9]. Three features of EEG sleep patterns have been established as the most frequently observed abnormalities in depressed patients, which include alterations in REM sleep, sleep continuity disturbances, and a marked reduction in slow-wave sleep. The two REM sleep measures receiving the greatest amount of attention have been the shortened REM latency, first observed in 1972 by Kupfer and Forster [10], and the abnormal distribution of REM sleep during the night characterized by the shift of REM sleep time and intensity to the earlier portion of the night [11].

In 1980, Vogel suggested a necessary association between depression [12] and high REM density. Shulz and Trojan found that while shortened REM latency was characteristic of depression and normalized with euthymia (i.e., normal nondepressed positive mood), increased REM density appeared to be a trait characteristic with only minor differences between bipolar and unipolar depression. For instance, bipolar patients have a tendency for longer sleep time and more fragmented REM sleep periods compared to unipolar ones. No difference in REM latency or other measures was found [13, 14] between unipolar and bipolar depression.

Since polysomnographic examinations are very difficult to be carried out in patients affected by mania, only few studies concerning sleep and mania are published in the literature. In 1986, Van Sweden [15], while studying two unmedicated severely manic patients, found that both of them showed stage 2 sleep within seconds of closing their eyes, contrary to the common assumption that manic patients are unable to sleep. Both normal [16] and shorter than normal [17] REM sleep density were found in manic patients. Moreover, Linkowski and colleagues [16] found that although manic patients spent less time asleep during the day and took longer to fall asleep

S. Dallaspezia (✉) · F. Benedetti
Department of Clinical Neurosciences, Scientific Institute and University Vita-Salute San Raffaele, Via Stamira d'Ancona 20, 20127, Milano, Italy
e-mail: dallaspezia.sara@hsr.it

than healthy subjects, they showed duration of time spent in any stage of sleep similar to the ones of unaffected people, and Hudson and colleagues [17] found a higher REM density in unmedicated manic patients compared to healthy subjects.

Sitaram and colleagues, recalling the cholinergic supersensitivity theory of depression and mania postulated by Janowsky et al. in 1972 [18], supposed that shortened REM latency could be explained by increased cholinergic activity coupled with decreased adrenergic activity [19]. The author in the early 1980s [20] first used the cholinergic REM induction test (CRIT) in patients affected by affective disorders which provides an experimental strategy for evaluating the hypothesis of the involvement of central nervous cholinergic neurotransmission in REM sleep. Patients affected with bipolar disorder showed a shortening of REM latency after cholinergic stimulation compared to healthy subjects. Cholinergic sensitivity was positively correlated with first REM period density, which was significantly higher than normal in both the depressed [21] and euthymic states [19]. These findings prompted Sitaram to hypothesize that increased cholinergic sensitivity and increased REM density may be biological markers of vulnerability to bipolar disorder. In agreement with these findings, other studies showed that the anticholinergic drug clomipramine suppressed initial REM sleep in depressed patients [22] and nortriptyline also produced REM sleep suppression [23].

Several circadian rhythm theories have been proposed to explain the observed links between sleep physiology and depression. Wehr and Goodwin in 1983 [24] proposed the phase advance theory postulating that depression is associated with an advance of certain circadian rhythms, including the REM sleep rhythm, relative to the other circadian rhythms, such as the sleep–wake activity rhythm. A related theory [25] suggests a "critical phase" in the circadian temperature rhythm. During depression, sleep overlaps the critical phase with resulting depressive symptoms and sleep disturbances.

In 1982, Borbely proposed a theory that served as the basis for circadian rhythm theories of sleep abnormalities in mood disorders: the two-process model of sleep regulation [26]. This theory postulates that sleep is regulated by the interaction of a homeostatic process S and a circadian process C. Sleep need is represented by process S and is reflected in EEG slow-wave activity. Sleep onset and sleep termination are determined by the level of S and by a gating system consisting of two thresholds under the control of circadian process C. Borbely and Wirz-Justice [27] suggested in their S-deficiency model that during depression there is a deficient buildup of the homeostatic process with process C remaining unaffected. Process S deficiency could be associated with re-duced slow-wave sleep, and indirectly, with reduced REM sleep latency observed during depression. This lack of homeostatic sleep pressure has however not been confirmed in experimental settings [28].

Several findings have suggested connections between sleep and mood in depression. In the early 1970s, Hauri and Hawkins [29] first observed a correlation between nightly fluctuations in phasic REM activity and daily fluctuations in self-rated mood in depressed patients, with a higher percentage of REM sleep with phasic activity being associated with worse mood ratings.

The study of sleep has contributed to our understanding of depression and bipolar disorder. Moreover, manipulation of sleep through sleep deprivation (SD) has been demonstrated to be useful in the treatment of bipolar depression [30].

Schulte [31] first suggested that SD might benefit depressed patients, basing on anecdotal reports from three depressed patients who "treated" themselves with accidental SD. Schulte's great contribution was to take these reports seriously and to prompt his collaborators Pflug and Tölle to carry out systematic investigations subsequently [32]. Initially, the use of SD was restricted to experimental settings aimed at increasing knowledge about the pathophysiology of mood disorders. Indeed, the observation that SD generally caused a transient antidepressant effect in most of the patients showing a relapse after a night of recovery sleep, even when a complete response had been achieved the evening before [33], discouraged the application of this treatment in common clinical practice. During subsequent years, different clinical strategies have been studied and developed to prevent the short-term relapse and to sustain the effects of SD over time [34]. The add-on of repeated SD plus light therapy along with antidepressant medication and lithium was also found to be useful in the treatment of drug-resistant bipolar patients, with an acute antidepressant response in the 44 % of patients who did not show a response to antidepressant drug.

Nowadays, SD has been proven to be a powerful clinical instrument for the treatment of depression in everyday clinical practice, with a rapid antidepressant effect which is highly reproducible and substantial making SD a potential first-line treatment for bipolar depression [30].

In conclusion, the future of sleep studies in bipolar disorder is likely to involve a shift from the early descriptive approach to the development of more and more reliable monitoring and treatment strategy. Focusing on the alteration of the wake–sleep rhythm and its manipulation as a therapy, it should be possible to find some responses about the nature of bipolar disorder, which is still an unsolved problem.

References

1. Bauer M, Glenn T, Whybrow PC, et al. Changes in self-reported sleep duration predict mood changes in bipolar disorder. Psychol Med. 2008;38:1069–71.

2. Bauer M, Grof P, Rasgon N, Bschor T, Glenn T, Whybrow PC. Temporal relation between sleep and mood in patients with bipolar disorder. Bipolar Disord. 2006;8:160–7.

3. Leibenluft E, Albert PS, Rosenthal NE, Wehr TA. Relationship between sleep and mood in patients with rapid-cycling bipolar disorder. Psychiatry Res. 1996;63:161–8.

4. Wehr TA, Sack DA, Norman E. Sleep reduction as a final common pathway in the genesis of mania. Am J Psychiatry. 1987;144:201–4.

5. Barbini B, Bertelli S, Colombo C, Smeraldi E. Sleep loss, a possible factor in augmenting manic episode. Psychiatry Res. 1996;15:121–5.

6. Akiskal HS, Benazzi F. Atypical depression: a variant of bipolar II or a bridge between unipolar and bipolar II? J Affect Disord. 2005;84:209–17.

7. Detre TP, Himmelhoch JM, Swartzburg M, Anderson CM, Byck R, Kupfer DJ. Hypersomnia and manic—depressive disease. Am J Psychiatry. 1972;128:1303–5.

8. Leibenluft E, Clark CH, Myers FS. The reproducibility of depressive and hypomanic symptoms across repeated episodes in patients with rapid-cycling bipolar disorder. J Affect Disord. 1995;33:83–8.

9. Benca RM, Obermeyer WH, Thisted RA, Gillin JC. Sleep and psychiatric disorders. A meta-analysis. Arch Gen Psychiatry. 1992;49:651–68; discussion 69–70.

10. Kupfer DJ, Foster FG. Interval between onset of sleep and rapid-eye-movement sleep as an indicator of depression. Lancet. 1972;2:684–6.

11. Kupfer DJ. REM latency: a psychobiologic marker for primary depressive disease. Biol Psychiatry. 1976;11:159–74.

12. Vogel GW, Vogel F, McAbee RS, Thurmond AJ. Improvement of depression by REM sleep deprivation. New findings and a theory. Arch Gen Psychiatry. 1980;37:247–53.

13. Giles DE, Rush AJ, Roffwarg HP. Sleep parameters in bipolar I, bipolar II, and unipolar depressions. Biol Psychiatry. 1986;21:1340–3.

14. Duncan WC, Jr., Pettigrew KD, Gillin JC. REM architecture changes in bipolar and unipolar depression. Am J Psychiatry. 1979;136:1424–7.

15. Van Sweden B. Disturbed vigilance in mania. Biol Psychiatry. 1986;21:311–3.

16. Linkowski P, Kerkhofs M, Rielaert C, Mendlewicz J. Sleep during mania in manic-depressive males. Eur Arch Psychiatry Neurol Sci. 1986;235:339–41.

17. Hudson JI, Lipinski JF, Frankenburg FR, Grochocinski VJ, Kupfer DJ. Electroencephalographic sleep in mania. Arch Gen Psychiatry. 1988;45:267–73.

18. Janowsky DS, el-Yousef MK, Davis JM, Sekerke HJ. A cholinergic-adrenergic hypothesis of mania and depression. Lancet. 1972;2:632–5.

19. Sitaram N, Nurnberger JI, Jr., Gershon ES, Gillin JC. Cholinergic regulation of mood and REM sleep: potential model and marker of vulnerability to affective disorder. Am J Psychiatry. 1982;139:571–6.

20. Sitaram N, Nurnberger JI, Jr., Gershon ES, Gillin JC. Faster cholinergic REM sleep induction in euthymic patients with primary affective illness. Science. 1980;208:200–2.

21. Foster FG, Kupfer DJ, Coble P, McPartland RJ. Rapid eye movement sleep density. An objective indicator in severe medical-depressive syndromes. Arch Gen Psychiatry. 1976;33:1119–23.

22. Hochli D, Riemann D, Zulley J, Berger M. Initial REM sleep suppression by clomipramine: a prognostic tool for treatment response in patients with a major depressive disorder. Biol Psychiatry. 1986;21:1217–20.

23. Kupfer DJ, Spiker DG, Rossi A, Coble PA, Shaw D, Ulrich R. Nortriptyline and EEG sleep in depressed patients. Biol Psychiatry. 1982;17:535–46.

24. Wehr TA, Goodwin FK. Biological rhythms in manic-depressive illness. In: Wehr TA, Goodwin FK, editors. Circadian rhythms in psychiatry. Pacific Groove: Boxwood; 1983. pp. 129–84.

25. Wehr TA, Wirz-Justice A. Circadian rhythm mechanisms in affective illness and in antidepressant drug action. Pharmacopsychiatria. 1982;15:31–9.

26. Borbely AA. A two process model of sleep regulation. Hum Neurobiol. 1982;1:195–204.

27. Borbely AA, Wirz-Justice A. Sleep, sleep deprivation and depression. A hypothesis derived from a model of sleep regulation. Hum Neurobiol. 1982;1:205–10.

28. Frey S, Birchler-Pedross A, Hofstetter M, et al. Young women with major depression live on higher homeostatic sleep pressure than healthy controls. Chronobiol Int. 2012;29:278–94.

29. Hauri P, Hawkins DR. Phasic REM, depression, and the relationship between sleeping and waking. Arch Gen Psychiatry. 1971;25:56–63.

30. Benedetti F, Colombo C. Sleep deprivation in mood disorders. Neuropsychobiology. 2011;64:141–51.

31. Schulte W. Zum Problem der Provokation und Kupierung von melancholischen Phasen. Schweizer Arch Neurol Neurochem Psychiatr. 1971;109:427–35.

32. Pflug B, Tolle R. Therapy of endogenous depressions using sleep deprivation. Practical and theoretical consequences. Nervenarzt. 1971;42:117–24.

33. Leibenluft E, Wehr TA. Is sleep deprivation useful in the treatment of depression? Am J Psychiatry. 1992;149:159–68.

34. Wirz-Justice A, Benedetti F, Terman M. Chronotherapeutics for affective disorders. A clinician's manual for light and wake therapy. Basel: Karger; 2009.

Part IX
Respiratory Diseases

A Short History of Obstructive Sleep Apnea Syndrome

Brendon Richard Peters and Christian Guilleminault

A comprehensive account of the history of OSA is a difficult endeavor, considering the long history of the entity and several misunderstandings that persist to this day. Our modern conceptualizations of the pathophysiology, epidemiology, and treatment have evolved, extending from its earliest description in literature from the nineteenth century with behavioral observation of abnormal breathing during sleep to scientific advances made over recent decades with recognition of different syndromes associated with abnormal breathing and sleep. There have been lessons on the nature of hypoventilation and sleepiness, the role of carbon dioxide retention and sleep fragmentation, increasingly sophisticated monitoring, nuanced redefinition of terms, debates on the underlying airway mechanics, new treatments, and recognition of the prevalence and long-term consequences. This knowledge serves as a cornerstone in the practice of sleep medicine, and a reflection on its history enhances the appreciation and understanding of the relationship between sleep and breathing.

One of the earliest literary accounts describing an obese subject prone to excessive daytime sleepiness exists in *The Pickwick Papers*, the first novel by Charles Dickens, published in 1837 [1]. Dickens gave a very vivid account of a well-studied character called "Joe." He is "a wonderfully fat boy...standing upright on the mat, with his eyes closed as if in sleep." Subsequently, several well-known medical authors, particularly Sir William Osler in 1837, used the term "Pickwickian" to describe obese and sleepy patients. In 1956, Burwell and colleagues published an article entitled "Extreme obesity associated with alveolar hypoventilation—A Pickwickian Syndrome," [2] reporting on an obese, sleepy patient. This report clearly emphasized the importance of "alvcolar hypoventilation," a concept overlooked by many thereafter. An important issue was further raised: How should one determine "hypoventilation"? Preceding the report of Burwell et al. [2], Auchincloss and colleagues [3], as well as Siekert et al. [4] described cases of obesity, hypersomnolence, and cardiopulmonary syndrome. Even before these reports, Kerr and Lagen in 1936 [5] reported a case that showed obesity could lead to significant cardiorespiratory failure.

To classically assess for hypoventilation, one does testing and gas challenges on a patient seated in a laboratory environment. Analysis of the response of breathing to inhalation of increasing levels of CO_2 occurs, using different techniques to avoid simultaneous hypoxemia. More sophisticated technical analyses were later developed, performing challenges while supine and awake and, finally, during nonrapid eye movement (NREM) and rapid eye movement (REM) sleep. Progressively, the notion that hypoventilation may occur during sleep, and sometimes only during REM sleep, emerged. This was well demonstrated, especially after subsequent investigation of patients with muscle and neuromuscular dysfunctions.

Simultaneously, researchers focused on investigations to better understand daytime sleepiness. In those early years, many patients were improperly called "narcoleptics," with the term used as a synonym for those who were "excessively sleepy" (forgetting the original description given by Jean Baptiste Edouard Gelineau [6]. In order to decipher the nature of sleepiness, neurophysiologists working in epilepsy differentiated between sleepiness unrelated and related to abnormal behaviors associated with seizure disorders. These investigators used a polygraph to monitor the brain, and after the discovery of REM sleep, added electrodes monitoring eye movement and chin muscle activity. In order to recognize specific electroencephalography (EEG) artifacts, they also often had one channel indicating heart rate and a respiratory belt. Therefore, early in the investigation of obstructive

C. Guilleminault (✉)
Sleep Medicine Division, Stanford University Outpatient Medical Center, 450 Broadway, Redwood City, CA 94063, USA
e-mail: cguil@stanford.edu

B. R. Peters
Stanford Sleep Medicine Center, Stanford School of Medicine, Redwood City, CA, USA

S. Chokroverty, M. Billiard (eds.), *Sleep Medicine*, DOI 10.1007/978-1-4939-2089-1_41,
© Springer Science+Business Media, LLC 2015

sleep apnea, a dichotomy emerged: Obese patients were seen either by an internist due to their obesity or by a neurologist or neurophysiologist due to their daytime sleepiness. In the modern era, the individuals who started the ball rolling and made the first new discoveries were Gerardy and colleagues from Germany. The first to record an obese and sleepy "Pickwickian" patient was Werner Gerardy [7], an internist at the Heidelberg University Hospital. The patient had come to the hospital for investigation of recurring morning headaches and was observed to have respiratory pauses during sleep with recovery breathing with a loud snore. A polygraphic investigation was performed to investigate the brain problem associated with the headaches. Gerardy, Herberg (head of the internal medicine department), and Kuhn studied another "obese–Pickwickian" before reporting their findings that recorded the following features during a daytime nap:

> After 10 min of recording, the patient presented periodic breathing, with short suspension of breathing with the tongue falling back at onset of the respiratory suspension, so there was no airflow despite increased movements of the thorax. Then the patient woke-up suddenly, the tongue moved forward and a second and a half later the first breath occurred. The heart rate during the suspension of breathing became slower and slower, but was greatly accelerated with renewal of breathing.

The working hypothesis was that the daytime sleepiness was related to CO_2 retention, an idea that was further tested by American researchers.

Two years later, a US team at the National Institutes of Health (NIH) studied an obese woman, not only performing brainwave analysis but also measuring blood gases looking at oxygen and CO_2. In their patient, Drachman and Gumnit [8] identified repetitive stoppage of air exchange despite persistence of thoracoabdominal movements. This was associated with bradycardia to 50 beats/min and tachycardia to 140 beats/min with resumption of breathing. They also documented an oxygen desaturation to 50% during the air-exchange arrest and a return to normal levels with resumption of respiration. The patient was placed on a strict diet and after a significant weight loss saw her sleepiness disappear. Both of these groups clearly described the tongue movements, the persistence of thoracoabdominal movements, and the repetitive awakenings to resume breathing with the cycle of bradytachycardia. Drachman and Gumnit also documented the associated important changes in blood gases, again attributing the daytime sleepiness to CO_2 retention.

This hypothesis was challenged by Kuhlo [9–11], an individual who may not have been recognized for his important role in this initial phase of the understanding of OSA due to his decision to change his name and publish reports under two names, often in German. He was director of the EEG unit in the neurophysiology department at Freiburg, led by the famous professor Richard Jung. He was very interested in the sleepiness of Pickwickian patients and he began

investigating obese patients with daytime sleepiness, monitoring them during nocturnal sleep. He demonstrated that the abnormal breathing was noted all night long, and resumption of breathing was associated with arousals, but most commonly there was no daytime CO_2 retention during wakefulness. Following his observations, he concluded that the sleepiness present in these patients was not due to increased CO_2, but he still thought that sleepiness may be related to a "central" component. His patients underwent weight reduction with a significant improvement in sleep and breathing functions, despite the fact that the syndrome did not disappear completely.

These discoveries were presented as an abstract at the winter conference of the European Neurological Society in 1964 in Oberstdorf, within the German Alps, and at the International Symposium on Sleep Mechanisms (in Zurich in September 1964 and in 1965) [8]. The presentations attracted the attention of two participants: Henry Gastaut from Marseille University, who for many years was an important member and prolific researcher of the European Neurophysiology Society. One of his old students who for many years collaborated with him and sent many fellows to be trained in Marseille was Elio Lugaresi from the University of Bologna. These universities would become central in the development of the understanding of abnormal breathing during sleep in obese subjects.

The contribution of Wolfgang Kuhlo did not end with these presentations, however, and he carried on investigating obese sleepy patients [10]. One of his patients had a gradually increasing depressed level of consciousness, needing an urgent and drastic treatment. To treat the patient's problem, he ordered a tracheostomy [11]. Before the tracheostomy, the patient had not only nocturnal blood gases drawn at different times during the night but also continuous measurement of pulmonary artery pressure. After the procedure, the patient had a very rapid disappearance of daytime sleepiness. This improvement persisted for 2.5 years at follow-up evaluation. In addition, the very abnormal pulmonary hypertension measured at baseline improved. In summary, by 1969, he had demonstrated that the sleepiness of Pickwickian patients was related to sleep disruption induced by abnormal breathing associated with obstruction of the upper airway. When this was bypassed by performing a tracheostomy, there was a clear impact on pulmonary pressure during sleep. These findings highlighted the important role of sleep fragmentation secondary to apnea. As the first to perform a tracheostomy for abnormal breathing during sleep, he also identified a potential treatment for the problem.

The seminal work and reports of Kuhlo had an important impact on his colleagues in Marseille and Bologna. In both places, research teams monitored "Pickwickian patients" with the goal of better understanding the underlying pathology leading to daytime sleepiness. There was a lot of interaction between these groups, particularly through an individual from Bologna doing research projects in Marseille, CA Tassinari. Critical input was provided by Bernard Duron, a pulmonary specialist in Marseille, and by two neurologists/anesthesiologists in Bologna: Giorgio Coccagna and Paola Verucci-Coccagna.

During this time, the monitoring of breathing during sleep in Pickwickian patients became more sophisticated. Thoracic and abdominal bands were used as was a thermocouple placed in a full-face mask. These technical changes allowed Duron and the Gastaut team to refine the evaluations performed by the German scientists [12, 13]. The polygraphic measurements permitted them to clearly identify three different abnormal breathing patterns during sleep with creation of the terms obstructive, mixed, and central apneas. Moreover, they could show that the majority of the apneas noted during sleep in Pickwickian patients were obstructive, despite the fact that central and mixed events were seen. Initially "mixed apnea" was called "complex apnea" and was described as a central segment usually followed by an obstructive component [13]. Lugaresi et al. added an esophageal catheter in 1968 to better define the different types of apneas [14].

These authors also observed that there was a difference in the duration and type of apneas based on sleep stage. The longest apneas occurred in REM sleep and the shortest apneas were of central type. It was also during this period that researchers led by Tassinari [15] in Marseille and Bologna indicated that the abnormal breathing events were most prominent in stages one and two NREM sleep and REM sleep, and that they may not be as prominent during stages three and four NREM sleep. Both in Marseille and Bologna, changes in EEG patterns before and after the occurrence of an apnea were observed, and the term "respiratory related arousal" was created by the Marseille school. The suggestion that the sleepiness seen in Pickwickian patients was related to this arousal pattern was made in 1966, before being affirmed with the results of tracheostomy later.

The discoveries surrounding abnormal breathing during sleep also led to investigation of normal breathing during sleep, particularly by Duron in Marseille [13], and the recognition that the most stable breathing during sleep was during slow-wave sleep. It was noted that there were periods of irregular breathing during REM sleep with the presence of short, central pauses. Investigation of the breathing patterns of Pickwickian patients during sleep extended to other university cities, including Strasbourg where it was found that some had only partial apnea events that were called "hypopnea" by Kurtz (a neurophysiologist) and Lonsdorfer (a pulmonary specialist) [16]. These authors believed that the hypopneas indicated a transitional form of the Pickwickian syndrome either toward greater or lesser severity. These very first observations of hypopneas were further investigated in the following years by a resident of Kurtz, Jean Krieger,

who showed that they were not necessarily an indication of a transitional form [17]. The initial breathing patterns during sleep, both in normal and Pickwickian patients, were described in Marseille by the Gastaut team and the successive contribution was made by the Lugaresi team who added more invasive monitoring approaches. With the help of the anesthesiologist Paola Verucci-Coccagna, vital functions were monitored with arterial lines. Beginning in 1970, studies using esophageal pressure and monitoring of systemic arterial pressure through radial and pulmonary artery catheters started. The conclusion from ten patients was that there was an increase in blood pressure and pulmonary artery pressure during sleep in association with apneic events. These increases were related to sleep stages, with the highest increases in REM sleep [18]. Following the report by Kuhlo [12] that tracheostomy had significantly helped Pickwickian patients with apnea during sleep, patients were submitted to similar treatment approaches and five of them were studied before and after tracheostomy with these invasive techniques during sleep. These studies occurred from 1970 to 1973, and other teams began performing similar investigations, particularly in Japan and in the USA. However, lung specialists were little involved in these studies performed mostly by neurophysiologists. In fact, what was behind the term "Pickwickian syndrome" was questioned by Douglas Carroll, a respected pulmonary specialist, who wrote in 1972 [19]:

> It is possible to identify a number of different syndromes which demonstrate either singly or in combination obesity, hypoventilation and hypersomnia. In the past many authors have referred to all these syndromes as Pickwickian Syndrome. It appears that the waste basket of Pickwickian syndrome can be broken.

To this end, Lugaresi hoped to break up this "syndrome" and organized a meeting in Rimini, Italy in 1972 attended by many researchers involved in the topic. Their report was published in a well-known scientific journal called *Bulletin de physio-pathologie respiratoire* (*Clinical Respiratory Physiology*), under the auspices of the French National Institute of Health and Medical Research. Soon thereafter, this journal merged with the *Scandinavian Respiratory Journal* to give birth to the *European Respiratory Journal*. But what ultimately came out of the symposium was a broken hope: Confusion remained with the term "OSA" used to describe entities that members of the symposium wanted to see separated.

Nevertheless, the Rimini Symposium was a landmark: For the first time, neurophysiologists and pulmonary specialists came together trying to differentiate the different sleep-related breathing disorders that had been lumped together. The participants attempted to parse out the different clinical presentations, daytime consequences, and the underlying contributions. The presence of three types of polygraphic patterns was confirmed when studying breathing during sleep. It was recognized that esophageal manometry was the most accurate way at the time to define these three patterns, which were named central, obstructive, and mixed—the names we still use today. It also became clear that there were incomplete patterns that were called "hypopneas" that required further study. Simple recognition of the presence of a pattern was not diagnostic: The three types of patterns could be seen with variable distribution in association with complaints of hypersomnia and obesity. Daytime testing for hypoventilation did not predict the presence or absence of hypoventilation during sleep. Carroll proposed that the term "Pickwickian" still be used, but that it should be subdivided based on findings obtained after nocturnal polygraphy.

At the same congress, the views on OSA as a pattern of Pickwickian syndrome were challenged. There were two different aspects brought up. Tammeling et al. presented a case report of OSA in an individual with a craniofacial malformation [20]. Guilleminault and colleagues [21] presented non-obese men with typical OSA and complaints of insomnia, and also cases of narcolepsy–cataplexy patients with sleep apnea. These presentations challenged the supposition that OSA only occurred in obese, Pickwickian-type patients.

Also, in 1973, Guilleminault et al. reported on pediatric cases of OSA [22]. This led these authors to describe an "obstructive sleep apnea syndrome" (OSAS) [23, 24] based on their studies of nonobese subjects. These studies indicated that daytime sleepiness and insomnia could represent sleep-related complaints in these subjects. Moreover, the same blood pressure and pulmonary artery pressure changes were noted [25, 26] as had been observed in obese patients. In addition, tracheostomy was as successful a treatment as in obese Pickwickian-type subjects, eliminating the hypertension noted at baseline [26].

During the following 3 years, investigations on the cardiovascular complications associated with OSA were undertaken. The typical bradytachycardia associated with OSA and the cyclic variation of heart rate were described. The Stanford group performed systematic investigation of the arrhythmias associated with OSA, indicating that asystole and atrial fibrillation were commonly seen in these patients [27]. A controversy arose between the team of Eliot Weitzman and the Stanford group on the underlying mechanism of the airway occlusion, the former suggested it was due to an active contraction of the upper airway muscles [28], while the latter indicated that there was an absence of sufficient contraction of these muscles [29]. This led to monitoring of the upper airway muscles in normal subjects and OSA patients with different wires, needle electrodes, and imaging investigations with fluoroscopy (in New York [28]) and direct filming through a fiberoptic scope (at Stanford [29]) of the events during sleep. Guilleminault et al. also published a series of OSA children and their response to treatment with complete elimination of daytime hypertension, describing OSAS in children [30].

By 1977, there was demonstration by the group in Bologna that adult Pickwickian syndrome patients not only presented with OSA but also their daytime sleepiness and day and night hypertension were eliminated with tracheostomy. There was growing evidence from studies by Guilleminault et al. that adult non-Pickwickian patients with OSAS presented with either excessive daytime sleepiness or insomnia complaints, hypertension, and cardiac arrhythmias [24]. The Stanford group showed these abnormalities were also eliminated by tracheostomy. They also further elucidated the cardiovascular problems in children as well as the impact on learning in school and the association with NREM parasomnias. All of these symptoms were again eliminated by tracheostomy [30, 31].

These advances were important and a new international meeting was planned by Guilleminault and Dement with the help of the Kroc Foundation in southern California in 1977. The subject was "sleep apnea syndrome," emphasizing the movement beyond the "Pickwickian syndrome" and the recognition of the condition's presence in nonobese subjects. One of the principal questions proposed at this meeting was: Why does obstruction occur during sleep? It was a consideration that guided the following years of research.

Sauerland and Harper studied the genioglossal muscles of normal subjects during wakefulness and sleep with a new technique involving a bipolar recording electrode. They showed that there was normally similar bursting during wakefulness and NREM sleep, but decreased tone during REM sleep [32]. The Stanford group recorded different upper airway muscles including the genioglossus and geniohyoid muscles with wire electrodes inserted into the muscles. They reported a drop in muscle tone during sleep, particularly in association with obstructive events [29]. These reports led to further investigation of the upper airway muscles during wakefulness and sleep.

As a result of the meeting in 1977, the following year the different presentations were published and the existence of the "OSAS" in adults was established [33]. In addition, the existence of cardiovascular comorbidity, specifically hypertension and cardiac arrhythmias were confirmed. These were shown to be directly related to the abnormal breathing during sleep and were eliminated by tracheostomy, bypassing the site of obstruction. The role of the upper airway dilator muscles in the collapse of the upper airway became apparent. In short, this meeting presented the initial evidence that would become the subject of many research projects over the following 20 years.

Remmers and colleagues following the studies of Sauerland and Harper, and the Stanford group recognized the critical role of the tongue muscles in the occurrence of occlusion of the upper airway during sleep [34]. They mentioned that with sleep onset there was a "critical" point when considering esophageal pressure and supraglottic pharyngeal pressure and genioglossal contraction. This critical point was when the pharyngeal pressure exceeded the genioglossal contraction force (which is lower during sleep than during wakefulness). Lugarsi and colleagues suggested that chronic snoring was the precursor of OSA [35]. There were also reports that patients with significant micrognathia also presented with OSAS, a fact already suggested in 1972 by Tammeling and colleagues [16] in three cases. This highlighted the potential role of the skeletal structures in the development of sleep apnea syndrome. The publication also emphasized the presence of sleep-disordered breathing in neurological disorders, particularly muscle diseases such as myotonic dystrophy and neuromuscular syndromes such as post-poliomyelitis syndrome and Shy–Drager syndrome (today referred to as "multiple system atrophy") The Stanford group presented these different associations in different reports [33] and emphasized the difference between OSAS and the abnormal breathing that was predominant during REM sleep in these syndromes. There was also demonstration of the association between OSA and chronic obstructive pulmonary disease (COPD) and improvement after tracheostomy [36, 37]. This initial report from Stanford led to a strong rebuttal in the UK published in the *Lancet* [38],but several years later the same UK team recognized its existence and described it as the "overlap syndrome" [39].

The most important event, however, occurred in 1981 when Colin Sullivan and colleagues [40] reported the very beneficial results obtained with home continuous positive airway pressure (CPAP) treatment in obstructive sleep apnea. Positive airway pressure had been used in neonatal intensive care, but Sullivan, using his mother's old vacuum cleaner, developed the equipment that eliminated the need to perform tracheostomy. It was a discovery that would ultimately benefit millions of patients. With less impact, Fujita and colleagues suggested performing palatal surgery with a procedure called "uvulopalatopharyngoplasty" (UPPP) [41], which is currently no longer recommended. It has been largely replaced by "pharyngoplasty" with or without tonsillectomy. The Stanford group performed the first maxilla and mandibular osteotomy to eliminate the need to perform tracheostomy [42]. In 1983, the first use of dental devices was reported [43]. Though early trials occurred in Marburg, Germany, around 1990, it would be a decade before a novel treatment was introduced: the successful use of electrical stimulation of the hypoglossal nerve in 2001 [44].

Moreover, by 1981, our understanding of OSAS in children was well advanced: It was clear that the syndrome had a pervasive detrimental impact. It not only led to cardiovascular dysfunction but there were also clear effects on alertness, learning, memory, school success, growth, abnormal behavior suggestive of attention deficit and hyperactivity

disorder (ADHD), and mood disorders such as depression and parasomnias (e.g., enuresis, sleepwalking, and night terrors) as reported by the Stanford group [45]. The Department of Otolaryngology in New York demonstrated that these symptoms could be relieved by adenotonsillectomy [46]. In the ensuing decades, attention turned to epidemiological and large cohort investigations. These included the San Marino cohort of Lugaresi et al. [47], the Wisconsin Sleep Cohort of Young et al. [48], and the Singapore study [49]. The Singapore study was the first to clearly indicate that Far East Asians had greater risks of developing OSA due to their anatomy than other ethnic groups [49]. These studies added important population information on the prevalence of obstructive sleep apnea.

Towards the end of last century work by several teams—and particularly by Frieberg and colleagues from Sweden [50]—indicated that sleep-disordered breathing induced destruction of mechano-(and perhaps other) receptors as well as damage to small motor fibers in the upper airway. This may be responsible for a local neuropathy that leads to abnormal contraction of the upper airway dilators during sleep, referring to the earlier question about the underlying pathophysiology that remains unresolved.

The development of the obesity epidemic in the recent past has rekindled the concepts of "Pickwickian syndrome." It is important to dissociate the role of obesity from the consequences of the occlusion of the upper airway during sleep: Obesity per se leads to the same cardiovascular morbidity and alertness changes without having to call upon the presence of OSA (as may be seen in individuals of normal weight with OSAS). Abdominal obesity contributes to a chest bellow syndrome during sleep, most prominent during REM sleep. Finally, obesity leads to hyperactivity of the adipocyte, a complex cell that controls many important peptides that regulate many metabolic functions. Obesity has also been shown by Schwab et al. [51] to secondarily enlarge the tongue, leading to obstructive sleep apnea. Understanding the historical narrative and the progressive advances made in the understanding of OSA and OSAS will be invaluable as we continue to unravel the different aspects of abnormal breathing during sleep in the years to come.

References

1. Dickens C. The posthumous papers of the Pickwick Club. London: Chapman and Hall; 1837.
2. Burwell CS, Robin ED, Whaley RD, Biskelmann AG. Extreme obesity associated with alveolar hypoventilation. A Pickwickian syndrome. Am J Med. 1956;21:811–8.
3. Auchincloss JH, Cook E, Renzetti AD. Clinical and physiological aspects of a case of obesity, polycythemia and alveolar hypoventilation. J Clin Invest. 1955:34:1537–45.

4. Sieker HO, Estes EH Jr., Kielser GA, McIntosh HD. A cardiopulmonary syndrome associated with extreme obesity. J Clin Invest. 1955;34:916

5. Kerr WJ, Lagen JB. The postural syndrome of obesity leading to postural emphysema and cardiorespiratory failure. Ann Intern Med. 1936;10:569–74.

6. Gelineau JB. De la narcolepsie. Gaz des Hôp (Paris) 1880; 83:626–28 and 84:635–37.

7. Gerardy W, Herberg D, Kuhn HM. Vergleichende untersuchungen der Lungfunktion und der Elektroencephalogramm bei zwei Patienten. Z Klin Med 1960;156:362–80.

8. Drachman DB, Gumnit RJ. Periodic alteration of consciousness in the Pickwickian syndrome. Arch Neurol. 1962;6:63–9.

9. Jung R, Kuhlo W. Neurophysiology studies of abnormal night sleep in the Pickwickian syndrome. In: Akert K, Bally C, Shade JP, editors. Progress in brain research: sleep mechanisms, vol. 18. Amsterdam: Elsevier; 1965. pp. 14–159.

10. Kuhlo W. Neurophysiologische und klinische untersuchungen beim Pickwick-Syndrom. Arch Psychiatr Nervenkr. 1968;211:170

11. Kuhlo W, Doll E, Franc MC. Exfolgreiche behandlung eines Pickwick Syndrom durch eine dauertracheal Kanule. Deutsch Med Wschr 1969;94:1286–90.

12. Gastaut H, Tassinari CA, Duron B. Polygraphic study of the episodic diurnal and nocturnal manifestations of the Pickwickian syndrome. Brain Res. 1966;1:167–86.

13. Duron B, Quichaud J, Fullana N. Nouvelles recherches sur le mécanisme des apnées du syndrome de Pickwick. Pathophysiol Respir. 1972;8:1277–88.

14. Lugaresi E, Coccagna G, Petrella A, Berti-Ceroni G, Pazzaglia P. Il disturb de sonno e del respire nella syndrome di Pickwick. Sist Nerv. 1968;1:38–50.

15. Tassinari CA, Dalla Bernardina D, Cirignota F. Apneoic periods and the respiratory related arousal patterns during sleep in the Pickwickian syndrome; a polygraphic study Bull. Pathophysiol Respir.1972;8:1087–102

16. Kurtz D, Meunier-Carus J, Baptst-Reiter J, Landsdorfer J, Micheletti G, Benignus E, Rohmer F. Problèmes nosologiques posés par certaines formes d'hypersomnie. Rev EEG Neurophysiol (French). 1971;1:227–30

17. Krieger J. les séquences hypno-apnéiques chez les sujets Pickwickiens: leur semeiologie et leur repartition. Strasbourg. Thèse de Médecine Faculté de Médecine de Strasbourg; 1975.

18. Coccagna G, Mantovani M, Brignani F, Parchi C, Lugaresi E. Continuous recording of pulmonary and systemic arterial pressure during sleep in syndromes of hypersomnia with periodic breathing. Bull Physiopathol Respir.1972;8:1159–72

19. Carroll D. Nosology of the Pickwickian syndrome. Bull Physiopathol Respir. 1972;8:1241–8.

20. Tammeling GJ, Blokzijl EJ, Boonstra S, Sluiter HJ. Micrognathia, hypersomnia and periodic breathing. Bull Physiopathol Respir. 1972;8(5):1229–38.

21. Guilleminault C, Eldridge FL, Dement WC. Insomnia, narcolepsy and sleep apneas. Bull Physiopathol Respir. 1972;8:1127–38.

22. Guilleminault C, Dement WC, Monod N. Syndrome 'mort subite du nourrisson': apnées au cours du sommeil. Nouvelle hypothèse. Nouv Presse Med.1973;2:1355–8

23. Guilleminault C, Eldridge FL, Dement WC. Insomnia with sleep apnea: a new syndrome. Science. 1973;181:856–8.

24. Guilleminault C, Tilkian A, Dement WC. The sleep apnea syndromes. Annu Rev Med. 1976;27:465–84.

25. Guilleminault C, Eldridge F, Simmons FB, Dement WC. Sleep apnea syndrome: can it induce hemodynamic changes? West J Med. 1975;123:7–16.

26. Tilkian AG, Guilleminault C, Schroeder JS, Lehrman KL, Simmons FB, Dement WC. Hemodynamics in sleep induced apnea: studies during wakefulness and sleep. Ann Intern Med. 1976;85:714–9

27. Tilkian AG, Guilleminault C, Schroeder JS, Lehrman KL, Simmons FB, Dement WC. Sleep induced apnea syndrome: prevalence of cardiac arrhythmias and their reversal after tracheostomy. Am J Med. 1977;63:348–58

28. Weitzman ED, Pollack CP, Borowiecki B, Shprintzen R, Rakoff S. The hypersomnia sleep apnea syndrome: site and mechanism of upper airway obstruction. In: Guilleminault C, Dement WC, editors. Sleep apnea syndrome. New York: AR Liss: 1988. pp. 235–48

29. Guilleminault C, Hill MW, Simmons FB, Dement WC. Obstructive sleep apnea: electromyographic and fiberoptic studies. Exp Neurol. 1978;62:48–67.

30. Guilleminault C, Eldridge F, Simmons F, Dement WC. Sleep apnea in eight children. Pediatrics. 1976;58:23–30.

31. Guilleminault C, Korobkin R, Winkle R. A review of 50 children with obstructive sleep apnea syndrome. Lung. 1981;159:275–87.

32. Sauerland EK, Harper RM. The human tongue during sleep: electromyographic activity of the genioglossus Muscle. Exp Neurol. 1976;51:160–70.

33. Guilleminault C, Dement WC, editors. Sleep apnea syndrome. New-York: AR Liss; 1978. pp. 1–372.

34. Remmers JE, de Groot WJ, Sauerland EK, Anch AM. Pathogenesis of upper airway occlusion during sleep. J Appl Physiol. 1978;44:931–8.

35. Lugaresi E, Coccagna G, Cirignotta F. Snoring and its clinical implications. In: Guilleminault C, Dement WC, editors. Sleep apnea syndrome. New-York: AR Liss; 1978. pp. 13–21.

36. Guilleminault C, Cummiskey J, Motta J. Chronic obstructive air flow disease and sleep studies. Am Rev Respir Dis. 1980;122:397–406.

37. Guilleminault C, Cummiskey J. Progressive improvement of apnea and ventilatory response to CO2 following tracheostomy in obstructive apnea syndrome. Am Rev Resp Dis. 1982;126:14–20.

38. Shapiro CM, Catteral JR, Oswald I, Flenley DC. Where are the British sleep apnoea patients? Lancet. 1981;318:523.

39. Flenley DC. Sleep in chronic obstructive lung disease. Clin Chest Med. 1985;6:651–61.

40. Sullivan CE, Berthon-Jones M, Issac FC, Eves L. Reversal of obstructive sleep apnea by continuous positive airway pressure applied through the nares. Lancet. 1981;1:862–5

41. Fujita S, Conway WA, Zorick R, Roth T. Evaluation of the effectiveness of uvulo-palato-pharyngo-plasty. Laryngoscope. 1985;95:70–4

42. Riley R, Powell N, Guilleminault C, Nino-Murcia G. Maxillary, mandibular, and hyoid advancement: an alternative to tracheostomy in obstructive sleep apnea syndrome. Otolaryngol Head Neck Surg. 1986;94:589–93.

43. Andrews JM, Guilleminault C, Holdaway RA. Use of a mandibular positioning device in obstructive sleep apnea: a case report. Bull Eur Physiopath Resp (Clin Resp Physiol). 1983;19:611.

44. Schwartz AR, Bennett ML, Smith PL, De Backer W, Hedner J, Boudewyns A et al. Therapeutic electrical stimulation of the hypoglossal nerve in obstructive sleep apnea. Arch Otolaryngol Head Neck Surg. 2001;127:1216–23.

45. Guilleminault C, Korobkin R, Winkle R. A review of 50 children with obstructive sleep apnea syndrome. Lung. 1981:159;275–87.

46. Kravath R, Pollak C, Borowiecki B. Hypoventilation during sleep in children who have lymphoid airway obstruction treated by a nasopharyngeal tube and tonsillectomy and adenoidectomy. Pediatrics. 1977;59:865–71.

47. Mondini S, Zucconi M, Cirignotta F, Aguglia U, Lenzi PL. Zauli C, Lugaresi E. Snoring as a risk factor for cardiac and circulatory problems: an epidemiologicoal study. In: Guilleminault C, Lugaresi E, editors. Sleep-wake disorders: epidemiology and long term follow-up. New-York: Raven; 1983. pp. 99–105.

48. Young T, Palta M, Dempsey J, Skatrud J, Weber S, Badr S. The occurrence of sleep-disordered-breathing among middle age adults. N Engl J Med 1993;328:1230–5.

49. Puvanendram K, Goh KL. From snoring to sleep apnea in the Singapore population. Sleep Res Online. 1999;2:11–4.

50. Frieberg D, Ansved T, Borg K, et al. Histological indications of a progressive snorers disease in an upper airway muscle. Am J Respir Crit Care Med. 1998;157:586–93.

51. Schwab RJ, Pasirstein M, Pierson R, Mackley A, Arens R, Maislin G, Pack AI. Identification of upper airway anatomic risk factors for obstructive sleep apnea with volumetric MRI. Am J Respir Crit Care Med. 2003;168:522–30.

Upper-Airway Resistance Syndrome: A Short History

Brandon Richard Peters and Christian Guilleminault

While investigating obstructive sleep apnea in children, Guilleminault learned in 1977 that snoring children had similar complaints and polysomnography-recorded tachypnea but not sleep apnea. The complaints and tachypnea resolved with adenotonsillectomy. Thereafter, all children with clinical symptoms and history of snoring during sleep were systematically studied with calibrated esophageal pressure monitoring to evaluate for the presence of abnormally increased respiratory effort, independent of the presence or absence of hypopnea and apnea during sleep. These investigations included, by necessity, the associated EEG during sleep.

Guilleminault et al. had well described the obstructive sleep apnea syndrome (OSAS) in children, emphasizing that cognitive dysfunction and abnormal behavior during sleep were important problems in this pediatric age group [1, 2]. However, the description did not fully cover the spectrum of abnormal breathing during sleep. In 1982, Guilleminault and colleagues published a case-series on children with similar clinical presentations to those with pediatric OSAS but with only abnormal flow limitation and abnormally increased effort during sleep, as demonstrated by esophageal manometry (Pes) measurement during sleep, and subsequent response to adenotonsillectomy [3]. Despite emphasizing the "resistive-load" as an important feature when investigating sleep-disordered breathing, nobody followed this lead and the Stanford Sleep Clinic was one of the places where children were systematically studied using Pes to monitor breathing during sleep.

Guilleminault asked Riccardo Stoohs, a young postgraduate fellow from Marburg, Germany, where Guilleminault had been on sabbatical, to investigate things further. Stoohs was enticed to come and perform postgraduate research at Stanford focusing on this abnormal breathing pattern that was now seen not only in children but also in teenagers and young adults. The studies were also performed in adults and for the first time the term "upper-airway resistance" was used and these adult cases were published [4]. These authors explained the reasons for arousal without hypopneas and oxygen de saturation but with significant daytime dysfunction. Unfortunately, these observations were neglected, and the scientific world had just barely accepted the notion of OSAS. The pulmonary specialists became interested in evaluating nocturnal oximetry and breathing during sleep, but investigation of subtle changes in the EEG was neglected.

The Stanford group was inspired by the observations of Toshiaki Shiomi that abnormal efforts during sleep with or without hypopnea or apnea had a clear impact on the intraventricular cardiac septum [5] and decided to investigate further. The same group coined the term "upper-airway resistance syndrome" or "UARS" to describe the condition of abnormal breathing pattern during sleep without necessarily having any oxygen de saturation. The clinical and polysomnographic features were published [6], following which the term UARS was finally accepted by individuals working in the field of sleep medicine.

Even with further evidence of the impact of such abnormal breathing patterns during sleep on cardiovascular variables [7], there was reluctance by sleep specialists to routinely use Pes during polysomnography. The Stanford group tried to see if other variables considered to be "less invasive" could be used, and for the first time, the term "flow limitation" was associated with UARS and "snoring intensity" was evaluated as an alternative [8]. However, the possible usage of "flow limitation" as an alternative to measurement of Pes was only considered when the "nasal cannula pressure transducer" was better defined [9–11]. In the prior physiological reports, the Stanford group had used a full-face mask with a

C. Guilleminault (✉)
Sleep Medicine Division, Stanford University Outpatient Medical Center, 450 Broadway, Redwood City, CA 94063, USA
e-mail: cguil@stanford.edu

B. R. Peters
Stanford Sleep Medicine Center, Stanford School of Medicine, Redwood City, CA, USA

S. Chokroverty, M. Billiard (eds.), *Sleep Medicine*, DOI 10.1007/978-1-4939-2089-1_42,
© Springer Science+Business Media, LLC 2015

tightly fitted valve, a pneumotachograph, and Pes for the calculation of flow and tidal volume. This equipment, though well-suited for research purposes, could not be easily transferred to clinical practice. One was left again with measurement of Pes.

In 1999, Housselet and colleagues [9] defined "flow limitation" in adults. Such a measurement provided ease of recognition of UARS, even if it does not always match Pes measurements. The first review on UARS was also published that year [12], and usage of nasal cannula to recognize UARS was emphasized by Epstein et al. [13]. It was clear that, depending on the authors, the term was being used a bit differently [14, 15]. To demonstrate that there was a difference between OSAS and UARS, the Stanford group published diverse investigations looking at the autonomic nervous system responses and brain disturbances [16, 17]. However, the demonstration that OSA could be associated with a local neuropathy was presented by Swedish investigators [18, 19]. Demonstration of progressive destruction of local upper-airway receptors provided evidence that the presence of a different syndrome may occur based on the presence or absence of these receptors which are required to respond quickly and appropriately to a challenge during sleep [20]. When they do not respond, completely different means are necessary to inform the brain to control the problem. This variance may lead to different types of comorbidities.

Gold et al. [21] further emphasized the difficulties of recognizing UARS. The Stanford group had shown that UARS can be an important factor in the occurrence of parasomnias in children and adults [22] and that it is often unrecognized in young individuals, particularly women [23]. To increase recognition, the condition has been studied using the cyclic alternating pattern (CAP) EEG scoring system [24]. The latest investigations have included calculation of the prevalence of UARS in the general population, derived from the Sao Paulo epidemiologic study. This study was led by Luciana Palombini and determined the prevalence to be about 15 % [25]. Despite the fact that UARS is still not often recognized and treated, this syndrome significantly impairs the well-being of many, and in 2011, a "lesson" was requested by the American College of Chest Physicians [26] to summarize the current findings.

References

1. Guilleminault C, Eldridge F, Simmons F, Dement WC. Sleep apnea in eight children. Pediatrics. 1976;58:23–30.
2. Guilleminault C, Korobkin R, Winkle R. A review of 50 children with obstructive sleep apnea syndrome. Lung. 1981;159:275–87.
3. Guilleminault C, Winkle R, Korobkin R, Simmons B. Children and nocturnal snoring: evaluation of the effects of sleep related respiratory resistive load and daytime functioning. Eur J Pediat. 1982;139:165–71.
4. Stoohs R, Guilleminault C. Obstructive sleep apnea syndrome or abnormal upper airway resistance during sleep? J Clin Neurophysiol. 1990;7:83–92.
5. Guilleminault C, Shiomi T, Stoohs R, Schnittger I. Echocardiographic studies in adults and children presenting with obstructive sleep apnea or heavy snoring. In: Gaultier C, Escourrou P, Curzi-Dascalova L, editors. Sleep and cardiorespiratory control. Paris: John Libbey; 1991. p. 95–104.
6. Guilleminault C, Stoohs R, Clerk A, Cetel M, Maistros P. A cause of excessive daytime sleepiness: the upper airway resistance syndrome. Chest. 1993;104:781–7.
7. Guilleminault C, Stoohs R, Shiomi T, Kushida C, Schnittger I. Upper airway resistance syndrome, nocturnal blood pressure monitoring, and borderline hypertension. Chest. 1996;109(4):901–8.
8. Stoohs R, Skrobal A, Guilleminault C. Does snoring intensity predict flow limitation or respiratory effort during sleep? Resp Physiol. 1993;92:27–38.
9. Hosselet JJ, Norman RG, Ayappa I, Rapoport D. Detection of flow limitation with nasal cannula/pressure transducer system. Am J Respir Crit Care Med. 1999;157:1461–7.
10. Aittokallio T, Saaresranta T, Polo-Kantola P, Nevalainen O, Polo O. Analysis of inspiratory flow shapes in patients with partial upper-airway obstruction during sleep. Chest. 2001;119:337–44.
11. Serebrisky D, Cordero R, Mandeli J, et al. Assessment of inspiratory flow limitation in children with sleep-disordered breathing by a nasal cannula pressure transducer system. Pediatric Pulmonol. 2002;33:380–7.
12. Exar EN, Collop NA. The upper airway resistance syndrome. Chest. 1999;115:1127–39.
13. Epstein MD, Chicoine SA, Hanumara RC. Detection of upper airway resistance syndrome using a nasal cannula/transducer. Chest. 2000;117:1073–7.
14. Wheatley J.R. Definition and diagnosis of upper airway resistance syndrome. Sleep. 2004;23:S193–6.
15. Bao G, Guilleminault C. The upper airway resistance syndrome—one decade later. Curr Opin Pulm Med. 2004;10:461–7.
16. Guilleminault C, Faul JL, Stoohs R. Sleep-disordered breathing and hypotension. Am J Respir Crit Care Med. 2001;164:1242–7.
17. Guilleminault C, Kim YD, Chowdhuri S, Horita M, Ohayon M, Kushida C. Sleep and daytime sleepiness in upper airway resistance syndrome compared to obstructive sleep apnea syndrome. Eur Respir J. 2001;17:1–10.
18. Friberg D. Heavy snorer's disease: a progressive local neuropathy. Acta Otolaryngol. 1999;119: 925–33.
19. Friberg D, Ansved T, Borg K, et al. Histological indications of a progressive snorer's disease in an upper-airway muscle. Am J Resp Crit Care Med. 1999;157:586–93.
20. Guilleminault C, Li K, Chen NH, Poyares D. Two-point palatal discrimination in patients with upper airway resistance syndrome, obstructive sleep apnea syndrome, and normal control subjects. Chest. 2002;122:866–70.
21. Gold AR, Dipalo F, Gold MS, O'Heam D. The symptoms and signs of upper airway resistance syndrome: a link to the functional somatic syndromes. Chest. 2003;123:87–95.
22. Guilleminault C, Kirisoglu C, Bao G, Arias V, Chan A, Li KK. Adult chronic sleepwalking and its treatment based on polysomnography. Brain. 2005;128:1062–9.
23. Tantrakul V, Pack SC, Guilleminault C. Sleep-disordered-breathing in premenopausal women: differences between younger (less than 30 years old) and older women. Sleep Med. 2012;13: 656–62.
24. Guilleminault C, Lopes MC, Hagen CC, Rosa da A. The cyclic alternating pattern demonstrates increased sleep instability and correlates with fatigue and sleepiness in adults with upper airway resistance syndrome. Sleep. 2007;30:641–7.
25. Palombini L Tufik, S, Rapoport D, Ayappa I, Guilleminault C, de Godoy L, Casto L, Bittencourt L. Inspiratory flow limitation in a normal population of adults in Sao Paolo, Brazil. Sleep. 2013; 36: 1663-68.
26. Ogunrrindi O, Hue HJ, Guilleminault C. Upper airway resistance PCCSU. Chest. 2011;25:lesson 13.

Restrictive and Obstructive Lung Diseases and Sleep Disorders

Vipin Malik and Teofilo Lee-Chiong

Sleep has several effects on the respiratory system and can influence airflow and gas exchange. The latter, in turn, can lead to sleep fragmentation and diminished sleep quality. Sleep disruption and nocturnal hypoxemia are particularly exaggerated in patients with pulmonary illnesses and can lead to increased morbidity and mortality.In this chapter, we discuss the evolution of our current understanding of how sleep and circadian rhythms affect respiratory physiology, and how this increased recognition is influencing current evaluation and management of pulmonary disorders. We, thus, review some of the earliest literature and determine how these tentative beginnings led to the most recent advances in our knowledge today.

Scientific Inquiries of Sleep and Respiration

Before attempting to explore the progress of our understanding of the relationship between sleep and respiration, starting from its earliest beginnings and spanning the several previous decades of scientific investigations, it is reasonable to start by asking why it took so long for the medical community to acknowledge the impact of sleep and biologic rhythms on the respiratory system and on pulmonary disorders. There are several possible explanations why early researchers and clinicians limited their queries and practice to the wake patient during the day and why changes in physiologic and pathologic processes resulting from sleep and circadian rhythm were often considered unimportant and, therefore, ignored (which Lee-Chiong had referred to previously as the "two-thirds science investigating a 2/3 person in a 2/3 world"). First, there was lack of resources to maintain 24-h research laboratories or to conduct research at night. Second, there

were no easily available technologies to conduct research on the sleeping person. Clearly, before the advent of polysomnography (PSG) and other techniques that objectively monitor the stages of wake and sleep, the only way to measure biologic parameters during "sleep" was through observation, which was, unfortunately, both unreliable and poorly sensitive and specific. Thus, progress in the field required parallel technological advances in noninvasive monitoring of sleep and pulmonary function. Digitization and computers have hastened this over the past 15 years. Finally, and most important, there was a lack of appreciation that human beings are not an 16-h species and that the 8-h sleep period has significant effects on the clinical manifestations, natural course, and outcomes of specific medical disorders, as exemplified by sleep-related oxygen desaturation in chronic obstructive pulmonary disease (COPD) and nocturnal exacerbations of asthma, and on the proper timing of therapy.

Respiratory Physiology during Sleep Mature

The study of respiratory physiology was confined, for many centuries, to the waking state. Our current knowledge of the profound changes in the respiratory system accompanying sleep took several decades of maturation. Even today, investigators continue to grapple with explanations for changes in respiratory mechanics, inflammation, control and compensatory processes, and aberrations during sleep.

Control of respiration, which relies on both metabolic (pH, PaO_2, and $PaCO_2$), and behavioral factors during wake, is under sole metabolic control during sleep. Behavioral influences on respiration end with the cessation of stimulating input from the waking state. Anatomical changes of the ribcage occurring during the supine position of sleep also result in significant alterations in respiratory mechanics [1].

Minute ventilation falls with the onset of sleep in response to decreased metabolism and decreased chemosensitivity to oxygen (O_2) and carbon dioxide (CO_2) [2, 3]. The decline in minute ventilation is mainly due to a decrease in tidal vol-

V. Malik (✉) · T. Lee-Chiong
Department of Medicine, National Jewish Health, University of Colorado Denver, M323, 1400 Jackson Street, Denver, CO 80130, USA
e-mail: malikv@njhealth.org

ume during non-rapid eye movement (NREM) sleep, especially stage N3 sleep as well as from a reduction in inspiratory drive. Consequently, end-tidal carbon dioxide ($ETCO_2$) during NREM sleep increases by 1–2 torr compared with the waking state. $ETCO_2$ rises by an additional 1–2 torr with the onset of rapid eye movement (REM) sleep.

Ventilatory responses to CO_2 and O_2 vary during REM and NREM sleep. Arousal thresholds for hypercapnia range between 56 and 65 torr and differ among the different sleep stages. In addition to a reduction in the slope of ventilatory response to PaCO2, the threshold of response to CO_2 is shifted upwards, with a higher $ETCO_2$ required to drive respiration in sleep [4]. More variable and less predictable changes in respiratory responses to hypoxia are seen in NREM sleep; these changes are further attenuated in REM sleep.

Activity of dilator muscles that maintain patency and prevent collapse of the upper airways during inspiration, i.e., genioglossus, tensor palatini, and sternohyoid, are reduced during sleep. Upper and lower airway resistances increase during sleep and can result in obstructive apnea in predisposed individuals [5, 6]. During wakefulness, upper airway muscles, especially genioglossus, respond briskly to increases in $PaCO_2$, elastic loading, and airway resistance, but this response is markedly diminished during sleep. During NREM sleep, an increase in resistance loads results in reduced tidal volumes and higher respiratory rates but no significant change in inspiratory time; this is in contrast to increases in duration of the respiratory cycle and tidal volume as well as decreases in respiratory rate and increases in minute ventilation during the wake state.

To improve ventilation, activity of accessory muscles of breathing is increased during NREM sleep. However, during REM sleep, ventilation is accomplished primarily by the diaphragm due to generalized skeletal muscle atonia. Predisposition to paradoxical chest wall motion, due to increased chest wall compliance from diminished intercostal tone, also increases during REM sleep. Positional changes during sleep also affect the mechanics of breathing significantly. Functional residual capacity decreases during sleep due to a change in the ribcage and lung recoil pressures; decrease in the ribcage volume from cephalad motion of the diaphragm; and central pooling of blood resulting from greater venous return [7].

Restrictive Lung Diseases

Pulmonary restriction, whether intra- or extra-thoracic, is associated with neurally mediated increase in ventilatory drive, increased work of breathing, and gas exchange abnormalities. Major symptoms in patients with chronic interstitial lung diseases include progressive breathlessness, fatigue,

dry cough, decreased activity levels with loss of independence, anxiety/depression, and decreased mobility. By the early 1980s, it was widely recognized that patients with a variety of interstitial lung disease can have fragmented sleep, with increased arousals, and greater percentage of stages N1 and N2 sleep along with less N3 and REM sleep [8]. In addition, early descriptions of the spectrum of breathing disorders associated with kyphoscoliosis included central and obstructive apneas/hypopneas [9, 10]. The first issue of the journal Sleep featured a report on the respiratory and hemodynamic parameters in patients with myotonic dystrophy during wakefulness and sleep [11].

Currently, treatment of restrictive lung diseases consists of oxygen supplementation to improve gas exchange and noninvasive mechanical ventilation for respiratory failure. Mean oxygen saturation (SaO_2) during sleep and sleep quality, including total sleep time, sleep efficiency, and frequency of awakenings, improve with noninvasive ventilation treatment in patients with chronic respiratory failure due to thoracic restriction.

Chronic Obstructive Pulmonary Disease

COPD involves progressive, not fully reversible, airflow limitation due to injury to the small airways and alveoli from noxious particles or gases. The term "COPD" encompasses several distinct disorders, including chronic bronchitis (clinically defined as chronic productive cough for 3 months in each of 2 successive years) and emphysema (anatomically defined as abnormal, permanent enlargement of the airspaces distal to the terminal bronchioles). Patients with COPD often present with complaints of dyspnea, chronic cough, or chest tightness.

Nighttime Symptoms

The prevalence of nighttime symptoms in COPD is not well understood. Although sleep quality is often poor in COPD patients, sleep disturbance is frequently unreported by the latter. Additionally, there is no uniform definition for "nocturnal symptoms." Despite these limitations, it has been suggested that the prevalence of nighttime symptoms and sleep disturbance may exceed 75 % in this population [12].

Nocturnal Oxygen Desaturation

Nocturnal hypoxemia can develop in moderate-to-severe COPD. As early as the late 1970s, researchers have demonstrated that episodes of sleep-related O_2 desaturation are more frequent, of greater duration, and more severe during REM sleep versus NREM sleep [13]. Nocturnal hypoxemia was also noted early on to be more common in blue bloaters than in pink puffers [14].

There are several mechanisms responsible for sleep-related hypoxemia, such as hypoventilation, ventilation–perfusion mismatching, and diminished lung volumes. Hypoventilation appears to be the most important factor and can produce both hypoxemia and hypercapnia. Oxygenation during wakefulness is the major predictor of mean and lowest SaO_2 during sleep in COPD. Several factors have been shown to predict nocturnal O_2 desaturation among stable COPD patients without daytime respiratory failure or obstructive sleep apnea (OSA). These included higher diurnal $PaCO_2$, lower daytime SaO_2, lung dynamic hyperinflation, lower inspiratory capacity, and smaller upper airway caliber (i.e., oropharyngeal junction area) [15].

Sleep Disturbance

There is a high prevalence of poor sleep quality among COPD patients. In an article published in 1983, 43 % of patients with COPD reported having sleep difficulties that occurred either "almost always" or "always" [16].

In the Tucson Epidemiologic Study of chronic lung disease, the prevalence of insomnia in COPD depended on number of symptoms (cough or wheezing)—28 % in asymptomatic patients, 39 % if either cough or wheezing is present, and 53 % if the patient has both symptoms [17]. The frequency of insomnia waxes and wanes in relation to respiratory symptoms. Persons with new or persistent respiratory symptoms, such as cough, dyspnea, or wheezing, are more likely to develop new insomnia, and have persistent sleep disturbance than those with no symptoms [18]. Not unlike in the general population, insomnia is more common in women and older adults [18].

Disturbed sleep predicts poor general health-related and disease-specific quality of life (QOL) in COPD patients. In one report, 70 % of patients with COPD described poor sleep quality (Pittsburgh Sleep Quality Index; PSQI > 5). Quality of sleep, along with severity of dyspnea (Modified Medical Research Council scale) and post-bronchodilator FEV_1, was significantly correlated with health-related (HR) QOL using the Saint George's Respiratory Questionnaire [19].

Etiology

There are multiple possible causes of sleep disturbance in COPD patients; these include demographic factors (e.g., aging); disease-specific factors (cough, dyspnea, hypoxemia, and acute exacerbations); pharmacotherapy; associated med-

ical disorders (depression or cardiovascular diseases); and presence of comorbid sleep disorders, such as OSA, primary insomnia, and restless legs syndrome (RLS). Depression may contribute to the development of sleep disturbance.

Predictors of poor sleep quality in COPD patients include daytime PaO_2, cough, dyspnea, COPD severity, need for medications and O_2, and hospital-based utilization [20]. Severity of airflow obstruction and thoracic hyperinflation may also be responsible for poor sleep quality in COPD patients.

Overlap Syndrome

During the early 1980s, investigators have noted that a substantial percentage of patients with obstructive lung disease who presented with complaints of daytime sleepiness had comorbid OSA [21]. The term "overlap syndrome" was first coined in 1985 to describe the presence of both COPD and OSA in the same individual [22]. The prevalence of OSA in COPD is similar to that in the general population, and vice versa. Decreased pulmonary function among COPD patients is not an independent risk factor for OSA. One report showed no correlation between FEV_1 % predicted and risk for OSA, total apnea–hypopnea index (AHI), oxygen desaturation index (ODI), % time with $SaO_2 < 90$ %, and mean SaO_2 [23]. However, because both conditions are highly prevalent, it is not uncommon for both disorders to be present in the same individual.

Compared to isolated COPD, patients with overlap syndrome tend to have lower PaO_2, higher $PaCO_2$, and more elevated pulmonary artery (PA) pressures. Furthermore, compared to patients with COPD alone, those with overlap syndrome not treated with continuous positive airway pressure (CPAP) have increased risk of death and hospitalization due to COPD exacerbation. More extensive right ventricular (RV) remodeling in patients with comorbid OSA and COPD compared to those with COPD alone might explain, at least in part, the higher cardiovascular mortality associated with the overlap syndrome [24]. Treatment with CPAP improved survival and decreased hospitalizations [25]. Finally, the presence of OSA results in an elevated economic burden in patients with COPD. Using Medicaid claims data, investigators noted that COPD beneficiaries with OSA had higher medical service claims, and higher medical costs than those without OSA [26].

Restless Legs Syndrome

RLS is common in patients with COPD. An estimated 29–36 % of COPD patients experience RLS-type symptoms. Prevalence of RLS may even be higher during acute exacerbations (up to 54 % in one study) [27]. In another study,

RLS was more prevalent (36 vs. 11%; $P<0.001$), more severe (International Restless Legs Syndrome Study; IRLSS severity scale score of 20.5 ± 2.8 vs. 18 ± 3.5; $P=0.016$), and associated with more severe daytime sleepiness (ESS score of 11.8 ± 1.1 vs. 8.6 ± 3.6; $P=0.009$) in COPD patients than in healthy individuals [28].

Evaluation

PSG is not routinely indicated in persons with COPD, but should be considered if there is clinical suspicion for OSA, if complications from unexplained hypoxemia are present, or if severity of pulmonary hypertension is out of proportion to the degree of airflow limitation. Patients with poorly controlled disease often demonstrate prolonged sleep onset latency, reduced sleep efficiency, decreased total sleep time, increased sleep stage changes, more frequent arousals and awakenings, and reduced REM sleep. Nevertheless, many patients with COPD may have normal sleep architecture during PSG. Portable sleep apnea testing is not recommended to diagnose OSA in COPD patients. Actigraphy may demonstrate lower sleep efficiency and shorter sleep duration in COPD patients with insomnia. Other actigraphic findings include prolonged sleep latency, increased mean activity, and more wake-after-sleep onset compared to healthy controls. One study noted that actigraphic measures of sleep efficiency, total sleep time, and sleep activity correlated with severity of dyspnea [29]. Overnight oximetry should be performed in patients presenting with daytime hypercapnia and/or hypoxemia, pulmonary and/or systemic hypertension, or right heart failure.

Treatment

Treatment of nocturnal symptoms consists of long-acting beta-agonists, theophylline or long-acting anticholinergic agents, but these agents have not been used consistently to improve nighttime sleep quality. Oxygen therapy is indicated for significant nocturnal O_2 desaturation. The beneficial effects of oxygen therapy on nocturnal oxygen desaturation in patients with COPD have been known for at least three decades. However, early investigators reported that nighttime oxygen supplementation does not diminish frequency of arousals in this population. Although arousals are strongly associated with periods of desaturation, O_2 therapy to correct nocturnal hypoxemia has no consistent effect on sleep quality or frequency of arousals [30, 31]. Both the US Nocturnal Oxygen Therapy Trial Group and the British Research Council Working Party established the scientific foundations for the use of long-term oxygen therapy for COPD in 1980 and 1981, respectively [32, 33].

Treatment of overlap syndrome consists of O_2 supplementation as needed, positive airway pressure (PAP) therapy, and nasal intermittent positive pressure ventilation (NIPPV). Treatment of OSA with CPAP in patients with overlap syndrome has beneficial effects on daytime PaO_2 and $PaCO_2$, nocturnal SaO_2, mean PA pressure, maximal inspiratory pressure and daytime sleepiness as measured by ESS [34]. More important, CPAP treatment of OSA improves survival of hypoxemic COPD patients. In a prospective, cohort study, survival was higher in patients with overlap syndrome receiving long-term O_2 therapy for chronic hypoxemia who were compliant with the CPAP therapy compared to patients who were non compliant with therapy (5-year survival rates of 71% vs. 26%; $P<0.01$). Patients who used CPAP had significantly lower risk of death (hazard ratio of death vs. nontreated patients of 0.19 [0.08–0.48]) [35].

Asthma

Asthma refers to reversible bronchoconstriction and airway hyperreactivity to specific and nonspecific stimuli. Main clinical features consist of episodic dyspnea, wheezing, and coughing.

Nocturnal Asthma Symptoms

Nocturnal asthma symptoms requiring rescue short-acting bronchodilator therapy are common in children with mild-to-moderate persistent asthma, despite controller therapy, and in one study was reported at least once in 72% of patients and occurred 13 or more times in 24% of patients. More important, nocturnal asthma symptoms were poor predictors of exacerbations [36]. In another study, involving children with persistent asthma, 41% had intermittent, 23% had mild persistent, and 36% had moderate-to-severe nocturnal asthma symptoms. The Children's Sleep Habits Questionnaire's average total sleep quality score indicated significant sleep disturbance, and were worse in those with more nocturnal asthma symptoms [37].

Sleep-Related Complaints

Sleep complaints, including insomnia, excessive sleepiness, and nocturnal hypoxemia, are common in nocturnal asthma. One study reported that asthma-related sleep difficulties occurred approximately four times per week in adults and approximately three times per week in children. Symptoms in the morning on awakening and feelings of tiredness and impaired activity on days after experiencing nighttime symptoms were more frequent in adults than children [38].

Sleep disturbance is more common among persons with uncontrolled versus controlled asthma and is indicative of poor asthma control. More patients with uncontrolled asthma described waking up at night with symptoms, using a rescue inhaler at night, having difficulty waking up in the morning and getting out of bed, and being overly tired all day [39].

Excessive daytime sleepiness is also strongly associated with asthma. In a study of school-aged children, the presence of asthma was among the strongest predictors of excessive daytime sleepiness, along with anxiety/depression and trouble falling asleep [40].

Causes of Sleep Disturbance

Causes of poor sleep quality include coughing, dyspnea, wheezing, and chest discomfort. Nocturnal asthma attacks are not specific to any sleep stage. Several mechanisms can account for nocturnal exacerbation of asthma-related symptoms. There is clearly a circadian influence on airflow with lowest levels in the early morning. This relationship between diurnal rhythms and airway obstruction was described in the 1970s and had since changed fundamentally our knowledge of the 24-h course of asthma morbidity [41]. Changes in the autonomic nervous system (i.e., increased parasympathetic tone and decreased sympathetic activity), lung capacity, and inflammatory mediators during sleep are also important pathophysiologic factors. At about the same time that circadian rhythm influences on nocturnal asthma were being described, other researchers have demonstrated that declines in airflow among asthmatic shift workers with varying sleep times correlated less to time of day than to time of sleep [42]. Lastly, other medical disorders, such as tonsillar hypertrophy, local and systemic inflammation, cardiac dysfunction, obesity, changes in airways related to leptin, and vascular endothelial growth factor-induced airway angiogenesis might worsen asthma control [43]. Nocturnal Gastroesophageal Reflux (GER), allergic rhinitis and OSA may either occur only during the sleep period or be worse at this time compared to the wake state; and depression may reduce asthma control, sleep quality and QOL.

Obstructive sleep apnea is both more prevalent and more severe in patients with severe asthma compared to those with more moderate asthma or without asthma. This pattern was confirmed in a study showing increasing prevalence of OSA (AHI $\geq$ 15 events per hour) in relation to the presence and severity of asthma, namely without asthma (31 %), with moderate asthma (58 %), and with severe asthma (88 %). When OSA was defined by an AHI of $\geq$ 5 events per hour, the prevalence of OSA among patients without asthma, with moderate asthma, or with severe asthma were 12, 23, and 50 %, respectively. OSA was more severe in patients with asthma compared with healthy controls [44]. Mechanical

strain on the airway can enhance airway hyperresponsiveness; this may explain why OSA exacerbates asthma symptoms as well as how CPAP therapy can reduce airway reactivity [45]. Conversely, asthma is also prevalent in patients with OSA. Investigators have reported a prevalence of 35 % of asthma with body mass index BMI (>35 kg/m^2) the only predictor for the latter [46]. This important observation regarding asthma and OSA needs to be emphasized. Poorly controlled asthma, itself, is a predictor of more severe OSA. OSA, in turn, may contribute to worse asthma control.

Finally, tonsillar hypertrophy was found more frequently in children with a history of wheezing compared to children who did not wheeze. It has been reported that a history of wheezing was significantly associated with tonsillar hypertrophy and snoring even after adjustments for age, gender, obesity, and passive exposure to smoking [47].

Diagnosis of Nocturnal Asthma

Diagnosis consists of confirming circadian variability in lung function. In nocturnal asthma, evening peak expiratory flow rates or FEV_1 values are often reduced compared to their daytime counterpart. PSG is not indicated; if performed for other indications, it commonly shows disturbed sleep that is correlated with disease severity (decreased sleep efficiency, reduced total sleep time, and increase in wake time after sleep onset). Several investigators have reported these PSG changes over a period of four decades [48, 49].

It has been suggested that patients with difficult-to-control asthma should be screened for the presence of comorbid OSA [50]. Predictors of OSA and habitual snoring in patients with asthma include severity of asthma, use of an inhaled corticosteroid, and presence of GER. Unlike in the general population, women had a 2.11 times greater odds for high OSA risk [51].

Therapy of Nocturnal Asthma

Nocturnal asthma symptoms indicate suboptimally treated asthma; thus, treatment should emphasize general control of the disorder rather than merely symptomatic management of nighttime complaints.

Various treatments for asthma have been proposed for hundreds of years. In early Egypt and China, herbs (some of which might have contained ephedrine or stramonium) have been administered to treat this condition. Galen, an ancient Greek physician, proposed using wine containing blood from owls. Pliny the elder, on the other hand suggested, eating millipedes soaked in honey. The rabbi Moses Maimonides (1135–1204 CE) added that chicken soup might be beneficial as well; more important, he recommended that asthma sufferers get plenty of sleep and rest.

Treatment of nocturnal asthma consists of long-acting bronchodilators, inhaled corticosteroids, or leukotriene inhibitors; avoidance of environmental precipitants in the bedroom; and control of comorbid conditions, such as GER, OSA, and allergic rhinitis, that might potentially worsen nocturnal asthma control. Short-acting beta-agonists are helpful for acute control. PAP therapy may reduce symptoms in certain patients with concurrent asthma and OSA by modifying airway smooth muscle function, suppression of gastroesophageal reflux, inhibition of local and systemic inflammation, improvements in cardiac function, reduction in leptin, better weight management, or restoration of normal sleep patterns [43]. Similarly, the improvement in asthma symptoms following adenotonsillectomy in children can result from beneficial changes in the upper and lower airways [52].

Summary

Many patients with restrictive and obstructive lung disease present with disturbances in duration, timing, or quality of sleep. Disturbed sleep is not merely a manifestation of poorly controlled disease or a contributor to diminished daytime functioning and QOL, it can also profoundly affect the natural course, symptom severity, and long-term outcomes of the comorbid disorder. Evaluation of sleep complaints is, therefore, essential and relies chiefly on a comprehensive sleep history. Frequent follow-up is recommended to determine response to therapy as well as development of new sleep complaints.

References

1. Tusiewicz K, Moldofsky H, Bryan AC, Bryan MH. Mechanics of the rib cage and diaphragm during sleep. J Appl Physiol: Respirat Environ Exerc Physiol. 1977;43:600–2.
2. Douglas NJ, White DP, Weil JV, et al. Hypoxic ventilatory response decreases during sleep in normal men. Am Rev Respir Dis. 1982;125(3):286–9.
3. Douglas NJ, White DP, Weil JV, et al. Hypercapneic ventilatory response in sleeping adults. Am Rev Respir Dis. 1982;126(5):758–62.
4. Berthon-Jones M, Sullivan CE: Ventilation and arousal responses to hypercapnia in normal sleeping humans. J Appl Physiol. 1984;57:59–67.
5. Hudgel DW, Martin RJ, Johnson BJ, Hill P. Mechanics of the respiratory system and breathing pattern during sleep in normal humans. J Appl Physiol: Respirat Environ Exerc Physiol. 1984;56:133–7.
6. Hetzel MR, Clark TJH. Comparison of normal and asthmatic circadian rhythms in peak flow rate. Thorax 1980;35:732–8.
7. Muller N, Volgyesi G, Becker L, Bryan MH, Bryan AC. Diaphragmatic muscle tone. J Appl Physiol: Respirat Environ Exerc Physiol. 1979;47:279–84.
8. Bye PT, Issa F, Berthon-Jones F, Sullivan CE. Studies of oxygenation during sleep in patientsc with interstitial lung disease. Am Rev Respir Med. 1984;129:27–32.

9. Guilleminault C, Kurland G, Winkle R, Miles LE. Severe kyphoscoliosis, breathing and sleep: the "Quasimodo" syndrome during sleep. Chest. 1981;76:626–30.
10. Meson BL, West P, Israels J, Kryger M. Sleep breathing abnormalities in kyphoscoliosis. Am Rev Respir Dis. 1980; 122:617–621.
11. Guilleminault C, Cummiskey J, Motta J, Lynne-Davies P. Respiratory and hemodynamic study during wakefulness and sleep in myotonic dystrophy. Sleep 1978;1:19–31.
12. Agusti A, Hedner J, Marin JM, Barbé F, Cazzola M, Rennard S. Night-time symptoms: a forgotten dimension of COPD. Eur Respir Rev. 2011 Sep 1;20(121):183–94.
13. Douglas NJ, Calverly PM, Leggett RJ, Brash HM, Flenley DC, Brezinova V. Transient hypoxaemia during sleep in chronic bronchitis and emphysema. Lancet 1979;1:1–4.
14. DeMarco FJ, Wynne JW, Block AJ, Boysen PG, Taasan VC. Oxygen desaturation during sleep as a determinant of the "blue and bloated" syndrome. Chest 1981;79:621–5.
15. Corda L, Novali M, Montemurro LT, La Piana GE, Redolfi S, Braghini A, Modina D, Pini L, Tantucci C. Predictors of nocturnal oxyhemoglobin desaturation in COPD. Respir Physiol Neurobiol. 2011;179(2–3):192–7.
16. Kinsman RA, Yaroush RA, Fernandez E, Dirks JF, Schocket M, Fukuhara J. Symptoms and experiences in chronic bronchitis and emphysema. Chest 1983;83(5):755–61.
17. Klink M, Quan SF. Prevalence of reported sleep disturbances in a general adult population and their relationship to obstructive airways diseases. Chest 1987;91(4):540–6.
18. Dodge R, Cline MG, Quan SF. The natural history of insomnia and its relationship to respiratory symptoms. Arch Intern Med. 1995;155(16):1797–800.
19. Nunes DM, Mota RM, de Pontes Neto OL, Pereira ED, de Bruin VM, de Bruin PF. Impaired sleep reduces quality of life in chronic obstructive pulmonary disease. Lung. 2009;187(3):159–63.
20. McSharry DG, Ryan S, Calverley P, Edwards JC, McNicholas WT. Sleep quality in chronic obstructive pulmonary disease. Respirology. 2012;17(7):1119–24.
21. Guilleminault C, Cummiskey J, Motta J. Chronic obstructive airflow disease and sleep studies. Am Rev Respir Dis. 1980;122(3):397–406.
22. Flenley DC. Sleep in chronic obstructive lung disease. Clin Chest Med. 1985;6(4):651–61.
23. Sharma B, Feinsilver S, Owens RL, Malhotra A, McSharry D, Karbowitz S. Obstructive airway disease and obstructive sleep apnea: effect of pulmonary function. Lung. 2011;189(1):37–41.
24. Sharma B, Neilan TG, Kwong RY, Mandry D, Owens RL, McSharry D, Bakker JP, Malhotra A. Evaluation of right ventricular remodeling using cardiac magnetic resonance imaging in co-existent chronic obstructive pulmonary disease and obstructive sleep apnea. COPD. 2013;10:4–10.
25. Marin JM, Soriano JB, Carrizo SJ, Boldova A, Celli BR. Outcomes in patients with chronic obstructive pulmonary disease and obstructive sleep apnea: the overlap syndrome. Am J Respir Crit Care Med. 2010;182(3):325–31.
26. Shaya FT, Lin PJ, Aljawadi MH, Scharf SM. Elevated economic burden in obstructive lung disease patients with concomitant sleep apnea syndrome. Sleep Breath. 2009;13(4):317–23.
27. Aras G, Kadakal F, Purisa S, Kanmaz D, Aynaci A, Isik E. Are we aware of restless legs syndrome in COPD patients who are in an exacerbation period? Frequency and probable factors related to underlying mechanism. COPD 2011;8(6):437–43.
28. Lo Coco D, Mattaliano A, Lo Coco A, Randisi B. Increased frequency of restless legs syndrome in chronic obstructive pulmonary disease patients. Sleep Med. 2009;10(5):572–6.
29. Nunes DM, de Bruin VM, Louzada FM, Peixoto CA, Cavalcante AG, Castro-Silva C, de Bruin PF. Actigraphic assessment of sleep in chronic obstructive pulmonary disease. Sleep Breath. 2013;17:125–32.

30. Calverly PM, Brezinova V, Douglas NJ, Catterall JR, Flenly DC. The effect of oxygenation on sleep quality in chronic bronchitis and emphysema. Am Rev Respir Dis. 1982;126:206–10.

31. Fleetham J, West P, Meson B, Conway W, Roth T, Kryger M. Sleep, arousals, and oxygen desaturation in chronic obstructive pulmonary disease: The effect of oxygen therapy. Am Rev Respir Dis. 1982;126:429–33.

32. Nocturnal Oxygen Therapy Trial Group. Continuous or nocturnal oxygen therapy in hypoxemic chronic obstructive lung disease: a clinical trial. Ann Intern Med. 1980;93:391–8.

33. Research Council Working Party. Long term domiciliary oxygen therapy in chronic hypoxic cor pulmonale complicating chronic bronchitis and emphysema. Lancet. 1981;1:681–6.

34. Toraldo DM, De Nuccio F, Nicolardi G. Fixed-pressure nCPAP in patients with obstructive sleep apnea (OSA) syndrome and chronic obstructive pulmonary disease (COPD): a 24-month follow-up study. Sleep Breath. 2010;14(2):115–23.

35. Machado MC, Vollmer WM, Togeiro SM, Bilderback AL, Oliveira MV, Leitão FS, Queiroga F Jr, Lorenzi-Filho G, Krishnan JA. CPAP and survival in moderate-to-severe obstructive sleep apnoea syndrome and hypoxaemic COPD. Eur Respir J. 2010;35(1):132–7.

36. Horner CC, Mauger D, Strunk RC, Graber NJ, Lemanske RF Jr, Sorkness CA, Szefler SJ, Zeiger RS, Taussig LM, Bacharier LB, Childhood Asthma Research and Education Network of the National Heart, Lung, and Blood Institute. Most nocturnal asthma symptoms occur outside of exacerbations and associate with morbidity. J Allergy Clin Immunol. 2011;128(5):977–82.

37. Fagnano M, Bayer AL, Isensee CA, Hernandez T, Halterman JS. Nocturnal asthma symptoms and poor sleep quality among urban school children with asthma. Acad Pediatr. 2011;11(6):493–9.

38. Lanier BQ, Nayak A. Prevalence and impact of nighttime symptoms in adults and children with asthma: a survey. Postgrad Med. 2008;120(4):58–66.

39. Dean BB, Calimlim BC, Sacco P, Aguilar D, Maykut R, Tinkelman D. Uncontrolled asthma among children: impairment in social functioning and sleep. J Asthma. 2010;47(5):539–44.

40. Calhoun SL, Vgontzas AN, Fernandez-Mendoza J, Mayes SD, Tsaoussoglou M, Basta M, Bixler EO. Prevalence and risk factors of excessive daytime sleepiness in a community sample of young children: the role of obesity, asthma, anxiety/depression, and sleep. Sleep. 2011;34(4):503–7.

41. Connolly CK. Diurnal rhythms in airway obstruction. Br. J Dis Chest. 1979.73:357–366.

42. Clark TJH, Hetzel MR. Diurnal variation in asthma. Br J Dis Chest. 1977;71:87–92.

43. Alkhalil M, Schulman E, Getsy J. Obstructive sleep apnea syndrome and asthma: what are the links? J Clin Sleep Med. 2009;5(1):71–8.

44. Julien JY, Martin JG, Ernst P, Olivenstein R, Hamid Q, Lemière C, Pepe C, Naor N, Olha A, Kimoff RJ. Prevalence of obstructive sleep apnea-hypopnea in severe versus moderate asthma. J Allergy Clin Immunol. 2009;124(2):371–6.

45. Teodorescu M, Polomis DA, Teodorescu MC, Gangnon RE, Peterson AG, Consens FB, Chervin RD, Jarjour NN. Association of obstructive sleep apnea risk or diagnosis with daytime asthma in adults. J Asthma. 2012;49(6):620–8.

46. Alharbi M, Almutairi A, Alotaibi D, Alotaibi A, Shaikh S, Bahammam AS. The prevalence of asthma in patients with obstructive sleep apnoea. Prim Care Respir J. 2009;18(4):328–30.

47. Kaditis AG, Kalampouka E, Hatzinikolaou S, Lianou L, Papaefthimiou M, Gartagani-Panagiotopoulou P, Zintzaras E, Chrousos G. Associations of tonsillar hypertrophy and snoring with history of wheezing in childhood. Pediatr Pulmonol. 2010;45(3):275–80.

48. Kales A, Beall GN, Bajor GF, Jacobson A, Kales JD. Sleep studies in asthmatic adults: Relationship of attacks to sleep stage and time of night. J Allergy. 1968;41:164–73.

49. Montplaisir J, Walsh J, Malo JL. Nocturnal asthma: Features of attacks, sleep and breathing patterns. Am Rev Respir Dis. 1982;125:18–22.

50. Teodorescu M, Polomis DA, Hall SV, Teodorescu MC, Gangnon RE, Peterson AG, Xie A, Sorkness CA, Jarjour NN. Association of obstructive sleep apnea risk with asthma control in adults. Chest. 2010;138(3):543–50.

51. Teodorescu M, Consens FB, Bria WF, Coffey MJ, McMorris MS, Weatherwax KJ, Palmisano J, Senger CM, Ye Y, Kalbfleisch JD, Chervin RD. Predictors of habitual snoring and obstructive sleep apnea risk in patients with asthma. Chest. 2009;135(5):1125–32.

52. Busino RS, Quraishi HA, Aguila HA, Montalvo E, Connelly P. The impact of adenotonsillectomy on asthma in children. Laryngoscope. 2010;120(Suppl 4):221.

NREM Arousal Parasomnias

Mark R. Pressman and Roger Broughton

The nonrapid eye movement (NREM) arousal parasomnias include some of the most well-known and misunderstood sleep disorders. They include sleepwalking, confusional arousals, and sleep terrors. A generally accepted definition of a parasomnia is:

> Parasomnias are undesirable physical events or experiences that occur during entry into sleep, within sleep or during arousals from sleep. (p. 137) [1]

Descriptions of sleepwalking and related disorders have been reported since at least the time of the ancient Greeks. However, prior to the first description of REM sleep in 1953 [2] and the first sleep laboratory studies of clinically diagnosed sleepwalkers in 1963 [3], the term sleepwalking might have been better replaced by that of "nocturnal wandering." Early historical reports of sleepwalking or somnambulism almost certainly included a number of different disorders and states such as epilepsy, fugue, rapid eye movement (REM), sleep behavior disorder (RBD), and dissociative disorder (see Table 44.1). However, these episodes almost certainly also included examples of NREM arousal parasomnias in the current diagnostic nosology that have similar signs, symptoms, and behaviors although described under a variety of labels [1] (see Table 44.2).

The availability of advanced diagnostic techniques and the start of the modern field of sleep medicine have resulted in ever-expanding and more specific differential diagnoses. His-

torical descriptions and interpretations of nocturnal wandering generally reflected the state of science, medicine, religious beliefs, and superstitions of that time. However, when the religious and superstitious aspects are removed, the "clinical" description of signs and symptoms in early reports of sleepwalkers is often quite close to current diagnostic descriptions.

There is a large number of case reports or stories of sleepwalkers going back centuries. They typically include elements consistent with current sleepwalking science and theory as well as other elements that are clearly not consistent with modern views. The following case of Negretti, aged 20 years, appears in several nineteenth-century books on sleep and sleepwalking. The common signs and symptoms of sleepwalking and related disorders in modern sleep medicine can be found in Table 44.3 for purposes of comparison and analysis.

> On the evening of the 16th of March, 1740, after going to sleep on a bench in the kitchen, he began first to talk, then walked about, went to the dining-room and spread a table for dinner, placed himself behind a chair with a plate in his hand, as if waiting on his master. After waiting until he thought his master had dined, he uncovered the table, put away all of the materials in a basket, which he locked in a cupboard. He afterwards warmed a bed, locked up the house, and prepared for his nightly rest. Being then awakened and asked if he remembered what he had been doing, he answered no. [4]

This case describes behaviors that may be too complex to meet current standards. However, if this was his usual routine, these activities might be considered "automatic behaviors" during an amnestic confusional arousal. His going to the dining room, setting the table, and so forth bears a passing resemblance to behaviors noted in sleep-related eating disorder, which is a variant of sleepwalking. The lack of recall of events would certainly be consistent.

A second case described in several nineteenth-century books is:

> A young ecclesiastic was in the habit of getting up during the night, in a state of somnambulism, of going to his room, taking pen, ink, and paper, and composing and writing sermons. When

M. R. Pressman (✉)
Sleep Medicine Services , Lankenau Medical Center/Lankenau Institute For Medical Research , Wynnewood , Pennsylvania , USA
e-mail: Sleepwake@comcast.net

Jefferson Medical College, Philadelphia, Pennsylvania, USA

Lankenau Institute For Medical Research, Wynnewood, Pennsylvania, USA

Villanova School of Law, Villanova, Pennsylvania, USA

R. Broughton
University of Ottawa , Ottawa , Canada

S. Chokroverty, M. Billiard (eds.), *Sleep Medicine,* DOI 10.1007/978-1-4939-2089-1_44,
© Springer Science+Business Media, LLC 2015

Table 44.1 List of probable disorders and states of consciousness labeled as sleepwalking prior to the 1950s–1960s

Epilepsy
Fugue state
Schizophrenia
Concussion
Dissociative disorder
REM behavior disorder
Nightmare
REM rapid eye movement

Table 44.2 List of terms used to describe sleepwalking prior to 1950

Oneirology
Somnolencia
Somnomania
Somnambulism
Somnolentia
Sleep drunkenness
Schlaftrunkenheit
l'ivresse du sommeil
Syndrome d'Elpenor
Oneirodynia
Noctambulism
Coma vigil
Somno-vigilia
Somnambulismus
Ecstatis or cataleptic somnambulism
Somnambulator

he had finished one page of the paper on which he was writing, he would read over what he had written and correct it.... In order to ascertain whether the somnambulist made any use of his eyes, the Archbishop held a piece of pasteboard under his chin, to prevent him from seeing the paper upon which he was writing; but he continued to write on, without appearing to be incommoded in the slightest degree.... He wrote pieces of music while in this state, and in the same manner, with his eyes closed. [5]

In current sleepwalking theories, sleepwalkers have impaired higher cognitive functions and should not be able to read, write, compose, or correct writings. Sleepwalkers are currently reported to perform their behaviors with eyes open. The report that this young cleric continued to write even when his line of sight was blocked is consistent with early theories attributing special visual abilities or supernatural powers such as clairvoyance to sleepwalkers who were thought to move about and perform various behaviors with eyes closed. Additional information that does not appear in this version of the case history is that his sleepwalking episodes only occurred during the month of March, and that he walked with his eyes closed and often bumped into walls and doors.

The following story appears in several nineteenth-century books [6], often with some details added or eliminated. It concerns complex apparently sleep-related behaviors described by an eyewitness, the prior of the convent where it occurred:

Very late one evening the monk entered the chamber of the Prior, his eyes were open but fixed, the light of two lamps made no impression upon him, his features were contracted, and he carried in his hand a large knife. Going straight to the bed, he appeared to examine if the Prior was there. He then struck 3 blows, which pierced the coverings and even a mat which served as the purpose of a mattress. In returning, his countenance was unbent and was marked by an air of satisfaction. The next day the Prior asked the monk what he had dreamed of the preceding night, and the latter answered that he had dreamed that his mother had been killed by the Prior, and that her ghost had appeared demanding vengeance, that at this sight he was so transported by rage that he had immediately run to stab the assassin of his mother; that a little while after, he awakened bathed in perspiration and very content to find he had only dreamed.

According to another account, thereafter, the monk slept in a locked room. It is quite curious that none of the accounts state whether the prior was actually in bed when the monk attacked with a knife. This story contains a number of elements that would not be considered consistent with sleepwalking in modern times. Sleepwalking with eyes open is consistent with current knowledge. Carrying a knife is also for unknown reasons fairly common in modern cases of sleepwalk

ing violence [7]. However, violent sleepwalkers do not seek out their victims [8]. Sleepwalking violence is thought to be defensive in nature. The victim almost always seeks out or encounters the sleepwalker. The very detailed description of the dream is inconsistent with an NREM arousal parasomnia such as sleepwalking. Sleep terrors are often associated with a frightening image, but these images tend to be static, without a story line. Dreaming, on the other hand, is typically associated with electromyographic (EMG) atonia so that the dreamer lacks the muscle tone to get up and act out his dream. In RBD, first described in 1986 [9], dreams may be enacted; this is due to the effects of neurodegenerative disease on areas of the brain that control EMG atonia during REM sleep. However, RBD patients rarely leave their own beds. Dreamers exist in their own dream world and have little or no knowledge of their location or the location of others. Based on current sleep science, an RBD patient should not be able to navigate from one room to another.

Thus, it can be seen that many early descriptions of "sleepwalking" may not be consistent at all with current definitions or theories. Nevertheless, an historical analysis shows the development or evolution of beliefs and knowledge of sleepwalking that still reflects on our modern views.

Early Greek Contributions

Some of the earliest descriptions of sleepwalking were by early Greek writers. As translated by Weinholt from Greek into German in his Seven Lectures on Somnambulism and to English by Colquhoun [5], a third-century BC Greek, Iamblichus wrote in his treatise *De Mysteriis Egyptiorum,*

On the approach of such a spirit of prophecy during sleep," says he, "the head begins to sink, and the eyes involuntarily close: It is, as it were, a middle state between sleeping and waking. In ordinary dreaming, we are fast and perfectly asleep; we cannot precisely distinguish our perceptions. But when our dreams are from God, we are not asleep—we exactly recognise all objects, and sometimes even more distinctly than when awake. And in this species of dreams prophecy has its foundation.

Table 44.3 Common signs and symptoms of sleepwalking in modern sleep medicine

1.	*Sleep stage and timing*: Sleepwalking occurs out of deep sleep (also known as slow-wave sleep or stage 3 or 4 sleep)—usually 40–90 min after sleep onset. Sleepwalking does not occur spontaneously from wakefulness
2.	*Arousal from deep sleep*: Not only must the sleepwalker be in deep sleep when the event is triggered but also a sudden arousal must occur while in deep sleep
3.	*Types of triggers*: Arousal can be caused by sound, touch, or some internal change or other things going bump in the night
4.	*Duration*: Typically last for short period of time—seconds or minutes although longer episodes have been reported
5.	*Deep sleep not dreaming sleep*: Sleepwalking is not associated with REM sleep dreaming
6.	*Proximity and provocation*: Violent sleepwalking behavior is defensive when another individual is in close proximity or is provocative
7.	*Violence*: Sleepwalkers do not seek out victims. Sleepwalking violence is defensive. Typically, victims seek out or encounter sleepwalkers
8.	*Higher level cognitive function*: Absence of planning, intent, and memory
9.	*Continuity*: Sleepwalking episodes are continuous. They do not usually wax and wane
10.	*Memory*: Sleepwalkers generally have complete amnesia for their episodes. The sleepwalker does not forget, but never stores the memory
11.	*Memory from before incident*: Sleepwalkers are unable to access memories formed to the immediate past
12.	*Memories formed during the incident*: Sleepwalkers are unable to form new memories during the sleepwalking episode itself
13.	*Ease of awakening*: Sleepwalkers are extremely hard to awaken
14.	*Situational stress*: Reports of stressful situation before episodes of sleepwalking are common—death in family, loss of job, etc.
15.	*Sleep deprivation*: Sleep deprivation for 1 or more days prior to sleepwalking episodes is often reported
16.	*Out-of-character behavior*: Violent sleepwalkers are almost always found to be nonviolent while awake
17.	*Social interaction*: Social interaction requires higher-level cognitive functioning not available to the sleepwalker
18.	Personal history of *NREM arousal parasomnias*
19.	Family history of *NREM arousal parasomnias*—familial pattern

Both Hippocrates and Aristotle are reported to have commented on sleepwalking. As cited and translated from the Greek by Tuke [6], Hippocrates wrote, "I have known many persons during sleep moaning and calling out…and others rising up, fleeing out of doors, and deprived of their reason until awake, and afterwards becoming well and rational as before, although they may be pale and weak." Aristotle noted "some are moved while they sleep, and perform many things which pertain to wakefulness, though not without a certain phantasm and a certain sense, for a dream is after a certain manner a sensible perception" (p. 5).

Diogenes Laertius, a biographer of Greek philosophers, is reported to have noted two cases of sleepwalking and he himself was reported to read, write, and make corrections to his books while asleep [4]. Many insights into the historical evolution of our understanding of sleepwalking come from court cases and are consistent with current legal concepts of automatism. The 1313 Council of Vienne [10] stated:

> If a child, madman or sleeper killed someone he was not culpable.

Fifteenth to Sixteenth Century

Levinus Lemnious (1505–1568) was concerned about the safety of sleepwalkers when he advised "not to call night-walkers by their proper name…whereas you must let them go as they will and retire again at pleasures."

Diego de Covarrubias (1512–1577) discussed when, and if, the violent actions of a sleeping individual would be considered a sin. Generally, the act of the sleeper would not be a sin, unless the sleeper somehow made prior arrangements to commit the violent act in his sleep. As translated from the Latin by Walker [11]:

> It follows of course…that a person who was asleep at the time of the homicide is not at fault, for the obvious reason that he was asleep when he killed his victim; such one lacks understanding and reason, and is like a madman…. For this reason the misdeed of a sleeper is not punished, unless it happens that in his waking state he knew very well that in his sleep he would seize weapons and attack people. For then if he did not take care to prevent himself from doing harm in his sleep to someone, certainly he should be punished, although not in the usual way.

King James I (1566–1625) is reported to have had a keen interest in sleepwalking [10]. He and his mother are said to have had paroxysms associated with loss of consciousness, large mood swings, and insomnia. The lay public during this period attributed nightmares and sleepwalking to the devil. Nightmares and sleepwalking were attributed to a "grave perturbation of spirit" and "ill-directed imagination outside of the control of reason."

Mathaeuss (1664) noted that a sleepwalker who committed a violent act should be punished if during wakefulness he had a grudge or complaint against the person [11]. McKenzie (1678), a Scottish jurist, noted in an early volume on criminal law [12] that "such as commit any crime whilst the sleep, are compared to infants."

A famous legal case of the time was that of Colonel Cheyney Culpeper in 1686 [11]. His brother Lord Culpeper was an important member of the court of King James II. Colonel Culpeper was reported to be a "famous dreamer" and apparently was well known to perform complex behaviors in his sleep. During a purported episode of dreaming, he shot a guardsman as well as the guardsman's horse. Put on trial for manslaughter, his defense was that he had been asleep when he shot the guardsman. He is reported to have produced 50 witnesses who testified to his complex behaviors during sleep. The jury initially returned a guilty verdict of manslaughter, but this verdict was apparently not accepted and the jury was sent out again. They returned with a special verdict of manslaughter while insane. In a few days, the instructions from the court of King James II delayed sentencing and within weeks he had been pardoned most likely resulting from the influence of his brother. This story was reprinted in altered form in at least two nineteenth-century books on sleep.

Seventeenth to Eighteenth Century

The description of sleepwalking as a state between sleep and waking was first put forth during this time period and would be understood and accepted by modern sleep medicine. However, it is confounded with religious beliefs, as well as the assumption that sleepwalkers are acting out dreaming. Starting in the eighteenth century, more physiological concepts of sleepwalking started to appear, whereas the more religious and supernatural views started to decline.

Nineteenth Century

1815: Polidori

The early nineteenth-century and late eighteenth-century views of sleepwalking—typically called oneirodynia—are summed up in a recently translated medical dissertation by John Williams Polidori published in Italian in 1815 [12]. Polidori was the personal physician to Lord Byron and an early writer of horror stories of some note. He shows a remarkable prescience for modern knowledge of sleepwalking. The term oneirodynia as translated from the Greek is literally "walking while in a dream." It is of interest that Polidori attributes the first use of the term "somnambulism" to Sauvages de la Croix in a medical nosology book, *Nosologia Methodica,* Amsterdam, Sumptibus Fratrum de Tournes, 1763. This term also appears in several nineteenth-century medical nosologies.

Polidori's definition of sleepwalking was "a hallucination in which dreamers rise from their bed and expose themselves

to various dangers." Undoubtedly, just as injuries or near misses related to sleepwalking are a fairly common reason for referral to a modern sleep disorders center, at the time only the more dangerous and bizarre episodes of sleepwalking were likely to come to public knowledge or be repeated in books or medical journals. Polidori's general description of sleepwalking is consistent with several currently accepted aspects of sleepwalking: the sudden arousal from sleep, performance of complex behaviors as if awake, and, most interesting, performance of behaviors that are often typical of wakefulness. This anticipates the concept of so-called automatic behaviors—behaviors that are performed repeatedly so that higher cognitive function becomes unnecessary:

> When we discuss [oneirodynia] in a medical context, however, it should be understood to refer not only to someone who walks while in a dream, but also to someone who appears to wake up while still asleep, and who performs actions or speaks as if he were awake. If I might offer a definition of this disease, it is the habit of doing something in sleep that is usually done by those who are awake…. There are as many types as there are distinctions observed in the disease. (p. 76)

> …though all passageways to the various senses are open in sufferers from oneirodynia, it appears nonetheless that they experience no sensations beyond those that pertain to the specific action they are performing.

Polidori also anticipates modern concepts of sleepwalking by suggesting it may require several factors to occur. Modern sleepwalking theory supposes that sleepwalking must have a predisposing factor (genetic), a priming factor (usually sleep deprivation and/or situational stress), and a provoking factor or trigger (often a sound, touch, or other form of stimulation) [13, 14]:

> We may say that there are three causes of diseases, namely the proximate [proxima], the remote [remota], and the predisposing [praedisponens]. The proximate is that cause from which the disease itself immediately arises; the remote is the cause that precedes the proximate; and the predisposing is the cause that makes men susceptible to a certain disease. But since we know nothing for sure regarding the proximate causes and can do nothing but relay hypotheses, I propose to pass over conjectures and subtle argumentation. And in the case of the other types of causes too we do not know much, whether because of a lack of clinical accounts, or because of the superficial scrutiny applied to old cases and more recent ones, or because of nature's own delay. The remote causes are varied, but they all seem to affect the brain in some fashion. Thus a wound to the head has at times induced oneirodynia, as may be seen in volume VIII no. xix of the notes of Lenadus. Moreover oneirodynia sometimes presents along with hysteria, epilepsy, and other diseases that arise from an affliction of the brain. This demonstrates plainly that oneirodynia is produced from an internal brain lesion. Yet it is much more typical for no clear cause to appear. The predisposing or determining [determinantes] causes are: intoxication, overeating, food that produces gas, use of too much bedding, placing the head lower than the body, lying on one's back, study, use of opium, and everything that moves blood to the brain. (p. 777)

Although Polidori lacked knowledge of modern sleep medicine, his model is very close to what is generally accepted today. Polidori is also one of the only writers prior to modern sleep medicine to offer suggestions for treatment. He anticipates current pharmacological and nonpharmacological treatments.

> The Curing of the Disease
> The health of those suffering from oneirodynia is usually sound, and the disease would pose no danger if it did not draw sufferers into dangerous places. Some authors say that this disease sometimes induces catalepsy [catalepsis] and madness [mania]. Thus we must do everything we can, but—as is generally the case—we do not know of anything to expel the disease.
> The indications to be followed are two.
> (1) To interrupt the progress of episodes that are underway.
> (2) To keep the episodes away once they have withdrawn.
> To follow the first indication, we can only remove the predisposing causes. In the case of a sleepwalker, drunkenness, study, and other things that stimulate the mind and afterwards weaken it must be avoided. Tonics may perhaps be given, such as Peruvian Bark, iron and similar things, yet how much and when may be known only through experience. But we must distract the sufferer's mind from serious matters as much as we are able. During the course of an episode, first of all doors and windows should be closed and every exit blocked. For a certain sleepwalker, believing that he saw Aristotle and other philosophers going out through a window, would have followed them if his friends had not held him back. Second, methods should be applied that may rouse the sufferer from sleep by terrifying him. Beatings, electricity, frigid baths—if they are placed in such a way that the sufferer may fall into them when he strays from his bed in the course of sleepwalking—will perhaps hinder the return of his episodes.

His first suggested treatment involves attempts to remove predisposing causes. In modern sleep medicine, sleepwalkers are often told to avoid sleep deprivation, increase their total sleep time, learn to reduce stress, and eliminate possible triggers with treatment of snoring or sleep apnea. Secondly, there is a suggestion that administration of apparently medicinal substances may reduce or eliminate sleepwalking, although the author admits a lack of knowledge as to dosage and timing of treatment. Finally, Polidori deals with the sleepwalker's safety. All doors and windows must be closed and exits blocked. The final suggestion of trying to awaken the sleepwalker during an episode would not be accepted currently. And the suggestion that "beatings, electricity or frigid baths" may be used to arouse the sleepwalker is quite inconsistent with current belief that family members speak simply and directly to the sleepwalker in an effort to return him or her to the bedroom. However, the drastic measures suggested by Polidori do suggest that the sleepwalker may be very hard to arouse, which is consistent with modern sleep science.

1835 : C. Prichard

C Prichard writing in the 1835 *Cyclopedia of Practical Medicine* strongly supported the relationship between dreaming and sleepwalking [4]:

> A somnombulator is a dreamer who is able to act out is dreams. (p. 21)

1838 : Isaac Ray

Isaac Ray, generally thought to be the first American forensic psychiatrist, was the author of *Treatise of Mental Jurisprudence of Insanity*. Remarkably, this volume contains three chapters on somnambulism [15]. For the most part, Ray's intention, as with Wharton, is to describe the legal evaluation of sleepwalking as a criminal defense. Anticipating many modern cases in which sleepwalking is presented as a defense for a criminal act, it includes a chapter on how to detect simulated somnambulism. Although he does not discuss etiology in any detail, it is clear he believes sleepwalking is related to dream enactment. However, he also appears to suggest that there is a physiological reason for its occurrence:

> § 508. As the somnambulist does not enjoy the free and rational exercise of his understanding, and is more or less unconscious of his outward relations, none of his acts, during the paroxysms, can rightfully be imputed to him as crimes. (p. 509)

Ray notes that there is no real physiological evidence that the sleepwalker's body is acting out thoughts occurring in the mind during sleep. He appears to reject more fanciful descriptions of sleepwalkers as possessing supernatural visual abilities:

> § 494. Whether this condition is really anything more than a cooperation of the voluntary muscles with the thoughts which occupy the mind during sleep, is a point very far from being settled among physiologists. While, to some, the exercise of the natural faculties alone seems to be sufficient to explain its phenomena, others have deemed it necessary to suppose that some new and extraordinary powers of sensation are concerned in its production, though unable to convey a very clear idea of their nature or mode of operation.

Ray further suggests that somnambulism is the result of some problem of the brain and that this is linked likely to general conditions that result in health problems:

> § 503. It now scarcely admits of a doubt, that somnambulism results from some morbid condition in the system, involving, primarily or secondarily, the cerebral organism…. The more active forms of sleep-walking seldom, if ever, exist, except in connection with those habits or conditions that deteriorate the general health.

1845 : Colquhoun and Weinholt

The attribution of sleepwalking or other complex behaviors in sleep to God, supernatural forces, or the devil continued well into the nineteenth century. J.C. Colquhoun in his introduction to the English translation of Arnold Weinholt's *Seven Lectures on Somnambulism* (1845) lamented the difficulty in shedding religious views of sleepwalking and demanding more scientific ones [5]:

The manifestations of this peculiar affection, however, seem to have always appeared so anomalous and incomprehensible, as to have excited religious veneration and awe, rather than to have been considered as a proper subject for philosophical contemplation. These manifestations, therefore, came to be generally regarded as the immediate consequence of Divine appointment, or as the effects of diabolical agency, according to the peculiar character which the affection might happen to assume, or the particular views entertained by the different observers. Similar notions, upon this subject, appear to have been almost universally entertained during the dark ages of Europe; and even long after science had begun to subject the actual phenomena of nature to the scrutiny of a more strict and searching analysis, somnambulism still continued to constitute a perplexing puzzle for the philosopher and the physician. A variety of instances of the affection, indeed, had been occasionally observed; but the explanation of the phenomena was long held to be a subject far too sacred for profane philosophical speculation; and it was, accordingly, consigned almost entirely to the province of the theologian. Ignorant and crafty men availed themselves of these facts and dispositions for the purpose of extending their influence by enlarging the boundaries of superstition and delusion. And so deeply rooted were these erroneous impressions in the minds of mankind, that even the attempts which have been made, in recent and more enlightened times, to extirpate these unphilosophical and pernicious notions, by explaining the natural causes of the phenomena in question, have been viewed by many as an impertinent and unhallowed inroad upon the sacred territory of the Divine, or as an iniquitous design to extend and perpetuate the empire of Satan. (p. 2)

Weinholt and Colquhoun were strong proponents of mesmerism [4]. The hypnotic state was conceived of as an artificial form of natural somnambulism. The ability to induce somnambulism during wakefulness artificially strongly suggested that it had nothing to do with religious belief but was due to some changes in physiology.

1855 : Francis Wharton

Francis Wharton was a lawyer, clergyman, expert in criminal law, and a forensic expert. In 1855, he published a "Monograph on Mental Unsoundness" [16] that would later appear as part of his *Treatise of Medical Jurisprudence* published with Dr. Moreton Stille. Although his terminology differs somewhat from other writers—he uses the term "sleep-drunkenness" to describe complex behavior after the sleepwalker arises—his general understanding of sleepwalking was quite advanced for the time:

Sleep-drunkenness may be defined as the lapping of a profound sleep on the domains of apparent wakefulness, producing an involuntary intoxication on the part of the patient, which destroys his moral agency. (p. 151)

As part of an effort to determine the legal responsibility of sleepwalkers who commit criminal acts he developed the following tests:

(a) A general tendency to deep and heavy sleep must be shown, out of which the patient could only be awakened by violent and convulsive effort;

This anticipates current knowledge that sleepwalking often occurs in the deep recovery sleep that follows sleep deprivation, and that sleepwalkers are very hard to awaken.

(b) Before falling asleep, circumstances must be shown producing disquiet which sleep itself does not entirely compose;

Modern concepts of sleepwalking suggest it is often preceded by situational stress.

(c) The act under examination must have occurred at the time when the defendant was usually accustomed to have been asleep;

To be sleepwalking, the patient must have actually been asleep. Sleepwalking does not occur directly from wakefulness. It most often occurs 1–4 h after sleep onset when deep sleep is most likely to occur.

(d) The cause of the sudden awakening must be shown. It is true that this cannot always happen, as sometimes the start may have come from a violent dream;

The trigger for an episode of sleepwalking is not always known, even when it occurs in the sleep laboratory. However, it is sometimes possible to correlate episodes with sleep disruption caused by a noise, sleep apnea, or periodic leg movements in sleep.

(e) The act must bear throughout, the character of unconsciousness

Current scientific evidence suggests that once an episode of sleepwalking is started, it continues until it is finished. There is usually little or no waxing and waning of symptoms.

(f) The actor himself, when he awakes, is generally amazed at his own deed, and it seems to him almost incredible. Generally speaking he does not seek to evade responsibility, though there are some unfortunate cases in which, the wretchedness of the sudden discovery, overcomes the party himself, who seeks to shelter himself from the consequences of a crime of which he was technically, though not morally, guilty. (p. 123)

It is generally accepted in modern sleep medicine that sleepwalkers who perform complex behaviors in their sleep will have no or very little recall of their actions. It is common for them immediately afterwards to be surprised or perplexed. Further, it is uncommon for sleepwalkers to evade responsibility. In several well-known sleepwalking criminal cases, the defendant, after fully awakening, alerted the police to the fact he must have killed or injured someone.

1869 : Hammond

Hammond was surgeon general of the Union Army during the American Civil War and the author of the first book on sleep written in the USA. Hammond anticipates the concept that sleepwalking is secondary to a deactivated brain with an "exalted" or activated spinal cord. He also suggests that, if the spinal cord is less excitable that, instead of sleepwalking, sleep talking might occur and if even less excitable, perhaps only movements of the head or body without complex behaviors [17]:

> Now in all sleep there is more or less somnambulism, because the brain, according as the sleep is more or less profound, is more or less removed from the sphere of action. If this quiescent state of the brain is accompanied, as it frequently is in nervous and excitable persons, by an exalted condition of the spinal cord, we have the higher order of somnambulic performance of complex and apparently systematic movements; if the sleep of the brain be somewhat less profound, and the spinal cord less excitable, the somnambulic manifestations do not extend beyond sleep talking; a still less degree of cerebral inaction and spinal irritability produces simply a restless sleep and a little muttering; and when the sleep is perfectly natural, and the nervous system of the person well balanced, the movements do not extend beyond changing the position of the head and limbs and turning over in bed. (pp. 217–218)

1878 : Fraser

One of the most famous cases of sleepwalking-related violence was reported by Yellowless [18]. HM Advocate v. Simon Fraser involved the death of the defendant's 18-month-old child. As described in court, Mr. Fraser was asleep in bed with his wife around 1 AM with his infant son nearby in a cradle. Mr. Fraser saw a "wild beast" come up through the floor and jump into bed with his child. He grabbed the wild beast and slammed it against the wall. His wife's screams finally caused him to awaken fully, when he found that he had actually picked up his son and killed him by smashing his head against the wall. Dr. Yellowless was one of the three experts called to testify and published his detailed case report the same year in the *Journal of Mental Science*. Mr. Fraser had an extensive history of prior episodes of sleepwalking, sleep talking, and sleep terrors. Family members as well as cell mates described violent attacks during sleep including attempting to strangle his sister and assaulting his father. He had also injured himself during episodes. Charged with murder, he famously pleaded by saying:

> I am guilty in my sleep, but not guilty in my senses.

Dr. Yellowless reports that the jury was so convinced by Mr. Fraser's personal history of violent sleepwalking episodes that they thought no further evidence was necessary and were ready to find him not responsible for his actions. Nevertheless, the testimony of three medical experts was heard. Dr. Yellowless is reported to define somnambulism as:

> a state of morbid activity of the brain coming on during sleep, of very varying intensity, sometimes little more than restless sleep, but sometime developing delusions and violence and amounting really to insanity.

Mr Fraser was described by Dr. Yellowless as "…unconscious of what he is doing, and has no true perception of the world around him, yet he has a kind of consciousness, a sort of mental activity going on, which is not consistent with ordinary sleep" (p. 455). Dr. Clouston, the expert witness for the defense, was not willing to say this episode was consistent with insanity because it had occurred in sleep. This attitude is remarkably similar to the opinion of the Canadian Supreme Court in R v. Parks when they confirmed his acquittal on the basis of sleepwalking in the murder of his mother-in-law [7]. Mr. Fraser was acquitted and allowed to return home only with his father, and his assurance that he would sleep in a separate room from other family members. The conclusion of the experts was that this episode was due to some morbid condition of the brain related to dreaming.

The mesmerism movement also contributed to the reduction of religious and supernatural explanations for sleepwalking [4, 6]. An altered state of consciousness most often labeled "artificial somnambulism similar to hypnosis" was said to result from the procedures that resembled hypnotism. That somnambulism could be induced ran counter to beliefs that episodes had a supernatural origin. The actual relationship between so-called natural somnambulism and artificial somnambulism is not known. However, in modern times, hypnotism has been used effectively to treat sleepwalking [19].

1884 : Tuke

During the nineteenth century, physiological explanations for sleepwalking increased although older theories did not disappear. In 1884, Tuke [6] published a volume devoted to sleepwalking and hypnotism. In discussing theories of sleepwalking, he appears to anticipate current theories that attribute sleepwalking to a dissociated state and a dysfunction of the brain stem and the cerebral cortex. Tuke wrote:

> In ordinary sleep-walking we see certain centres or tracts of the encephalon in functional activity while others are asleep, profoundly asleep, and temporarily paralysed; or, to adopt the language of Heidenhain, the ganglion cells of certain regions of the cerebral cortex are inhibited. (p. 4)

Dr. Tuke was also the first to conduct scientific research on sleepwalking in the form of a survey. In his book, he describes creating a "Circular of Inquiry" containing 25 questions about sleepwalking with documentation of age, sex, and occupation. These were distributed in an unspecified manner and returned to Dr. Tuke for analysis. The questions concerned, among others, family history, age of onset of sleepwalking, presence or absence of amnesia after episodes, any successful treatment, or awaken spontaneously. Question 20 was:

> Have you noticed whether you are especially apt to walk in your sleep after any particular event or condition? (e.g, late supper, fatigue, illness)

Early Twentieth-Century Freudian and Other Psychodynamic Approaches

Freud in his *Interpretation of Dreams* suggests a link between psychosis and somnambulism involving an expression of suppressed unconscious impulses and motor activity. Other psychodynamic theorists suggested that somnambulism involves a wish to avoid a threat or to seek out an object relation. Sours et al. [20] presented a list of different psychodynamic models or explanations for somnambulism, which were published between 1945 and 1958. They included: (1) "Flight from oedipal temptation as a defense against castration anxiety," (2) "Aggressive and sexual motor activity aimed primarily at the fear-inspiring father, inability to express resent and aggression to father," (3) "Homosexual, passive-receptive identification and strivings towards oedipal wishes," (4) "Attempts to solve problems through safe channels…to resolve oedipal indecision," (5) "Conflict around masculine identification, fears of passive-feminine dependent striving, and unconscious fantasies of homosexual attack," (6) "Overprotected, babied adult…arrested at homosexual level of psychosexual development," (7) "Breakthrough of infantile, erotic attitudes," and (8) "Intense fear of loss of control over forbidden hostile or sexual impulses" (p. 120).

Transition to Modern Sleep Medicine and Concepts of Sleepwalking

The process of transitioning to modern sleep medicine and its concepts of sleepwalking, sleep terrors, and confusional arousals includes progress in understanding both their physiology and etiology. Sleepwalking as dream enactment and with a purely psychological etiology becomes progressively abandoned and replaced by laboratory-based physiology and, for the most part, by nonpsychological etiologies and triggers.

Modern sleep medicine is generally considered to begin with, and be dependent upon, the discovery of REM sleep by Aserinsky and Kleitman in 1953 [2] and the subsequent finding that REM sleep is closely associated with reports of dreaming [21]. The development of the EEG-based technology required to record sleep objectively for extended periods was equally important. However, initially, there was significant overlap between older theories and the newer data based on sleep laboratory recordings.

The first published sleep laboratory recordings of sleepwalking and related disorders occurred in the Marseille laboratory of French neurologist Henri Gastaut whose specialty was epilepsy. The earliest studies were completed in 1962 and 1963 and were done to distinguish whether parasomnias in epileptic children were usually nonepileptic or epileptic in mechanism, as the findings would affect choice of treatment.

This led to studies of the parasomnias in nonepileptic children and adults. In 1963, Gastaut and Broughton [3] reported five children and two adults studied polygraphically. They recorded ten episodes of parasomnia of which eight were associated with slow-wave sleep (SWS) and two with REM sleep. The SWS-associated complex behaviors included five confusional arousals, two sleep terrors, and one episode of sleepwalking. The other episode of sleepwalking occurred during a transition from stage 2 to REM sleep, a pattern not encountered or reported later. The SWS episodes were associated with amnesia. Anticipating modern theories of sleepwalking, they concluded that:

> These paroxysms appear best considered as phenomena of dissociation (between behavior and EEG).

This study overlapped with the last major scientific publication concerning somnambulism published prior to the start of modern sleep medicine and sleepwalking. Sours et al. [20] in the *Archives of General Psychiatry* in 1963 summarized the prevailing views up to that time. In the introduction, it is noted that "Sleepwalking is attributed to acting out a dream or fantasy or re-enactment of an earlier trauma." The authors were three Navy psychiatrists whose interest in sleepwalking was related to the safety of active duty sailors and soldiers who might be endangered were they to sleepwalk on a ship or in a battle zone. Sours et al. studied 14 sailors referred for psychiatric evaluation due to sleepwalking. Of these, 11 had documented episodes of sleepwalking while in service. All subjects underwent a neurological and psychiatric evaluation. Additionally, an EEG that included sleep was performed. Many of the subjects in this study had signs and symptoms of sleepwalking that would be consistent with modern views. Most had onset of episodes around 11 years of age. In 7 of 14 subjects, episodes were associated with stress or conflict. Four of the fourteen subjects first exhibited sleepwalking in boot camp most likely secondary to sleep deprivation and stress. However, this study differed significantly from modern concepts in that significant psychopathology was reported. The report concluded that 35 % of their sleepwalking subjects were "overt schizophrenics" and 28 % had schizoid personalities. The remaining sailors were found to have neurotic character disorders. All received at least one psychiatric diagnosis. Sour et al. approached interpretation of the psychiatric evaluation from a decidedly psychodynamic point of view. Thus, their results are consistent with a confirmation basis. The diagnostic EEG studies were reported as negative, although 2 of the 14 subject's records contained "slow burst activity." It is not made clear if this occurred during sleep or not or if this was read as epileptic. Even though this study was published in 1963, there is no mention of REM sleep in the article [2].

The first full descriptions of sleepwalking and sleep terrors in a sleep laboratory were published in the 1960s [3, 22–24]. The Marseille group including Gastaut and Broughton produced a number of publications. Their results on sleepwalking were confirmed by researchers at the University of California, Los Angeles (UCLA) including Alan Jacobson [25] and Anthony Kales [26], and on sleep terrors by Charles Fisher et al. at Mt. Sinai Hospital in New York City [27].

After their report in 1965, Gastaut and Broughton in 1965 published a wide-ranging and detailed description of "episodic phenomena" during sleep which included early polysomnographic (PSG) illustrations of sleepwalking, sleep terrors, and confusional arousals [28]. They emphasized that somnambulism should not be confused with psychomotor epileptic seizures or attacks of hysteria. They provided detailed descriptions of somnambulism especially in children that confirmed that these episodes are associated with eyes being open, severe difficulty in arousing, limited or absent social interaction during an episode, and complete amnesia the morning afterwards. They reported the results of sleep studies in 8 patients with sleepwalking (3 children, 5 adults) of 30 subjects with daily episodes at home and who had episodes of somnambulism recorded in the sleep laboratory whereas 24 patients did not. The authors noted that these episodes always began during slow-wave EEG activity, most often during stage 4 (phase IV) which is currently combined with previous stage 3 as stage N3 sleep following an "intense awakening EEG reaction" that occurred concurrently or seconds before. They also pioneered the method of provoking episodes of confusional arousals and sleepwalking in children with a clinical history of this disorder. The method was to record the sleep EEG in children and await entry into deep sleep—stage 3 or 4 sleep (now N3)—as defined by high-amplitude delta waves. The child was then literally picked up and placed on his or her feet. Typically, the patient had to be supported for a variable time, but muscle tone then returned. As monitoring continued via long cables or telemetry with the eyes typically open, the child then walked about and then most often returned to bed. Gastaut and Broughton noted that, of the wide range of sleep automatisms they studied, almost none occurred in REM sleep. Their research strongly suggested that:

> Somnambulism may therefore be considered as an ambulatory automatism related to sudden arousal, usually from slow-wave sleep.

These findings in sleep recordings of sleepwalking were confirmed by a UCLA-based group including Allan Jacobson and Anthony Kales who used long cables to permit subjects to move around more freely [25]. In their initial study in 1965, they studied nine frequent sleepwalkers aged 9–23 years for a total of 47 nights. They noted 74 episodes including 9 episodes of sleepwalking and 65 episodes in which the subjects sat up suddenly but did not leave the bed. They noted that all episodes began during SWS. This occurred of either stage 3 or 4. This occurred predominantly during the first quarter of the night and was not related to REM sleep. The sleepwalkers were described as being "aware of their environment, but indifferent to it." Eyes were reported to be open, but the "expressions blank" and movements "somewhat rigid." They reported complete amnesia for these episodes upon awakening in the morning.

A second UCLA study published the next year [26] involved two groups of patients consisting of four known sleepwalkers aged 9–11 years and four normal controls aged 7–11 years. Additionally, a single 27-year-old sleepwalker was studied separately. Each subject underwent two types of studies. The first study night allowed for uninterrupted sleep in the sleep laboratory. The second study night involved attempts to provoke sleepwalking by either: (1) standing subjects up or (2) attempting to arouse them by calling them by name or using meaningless loud noise. During the uninterrupted nights of the child sleepwalkers, 15 episodes were noted including 2 sleepwalking episodes and 13 episodes of sitting up or crawling around the bed. All incidents occurred during deep NREM sleep. No episodes were noted in the 27-year-old sleepwalker or for the child normal controls.

During the provocation nights, the experimenters were generally unsuccessful in inducing sleepwalking or any related behavior from deep sleep by calling their names or using loud sounds. Only one of the child somnambulists responded to calling of his name by sleepwalking on two occasions. On the other hand, making child somnambulists stand up was much more effective and provoked episodes during 7 of the 38 attempts. None of the normal controls had any episodes using this technique. The experimenters noted that the frequency of sleepwalking episodes in the laboratory was far less than reported at home. Kales et al. concluded that sleepwalking was related to deep NREM sleep but not REM sleep.

These studies were followed by a seminal article in the journal *Science* in 1968 by Broughton in which he formally defined somnambulism, sleep terrors, and confusional awakenings as "disorders of arousal" [29]. The article clarifies that the reason for this is not because an arousal occurs, but that in afflicted patients, arousal from SWS is abnormal. This is shown by the fact that the attacks may be triggered experimentally by forced arousal, whereas in normal subjects lacking these parasomnias, forced arousal does not precipitate an attack. It is therefore the arousal process which is abnormal. This ability to induce episodes in patients by forced arousal also excludes their episodes necessarily being generated by dreaming or other mental activity in sleep. Otherwise, it would be a remarkable coincidence that the externally induced forced arousal occurred at the precise moment when internal mentation, unknown to the investigator, was about to lead to an attack. Since the publication of this article, the *International Classification of Sleep Disorders* (ICSD-1 and

ICSD-2) groups sleepwalking, sleep terrors, and confusional arousals as disorders of arousal [1].

Broughton also made it very clear that these disorders do not occur in REM sleep. Furthermore, he provides a list of six symptoms, which to this day are consistent with current nosologies and are essential for proper differential diagnosis. They are:

1. mental confusion and disorientation
2. automatic behavior
3. relative nonreactivity to external stimuli
4. poor response to efforts to provoke behavioral wakefulness, where provoking awakening from REM sleep was, by comparison quite easy
5. retrograde amnesia for many intercurrent events (an entire sleepwalking episode, the activity of the investigators, and so on)
6. only fragmentary recall of apparent dreams, or none at all

Although this article forms the basis of our modern conceptualization of sleepwalking and its related disorders, our knowledge has been greatly expanded since that time and in many aspects. Some of these areas are as follows.

An early report of a recorded patient with sleep terrors was by Gastaut et al. in 1962 [30]. Sleepwalking associated with violence was reported in Ottawa in 1978 [31–33]. In a more recent publication [34], Brougton provides a review of the history of research by the Marseilles group including the common and related parasomnia of bedwetting (enuresis nocturna). It, as mentioned earlier [7], describes the existence of the so-called hybrid or compound attacks in which, for example, sleep terrors immediately evolve in sleepwalking. Tassinari et al. [35] showed that in epileptic children with sleep terrors the latter were essentially always of non-epileptic origin, confirming earlier reports of Broughton and Gastaut for enuresis in epileptic children.

Tonic EMG Levels in Recording

Measurement of EMG levels from the mentalis or submentalis muscles on the chin is now routine and required element for sleep scoring to distinguish a REM sleep from NREM sleep. EMG atonia is now considered to be a normal component of REM sleep. It is notable that submental EMG recording was absent in the original studies of Aserinsky, Kleitman, Dement, and others [2]. Thus, REM sleep atonia was not an original requirement for the scoring of REM sleep. Later, Jouvet [36] noted the absence of tonic EMG during REM sleep in cats, and Hodes and Dement [37] and Berger [38] confirmed that the same was true in humans. However, Jacobson et al. are generally credited with establishing EMG atonia as a required element of REM sleep [39]. This study was later cited in the Rechtshaffen and Kales (R&K) manual

[40]. Submental EMG was not included as part of the scoring rules in Dement and Kleitman initial sleep scoring criteria [41]. And EMG was also not included in the modification of Dement and Kleitman by Williams et al. and best found in their 1974 book *The EEG of Human Sleep* [42]. They continued to use this method well into the 1970s even after the 1969 R&K manual became standard. The R&K scoring manual has continued to be used until recently in the USA and continues to be widely used elsewhere. This delay in accepting EMG atonia as an essential component of normal REM sleep was important in that, prior to this, it could not have been known that during REM sleep the presence of EMG atonia and paralysis would prevent dreamers from enacting their dreams.

Hypersynchronous Delta Waves and Increased Slow-Wave Arousals

These EEG signs were reported by researchers as common and even diagnostic for sleepwalking and related disorders [25]. Sensitivity is a term used to describe if a test is regularly positive for the disorder it is intended to test. Specificity is a term that is used to describe if a test is positive in disorders for which it was not intended to test. Published research shows the sensitivity of hypersynchronous delta waves (HDWs) is less than 100 % and indeed may not occur even in patients who have full-blown episodes in the sleep laboratory. Further, the specificity is very low. Recent studies have reported that it frequently occurs in patients with obstructive sleep apneas who have no history or other symptoms of any disorders of arousal [43]. Additionally, arousals from SWS are also common in patients with obstructive sleep apnea. Thus, in the absence of a positive clinical history, these EEG signs are not thought to be reliable for diagnosis.

Polysomnography

Gastaut and Broughton [28] and Jacobson et al. [25] noted on several occasions that the frequency of episodes in the sleep laboratory was far less than what was reported at home. This is consistent with the reports that patients being evaluated in clinical sleep centers for sleepwalking almost never have a spontaneous episode. It may be that the novel environment or disturbances from electrodes and sensors somehow interfere with their occurrence. As a result of the lack of specificity and reliability of EEG signs, and the very poor chance an actual episode of sleepwalking will occur in the sleep laboratory, sleepwalking is one of the few sleep disorders listed in the ICSD-3 in which a sleep study is neither recommended nor needed for diagnosis.

Radio Telemetry

Both Gastaut and Broughton [28] and Kales et al. [26] made use of radio telemetry to allow sleepwalkers to leave the bed unencumbered. Although the technology available has greatly improved since the 1960s, no subsequent telemetry-based studies of these parasomnias have been reported.

Video PSG

Video PSG has become a standard technique to supplement traditional PSG. Currently, digital video is time-locked to physiological signals so it can be determined if movements and behaviors are related to changes in the EEG and vice versa. Additionally, the capacity of modern polysomnographs allows the simultaneous measurement of 32 or more channels. Measurement of physiological signals other than EEG, EOG, and submental EMG needed to stage sleep are almost routinely supplemented by ECG, chest movement, upper airway airflow, oxygen saturation, and arm and leg EMG for movements.

Provocation

Studies from the Montreal group have shown that 24–36 h of experimental sleep deprivation generally increases the number and complexity of behaviors during SWS in young, healthy adult sleepwalkers [44, 45]. This has been shown to have high sensitivity in sleepwalkers, but the specificity of this method is not known, limiting its diagnostic usefulness. Pilon et al. have further developed provocation techniques by adding acoustic arousals to the sleep deprivation protocol to further increase the number and complexity of behaviors from sleep. They are now using a research protocol in which the subject stays up all night and sleeps in the daytime during which the acoustic arousals are administered. This protocol has almost a 100 % success rate in clinically diagnosed, young, healthy sleepwalkers. Its usefulness as a diagnostic tool remains to be determined.

Genetics

Even prior to the 1960s, it was known that sleepwalking and related disorders ran in families. Published studies of sleepwalking genetics have identified several potential different loci [46, 47]. Different models of the mode of inheritance have been proposed including multifactorial, recessive with incomplete penetrance, and autosomal dominant trait with reduced penetrance. Furthermore, it is not known in what way a genetic predisposition contributes to their occurrence.

Familial studies of sleepwalking found that having a first-degree relative with a history of sleepwalking increases the chance of a descendent developing sleepwalking by a factor of 40 [46]. Unfortunately, the sensitivity and specificity of these markers are insufficiently high for use as a genetic diagnostic test.

Treatment

Medication

Although a number of treatments for sleepwalking and sleep terrors had been in use prior to the 1960s to the 1970s, none were reported as consistently effective and none had been subjected to experimental validation. In 1973, Fisher et al. were the first to administer a benzodiazepine sedative, diazepam (Valium), to patients clinically diagnosed with night terrors [27]. Fisher et al. had noted the strong relationship reported between the amount of SWS and the intensity of night terrors. Benzodiazepines had been previously reported to suppress SWS without any side effects. Fisher et al. hypothesized that, by administering diazepam, SWS could be suppressed and thus night terrors would be eliminated. They studied six subjects ranging in age from 27 to 34 years who complained of frequent episodes. They conducted nine experiments for a total of 296 nights with various combinations and dosages of diazepam compared to placebo. Diazepam was reported to reduce the percentage of stage 4 sleep by a mean of 90.4 %. The number of night terrors was reduced by a mean of 80.5 %. Since that time, benzodiazepines or similar sedative/hypnotics have been shown to be effective treatments for both sleepwalking and sleep terrors and for sustained periods of time [48]. Clonazepam has become the drug of choice [49]. Some patients have been helped using tricyclic antidepressants, especially chlorimipramine. And isolated cases have been reported to respond to trazodone or paroxetine [50].

Other

Some patients with a disorder of arousal have a coexistent sleep disorder or medical, neurological, or psychiatric disorder, and these should be treated independently.

Identification and Elimination of Potential Triggers

The rapid expansion of research in this area has identified a number of priming and provoking factors.

Sleep Deprivation

Anecdotal reports after the 1960s, have increasingly linked prior sleep deprivation with the occurrence of sleepwalking. A night of total sleep deprivation is well established to lead to the rebound of SWS (an increased percentage of SWS) on the next night [44, 45]. The Montreal group led by Montplaisir and Zadra has conducted a number of sleep-laboratory-based experiments of 24–36 h of sleep deprivation in young, otherwise healthy sleepwalkers. Sleep deprivation has been shown to increase the number of episodes in the sleep laboratory. This finding suggests both the importance of avoiding periods of sleep deprivation and of extending the hours in bed and hours of sleep in sleepwalkers.

Sleep Fragmentation

An increase in arousals, especially from slow wave sleep, is well established in sleepwalking [50, 51] and in sleep terrors [52]. In the modern sleep era, the most common sources of sleep fragmentation are coexistent sleep disorders such as sleep apnea. Sleep apnea consists of repeated interruptions of upper airway airflow and in obstructive apneas each event is associated with an arousal from sleep. Recent research has demonstrated that these sleep apnea-related arousals are often the proximal trigger for sleepwalking, night terrors, and confusional arousals in both children and adults [53, 54]. This is supported by research that shows that effective treatment of sleep apnea and its associated arousals by continuous positive airway pressure (CPAP) or surgery lead to a significant reduction or elimination of sleepwalking in patients with coexistent obstructive sleep apneas [55].

Mentation

Although research has conclusively indicated that sleepwalking is not related to REM-sleep-related dreaming, recent research has suggested that some types of mentation do continue during NREM sleep and may be associated with sleepwalking and sleep terrors and may possibly initiate some episodes. Sleep terrors have long been known to start with a vivid, often frightening image—house on fire, intruder in bedroom, and so forth. However, the reported mental activity has in general lacked the hallucinatory complexity of what we usually call dreams and that are typically associated with REM sleep. Recently, several reports have been published suggesting that sleepwalking as well as confusional arousals may be associated with similar imagery. Many of the earlier reports were based upon questioning the patient the following morning. Questioning the patient seconds or minutes after the occurrence of the episode appears to be

necessary. Just as with dreams, this type of mentation may be hard for the patient to retain in memory.

Differential Diagnosis

Nightmares

Sleep terrors must be distinguished from REM nightmares. The discovery of REM sleep and the association of the onset of night terrors with deep NREM sleep led Fisher et al. to conclude that episodes of "anxiety arousals" occurring in REM and NREM sleep, although superficially similar, have quite different etiologies [56]. They suggested limiting the term "nightmare" to episodes occurring in REM sleep and night terror (sleep terror) for episodes beginning in deep NREM sleep. Sleep terrors are consequently common early in the sleep period while nightmares occur more often in the early morning hours, where REM sleep is greatly increased.

With the expanded research and the development of clinical sleep medicine, a number of common subtypes or variants of sleepwalking were described and added to nosologies. Many of these variants appear to reflect basic human drives such as eating, sex, and violence.

Sleep Eating

Patients with this disorder typically arouse and make their way to the kitchen where they may eat unusual combinations of food. As with sleepwalking, it is typically followed by amnesia although scraps of food in the bed or a very disordered kitchen in the morning may provide clues to the diagnosis

Sleep Sex

First described in 2003 by Shapiro et al. [57], such patients typically initiate sex with their usual bed partners while in a state similar to sleepwalking. They usually have no memory of their sexual behaviors in the morning [58].

Sleep Violence

Episodes of violence while sleepwalking have been reported and occasionally result in criminal charges [7]. Violence most often results when family members or friends try to block or impede the behavior of a sleepwalker. With the cortex deactivated, the sleepwalker is unable to understand the situation or recognize family members, Instead, he responds with defensive aggressiveness. He may hit, punch, or kick. Sleepwalkers do not seek out their victims but may encounter them during sleepwalking episodes [33].

REM Sleep Behavior Disorder

The discovery of RBD in 1986 [9] was arguably as important to modern sleep medicine as the pathophysiological description of sleepwalking and sleep terrors as disorders of arousal. RBD occurs when the mechanisms responsible for REM sleep atonia and paralysis fail to function properly. With tonic EMG present, patients can and do behaviorally act out their dreams. Thus, this disorder has most of the characteristics that almost everyone attributed to sleepwalking prior to the 1960s. Its clinical significance is great as it often precedes the onset of Parkinson's disease [59].

Nocturnal Frontal Lobe Epilepsy

These seizures consist of stereotypical dyskinetic movements of varying intensity with vocalization arising in NREM sleep and without postseizure mental confusion. Due to the vocalization, these epileptic seizures are most often confused with sleep terrors, but their stereotyped symptomatology and lack of massive sympathetic discharge with marked increase in heart rate makes clinical differentiation easy. The scalp EEG during the seizures does not show an ictal discharge. The condition is sometimes referred to as nocturnal paroxysmal dystonia [60, 61]. MRI lesions in the frontal lobe have been reported [62] and the seizures are generally thought to arise from the mesial frontal or orbitofrontal cortices. This would explain the absence of a discharge on scalp EEG. However, stereotactic intra-cerebral electrodes have confirmed epileptogenic foci in the areas involved. Treatment is typically neurosurgical removal of the epileptogenic foci plus anticonvulsant medication. Halasz et al. [63] have proposed the existence of an overlap of mechanisms of these seizures with the NREM arousal parasomnia. But given the lack of evidence that the seizures can be provoked by forced arousal plus the variable behavior from attack to attack of the NREM arousal parasomnias versus the stereotypical nature of the seizures an overlap of mechanisms seems unlikely.

Nocturnal Temporal and Frontal Lobe Seizures

Mainly studied in the 1960s and 1970s by the Montpellier group led by Pierre Passouant, these epileptic seizures can lead to nocturnal wanderings which can be very difficult to distinguish clinically from sleepwalking. They are, however, almost always associated with discharge on scalp EEG over the area of the epileptogenic focus [60], they mainly take place in REM sleep in the second half of the night [65], more or less similar seizures and discharges are usually present in wakefulness [64, 66], and they usually respond well to anti-epileptic medication.

Theory

Advances in the neurosciences and new imaging technologies have in the last few years led to conceptualization of sleepwalking as a disorder of dissociation. This is, however, not a new concept. Early reports have stressed the dissociations inherent in the episodes (mind asleep, body awake; EEG showing light sleep, behavior suggesting wakefulness). In support of the importance of dissociation, Bassetti et al. [67] captured a sleep terror episode in a 17-year-old during single-photon emission computed tomography (SPECT) imaging. They found that the cortex and, in particular, the frontal lobes were deactivated as is typical during normal NREM sleep, but the ascending stimuli that should have been blocked at the level of the thalamus were not blocked and continued on to the cortex. Without the frontal lobes to inhibit behaviors, sleepwalking was possible. Other researchers have pointed out that sleep and wake are not unitary states. Instead, it has been determined that some areas of the brain may be asleep while others are awake as was already believed, as mentioned earlier by nineteenth century writers, Warton (1855) and Tuke (1884). "Local sleep" may well be the basis of sleepwalking as it is also supported by behavioral and perceptual dissociations and by electrophysiological evidence including the absence of blocking of the alpha rhythm to very intense floodlights used for filming during sleepwalking episodes monitored by telemetry [28] and by the presence in visual evoked potential during induced confusional arousals of the coexistence of VEP components characteristic of NREM sleep and others characteristic of wakefulness [29].

References

1. American Academy of Sleep Medicine. ICSD-2—International Classification of Sleep Disorders, 2nd ed. Diagnostic and Coding Manual. Westchester: American Academy of Sleep Medicine; 2005.
2. Aserinsky E, Kleitman N. Regularly occurring periods of eye motility, and concomittant phenomena, during sleep. Science 1953;118:273–4.
3. Gastaut H, Broughton R. Paroxysmal psychological events and certain phases of sleep. Percept Mot Skills. 1963;17:362. (Epub 1963/10/01).
4. Prichard JC. Somnambulism and animal magnetism. In Forbes JT, Tweedie A, Conolly J, editors. The Cyclopaedia of practical medicine. London: Whittaker, Treacher and Company; 1835. p. 21–39.
5. Colquhoun JC. Introduction. Edinburgh: Adam and Charles Black; 1845.
6. Tuke D. Sleep-walking and hypnotism. Philadelphia: P. Blakiston; 1884.
7. Broughton R, Billings R, Cartwright R, Doucette D, Edmeads J, Edwardh M, et al. Homicidal somnambulism: a case report. Sleep 1994;17(3):253–64.
8. Pressman MR. Disorders of arousal from sleep and violent behavior: the role of physical contact and proximity. Sleep 2007;30(8):1039–47.

9. Schenck CH, Bundlie SR, Ettinger MG, Mahowald MW. Chronic behavioral disorders of human REM sleep: a new category of parasomnia. Sleep 1986;9(2):293–308.

10. Pady DS. The medico-psychological interests of King James I. Clio Medica. 1984;19(1–2):22–31.

11. Walker N. Crime and insanity in England. Edinburgh: Edinburgh University Press; 1968. p. 302.

12. Petrain D. An English translation of John William Polidori's (1815) medical dissertation on Oneirodynia (Somnambulism). Eur Rom Rev 2010;21:775–88.

13. Broughton RJ. NREM arousal parasomnias. In: Kryger MH, Roth T, Dement WC, editors. Principles and practice of sleep medicine. 3rd ed. Philadelphia: W. B. Saunders Company; 2000. p. 1336.

14. Pressman MR. Factors that predispose, prime and precipitate NREM parasomnias in adults: clinical and forensic implications. Sleep Med Rev. 2007;11(1):5–30.

15. Ray I. A treatise on the medical jurisprudence of insanity. Boston: Charles C. Little and James Brown; 1838.

16. Wharton F. A monograph on mental unsoundness. Philadelphia: Kay and Brother; 1855. p. 228.

17. Hammond W. Sleep and its derangements. Philadelphia: Lippincott; 1869.

18. Yellowless, D. Homicide by somnabulist. J Ment Scie 1878;24:451–8.

19. Hurwitz TD, Mahowald MW, Schenck CH, Schluter JL, Bundlie SR. A retrospective outcome study and review of hypnosis as treatment of adults with sleepwalking and sleep terror. J Nerv Ment Dis. 1991;179(4):228–33.

20. Sours JAF, Frunkin P, Indermill RR. Somnambulism: its clinical significance and dynamic meaning in late adolescence and adulthood. Arch Gen Psychiatry. 1963;9:400–13.

21. Dement WC, Kleitman N. The relation of eye movements during sleep to dream activity: an objective method for the study of dreaming. J Exp Psychol. 1957;53(5):339–46.

22. Gastaut H, Batini C, Broughton R, Fressy J, Tassinari CA. Etude électroencéphalographique des manifestations paroxystiques non-épileptiques au cours du sommeil nocturne. Rev Neurol. 1964;110:309–10.

23. Gastaut H, Batini C, Broughton R, Fressy J, Tassinari CA. Etude électroencéphalographique des phénomènes non-épileptiques au cours du sommeil. In: Fischgold H, editor. Le sommeil de nuit normal et pathologique: Etudes électroencéphalographiques. Paris: Masson; 1965, p. 215.

24. Broughton R, Gastaut H. Recent sleep research on enuresis nocturna, sleep walking, sleep terrors and confusional arousals: a review of dissociative awakening disorders in slow wave sleep. In: Levin P, Koella W, editors. Sleep 1974. Karger: Basel; 1975. p. 82–91.

25. Jacobson A, Kales A, Lehmann D, Zweizig J. Somnambulism: all-night electroencephalographic studies. Science. 1965:975–7.

26. Kales A, Jacobson A, Paulson MJ, Kales JD, Walter RD. Somnambulism: psychophysiological correlates. I. All-night EEG studies. Arch Gen Psychiatry. 1966;14:586–94.

27. Fischer C, Kahn E, Edwards A, David DM. A psychophysiological study of nightmares and night terrors. The suppression of stage 4 night terrors with diazepam. Arch Gen Psychiatry. 1973;28:252–9.

28. Gastaut H, Broughton R. A clinical and polygraphic study of episodic phenomena during sleep. In Wortis J, editor. Recent advances in biological psychiatry (Vol 7). New York: Plenum; 1965. p. 197–221.

29. Broughton RJ. Sleep disorders: disorders of arousal? Enuresis, somnambulism, and nightmares occur in confusional states of arousal, not in "dreaming sleep". Science. 1968;159:1070–8.

30. Gastaut H, Dongier M, Batini C, Rhodes J. Etude électroencéphalographique des terreurs nocturnes et diurnes chez un névrosé. Rev Neurol. 1962;107:277–99.

31. Broughton R. Aggression during sleepwalking: a case report. Sleep Res. 1978;7:215.

32. Broughton R, Warnes H. Violence in sleep: eleven cases. Sleep Res. 1989;18:205.

33. Broughton R, Shimizu T. Sleep-related violence: a medical and forensic challenge. Sleep. 1995;18:727–30.

34. Broughton R. Pathophysiology of enuresis nocturna, sleep terrors and sleep walking: current status and the Marseilles contribution. In: Broughton R, editor, Henti Gastaut and the Marseilles contribution to the Neurosciences. Amsterdam: Elsevier; 1982. p. 401.

35. Tassinari CA, Mancia D, Della Bernardina B, Gastaut H. Pavor nocturnus of non-epileptic nature in epileptic children. Electroenceph Clin Neurophysiol. 1972;33:603–7.

36. Jouvet M. Research on the neural structures and responsible mechanisms in different phases of physiological sleep. Arch Ital Biol. 1962;100:125–206.

37. Hodes RD, Dement WC, editors. Abolition of electrically induced reflexes during rapid eye movement (REM) periods of sleep in normal subjects (preliminary report). Brooklyn: Association for the psychophysiology of sleep (APSS). 1963.

38. Berger R. Tonus of extrinsic laryngeal muscles during sleep and dreaming. Science. 1961;134:840.

39. Jacobson A, Kales A, Lehmann D, Hoedemaker FS. Muscle tonus in human subjects during sleep and dreaming. Exp Neurol. 1964;10:418–24.

40. Rechtschaffen A, Kales A, editors. A manual of standardized terminology, techniques, and scoring system for sleep stages of human subjects. Los Angeles. Brain Information Service/Brain Research Institute. 1968.

41. Dement W, Kleitman N. Cyclic variations in EEG during sleep and their relationship to eye movements, body motility and dreaming. Electroencephalogr Clin Neurophysiol. 1957;9:673–90.

42. Williams RL, Karacan I, Hursch C. EEG of human sleep: clinical applications. New York: Wiley; 1974.

43. Pressman MR, Hypersynchronous delta sleep EEG activity and sudden arousals from slow-wave sleep in adults without a history of parasomnias: clinical and forensic implications. Sleep. 2004;27:706–10.

44. Joncas S, Zadra A, Montplasir J. Sleep deprivation increases the frequency and complexity of behavioral manifestations in adult sleep walkers. Sleep. 2000;23(Suppl. 2):A14.

45. Joncas S, Zadra A, Paquet J, Montplaisir J. The value of sleep deprivation as a diagnostic tool in adult sleepwalkers. Neurology. 2002;58:936–40.

46. Lecendreux M, Bassetti C, Dauvilliers Y, Mayer G, Neidhart E, Tafti M. HLA and genetic susceptibility to sleepwalking. Mol Psychiatry. 2003;8:114–7.

47. Licis AK, Desruisseau DM, Yamada KA, Duntley SP, Gurnett CA. Novel genetic findings in extended family pedigree with sleepwalking. Neurology. 2011;76:49–52.

48. Schenck CH, Mahowald MW. Long-term, nightly benzodiazepine treatment of injurious parasomnias and other disorders of disrupted nocturnal sleep in 170 adults. Am J Med. 1996;100:333–7.

49. Harris M, Grundstein RR. Treatments for somnambulism in adults: assessing the evidence. Sleep Med Rev. 2009;13:295–7.

50. Broughton R, Mullington J. Polysomnography: principles and applications in sleep and arousal disorders. In: Niedermeyer E, Lopes da Silva E, editors. Electroencephalography: basic principles. Clinical applications and related fields. Baltimore: Williams and Wilkens; 2004. p. 899.

51. Boucher B, Broughton R. Sleep architecture differences between sleep terror and sleepwalker patients and matched controls. J Sleep Res. 2000;9(Suppl 1):23.

52. Broughton RJ. Phasic and dynamic aspects of sleep: a symposium review and synthesis. In: Terzano MG, Halasz P, Declerck AC, editors. Phasic and dynamic aspects of sleep. New York: Raven; 1991. p. 185.

53. Guilleminault C, Palombini L, Pelayo R, Chervin RD. Sleepwalking and sleep terrors in prepubertal children: what triggers them? Pediatrics. 2003;111:17–25.

54. Guilleminault C, Kirisoglu C, Bao G, Arias V, Chen A, Li KK. Adult chronic sleepwalking and its treatment based on polysomnography. Brain. 2005;12:1062–9.

55. Guilleminault C, Kirisoglu C, da Rosa AC, Lopez C, Chen A. Sleepwalking, a disorder of NREM sleep instability. Sleep Med. 2006;7:163–70.

56. Fisher C, Byrne J, Edwards A, Kahn E. REM and NREM nightmares. Int Psychiat Clin. 1970;7:183–7.

57. Shapiro CM, Trajanovic NN, Fedoroff JP. Sexsomnia- a new parasomnia? Can J Psychiatry-Rev Can Psychiatrie. 2003;48:311–7.

58. Guilleminault C, Moscovitch A, Yuen K, Poyares D. Atypical sexual behavior during sleep. Psychosom Med. 2002;64:328–36.

59. Arnulf I, Neutel D, Herlin B, Golmard JL, Leu-Semenescu S, de Cock VC, Vidailhet M. Sleepiness in idiopathic REM sleep behavior disorder and Parkinson disease. Sleep. 2015. Pii:sp-00663-14 (Epub ahead of print).

60. Lugaresi E, Cirignotta F. Hypnogenic paroxysmal dystonia: epileptic scizures or new syndrome? Sleep. 1981;4:129–38.

61. Lugaresi E, Cirignotta F, Montagna P. Nocturnal paroxysmal dystonia. J Neurol Neurosurg Psychiatry. 1986;49:375–80.

62. Provini F, Piazzi G, Lugaresi E. From nocturnal paroxysmal dystonia to frontal lobe epilepsy. J Clin Neurophysiol. 2000;111:52–8.

63. Halasz P, Kelemen A, Szucs A. Physiopathogenetic interrelationship between nocturnal frontal lobe epilepsy and NREM arousal parasomnia. Epilepsy Res Treat. 2012;12:312–93.

64. Passouant P, Latour H, Cadilhac J. L'épilepsie morphéique. Ann Med Psychol. 1961;109:529–41.

65. Cadilhac J, Vlahovitch B, Delange-Walter C. Considérations sur les modifications des décharges épileptiques au cours de la période des mouvements oculaires. In: Fischgold H, editor. Le sommeil de nuit normal et pathologique. Paris: Masson; 1965.

66. Gastaut H, Broughton R. Epileptic seizures: clinical and electrographic features, diagnosis and treatment. Sringfield: Charles C Thomas; 1972, 286 pp.

67. Bassetti C, Vela S, Donati I, Weber H. SPECT during sleepwalking. Lancet. 2000;356:484–5.

REM Sleep Behavior Disorder

Carlos H. Schenck

...he was thrusting his sword in all directions, speaking out loud as if he were actually fighting a giant. And the strange thing was that he did not have his eyes open, because he was asleep and dreaming that he was battling the giant... He had stabbed the wine skins so many times, believing that he was stabbing the giant, that the entire room was filled with wine.... [1]

Personal Experiences with Rapid Eye Movement Sleep Behavior Disorder in Patients and Spouses

Although rapid eye movement (REM) sleep behavior disorder (RBD), featuring its quintessential violent dream-enacting behaviors, was described in the world literature by Cervantes as early as 1605, it was not until 1986–1987 that RBD was formally identified and named [2, 3]. RBD was included in the international classification of sleep disorders (ICSD) in 1990, with diagnostic criteria being established, and with updates in the ICSD-2 in 2005 [4] and in the ICSD-3 in 2014. RBD emerges during loss of the mammalian generalized skeletal muscle atonia of REM sleep, a pathological state known as REM without atonia (RWA).

The index patient aptly described his RBD as "violent moving nightmares" [2]. The report of his case illustrated many common features of RBD: "Patient 1. A 67-year-old dextral man was referred because of violent behavior during sleep.... He had slept uneventfully through adolescence in a small room with three brothers. But on his wedding night, his wife was 'scared with surprise' over his sleep talking, groaning, tooth grinding, and minor body movements. This

persisted without consequence for 41 years until one night, 4 years before referral, when he experienced the first 'physically moving dream' several hours after sleep onset; he found himself out of bed attempting to carry out a dream. This episode signaled the onset of an increasingly frequent and progressively severe sleep disorder; he would punch and kick his wife, fall out of bed, stagger about the room, crash into objects, and injure himself. These harmful behaviors, most prominent every tenth night, typically appeared several hours after sleep onset and never within the first hour... he quickly became alert with each awakening. In search of sound sleep, his wife began to sleep in another room 2 years before referral. They remain happily married, believing that these nocturnal behaviors are out of his control and discordant with his waking personality."

"An example of a recurring RBD dream consisted of his delivering a speech and emphasizing certain points with his right hand from which he awakened sitting up with right arm outstretched and fingers pointing in a manner consistent with the dream action. Another time 'I was on a motorcycle going down the highway when another motorcyclist comes up alongside me and tries to ram me with his motorcycle. Well, I decided I'm going to kick his motorcycle away and at that point my wife woke me up and said, 'What in heavens are you doing to me?', because I was kicking the hell out of her'." Both of these episodes exemplify an "isomorphism" between the dream action and the enacted behaviors (e.g., kicking)."

His most vivid and violent dream, which prompted referral, was described in a National Geographic magazine article, "What Is This Thing Called Sleep?," Dec. 1987, p. 787: "The crowd roared as running back Donald Dorff, age 67, took the pitch from his quarterback and accelerated smoothly across the artificial turf. As Dorff braked and pivoted to cut back over tackle, a huge defensive lineman loomed in his path. One hundred twenty pounds of pluck, Dorff did not hesitate. But let the retired grocery merchandiser from Golden Valley, Minnesota, tell it: 'There was a 280-pound tackle waiting for me, so I decided to give him my shoulder. When I came

C. H. Schenck (✉)
Minnesota Regional Sleep Disorders Center, Minneapolis, USA
e-mail: schen010@umn.edu

Department of Psychiatry, Hennepin County Medical Center, Minneapolis, USA

Department of Psychiatry, University of Minnesota Medical School, Minneapolis, MN, USA

S. Chokroverty, M. Billiard (eds.), *Sleep Medicine,* DOI 10.1007/978-1-4939-2089-1_45,
© Springer Science+Business Media, LLC 2015

to, I was on the floor in my bedroom. I had smashed into the dresser and knocked everything off it and broke the mirror and just made one heck of a mess. It was 1:30 a.m.'"

Patient #4 in the original series of RBD patients [2] had a notorious deer-hunting dream-enacting episode, in which he nearly strangled his wife to death in bed, that was described as "Hunting Deer Under the Blanket" (Stern magazine, Germany, March 24, 1988), and as "The Man Who Mistook His Wife For A Deer" (New York Times Sunday magazine cover story, February 2, 2003). "Mel Abel's eyes brim with tears when he tells how criminally close he came to harming his wife, Harriet. He was struggling with a deer whose head he was trying to snap when he discovered he was actually home in bed with his hands on Harriet's head and chin. Harriet woke him up, hollering, 'Mel, what in the world are you trying to do?'" (p. 36). "I started to cry and I said, 'Oh my God, am I glad you woke me up!' Another minute, you know, and I give a snap, and it might have broke her neck [5] (p. 51)." Figure 45.1 shows his desperate, often ineffective and at times harmful, self-remedy for control of the RBD.

Table 45.1 lists descriptions of sleeping and living with RBD by a group of 26 patients and their spouses that signal the dangers of sleeping with RBD [5]. Extreme force can be generated in RBD that rapidly produces life-threatening situations. The wives were convinced that their husbands were fully asleep while having prominent, excessive body movements throughout the night: "He is sleeping and his body is in motion" (p. 132). The assumption often expressed by patients and spouses was that RBD was caused by work stress

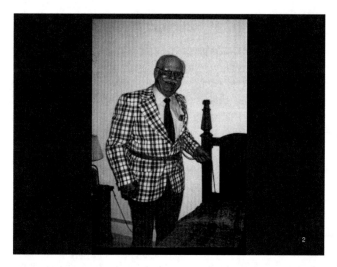

Fig 45.1 Patient #4 from the original reported series of RBD cases in 1986 [2] demonstrates a "home remedy" he resorted to using in desperation to prevent himself from leaping or falling out of bed and injuring himself. He wore a belt around his pajamas and then tied a rope around the belt on one end while tying the other end of the rope around the headboard of the bed. He engaged in this bedtime tethering ritual every night for 5 years before finding out about RBD in a news report and then presenting for evaluation at the sleep center

that would resolve with retirement turned out to be false, much to their chagrin. Another common assumption was that RBD was "part of getting old" and "it simply became routine," [5] (p. 125); these couples became resigned to live with this new late-life "normality"—until they heard about RBD and its successful therapy, usually from media reports.

Historical Background of RBD: 1966–1985

Various polysomnography (PSG) and clinical aspects of human RBD were described since 1966 by investigators from Europe, Japan, and North America, almost exclusively in neurologic settings, as reviewed [2, 6, 7]. Two groups of pioneering investigators should be recognized [6]: (i) Passouant et al. from France in 1972 first identified a dissociated state of REM sleep with tonic muscle activity induced by tricyclic antidepressant medication. (ii) Tachibana et al. from Japan in 1975 named "stage 1-REM sleep" as a peculiar sleep stage characterized by muscle tone during an REM sleep-like state that emerged during acute psychoses related to alcohol and meprobamate abuse. Also, clomipramine therapy of cataplexy in a group of patients with narcolepsy commonly produced RWA in a study from 1976 by Guilleminault et al. [8]. Elements of both acute and chronic RBD manifesting with "oneirism" were represented in the early literature, along with RWA without clinical correlates: Delirium Tremens (DTs) and other sedative and narcotic withdrawal states, anticholinergic use, spinocerebellar and other brainstem neurodegenerative disorders; the "REM rebound and REM intrusion" theories were proposed and discussed in many of these early reports. The 1986 report in SLEEP firmly established that RBD is a distinct parasomnia, which occurs during unequivocal REM sleep, and which can be idiopathic or symptomatic of a neurologic disorder [2]. Although there is a variable loss of the customary, generalized muscle paralysis of REM sleep, all other major features of REM sleep remain intact in RBD, such as REM latency, REM percent of total sleep time, number of REM periods, and REM/nonrapid eye movement (NREM) cycling. PSG monitoring of these patients established that RBD did not emerge from a "stage-1 REM sleep" that was separate from REM sleep, nor did RBD emerge from a poorly defined variant of REM sleep, or from an unknown or "peculiar" stage of sleep, or during "delirious" awakenings from sleep—all of which had been mentioned in the literature. The 1986 SLEEP report also called attention to generalized motor dyscontrol across REM and NREM sleep, manifesting as increased muscle tone and/or excessive phasic muscle twitching in REM sleep, along with periodic limb movements and excessive nonperiodic limb twitching in NREM sleep [2]. A lengthy prodrome in

Table 45.1 RBD behaviors causing imminent danger: patient and spouse comments[a]

A. Comments by RBD Patients

1	"It seems that I am extra strong when I am sleeping." (p. 142)
2	"I ran right smack into the wall, an animal was chasing me. I think it was a big black dog." (p. 157)
3	"And the last time that happened, I didn't remember the dream because I knocked myself out." (p. 149)
4	"I thought I was wrestling someone and I had her by the head." (p. 136)
5	"Pounding through the curlers into her head." (p. 157)
6	"What scares me is what a catastrophe that would be to wake up and find that I had broken her neck." (p. 137)
7	"I have hit her in the back too, and she has had a couple of (vertebral) disc operations." (p. 143)
8	"One night I woke up as I was beating the hell out of her pillow…that's when I realized that I had a problem." (p. 106)
9	"Just recently, I rammed into her pelvis with my head…during a dream." (p. 93)

B. Comments by the Wives

1	"It's amazing. You should see the energy behind that activity, oh, it's unreal."(p. 107)
2	"He literally just kind of flew out of bed and landed on the floor with tremendous strength" (p. 53)
3	"It almost seems like a force picks him up." (p. 130)
4	"His legs go so fast, just like he's running" (p. 155)
5	"It is his kicking, violent kicking, his feet are just like giant hammers when they hit you over and over again." (p. 73)
6	"I felt that kick on the ankle for two months afterwards." (p. 82)
7	"That's the reason we got the waterbed—because he was wrecking his hands on the wooden bed." (p. 111)
8	"Oh, yes, there were always bloody sheets." (p. 105)
9	"Roaring like a wounded wild animal: he roared, he crouched, he punched." (p. 75)
10	"I told him I'd have one devil of a time explaining how I got a broken arm in bed with both of us asleep." (p. 126)
11	"What happens to people like my husband who don't get diagnosed? Do they kill their wives in these experiences, do we know?" (p. 139)

[a] From [5] a book based on audio-recorded interviews of a series of older male patients with RBD and their wives from the Minnesota Regional Sleep Disorders Center, with signed permission by the patients and spouses

RBD was also described; a characteristic dream disturbance was identified; and a successful treatment with bedtime clonazepam was empirically discovered.

Animal Models of RBD

An experimental animal model of RBD was first reported in 1965 by Jouvet and Delorme from the Claude Bernard University in Lyons, France [6, 9], which was produced by brainstem lesions in the peri-locus ceruleus area that released a spectrum of "oneiric" behaviors during REM sleep (called paradoxical sleep and active sleep by basic scientists). These oneiric behaviors in cats closely match the repertoire of RBD behaviors in humans. Research on animal models of RBD (that now include cats, rats (brainstem lesion models), and mice (transgenic mouse model with impaired GABA and glycine transmission) [6, 9–11] and on the neuroanatomy and neurochemistry subserving REM-atonia and the phasic motor system in REM sleep has progressed considerably in recent years.

Ramaligam et al. [12] summarize research from the past five decades on the neural circuitry regulating REM-atonia, and identify REM-active glutamatergic neurons in the pontine sublaterodorsal (SLD) nucleus as being a critical area, as descending projections from the SLD activate neurons in the ventromedial medulla (VMM), from where inhibitory descending projections to the spinal cord ultimately produce the REM atonia. Damage to the SLD appears critical for triggering RBD in humans, based on neuropathological findings in humans with neurodegenerative disorders. Luppi et al. focus on the potential roles of brainstem glutamate, GABA, and glycine dysfunction in the pathophysiology of RBD, and propose alternative explanations for RBD apart from SLD damage [13]. A new study by Hsieh et al. [14] found that yet another brainstem region may be implicated in human RBD, involving GABA-B receptor mechanisms in the external cortex of the inferior colliculus. Therefore, REM sleep has an intrinsically programmed, brain-generated, active motor-inhibitory system, and not a passive withdrawal of motor activity. The atonia of REM sleep is briefly interrupted by excitatory inputs which produce the REMs and the muscle jerks and twitches characteristic of REM sleep.

All categories of behaviors found in human RBD are mirrored in an experimental animal model of RBD produced by pontine tegmental lesions [6, 9]. The pathophysiology of human RBD is presumed to correspond to the findings from an animal model of RBD in regard to interruption of the REM-atonia pathways and/or disinhibition of brainstem motor pattern generators.

Finally, naturally occurring, congenital, and adult-onset RBD in cats and dogs has been reported, with effective

Table 45.2 Early historical milestones in RBD[a]

1986–1987	Formal description, naming, and treatment of RBD [2, 3]
1989	RBD in the differential diagnosis of sleep-related injury [15]
1990	Forensic aspects of RBD [16]
1991	Status dissociatus [17]
1992	Medication-induced RBD [18]
1992	Narcolepsy-RBD [19]
1996	Delayed emergence of parkinsonism in RBD [20]
1996	Association of RBD with specific HLA haplotypes [21]
1997	Parasomnia overlap disorder [22]

[a] From the Minnesota Regional Sleep Disorders Center, Minneapolis, Minnesota, USA

therapies being identified (as reviewed [5, p. 415–6], [6]). This reflects an intriguing animal–human reciprocity, as the experimental animal model of RBD facilitated the understanding of human RBD and its effective therapy with clonazepam, which in turn facilitated awareness of naturally occurring RBD in dogs and cats and use of effective therapy with clonazepam.

Early Historical Milestones of RBD: 1986–1997

Among the ten patients in the original series, five had diverse neurologic disorders etiologically linked with RBD, and five were idiopathic [2, 3]. As a larger group of idiopathic RBD (iRBD) patients was gathered and followed longitudinally at our center, a surprisingly strong and specific association with eventual parkinsonism and dementia became apparent [20, 23], which has spurred a major, growing, multinational research effort [24, 25], including the formation of the International RBD Study Group (IRBD-SG) [10]. Many other important clinical associations with RBD have been identified, such as the strong link with narcolepsy [19, 26]. RBD is situated at a strategic crossroad of sleep medicine, neurology, and the neurosciences. The literature on RBD has continued to grow exponentially in breadth and depth [27]. RBD publications have now exceeded 100 per year. The "RBD odyssey" [28] exemplifies the strong cross-linkage between the basic science underlying REM sleep and the clinical features of RBD, and the close correspondences between animal models of RBD and clinical RBD. Table 45.2 presents early RBD historical milestones [2, 3, 20, 19, 15–18, 21, 22], with elaboration below.

Clinical and PSG Findings in RBD

There are two essential diagnostic hallmarks of RBD, involving clinical and PSG components [4]. The clinical component involves either (i) a history of abnormal sleep-related behaviors that are often dream-enacting behaviors, and/or emerge during the second half of the sleep cycle when REM sleep predominates compared to the first half of the sleep cycle, and/or (ii) abnormal REM sleep behaviors documented during video-PSG in a sleep laboratory, which are often manifestations of dream enactment. It is important to note that the diagnosis of RBD does not require dream enactment [4], since about 30 % of reported RBD cases in the world literature do not have dream enactment (usually in patients with neurodegenerative disorders, including dementia), as reviewed [29]. The PSG hallmark of RBD consists of electromyographic (EMG) abnormalities during REM sleep, referred to as "loss of REM-atonia," or "RWA," featuring increased muscle tone and/or increased phasic muscle twitching [4]. Figures 45.2, 45.3, 45.4a, b depict examples of PSG findings in RBD.

RBD represents how one of the defining features of mammalian REM sleep, viz. generalized skeletal muscle atonia—"REM-atonia"—can be partially or completely eliminated, resulting in a major clinical disorder. RBD is the only parasomnia in the ICSD-2 [4] and ICSD-3 that requires PSG confirmation. There are three reasons for this requirement: first, the core EMG abnormalities of RBD are present every night (given a sufficient amount of REM sleep); second, RBD is not the only dream-enacting disorder in adults, and so objective confirmation is highly desirable; third, given the strong probability of future parkinsonism in males ≥ 50 years of age initially diagnosed with idiopathic RBD, it is imperative to diagnose RBD objectively so that affected males (and their families) can be properly informed and be encouraged to plan for the future accordingly.

Some patients almost exclusively have arm and hand behaviors during REM sleep, indicating the need for both upper and lower extremity EMG monitoring in fully evaluating for RBD. Some patients preserve most of their REM-atonia, but have excessive EMG twitching during REM sleep. Autonomic nervous system activation (viz. tachycardia) is uncommon during REM sleep motor activation in RBD, in contrast to the disorders of arousal. Periodic limb movements (PLMs) during NREM and REM sleep are very common with RBD, and may disturb the sleep of the bed partner. These PLMs are rarely associated with electroencephalogram (EEG) signs of arousal. Increased percentages of slow-wave sleep and increased delta power in RBD have been found in controlled and uncontrolled studies, but this can be a highly variable

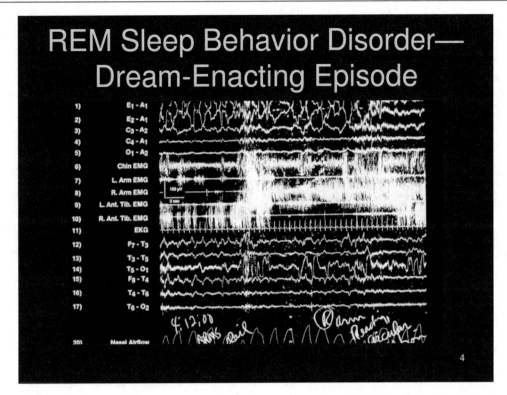

Fig 45.2 Dream-enacting episode during REM sleep in a 62-year-old man with RBD. As the sleep technologist noted the episode on the PSG tracing, the man was dreaming that he was on a boat on Lake Superior, by Duluth, Minnesota. The boat was rocking violently in the water, and he was on the main deck urgently reaching for the handrail with his right hand in circular motions to grab hold of the handrail and stabilize himself—and avoid being thrown down into the hold of the ship where menacing skeletons were beckoning at him. When he woke up, he instantly became alert and oriented, and relayed the dream to the technol-ogist, who acknowledged that the observed behavior closely matched the dream sequence, an example of "isomorphism." There is complete obliteration of "REM-atonia" in this tracing, with continuous increase of chin muscle tone, and tremendous phasic EMG activation of the chin and both upper and lower extremities. Despite the intense, generalized phasic motor activation and concomitant behavioral release, the EKG rate remains constant, without acceleration, which is typical of RBD and in sharp contrast to the disorders of arousal from slow-wave sleep.

Fig 45.3 Same-patient and same-night PSG as in Fig. 45.2. This tracing during REM sleep shows REMs in the top two channels, nearly complete loss of REM-atonia, with brief restoration of normal REM-atonia in the chin EMG towards the end of the tracing. The upper extremities show robust phasic EMG twitching, in sharp contrast to the virtual lack of phasic EMG activity in the lower extremities, thus calling attention to the recommended EMG montage in evaluating for RBD that should include bilateral upper extremity EMG monitoring, besides lower extremity and chin EMG monitoring

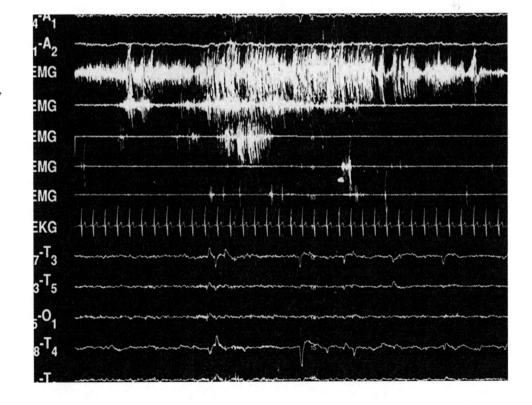

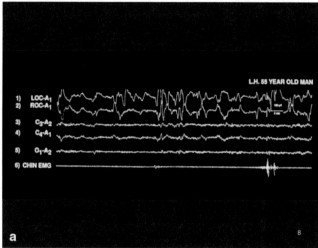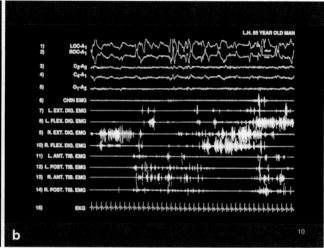

Fig 45.4 a PSG tracing of RBD, with REMs, an activated EEG, and continuously preserved REM-atonia, with normal, brief phasic twitching of the chin EMG **b** Expanded montage. Note the excessive phasic EMG twitching of opposing flexor and extensor muscles in both the upper and lower extremities, in the context of preserved REM-atonia shown by the chin EMG. This exemplifies the need for an expanded EMG montage in the evaluation of RBD. Also, the phasic coactivation of opposing muscle groups, viz. right flexor and right extensor digito-

rum muscles (robust in this tracing), is a common finding during REM sleep in RBD, which ordinarily is not present in wakefulness, since it would be completely dysfunctional (usually there is reciprocal inhibition of an opposing muscle group when one muscle group is activated for a functional purpose). This tracing exemplifies a subtype of motor dyscontrol in RBD in which there is excessive extremity phasic EMG twitching with preserved background atonia shown in the chin EMG

finding in RBD, depending on the clinical population. Sleep architecture and the customary cycling among REM and NREM sleep stages are usually preserved in RBD, although some patients show a shift toward N1 sleep (particularly in neurodegenerative disorders).

There has been an advance over time from the qualitative determination of RWA to a more rigorous, quantitative determination of RWA, to assist with the diagnosis of RBD. The most current evidence-based objective data provide the following guidelines for detecting RWA and guidelines for their interpretation supporting the diagnosis of RBD:

1. RWA is supported by the PSG findings of either: (i) tonic chin EMG activity in ≥30 % of REM sleep; or (ii) phasic chin EMG activity in ≥15 % REM sleep, scored in 20 s epochs [30].
2. Any (tonic/phasic) chin EMG activity combined with bilateral phasic activity of the flexor digitorum superficialis muscles in ≥27 % of REM sleep, scored in 30 s epochs [31].
3. Automated quantification methods have been developed for generating the "REM sleep atonia index" with scores ranging from 0 (complete loss of REM-atonia) to 1 (complete preservation of REM-atonia); cut-score for RSWA is atonia index <0.9 [32].

As demonstrated by RBD, REM-atonia serves an important protective function, as it allows the dreaming human or other mammal to engage in a full spectrum of physically active dreams while being simultaneously paralyzed and thus unable to actually move while having active dreams. A person

with RBD moves with eyes closed and with complete unawareness of the actual surroundings—a highly vulnerable state for the dreamer [5, 15, 16]. The clinical manifestation of RBD is usually (but not necessarily) dream-enacting behavior. Injury to oneself or bed partner is common in RBD. Typically, at the end of an episode, the individual awakens quickly, becomes rapidly alert, and reports a dream with a coherent story, with the dream action corresponding to the observed sleep behaviors. This phenomenon is called "isomorphism" with examples provided in the previous section. After awakenings from RBD episodes, behavior and social interactions are appropriate, mitigating against either an NREM sleep phenomenon, delirious state, or an ictal phenomenon.

Sleep and dream-related behaviors reported by history and documented during video PSG include both violent and (less commonly) nonviolent and even pleasant behaviors [6, 33]: talking, smiling, laughing, singing, whistling, shouting, swearing profanities, crying, chewing, gesturing, reaching, grabbing, arm flailing, clapping, slapping, punching, kicking, sitting up, looking around, leaping from bed, crawling, running, dancing, and searching for a treasure or other objects. Walking, however, is quite uncommon with RBD, and leaving the room is especially rare, and probably accidental. Rarely there can be smoking a fictive cigarette; masturbation-like behavior; pelvic thrusting; and mimics of eating, drinking, urinating, and defecating. Since the person is attending to the dream action with eyes closed, and not attending to the actual environment with eyes open, this is a major reason for the high rate of injury in RBD, besides the aggressive and violent behaviors.

Sleep talking with RBD runs the spectrum from short and garbled to long-winded and clearly articulated speech. Angry speech with shouting and profanity, and also humorous speech with laughter, can emerge.

One recent study found that of 14 RBD patients with repeated laughing during REM sleep documented by video-PSG, 9 were clinically depressed during the daytime, indicating a state-dependent dissociation between waking versus REM sleep emotional expression in RBD [34].

As RBD occurs during REM sleep, it usually appears at least 90 min after sleep onset, unless there is a coexisting narcolepsy, in that case RBD can emerge shortly after sleep onset during a sleep-onset REM period (SOREMP). Although irregular jerking of the limbs may occur nightly (comprising the "minimal RBD syndrome"), the major behavioral episodes appear intermittently with a frequency minimum of usually once every 1–2 weeks up to a maximum of four times nightly on ten consecutive nights [5, 6].

Chronic RBD may be preceded by a lengthy prodrome (in one series it was 25 %) consisting of prominent limb and body movements during sleep and new-onset sleep talking [35]. RBD is usually a chronic progressive disorder, with increasing complexity, intensity, and frequency of expressed behaviors. Spontaneous remissions are very rare. RBD, however, may subside considerably during the later stages of an underlying neurodegenerative disorder. Although the prevalence of RBD is not known, surveys have estimated a prevalence of 0.38–0.5 % [4]. The prevalence of RBD in older adults is probably considerably higher [36].

Most patients with RBD who present for clinical evaluation complain of sleep injury and rarely of sleep disruption. Daytime tiredness or sleepiness is uncommon, unless narcolepsy is also present, or there is coexisting obstructive sleep apnea (OSA). There is typically no history of irritable, aggressive, or violent behavior during the day. One study of consecutive referrals to a sleep center found that the majority of patients diagnosed with RBD reported symptoms on specific questioning only, underlining the importance of eliciting a comprehensive history for the diagnosis of RBD [37].

Documented injuries to the patient and bed partner resulting from RBD include: bruises; subdural hematomas; lacerations (including arteries, nerves, tendons); fractures (including high cervical fractures); dislocations, sprains, abrasions, rug burns; tooth chipping; scalp injury from hair pulling. The published cases of RBD (as of 2010 [38]), associated with potentially lethal behaviors include: choking/headlock ($n=22$–24), diving from bed ($n=10$), defenestration ($n=7$), and punching a pregnant bed partner ($n=2$). The potential for injury to self or bed partner raises important and challenging clinical issues (such as in ICU settings [39, 40]) and forensic medicine issues [16], including "parasom-nia pseudo-suicide" [41] and inadvertent murder; guidelines have been developed to assist experts in forensic parasomnia cases [16, 42].

There has only been one reported case of marital separation or divorce related to RBD, in a recently married young adult with narcolepsy-RBD [43], this probably reflects the many decades of marriage prior to the onset of typical RBD, and so the wives of men with RBD understand that the violent dream-enacting behaviors are completely discordant from the usual pleasant-waking personality [5]. Nevertheless, RBD can pose serious risks to a marriage. A recently married, young adult Taiwanese woman with RBD attempted suicide because her husband would not sleep with her at night, since he complained that her RBD disrupted his sleep excessively and compromised his work productivity [44]. Fortunately, once her RBD was diagnosed and effectively treated with clonazepam, the husband resumed sleeping in their conjugal bed, and their marriage was preserved.

Finally, there is an acute form of RBD that emerges during intense REM sleep rebound states, such as during withdrawal from alcohol and sedative–hypnotic agents, with certain medication use, drug intoxication, or relapsing multiple sclerosis [45].

RBD and Dreaming

In typical RBD affecting middle-aged and older men, the enacted dreams are often vivid and action-filled with unpleasant ("nightmarish") scenarios involving confrontation, aggression, and violence with unfamiliar people and animals, and the dreamer is rarely the instigator. In fact, the dreamer is often defending his wife in a dream while actually beating her in bed. There can also be culture-specific sports dreams, such as American football, Irish rugby, or Canadian ice hockey. Some patients experience recurrent dreams (with enactment) with presumed vestibular activation, involving spinning objects or angular motion with acceleration (e.g., a car speeding down a steep hill); other patients experience atonia suddenly intruding into their dream-enacting episodes, and fall down while dreaming of suddenly becoming stuck in mud or trapped in deep snow.

The abnormal dreams of RBD typically emerge in tandem with the release of dream-enacting behaviors, and over time, they can progress and intensify in tandem, and ultimately both of these basic components of RBD usually resolve in tandem with clonazepam therapy [6]. This link suggests a mutual pathophysiology of behavioral and dream dyscontrol in RBD (with "isomorphism" in dream-enactment, as described in the first section). There is a focus on brainstem motor pattern generators, as extracted from Hobson and McCarley's "activation-synthesis model" of dream generation [46]. Also, temporary or sustained relapse of abnormal dreaming and RBD behaviors often emerge in tandem (such as when a patient forgets to bring clonazepam on a trip), which also suggests a mutual pathophysiology.

A controlled study found that untreated men with RBD had more aggressive (and less sexual) dreams than controls, but did not have any increased tendency for aggressiveness in their waking lives [47]. A more recent study has challenged the universality of this finding in RBD [48], but most patients in a latter study were being treated with clonazepam, a highly effective therapy of both the disordered behaviors and disturbed dreaming in RBD, thus raising serious questions about the validity of the study [49, 50].

Atypical dream-enacting behaviors in RBD have been reported in a group of patients from three countries [51]: (i) retaliation dreams, related to prior verbal/physical abuse (USA); (ii) culture-specific dreams, involving Samurai warrior combat (Japan); (iii) religion-specific dreams (Taiwan). These cases encourage further search for atypical dream enactment in RBD, including across cultures.

Predisposing and Precipitating Factors

The major predisposing factors are male gender, age 50 years or older, and an underlying neurological disorder, particularly parkinsonism, multiple system atrophy (MSA), dementia with Lewy bodies (DLB), narcolepsy, and stroke [6, 45]. A recent, multicenter case-control study of environmental risk factors of RBD found that smoking, head injury, pesticide exposure, and farming were significant risk factors [52, 53]. An increasingly recognized precipitating factor involves medication-induced RBD, particularly the antidepressants venlafaxine, serotonin-specific reuptake inhibitors (SSRIs), mirtazapine, tricyclic antidepressants (TCAs), monoamine oxidase inhibitors (MAOIs), but not bupropion, trazodone, or nefazadone [45]. Beta blockers (bisoprolol, atenolol), anticholinesterase inhibitors, and selegiline can also trigger RBD, along with excess use of caffeine and chocolate. Psychiatric disorders involving depression (that require antidepressant pharmacotherapy) may comprise a predisposing factor, particularly in adults under 50 years of age [54, 55]; in fact, the Lam and Wing group in Hong Kong proposed that there is a "complex relationship of RBD, depression, and antidepressant usage" and discussed this topic from a variety of emerging data-based perspectives [56–58]. Also, RBD may be associated with some cases of post-traumatic stress disorder [45].

The overwhelming male predominance in RBD begs the question of hormonal influences, as suggested in male-aggression studies in both animals and humans. However, serum sex hormone levels are normal in idiopathic RBD or in RBD associated with Parkinson's disease (PD) [59, 60].

Another possible explanation for the male predominance is sex differences in brain development and aging.

Narcolepsy-RBD

RBD can be strongly linked with narcolepsy (almost always narcolepsy-cataplexy [NC]), as another form of REM sleep motor-behavioral dyscontrol, and may also be precipitated or worsened by the pharmacologic treatment of cataplexy with TCAs, SSRIs, and venlafaxine [19, 26, 45], but not with sodium oxybate therapy. The demographics (age and sex) of RBD in narcolepsy conform to those of narcolepsy (i.e., younger adults, and nonmale predominant), indicating that RBD in these patients is yet another manifestation of state boundary dyscontrol (primarily REM sleep-wakefulness boundaries) seen in narcolepsy [26]. RBD associated with narcolepsy is now considered to be a distinct phenotype of RBD, characterized by lack of gender predominance, less complex and more elementary movements in REM sleep, less violent behavior in REM sleep, earlier age of onset, and hypocretin deficiency (that is typical of NC, and not found in RBD [26]). In children, RBD can sometimes emerge months before the appearance of classic symptoms of NC. RBD is present in over half of patients with narcolepsy, and may be a presenting symptom in narcolepsy, including childhood narcolepsy. It is intriguing to note the pathological reverse images in motor dyscontrol involved with cataplexy, with sudden atonia during wakefulness precipitated by emotional triggers, and with RBD, with increased muscle tone and behavioral release associated with emotionally charged dreams during REM sleep. Also, a case of presumed RBD arising from cataplexy and wakeful dreaming has been reported [61].

Other reported etiologic associations of RBD with neurologic disorders include ischemic or hemorrhagic cerebrovascular disease, multiple sclerosis, Guillain–Barré syndrome, brainstem neoplasms (including cerebellopontine angle tumors), Machado–Joseph disease (spinocerebellar ataxia type 3), mitochondrial encephalo-myopathy, normal pressure hydrocephalus, Tourette's syndrome, group A xeroderma, autism, oneiric dementia, etc. [45].

Association of RBD with Specific Human Leukocyte Antigen Haplotypes

RBD, like narcolepsy, is a prominent disorder of REM sleep and REM sleep motor dysregulation. Narcolepsy has a very strong association with human leukocyte antigen (HLA) class II genes, with the DQB1*0602 (DQw1 group) allele being expressed in nearly all cases. Our center performed a study of HLA class II antigen phenotyping in a group of 25 Caucasian males who had RBD but not narcolepsy: 84% (*N*=21) were DQw1 (DQB1*0506) positive (and 28% (*N*=7) were DR2-positive); DQB1*0501 (*N*=9) and DQB1*0602 (*N*=7) were the most common phenotypes [21]. The 84% DQw1 rate in RBD was significantly greater (*p*=.015) than the 56% DQw1 rate found in a local Caucasian comparison group (*N*=66), and was greater than the 39–66% DQw1 rates in 12 published Caucasian groups (*N*=40–418 per group). In contrast to the nearly 100% DQw1–DR2 linkage in narcolepsy, only 28% of RBD patients in this report were DR2-positive. The strong dissociation between DQw1 and DR2 in RBD can be contrasted with the very strong DQw1–DR2 association in narcolepsy. Narcolepsy and RBD, therefore, have strikingly convergent (DQw1) and divergent (DR2) HLA findings.

These data raise the question of whether RBD is, in part, an autoimmune disorder, analogous to NC that is presumed to be an autoimmune disorder [26]. The question of an autoimmune basis of RBD has been reinforced by the documented series of cases of RBD emerging in tandem with autoimmune limbic encephalitis, and with a shared therapeutic response to autoimmune therapy [62].

RBD in Children and Adolescents

RBD is uncommon in childhood and adolescence, and idiopathic RBD in children is especially rare, and when present, it can be an initial manifestation of NC lasting for months before the frank emergence of NC. RBD in this age group is most commonly found in association with NC or is psychotropic medication-induced (as therapy of cataplexy or depression/anxiety), related to brainstem tumor, or to a variety of rare conditions [6, 63]. Therapy with clonazepam is often effective, as with adults. There can be some atypical features, such as a predominant complaint of "scary dreams" that could delay diagnosis. Developmental considerations in juvenile RBD have been discussed [6].

Younger Versus Older Adult-Onset RBD

Classic RBD is a male-predominant disorder that usually emerges after the age of 50 and that usually signals the future emergence of parkinsonism/dementia [23]. However, any age group, from early childhood to 88 years of age, can be affected by RBD [6, 64]. RBD emerging in adults before 50 years of age is now recognized to comprise a subgroup of RBD patients with different demographics and associated features, including greater gender parity and increased rates of idiopathic cases, parasomnia overlap disorder (POD) cases, narcolepsy cases, antidepressant medication use, and possibly autoimmune diseases [65]. Also, the clinical presentation of RBD in younger adults differs from that in older adults in being less aggressive and violent on the basis of greater female representation and narcolepsy representation that manifest with more mild RBD behaviors. Otherwise, RBD associated with neurologic disorders and other symptomatic forms of RBD are as male-predominant as idiopathic RBD, with the exception of narcolepsy, as already described.

Parasomnia Overlap Disorder

POD is a variant of RBD that consists of RBD combined with a disorder of arousal (confusional arousals, sleepwalking, and sleep terrors) [4, 6, 22, 66], although it is now known to also consist of RBD combined with sleep-related eating disorder, sexsomnia, or rhythmic movement disorder [66]. Diagnostic criteria for both RBD and a disorder or disorders of arousal, or for both RBD and one of the other disorders just mentioned, must be met [4]. POD is male-predominant but less so than RBD. Most cases begin during childhood or adolescence. Virtually all age groups can be affected. It can be idiopathic or symptomatic of a broad set of disorders, including narcolepsy, multiple sclerosis, brain tumor (and therapy), rhombencephalitis (right pontine tegmentum/medullary lesion), brain trauma, congenital Mobius syndrome, Machado–Joseph disease, indeterminate neurologic disorder, nocturnal paroxysmal atrial fibrillation, various psychiatric disorders and their pharmacotherapies, and substance-abuse disorders and abstinence states, and the other conditions described in a recent update of POD [22, 66].

These cases demonstrate motor-behavioral dyscontrol extending across NREM and REM sleep, in addition to the usual findings in RBD of increased PLMs and nonperiodic limb movements during NREM sleep. These cases also suggest a possible unifying hypothesis for disorders of arousal and RBD: the primary underlying feature is motor disinhibition during sleep—when it predominately occurs during NREM sleep, it manifests as a disorder of arousal; and when it predominately occurs during REM sleep, it manifests as RBD—with the POD occupying an intermediate or mixed position, with features of both. Furthermore, developmental considerations may play a crucial role with a postulated evolution in POD, with the NREM parasomnia component predominating during earlier life stage, with a shift toward RBD predominance during middle and later life stages. In the original reported series of 33 patients [22], the mean age of parasomnia onset was 15 years (range: 1–66); and 70% (*N*=23) were males. An idiopathic subgroup (*N*=22) had a significantly earlier mean age of parasomnia onset (9 years; range: 1–28) than a symptomatic subgroup (*N*=11; 27 years; range: 5–66).

Status Dissociatus

…When I have seen the hungry Ocean gain
Advantage on the Kingdom of the shore,
And the firm soil win of the watery main,
Increasing store with loss, and loss with store; When I have seen
such interchange of state, Or state itself confounded to decay….
(excerpt from a Shakespeare Sonnet)

Status dissociatus (SD) is classified as a subtype of RBD that manifests as an extreme form of state dissociation without identifiable sleep stages, but with sleep- and dream-related behaviors that closely resemble RBD [4, 17]. SD represents a major breakdown of the PSG markers for REM sleep, NREM sleep, and wakefulness, with admixtures of these states being present, but with conventional sleep stages not being identifiable during PSG monitoring. There is abnormal behavioral release that can be associated with disturbed dreaming that closely resembles RBD. Not uncommonly, however, the individual thinks he is awake when observers presume he is asleep and attempting to act out a dream, or vice versa. An underlying neurologic or medical condition is virtually always present; reported cases can be classified as follows [66]: (i) proteopathies (synucleinopathies: PD, MSA, DLB; tauopathies: frontotemporal dementia; prion protein: fatal familial insomnia; ataxin: spinocerebellar ataxia); (ii) anoxic (cardiogenic CNS anoxia); (iii) lesional; (iv) autoimmune (Morvan's syndrome, Guillain–Barré syndrome, voltage-gated potassium channel autoimmune encephalitis), (v) infectious (brainstem involvement of HIV infection), (vi) mixed disorders/pharmacotherapy/ alcohol abuse NC and its pharmacotherapy; OSA/NC, and its pharmacotherapy; chronic severe alcohol abuse and acute withdrawal (delirium tremens); (vii) Mulvihill–Smith syndrome; (viii) Harlequin syndrome.

RBD and Neurodegenerative Disorders

As stated previously, a full range of neurologic disorders, including neurodegenerative disorders, can be etiologically linked with the onset of RBD, and most likely reflects the neuroanatomical location of the lesion that disrupts the brainstem nuclei and/or pathways subserving REM-atonia and the customary inhibition of motor-behavioral patterns during REM sleep [29, 67]. However, a selective and very strong association of RBD with the alpha-synuclein neurodegenerative disorders (PD, MSA, DLB) is now recognized. This area of clinical medicine and scientific research (both clinical and basic) is the subject of intense multidisciplinary research on a global scale, with an exponential growth of publications, and has culminated in the formation of the IRBD-SG [10]. RBD can precede, emerge concurrently with, or develop after the emergence of an alpha synucle-

inopathy [68]. The synucleinopathies comprise a set of neurodegenerative disorders that share a common pathologic lesion composed of aggregates of insoluble alpha-synuclein protein in selectively vulnerable populations of neurons and glial cells. These pathologic aggregates appear to be closely linked to the onset and progression of clinical symptoms and the degeneration of affected brain regions in neurodegenerative disorders [69].

Delayed emergence of a neurodegenerative disorder, often more than a decade after the onset of idiopathic RBD, is very common in men who are 50 years of age and older [20, 24, 25]. One recently reported series from our center found an eventual conversion rate from iRBD to parkinsonism/dementia of 81 %, with a mean interval of 14 years from the onset and range extending to 29 years [23]. These data comprise a 16-year extension of previously published data indicating a 38 % rate of eventual emergence of parkinsonism in our series of male RBD patients. Identical findings, with an 82 % conversion rate, were recently reported by the Barcelona group of Iranzo et al. [70]. Furthermore, a retrospective study found that the interval from onset of iRBD to parkinsonism can extend up to 50 years [71]. Conversely, RBD is present in >90 % of the reported cases of MSA, and in approximately 50 % of the reported cases of PD and DLB, as reviewed [29, 69, 72, 73].

Combined animal and human studies have identified physiological and anatomical links between RBD and neurodegenerative disorders, leading to the proposal that neurodegeneration can begin in either the rostroventral midbrain or the ventral mesopontine junction and progressively extend to the rostral or caudal part of the brainstem, as reviewed [68, 74]. When the lesion starts in the ventral mesopontine region, RBD will develop first, but when the lesion initially involves the rostroventral midbrain, PD will be the initial manifestation. Also, midbrain degeneration may produce RBD and PD simultaneously, with support of this scenario coming from the lack of PLMs in NREM sleep in rats with lesions to the subceruleus region [75]. Perhaps mild damage produces RBD, and severe damage produces PD.

The link between PD and RBD is supported by the fact that impaired olfactory and color discrimination is common to both [76]. Also, the presence of cognitive deficits and slowing in the waking EEG in idiopathic RBD share common features with DLB disease [77]. Interestingly, there is a striking male predominance in patients with PD who display REM sleep behavior disorder [29, 69], although somewhat less than the male predominance found in idiopathic RBD. Additionally, two studies found that PD patients with RBD mostly had the nontremor subtype of PD [78, 79]. Also, RBD precedes PD only if PD starts after age 50 years [78].

Neuroimaging studies indicate dopaminergic abnormalities in RBD that are less severe forms of the same abnormalities found in PD. Single-photon emission computerized tomography (SPECT) and positron emission tomography (PET) studies have found reduced striatal dopamine transporters, and decreased striatal dopaminergic innervations [80–83]. PET and SPECT studies have revealed decreased nigrostriatal dopaminergic projections in patients with MSA and RBD, as reviewed [69]. Impaired cortical activation as determined by EEG spectral analysis in patients with idiopathic RBD supports the relationship between RBD and neurodegenerative disorders [76, 84]. An increasing number of brain-based tests across many dimensions in iRBD patients have consistently revealed abnormal findings in RBD that are commonly seen in PD. Therefore, the brains of iRBD patients closely resemble the brains of PD patients despite the absence of clinical PD signs and symptoms. In this regard, it is notable and not surprising that the only two brain postmortem cases published to date on iRBD found extensive Lewy body pathology in the brainstem [85, 86]. In fact, iRBD is now being called "cryptogenic RBD" [87] because of the seeming inevitability of the eventual emergence of parkinsonism or dementia in middle-aged and older adults. iRBD is also considered to be the first manifestation of Lewy body disease (LBD), and there are compelling reasons to support this position [68].

Another important set of findings indicates that the presence of RBD in PD confers increased morbidity across virtually all dimensions tested, compared to PD without RBD, including higher Hoehn and Yahr stages, more falls, more fluctuations, more visual hallucinations, greater cognitive decline, greater psychiatric morbidity, and greater life burden [69, 72]. On the other hand, movements and speech in patients with RBD-PD and with RBD-MSA improve substantially during REM sleep compared to wakefulness, as carefully documented in two studies [88, 89]. There was restoration of normal motor control in REM sleep, in sharp contrast to the compromised movements and speech in wakefulness from these extrapyramidal disorders. In REM sleep, the movements became faster, smoother, stronger, with normalized facial expressions, and speech became louder and better articulated. The rate of these improvements was higher in PD than in MSA. Clearly, during REM sleep in PD and MSA, the extrapyramidal system is bypassed, thus facilitating the normalization of movements and speech. This is a striking example of how within a distinctly abnormal motor-behavioral state, i.e., RBD (produced by the abnormal wakeful motor state of PD or MSA), there can be substantial normalization of motor-behavioral functions in movements, facial expression, and speech.

A large, multicenter postmortem brain autopsy study of RBD has recently been published [90]. Of the 172 cases, 83% were men, with mean ± SD age of RBD onset of 62 ± 14 years (range 20–93). RBD preceded the onset of cognitive impairment, parkinsonism and/or autonomic dysfunction in 51% of patients by 10 ± 12 (range 1–61) years. The predominant neuropathologic diagnoses were LBD ($n=77$), combined LBD and Alzheimer's Disease ($n=59$), and MSA ($n=19$). Among the neurodegenerative disorders associated with RBD ($n=170$), 160 (94%) were synucleinopathies. The RBD-synucleinopathy association was particularly high when RBD preceded the onset of other neurodegenerative syndrome features. The pathophysiology of RBD in neurodegenerative diseases has been examined comprehensively [91].

Differential Diagnosis

RBD is one of several disorders that can manifest as complex, injurious, and violent sleep-related and dream-related behaviors in adults, and it is one of various disorders that can disrupt the sleep of children [6, 15, 45]. Table 45.3 lists the main differential diagnoses. In general, RBD involves attempted enactment of altered dreams, and rapid awakening from an episode that usually occurs 2 h or more after sleep onset. In contrast, sleepwalking and sleep terror episodes often emerge within 2 hours after sleep onset, are not usually associated with rapid alertness, and are rarely associated with dreaming in children. Adults can have associated dreaming, but it is usually more fragmentary and limited than RBD dreams. "OSA pseudo-RBD" presents with severe OSA/hypopnea-induced arousals with dream enactment, together with loud snoring and daytime sleepiness, and responds to continuous positive airway pressure (CPAP) therapy [92]. Sleep-related seizures usually present with repetitive, stereotypical behaviors, with or without associated dreaming. Sleep-related dissociative disorders can present with dreaming during the abnormal nocturnal behaviors, but the "dreaming" represents dissociated memories of past abuse occurring during wakefulness. Malingering should always be considered in the differential diagnosis of RBD and other parasomnias [93].

Table 45.3 Differential diagnosis of dream-enacting behaviors in adults

1	REM sleep behavior disorder
2	Sleepwalking and sleep terrors
3	Obstructive Sleep Apnea ("OSA Pseudo-RBD")
4	Nocturnal seizures
5	Sleep-related dissociative disorders
6	Malingering

Treatment of RBD

Maximizing the safety of the sleeping environment is imperative. Clonazepam is the established primary pharmacotherapy of RBD in most cases, with a typical dose of 0.25–2.0 mg at bedtime, and is usually well tolerated [35, 94–96]. A number of large case series totaling >250 RBD patients have reported a response rate to clonazepam therapy of 87–90% [6]. Clonazepam is not usually associated with dosage tolerance (habituation effect), despite years of nightly therapy [43, 95], as shown in Table 45.4. The mechanism of action appears to be suppression of the excessive phasic motor-behavioral activity rather than restoration of REM-atonia [94, 97].

A recent PSG study of RBD found no objective effects of clonazepam on REM sleep parameters, and an analysis of NREM sleep parameters found beneficial effects from clonazepam in these RBD patients [98, 99]. To date, there have been no double blind, controlled, randomized trials of clonazepam (or other) therapy of RBD. The therapies of RBD have been reviewed [100–102]. The American Academy of Sleep Medicine has recently published best practice guidelines for the treatment of RBD [103].

A recognized [103], co-first-line therapy of RBD is bedtime melatonin at robust pharmacologic doses ranging from 3 to 15 mg. The mechanism of action appears to be partial restoration of REM-atonia [102].

Tertiary pharmacotherapies of RBD include pramipexole, acetylcholinesterase inhibitors (which can also trigger RBD), desipramine/ imipramine (TCAs that can also trigger or aggravate RBD), paroxetine (in Japanese patients), monoamine oxidase inhibitors, clonidine, carbamazepine, gabapentin, zopiclone, temazepam, and sodium oxybate. The finding that paroxetine, an SSRI that can trigger or aggravate RBD in Caucasians, was effective in controlling RBD in Japanese patients [60, 61, 104] raises questions about racially mediated, divergent pharmacologic responses in RBD. Also, the herbal preparation *Yi-Gan San*, approved for treating insomnia in Japan, was reported to be effective in RBD in three cases from Japan [105]. Immunosuppressive therapy induced complete resolution of RBD in tandem with remission of autoimmune limbic encephalitis in three patients with potassium channel antibody-associated limbic encephalitis [62].

Table 45.4 Long-term nightly clonazepam therapy of RBD without dosage tolerance [90]

Paired *t*-test (N-49)	
1	Initial nightly dose: 0.63 ± 0.40 mg
2	Latest follow-up dose: 0.97 ± 0.89 mg
3	Paired *t*-test: no significant difference
4	Duration of treatment: 3.7 ± 2.3 years

The International RBD Study Group

The IRBD-SG was formed in 2007 and legally incorporated in Marburg, Germany, in 2009. It is comprised of an international team of leading basic science and clinical RBD researchers from 13 countries representing Europe, North America, and Asia [10]. The IRBD-SG has held eight symposia by September 2014 in Germany, Canada, Japan, France, and Spain and Finland. Objectives of the IRBD-SG are the promotion of international scientific research in the field of RBD and related fields (such as PD), and the optimization of medical care for patients by improving diagnostic and therapeutic measures. Given the relatively low number of patients with RBD identified at individual RBD research centers, a major focus of the IRBD-SG is to facilitate multicenter studies. One multicenter study identified familial RBD [106]. Also, there is an urgent need to test promising neuroprotective agents in controlled studies of high-risk groups of patients for imminent parkinsonism/dementia (i.e., within 5 years). such groups have been identified, consisting of iRBD patients with either decreased striatal dopamine transporter uptake and substantia nigra hyperechogenicity [82], or iRBD patients with olfaction and color vision impairment [107]. An overarching aim of the IRBD-SG is to enhance professional and public awareness of the field of RBD and associated fields, and to foster cooperation among physicians, scientists, and patients along with their family members.

Conclusions

RBD is an "experiment of Nature" that reveals a spectrum of brain mechanisms of motor dyscontrol and other disturbed functions in REM and NREM sleep, and its relation to neurologic disorders, antidepressant medications, and many other areas of neuroscience and clinical (sleep) medicine. RBD also provides a compelling example of the important and pervasive phenomenon of state dissociation [17, 108–111].

Finally, RBD was depicted in Disney animated films long before the formal identification of RBD in humans in 1986 [112]. In *Cinderella* (1950), a dog had nightmares with dream enactment, and three additional dogs with presumed RBD appeared in *Lady and the Tramp* (1955), *The Fox and the Hound* (1981), and in the short film *Pluto's Judgment Day* (1935). These dogs were elderly males who would pant, whine, snuffle, howl, laugh, paddle, kick, and propel themselves while dreaming that they were chasing someone or running away. Moreover, in *Lady and the Tramp*, the dog was also losing his sense of smell and his memory, two prominent associated features of human RBD, and very frequent findings in PD. The Disney screenwriters were clearly astute observers of sleep and its disorders, including RBD. To quote Walt Disney, "Sometimes we can recognize our-

Fig 45.5 Mark W. Mahowald, M.D., director of the Minnesota Regional Sleep Disorders Center, Hennepin County Medical Center, Minneapolis, Minnesota, USA, from 1986 to 2010

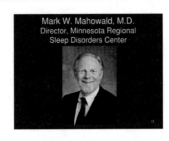

selves in animals. That's what makes them so interesting." Disney's words also conveyed scientific prescience.

Acknowledgment Special gratitude goes to my longstanding collaborator, Mark W. Mahowald, M.D. (Fig. 45.5), founding codirector (1978) and director of the Minnesota Regional Sleep Disorders Center from 1986 to 2010, who considered RBD to be a prime example of a dissociated state of sleep that represented important common ground for cross-fertilization among basic researchers and sleep clinicians.

References

1. de Cervantes M. Don Quijote de La Mancha. 1995 edition. Barcelona: Editorial Juventud;1605. p. 364. (author's translation).
2. Schenck CH, Bundlie SR, Ettinger MG, Mahowald MW. Chronic behavioral disorders of human REM sleep: a new category of parasomnia. Sleep. 1986;9:293–308.
3. Schenck CH, Bundlie SR, Patterson AL, Mahowald MW. Rapid eye movement sleep behavior disorder. A treatable parasomnia affecting older adults. JAMA. 1987;257:1786–9.
4. American Academy of Sleep Medicine. International classification of sleep disorders: diagnostic and coding manual. 2nd ed. Westchester: American Academy of Sleep Medicine; 2005.
5. Schenck CH. Paradox lost. Midnight in the battleground of sleep and dreams. Minneapolis: Extreme-Nights, LLC; 2005.
6. Schenck CH, Mahowald MW. REM sleep behavior disorder: clinical, developmental, and neuroscience perspectives 16 years after its formal identification Sleep. 2002;25:120–38.
7. Shimizu T, Inami Y, Sugita Y, et al. REM sleep without muscle atonia (stage 1-REM) and its relation to delirious behavior during sleep in patients with degenerative diseases involving the brainstem. Jpn J Psychiatry Neurol. 1990;44:681–92.
8. Guilleminault C, Raynal D, Takahashi S, Carskadon M, Dement W. Evaluation of short-term and long-term treatment of the narcolepsy syndrome with clomipramine hydrochloride. Acta Neurol Scand. 1976;54:71–87.
9. Jouvet M, Delorme F. Locus coeruleus et sommeil paradoxal. CR Soc Biol. 1965;159:895–9.
10. Schenck CH, Montplaisir JY, Frauscher B, et al. REM sleep behavior disorder (RBD): devising controlled active treatment studies for symptomatic and neuroprotective therapy—a consensus statement by the International RBD Study Group. Sleep Med. 2013. ;14:795–806.
11. Brooks PL, Peever JH. Impaired GABA and glycine transmission triggers cardinal features of rapid eye movement sleep behavior disorder in mice. J Neurosci. 2011;31:7111–21. (Erratum in: J Neurosci 2011; 31: 9440).
12. Ramaligam V, Chen MC, Saper CB, Lu J. Perspectives on the rapid eye movement sleep switch in rapid eye movement sleep behavior disorder. Sleep Med. 2013;14:707–13.
13. Luppi P-H, Fort P, Clement O, Valencia Garcia S, et al. New aspects in the pathophysiology of rapid eye movement sleep behavior disorder: the potential role of glutamate, gama-aminobutyric acid, and glycine. Sleep Med. 2013;14:714–8.
14. Hsieh KC, Nguyen D, Siegel JM, Lai YY. Lai YY, Nguyen D, Siegel JM. New pathways and data on rapid eye movement sleep behavior disorder in a rat model. Sleep Med.2013;14:719–28.
15. Schenck CH, Milner DM, Hurwitz TD, Bundlie SR, Mahowald MW. A polysomnographic and clinical report on sleep-related injury in 100 adult patients. Am J Psychiatry. 1989;146:1166–73.
16. Mahowald MW, Bundlie SR, Hurwitz TD, Schenck CH. Sleep violence–forensic science implications: polygraphic and video documentation. J Forensic Sci. 1990;35:413–32.
17. Mahowald MW, Schenck CH. Status dissociatus—a perspective on states of being. Sleep. 1991;14:69–79.
18. Schenck CH, Mahowald MW, Kim SW, O'Connor KA, Hurwitz TD. Prominent eye movements during NREM sleep and REM sleep behavior disorder associated with fluoxetine treatment of depression and obsessive-compulsive disorder. Sleep. 1992;15:226–35.
19. Schenck CH, Mahowald MW. Motor dyscontrol in narcolepsy: rapid-eye-movement (REM) sleep without atonia and REM sleep behavior disorder. Ann Neurol. 1992;32:3–10.
20. Schenck CH, Bundlie SR, Mahowald MW. Delayed emergence of a parkinsonian disorder in 38 % of 29 older men initially diagnosed with idiopathic rapid eye movement sleep behaviour disorder. Neurology. 1996;46:388–93.
21. Schenck CH, Garcia-Rill E, Segall M, Noreen H, Mahowald MW. HLA class II genes associated with REM sleep behavior disorder. Ann Neurol. 1996;39:261–3.
22. Schenck CH, Mahowald MW. A parasomnia overlap disorder involving sleepwalking, sleep terrors and REM sleep behavior disorder: report in 33 polysomnographically confirmed cases. Sleep. 1997;20:972–81.
23. Schenck CH, Boeve BF, Mahowald MW. Delayed emergence of Parkinsonism or dementia in 81 % of older males originally diagnosed with idiopathic rapid eye movement sleep behavior disorder: 16 year update on a previously reported series. Sleep Med. 2013;14:744–48.
24. Iranzo A, Molinuevo JL, Santamaria J, Serradell M, Marti MJ, Valldeoriola F, et al. Rapid-eye-movement sleep behaviour disorder as an early marker for a neurodegenerative disorder: a descriptive study. Lancet Neurol. 2006;5:572–7.
25. Postuma RB, Gagnon JF, Vendette M, Fantini ML, Massicotte-Marquez J, Montplaisir J. Quantifying the risk of neurodegenerative disease in idiopathic REM sleep behavior disorder. Neurology. 2009;72:1296–300.
26. Dauvilliers Y, Jennum P, Plazzi G. rapid eye movement sleep behaviour and rapid eye movement sleep without atonia in narcolepsy. Sleep Med. 2013;14:775–81.
27. Turek FW, Dugovic C. RBD–an emerging clue to neurodegenerative disorders. Sleep. 2005;28:920–1.
28. Mahowald MW, Schenck CH. The REM sleep behavior disorder odessey (editorial). Sleep Med Rev. 2009;13:381–4.
29. Iranzo A, Santamaria J, Tolosa E. The clinical and pathophysiological relevance of REM sleep behavior disorder in neurodegenerative diseases. Sleep Med Rev. 2009;13:385–401.
30. Montplaisir J, Gagnon JF, Fantini ML, Postuma RB, Dauvilliers Y, Desautels A, et al. Polysomnographic diagnosis of idiopathic REM sleep behavior disorder. Mov Disord. 2010;25:2044–51.
31. Frauscher B, Iranzo A, Gaig C, et al. Normative EMG values during REM sleep for the diagnosis of REM sleep behavior disorder. Sleep. 2012;35:835–47.
32. Ferri R, Rundo F, Manconi M, Plazzi G, Bruni O, Oldani A, et al. Improved computation of the atonia index in normal controls and patients with REM sleep behavior disorder. Sleep Med. 2010;11:947–9.
33. Oudiette D, De Cock VC, Lavault S, Leu S, Vidailhet M, Arnulf I. Nonviolent elaborate behaviors may also occur in REM sleep behavior disorder. Neurology. 2009;72:551–7.

34. Siclari F, Wienecke M, Poryazova R, Bassetti CL, Baumann CR. Laughing as a manifestation of rapid eye movement sleep behavior disorder. Parkinsonism Relat Disord. 2011;17:382–5.

35. Schenck CH, Hurwitz TD, Mahowald MW. Symposium: normal and abnormal REM sleep regulation: REM sleep behaviour disorder: an update on a series of 96 patients and a review of the world literature. J Sleep Res. 1993;2:224–31.

36. Boot BP, Boeve BF, Roberts RO, et al. Probable rapid eye movement sleep behavior disorder increases risk for mild cognitive impairment and Parkinson disease: a population-based study. Ann Neurol. 2012;71:49–56.

37. Frauscher B, Gschliesser V, Brandauer E, Marti I, Furtner MT, Ulmer H, et al. REM sleep behavior disorder in 703 sleep-disorder patients: the importance of eliciting a comprehensive sleep history. Sleep Med. 2010;11:167–71.

38. Schenck CH, Lee SA, Bornemann MA, Mahowald MW. Potentially lethal behaviors associated with rapid eye movement sleep behavior disorder: review of the literature and forensic implications. J Forensic Sci. 2009;54:1475–84.

39. Schenck CH, Mahowald MW. Injurious sleep behavior disorders (parasomnias) affecting patients on intensive care units. Intensive Care Med. 1991;17:219–24.

40. Cochen V, Arnulf I, Demeret S, Neulat ML, Gourlet V, Drouot X, et al. Vivid dreams, hallucinations, psychosis and REM sleep in Guillain-Barré syndrome. Brain. 2005;128(Pt 11):2535–45.

41. Mahowald MW, Schenck CH, Goldner M, Bachelder V, Cramer-Bornemann M. Parasomnia pseudo-suicide. J Forensic Sci. 2003;48:1158–62.

42. Mahowald MW, Schenck CH. Parasomnias: sleepwalking and the law. Sleep Med Rev. 2000;4:321–39.

43. Ingravallo F, Schenck CH, Plazzi G. Injurious sleep behaviour disorder in narcolepsy with cataplexy contributing to criminal proceedings and divorce. Sleep Med. 2010;11:950–2.

44. Yeh S-B, Schenck CH. A case of marital discord and secondary depression with attempted suicide resulting from REM sleep behavior disorder in a 35-year-old woman. Sleep Med. 2004;5:151–4.

45. Mahowald MW, Schenck CH. REM sleep parasomnias. In: Kryger MH, Roth T, Dement WC, editors. Principles and practice of sleep medicine, 5th ed. Philadelphia: Elsevier Saunders; 2010. pp. 1083–97.

46. Hobson JA, McCarley RW. The brain as a dream state generator: an activation-synthesis hypothesis of the dream process. Amer J Psychiatry. 1977;134:1335–48.

47. Fantini ML, Corona A, Clerici S, Ferini-Strambi L. Aggressive dream content without daytime aggressiveness in REM sleep behavior disorder. Neurology. 2005;65:1010–5.

48. D'Agostino A, Manni R, Limosani I, Terzaghi M, Cavallotti S, Scarone S. Challenging the myth of REM sleep behavior disorder: no evidence of heightened aggressiveness in dreams. Sleep Med. 2012;13:714–9.

49. Fantini ML, Ferini Strambi L. Dream content in RBD: effect of clonazepam. Sleep Med. 2012;13:1110.

50. D'Agostino A, Manni R, Limosani I, Terzaghi M, Cavallotti S, Scarone S. Response to "dream content in RBD: effect of clonazepam". Sleep Med. 2012;13:1110–1.

51. Schenck CH, Mahowald MW, Tachibana N, Tsai C-S. Atypical dream-enacting behaviors in REM sleep behavior disorder (RBD), involving abuse-retaliation dreams, culture-specific dreams, and religion-specific dreams. Sleep. 2008;31(Suppl.):A263–A4.

52. Postuma RB, Montplaisir JY, Wolfson C, Pelletier A, Dauvilliers Y, Oertel W, et al. Environmental risk factors for REM sleep behavior disorder-a multicenter case-control study. Neurology. 2012;79:428–34.

53. Sullivan SS, Schenck CH, Guilleminault C. Hiding in plain sight: risk factors for REM sleep behavior disorder. Neurology. 2012;79:402–3.

54. Schenck CH, Hurwitz TD, Mahowald MW. REM sleep behavior disorder. Am J Psychiatry. 1988;145:652.

55. Lam S-P, Li SX, Chan JWY, et al. Does rapid eye movement sleep behavior disorder exist in psychiatric populations? A clinical and polysomnographic case-control study. Sleep Med. 2013;14:788–94.

56. Lam SP, Li SX, Mok V, Wing YK. Young-onset REM sleep behavior disorder: beyond the antidepressant effect. Sleep Med. 2012;13:211.

57. Lam SP, Fong SYY, Ho CKW, Yu MWM, Wing YK. Parasomnia among psychiatric outpatients: a clinical, epidemiologic, cross-sectional study. J Clin Psychiatry. 2008;69:1374–82.

58. Lam SP, Zhang J, Tsoh J, Li SX, Ho CK, Mok V, et al. REM sleep behavior disorder in psychiatric populations. J Clin Psychiatry. 2010;71:1101–3.

59. Iranzo A, Santamaria J, Vilaseca I, de Osaba MJ. Absence of alterations in serum sex hormone levels in idiopathic REM sleep behavior disorder. Sleep. 2007;30:803–6.

60. Chou KL, Moro-De-Casillas ML, Amick MM, Borek LL, Friedman JH. Testosterone not associated with violent dreams or REM sleep behavior disorder in men with Parkinson's. Mov Disord. 2007;22:411–4.

61. Attarian HP, Schenck CH, Mahowald MW. Presumed REM sleep behavior disorder arising from cataplexy and wakeful dreaming. Sleep Med. 2000;1:131–3.

62. Iranzo A, Graus F, Clover L, Morera J, Bruna J, Vilar C, et al. Rapid eye movement sleep behavior disorder and potassium channel antibody-associated limbic encephalitis. Ann Neurol. 2005;59:178–82.

63. Lloyd R, Tippmann-Peikert M, Slocumb N, Kotagal S. Characteristics of REM sleep behavior disorder in childhood. J Clin Sleep Med. 2012;8:127–31.

64. Yeh SB, Yeh PY, Schenck CH. Rivastigmine-induced REM sleep behavior disorder (RBD) in a 88-year-old man with Alzheimer's disease. J Clin Sleep Med. 2010;6:192–5.

65. Ju Y-E. rapid eye movement sleep behavior disorder in adults younger than 50 years of age. Sleep Med 2013;14:768–74.

66. Schenck CH, Howell MJ. Spectrum of rapid eye movement sleep behavior disorder (overlap between rapid eye movement sleep behavior disorder and other parasomnias). Sleep Biol Rhythms. 2013;11(suppl. 1):27–34.

67. Iranzo A, Aparicio J. A lesson from anatomy: focal brain lesions causing REM sleep behavior disorder. Sleep Med.2009;109–12.

68. Schenck CH, Boeve BF. The strong presence of REM sleep behavior disorder in PD: clinical and research implications (editorial). Neurology. 2011;77:1030–2.

69. Boeve BF. REM sleep behavior disorder: updated review of the core features, the REM sleep behavior disorder-neurodegenerative disease association, evolving concepts, controversies, and future directions. Ann N Y Acad Sci. 2010;1184:15–54.

70. Iranzo A, Tolosa E, Gelpi E, et al. Neurodegenerative disease status and post-mortem pathology in idiopathic rapid eye movement sleep sleep behavior disorder: an observational cohort study. Lancet Neurol. 2013; 12:443–53.

71. Claassen DO, Josephs KA, Ahlskog JE, Silber MH, Tippmann-Peikert M, Boeve BF. REM sleep behavior disorder preceding other aspects of synucleinopathies by up to half a century. Neurology. 2010;75:494–9.

72. Sixel-Döring FTE, Mollenhauer B, Trenkwalder C. Associated factors for REM sleep behavior disorder in Parkinson disease. Neurology. 2011;77:1048–54.

73. Postuma RB, Gagnon JF, Montplaisir JY. REM sleep behavior disorder: from dreams to neurodegeneration. Neurobiol Dis. 2012;46:553–8.

74. Lai YY, Siegel JM. Physiological and anatomical link between Parkinson-like disease and REM sleep behavior disorder. Mol Neurobiol. 2003;27:137–52.

75. Lu J, Sherman D, Devor M, Saper CB. A putative flip-flop switch for control of REM sleep. Nature. 2006;441:589–94.

76. Postuma RB, Gagnon JF, Vendette M, Montplaisir JY. Markers of neurodegeneration in idiopathic rapid eye movement sleep behaviour disorder and Parkinson's disease. Brain. 2009;132(Pt 12):3298–307.

77. Gagnon JF, Postuma RB, Mazza S, Doyon J, Montplaisir J. Rapid-eye-movement sleep behaviour disorder and neurodegenerative diseases. Lancet Neurol. 2006;5:424–32.

78. Kumru H, Santamaria J, Tolosa E, Iranzo A. Relation between subtype of Parkinson's disease and REM sleep behavior disorder. Sleep Med. 2007;8:779–83.

79. Postuma RB, Gagnon JF, Vendette M, Charland K, Montplaisir J. REM sleep behaviour disorder in Parkinson's disease is associated with specific motor features. JNNP. 2008;79:1117–21.

80. Eisensehr I, Linke R, Noachtar S, Schwarz J, Gildehaus FJ, Tatsch K. Reduced striatal dopamine transporters in idiopathic rapid eye movement sleep behaviour disorder. Comparison with Parkinson's disease and controls. Brain. 2000;123:1155–60.

81. Eisensehr I, Linke R, Tatsch K, Kharraz B, Gildehaus FJ, Wetter CT, et al. Increased muscle activity during rapid eye movement sleep correlates with decrease of striatal presynaptic dopamine transporters. IPT and IBZM SPECT imaging in subclinical and clinically manifest idiopathic REM sleep behavior disorder, Parkinson's disease, and controls. Sleep. 2003;26:507–12.

82. Iranzo A, Lomena F, Stockner H, Valldeoriola F, Vilaseca I, Salamero M, et al. Decreased striatal dopamine transporter uptake and substantia nigra hyperechogenicity as risk markers of synucleinopathy in patients with idiopathic rapid-eye-movement sleep behaviour disorder: a prospective study (corrected). Lancet Neurol. 2010;9:1070–7.

83. Albin RL, Koeppe RA, Chervin RD, Consens FB, Wernette K, Frey KA, et al. Decreased striatal dopaminergic innervation in REM sleep behavior disorder. Neurology. 2000;55:1410–2.

84.. Fantini ML, Gagnon J-F, Petit D, Rompre S, Decary A, Carrier J, et al. Slowing of electroencephalogram in rapid eye movement sleep behavior disorder. Ann Neurol. 2003;53:774–80.

85. Uchiyama M, Isse K, Tanaka K, Yokota N, Hamamoto M, Aida S, et al. Incidental Lewy body disease in a patient with REM sleep behavior disorder. Neurology. 1995;45:709–12.

86. Boeve BF, Dickson DW, Olson EJ, Shepard JW, Silber MH, Ferman TJ, et al. Insights into REM sleep behavior disorder pathophysiology in brainstem-predominant Lewy body disease. Sleep Med. 2007;8:60–4.

87. Ferini-Strambi L, DeGioia MR, Castronovo VE, Oldani A, Zucconi M, Cappa S. Neuropsychological assessment in idiopathic REM sleep behavior disorder (RBD). Does the idiopathic form of RBD really exist? Neurology. 2004;62:41–5.

88. De Cock VC, Vidailhet M, Leu S, Texeira A, Apartis E, Elbaz A, et al. Restoration of normal motor control in Parkinson's disease during REM sleep. Brain. 2007;130:450–6.

89. Cochen De Cock VC, Debs R, Oudiette D, et al. The improvement of movement and speech during rapid eye movement sleep behaviour disorder in multiple system atrophy. Brain. 2011;134(Pt 3):856–62.

90. Boeve BF, Silber MH, Ferman TJ, et al. Clinicopathologic correlations in 172 cases of rapid eye movement sleep behavior disorder with or without a coexisting neurologic disorder. Sleep Med. 2013;14:754–62.

91. Boeve BF, Silber MH, Saper CB, Ferman TJ, Dickson DW, Parisi JE, et al. Pathophysiology of REM sleep behaviour disorder and relevance to neurodegenerative disease. Brain. 2007;130:2770–88.

92. Iranzo A, Santamaria J. Severe obstructive sleep apnea/hypopnea mimicking REM sleep behavior disorder. Sleep. 2005;28:203–6.

93. Mahowald MW, Schenck CH, Rosen GR, Hurwitz TD. The role of a sleep disorders center in evaluating sleep violence. Arch Neurol. 1992;49:604–7.

94. Schenck CH, Mahowald MW. Polysomnographic, neurologic, psychiatric, and clinical outcome report on 70 consecutive cases with REM sleep behavior disorder (RBD): sustained clonazepam efficacy in 89.5 % of 57 treated patients. Cleve Clin J Med. 1990;57 (Suppl):S9–23.

95. Schenck CH, Mahowald MW. Long-term, nightly benzodiazepine treatment of injurious parasomnias and other disorders of disrupted nocturnal sleep in 170 adults. Am J Med. 1996;100:333–7.

96. Olson EJ, Boeve BF, Silber MH. Rapid eye movement sleep behaviour disorder: demographic, clinical and laboratory findings in 93 cases. Brain. 2000;123:331–9.

97. Lapierre O, Montplaisir J. Polysomnographic features of REM sleep behavior disorder: development of a scoring method. Neurology. 1992;42:1371–4.

98. Ferri R, Marelli S, Ferini-Strambi L, Oldani A, Colli F, Schenck CH, et al. An observational clinical and video-polysomnographic study of the effects of clonazepam in REM sleep behavior disorder. Sleep Med. 2013;14:24–9.

99. Ferri R, Marelli S, Ferini-Strambi L, Plazzi G, Schenck CH, Zucconi M. Effects long-term use of clonazepam on NREM sleep patterns in rapid eye movement sleep behavior disorder. Sleep Med. 2013;14:399–406.

100. Gagnon JF, Postuma RB, Montplaisir J. Update on the pharmacology of REM sleep behavior disorder. Neurology. 2006;67:742–7.

101. Gugger JJ, Wagner ML. Rapid eye movement sleep behavior disorder. Ann Pharmacother. 2007;41:1833–41.

102. Schenck CH, Mahowald MW. REM sleep parasomnias in adults: REM sleep behavior disorder (RBD), isolated sleep paralysis and nightmare disorder. In: Barkoukis TJ, Matheson JK, Ferber RF, Doghramji K, editor. Therapy in sleep medicine. Philadelphia: Elsevier; 2011. pp. 549–558.

103. Aurora RN, Zak RS, Maganti RK, Auerbach SH, Casey KR, Chowdhuri S, et al. Best practice guide for the treatment of REM sleep behavior disorder (RBD). J Clin Sleep Med. 2010;6:85–95.

104. Yamamoto K, Uchimura N, Habukawa M, Takeuchi N, Oshima H, Oshima N, et al. Evaluation of the effects of paroxetine in the treatment of REM sleep behavior disorder. Sleep Biol Rhythms. 2006;4:190–2.

105. Shinno H, Kamei M, Nakamura Y, Inami Y, Horiguchi J. Successful treatment with Yi-Gan San for rapid eye movement sleep behavior disorder. Prog Neuropsychopharmacol Biol Psychiatry. 2008;32:1749–51.

106. Dauvilliers Y, Postuma RB, Ferini Strambi L, et al. Familial history of idiopathic REM behavior disorder: a multicenter case-control study. Neurology. 2013;80:2233–5.

107. Postuma RB, Gagnon JF, Vendette M, Desjardins C, Montplaisir J. Olfaction and color vision identify impending neurodegeneration in idiopathic REM sleep behavior disorder. Ann Neurol. 2011;69:811–8.

108. Mahowald MW, Schenck CH. Dissociated states of wakefulness and sleep. Neurology. 1992;42:44–52.

109. Mahowald MW, Schenck CH. Evolving concepts of human state dissociation. Archives Italiennes de Biologie. 2001;139:269–300.

110. Mahowald MW, Cramer BMA, Schenck CH. State dissociation, human behavior, and consciousness. Curr Top Med Chem. 2011;11:2392–402.

111. Mahowald MW, Schenck CH. Insights from studying human sleep disorders. Nature. 2005;437:1279–85.

112. Iranzo A, Schenck CH, Fonte J. REM sleep behavior disorder and other sleep disturbances in Disney animated films. Sleep Med. 2007;8:531–6.

Chronobiology and Sleep

Juergen Zulley and Scott S. Campbell

Introduction

The interrelationship between night sleep and daytime activity has been recognized for decades. Yet, this complex interaction between sleep and waking was, for many years, largely ignored in the fields of sleep research and sleep disorders medicine. As a result, the vast majority of sleep research experiment and sleep disorders diagnosis was based purely on night-time sleep recording.

Despite this neglect of a fundamental aspect of sleep behaviour and physiology by sleep scientists, an independent research area, known as chronobiology, had long focussed on this relationship, though almost exclusively in non-human species, and with a general disregard for the internal structure of sleep. To view sleeping and waking as part of a fundamental biological rhythm which controls almost all living organisms is a primary focus of chronobiology, the scientific study of rhythmic biological and behavioural processes over time. This research discipline examines if and how various functions exhibit rhythmic patterns and how they interact with each other. It also examines how external factors influence these periodic processes and, as a major task, what is the origin of the rhythms. Do they depend wholly on extrinsic factors, or do organisms have "internal clocks" governing such rhythms? Clearly, the alternation of day and night—light and darkness—is one of the most potent rhythmic patterns which shows a close relationship to human sleeping and waking, an obvious hint about the significance of chronobiology for sleep research. Yet, surprisingly, early chronobiology developed in the absence of sleep research.

The Roots of Chronobiology

As early as 1793, the physicist Georg Christoph Lichtenberg from Goettingen proposed the existence of an "internal clock" that regulates numerous human functions. He stated that "so-called 'people of the clock' normally live to be old", and concluded that there must be such a thing as an internal clock: "Behaving by the clock is however dictated by an intrinsic clock-following predisposition". A few years later, the Tuebingen physician Johann Heinrich Ferdinand Autenrieth concluded in his manual of empirical human physiology: "Even in a constitution of good health, and oft-times with more intensity despite diminished vitality, the whole body does therefore seem to undergo lively oscillation, independent of circulation". Similarly, in 1811, the neurophysiologist Karl-Friedrich Burdach discussed in his book *Dietetics for the Healthy* links between the time of day and bodily functions. He describes "slow and strong heartbeat and breathing" in the early hours of the day when "powers of judgement and reason predominate over other powers". Furthermore, he observed "almost fever-pitch pulse rates in the evenings, dedicated to convivial pleasures and the jovial games of fantasy". He concluded that "people are different, depending on the time of day...". These European scientists were among the first to postulate the existence of "internal clocks", though it would take well over a century for this hypothesis to be verified [1].

At about the same time that these scientists were speculating about the existence of an internal biological clock, others focused on what they viewed as evidence for temporal aspects in clinical practice. In 1800, Claude Bernard described in his Sorbonne dissertation that within the human organism the systematic oscillation of various functions helped to sustain balance. In Stockholm, Johanson demonstrated that the effectiveness of quinine varied according to the time of day

J. Zulley (✉)
Andreasstr. 2, 93059 Regensburg, Germany
e-mail: juergen@zulley.de

J. Zulley
Department of Psychology, University of Regensburg, Regensburg, Germany
e-mail: juergen@zulley.de

S. S. Campbell
64 Cabin Ridge Road, 10514 Chappaqua, NY, USA

S. Chokroverty, M. Billiard (eds.), *Sleep Medicine,* DOI 10.1007/978-1-4939-2089-1_46,
© Springer Science+Business Media, LLC 2015

it was taken. Herrmann von Helmholtz wrote in 1848 about the rhythmic development of various bodily functions, and Arthur Jores discovered that liver activity adheres to a daily rhythm. Also around 1850, the idea of bodily rhythms first appeared in textbooks. The physician Johannes Mueller suggested that the functions of the entire human organism were rhythmical [1].

Despite these early observations and speculations, the true beginning of human chronobiology as a research area might be said to coincide with a conference held in Ronneby in South Sweden in 1937. Among the participants was Franz Halberg who is credited with coining the term "circadian". At that meeting, the "International Society for Biological Rhythms" was established, with Erik Forsgren named as the first chairman. In 1917, at the University of Stockholm, Forsgren had described the rhythmic pattern of liver function. He found that the liver cannot produce glycogen and bile simultaneously, and that it was mainly the time of day that controls the production of the different substances. Until that time, it was assumed that the activity of the liver was triggered by the time of food intake. The majority of attendees at the 1937 conference were focused mainly on pathological functioning and in 1947 the internist Ludwig R Grote used the term "chronopathology" to describe specifically the rhythmical aspects of certain human disorders. As a consequence, rhythm researchers could develop practical hints for everyday medical practice with a special focus on the concept that the human body functions are in a rhythmic way related to time of day [1].

Pioneers in Chronobiology

During the rhythm research of the clinical experts, the question regarding the origin of the periodic fluctuations had taken a back seat; such a question was addressed in the 1950s when physiologists began the search of the internal clock in humans. The only exception, back in 1920, was Nathaniel Kleitman (1895–1999) from Chicago, who was not only a chronobiologist but also a sleep researcher and who wrote the fundamental book *Sleep and Wakefulness* [2]. Besides Nathaniel Kleitman, the pioneers of chronobiology in the USA were Franz Halberg from Minnesota and Colin Pittendrigh from California. The scientific basis of chronobiology in Europe was addressed by notable scientists such as Jürgen Aschoff (1913–1998) in Andechs, near Munich, and Gunther Hildebrandt (1924–1999) in Marburg.

In Search of the Internal Clock in Humans— Isolation Studies

There is little question that Jürgen Aschoff had the greatest early impact on the search for empirical evidence of the "internal clock" in humans. Together with the physicist Rütger

Wever (1923–2010) he established in 1963 an underground isolation facility to examine the endogenous origins of biological rhythms, in the absence of any external time cues [3, 4]. Prior to this, several isolation studies were conducted in Munich, where Aschoff himself was a subject in order to establish the feasibility of such studies. The first paper was published in 1962 on the spontaneous periodicity of humans in the absence of time cues [5]. Shortly afterwards, isolation experiments were conducted in England and France, though under very different conditions such as being isolated in a natural cave [6]. Outside of Europe, the first isolation studies were conducted in 1976, in New York, by Elliot Weitzman and co-workers [7].

At the facility of the Max-Planck Institute for Behavioural Physiology in Andechs, Germany—which became known informally as "the bunker"—human subjects lived singly, in complete isolation from external time cues, for periods averaging about 4 weeks. The subjects had no information about the time of day and could go to sleep whenever they wanted to. They had to prepare their own meals, had no social contacts, and were instructed to turn the lights off when they decided to sleep. In addition, further experiments had been carried out, in which the degree of monotony as well as light condition had been varied [8]. Besides a variety of physiological and psychological variables, the state of activity and rectal temperature were recorded continuously. In 1974, the first polysomnographic recordings under such experimental condition were performed by Zulley [9]. Overall, between 1964 and the end of the Andechs studies in 1989 about 450 volunteers "went underground" [10].

In these experiments, the rest–activity cycle was totally self-selected by the subjects and in the vast majority of the experiments this remained remarkably regular. Since the resulting rhythm of rest and activity as well as the physiological and psychological functions had no external influences, such rhythms were referred to as "free-running" or "autonomous" rhythms. The mean periodicity of all experiments was longer than 24 h, on the average of about 25 h. Such periodicities were described as circadian (from the Latin *circa*: about; *dies*: day) rhythms. Since such a periodicity is not known in the natural world, it was assumed that these circadian rhythms were governed by an "internal clock" [4]. This conclusion is still valid although later studies have shown that the free-running rhythm of most humans is very close to 24 h [11].

Following the discovery that humans exhibit behavioural and physiological rhythms consistent with the existence of an internal clock, researchers began to investigate possible external factors that might influence the internal clock. Because we live in a 24-h day, and because our internal clocks run at a slightly different periodicity, the internal clock must be synchronized, or entrained, to the natural day. The question facing researchers, then, was which regularly occurring external stimuli, time cues, or "Zeitgebers" (the term was incorporated into English unchanged) were relevant for the endogenous rhythms and had the capacity to synchronize those rhythms. Since the daily light/dark cycle seemed to be a logical candidate, experiments with artificial alternation of darkness and light were conducted. In addition, regular signals or timing of meal times were examined as a zeitgeber.

The first experiments showed that the simple alternation of darkness with normal indoor lighting (about 400 lx) is not sufficient to entrain the normal daily rhythm in humans, in contrast to animals. Later studies found that higher light intensity, with more than 2000 lx, was an effective zeitgeber in humans [12]. In addition to light/dark cycles, researchers demonstrated that other cues such as the regular timing of meals, as well as scheduled motor activity and social contacts were also effective zeitgebers, though significantly less effective than light/dark cycles.

Yet, there were limits to which zeitgebers could synchronize circadian rhythms. External time cues could reach values beyond which the rest–activity cycle and/or physiological rhythms (e.g. body core temperature) could not be synchronized. These time cues were said to be out of the "range of entrainment". Such a state did lead to a disturbance of the circadian system referred to as desynchronization. Desynchronization could be elicited either by an induced sleep–wake cycle ("forced desynchronization") or, very rarely, desynchronization in which the rest/activity cycle and the rhythm of body core temperature ran at different periodicities, was observed to occur spontaneously ("spontaneous internal desynchronization"). Such a state could occur in the temporal isolation experiments whereby spontaneous rest–activity cycles showed periods between 17 and 50 h, while the rhythm of body temperature remained between 23 and 27 h. Such observations led to the notion that separate internal oscillators were governing the periodicities of these functions. Wever [4] was the most outspoken proponent of this notion and developed a mathematical model describing the hypothesis. The empirical evidence and assumptions underlying the two-oscillator model was later brought into question [13].

Ultradian Rhythms

In addition to circadian cycles, with one oscillation occurring each day, shorter periodicities have also been observed consisting of more than one maximum and minimum during the day. These oscillations are referred to as ultradian rhythms. Such rhythms have been found in numerous vigilance and neurobehavioural performance parameters, as well as, in a majority of physiological and psychological functions. In contrast, human sleep/wake patterns were long thought to be strictly circadian in nature: Typically, we sleep for about 8 h at night and maintain 16 h of wakefulness during the day. If the human sleep system is, indeed, monophasic in nature, it

would stand out as the sole exception to the rule of ultradian sleep patterns in every other animal studied. Yet, in the earlier studies on circadian rhythms, subjects were instructed not to nap but instead to have one major sleep episode per day. Later experiments in which subjects were permitted to sleep whenever they desired showed most of the time a strong tendency to have one or more short sleep episode(s) between their long major sleep phases [13, 14]. Such short sleep episodes correspond to the "siesta" in many cultures around the world. The need for this additional sleep episode is obviously less robust than during the night. This holds true, as well, for the ultradian course of the other variables like vigilance or body temperature. Such a second preferred phase for sleep may become relevant in situations where the normal course of sleeping and waking is disrupted or the need for sleep is intensified (e.g. shift work or jetlag).

In conditions, where the need or opportunity for sleep is even higher, more preferred phase positions for sleep become obvious. In the so-called bed-rest studies [8], a study design which has been called by others "constant-routine protocol", the occurrence of sleep was more frequent with regular sleep periods at approximately 4-h intervals. Overall, in the studies in time-free environments, it could be shown that with an increase in sleep propensity a monophasic (circadian) sleep pattern could switch into a biphasic (ultradian) pattern with two sleep episodes during a day and with further increase into a polyphasic sleep pattern with one major and three shorter sleep episodes. Again, within such an ultradian pattern the circadian influence remains more robust, as shown in the "chronochaos" and disentrainment experiments [10, 11].

Sleep Research Within Chronobiological Settings

Traditionally, chronobiologists used the term rest–activity instead of sleep–wakefulness, because sleep had not been measured electrographically. In 1974, the first polysomnographic recordings in an isolation study were undertaken by Zulley [9]. This may be considered as the beginning of the integration of human chronobiology and sleep research. At about the same time, Czeisler and co-workers in the USA were performing similar sleep studies in time-free environments and both studies came to the same conclusion: There is an interdependence between sleep architecture and the circadian system [7, 15, 16].

Prior to these studies, polysomnography had been performed in major sleep episodes either at night, at different, specified times of day [17, 18] or at different phase positions in the circadian temperature cycle [19, 20]. In contrast, isolation studies permitted sleep structure of the major sleep episodes to be measured during free-running circadian cycles, independent from time of day. In addition, the increased variability of the timing of sleep episodes in the state of desynchronization allowed much more detailed analyses of the relationship between circadian phase and sleep timing and structure. Specifically, they allowed differentiating between time of day, length of day, and circadian influences. With regard to the timing of sleep, it was found that spontaneous sleep onset, sleep duration and, hence the spontaneous termination of sleep, are all under strong control by the internal clock [16]. Furthermore, certain aspects of sleep stage structure were found to be strongly influenced by the circadian system [15]. For example, the duration of rapid eye movement (REM) sleep periods showed a pronounced circadian rhythmicity. Thus, the normally short REM sleep episodes observed in the beginning of a normal night's sleep are strictly a result of the fact that we typically go to bed at a particular circadian phase which is normally in synchrony with the 24-h day. If a sleep episode is initiated at, say, 11 a.m. instead of 11 p.m., the distribution of REM period duration is entirely different.

Sleep Models and Further Research

With regard to basic research within sleep and chronobiology, the findings regarding circadian aspects of the timing of sleep and the sleep stage structure led to new insight into the theoretical aspects of concepts of sleep regulation and the internal clock. In 1980, a new movement started, initiated by the presentation of the new results regarding chronobiological aspects of sleep. Specifically, Alex Borbely from Zürich [21] and Serge Daan from Groningen [22] presented a two-process model to predict the timing of sleep and the sleep stage structure by a single circadian oscillator (process C), and an interacting homeostatic process which represented the rising sleep pressure with duration of wakefulness (process S). This model removed earlier concepts of dual oscillators [4] and is still part of the ongoing research.

A different approach was the search for genetic factors within the framework of sleep and chronobiology. Here, it was the identification of a PER2 mutation in circadian sleep disorders which opened the field to the discovery of the role of clock genes. Studies with knockout mutant mice led to a further understanding of the role of genetic factors. In addition, the identification of further clock mutants in animals and humans opened the field for the search of the "internal clocks" and the understanding of homeostatic and circadian regulation [23, 24].

Besides the analyses of the central origin of the rhythms, additional findings with respect to external factors provided additional insight influences on the circadian system. One of the most important findings was that the human circadian rhythms are significantly impacted by the major zeitgeber which had been found for animals—light. The first attempts to entrain rhythms with light of relatively low intensity (about 200–500 lx) were not successful. However, in 1980, Lewy et al. demonstrated that exposure to a brighter light source (more than 2500 lx) resulted in the suppression of melatonin production [25]. This finding found strong interest in the field of chronobiology and Wever published a paper with the title "Bright Light Affects Human Circadian Rhythms" [12] which opened the field for research on the most effective time cue in humans. It was subsequently established that the daily timing of melatonin production is an important marker of circadian rhythms and that exogenous administration of the hormone can result in phase shift of the rhythms [26]. This has been applied in cases of circadian rhythm disorder including jetlag and shift work. Furthermore, the research on melatonin could identify the pathways through which this hormone is acting and its connection to the environmental light. A third group of photosensitive retinal ganglion cells were identified containing melanopsin, which is responsible for the suppression of melatonin and hence acts as a circadian photopigment. With this newly discovered connection of natural light input via the retina, nucleus suprachiasmaticus, and the pineal organ which regulates the secretion of melatonin, more details became obvious such as showing that blue light within the range of short wavelength light is most effective in suppressing melatonin [27].

Concluding Remarks

The union of the fields of sleep research and chronobiology has had a significant positive impact for both fields. It has provided new insight into circadian and ultradian rhythms on one hand and on sleep regulation on the other hand. New concepts could be developed to describe basic mechanisms of sleep–wake regulation and external influences. There are further opportunities to apply results from chronobiology and sleep research in our daily lives.

References

1. Menzel W. Clinical roots of biological rhythms research (Chronobiology). In: Hildebrandt G, Moog R, Raschke F, editors. Chronobiology and chronomedicine. Frankfurt: Peter Lang; 1987. pp. 277–87.
2. Kleitman N. Sleep and wakefulness. Chicago: University of Chicago Press; 1963.
3. Aschoff J. Circadian rhythms in man. Science. 1965;148:1427–32.
4. Wever R. The circadian system of man. Berlin: Springer; 1979.
5. Aschoff J, Wever R. Spontanperiodik des Menschen bei Ausschluss aller Zeitgeber. Naturwissenschaften. 1962;49:337–42.
6. Siffre M. Hors du temps. Paris: Julliard; 1963.
7. Czeisler CA, Weitzman ED, Moore-Ede MC, Zimmermann JC, Knauer RS. Human sleep: its duration and organization depend on its circadian phase. Science. 1980;210:1264–7.

8. Zulley J. Day and night sleep: the bedrest condition. In: Horne JA, editor. SLEEP '90. Bochum: Pontenagel Press; 1990. pp. 319–23.

9. Zulley J (1976) Schlaf und Temperatur unter freilaufenden Bedingungen. In: WH Tack (Ed) Ber 30. Kongr Dtsch Ges Psychol. Hogrefe, Göttingen, pp 398–399.

10. Zulley J. Schlafen und Wachen als biologischer Rhythmus. Regensburg, Roderer 1993. Available from: http://www.zulley.de/dokumente/SchlafenundWachen.pdf Accessed 15 December 2014.

11. Campbell SS, Dawson D, Zulley J. When the human circadian system is caught napping: evidence for endogenous rhythms close to 24 hours. Sleep. 1993;16:638–40.

12. Wever RA, Polasek J, Wildgruber CM. Bright light affects human circadian rhythms. Pflügers Arch. 1983;391:85–7.

13. Zulley J, Campbell S. Napping behavior during "spontaneous internal desynchronization": sleep remains in synchrony with body temperature. Human Neurobiol. 1985;4:123–6.

14. Campbell SS, Zulley J. Napping in time-free environments. In: Dinges DF, Broughton RJ, editors. Sleep and alertness: chronobiological, behavioral, and medical aspects of napping. New York: Raven Press; 1989. pp. 121–38.

15. Zulley J. Distribution of REM sleep in entrained 24 hour and free-running sleep-wake cycles. Sleep. 1980;2:377–89.

16. Zulley J, Wever R, Aschoff J. The dependence of onset and duration of sleep on the circadian rhythm of rectal temperature. Pflügers Arch. 1981;391:314–8.

17. Bryden G, Holdstock TL. Effects of night duty on sleep patterns of nurses. Psychophysiol. 1973;10:205–10.

18. Webb WB, Agnew HW, Williams RL. Effects on sleep of a sleep period time displacement. Aerospace Med. 1971;42:152–5.

19. Karacan I, Finley WW, Williams RL, Hursch CJ. Changes in stage 1-REM and stage 4 sleep during naps. Biol Psychiat. 1970;2:261–5.

20. Moses JM, Hord DJ, Lubin A, Johnson LC, Naitoh P. Dynamics of nap sleep during a 40 hour period. Electroencephal Clin Neurophysiol. 1975;39:627–33.

21. Borbely AA. A two process model of sleep regulation. Human Neurobiol. 1982;1:194–204.

22. Daan S, Beersma DG, Borbely AA. Timing of human sleep: recovery process gated by a circadian pacemaker. Am J Physiol. 1984;246:R161–R84.

23. Dudley C, Erbel-Sieler C, Estill SJ, Reick M, Franken P, Pitts S, et al. Altered patterns of sleep and behavioral adaptability in NPAS2-deficient mice. Science 2003;301:379–83.

24. Dunlap JC, Loros JJ, De Coursey PJ. Chronobiology: biological timekeeping. Sunderland: Sinauer; 2004.

25. Lewy AJ, Wehr TA, Goodwin FK, Newsome DA, Markey S. Light suppresses melatonin secretion in humans. Science 1980;210:1267–9.

26. Arendt J, Skene DJ. Melatonin as a chronobiotic. Sleep Med Rev. 2005;9:25–39.

27. Thapan K, Arendt J, Skene DJ. An action spectrum for melatonin suppression: evidence for a novel non-rod, none-cone photoreceptor system in humans. J Physiol. 2001;535:261–7.

Cardiovascular Disease and Sleep Dysfunction

Thomas Penzel and Carmen Garcia

Introduction

Investigations of sleep and sleep disorders always have been part of neurology, neurophysiology, and psychiatry. In the beginning of sleep medicine as a discipline of its own, little attention was given by medical departments to sleep-related disorders compared to neurology and psychiatry departments. Some case reports and few dedicated studies were published on effects of sleep on cardiovascular diseases [1, 2]. These studies with origin in neurophysiology/psychophysiology investigated sleep stage changes after the detection of rapid eye movement (REM) sleep. The studies looked for the specific effects of cardiovascular parameters during non-REM and REM sleep and compared these to wakefulness. Snyder looked at respiration, heart rate, and blood pressure in 12 young healthy subjects by using a new method to record blood pressure. An inflatable cuff was placed on the lower leg in order to get a high-resolution time profile. He found irregularities in all three parameters during REM sleep. As a consequence, he classified sleep into undisturbed sound sleep with a decrease in blood pressure and heart rate and into disturbed sleep with dreams and very high rises in blood pressure, and heart rate with remarkable irregularities [2]. Another early study focused on heart rate and blood pressure. Bristow investigated baroreflex sensitivity changes in addition to heart rate and blood pressure and compared normotensive and hypertensive subjects during wakefulness and sleep. He found a similar reduction of blood pressure and heart rate in both groups during sleep compared to wakefulness [1].

The attention in medical departments on sleep-related cardiovascular disorders changed substantially with the description of sleep apnea, recognition of the prevalence and clinical importance of sleep-disordered breathing, and the associated cardiovascular consequences. After a long period of ignoring the topic, sleep-related cardiovascular disorders are now about to make their way into guidelines and recommendation papers [3].

Additional insight was gained through application of new technologies for the recording of blood pressure, description of pathologies (sleep-disordered breathing), and a better understanding of physiology during sleep and different sleep stages. This resulted in a provocative statement that sleep might be regarded as an autonomic stress test for the heart [4]. Two pathways had advanced the knowledge on cardiovascular diseases and sleep dysfunctions. One was methodological development and the other was epidemiological research which was often related to sleep-disordered breathing [5]. Both pathways were complemented by studies on physiology of cardiovascular changes during sleep and studies on pathophysiology of cardiovascular diseases during sleep and sleep disorders. The pathway of methods is presented first followed by the pathway of epidemiological studies.

Methods for Cardiovascular Disease Assessment

Zemaityte et al. [6] investigated 20 healthy subjects and 75 subjects with ischemic heart disease during wakefulness and sleep. They distinguished the heart rate variability in different sleep stages and looked for overall heart rate variability including low-, middle-, and high-frequency components. Patients with heart disease had a lower heart rate variability during wakefulness and different sleep stages due to a lower high- and middle-frequency component.

Peng et al. [7] investigated Holter electrocardiogram (ECG) for 24-h recordings in ten healthy subjects and ten patients with heart failure for heart rate variability and found no difference in heart rate variability when summing up over the entire recording time. Therefore, they applied a new method which looked for beat-to-beat variability in terms

T. Penzel (✉) · C. Garcia
Interdisciplinary Sleep Medicine Center,
Charité—Universitätsmedizin Berlin,
Charitéplatz 1, 10117 Berlin, Germany
e-mail: thomas.penzel@charite.de

S. Chokroverty, M. Billiard (eds.), *Sleep Medicine,* DOI 10.1007/978-1-4939-2089-1_47,
© Springer Science+Business Media, LLC 2015

415

of short-range and long-range correlations. This technique had been developed in the field of statistical physics in order to investigate natural random processes like particle transmission trough a wall or fractal growth of ice blossoms on a window. There are different types of random behavior in nature. Using this analysis technique, it was possible to find remarkable differences between healthy persons and patients with heart failure. Patients with heart failure showed a breakdown of long-range correlations in heart rate variability. The new analysis technique was applied to sleep apnea by Ivanov et al. [8] using 18 healthy subjects and 16 sleep apnea subjects. This study showed that the beat-to-beat variability in sleep apnea was remarkably impaired; however, different sleep stages were not considered in this study. When investigating heart rate variability with this method for the effect of different sleep stages, big differences in correlation behavior were found in 15 healthy and 26 sleep apnea subjects independent of the sleep dysfunction [9]. During REM sleep, a strong long-term correlation behavior was found similar to wakefulness and in contrast to that no long-term correlations were found for light sleep and slow-wave sleep. On the basis of these results, many studies in heart rate and sleep stages were undertaken by biomedical engineers resulting in the development of many algorithms and software tools to detect sleep-disordered breathing and sleep stages from the ECG alone [10]. Besides heart rate being regulated by the autonomous nervous system activity, the ECG reflects also mechanical components of respiratory effort. ECG waveform is modulated by respiration and respiratory effort-related intrathoracic pressure does influence the amplitude of the R-wave and the T-wave. With that, it is possible to derive respiration from the ECG waveform. This derived signal is called ECG-derived respiration (EDR). The new algorithms show good results in recognizing both sleep stages and sleep-disordered breathing. They are currently prospectively evaluated for their use as a simple screening tool for upcoming epidemiological studies and for a risk assessment in populations such as professional drivers.

Blood pressure was much more difficult to investigate during sleep. The measurement of blood pressure using intermittent cuff-based methods tends to disturb sleep and in the worst case even interrupt sleep leading to useless values. As explained earlier, Bristow [1] used a cuff measurement technology during sleep with blood pressure determined every 5 min on the lower leg. With this high-resolution technique, he could demonstrate sleep-stage-dependent differences in blood pressure regulation. Recommendations today specify the measurement interval for cuff inflations during sleep to be 30 min. This is far too low to see effects related to sleep stage or sleep-related pathologies. Blood pressure changes quickly with sleep stages because blood pressure reflects changes in the autonomic nervous system tone. Due

to these rapid changes, only continuous blood pressure recording methods can adequately reflect the changes during sleep. Invasive blood pressure recording methods had been used in the beginning of this research but due to the potential complications this method had been abandoned later. Noninvasive continuous blood pressure recording techniques, such as the photo-finger-plethysmography (Finapres and Portapres), allow sleep studies with parallel recording of blood pressure. This method is able to track beat-to-beat changes in blood pressure. Thereby the method allows recording of abrupt changes as can be observed at sleep stage transitions and central nervous activations (arousals).

New technologies try to derive blood pressure from the finger pulse, more specifically from pulse transit time (PTT). The PTT, the time from the opening of the aortic valve to the time when the pulse wave is detected in the periphery (typically the finger), is measured by using ECG and finger pulse from an oximetry sensor [11]. This signal is strongly correlated with blood pressure. The shorter the time, the stiffer are the vessels and thus higher is the blood pressure. With this relationship, the signal can serve as a marker for blood pressure over considerable time periods. However, it cannot replace blood pressure due to severe limitations [12]. One of which is that only relative changes in blood pressure are recorded and the PTT signal needs to be calibrated.

Baroreceptor sensitivity as a marker for cardiovascular function is derived from calculations using both blood pressure and heart rate signals. Bristow [1] presented the first data on baroreceptor sensitivity during sleep. Many studies have shown an impaired baroreceptor sensitivity in cardiovascular diseases. This impairment was later also found in patients with sleep-disordered breathing [13] which recovered partially after treatment with continuous positive airway pressure (CPAP) [13].

Epidemiological Study Assessment

Several epidemiological studies have investigated the prevalence of sleep-disordered breathing and its cardiovascular consequences. Prevalence of sleep-related cardiovascular disorders independent from sleep-disordered breathing was not determined. Therefore, most results relate to cardiovascular disorders associated with sleep apnea. A well-known study in this field is the Sleep Heart Health Study [14]. This study estimated odds ratios for cardiovascular complications in patients with sleep apnea [15] which are presented in Table 47.1. With these data, it is evident that the risk for general mortality is increased, and atrial fibrillation and heart failure have the highest odds ratios. Results are all based on large and carefully conducted studies so that the odds ratios can be regarded as reliable.

Table 47.1 Odds ratio of cardiovascular diseases in patients with sleep-disordered breathing. (Data are taken from [15, 16].

Cardiovascular disease	Odds ratio (confidence interval 95%)
Arterial hypertension	1.37 (1.03–1.83)
Heart failure	2.38 (1.22–4.62)
Ischemic heart failure	1.27 (0.99–1.62)
Ischemic stroke	1.58 (1.02–2.46)
Atrial fibrillation	4.02 (1.03–15.5)
Pulmonary hypertension	1.4 (1.1–2.8)
General mortality	6.24 (2.01–19.4)

A large cohort study in Spain also investigated cardiovascular risk and outcome in patients with sleep-related breathing disorders. The study compared snoring, different severities of sleep apnea, and treated versus untreated patients with sleep-disordered breathing [17]. An increased mortality and an increased risk for cardiovascular incidents in patients with sleep apnea depending on severity were shown.

Patients with an apnea–hypopnea index (AHI) above 30 events per hour have an approximately twofold higher risk for fatal and nonfatal cardiovascular events as well as for developing arterial hypertension [17]. Patients with a regular use of CPAP therapy had a comparable mortality and cardiovascular outcome as in healthy subjects.

New population-based cohort studies including sleep investigations can clarify if sleep-related cardiovascular disorders and sleep-disordered breathing are linked or independent of each other. These new studies are currently ongoing. The Framingham study plans to add a sleep module. The study of health in Pomerania, a region in northern Germany with a high prevalence of arterial hypertension did add a sleep module with cardiorespiratory polysomnography for one night; 1269 out of more than 6700 randomly selected participants underwent a night in the sleep laboratory [18].

Sleep and the Autonomous Nervous System

From physiological investigations, we know that during non-REM and REM sleep autonomic controls are different [19]. During non-REM sleep, sympathetic activity decreases and is lowest during slow-wave sleep. In contrast, the vagal component is highest during slow-wave sleep with a decreased heart rate and blood pressure under normal conditions. During REM sleep, sympathetic activity is variable with intermittent high surges of activity followed by cessations. The average sympathetic activity recorded during REM sleep by neurography on the peroneal nerve is similar to that during wakefulness but higher than during non-REM sleep. Vagal activity during REM sleep is not as high as during slow-wave sleep. For vagal activity, only indirect parameters (e.g., derived from heart rate variability) are taken and no direct continuous variable was assessed so far.

Sleep-disordered breathing is accompanied by cyclical variation of heart rate (Fig. 47.1). This cyclical variation of heart rate had been described very early, shortly after the description of sleep apnea [20]. This cyclic heart rate variation is so typical, that it can be used to diagnose sleep apnea from the heart rate pattern alone [10]. Combining the results of previous studies, it is even possible to distinguish sleep stages and the severity of sleep apnea to some degree [21].

The autonomous nervous system also acts on the vascular tone during sleep. During REM sleep with a higher activity of sympathetic tone, a higher vascular tone resulting in a higher blood pressure is the consequence. If blood pressure is recorded with a sufficiently high resolution in amplitude and time, REM sleep can be identified in healthy subjects. Besides blood pressure, a couple of years ago a new technique was introduced to record vascular tone noninvasively and continuously. This is called peripheral arterial tonometry (PAT) [22]. Many studies had been conducted and the signal had proven to be a very useful marker in the recognition of sleep-disordered breathing through the autonomic responses [23]. Based on arterial tone, it is possible to detect arousals and differentiation between non-REM sleep and REM sleep [24].

Sleep and the Heart

Heart rate is regarded as a direct mirror to sympathetic activity. A decrease in heart rate during slow-wave sleep and a higher heart rate variability during REM sleep reflects up- and downregulation of sympathetic activity and corresponds to arrhythmias observed during sleep. Rhythm-related problems during sleep can be bradycardia, heart block of different types, and atrial fibrillation. Most often, arrhythmias are related to other underlying cardiac disorders and they have their specific expression during sleep as well. Some arrhythmias are related to specific sleep stages. During sleep-disordered breathing, one can observe bradycardia, other low-frequency arrhythmias, or even heart block at the end of apneic events. An impressive example of sleep-related arrhythmia of this type is depicted in Fig. 47.2. No direct or causal relationship amongst arrhythmias, sleep stages, and apneic events has been shown statistically, because these arrhythmias are rare events.

Heart failure has a high prevalence in persons above the age of 45 in Western countries [25]. Systolic and diastolic left ventricular dysfunctions are reported with prevalence between 5 and 20%. Mortality of heart failure is high. Sleep stages and altered regulation have a strong impact on heart function during the night. This is important in patients with heart failure because sleep apnea can trigger a reduction in the ejection fraction of the left ventricle.

Fig. 47.1 Holter ECG recording of a patient with sleep apnea and an extremely high variability of heart rate during the night. The ECG recording and the tape analysis were performed in spring 1982. At the time of recording, it was common to visualize 1-h distributions of RR intervals. The comparison of the two 1-h histograms shows an episode of regular sleep with low variability (22–23 h) and an episode with very high variability just 2 h later (0–1 h). *ECG* electrocardiogram

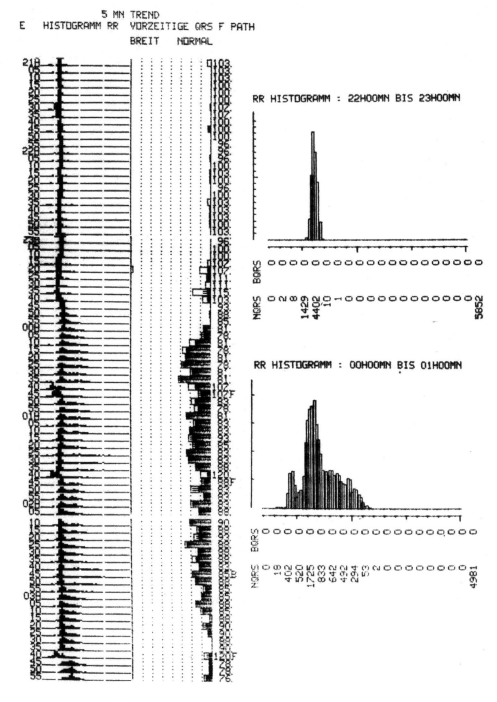

The prevalence of sleep-disordered breathing is very high in patients with heart failure [26]. Studies report between 30 and 50 % of the patients suffering from Cheyne–Stokes breathing and central sleep apnea. The Cheyne–Stokes breathing is characterized by a waxing and waning of respiratory amplitude which may assume very low amplitudes resembling just central apnea events. Another 20–40 % suffer from obstructive sleep apnea [27]. There are several potential mechanisms which link heart failure and sleep-disordered breathing. Heart failure, whether systolic or diastolic, increases the risk for central respiratory events, creating a

vicious cycle between sleep apnea and heart failure. Whether treatment of apnea with CPAP lowers mortality in these patients is not finally clarified. A large study did not show a beneficial effect regarding mortality [28]. A post hoc substudy analysis did show, however, a beneficial effect on patients in lowering central apnea in heart failure and increasing left ventricular ejection fraction [29]. Further investigation is needed to identify subpopulations who might benefit from treatment with CPAP.

Ischemic heart disease appears to be increased in patients with sleep-disordered breathing [30]. Hypoxemia during

Fig. 47.2 The ECG recording in the sleep laboratory during the 1980s shows a cardiac arrest with 15.6 s within one supraventricular beat and one ectopic beat observed. This was observed at the end of an obstructive apnea event and during REM sleep. *ECG* electrocardiogram, *REM* rapid eye movement

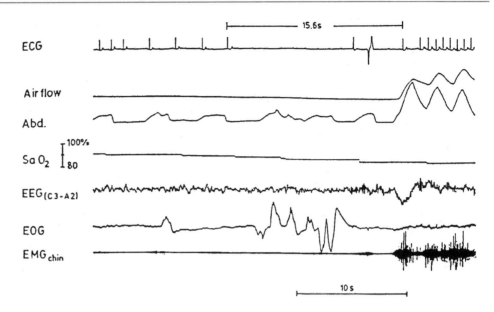

apnea events presents the pathophysiological mechanism of this complication. It is not clarified whether hypoxemia leads to a cumulative or an acute effect on the coronary vessels. It is even thought that re-oxygenation after each single apnea event might present an even more severe stress to the vessels. However, this association is not fully explored, neither by epidemiological studies nor by pathophysiological studies.

Sleep and the Vascular System

The association which has been found most consistently over a large number of studies is the association between sleep-disordered breathing and hypertension. [31–33]. In various well-designed placebo-controlled studies, the treatment of obstructive sleep apneas could show a modest but significant reduction in diurnal and nocturnal systolic and diastolic blood pressure [34, 35]. Meta-analyses on treatment studies also did show a great variety of effects on blood pressure, and therefore subgroups of sleep apnea patients who might benefit most have to be defined. Therapy-resistant arterial hypertension showed a significant reduction after treatment and this is important as more than 90 % of men and 60 % of women with a resistant hypertension have a sleep apnea syndrome [36]. In this group, CPAP seems to be more effective in lowering systolic blood pressure by 15 mmHg and diastolic blood pressure by 8 mmHg. Knowing that a reduction in systolic blood pressure by 10 mmHg lowers the risk of coronary artery disease by 22 % and risk of stroke by 41 %, physicians, cardiologists particularly should be aware of this relationship. A recognition of this led to the adoption of guidelines for the management of hypertension [3]. Besides this clear evidence, there are a number of other factors which are worth noting. Blood pressure increases during prolonged

episodes of apnea leading to dangerous situations with very high blood pressure peaks (Fig. 47.3). There seem to be cumulative effects of successive apnea and hypopnea events which can cause hypertensive crisis at the end. This may be a potential mechanism for sudden cardiac death in these patients. Another mechanism is the role of non-REM and REM sleep transitions with a sudden rise in blood pressure. This rise in blood pressure is observed in both systolic and diastolic values (Fig. 47.4). The rise of blood pressure is so clearly linked to the onset of REM sleep that this can be only explained by an immediate change of vascular resistance with the changed level of sympathetic activity. This supports the finding that PAT, which just reflects vascular tone, can be used very reliably to detect REM sleep. It would be challenging to investigate in how far this effect of activation is lost in patients with autonomic neuropathy or in patients with diabetes with blunted autonomic nervous system activity. Since we know that sleep apnea impairs autonomic responses, one might expect that this non-REM/REM transition response is impaired. But in general this does not seem to be the case. Possibly different degrees of disease progression might be distinguished by testing this change in autonomic nervous system response to sleep stage changes.

Pulmonary hypertension is reported to be found in 20 % of patients with obstructive sleep apnea syndrome. Prevalence values differ across studies due to different patient selection and different methods applied. Pulmonary hypertension is associated with obesity, poor lung function, and hypoxia in these patients. During the intrathoracic pressure changes accompanying apnea events, large swings in pulmonary pressure were observed. Consequently, a strong relationship between sleep apnea and pulmonary hypertension was assumed. This does not seem to be a simple linear relationship as far as daytime pulmonary hypertension is con-

Fig. 47.3 The recording shows a 5-min period with very high blood pressure peaks during REM sleep at the end of apnea events. The patient was a 70-year-old woman with treated hypertension, obstructive sleep apnea, and restless legs syndrome. The episodes of apnea are accompanied by excessive blood pressure peaks

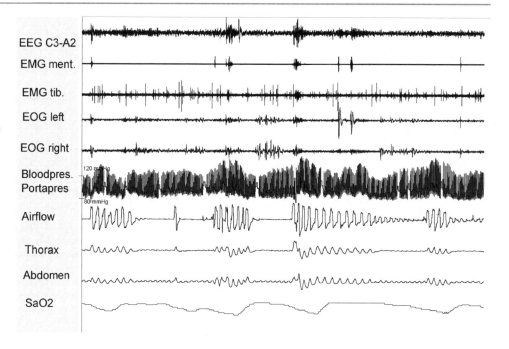

Fig. 47.4 The recording with invasive blood pressure recording during the 1990s shows high elevations of systolic blood pressure after each apnea event. The recording demonstrates also a sudden increase in diastolic and systolic blood pressure at the transition from non-REM sleep to REM sleep (see the eye blinks in the EOG trace and the lower EEG amplitude). This transition occurs in the middle of an apnea event. At the same time, the oxygen desaturation shows faster drops. One can even see how the slope changes during the time course of the apnea where REM begins. *REM* rapid eye movement, *EOG* electrooculogram, *EEG* electroencephalogram

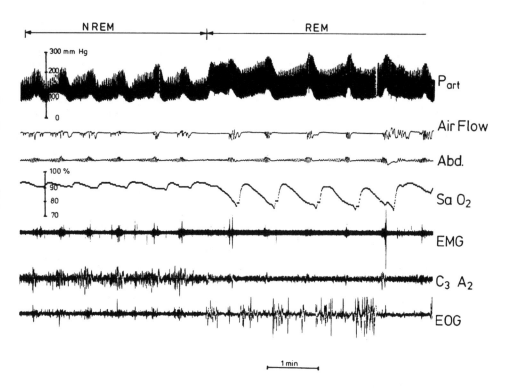

cerned. Apparently, pulmonary hypertension is not related to the severity of sleep-disordered breathing [37].

Nocturnal hypoxia, the recurrent reoxygenations at the end of apnea events causing oxidative stress and decreased antioxidant capacity may be a mechanism for arteriosclerosis [38]. Savransky and his group showed in rats that intermittent hypoxia is an independent risk factor for hypercholesterolemia [39]. The same group did show in arteriosclerosis-resistant mice that sleep apnea and high levels of

cholesterol lead to arteriosclerosis [39]. Mechanical factors of shear stress had also been discussed as potential contributing factors. Systemic or local inflammation may contribute to arteriosclerosis as well. C-reactive protein levels are elevated in persons with sleep apnea. Clinical findings suggest a direct role of sleep-disordered breathing in the development of arteriosclerosis. Patients with sleep apnea exhibit a thicker carotid wall. Experimental studies also suggest a direct relationship between sleep apnea, hypertension, and arteriosclerosis. Some studies indicate that CPAP treatment reverses some of these effects by lowering plasma levels of various adhesion molecules.

In summary, many cardiovascular consequences of sleep-disordered breathing are described. In patients with cardiovascular problems, very often, sleep-disordered breathing is also observed [40]. To what extent sleep-disordered cardiovascular problems constitute an entity without additional sleep-disordered breathing remains open; previous studies described patients with sleep-related hypertension and sleep-related arrhythmias. These patients need to be studied with well-defined inclusion and exclusion criteria. Otherwise, these subjects remain to be unusual cases only.

Acknowledgment The figures have been taken from recordings of the sleep laboratory at the University Marburg, Department for Internal Diseases. The sleep center at Marburg is acknowledged for these recordings performed in the 1980s and 1990s.

References

1. Bristow DJ, Honour AJ, Pickering TG, et al. Cardiovascular and respiratory changes during sleep in normal and hypertensive subjects. Cardiovasc Res. 1969;3:476–85.
2. Snyder F, Hobson JA, Morrison DF, et al. Changes in respiration, heart rate, ad systolic blood pressure in human sleep. J Appl Physiol. 1964;19:417–22.
3. Somers VK, White DP, Amin R, et al., American Heart Association Council for High Blood Pressure Research Professional Education Committee, Council on Clinical Cardiology; American Heart Association Stroke Council; American Heart Association Council on Cardiovascular Nursing; American College of Cardiology Foundation. Sleep apnea and cardiovascular disease: an American Heart Association/American College Of Cardiology Foundation Scientific Statement from the American Heart Association Council for High Blood Pressure Research Professional Education Committee, Council on Clinical Cardiology, Stroke Council, and Council On Cardiovascular Nursing. In collaboration with the National Heart, Lung, and Blood Institute National Center on Sleep Disorders Research (National Institutes of Health). Circulation. 2008;118:1080–111.
4. Verrier RL, Muller JE, Hobson JA. Sleep, dreams, and sudden death: the case for sleep as an autonomic stress test for the heart. Cardiovasc Res. 1996;31:181–211.
5. Young T, Peppard P. Sleep-disordered breathing and cardiovascular disease: epidemiologic evidence for a relationship. Sleep. 2000;23 (Suppl. 4): S122–6.
6. Zemaityte D, Varoneckas G, Plauska K, et al. Components of the heart rhythm power spectrum in wakefulness and individual sleep stages. Int J Psychophysiol. 1986;4:129–41.
7. Peng CK, Mietus J, Hausdorff JM, et al. Long-range anticorrelations and non-Gaussian behavior of the heart beat. Phys Rev Lett. 1993;70:1343–6.
8. Ivanov PC, Rosenblum MG, Peng CK, et al. Scaling behaviour of heartbeat intervals obtained by wavelet-based time-series analysis. Nature. 1996;383:323–7.
9. Bunde A, Havlin S, Kantelhardt JW, et al. Correlated and uncorrelated regions in heart-rate fluctuations during sleep. Phys Rev Lett. 2000;85:3736–9.

10. Penzel T, McNames J, de Chazal P, et al. Systematic comparison of different algorithms for apnoea detection based on electrocardiogram recordings. Med Biol Eng Comput. 2002;40:402–7.
11. Smith RP, Argod J, Pepin JL, et al. Pulse transit time: an appraisal of potential clinical applications. Thorax. 1999;54:452–8.
12. Payne RA, Symeonides CN, Webb DJ, et al. Pulse transit time measured from the ECG: an unreliable marker of beat-to-beat blood pressure. J Appl Physiol. 2006;100:136–41.
13. Bonsignore MR, Parati G, Insalaco G, et al. Baroreflex control of heart rate during sleep in obstructive sleep apnoea: effects of acute CPAP. Eur Resp J. 2006;27:128–35.
14. Nieto FJ, Young TB, Lind BK, et al. Association of sleep-disordered breathing, sleep apnea, and hypertension in a large community-based study. Sleep heart health study. JAMA. 2000;283:1829–36.
15. Shahar E, Whitney CW, Redline S et al. Sleep-disordered breathing and cardiovascular disease: cross-sectional results from the sleep heart health study. Am J Respir Crit Care Med. 2001;163:19–25.
16. Lavie P, Lavie L, Herer P. All-cause mortality in men with sleep apnea syndrome: declining mortality rates with age. Eur Respir J. 2005;27:1–7.
17. Marin JM, Carrizo SJ, Vicente E, et al. Long-term cardiovascular outcomes in men with obstructive sleep apnoea-hypopnoea with or without treatment with continuous positive airway pressure: an observational study. Lancet. 2005;365:1046–53.
18. Völzke H, Alte D, Schmidt CO, et al. Cohort profile: the study of health in Pomerania. Int J Epidemiol. 2011;40:294–307.
19. Somers VK, Dyken ME, Mark AL, et al. Sympathetic nervous system activity during sleep in normal subjects. N Engl J Med. 1993;328:303–7.
20. Guilleminault C, Connolly S, Winkle R, et al. Cyclical variation of the heart rate in sleep apnoea syndrome. Mechanisms, and usefulness of 24 h electrocardiography as a screening technique. Lancet. 1984;1(8369):126–31.
21. Penzel T, Kantelhardt JW, Grote L, et al. Comparison of detrended fluctuation analysis and spectral analysis for heart rate variability in sleep and sleep apnea. IEEE Trans Biomed Eng. 2003;50:1143–51.
22. Schnall R, Shlitner A, Sheffy J, et al. Periodic profound peripheral vasoconstriction: a new marker of obstructive sleep apnea. Sleep. 1999;22:939–46.
23. Penzel T, Kesper K, Pinnow I, et al. Peripheral arterial tonometry, oximetry and actigraphy for ambulatory recording of sleep apnea. Physiol Meas. 2004;25:1025–36.
24. Lavie P, Schnall RP, Sheffy J, et al. Peripheral vasoconstriction during REM sleep detected by a new plethysmographic method. Nat Med. 2000;6:606.
25. Levy D, Kenchaiah S, Larson MG, et al. Long-term trends in the incidence of and survival with heart failure. N Engl J Med. 2002;347:1397–402.
26. Naughton MT, Lorenzi-Filho G. Sleep in heart failure. Prog Cardiovasc Dis. 2009;51:339–49.
27. Sin DD, Fitzgerald F, Parker JD, et al. Risk factors for central and obstructive sleep apnea in 450 men and women with congestive heart failure. Am J Respir Crit Care Med. 1999;160:1101–6.
28. Bradley TD, Logan AG, Kimoff RJ, et al. Continuous positive airway pressure for central sleep apnea and heart failure. N Engl J Med. 2005;353:2025–33.
29. Arzt M, Floras JS, Logan AG, et al. Suppression of central sleep apnea by continuous positive airway pressure and transplant-free survival in heart failure: a post hoc analysis of the Canadian continuous positive airway pressure for patients with central sleep apnea and heart failure trial (CANPAP). Circulation. 2007;115:3173–80.

30. Lüthje L, Andreas S. Obstructive sleep apnea and coronary artery disease. Sleep Med Rev. 2008;12:19–31.
31. Grote L, Ploch T, Heitmann J, Knaack L, et al. Sleep-related breathing disorder is an independent risk factor for systemic hypertension. Am J Respir Crit Care Med. 1999;160:1875–82.
32. Marin JM, Agusti A, Villar I, et al. Association between treated and untreated obstructive sleep apnea and risk of hypertension. JAMA. 2012;307:2169–76.
33. Peppard PE, Young T, Palta M, et al. Prospective study of the association between sleep-disordered breathing and hypertension. N Engl J Med. 2000;342:1378–84.
34. Becker HF, Jerrentrup A, Ploch T, et al. Effect of nasal continuous positive airway pressure treatment on blood pressure in patients with obstructive sleep apnea. Circulation. 2003;107:68–73.
35. Montesi SB, Edwards BA, Malhotra A, et al. The effect of continuous positive airway pressure treatment on blood pressure: a systematic review and meta-analysis of randomized controlled trials. J Clin Sleep Med. 2012;8:587–96.
36. Calhoun DA. Obstructive sleep apnea and hypertension. Curr Hypertens Rep. 2010;12:189–95.
37. Selim B, Won C, Yaggi HK. Cardiovascular consequences of sleep apnea. Clin Chest Med. 2010;31:203–20.
38. Wolk R, Somers VK. Cardiovascular consequences of obstructive sleep apnea. Clin Chest Med. 2003;24:195–205.
39. Savransky V, Nanayakkara A, Li J, et al. Chronic intermittent hypoxia induces atherosclerosis. Am J Respir Crit Care Med. 2007;175:1290–7.
40. Martinez-Garcia MA, Serra PC. Is sleep apnoea a specialist condition? The role of general practitioners. Breathe. 2010;7:145–56.

Nonrestorative Sleep, Musculoskeletal Pain, Fatigue in Rheumatic Disorders, and Allied Syndromes: A Historical Perspective

48

Harvey Moldofsky

Introduction

The idea that the sleeping–waking brain is intimately related to complaints of unrefreshing sleep, musculoskeletal pain, fatigue, and suffering is not a novel notion. Its origins are found in the remote past. Over the millennia, its origins and significance have been immersed in religious beliefs in evil thoughts or sinful human behavior with special opportunities for redemption through rituals performed by healers, by sacrifice, or by prayer. Consequently, medical attempts have evaded our understanding. Even to this day, rheumatologists, who are often asked to assess and manage such afflicted patients, say that they have no relevance to their focus of interest in people with discernible objective evidence for arthritic or immunological disease pathology. Even though such patients search for understanding and help with their affliction and suffering, they may face rejection by physicians or exploitation by remedies that do not improve their sleep or cure them of their bodily complaints. This matter of despair and hopelessness is clearly and simply described in *Ecclesiastes* 2:23, "All their days their work is grief and pain; even at night their minds do not rest. This too is meaningless." Despite *Ecclesiastes*, a pessimistic perspective on the troubles of mankind, this chapter focuses on our efforts to bring scientific understanding to how the physiology of sleeping–waking brain allows us to better understand the origins and management of their widespread pain, suffering, and disability.

Such people have acquired a variety of diagnostic labels by various medical disciplines, as though a mere diagnosis provides both understanding and treatment. At the turn of the

last century, such people were given the label, "fibrositis" by an English neurologist, William Gower. He believed that the basis of his patients' painful limbs and backs were the result of inflammation of fibrous tissue. When systematic studies of infectious or disease pathology could not be verified, the term became a wastebasket diagnosis used by rheumatologists to differentiate these patients from those with similar symptoms but having objective evidence for disease pathology. Other medical specialists, to whom such afflicted people would visit, applied explanations that relate to their specialty's focus of interest. See Table 48.1 for such a list of health-care specialist providers, their areas of interest, and diagnostic labels that are provided to such patients.

The medical field becomes more complicated when such symptoms are found in patients with a known disease. Even though the disease is successfully treated by well-established disease-modifying substances, they may remain chronically ill with unrefreshing sleep, widespread pain, tenderness, chronic fatigue, and psychological distress. These features often occur in patients with systemic lupus erythematosis and rheumatoid arthritis. Without the objective evidence for arthritic, neuroendocrine, or immunological disease pathology, the community of rheumatologists abandoned the term of ill-understood "fibrositis" and adopted the now-popular descriptive diagnosis, "fibromyalgia" (FM) or "fibromyalgia syndrome" (FMS). The formalization of criteria for the diagnosis approved by the American College of Rheumatology in 1991 [1] permitted epidemiological studies to determine the prevalence of the syndrome. Subsequently, approximately 2% of the US population (3.4% women, 0.5% men) were found to be affected [2]. Those with the diffuse musculoskeletal pains and debilitating fatigue in five European countries (France, Germany, Italy, Portugal, and Spain) affected 2.9% of the population (3.6% women and 2.1% men) [3], making this rheumatic disorder the second most common rheumatic ailment after osteoarthritis.

About the same time, infectious disease experts noted that pain and fatigue symptoms prevailed long after an acute infectious disease had past. They variously diagnosed such

H. Moldofsky (✉)
Centre for Sleep and Chronobiology Research, 951 Wilson Ave, Unit 15B, M3K 2A7 Toronto, ON, Canada
e-mail: h.moldofsky@utoronto.ca

Department of Psychiatry, Faculty of Medicine, University of Toronto, Toronto, ON, Canada

Toronto Psychiatric Research Foundation, North York, Canada

patients as having a post-infectious or post-viral syndrome, myalgic encephalomyelitis (ME), and Epstein virus syndrome. Where a sporadic cluster of such mysterious ailments appeared, diagnostic labels were attributed to geographic locations, e.g., in 1934, Los Angeles County Hospital disease also known at the time as "atypical poliomyelitis"; in 1948–1949, Akureyri disease (also called Iceland disease); and in 1955, London's Royal Free (Hospital) disease, which subsequently was thought to be a form of mass hysteria. The absence of any verifiable evidence for any specific infectious agent or inflammatory disease pathology proved perplexing for infectious disease specialists. The lack of objective evidence for a specific virus or specific infectious disease led to a committee of advisory experts to the US Centre for Disease Control to formalize criteria. The current diagnosis, chronic fatigue syndrome (CFS), came into existence [4]. This vague descriptive label emerged in 1994 much to the chagrin of affected American patients who advocate for special recognition by government health agencies for their preferred term "chronic immune deficiency syndrome." In the UK, the label chronic infectious neuromyasthenia encephalitis is preferred. Often, there is an overlap among the variable clinical criteria adopted by committees of the various medical disciplines so that some authors have referred to such patients as coming under an umbrella of a cluster of overlapping ailments (see Table 48.1). The overriding common feature is the absence of any known clinical features of disease or signs of any abnormalities in any radiological, hematological, histological, chemical, metabolic, or immunological tests. Nevertheless, the hunt for a viral etiology persists with the most current being the 1990 report in *Science* on the prevalence of a retrovirus, xenotropic murine leukemia virus-related virus (XMRV) finding in more than 60 % of the patients with CFS. Two years of several scientific reports of failures to replicate the initial findings led to a formal retraction by this journal

in November 2011 [5]. A viral etiology, however, remains relevant in selected populations with post-febrile persistent chronic fatigue and diffuse myalgia. For example, following an outbreak in Toronto of severe acute respiratory syndrome (SARS), those who had survived and had no residual respiratory disease 1–3 years later had persistent diffuse myalgia, disabling fatigue, weakness with unrefreshing sleep, and anomalous increased sleep EEG alpha and the EEG sleep cyclical alternating pattern (CAP) in non-REM sleep. The possibility that the SARS coronavirus, which is known to enter the brain during the acute phase, may have a continuing adverse influence on the sleeping waking brain with associated physical and behavioral symptoms [6].

In the absence of medical disease, these people with ill-understood poor sleep quality, chronic pain, and fatigue tend to be cast into the dark chasm of vague psychiatric labels. The psychiatric diagnostic labels have changed over the course of five revisions of the American Psychiatric Association (APA) *Diagnostic and Statistical Manual of Mental Disorders* (DSM). They range from neurasthenia and hysterical conversion disorder to somatoform pain disorder, somatization disorder, and now the DSM-5 feckless diagnosis, "somatic symptom disorder" [7]. This chain of psychiatric labels represents a history of collective transient agreements by generations of US psychiatric committees that have applied some form of presumed scientific explanations to bodily complaints and sickness where there is no satisfactory medical or psychological explanation. Now, most of these earlier psychiatric diagnoses have been abandoned, in favor of an empirical, presumably less controversial, descriptive label. As seen in Table 48.1, the diagnostic labels adopted by various groups of health specialists are afflicted with similar scientific explanatory dilemmas.

In the prescientific evolution of knowledge, such people and their ailments were given various religious or spiritual

Table 48.1 Medical specialties and their diagnoses of patients with chronic widespread pain, fatigue, unrefreshing sleep, psychological distress, and no medical pathology

Health specialists	Symptom interest, no pathology	Diagnosis
Rheumatologists	Pain, mobility, fatigue	Fibromyalgia
Physiatrists	Pain, mobility, fatigue	Regional pain
Orthopedists	Pain, mobility, fatigue	Chronic pain syndrome
Chiropractors	Pain, mobility, fatigue	Faulty spinal alignment
Infectious disease allergists and environment medicine	Fatigue, pain Hypersensitivities	Myalgic encephalomyelitis, CFS Multiple chemical sensitivity, SBS
Psychiatrists/psychologists	Behavior, mood, cognition	Somatoform or mood disorder
Neurologists	Headache, fatigue, behavior	Tension headache
Gynecologists	Abdominal and pelvic pain	Chronic pelvic pain, dyspareunia
Gastroenterologists	Abdominal pain, GI disorder, fatigue	Irritable bowel syndrome
Urologists	Urinary tract pain and frequency	Interstitial cystitis/irritable bladder
Dentists	Jaw pain with movement	TMJ disorder
Cardiologists	Chest pain, fatigue	Atypical chest pain

GI gastrointestinal, *CFS* chronic fatigue syndrome, *SBS* sick building syndrome, *TMJ* temporomandibular joint

explanations. Remedies stem from particular prayers, rituals, and/or special natural remedies. In non-Western societies, the systems of beliefs, their respective special names, and remedial methods are deemed to be features of culture-bound syndromes. For example, *hwa-byung*, a Korean folk illness is characterized by insomnia, pains, fatigue, weakness, gastrointestinal symptoms, and emotional distress. Chinese patients who have sleep difficulties, headaches, various pains, fatigue, and sexual dysfunction are termed *shenjing shuairuo*. Their society's belief is that the affected people's vital essence is being lost and life threatening. In the Indian society, the term is *dhat*, where Hindus have a similar belief in the dangers to self of the loss of essential sexual fluids. In Latin-American societies, such frightened and emotionally distressed people with similar sleep and somatic symptoms are considered to be afflicted with *susto* or "soul loss." Even now in the Western society, where there is no clear medical understanding of the cause or treatment of such ill-defined symptoms, these culture-bound belief systems and methods for treating these illnesses continue to prevail in our societies. Hence, there is a large industry of purveyors of herbal substances, acupuncture, moxibustion procedures, and useless remedies of various vitamins and minerals. Where there is a lack of faith in medical explanations, there is the hope that nontraditional methods would remedy the mysterious rheumatic symptoms.

Rather than focusing on traditional rheumatic interests in joints, connective tissue, and muscles, current interest has shifted to the central nervous system as the source of hypersensitivity with application of pressure to various predesignated regions of the body and pain behavior that are readily observed by rheumatologists in examining their patients' musculoskeletal system. Based upon experimental evidence, Moldofsky proposed the hypothesis that the sleeping/waking brain is integral to the somatic and behavioral symptoms of these ill-understood painful, fatiguing, distressing, and often disabling chronic illnesses [8]. This hypothesis gives rise to the following questions:

1. How does the sleeping–waking brain connect to these poorly understood somatic and behavioral symptoms?
2. Does an understanding of the disturbances in the sleeping/waking brain favorably influence the management of these suffering patients?

This chapter reviews advances in our scientific understanding of how the sleeping–waking brain is intimately connected to the widespread musculoskeletal pain, fatigue, and psychologically distressing symptoms of previously presumed to be unexplained medical illnesses, which have led to the current advances in their management.

Review of EEG Sleep, Pain, and Fatigue

The pioneering work of Moldofsky and colleagues yielded two critically important findings with regard to the relationship of sleep to widespread musculoskeletal pain and fatigue in rheumatological patients without known medical disease:
1) EEG sleep is disturbed in more than 90 % of FM patients who report persistently poor sleep quality and impaired quality of life [9, 10].
2) Experimental sleep disturbance in healthy individuals can induce FM-like musculoskeletal pain and tenderness [11].

Manifestations of disturbed sleep typically comprise the experience of light and unrefreshing sleep, nocturnal restlessness with frequent awakenings, and at times, sleep-related loud snoring and breathing problems, or periodic involuntary leg movements. Typically, there is a variation in the diurnal pattern of symptoms. Upon awakening from their poor quality of sleep, patients usually experience generalized muscular stiffness, diffuse pain, and profound fatigue, which are unchanged or even increased compared to the previous evening. They report improvement in symptoms with improved energy from late morning to mid-afternoon; then, thereafter there is a downhill course in symptoms as the day progresses. The narrower the period of improvement, the more disabled is the patient. On the rare occasion, they might achieve a restful night of sleep and improved symptoms on the following day. Indeed, unrefreshing or nonrestorative sleep is closely correlated to the widespread pain and tender points in FM while psychological distress is not [12]. FM subjects with light unrefreshing sleep have diurnal impairment in speed of performance on complex cognitive tasks, which are accompanied by sleepiness, fatigue, and negative mood. Such psychological impairment could account for the functional disabilities that are encountered in a work environment and in social behavior. There may be an associated predisposition to emotional hypersensitivity resulting from distrust and insecure attachment in their personality, which is shown to be associated with the alpha-EEG anomaly during sleep [13].

These disabling behavioral symptoms are commonly associated with disturbances in the physiology of sleep [8, 9]. How these FM symptoms are linked to the subjective poor sleep quality and objective PSG measures continues to be of considerable interest in determining the pathophysiology of this illness. Early on, aspects of anomalous changes in EEG sleep physiology were identified in FM patients that were considered to be consistent with subjective poor quality of sleep. Nocturnal polysomnography (PSG) shows a prominent EEG alpha frequency (8–12 Hz) rhythm in the central EEG regions during stages 2 and slow-wave sleep (SWS) NREM sleep (see Fig. 48.1) but less frequently in patients with severely diminished or absent delta SWS [8]. As Hauri and Hawkins had noticed this alpha EEG anomaly to

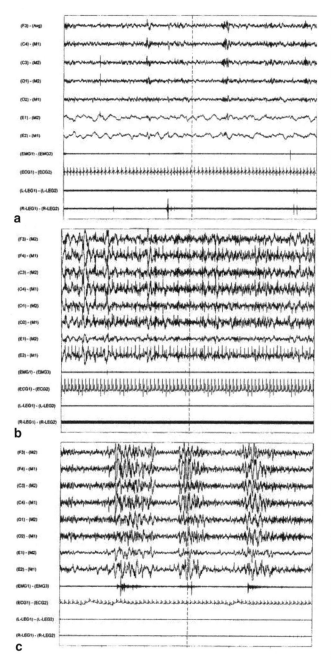

Fig. 48.1 Examples of 60-s stage 2 non-REM sleep EEG and electromyography (*EMG*) and electrocardiographic (*EKG*) recordings. **a** Normal, **b** α-EEG sleep, **c.** Cyclic alternating pattern (*CAP*) sleep EEG: subtype CAP A3 with periodic bursts of polyphasic EEG and coincident bursts of submental EMG activity. *REM* rapid eye movement, *EEG* electroencephalogram. (From [24] The Journal of Rheumatology 38:10; 2011)

coincide with the delta frequency (0–<4 Hz) slow waves of SWS, they coined the term alpha–delta sleep, which they described in a small group of not depressed psychiatric patients with poorly understood illness who complained of chronic,

somatic malaise, and fatigue [14]. Subsequently, Moldofsky and colleagues reported this anomaly in patients with so-called fibrositis [11], later considered by rheumatologists to be a wastebasket diagnosis because of the lack of replicated evidence of presumed inflammation of fibrous tissue. Subsequently, the symptoms were relabeled as FM or FMS. This anomalous alpha EEG sleep is seen predominantly in the frontal–central brain area in contrast to the alpha EEG frequency occurring in quiet wakefulness that is localized in the occipital region [15, 16]. Subsequently, reports of this anomalous increased alpha EEG activity in NREM sleep were reported in FM patients [8, 17–21]. Patients with FMS, however, are heterogeneous with respect to exhibiting the alpha anomaly [21]. This alpha activity in NREM sleep is not specific to FM, since it occurs in patients with other painful rheumatic diseases. Moreover, it is described to occur in patients with primary insomnia [22]. As EEG alpha-like rhythm is associated with mentation [16, 18], alpha occurring in NREM sleep may represent a vigilant arousal state that interferes with bodily restorative functions [8]. This abnormal EEG sleep feature may account for a common aspect of impaired sleep quality with symptoms of light sleep and sleep mentation with external environmental awareness and internal self-awareness of subjective discomfort. This sense of vigilance is shown to be associated with an underlying faulty personality characteristic in such people with the prominent alpha EEG sleep anomaly and physical illness which stems from a faulty interactional pattern of childhood personality development. In formal personality testing of such people with the alpha EEG sleep anomaly, most of whom have FMS, they show a pattern of overall distrust and insecurity in interpersonal relationships. Consequently, this pervasive sense of insecurity and distrust, which are ingrained in their personalities, is thought to make them difficult to accept any medical therapeutic effort that results in perpetuation of chronic physical illness behavior [13].

A second physiological component of impaired sleep quality is thought to be a specific EEG pattern that contributes to unstable or nonrestorative sleep, a major diagnostic feature of FMS and CFS. This objective physiological feature in the sleep EEG sleep comprises a high frequency of the CAP. The CAP phenomenon occurs variably throughout NREM sleep characterized by a frequency of approximately 20–30 cycles per second (see Fig. 48.1). The specific type of CAP is reported to reflect a measure of relative stable–unstable sleep. In patients with FMS and CFS where unstable or nonrestorative sleep is commonly reported, there is an increase of CAP activity. The sleep EEG dominant rhythm of CAP A1 and no significant ancillary increase in autonomic or peripheral EMG activity, as seen in CAP A2 and increased in CAP A3, is associated with sleep stability that is commonly found in young asymptomatic healthy people. In the subgroup CAP A2 and CAP A3, there is physiological evidence for progressive increases in sleep instability [23–25]. This high amount of CAP correlates with the severity of pain as measured by the number of tender points in FMS [23]. The EEG CAP A2 and especially CAP A3 are associated with pathological sleep characterized by physiological evidence of motor and autonomic nervous system abnormalities, e.g., periodic limb movement (PLM) and sleep apnea disorders [24, 26]. Such clinically significant periodic PSG sleep disorders are found in a large sample of US patients with FMS. In this multicenter PSG study of more than 200 FMS patients, 94% were female, with a mean body mass index of about 30 who had FMS for more than 5 years. Approximately 15% had moderate to severe apnea–hypopnea respiratory index and 20% had PLM disorder [24]. Their sedentary behavior with resultant weight gain and obesity may have promoted the sleep apnea disorder and the coincident CAP A2 and A3 EEG unstable and nonrestorative sleep.

Another feature of sleep EEG disturbance, which is reported in FMS, is a decrease in stage 2 EEG sleep spindles [27]. The presence of EEG sleep spindles, a characteristic of this stage of NREM sleep, is hypothesized to be a physiological feature of sleep stability. This hypothesis is supported by the shorter duration of stage 2 sleep periods, which is normally dominated by CAP A1. In addition, there is increased frequency of EEG sleep stage shifts [28], increased sleep awakenings, and decreased sleep efficiency (ratio of time asleep/time in bed) [23, 29].

Moreover, there is a reduction of SWS in FM patients [11, 19–21, 29]. One such study showed that decreased SWS is correlated with high-phasic EEG alpha rhythm [21]. The finding of reduced SWS in FMS patients also coincides with nocturnal neuroendocrine abnormalities of increased nocturnal cortisol levels and decreased release of growth hormone (GH) [30]. Quantitative studies suggest that the duration of SWS serves to regulate homeostasis and is correlated with the amount of prior waking. That is, SWS increases following extended wakefulness and is decreased during nocturnal sleep following a daytime nap containing SWS [31]. This decreased amount of SWS in FM might indicate an impairment of the SWS homeostatic drive.

Some sleep abnormalities in FM patients have not been consistently reported. In some studies, for example, FM patients are reported to be not significantly different from controls with respect to alpha sleep EEG activity or the duration of SWS [28, 32]. It is unclear whether these discrepancies result from heterogeneity of sleep pathology in FM patients, technical considerations such as differences in scoring of sleep EEG alpha anomalies, or the night-to-night variability in many sleep measures, including SWS [33].

Relationship Between Sleep and Pain Processing

Epidemiological Studies

Among patients with FMS, poor sleep quality is shown to be a key in the vicious cycle of feeling unrefreshed after sleep, morning aching/stiffness, fatigue, and dyscognition. Several prospective clinical studies report a correlation between poor sleep quality and FM symptoms. A statistical path analysis of a large population of FM patients found that a night of increased sleep disturbance correlates with increased pain, which predicted poorer physical functioning and subsequently greater depression [9]. In another study, poor sleep quality mediates the impact of increased pain upon fatigue [34]. These studies extend previous findings that a night of poor sleep is followed by a day of increased pain [35]. Moreover, after accounting for the effects of positive and negative events and pain on daily mood ratings, sleep duration and quality are prospectively related to affect and fatigue. Inadequate sleep has a cumulative effect on negative affect and prevents mood recovery from days with a high number of negative events [36].

Clinical Experimental Studies

As described above, Moldofsky and colleagues were the first to attribute functional disturbances in the sleeping–waking brain to the etiological core of promoting FM symptoms. In 1975 and 1976 publications, they showed that by interrupting SWS with auditory stimuli, an FM-like state including variable aching, fatigue, and increased sensitivity to pain pressure could be induced in healthy normal nonathletic subjects [11, 37]. They also showed in a small pilot study that under similar experimental prospective sleep and symptom test circumstances, several members of the University of Toronto track team did not experience such pain and fatigue symptoms. This preliminary finding suggests that aerobic physical fitness is involved in preventing or reducing the emergence of these symptoms. Since then, other researchers have confirmed that selective deprivation or disruption of sleep induces increased bodily sensitivity, decreased pain threshold, and reports of nonrestorative sleep [8, 38–42]. One study involving presumably fit US military men found a reduction of pain threshold, albeit not significantly different from controls [42]. Another experimental clinical study of sleep deprivation does not alter somatosensory (nonnociceptive) functions [39]. Furthermore, the effects of interruptions of SWS increases sensitivity to both painful and nonpainful stimuli, such as bright light, loud sounds, and strong odors [40]. In this study, selective sleep deprivation of middle-aged, sedentary women (similar to the major demographic population of FM patients) also produced impairment in diffuse noxious inhibitory controls (DNIC), similar to that observed in FM patients [40]. Recovery after sleep deprivation results in increased amounts of SWS and normalization of pain threshold [8]. The importance of SWS in maintaining homeostatic properties of the CNS is purported to involve downregulation of synapses [43, 44].

Synaptic upregulation, a feature of a state of central sensitization and pain augmentation, may be caused by disturbances in the physiology of sleep that leads to impaired sleep quality and nonrestorative sleep symptoms. Consequently, total sleep deprivation and REM sleep deprivation adversely affects pain threshold and pain behavior [40], which also occurs as the result of the experimental induced loss of the terminal four hours of sleep with its REM and non-REM sleep [45].

Disordered Metabolic Functions

Despite the absence of specific structural pathology, there is evidence for disordered metabolic functions that involve the sleeping/waking brain. These include a decrease in sleep-related prolactin, decrease in GH and its metabolites, disturbances in the hypothalamic-cortical adrenal axis, and elevation of cerebral spinal fluid substance P (SP) [46–53]. Furthermore, specific dysfunctions in neurotransmitter functions are shown to contribute to bodily sensitivity and disordered sleep. For example, inhibition of serotonin (5HT) synthesis by p-chlorophenylalanine induces insomnia and a hyperalgesic state in animals and humans [54]. The increased levels of SP that are found in the CSF of FMS patients led to experimental studies that demonstrated that SP operates through a neurokinin (NK) pathway to influence nociception and sleep. Intracerebral ventricular administration of SP in sufficient quantities that did not induce nociceptive response in mice delayed onset of sleep and provoked awakenings from sleep. An NK-1 receptor antagonist reversed the interfering effect upon sleep by SP [55]. This research demonstrates that the blocking of the SP-induced insomnia by prior treatment of the mice with NK1 receptor antagonist provides support to the notion of the arousing effect of increased SP on the sleeping/waking brain. Moreover, this research provides an experimental animal model for studying sleep disturbances and musculoskeletal pain.

Functional neuroimaging of FMS patients support the hypothesis of deficits in CNS inhibition and central pain augmentation. FMS patients are reported to have a premature decrease in gray matter volume in the cingulate, insular, medial frontal cortices, and parahippocampal gyri, which may be associated with affective disturbances and chronic widespread pain [56]. Whereas the duration of pain or functional pain disability was not related with gray matter vol-

umes, there is the suggestion that there is a trend of reduction in the anterior cingulate cortex (ACC) gray matter volume. In another brain imaging study, FM patients showed lower ACC connectivity to the bilateral hippocampi, amygdala, brainstem, and rostral ventromedial medulla, which are brain areas involved in the descending inhibitory modulation of pain and increased central nervous system sensitization [57]. Furthermore, sleep deprivation that has an adverse effect on pain perception and cognitive functioning alters dopamine metabolism (D2 receptor) in the striatum, which merits further study because of this neurotransmitter involvement in sleep/wake mechanisms [58].

Increased overnight sympathetic activity using electrocardiographic methodology is consistent with the notion of circadian autonomic metabolic dysfunction associated with an arousal disturbance during the sleep of patients with FM [59].

In conclusion, the continuing search for biological and behavioral etiological factors has resulted in the absence of a specific triggering event to the onset of symptoms. This absence of a medically explanatory specific triggering etiological agent has led to the belief in a combined genetic and environmental predisposition to these pain and fatigue syndromes. Accordingly, a pattern of specific genes may become activated by a variety of noxious triggering influences. Examples include industrial or motor vehicle accidents, psychologically traumatic events (e.g., posttraumatic stress injury), and viral infection with a consequent chronic M.E. or post viral CFS, e.g., post-viral SARS [6]. These potential triggering events may adversely affect the operations of the sleeping/waking brain with associated abnormal metabolic and neurophysiologic functions. The resulting neurophysiological dysfunctions affect inhibitory and reciprocal excitability sensory operations, which clinically manifest as hypersensitivities to various external noxious stimuli, e.g., application of pressure, loud noise, bright light, or unpleasant odors. Organ sensory dysfunctions may be affected with reactive hypermotility (e.g., irritable bowel or bladder syndromes). Such clinical experiences may evolve into a psychological distressing pattern of self-perpetuating chronic unrefreshing sleep, widespread pain, fatigue, and psychosocial behavioral problems. In their search for help, those affected (often females) are labeled with diagnoses that reflect the education, special focus of interest, and belief system in particular methods of treatments employed by health professionals in their practices (see Table 48.1).

Management

Currently, although no cure is on the horizon, the awareness, research, and improved knowledge of FMS are benefitting the development of methods of management of the illness.

Nonspecific sleep and behavioral measures such as sleep hygiene, gentle aerobic fitness, and cognitive behavioral techniques, together with a variety of sleep-promoting sedative, analgesic, and antidepressant remedies are being employed to treat pain symptoms. These include reports of experimental trials of medications, various remedies, and behavioral procedures based upon various ideas about mechanisms involved in the promotion of pain and fatigue symptoms. Some have resulted in the government approval of pharmaceutical agents. Some have been rejected for a variety of reasons and some are in various phases of experimental trials. These are briefly reviewed below.

Approved Neuroregulatory Drugs

Over the past several years, three CNS drugs, pregabalin (a drug with anticonvulsant properties), duloxetine, and milnacipran (drugs initially marketed as antidepressants), have been approved for the treatment of FM by the US Food and Drug Administration (FDA). Pregabalin and duloxetine are approved by Health Canada, but none of these drugs are approved by the European Medicines Agency. The neurotransmitter modulatory agent pregabalin, which is an alpha$_2$–delta ligand that causes increased cellular expression of calcium channels, reduces the expression of SP and noradrenaline. Studies show that this drug improves the pain, quality of sleep, and fatigue in FMS. Duloxetine and milnacipran are noradrenaline–serotonin reuptake inhibitors, which are known to be helpful in improving mood and also benefit pain and sleep in animal studies and neuropathic pain in humans.

Unapproved Randomized Control Trials of Neuroregulatory Medicinal Agents

A US multicenter randomized placebo-controlled 8-week trial (RCT) with sodium oxybate given in a 4.5- or 6-g qhs dose improved sleep physiology with reduced percent CAP A2/A3 rate and increased SWS in addition to improvement of the self ratings of quality of sleep and reduction of pain and fatigue in FMS patients [24].

A meta-analysis of five RCT trials with 10–40 mg cyclobenzaprine, given at variable times during the day, showed an overall global improvement in FM, a short-term modest improvement in pain, moderate improvement in sleep, and no improvement in fatigue or tender points. However, 85 % of patients experienced untoward effects, commonly drowsiness, dizziness, and dry mouth [60]. A recent two-site RCT of 1–4 mg cyclobenzaprine at bedtime (mean dose of about 3 mg) showed improved pain, tenderness, depression, and sleep quality or sleep stability as measured with sleep EEG CAP. More subjects taking the low dose of cyclobenzaprine

versus the placebo group had more nights of restorative sleep which was accompanied by improved fatigue and depression [25].This drug is under further FDA development.

Some effort has been directed to remedying aspects of abnormal neuroendocrine function, e.g., about one third of patients with low levels of insulin-like growth factor 1 (IGF-1), a surrogate marker for low GH secretion, have been treated with daily injections of GH. In a 9-month randomized, placebo-controlled, double-blind study, there was an increase in IGF-1, and a reduction in pain and tenderness. On the other hand, GH, which is reduced in patients with FMS, improved symptoms, but its high cost and the need for daily injections make its use impractical [61].

A single non-RCT of pramipexole, a dopamine agonist, is reported to be helpful for pain, fatigue, and overall function in a subset of FMS patients, half of whom were also taking narcotics [62].

No consistent abnormalities have been reported in the secretion of melatonin in patients with either CFS or FMS, nor has its administration been found to be useful in controlled studies [63]. Furthermore, the use of morning bright light treatment, which tends to modify the timing of the nocturnal secretion of melatonin and is helpful in seasonal affective disorder, does not benefit sleep, pain, or mood symptoms in patients with FMS [64].

Finally, patients with primary sleep disorders such as restless legs/PLM disorder and sleep apnea have not as yet been subject to RCT for pain and fatigue with the well-established remedies for such conditions. In particular, a further study of pramipexole (and similar dopamine agonist) is required to determine whether the improvement noted in some patients [62] may be related to the reduction in restless legs/PLM sleep disorder that occur in some patients.

In conclusion, advances in our scientific understanding of how the sleeping–waking brain is intimately connected to the widespread musculoskeletal pain, fatigue, and psychologically distressing symptoms of previously presumed to be unexplained medical illnesses, and current advances in medical knowledge is leading to the improved management of the FMS and similar pervasive syndromes with chronic unrefreshing sleep, diffuse myalgia, fatigue, and psychological distress.

References

1. Wolfe F, Smythe HA, Yunus MB, Bennett RM, Bombardier C, Goldenberg DL, et al. The American College of Rheumatology 1990 criteria for the classification of fibromyalgia. Report of the Multicenter Criteria Committee. Arthritis Rheum. 1990;33(2):160–72.
2. Wolfe F, Ross K, Anderson J, Russell IJ, Hebert L. The prevalence and characteristics of fibromyalgia in the general population. Arthritis Rheum. 1995;38(1):19–28.

3. Branco JC, Bannwarth B, Failde I, Abello Carbonell J, Blotman F, Spaeth M, et al. Prevalence of fibromyalgia: a survey in five European countries. Semin Arthritis Rheum. 2010;39(6):448–53.

4. Fukuda K, Straus SE, Hickie I, Sharpe MC, Dobbins JG, Komaroff A. The chronic fatigue syndrome: a comprehensive approach to its definition and study. Annals Internal Med. 1994;121(12):953–9.

5. Simmons G, Glynn SA, Komaroff AL, Mikovits JA, Tobler LH, Hackett J Jr, et al. Failure to confirm XMRV/MLVS in the blood of patients with chronic fatigue syndrome: a multi-laboratory study. Science. 2011;334(6057):814–7.

6. Moldofsky H, Patcai J. Chronic widespread musculoskeletal pain, fatigue, depression and disordered sleep in chronic -post-SARS syndrome; a case-controlled study. BMC Neurol. 2011;11:37.

7. American Psychiatric Association. Diagnostic and statistical manual of mental disorders (5th ed.). Washington, DC. (2013).

8. Moldofsky H. The significance of the sleeping-waking brain for the understanding of widespread musculoskeletal pain and fatigue in fibromyalgia syndrome and allied syndromes. J Joint Bone Spine. 2008;75(4):397–402. (Simultaneously published in French: Importance du cycle veille-sommeil dans la compréhension des douleurs musculosquelettiques diffuses et de la fatigue au cours de la fibromyalgie et des syndromes apparentés. Rev Rhum. 2008;75(7):582–9).

9. Bigatti SM, Hernandez AM, Cronan TA, Rand KL. Sleep disturbances in fibromyalgia syndrome: relationship to pain and depression. Arthritis Rheum. 2008;59(7):961–7.

10. Russell IJ, Bieber CS. Myofascial pain and fibromyalgia syndrome. In: McMahon SB, Koltzenburg M, editors. Wall and Melzack's textbook of pain. 5th edn. London: Elsevier; 2006. pp. 669–82.

11. Moldofsky H, Scarisbrick P, England R, Smythe H. Musculosketal symptoms and non-REM sleep disturbance in patients with "fibrositis syndrome" and healthy subjects. Psychosom Med. 1975;37(4):341–1.

12. Yunus MB, Ahles TA, Aldag JC, Masi AT. Relationship of clinical features with psychological status in primary fibromyalgia. Arthritis Rheum. 1991;34(1):15–21.

13. Sloan E, Maunder R, Hunter J, Moldofsky H. Insecure attachment is associated with the alpha-EEG anomaly during sleep. BioPsychoSocial Med. 2007;1:20. doi:10.1186/1751-0759-1-20.

14. Hauri P, Hawkins DR. Alpha-delta sleep. Electroencephalogr Clin Neurophysiol. 1973;34(3):233–7.

15. Benca RM, Obermeyer WH, Larson CL, Yun B, Dolski I, Kleist KD, et al. EEG alpha power and alpha power asymmetry in sleep and wakefulness. Psychophysiology. 1999;36(4):430–6.

16. Cantero JL, Atienza M, Salas RM. Human alpha oscillations in wakefulness, drowsiness period, and REM sleep: different electroencephalographic phenomena within the alpha band. Neurophysiol Clin. 2002;32(1):54–71.

17. Horne JA, Shackell BS. Alpha-like EEG activity in non-REM sleep and the fibromyalgia (fibrositis) syndrome. Electroencephalogr Clin Neurophysiol. 1991;79(4):271–6.

18. Anch AM, Lue FA, MacLean AW, Moldofsky H. Sleep physiology and psychological aspects of the fibrositis (fibromyalgia) syndrome. Can J Psychol. 1991;45(2):179–84.

19. Branco J, Atalaia A, Paiva T. Sleep cycles and alpha-delta sleep in fibromyalgia syndrome. J Rheumatol. 1994;21(6):1113–7.

20. Drewes AM, Nielsen KD, Taagholt SJ, Bjerregard K, Svendsen L, Gade J. Sleep intensity in fibromyalgia: focus on the microstructure of the sleep process. Br J Rheumatol. 1995;34(7):629–35.

21. Roizenblatt S, Moldofsky H, Benedito-Silva AA, Tufik S. Alpha sleep characteristics in fibromyalgia. Arthritis Rheum. 2001;44(1):222–30.

22. Schneider-Helmert D, Kumar A. Sleep, its subjective perception, and daytime performance in insomniacs with a pattern of alpha sleep. Biol Psychiatry. 1995;37(2):99–105.

23. Rizzi M, Sarzi-Puttini P, Atzeni F, Capsoni F, Andreoli A, Pecis M, et al. Cyclic alternating pattern: a new marker of sleep alteration in patients with fibromyalgia? J Rheumatol. 2004;31(6):1193–9.

24. Moldofsky H, Inhaber NH, Guinta DR, Alvarez-Horine SB. The effects of sodium oxybate on sleep physiology and sleep/wake-related symptoms in patients with fibromyalgia syndrome: a double-blind, randomized, placebo-controlled study. J Rheumatol. 2010;37(10):2156–66. Epub 2010 Aug 3.

25. Moldofsky H, Harris HW, Archambault T, Kwong T, Lederman S. Effects of bedtime very low dose (VLD) cyclobenzaprine (CBP) on symptoms and sleep physiology in patients with fibromyalgia syndrome (FM): a double-blind, randomized, placebo-controlled study. J Rheumatol. 2011;38(12):2653–63. Epub 2011 Sep 1.

26. Thomas RT. Sleep as a window into the world of fibromyalgia syndrome. J Rheumatol. 2011;38(12):2499–500.

27. Landis CA, Lentz MJ, Rothermel J, Buchwald D, Shaver JL. Decreased sleep spindles and spindle activity in midlife women with fibromyalgia and pain. Sleep. 2004;27(4):741–50.

28. Chervin RD, Teodorescu M, Kushwaha R, Deline AM, Brucksch CB, Ribbens-Grimm C, et al. Objective measures of disordered sleep in fibromyalgia. J Rheumatol. 2009;36(9):2009–16.

29. Sergi M, Rizzi M, Braghiroli A, Sarzi Puttini P, Greco M, Cazzola M, et al. Periodic breathing during sleep in patients affected by fibromyalgia syndrome. Eur Respir J. 1999;14(1):203–8.

30. Van Cauter E, Spiegel K, Tasali E, Leproult R. Metabolic consequences of sleep and sleep loss. Sleep Med. 2008;9(Suppl 1): S23–8.

31. Dijk DJ. Regulation and functional correlates of slow wave sleep. J Clin Sleep Med. 2009;5(Suppl 2):S6–15.

32. Burns JW, Crofford LJ, Chervin RD. Sleep stage dynamics in fibromyalgia patients and controls. Sleep Med. 2008;9(6):689–96.

33. Larsen LH, Moe KE, Vitiello MV, Prinz PN. A note on the night-to-night stability of stages 3+4 sleep in healthy older adults: a comparison of visual and spectral evaluations of stages 3+4 sleep. Sleep. 1995;18(1):7–10.

34. Nicassio PM, Moxham EG, Schuman CE, Gevirtz RN. The contribution of pain, reported sleep quality, and depressive symptoms to fatigue in fibromyalgia. Pain. 2002;100(3):271–9.

35. Affleck G, Urrows S, Tennen H, Higgins P, Abeles M. Sequential daily relations of sleep, pain intensity, and attention to pain among women with fibromyalgia. Pain. 1996;68(2–3):363–8.

36. Hamilton NA, Affleck G, Tennen H, Karlson C, Luxton D, Preacher KJ, et al. Fibromyalgia: the role of sleep in affect and in negative event reactivity and recovery. Health Psychol. 2008;27(4):490–7.

37. Moldofsky H, Scarisbrick P. Induction of neurasthenic musculo-skeletal pain syndrome by selective sleep stage deprivation. Psychosom Med. 1976;38(1):35–44.

38. Lentz MJ, Landis CA, Rothermel J, Shaver JL. Effects of selective slow wave sleep disruption on musculoskeletal pain and fatigue in middle aged women. J Rheumatol. 1999;26(7):1586–92.

39. Kundermann B, Spernal J, Huber MT, Krieg JC, Lautenbacher S. Sleep deprivation affects thermal pain thresholds but not somatosensory thresholds in healthy volunteers. Psychosom Med. 2004;66(6):932–7.

40. Smith MT, Edwards RR, McCann UD, Haythornthwaite JA. The effects of sleep deprivation on pain inhibition and spontaneous pain in women. Sleep. 2007;30(4):494–505.

41. Onen SH, Alloui A, Gross A, Eschallier A, Dubray C. The effects of total sleep deprivation, selective sleep interruption and sleep recovery on pain tolerance thresholds in healthy subjects. J Sleep Res. 2001;10(1):35–42.

42. Older SA, Battafarano DF, Danning CL, Ward JA, Grady EP, Derman S, et al. The effects of delta wave sleep interruption on pain thresholds and fibromyalgia-like symptoms in healthy subjects; correlations with insulin-like growth factor I. J Rheumatol. 1998;25(6):1180–6.

43. Tononi G, Cirelli C. Sleep and synaptic homeostasis: a hypothesis. Brain Res Bull. 2003;62(2):143–50.

44. Tononi G. Slow wave homeostasis and synaptic plasticity. J Clin Sleep Med. 2009;5(Suppl 2):S16–9.

45. Roehrs T, Hyde M, Blaisdell B, Greenwald M, Roth T. Sleep loss and REM sleep loss are hyperalgesic. Sleep. 2006;29(2):145–51.

46. Landis CA, Lentz MJ, Rothermel J, Riffle SC, Chapman D, Buchwald D, et al. Decreased nocturnal levels of prolactin and growth hormone in women with fibromyalgia. J Clin Endocrinol Metab. 2001;86:1672–8.

47. Paiva ES, Deodhar A, Jones KD, Bennett RY, et al. Impaired growth hormone secretion in fibromyalgia patients: evidence for augmented hypothalamic somatostatin. Arthritis Rheum. 2002;46:440–50.

48. Bennett RM. Adult growth hormone deficiency in patients with fibromyalgia. Curr Rheumatol Rep. 2002;4:306–12.

49. Bennett RM, Clark SC, Campbell SM, Burckardt CS, et al. Low levels of somatomedin C in patients with the fibromyalgia syndrome: a possible link between sleep and muscle pain. Arthritis Rheum. 1992;35:1113–6.

50. Demitrack MA, Crofford LJ. Evidence for and pathophysiologic implications of the hypothalamic-pituitary-adrenal axis dysregulation in fibromyalgia and chronic fatigue syndrome. Ann N Y Acad Sci. 1998;840:684–97.

51. Adler GK, Kinsley BT, Hurwitz S, Mossey CJ, Goldenberg DL, et al. Reduced hypothalamic-pituitary-adrenal and sympathoadrenal responses to hypoglycemia in women with fibromyalgia syndrome. Am J Med. 1999;106:534–43.

52. Klerman EB, Goldenberg DL, Brown EN, Maliszewski AM, Adler GK, et al. Circadian rhythms of women with fibromyalgia. J Clin Endocrinol Metab. 2001;86:1034–9.

53. Russell IJ. The promise of substance P inhibitors in fibromyalgia. Rheum Dis Clin North Am. 2002;28(2):329–42.

54. Moldofsky H. Rheumatic pain modulation syndrome: the interrelationships between sleep, central nervous system serotonin, and pain. In: Critchley M, Freedman AP, Sicuteri F, editors. Advances in neurology, vol. 33. New York: Raven; 1982. pp. 51–7.

55. Andersen ML, Nascimento DL, Machado RB, Roizenblatt S, Moldofsky H, Tufik S, et al. Sleep disturbance induced by substance P in mice. Behav Brain Res. 2006;167:212–8.

56. Kuchinad A, Schweinhardt P, Seminowicz DA, Wood PB, Chizh BA, Bushnell MC. Accelerated brain gray matter loss in fibromyalgia patients: premature aging of the brain? J. Neurosci. 2007;27(15):4004–7.

57. Carville S, Choy E, Fransson P, Gollub R, Gracely RH, Ingvar M, et al. Patients with fibromyalgia display less functional connectivity in the brain's pain inhibitory network. Mol Pain. 2102;8:32.

58. Volkow ND, Tomasi D, Wang GJ, Telang F, Fowler JS, Wang RL. Hyperstimulation of striatal D2 receptors with sleep deprivation: Implications for cognitive impairment. Neuroimage. 2009;45(4):1232–40.

59. Lerma C, Martinez A, Ruiz N, Vargas A, Infante O, Martinez-Lavin M. Nocturnal heart rate variability parameters as potential fibromyalgia biomarker: correlation with symptoms severity. Arthritis Res Ther. 2011;13(6):R185.

60. Tofferi JK, Jackson JL, O'Malley PG. Treatment of fibromyalgia with cyclobenzaprine: a meta-analysis. Arthritis Rheum. 2004;51(1):9–13.

61. Bennett RM, Clark SC, Walczyk J. A randomized, double-blind, placebo-controlled study of growth hormone in the treatment of fibromyalgia. Am J Med. 1998;104(3):227–31.

62. Holman AJ, Myers RR. A randomized, double-blind, placebo-controlled trial of pramipexole, a dopamine agonist, in patients with fibromyalgia receiving concomitant medications. Arthritis Rheum. 2005;52(8):2495–505.

63. Geenen R, Jacobs JW, Bijlsma JW. Evaluation and management of endocrine dysfunction in fibromyalgia. Rheum Dis Clin North Am. 2002;28:389–404.

64. Pearl SJ, Lue F, MacLean AW, Heslegrave RJ, Reynolds WJ, Moldofsky H. The effects of bright light treatment on the symptoms of fibromyalgia. J Rheumatol. 1996;23:896–902.

Sleep and Pain: Milestones and Advances from Research

Carol A. Landis

Introduction

Sleep is a behavioral state that usually occurs naturally every day. Pain is a common experience but, unlike sleep, does not necessarily occur on a daily basis. Acute pain is a warning signal of potential, impending, or actual tissue injury. Chronic or pathologic pain is quite different. Accumulating evidence in pain science attests to the unique reorganization of pain pathways and ongoing plasticity within the brain that are distinctly associated with different chronic pain conditions (e.g., musculoskeletal, neuropathic) [1]. From elegant research in preclinical models and clinical studies, chronic pain is characterized by altered functioning of pain transduction, transmission, and modulation pathways in the central nervous system (CNS) such that nociceptive stimuli and tissue injury are no longer required for pain to be perceived. Episodes of spontaneous pain arise, non-nociceptive stimuli evoke pain sensations, and pain is perceived long after tissues have healed [2].

Regardless of whether pain is acute or chronic, there is a common expectation that pain will lead to disturbed sleep. Indeed, surveys attest to the prevalence of sleep problems in chronic pain conditions. Less than 20 years ago, the National Sleep Foundation conducted one of the first surveys on pain-related sleep disturbance in the USA [3]. This poll found that > 50 % of respondents from a large sample of adults reported nighttime pain; nearly half of the sample reported short sleep duration of ≤ 6 h. A recent survey of sleep and mental health from community-based samples in five European countries found a 17.1 % prevalence of a painful physical condition and a 10.3 % prevalence of insomnia symptoms (e.g., difficulty in falling asleep, staying asleep, or waking up early in the morning and unable to fall back to sleep) [4]. In this study, more than 20 % of individuals

with a chronic pain condition reported insomnia, but strikingly 40.2 % of individuals reporting insomnia also reported chronic pain. Sleep disturbances and insomnia were the most frequent comorbidities reported in a large Internet survey of adults with chronic pain from five Western European countries [5], and the prevalence of insomnia was higher in individuals self-reporting neuropathic pain (46 %) compared to other types of chronic pain (30 %). Sleep disturbance in chronic pain conditions varies considerably from 40 % to over 85 % depending upon the clinic population studied and methods used to measure sleep [6–10]. Sleep disturbance is common in the elderly [11] and also in children and adolescents [12]; over 50 % of youth with chronic pain conditions report symptoms consistent with insomnia [13]. Despite the prevalence of pain-related sleep problems, research on the best methods for treating pain and improving sleep, or for improving sleep and reducing pain, is quite limited. The evidence base for the clinical management of sleep problems in chronic pain conditions has just begun to appear in the literature and much more research is needed [9, 14]. Pain and coexisting sleep disturbance complaints are common, a large number of people worldwide are affected, and have serious negative consequences on health, quality of life, and work productivity as well as the rising costs of health care.

Since one of the first polysomnographic studies of sleep reported by Wittig and colleagues in 1982 [15], research on interactions between sleep and pain has grown considerably. Based on recent review of PUBMED under a broad search of "sleep and pain," 102 published references were accessible in 1992; 693 in 2012. Given the growing literature on the interaction of the problem of sleep disturbance in patients with pain, what do we know about the extent to which pain is associated with or leads to disturbed sleep? What do we know about the extent to which disturbed sleep modulates pain? Finally, what is the evidence that improving sleep relieves pain or vice versa? Considerable advances in pain science have been made in the past decade, especially in the use of brain imaging techniques applied to studies of individuals with chronic pain, and such advances have important impli-

C. A. Landis (✉)
Department of Biobehavioral Nursing and Health Systems, University of Washington, 1959 NE Pacific, Health Sciences, T-611C, Box 357266, 98195-7266 Seattle, WA, USA
e-mail: calandis@uw.edu

cations for understanding the impact of pain on sleep. However, a discussion of milestones in pain science is beyond the scope of this review [1]. The purposes of this chapter are to summarize the milestones and provide a critical commentary on the progress of generating research evidence on interactions of pain and sleep. This review includes selected preclinical studies, experimental human and clinical studies, as well as recent studies focused on interventions designed to improve sleep and reduce pain in people with chronic pain.

Sleep and Pain Interaction

A current view of sleep and pain has evolved to a bidirectional model stipulating that disturbed sleep is a consequence of presleep pain intensity and disturbed sleep leads to enhanced post-sleep pain (Fig. 49.1a). This bidirectional model has roots in a circular model originally proposed by Moldofsky and colleagues [16] in pioneering studies of sleep disturbance in fibromyalgia. Moldofsky proposed that disturbed sleep did not *cause* pain, but that, once pain was manifest, disturbed sleep followed leading to a continuous cycle of pain, poor sleep, and amplified pain (Fig. 49.1b). The idea that sleep disturbance or sleep loss can amplify pain and feelings of discomfort has roots in common experience and findings from research. Sleep deprivation (SD) studies conducted in the 1930s, first, showed that 2 days of total sleep loss reduced the pain (nociceptive) threshold [17]. A more recent study has shown that sleep loss of only 4 h and specific loss of rapid eye movement (REM) sleep evoked hyperalgesia, but the mechanisms underlying the exaggerated responses to noxious stimuli remain unknown [18]. Although intuitively appealing and parsimonious, a bidirectional, linear model of pain leading to disturbed sleep and disturbed sleep leading to

amplified pain is probably too simplistic. Likewise, a simple vicious cycle of pain-disturbed sleep pain fails to take into account other factors before, during, and after sleep that affect the interaction of pain and sleep (Fig. 49.1b).

Chronic pain patients are heterogeneous, and all pain is not the same. Chronic pain is associated with many comorbidities including anxiety, depression, specific sleep disorders, poor sleep hygiene, and symptoms associated with source of the pain, such as musculoskeletal disorders [1, 19], depression [20], or neuropathic pain [1]. These patients are also at risk for undergoing multiple surgeries or other types of invasive treatments. They often consume many types of prescription and over-the-counter medications with adverse and unpredictable effects upon sleep. Further, sleep quality and duration are influenced by physical activity, fatigue, daytime naps, and lifestyle behaviors such as smoking and the consumption of caffeine and alcoholic beverages. These factors have not been assessed or accounted for in the statistical analysis in many research studies. Finally, gender differences have been observed in sleep [21] and in the prevalence of clinical pain syndromes [22]; these differences have only begun to be studied in a systematic way in patients with chronic pain [23].

Does Pain Lead to Disturbed Sleep?

Pain is a unique, personal, and subjective unpleasant experience with a combination of sensory, affective, and behavioral dimensions, most often, associated with actual or potential tissue damage [24]. From studies of preclinical pain models, considerable evidence has accumulated about the plasticity and heightened sensitivity of pain transduction, transmission, and modulation processes in peripheral nerves [25], neurons, and synapses in the CNS [2] in response to various types of nociceptive stimuli. Evidence from clinical studies suggests that peripheral and central sensitization contributes to pain in arthritis, temporomandibular disorders, fibromyalgia, headache, complex regional pain syndrome, visceral pain, and post-surgical pain [2].

The models used to study pain processing have been categorized into three phases representative of the type of nociceptive stimulus and the extent of tissue injury [26], and is a useful framework to assess the impact of pain on sleep. Phase 1 pain involves the transient application of a nociceptive stimulus, which produces a minimal inflammatory reaction and brief vocal (cry, ouch), behavioral (reflex withdrawal, body movement), or physiological (altered neuronal activity) responses. Phase 2 pain occurs as a result of the application of substances that induce tissue damage and inflammation that persist for varying periods of time depending upon the agent used. Phase 2 pain is associated with release of mediators in tissues from damaged cells, blood vessels, and

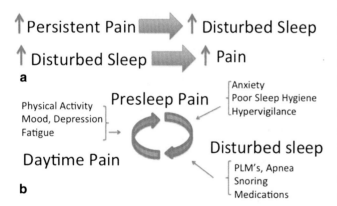

Fig. 49.1 a A bidirectional model assumes that higher pain intensity prior to sleep onset will lead to greater disturbed sleep; and greater disturbed sleep will lead to increased pain. **b** A circular model assumes that pain disturbs sleep and subsequently poor sleep affects pain. Various factors likely impact both pain and sleep and the interaction such that neither a linear nor a circular model fully accounts for the complexity of pain-related sleep disturbance

activated peripheral nociceptors. These chemical mediators directly activate or sensitize primary afferent nerve fibers to increase transmission of nociceptive information to the spinal cord invoking hyperactive neuronal responses that underlie the development of hyperalgesia (exaggerated response to nociceptive stimuli) and allodynia (pain-related response to non-nociceptive stimuli). Phase 3 pain involves damage specifically to neurons and nerve fibers. Behavioral signs of spontaneous and evoked pain responses persist for varying periods of time as do changes in the functional properties of CNS neurons and synapses. Peripheral and central sensitization is associated with a change in the gain of pathways involved in pain transduction, transmission, and modulation such that nociceptive stimuli or tissue injury are no longer necessary for pain to be perceived.

Phase 1 Pain Studies

Studies of phase 1 pain applied to animals or human volunteers during sleep yield evidence of transient sleep disturbance. In all of the studies, the experimenter [27] or subjects reported at least moderate-level pain to nociceptive stimuli (e.g., saline infusions into muscle, finger joint pressure, cutaneous laser heat) when they were awake [28–30]. In animal studies, behavioral withdrawal responses to the application of phase 1 laser heat pain were faster during slow-wave sleep (SWS) compared to waking. The animals fell back to sleep quickly when stimulated during sleep, and showed more prolonged pain-related responses (orienting to the site, licking the paw, changing body position) and took a longer time to return to sleep during waking compared to sleep [27]. These results were interpreted as evidence of a lower-pain threshold during SWS that were attributable to disinhibitory neuronal processes known to occur during sleep.

In studies with human volunteers, application of phase 1 pain stimuli leads to electroencephalographic (EEG) cortical arousal responses or brief awakenings during sleep [28–30]. It is difficult to compare results across studies because the type, duration, and intensity of nociceptive stimuli and protocols used in each study were quite different. Cutaneous heat of moderate [30] or high intensity [28] produced more frequent cortical arousals from non-REM (NREM) stage 2 compared to SWS and REM sleep, yet subjects reported the following morning minimal awareness of having been aroused or awakened during sleep. Nociceptive and non-nociceptive stimuli both produced a similar number of awakening responses from NREM stage 2 sleep and to reduced amounts of SWS and REM sleep obtained on experimental nights [31]. Findings from a laboratory study of sleep inertia (a transitional state of lower arousal) showed a large reduction in the perception of pain immediately after subjects were awakened from REM sleep, compared both to SWS

and wake [32]. In a study of laser heat stimuli applied during sleep, investigators observed arousals to 31 % of the stimuli, and 53 % of these were associated with visual motor reactions on the polysomnogram. No reductions in the latency to the first component (N2) of the cortical EEG-evoked potential were observed, but the latency to the second component (P2) was shorter, and the evoked potential amplitude was reduced during both NREM stage 2 and REM sleep [33]. Evoked potentials measured over the frontal cortex were attenuated in REM sleep, although overall morphology of the response was similar to wakefulness. Non-nociceptive stimuli give rise to similar EEG-evoked potentials over the cortex such that specificity of nociception is inferred from the nature of the stimuli applied, not from the EEG response. Further studies are warranted to determine whether patients with chronic pain are more susceptible to nociceptive stimuli during sleep. However, responses to nociceptive and non-nociceptive stimuli in patients with chronic pain are quite different from that of healthy volunteers as brain activity could be distorted by changes already present in the CNS associated with the particular chronic pain condition [1]. Given these observations, comparisons between patients with different types of chronic pain may be more informative compared to healthy controls.

Phase 2 and 3 Pain Studies

Experimentally induced preclinical studies of phase 2 and 3 pain (systemic arthritis and sciatic nerve damage) show physiological changes in sleep architecture indicative of sleep disturbance and provide evidence that pain leads to disturbed sleep, but findings are not consistent for all types of pain models tested. Sleep in arthritic animals is highly fragmented [34, 35] with increased wakefulness during the inactive and increased sleep during the active periods of the diurnal cycle [36]. Sleep disturbance was most prominent during the acute inflammatory phase of arthritis [35–37] or during the acute postoperative period following nerve injury [38, 39]. A recent study in mice found a statistically significant small amount of increased wakefulness and reduced NREM sleep at 7 days and again at 28 days post-sciatic nerve injury [40]. Disease severity was associated with greater sleep disturbance and *less* wakefulness with increased delta activity during sleep in the active period in arthritic animals [36]. Although neuropathic pain models induce persistent peripheral nerve denervation along with long-lasting changes in gene expression in the CNS and behavioral signs of hyperalgesia and allodynia, no changes in EEG spectral power were observed in animals for over four months after injury [39]. Preclinical neuropathic pain models are produced by a variety of types of nerve injury that could lead to distinct differences in disease severity and differential impact on sleep and changes in EEG frequency patterns during sleep.

Findings from these studies of phase 2 and phase 3 pain provide evidence of disturbed sleep, but isolating pain, as the "cause" of disturbed sleep, is difficult to ascertain. Systemic arthritis evokes systemic inflammation, increases body temperature, and elicits a variety of "sickness behaviors." Signs of disturbed sleep in peripheral nerve injury are most prominent in the acute postoperative period when systemic neuroendocrine responses to tissue injury, presumably, also are present. The most parsimonious explanation of these findings is an inability to sustain uninterrupted sleep episodes. Such changes could be related to persistent altered functioning of pain pathways, attributable to peripheral and central sensitization, that are more sensitive to slight bodily movements, or to environmental stimuli. Future studies of recently developed animals' models of stress-induced generalized pain [41], and of combined inflammation and neuropathic injury [42], have potential to advance understanding of mechanisms involved in chronic pain effects on sleep.

Clinical Studies in Chronic Pain

Most studies of pain and sleep in clinical populations have been cross-sectional observational studies comparing self-reported pain and sleep disturbance in patients with different chronic pain conditions or controls without pain. Chronic pain has well-recognized disturbing effects on *self-reports* of sleep quality and disturbance, but subjects often are asked about how much pain interferes with sleep, or are given a list of factors or symptoms and asked to indicate which ones they attribute to disturbing their sleep [43]. Thus, studies may be biased toward finding false-positive reports of pain-related sleep disturbance. The majority of clinical studies that have used both subjective and objective measures of sleep have been conducted on patients with musculoskeletal conditions, and most of these involved patients with fibromyalgia. Chronic pain has not been consistently associated with disturbed sleep as measured by polysomnography (PSG) or actigraphy [44–47]. In these studies, often the self-report of poor sleep quality is out of proportion to modest changes in PSG indicators of sleep [9], especially when patients are compared to sedentary control subjects of similar age [45].

Sleep studies of patients with other types of chronic pain, in particular neuropathic pain, back pain, and chronic regional pain syndrome, are few in number. A recent review of the literature in patients with chronic low back pain found self-reported generalized sleep disturbance, reduced sleep duration, quality, and satisfaction, with increased sleep latency, and problems functioning in the daytime [48]. Of note, this evidence-based review included only two studies (meeting investigator inclusion criteria) that used PSG or actigraphy

sleep measures, and only in < 10 patients in each study [49, 50]. A recent small clinical study of 16 patients with chronic low back pain yielded significant differences in self-reports of sleep disturbance compared to 16 control subjects, but no differences in sleep measures obtained from actigraphy [51]. It has been estimated that nearly 80 % of adults will, at some time, eventually experience back pain and metabolic biomarkers of brain function that correlate with clinical measures of chronic back pain [1]. We need PSG and nociceptive response studies during sleep in these clinical populations.

Investigators who preformed a structured evidence-based review of the literature (41 studies of good quality) on a variety of chronic pain conditions, that included some type of sleep measure, concluded that there is strong and consistent evidence to support an *etiological* role of pain with sleep disturbance due to a medical condition [7]. Of these, 77 % of 21 studies showed, through statistical modeling, that pain predicted the occurrence of a sleep problem, but only three of these studies were based on prospective analysis. Studies of daily temporal associations between pain and sleep with multilevel statistical modeling techniques have advanced our knowledge about pain–sleep interactions [9]. One of the first reports of a bidirectional relation between pain and sleep was derived from a prospective study in women with fibromyalgia [52]. Based on daily diary recordings over 30 days, a night of poor sleep was followed by more pain the next day; more pain during the day was followed by night of poorer sleep. Data on reports of nighttime sleep and pain for 8 days, from a large nationally representative sample of middle-aged adults in the USA, found that hours of sleep predicted subsequent frequency of pain and pain predicted subsequent hours of sleep, but the effect of sleep on pain was stronger than the effect of pain on sleep [53].

Recent studies of temporal associations between pain and sleep provide interesting and novel findings about the complexity of pain–sleep interactions. In a laboratory study of 75 children with juvenile arthritis, age, medications, anxiety, and evening pain explained 18 % of variance in subsequent EEG sleep arousals, but neither anxiety nor pain had a significant effect on sleep microstructure [54]. In a study of 97 adolescents with chronic pain or intermittent pain (healthy subjects), actigraphy-derived estimates of sleep duration and amount of wake after sleep onset, but not sleep efficiency or self-reported sleep quality, predicted next-day pain; daytime pain intensity did not predict subsequent nighttime sleep disturbance [12]. In a study of a group of 107 heterogeneous adult chronic pain patients (74 % women), both with moderate pain and insomnia severity scores, *presleep mood and cognitive arousal,* but not pain, predicted subsequent self-reported sleep quality; cognitive and somatic arousal predicted actigraphy-derived sleep efficiency [55]. Self-reported sleep quality and efficiency and actigraphy-derived sleep efficiency predicted next pain upon awakening, but predictors of pain in the first half or second half of the day varied. In post-hoc analysis, depression emerged as a significant predictor of self-reported sleep quality, along with presleep arousal. Thus, although relieving pain has potential to improve sleep, at the present time, it is not clear that pain is the most salient symptom to target in planning treatments to improve sleep in patients with chronic pain. Presleep arousal is an important factor influencing sleep quality and duration in insomnia [56], and therapies addressing arousal and mood [20] could be an important target for improving sleep in chronic pain patients.

Milestones: pain to sleep interactions

- Advances in pain research have established that chronic pain is characterized by altered functioning in pain transduction, transmission, and modulation pathways in the brain leading to persistent heightened sensitivity to pain and the perception of pain after tissues have healed.
- In animals, reflex withdrawal responses to pain stimuli are faster during NREM sleep and somewhat attenuated during REM sleep.
- In humans, pain stimuli, applied during sleep, leads to transient arousals and sometimes brief awakenings but in healthy subjects awakenings are rarely remembered the next morning.
- Substantial evidence exists to support pain in the etiology of *self-reported,* but not objective, measures of sleep disturbance in chronic pain.
- Presleep arousal and mood, along with pain, have emerged as important factors associated with subsequent sleep disturbance.

Does Sleep Modulate Pain?

Sleep Effects on Pain

During sleep, an individual is unaware of environmental surroundings with reduced responsiveness to sensory stimuli. Arousal thresholds and response duration vary as a function of stimulus type and strength, sleep stage, time of night, age, and other factors. The literature on sleep modulation of sensory stimuli was reviewed previously and suggested that responses to nociceptive stimuli are preserved during NREM sleep, but gated to some extent during REM sleep [57]. In that review, reference was made to a series of studies of brainstem neurons in the region of the ventromedial reticular formation that previously had been implicated as one of the important sources for the mediation of descending nociceptive (pain) modulation or facilitation and hypothesized to inhibit nociception during sleep [58]. Research on brainstem neurons, OFF cells (anti-nociceptive) and ON cells (pronociceptive) have shown distinct patterns of spontaneous

activity during waking, NREM, and REM sleep in rats [59] and more recently in mice [60]. OFF cells are continuously active during NREM sleep, sporadically active in wakefulness, and silent during REM sleep. ON cells are continuously active during waking, virtually silent during NREM sleep, and most active during REM sleep. Based on these response properties, one would expect that behavioral responses to noxious stimuli would be reduced during NREM sleep compared to wakefulness. However, paw withdrawal latencies to a radiant heat stimulus were faster during NREM sleep compared to wakefulness, and behavioral responses (e.g., licking the paw, moving about the cage) were suppressed during NREM sleep and exaggerated during waking [27]. In a recent study in mice [60], paw withdrawals to nociceptive heat were more reliably observed during sleep compared to wakefulness and associated with greater phasic activity of OFF cells prior to motor responses. Thus, rather than suppressing nociception, OFF cells appear to facilitate reflex motor protective withdrawal responses. However, how these neurons and others implicated in suppressing or facilitating pain responses would respond in the context of chronic pain has not been reported.

Sleep Loss Effects on Pain

Selective REM SD was one of the first types of sleep loss effects on pain studied. These experiments in rodents consistently have shown faster withdrawal latencies to noxious stimuli interpreted as reduced "pain" thresholds during [61], immediately after several days of deprivation [62–64], and after several days of recovery sleep [65]. Some evidence exists for reduced efficacy of opioid-mediated descending pain modulation in REM SD [66].

Increased pain perception or sensitivity has been observed in most experimental sleep loss studies in human volunteers, but such changes have not been consistently observed across studies involving the same type of nociceptive stimulus or similar SD protocols. One of the first total sleep deprivation (TSD) studies in human volunteers showed a progressive decrease in the threshold to pressure (von Frey hair), but not non-nociceptive stimuli [17]. One recent study has shown that the threshold to radiant heat pain was reduced after each of two nights of TSD compared to control subjects permitted usual sleep [67]; while the perception of reported pain on a visual analog scale was increased, the pain threshold was not altered after TSD in another study [68]. Selective SWS deprivation for three nights has been shown to increase muscle tenderness and reduce the threshold to pressure stimuli compared to baseline in young, primarily male, [69] and middle aged, female, subjects [70], but this change was not observed in another study [71]. Shorter latencies to radiant heat stimulus of 32 % have been observed after a single night of total sleep loss, after 4-h sleep loss, and after selective REM SD compared to non-REM deprivation [18]. Onen and colleagues [72] studied pain tolerance after one night of TSD followed by two consecutive nights of selective interruption of SW or REM sleep in counterbalanced order and a night of recovery sleep. Pressure, but not thermal, pain tolerance thresholds were reduced significantly after one night of TSD and remained lower after both SWS and REM sleep interruption nights, although the scores were not statistically different compared to baseline. After recovery sleep, there was a large increase in pressure pain tolerance scores, which was correlated with the amount of SWS during recovery. In one of the only reports of TSD in patients with chronic somatoform pain (e.g., without physical etiology) investigators reported increased pain perception, but without any change in pain thresholds to heat or pressure stimuli [73].

Compared to TSD, or selective sleep stage deprivation, inadequate or insufficient sleep is more common; one in three adults is estimated to sleep < 7 h per night [74]; thus, experimental studies of short sleep duration may provide data more applicable to sleep experienced in chronic pain conditions. In one of the few experimental studies of only women volunteers, neither three nights of interrupted sleep nor three nights of restricted, yet consolidated, sleep, both followed by a night of total sleep loss, led to any reliable group differences in pressure pain thresholds despite a 50 % reduction in total sleep time and increased sleepiness in both groups [75]. This study also assessed spontaneous pain symptoms and pain inhibitory processes using a test of diffuse noxious inhibitory controls (DNIC). In DNIC, the perception of a second nociceptive stimulus (e.g., pressure) is inhibited by the previous application of a nociceptive stimulus (cold) at a distant site. Only the group subjected to interrupted sleep showed an increase in spontaneous reports of pain symptoms and reduced pain inhibition. Another study involving assessment of endogenous pain-inhibitory processes after one night of experimental 4-h sleep restriction showed a 30 % increase in pain ratings, while reductions were observed in the amplitudes of laser-evoked EEG potentials; subjects were less able to inhibit pain when their attention was not focused on pain stimulus [76]. In a similar study of pain distraction, healthy individuals who habitually slept < 6.5 h, in the month preceding testing, had reduced pain inhibition, while playing video games, but they showed increased skin flare and augmented hyperalgesic responses to a heat-capsaicin stimulus compared to those who slept > 6.5 h [77]. In one of the only sleep restriction studies, found in the literature of patients with chronic pain, compared to control subjects, one night of 4-h sleep restriction augmented pain perception along with an increase in the number of painful arthritic joints, but fatigue, depression, and anxiety were also increased the next day [65]. With mild sleep loss, pain perception is augmented, both in healthy subjects and in patients with chronic pain, but increased pain perception is not always accompanied by evidence of altered pain thresholds. Such an increase in pain perception might be related to reduced functioning of pain-inhibitory processing.

Sleep Disorders and Pain

Sleep disorders often are associated with disturbed and fragmented sleep, and, in the case of insomnia, with short sleep duration, but few studies have measured pain perception or responses to nociceptive stimuli. Following the report of chronic pain by Ohayon [4] in a large percentage of people with insomnia, there is increased interest studying pain in primary and comorbid insomnia. Haack and colleagues [78] recently have shown that patients with primary insomnia reported twice as many days of spontaneous pain, showed reduced thresholds to heat and pressure pain, and both reduced pain facilitation and inhibition compared to control subjects. The results from this study were interpreted as evidence of subclinical pain and chronic activation of pain inhibitory mechanisms that produced a ceiling effect under challenging conditions. Additional research is necessary to confirm or refute this hypothesis.

Possible Mechanisms of Sleep Effects on Pain

Few studies have examined mechanisms that might underlie changes in pain perception with sleep loss [20]. Activation of inflammatory processes with increased circulating proinflammatory cytokines is one plausible mechanism that has been studied after sleep loss [79]. Increased C-reactive protein, an inflammatory biomarker of cardiovascular disease risk, was observed both after total sleep loss of 88 h or after 10 consecutive days of sleep restricted to 4 h nightly [80]. Increased plasma levels of interleukin-6, but not that of tumor necrosis factor alpha, have been observed following 10 days of 4-h sleep restriction [81], and increased urinary metabolites of prostaglandin E2 (PGE2) have been observed after 3 days of TSD [82]. In both studies, subjects reported spontaneous increased pain symptoms after several days of sleep loss. PGE2 is an important mediator of inflammation in peripheral tissues, capable of increasing peripheral nerve sensitivity [25] and neuron excitability in the spinal cord [83]. Proinflammatory cytokines released from circulating lymphocytes lead to release of cytokines by glia, in the spinal cord, and an increase in chemical mediators (e.g., excitatory amino acids, prostaglandins, nerve growth factors, and nitric oxide) that facilitate nociception and pain processing in the CNS [84]. Glia, rather than neurons, may be the biological basis of sickness behavior and therapies directed toward the upregulation of anti-inflammatory cytokines have been shown to reduce pain in animal studies [84].

Based on the results of the studies reviewed, it is not clear whether changes in pain perception and nociceptive thresholds with experimental sleep loss are attributable to total sleep loss, selective loss of a particular stage, restricting hours of sleep, or to sleepiness that inevitably accompanies sleep loss [85]. Sleepiness is one of the most reliable effects of experimental sleep loss. In fact, compared to well rested subjects, sleepy (as determined by multiple sleep latency tests) healthy subjects, after 8 h of sleep, showed increased pain sensitivity [86] and in a subsequent study, when subjects had extended time in bed, increased total sleep time correlated with reduced sleepiness and pain sensitivity [87]. As noted above, protective withdrawal reflexes to nociceptive stimuli are faster during NREM sleep and after experimental sleep loss when animals arc "sleepiest." Cytokines participate in the regulation of physiological sleep and are released after tissue injury, infection, and sleep loss [88]. Cytokines have a clear diurnal rhythm and reach the highest circulating levels during sleep [79]. It is possible that activation of cytokines during physiological sleep could participate in disinhibitory processes in the brainstem, which facilitate reflex withdrawal responses, yet protect sleep by not engaging sustained arousal responses? In addition to pain and sleepiness, cytokines have been associated with depressed mood, fatigue, impaired cognition, and memory—all symptoms that manifest with sleep loss. Thus, although activation of inflammatory processes is a plausible mechanism for increased pain sensitivity with sleep loss, further research is required to ascertain the role of cytokines and other inflammatory biomarkers to explain heightened pain following a night of disturbed sleep in patients with chronic pain, and in relation to levels of sleepiness.

Milestones: sleep to pain interactions.

- Latencies to EEG cortical responses to pain stimuli remain intact during sleep, although the amplitude of evoked potentials is attenuated, and reduced during REM sleep.
- In animals, REM SD is associated with reduced pain thresholds, possibly associated with reduced pain inhibitory processes.
- In humans, increased perception of pain is associated with loss of total sleep, selective stages of sleep, or reduced sleep amounts.
- Increased pain perception varies by type of pain stimulus (heat vs. pressure) and is not consistently accompanied by changes in pain threshold or physiological responses (e.g., changes in EEG-evoked potentials).
- Sleep loss may reduce pain inhibitory processes.
- Insomnia is associated with heightened pain sensitivity.

- Increased sleep reduces daytime sleepiness and pain sensitivity.
- Activation of inflammatory processes might be one mechanism underlying increased pain after sleep loss and with increased sleepiness.

Do Treatments for Sleep Modulate Pain?

In patients with chronic pain, pain is associated with disturbed sleep, and disturbed sleep augments pain. A recent evidence-based review concluded that pain is important in the etiology of sleep disturbances in patients with chronic pain and advocated that therapies to reduce pain ought to improve sleep [7]. Although treatments to reduce pain have potential to improve sleep, many medications commonly used to manage pain (opioids, antidepressants, anticonvulsants) have untoward and unpredictable effects on sleep [43, 89, 90]. Further, many of these medications produce sedation along with reducing pain, and, thus, attempts to assess the impact of such treatments on pain and sleep are complicated and potentially confounded [43]. In addition, many studies focused on managing pain, including studies of cognitive behavioral therapy specifically for pain, only focus on pain as an outcome and not on valid and reliable measures of sleep [9].

In the past few years, there is increased interest in studying the impact of treatments targeting sleep, and measuring pain outcomes [14]. Such efforts are supported by observations that reduced complaints of non-restorative sleep predicted reduced pain in a community sample of patients with chronic pain [91], and increased sleep time has been shown to lower pain sensitivity in experimental studies of sleep extension [87]. A recent review of selected clinical studies revealed that pharmacological management of insomnia with hypnotics (four studies of benzodiazepine receptor agonists; one study of benzodiazpene) improved sleep, but did not necessarily reduce pain in patients with fibromyalgia or arthritis [14]. In this review, three studies had been published on effects of cognitive-behavioral therapies for insomnia (CBT-I) in patients with nonmalignant chronic pain, fibromyalgia, and osteoarthritis with mixed results; sleep improved but pain was not reduced in all studies compared to control subjects. A more recent study evaluated the effect of CBT-I on sleep measures and on pain severity and interference with daytime functioning in a sample of middle-aged adults with nonmalignant chronic neck or back pain who developed insomnia after the onset of pain [92]. Self-reported sleep efficiency improved and sleep latency and wake after sleep onset were reduced, but total sleep time was unchanged after 8 weeks of therapy compared to attention controls. Pain severity and interference with daytime functioning were both reduced after 6 weeks compared to baseline, but pain severity was not statistically significantly different compared to controls. No follow-up data were reported. A major component of CBT-I is restricting time in bed to the reported time the patient actually reports sleeping. The amount of time in bed is advanced as total sleep time and sleep efficiency improve. CBT-I has shown improvements in self-reported and actigraphy measures of sleep quality and efficiency in fibromyalgia [93] but no changes in pain were reported. In patients with chronic pain, restricting sleep augments pain perception as shown by experimental studies noted above. CBT-I has long-lasting durable effects on sleep in primary and comorbid insomnia, and it is plausible, that only with sufficient practice over time would pain intensity subside as sleep time and quality increased. Notably, in the secondary analysis of the primary data from older adults with osteoarthritis at 1-year follow-up, CBT-I was associated with sustained improved sleep and reduced pain [94]. Thus, it has been hypothesized that sleep could be analgesic [94]. However, rather than being directly "analgesic," sleep might assist in the maintenance or resetting of pain inhibitory processes, which apparently can be reduced in association with experimental sleep restriction or associated with habitual short sleeping.

At this time, perhaps the major milestone in research, about whether improving sleep can reduce pain, is the recognition that interventions targeting only pain or only sleep and subsequently only measuring pain or sleep outcomes, respectively, are *inadequate* to address both comorbidities. To that end, the results of a pilot study have shown feasibility for combining CBT for pain with CBT-I in patients with chronic pain and insomnia. Preliminary results did not support the superiority of the combined approach over CBT-I for improving sleep, fatigue and mood, or for CBT for improving pain outcomes [95]. Based only on findings of a single small feasibility study, it is premature to evaluate whether a combination of CBT-pain and CBT-I will improve outcomes, but such studies do hold promise for future research. However, given observations above in patients with chronic pain, combination therapies addressing presleep arousal and mood, are likewise important to consider in future studies. Although there are few milestones to acknowledge about therapies for sleep having a positive impact on pain perception, there is increasing interest among investigators from many disciplines in addressing this question.

Summary and Recommendations

Evidence from self-reported data support a cyclical model of pain-poor sleep pain in chronic pain, but data from objective measures of sleep are less convincing. More research is required to elucidate the nature of sleep disturbance and pain using both self-report and objective measures of sleep and baseline and evoked measures of pain in patients with different types of chronic pain. Far less is known about the nature and extent of sleep disturbance, for example, in chronic back pain, chronic neuropathic pain, complex regional pain syndrome, and even in sleep disturbance pain in cancer survivors. There is increasing evidence that patients with some types of chronic pain show evidence of brain degeneration and atrophy [1], which would make the design of interventions to improve sleep and pain more complex and challenging. Studies are needed that test the efficacy of interventions focused on both reducing pain and improving sleep with a goal of improving functional health outcomes in patients with these comorbidities.

References

1. Apkarian AV, Baliki MN, Geha PV. Towards a theory of chronic pain. Prog Neurobiol. 2009;87:81–97.
2. Woolf CJ. Central sensitization: implications for the diagnosis and treatment of pain. Pain. 2011;152:S2–15.
3. National Sleep Foundation. Adult public's experiences with night-time pain. Princeton: Gallup Organization; 1996.
4. Ohayon MA. Relationship between chronic painful physical condition and insomnia. J Psychiatric Res. 2005;39:151–9.
5. Langley PC, Van Litsenburg C, Cappelleri JC, Carroll D. The burden associated with neuropathic pain in Western Europe. J Med Econ. 2013;16:85–95.
6. Becker N, Thomsen AB, Olsen AK, Sjogren P, Bech P, Eriksen J. Pain epidemiology and health related quality of life in chronic non-malignant pain patients referred to a Danish multidisciplinary pain center. Pain. 1997;73:393–400.
7. Fishbain DA, Cole B, Lewis JE, Gao J. What is the evidence for chronic pain being etiologically associated with the DSM-IV category of sleep disorder due to general medical condition? A structured evidence-based review. Pain Med. 2010;11:158–79,
8. Morin CM, Gibson D, Wade J. Self-reported sleep and mood disturbance in chronic pain patients. Clin J Pain. 1988;14:311–4.
9. Okifuji A, Hare BD. Do sleep disorders contribute to pain sensitivity? Curr Rheumatol Rep. 2011;13:528–34.
10. Pilowsky I, Crettenden I, Townley M. Sleep disturbance in pain clinic patients. Pain. 1985;23:27–33.
11. Chen Q, Hayman LL, Shmerling RH, Bean JF, Leveille SG. Characteristics of chronic pain associated with sleep difficulty in older adults: the maintenance of balance, independent living, intellect, and zest in the elderly (MOBLIZE) Boston study. J Am Geriatr Soc. 2011 59;1385–92.
12. Lewandowski AS, Palermo TM, de la Motte S, Fu R. Temporal daily associations between pain and sleep in adolescents with chronic pain versus healthy adolescents. Pain. 2010;151:220–5.
13. Palermo TM, Law E, Churchill SS, Walker A. Longitudinal course and impact of insomnia symptoms in adolescents with and without chronic pain. J Pain. 2012;13:1099–106
14. Roehrs T. Does effective management of sleep disorders improve pain symptoms? Drugs. 2009;69(Suppl 2):5–11.
15. Wittig RM, Zorick FJ, Blumer D, Heilbronn M, Roth T. Disturbed sleep in patients complaining of chronic pain. J Nerv Ment Dis. 1982;170:429–31.
16. Moldofsky H, Scarisbrick P, England R, Smythe HA. Musculoskeletal symptoms and non-REM sleep disturbance in patients with fibrositis syndrome and healthy subjects. Psychosom Med. 1975;37:341–51.

17. Cooperman NR, Mullin FJ, Kleitman N. Studies of the physiology of sleep XI. Further observations on the effects of prolonged sleeplessness. Am J Physiol. 1934;107:589–93.

18. Roehrs T, Hyde M, Blaisdell B, Greenwald M, Roth T. Sleep loss and REM sleep loss are hyperalgesic. Sleep. 2006;29:145–51.

19. Lavigne GJ, Nashed A, Manzini C, Carra MC. Does sleep differ among patients with common musculoskeletal pain disorders? Curr Rheumatol Rep. 2011a;13:535–42.

20. Finan PH, Smith MT. The comorbidity of insomnia, chronic pain, and depression: dopamine as a putative mechanism. Sleep Med Rev. 2012;doi:10.1016/j.smrv.2012.03.003.

21. Mong JA, Baker FC, Mahoney MM, Paul KN, Schwartz MD, Semba K, et al. Sleep, rhythms, and the endocrine brain: influence of sex and gonadal hormones. J Neurosci. 2011;31:16107–16.

22. Manson JE. Pain: sex differences and implications for treatment. Meta Clin Exper. 2010;59:S16–20.

23. Lavigne GJ, Okura K, Abe S, Colombo R, Huynh N, Montplaisir JY, et al. Gender specificity of the slow wave sleep lost in chronic widespread musculoskeletal pain. Sleep Med. 2011b;12:179–85.

24. Basbaum AI, Jessell TM. The perception of pain. In: Kandel ER, Schwartz JA, Jessell TM, editors. Principles of neural science. 4th edn. New York: McGraw-Hill; 2000. p. 474–91.

25. Reichling DB, Levine JD. Critical role of nociceptor plasticity in chronic pain. TINS. 2009;32:611–8.

26. Jeong Y, Holden JE. Commonly used preclinical models of pain. West. J Nurs Res. 2008;30: 350–64.

27. Mason P, Escobebo I, Gurgin C, Bergan J, Lee JH, Last EJ, et al. Nociceptive responsiveness during slow-wave sleep and waking in the rat. Sleep. 2001;24:32–8.

28. Bentley AJ, Newton S, Zio CD. Sensitivity of sleep stages to painful thermal stimuli. J Sleep Res. 2003;12:143–7.

29. Drewes AM, Nielsen KD, Arendt-Nielsen L, Birket-Smith L, Hansen LM. The effect of cutaneous and deep pain on the electroencephalogram during sleep—an experimental study. Sleep. 1997;20:632–40.

30. Lavigne G, Zucconi M, Castronovo C, Manzini C, Marchettini P, Smirne S. Sleep arousal response to experimental thermal stimulation during sleep in human subjects free of pain and sleep problems. Pain. 2000;84:283–90.

31. Lavigne GJ, Brousseau M, Kato T, Mayer P, Manzini C, Guitard F, Montplaisir J. Experimental pain perception remains equally active over all sleep stages. Pain. 2004;110: 646–55.

32. Daya VG, Bentley AJ. Perception of experimental pain is reduced after provoked waking from rapid eye movement sleep. J Sleep Res. 2010;19:317–22.

33. Bastuji H, Perchet C, Legrain V, Montes C, Garcia-Larrea L. Laser evoked responses to painful stimulation persist during sleep and predict subsequent arousals. Pain. 2008;137:589–99.

34. Andersen ML, Tufik S. Altered sleep and behavioral patterns of arthritic rats. Sleep Res Online. 2000;34:161–7.

35. Landis CA, Robinson CR, Levine JD. Sleep fragmentation in the arthritic rat. Pain. 1988;34:93–9.

36. Landis CA, Levine JD, Robinson CR. Decreased slow-wave and paradoxical sleep in a rat model of chronic pain. Sleep. 1989;12:167–77.

37. Colpaert FC. Evidence that adjuvant arthritis in the rat is associated with chronic pain. Pain. 1987;28:201–22.

38. Andersen ML, Tufik S. Sleep patterns over 21-day period in rats with chronic constriction of sciatic nerve. Brain Res. 2003;984:84–92.

39. Kontinen VK, Ahnaou A, Drinkenburg WH, Meert TF. Sleep and EEG patterns in the chronic constriction injury model of neuropathic pain. Physiol Behav. 2003;78:241–6.

40. Narita M, Nikura K, Nanjo-Niikura K, Narita M, Furuya M, Yamashita A, et al. Sleep disturbances in a neuropathic pain-like

condition in the mouse are associated with altered GABAergic transmission in the cingulate cortex. Pain. 2011;153:1358–72

41. Green PG, Alvarez P, Gear RW, Mendoza D, Levine JD. Further validation of a model of fibromyalgia syndrome in the rat. J Pain. 2011;12:811–8.

42. Allchornea AJ, Goodinga HL, Michellb R, Fleetwood-Walkera SM. A novel model of combined neuropathic and inflammatory pain displaying long-lasting allodynia and spontaneous pain-like behavior. Neurosci Res. 2012;74:230–8.

43. Smith MT, Haythornthwaite JA. How do sleep disturbance and chronic pain inter-relate? Insights from the longitudinal and cognitive-behavioral clinical trials literature. Sleep Med Rev. 2004;8:119–32.

44. Carette S, Oakson G, Guimont C, Steriade M. Sleep electroencephalography and the clinical response to amitriptyline in patients with fibromyalgia. Arthritis Rheum. 1995;38:1211–7.

45. Landis CA, Lentz MJ, Tsuji J, Buchwald D, Shaver JLF. Pain, psychological variables, sleep quality and natural killer cell activity in midlife women with and without fibromyalgia. Brain Behav Immun. 2004;18:304–13.

46. Leventhal L, Freundlich B, Lewis J, Gillen K, Henry J, Dinges D. Controlled study of sleep parameters in patients with fibromyalgia. J Clin Rheumatol. 1995;1:110–3.

47. Menefee LA, Cohen MJM, Anderson WR, Doghramji K, Frank ED, Lee H. Pain Med. 2000;1:156–72.

48. Kelly GA, Blake C, Power CK, Keeffe DO, Fullen BM. The association between chronic low back pain and sleep: a systematic review. Clin J Pain. 2011;27:169–81.

49. Harmon K, Pivik RT, D'Eon JL, Wilson KG, Swenson JR, Matsunaga L. Sleep in depressed and nondepressed participants with low back pain: electroencephalographic and behavior findings. Sleep. 2002;25:775–83.

50. Lavie P, Epstein R, Tzischinsky O, Gilad D, Nahir M, Lorber M, et al. Actigraphic measurements of sleep in rheumatoid arthritis: comparison of patients with low back pain and healthy controls. J Rheumatol. 1992;19:362–5.

51. Van de Water AT, Eadie J, Hurley DA. Investigation of sleep disturbance in chronic low back pain: an age-and gender-matched case-control study over a 7-night period. Man Ther. 2011;16:550–6.

52. Affleck G, Urrows S, Tennen H, Higgins P, Abeles M. Sequential daily relations of sleep, pain intensity, and attention to pain among women with fibromyalgia. Pain. 1996;68:363–8.

53. Edwards RR, Almeida DM, Klick B, Haythornthwaite JA, Smith MT. Duration of sleep contributes to next-day pain report in the general population. Pain. 2008;37:202–7.

54. Ward TM, Brandt PA, Archbold KH, Lentz MJ, Ringold S, Wallace CA, et al. Polysomnography and self-reported sleep, pain, fatigue, and anxiety in children with active and inactive juvenile rheumatoid arthritis. J Ped Psychol. 2008;33:232–41.

55. Tang NKY, Goodchild CE, Sanborn AN, Howard J, Salkovskis PM. Deciphering the temporal link between pain and sleep in a heterogeneous chronic pain patient sample: a multilevel daily process study. Sleep. 2012;35:675–87.

56. Harvey AG. A cognitive model of insomnia. Behav Res Ther. 2002;40:869–93.

57. Landis CA. Sleep, pain, fibromyalgia and chronic fatigue syndrome. In: Montagna P, Chokroverty S, editors. Handbook of clinical neurology, vol 38 Sleep disorders, Part 1. Edinburgh: Elsevier; 2011. p. 613–37.

58. Foo H, Mason P. Brainstem modulation of pain during sleep and waking. Sleep Med Rev. 2003;7:145–54.

59. Leung CG, Mason P. Physiological properties of medullary raphe neurons during sleep and waking. J Neurophysiol. 1999;81:584–95.

60. Hellman KM, Mason P. Opioids pro-nociceptive modulation mediated by raphe magnus. J Neurosci. 2012; 32:13668–78.

61. Onen S, Alloui A, Jourcan D, Eschalier A, Dubray C. Effects of rapid eye movement (REM) sleep deprivation on pain sensitivity in the rat. Brain Res. 2001b;900:261–7.

62. Hicks RA, Moore JD, Findley P, Hirshfield C, Humphrey V. REM sleep deprivation and pain thresholds in rats. Percep Motor Skills. 1978;47:848–50.

63. Hicks RA, Coleman DD, Ferrante F, Sahatjian M, Hawkins J. Pain thresholds in rats during recovery from REM sleep deprivation. Percep Motor Skills. 1979;48:687–90.

64. May ME, Harvey MT, Valdovinos MG, Kline IV, RH, Wiley RG, Kennedy CH. Nociceptor and age specific effects on REM sleep deprivation induced hyperalgesia. Behav Brain Res. 2005;159:89–94.

65. Irwin MR, Olmstead R, Carrillo C, Sadeghi N, FitzGerald JD, Ranganath VK, et al. Sleep loss exacerbates fatigue, depression, and pain in rheumatoid arthritis. Sleep. 2012;35:537–43.

66. Ukponmwan OE, Rupreht J, Dzoljic MR. REM sleep deprivation decreases the antinociceptive property of enkephalinase-inhibition, morphine, and cold-water swim. Gen Pharmac. 1984;15:255–8.

67. Kunderman B, Spernal J, Huber MT, Krieg JC, Lautenbacher S. Sleep deprivation affects thermal pain thresholds but not somatosensory thresholds in healthy volunteers. Psychosom Med. 2004;66:932–7.

68. Azevedo E, Manzano GM, Silva A, Martins R, Andersen ML, Tufik S. The effects of total and REM sleep deprivation on laser evoked potential threshold and pain perception. Pain. 2011;152:2052–8.

69. Moldofsky H, Scarisbrick P. Induction of neurasthenic musculoskeletal pain syndrome by selective sleep stage deprivation. Psychosom Med. 1976;38:35–43.

70. Lentz MJ, Landis CA, Rothermer J, Shaver JLF. Effects of selective slow wave sleep disruption on musculoskeletal pain and fatigue in middle-aged women. J Rheumatol. 1999;26:1586–92.

71. Older SA, Battafarano DF, Canning CA, Ward JA, Grady EP, Derman S, et al. The effects of delta wave sleep interruption on pain thresholds and fibromyalgia-like symptoms on healthy subjects; correlations with insulin-like growth factor I. J Rheumatol. 1999;25:1180–6.

72. Onen S, Alloui A, Gross A, Eschallier A, Dubray C. The effects of total sleep deprivation, selective sleep interruption and sleep recovery on pain tolerance thresholds in healthy subjects. J Sleep Res. 2001a;10:35–42.

73. Busch V, Hass J, Cronlein T, Pieh C, Geisler P, Hajak G, et al. Sleep deprivation in chronic somatoform pain—effects on mood and pain regulation. Psychiatry Res. 2012;195:134–43.

74. McKnight-Eily, LR, Liu Y, Perry GS, Presley-Cantrell LR, Strine TW, Lu H, et al. Perceived insuffi cient rest or sleep among adults—United States, 2008. Atlanta: Div of Adult and Community Health, National Center for Chronic Disease Prevention and Health Promotion, CDC. 2008.

75. Smith MT, Edwards RR, McCann UD, Haythornthwaite JA. The effects of sleep deprivation on pain inhibition and spontaneous pain in women. Sleep. 2007;30:494–505.

76. Tiede W, Mageri W, Baumgartner U, Durrer B, Ehlert U, Treede R-D. Sleep restriction attenuates amplitudes and attentional modulation of pain-related evoked potentials, but augments pain ratings of healthy volunteers. Pain. 2010;148:36–42.

77. Campbell CM, Bounds SC, Simango MB, Witmer KR, Campbell JN, Edwards RR, et al. Self-reported sleep duration associated with distraction analgesia, hyperemia, and secondary hyperalgesia in the heat-capsaicin nociceptive model. Euro J Pain. 2011;15:561–7.

78. Haack M, Scott-Sutherland J, Santangelo G, Simpson NS, Sethna N, Mullington JM. Pain sensitivity and modulation in primary insomnia. Eur J Pain. 2012;16:522–33.

79. Simpson N, Dinges DF. Sleep and inflammation. Nut Rev. 2007;11:S244–52.

80. Meier-Ewert HK, Ridker PM, Rifai R, Regan MM, Price NJ, Dinges DF, et al. Effect of sleep loss on C-reactive protein, an inflammatory marker of cardiovascular risk. J Am Coll. Card. 2004;43:678–83.

81. Haack M, Sanchez E, Mullington JM. Elevated inflammatory markers in response to prolonged sleep restriction are associated with increased pain experience in healthy volunteers. Sleep. 2007;30:1145–52.

82. Haack M, Lee E, Cohen DA, Mullington JA. Activation of the prostaglandin system in response to sleep loss in healthy humans: potential of increased spontaneous pain. Pain. 2009;145:136–41.

83. Fornasari D. Pain mechanisms in patients with chronic pain. Clin Drug Investig. 2012;32(Suppl 1):45–52.

84. Watkins LR, Maier S. Immune regulation of central nervous system functions: from sickness responses to pathological pain. J Int Med. 2005;257:139–55.

85. Roehrs T, Roth T. Sleep and pain: interaction of two vital functions. . Sem Neurol. 2005;25:106–16. (In: Roos KL, Avidan AY, editors).

86. Chhangani BS, Roehrs TA, Harris EJ, Hyde M, Drake C, Hudgel DW, et al. Pain sensitivity in sleepy pain-free normals. Sleep. 2009;32:1011–7.

87. Roehrs T, Harris E, Randall S, Roth T. Sensitivity and recovery from mild chronic sleep loss. Sleep. 2012;35:1667–72.

88. Clinton JM, Davis CJ, Zielinski MR, Jewett KA, Krueger JM. Biochemical regulation of sleep and sleep biomarkers. J Clin Sleep Med. 2011;7:S38–42.

89. Mystakidou K, Clark AJ, Fischer J, Lam A, Pappert K, Richarz U. Treatment of chronic pain by long-acting opioids and effects on sleep. Pain Practice. 2011;3:282–9.

90. Turk DC, Cohen MJM. Sleep as a marker in the effective management of chornic osteoarthritis pain and opioid analgesics. Semin Arthritis Rheum. 2010;39:477–90.

91. Davies KA, Macfarlane GJ, Nicholl BI, Dickens C, Morriss R, Day D, et al. Restorative sleep predicts the resolution of chronic widespread pain: results from the EPIFUND study. Rheumatology. 2008;47:1809–13.

92. Jungquist CR, O'Brien C, Matteson-Rusby S, Smith MT, Pigeon W, Xia Y, et al. The efficacy of cognitive behavioral therapy for insomnia in patients with chronic pain. Sleep Med. 2010;11:302–9.

93. Edinger JD, Wohlegemuth WK, Krystal AD, Rice JR. Behavioral insomnia therapy for fibromyalgia patients: a randomized clinical trial. Arch Int Med. 2005;165:2527–35.

94. Vitiello MV, Rybarczyk B, Von Korff M, Stepanski EJ. Cognitive behavioral therapy for insomnia improves sleep and decreases pain in older adults with co-morbid insomnia and osteoarthritis. J Clin Sleep Med. 2009;5:355–62.

95. Pigeon WR, Moynihan J, Matteson-Rusby S, Jungquist CR, Xia Y, Tu X, et al. Comparative effectiveness of CBT interventions for co-morbid chronic pain and insomnia: a pilot study. Beh Res Ther. 2012;50:685–9.

Endocrine–Metabolic Disorders and Sleep Medicine

50

Rachel Leproult and Georges Copinschi

Introduction

Despite the fact that some decades ago sleep was recognized as a strong modulator of hormonal secretions and glucose production, voluntary long-term sleep restriction, a phenomenon frequently encountered in our society, was long thought to have only consequences on the brain and not on the body. However, over the past 15 years, epidemiological and laboratory studies, as well as clinical investigations in patients with sleep disorders, have provided evidence for a considerable impact of sleep loss on bodily functions. In particular, it is now clear that sleep loss plays a major role in endocrine–metabolic disorders such as type II diabetes and obesity.

Following an overview of major chronological steps that evidenced the relationship between sleep architecture on the one hand, and the regulation of glucose metabolism and two major insulin counter-regulatory hormones (growth hormone (GH) and cortisol) on the other hand, this chapter traces the history of the effects of sleep loss on glucose metabolism and on appetite regulation in adults, as evidenced by epidemiological studies, experimental laboratory studies, and sleep disorders.

Sleep Physiology and Endocrine–Metabolic Function (Table 50.1)

Until the second half of the twentieth century, no method was available to estimate hormone levels, and the existence of possible relationships between sleep and endocrine–metabolic function was never mentioned . At the end of the 1950s,

a presentation by Yalow and Berson [1, 2] of a sensitive and specific radioimmunoassay, capable of measuring with a high degree of precision the insulin concentrations present in the circulation, opened a new and immense field for hormonal investigations. In 1959, it had also been shown that, despite prolonged fasting, glucose levels remain stable during sleep [3]. For years, however, no attempt was made to explore possible relationships between sleep and endocrine–metabolic function. In 1966, a first study [4] reported that, as judged from observations recorded in the diary, nocturnal GH peaks were regularly observed at times of likely deep sleep, leading the authors to hypothesize possible relations between GH secretion and sleep. A temporal association between slow-wave sleep (SWS) and elevated GH levels was evidenced in several studies [5–8], but other authors claimed that this relationship was fortuitous [9–11]. In the beginning of the 1990s, a new deconvolution procedure eventually allowed to determine with an extreme precision the amplitude and the temporal limits of GH secretory pulses and to unequivocally demonstrate the existence of a close temporal and quantitative relationship between SWS or slow-wave activity (SWA) and GH secretion [12, 13]. It was later shown that the age-related decrease in GH secretion during sleep occurs in parallel with the decline in SWS [14, 15].

For the past 20 years, the interrelations between GH and sleep have been extensively investigated and it is now well established that sleep is the major determinant of GH secretion in man. Conversely, GH-releasing hormone (GHRH) has been shown to stimulate SWS in animals [16–19] and in humans [16, 19]. Moreover, it was shown that SWS and SWA are increased in GH deficiency of primary pituitary origin [20]. Major steps are summarized in Table 50.1.

Meanwhile, the influence of the sleep–wake homeostasis on endocrine–metabolic regulation was progressively evidenced in many other fields. Two examples are illustrated in Table 50.1. In 1983, a first study showed that the 24-h rhythm of cortisol, though primarily driven by the circadian pacemaker [39], is also modulated by the sleep–wake cycle, since sleep onset is consistently followed by a drop in cir-

R. Leproult (✉)
Unité de Recherches en Neuropsychologie et Neuroimagerie Fonctionnelle (UR2NF), Université Libre de Bruxelles, Campus du Solbosch, CP 191, Avenue F.D. Roosevelt 50, 1050 Brussels, Belgium
e-mail: Rachel.Leproult@ulb.ac.be

G. Copinschi
Laboratory of Physiology and Physiopathology, Université Libre de Bruxelles, Brussels, Belgium

S. Chokroverty, M. Billiard (eds.), *Sleep Medicine,* DOI 10.1007/978-1-4939-2089-1_50,
© Springer Science+Business Media, LLC 2015

Table 50.1: Physiology of interrelationships between sleep and endocrine–metabolic function

Years	Relationship sleep–GH	Relationship sleep–cortisol	Relationship sleep–glucose
1959–1969	Temporal association between SWS and elevated GH levels (even if sleep is delayed or sleep–wake cycles are reversed or modified). SWS deprivation decreases GH levels [4–8]		During sleep, hourly glucose levels exhibit stable concentrations in nondiabetics [3]
1983–1989	*GHRH enhances NREM sleep and weakly increases REM sleep* [21, 22]	Temporal association between sleep onset and inhibition of cortisol secretion (even if sleep is delayed or sleep–wake cycles are reversed or modified) [23]	Glucose levels increase until mid-sleep under constant glucose infusion [24]
1990–1994	– Close temporal and quantitative relationship between SWS or SWA and GH secretion (estimated by deconvolution). GH response to GHRH is enhanced during SWS and inhibited by awakenings [12, 13] – *GHRH inhibition suppresses sleep* [17, 25] – *GHRH stimulates SWS* [16, 19]	– Inhibitory effect of sleep is related to SWS [26] – Awakenings trigger cortisol secretion [26–29]	Constant caloric intake results in increased glucose levels during the first part of a nocturnal or diurnal sleep period [29, 30]
1995–2000	– *GHRH stimulates NREM sleep in intact and hypophysectomized rats, but stimulates REM sleep only in intact animals* [18] – Pharmacological stimulation of SWS and SWA stimulates GH release [31, 32] – Age-related changes in SWS and GH levels occur with identical chronology [14, 15]	– Temporal coupling between EEG markers of alertness and cortisol secretion [33] – Age-related changes in REM sleep and evening cortisol levels occur with identical chronology [15]	Glucose utilization is lower during the first part of the night (rich of SWS) and higher during the second part of the sleep period (rich of REM sleep) [34–36]
2004–2010	SWS and SWA are increased in GH deficiency of primary pituitary origin [20]		Brain glucose consumption represents 30–50 % of total body glucose utilization [37, 38]

Italics denote studies performed on animals
SWS slow-wave sleep, *GH* growth hormone, *GHRH* GH-releasing hormone, *REM* rapid eye movement, *NREM* non-REM, *SWA* slow-wave activity

culating levels of the hormone [23]. About 10 years later, it was shown that this decrease is related to SWS [26], and conversely that transient awakenings during the sleep period, as well as the final awakening at the end of a sleep period, trigger cortisol secretion [26–29]. A few years later, in 1998, it was shown that during the waking period, there is a temporal coupling between cerebral alertness and cortisol secretion [33]. In 2000, it was evidenced that the age-related increase in evening cortisol levels occurs as a mirror image to the decline in rapid eye movement (REM) sleep [15].

Sleep modulates glucose production as well. A number of studies confirmed the 1959 finding [3] reporting stable glucose levels during the sleep period in healthy subjects [40–45]. In the 1980s/1990s, constant glucose infusion [29, 24] or constant enteral nutrition [30] appeared to result in increased glucose levels during the first part of a nocturnal [24, 29, 30] or diurnal [29, 30] sleep period. A few years later, constant glucose infusion [36] and positron emission tomography [34, 35] studies showed temporal associations between reduced glucose utilization and a high amount of SWS during the first part of the sleep period, and between enhanced glucose utilization and high amounts of REM sleep during the second part of the sleep period [34–36]. Noteworthy, it was discovered that the brain is a glucose guzzler as its consumption is estimated as 30–50 % of the total body glucose utilization [37, 38].

Sleep Loss and Endocrine–Metabolic Function (Table 50.2)

During the past decade, multiple epidemiological studies have documented a cross-sectional association between short sleep duration and increased risk for diabetes [46–54].

A number of prospective epidemiologic studies, more suitable at providing a direction of causality, have also examined the association between short sleep duration and diabetes prevalence [46, 55–65]. Many of them indicated a relationship between short sleep duration and diabetes prevalence [46, 55, 57, 58, 61, 64, 65], while others demonstrated a relationship between poor sleep quality and diabetes incidence [59, 60, 62, 63]. Only one study did not find any of these associations [56]. However, a meta-analysis [66] examining ten of these prospective studies reconciled the results to an association between short sleep duration and sleep disturbances, on the one hand, and the risk of developing diabetes, on the other hand. This association appeared to be stronger for men than for women [66].

The relationship between sleep loss and diabetes risk was also investigated in well-controlled laboratory studies. An alteration of glucose metabolism after total sleep deprivation had already been demonstrated in 1969 [78] and was confirmed later on by various groups [74–77]. Only one study

Table 50.2: Effects of sleep loss on glucose metabolism and appetite regulation

Studies	Sleep loss and glucose metabolism	Sleep loss and appetite regulation
Prospective population-based studies	– Short sleep duration predicts the risk of developing diabetes [46, 55, 57, 58, 61, 64, 65] – Difficulty in initiating and/or maintaining sleep [59, 60, 62], in falling asleep or using sleeping pills [63] predicts the risk of developing diabetes – Meta-analysis [66]: association between inadequate sleep and diabetes incidence	Short sleep duration is associated with weight gain [67–73]
Laboratory studies *Total sleep deprivation*	Increased glucose levels [74, 75] and increased insulin response to glucose [76]. Decreased insulin sensitivity [77] and glucose tolerance [78]	Decreased diurnal rhythm amplitude of leptin [79] and hunger [80]
Laboratory studies *Partial sleep restriction*	Altered glucose metabolism [81]. Decreased insulin sensitivity [82–89]	– Decreased leptin levels [90–92], increased ghrelin levels [92], increased hunger and appetite [92] – Increased caloric intake [93–96], increased caloric intake for snacks [95] increased caloric intake from an ad libitum buffet [97, 98] – Muscle (rather than fat) loss under caloric restriction [99]
Laboratory studies *Sleep quality alterations*	Increased insulin resistance after SWS suppression [100] and sleep fragmentation [101]	

SWS slow-wave sleep

[102] did not find any effect of one night of total sleep deprivation on glucose metabolism.

At the very end of the past century, exploration of bedtime curtailment, a phenomenon closer to everyday life, was initiated in laboratory studies. A pioneering study looking at the metabolic consequences of a semi-chronic sleep restriction was published in 1999 by Spiegel et al. [81], and rapidly became a "citation classic" (more than 1000 citations). Normal young men were submitted to 6 days of sleep restriction (4 h in bed), followed by 6 days of sleep extension (12 h in bed): sleep restriction (with partial preservation of SWS) led to alterations in glucose metabolism [81], together with higher evening cortisol levels [81] and elevated GH concentrations during the waking period [103]. Ten years later, the impact of a semi-chronic sleep restriction on glucose metabolism was confirmed in middle-aged men and women submitted to 2 weeks of reduced sleep by 1.5 h daily compared to 2 weeks of extended sleep by 1.5 h daily [86], and in young men submitted to 1 week of 5-h bedtimes in a study that used a euglycemic–hyperinsulinemic clamp, the gold standard method to evaluate insulin sensitivity [82].

In the meantime, additional laboratory studies had examined the impact of partial sleep restriction on glucose metabolism. Most of them found that partial sleep restriction, for 1–7 days, resulted in increased insulin resistance [84, 85, 87–89]. Another study did not find any effect on glucose tolerance after 8 weeks of bedtime restriction in self-reported long sleepers [104] but the sleep-restricted group averaged more than 6.5 h of sleep at the end of the restriction period and slept only 16 min less than the control group [105]. Glucose tolerance remained stable in a study of a 4-day pro-

gressive sleep restriction from 7 to 4 h of sleep per night in women [93]. Recently, it was shown that individuals with a parental history of type 2 diabetes have a higher risk of developing diabetes if they are short sleepers [83].

Not only does sleep duration play a major role in the endocrine–metabolic function but sleep quality appears to be important as well. Using sound delivery to perturb sleep, a study has elegantly demonstrated that SWS suppression results in reduced glucose tolerance and increased diabetes risk, despite preservation of sleep duration and REM sleep [100]. Consistent with these results, sleep fragmentation markedly reducing SWS together with a small decrease in REM sleep without changing sleep duration also resulted in reduced glucose tolerance [101].

Sleep Loss and Appetite Regulation (Table 50.2)

Over the past decade, numerous cross-sectional studies have provided accumulating evidence for a robust association between short sleep duration and increased body mass index (BMI). Here, we cite the most important publications from 2000 to 2005 [106–112] but the number of references has grown tremendously. In 2008, a meta-analysis including more than 600,000 adults confirmed this relationship [113]. Although cross-sectional studies have mostly used self-reported sleep duration, the few that have measured sleep objectively via wrist activity monitoring [114, 115] and polysomnography [116, 117] found the same association between short sleep duration and the risk of obesity.

Most prospective studies [67–73], but not all [114, 118], including observations over 6 months to over 16 years suggested that sleep restriction predicts the incidence of obesity.

The mechanisms involved in the association between sleep duration and obesity were explored in well-controlled laboratory studies. Total sleep deprivation was found to result in decreased amplitude of diurnal variations of leptin (an anorexigenic hormone principally secreted by fat cells) [79] and in increased subjective hunger on the morning that followed a night of sleep loss [80]. In 2003–2004, studies consistently found that two [92], six [91], or seven [90] nights of partial sleep restriction (4 h in bed per night) resulted in a decrease in circulating levels of leptin [90–92] and a concomitant increase in circulating levels of ghrelin (an orexigenic hormone mainly secreted by gastric cells) [92], together with an increase in hunger and appetite [92]. Around the same time, two epidemiological studies [110, 119] extended these findings to long-term sleep loss, showing an upregulation of appetite with chronic sleep loss, controlling for BMI. Altogether, these findings suggest that sleep restriction is likely to result in increased food consumption. In fact, more recently, an increase in caloric intake was observed after four nights of progressively increasing partial sleep curtailment [93], after five nights of 4-h bedtimes [96], and after one night of 4-h bedtimes [94]. In addition, 14 days of sleep restriction (5.5 h in bed per night) versus 14 days of sleep extension (8.5 h in bed per night) with ad libitum access to food resulted in an increased intake of calories from snacks [95]. Three of these studies [93, 95, 96] obtained measurements of resting and/or total energy expenditure and showed no change in energy need with sleep loss, indicating that sleep restriction results in energy intake in excess. Preliminary data obtained in normal [98] and in obese subjects [97] indicate that caloric intake during an ad libitum buffet was increased after sleep restriction. In a crossover study comparing 5.5 h in bed per night versus 8.5 h for 2 weeks in overweight subjects, moderate caloric restriction resulted in similar total weight loss in both conditions, but sleep restriction was associated with increased hunger, decreased loss of fat mass, and increased loss of fat free mass [99]. Recently, a population-based study in 1088 pairs of twins showed that longer sleep duration was associated with decreased BMI and that shorter sleep duration could increase expression of genetic risks for high body weight [120].

Sleep Disorders

Obstructive sleep apnea (OSA) is one of the most common sleep disorders involving reduced total sleep time, sleep fragmentation, and low levels of SWS. Its incidence is rising rapidly, in relation with the epidemic of obesity. Noteworthy, the prevalence of OSA in morbidly obese subjects is estimated at 50–98 % [121]. It was shown in the 1990s that nocturnal re-

lease of the two pituitary hormones whose secretion is markedly stimulated by sleep (GH and prolactin) is decreased in OSA [122–124]. GH secretion during the first few hours of sleep [122, 123] and the frequency of prolactin pulses [124] are partially restored under treatment with continuous positive airway pressure (CPAP). Years later, it was found that nocturnal luteinizing hormone (LH) and testosterone secretions were also decreased in OSA and partially corrected under CPAP treatment [125], and that adrenocorticotropic hormone (ACTH) and cortisol secretions were elevated in OSA and partially corrected by CPAP treatment [126, 127].

While obesity constitutes a major risk for OSA, OSA per se, independently of BMI, constitutes a risk for insulin resistance and therefore for diabetes: in 1993, a population-based study reported an association between snoring and abnormal glucose tolerance after adjustment for gender, BMI, physical activity, and alcohol and tobacco use [128], and a clinic-based study reported an association between the severity of OSA defined by polysomnography and insulin resistance [129]. In 1994, an improvement in insulin sensitivity was found in severely obese diabetic patients after 4 months of CPAP therapy [130]. Despite conflicting results (which can be due to differences in populations, selection of subjects, duration of therapy, variable compliance, etc.), there is now accumulating evidence suggesting that metabolic glucose abnormalities can be partially corrected under CPAP treatment, which is consistent with the concept of a causal link between OSA and altered glucose control (reviewed in [131, 132]).

Conclusions

Over the past 15 years, a large number of well-controlled studies have provided consistent evidence that partial sleep curtailment, a hallmark of modern society, increases the risk for obesity and diabetes. Given the morbidity and mortality associated with these diseases, the identification of novel potentially modifiable risk factors is particularly important. Future large field and interventional studies, incorporating objective measures of sleep duration and quality, should explore the potential benefits of sleep extension in short sleepers as a simple tool to reverse the adverse effects of sleep loss on diabetes and obesity risks.

References

1. Yalow RS, Berson SA. Assay of plasma insulin in human subjects by immunological methods. Nature. 1959; 184(Suppl 21):1648–9.
2. Yalow RS, Berson SA. Immunoassay of endogenous plasma insulin in man. J Clin Invest. 1960;39:1157–75.
3. Robin ED, Travis DM, Julian DG, et al. Metabolic patterns during physiologic sleep. I. Blood glucose regulation during sleep in normal and diabetic subjects. J Clin Invest. 1959;38:2229–33.

4. Quabbe HJ, Schilling E, Helge H. Pattern of growth hormone secretion during a 24-hour fast in normal adults. J Clin Endocrinol Metab. 1966;26:1173–7.

5. Honda Y, Takahashi K, Takahashi S, et al. Growth hormone secretion during nocturnal sleep in normal subjects. J Clin Endocrinol Metab. 1969;29:20–9.

6. Sassin JF, Parker DC, Johnson LC, et al. Effects of slow wave sleep deprivation on human growth hormone release in sleep: preliminary study. Life Sci. 1969;8:1299–307.

7. Sassin JF, Parker DC, Mace JW, et al. Human growth hormone release: relation to slow-wave sleep and sleep-walking cycles. Science. 1969;165:513–5.

8. Takahashi Y, Kipnis DM, Daughaday WH. Growth hormone secretion during sleep. J Clin Invest. 1968;47:2079–90.

9. Born J, Muth S, Fehm HL. The significance of sleep onset and slow wave sleep for nocturnal release of growth hormone (GH) and cortisol. Psychoneuroendocrinology. 1988;13:233–43.

10. Jarrett DB, Greenhouse JB, Miewald JM, et al. A reexamination of the relationship between growth hormone secretion and slow wave sleep using delta wave analysis. Biol Psychiatry. 1990;27:497–509.

11. Steiger A, Herth T, Holsboer F. Sleep-electroencephalography and the secretion of cortisol and growth hormone in normal controls. Acta Endocrinol (Copenh). 1987;116:36–42.

12. Holl RW, Hartman ML, Veldhuis JD, et al. Thirty-second sampling of plasma growth hormone in man: correlation with sleep stages. J Clin Endocrinol Metab. 1991;72:854–61.

13. Van Cauter E, Kerkhofs M, Caufriez A, et al. A quantitative estimation of growth hormone secretion in normal man: reproducibility and relation to sleep and time of day. J Clin Endocrinol Metab. 1992;74:1441–50.

14. Plat L, Van Cauter E. Differential effects of aging on human growth hormone and cortisol secretion during wake and during sleep in the course of aging. 77th Annual Meeting of the Endocrine Society. 1995;P 3:152.

15. Van Cauter E, Leproult R, Plat L. Age-related changes in slow wave sleep and REM sleep and relationship with growth hormone and cortisol levels in healthy men. JAMA. 2000;284:861–8.

16. Kerkhofs M, Van Cauter E, Van Onderbergen A, et al. Sleep-promoting effects of growth hormone-releasing hormone in normal men. Am J Physiol. 1993;264:E594–8.

17. Obal F, Jr., Payne L, Opp M, et al. Growth hormone-releasing hormone antibodies suppress sleep and prevent enhancement of sleep after sleep deprivation. Am J Physiol. 1992;263:R1078–85.

18. Obal F, Jr., Floyd R, Kapas L, et al. Effects of systemic GHRH on sleep in intact and hypophysectomized rats. Am J Physiol. 1996;270:E230–7.

19. Steiger A, Guldner J, Hemmeter U, et al. Effects of growth hormone-releasing hormone and somatostatin on sleep EEG and nocturnal hormone secretion in male controls. Neuroendocrinology. 1992;56:566–73.

20. Copinschi G, Nedeltcheva A, Leproult R, et al. Sleep disturbances, daytime sleepiness, and quality of life in adults with growth hormone deficiency. J Clin Endocrinol Metab. 2010;95:2195–202.

21. Ehlers CL, Reed TK, Henriksen SJ. Effects of corticotropin-releasing factor and growth hormone-releasing factor on sleep and activity in rats. Neuroendocrinology. 1986;42:467–74.

22. Obal F, Jr., Alfoldi P, Cady AB, et al. Growth hormone-releasing factor enhances sleep in rats and rabbits. Am J Physiol. 1988;255:R310–6.

23. Weitzman ED, Zimmerman JC, Czeisler CA, et al. Cortisol secretion is inhibited during sleep in normal man. J Clin Endocrinol Metab. 1983;56:352–8.

24. Van Cauter E, Desir D, Decoster C, et al. Nocturnal decrease in glucose tolerance during constant glucose infusion. J Clin Endocrinol Metab. 1989;69:604–11.

25. Obal F, Jr., Payne L, Kapas L, et al. Inhibition of growth hormone-releasing factor suppresses both sleep and growth hormone secretion in the rat. Brain Res. 1991;557:149–53.

26. Follenius M, Brandenberger G, Bandesapt JJ, et al. Nocturnal cortisol release in relation to sleep structure. Sleep. 1992;15:21–7.

27. Spath-Schwalbe E, Gofferje M, Kern W, et al. Sleep disruption alters nocturnal ACTH and cortisol secretory patterns. Biol Psychiatry. 1991;29:575–84.

28. Van Cauter E, van Coevorden A, Blackman JD. Modulation of neuroendocrine release by sleep and circadian rhythmicity. In: Yen S VW, editor. Advances in neuroendocrine regulation of reproduction. Norwell: Serono Symposia USA. 1990. p. 113–22.

29. Van Cauter E, Blackman JD, Roland D, et al. Modulation of glucose regulation and insulin secretion by circadian rhythmicity and sleep. J Clin Invest. 1991;88:934–42.

30. Simon C, Brandenberger G, Saini J, et al. Slow oscillations of plasma glucose and insulin secretion rate are amplified during sleep in humans under continuous enteral nutrition. Sleep. 1994;17:333–8.

31. Gronfier C, Luthringer R, Follenius M, et al. A quantitative evaluation of the relationships between growth hormone secretion and delta wave electroencephalographic activity during normal sleep and after enrichment in delta waves. Sleep. 1996;19:817–24.

32. Van Cauter E, Plat L, Scharf MB, et al. Simultaneous stimulation of slow-wave sleep and growth hormone secretion by gamma-hydroxybutyrate in normal young Men. J Clin Invest. 1997;100:745–53.

33. Chapotot F, Gronfier C, Jouny C, et al. Cortisol secretion is related to electroencephalographic alertness in human subjects during daytime wakefulness. J Clin Endocrinol Metab. 1998;83:4263–8.

34. Maquet P. Positron emission tomography studies of sleep and sleep disorders. J Neurol. 1997;244:S23–8.

35. Maquet P. Functional neuroimaging of normal human sleep by positron emission tomography. J Sleep Res. 2000;9:207–31.

36. Scheen AJ, Byrne MM, Plat L, et al. Relationships between sleep quality and glucose regulation in normal humans. Am J Physiol. 1996;271:E261–70.

37. DeFronzo RA. Pathogenesis of type 2 diabetes mellitus. Med Clin North Am. 2004;88:787–835, ix.

38. Magistretti PJ. Neuron-glia metabolic coupling and plasticity. J Exp Biol. 2006;209:2304–11.

39. Copinschi G, Turek FW, Van Cauter E. Endocrine rhythms, the sleep-wake cycle and biological clocks. In Jameson LJ, DeGroot LJ, editors. Endocrinology. 6th ed. Philadelphia: Elsevier-Saunders; 2010. p. 199–229.

40. Clore JN, Nestler JE, Blackard WG. Sleep-associated fall in glucose disposal and hepatic glucose output in normal humans. Putative signaling mechanism linking peripheral and hepatic events. Diabetes. 1989;38:285–90.

41. Garvey WT, Olefsky JM, Rubenstein AH, et al. Day-long integrated serum insulin and C-peptide profiles in patients with NIDDM. Correlation with urinary C-peptide excretion. Diabetes. 1988;37:590–9.

42. Kern W, Offenheuser S, Born J, et al. Entrainment of ultradian oscillations in the secretion of insulin and glucagon to the nonrapid eye movement/rapid eye movement sleep rhythm in humans. J Clin Endocrinol Metab. 1996;81:1541–7.

43. Levy I, Recasens A, Casamitjana R, et al. Nocturnal insulin and C-peptide rhythms in normal subjects. Diabetes Care. 1987;10:148–51.

44. Polonsky KS, Given BD, Van Cauter E. Twenty-four-hour profiles and pulsatile patterns of insulin secretion in normal and obese subjects. J Clin Invest. 1988;81:442–8.

45. Simon C, Brandenberger G, Follenius M. Absence of the dawn phenomenon in normal subjects. J Clin Endocrinol Metab. 1988;67:203–5.

46. Beihl DA, Liese AD, Haffner SM. Sleep duration as a risk factor for incident type 2 diabetes in a multiethnic cohort. Ann Epidemiol. 2009;19:351–7.

47. Buxton OM, Marcelli E. Short and long sleep are positively associated with obesity, diabetes, hypertension, and cardiovascular disease among adults in the United States. Soc Sci Med. 2010;71:1027–36.

48. Chaput JP, Despres JP, Bouchard C, et al. Association of sleep duration with type 2 diabetes and impaired glucose tolerance. Diabetologia. 2007;50:2298–304.

49. Gottlieb DJ, Punjabi NM, Newman AB, et al. Association of sleep time with diabetes mellitus and impaired glucose tolerance. Arch Intern Med. 2005;165:863–7.

50. Kim J, Kim HM, Kim KM, et al. The association of sleep duration and type 2 diabetes in Korean male adults with abdominal obesity: the Korean National Health and Nutrition Examination Survey 2005. Diabetes Res Clin Pract. 2009;86:e34–6.

51. Knutson KL, Ryden AM, Mander BA, et al. Role of sleep duration and quality in the risk and severity of type 2 diabetes mellitus. Arch Intern Med. 2006;166:1768–74.

52. Nakajima H, Kaneita Y, Yokoyama E, et al. Association between sleep duration and hemoglobin A1c level. Sleep Med. 2008;9:745–52.

53. Shankar A, Syamala S, Kalidindi S. Insufficient rest or sleep and its relation to cardiovascular disease, diabetes and obesity in a national, multiethnic sample. PLoS ONE. 2010;5:e14189.

54. Zizi F, Pandey A, Murrray-Bachmann R, et al. Race/ethnicity, sleep duration, and diabetes mellitus: analysis of the National Health Interview Survey. Am J Med. 2012;125:162–7.

55. Ayas NT, White DP, Al-Delaimy WK, et al. A prospective study of self-reported sleep duration and incident diabetes in women. Diabetes Care. 2003;26:380–4.

56. Bjorkelund C, Bondyr-Carlsson D, Lapidus L, et al. Sleep disturbances in midlife unrelated to 32-year diabetes incidence: the prospective population study of women in Gothenburg. Diabetes Care. 2005;28:2739–44.

57. Chaput JP, Despres JP, Bouchard C, et al. Sleep duration as a risk factor for the development of type 2 diabetes or impaired glucose tolerance: analyses of the Quebec Family Study. Sleep Med. 2009;10:919–24.

58. Gangwisch JE, Heymsfield SB, Boden-Albala B, et al. Sleep duration as a risk factor for diabetes incidence in a large U.S. sample. Sleep. 2007;30:1667–73.

59. Hayashino Y, Fukuhara S, Suzukamo Y, et al. Relation between sleep quality and quantity, quality of life, and risk of developing diabetes in healthy workers in Japan: the high-risk and population strategy for occupational health promotion (HIPOP-OHP) study. BMC Public Health. 2007;7:129.

60. Kawakami N, Takatsuka N, Shimizu H. Sleep disturbance and onset of type 2 diabetes. Diabetes Care. 2004;27:282–3.

61. Mallon L, Broman JE, Hetta J. High incidence of diabetes in men with sleep complaints or short sleep duration: a 12-year follow-up study of a middle-aged population. Diabetes Care. 2005;28:2762–7.

62. Meisinger C, Heier M, Loewel H. Sleep disturbance as a predictor of type 2 diabetes mellitus in men and women from the general population. Diabetologia. 2005;48:235–41.

63. Nilsson PM, Roost M, Engstrom G, et al. Incidence of diabetes in middle-aged men is related to sleep disturbances. Diabetes Care. 2004;27:2464–9.

64. Xu Q, Song Y, Hollenbeck A, et al. Day napping and short night sleeping are associated with higher risk of diabetes in older adults. Diabetes Care. 2010;33:78–83.

65. Yaggi HK, Araujo AB, McKinlay JB. Sleep duration as a risk factor for the development of type 2 diabetes. Diabetes Care. 2006;29:657–61.

66. Cappuccio FP, D'Elia L, Strazzullo P, et al. Quantity and quality of sleep and incidence of type 2 diabetes: a systematic review and meta-analysis. Diabetes Care. 2010;33:414–20.

67. Chaput JP, Despres JP, Bouchard C, et al. The association between sleep duration and weight gain in adults: a 6-year prospective study from the Quebec family study. Sleep. 2008;31:517–23.

68. Chaput JP, Leblanc C, Perusse L, et al. Risk factors for adult overweight and obesity in the Quebec family study: have we been barking up the wrong tree? Obesity (Silver Spring). 2009;17:1964–70.

69. Gunderson EP, Rifas-Shiman SL, Oken E, et al. Association of fewer hours of sleep at 6 months postpartum with substantial weight retention at 1 year postpartum. Am J Epidemiol. 2008;167:178–87.

70. Hairston KG, Bryer-Ash M, Norris JM, et al. Sleep duration and five-year abdominal fat accumulation in a minority cohort: the IRAS family study. Sleep. 2010;33:289–95.

71. Hasler G, Buysse DJ, Klaghofer R, et al. The association between short sleep duration and obesity in young adults: a 13-year prospective study. Sleep. 2004;27:661–6.

72. Nishiura C, Noguchi J, Hashimoto H. Dietary patterns only partially explain the effect of short sleep duration on the incidence of obesity. Sleep. 2010;33:753–7.

73. Patel SR, Malhotra A, White DP, et al. Association between reduced sleep and weight gain in women. Am J Epidemiol. 2006;164:947–54.

74. Benedict C, Hallschmid M, Lassen A, et al. Acute sleep deprivation reduces energy expenditure in healthy men. Am J Clin Nutr. 2011;93:1229–36.

75. Vondra K, Brodan V, Bass A, et al. Effects of sleep deprivation on the activity of selected metabolic enzymes in skeletal muscle. Eur J Appl Physiol Occup Physiol. 1981;47:41–6.

76. VanHelder T, Symons JD, Radomski MW. Effects of sleep deprivation and exercise on glucose tolerance. Aviat Space Environ Med. 1993;64:487–92.

77. Gonzalez-Ortiz M, Martinez-Abundis E, Balcazar-Munoz BR, et al. Effect of sleep deprivation on insulin sensitivity and cortisol concentration in healthy subjects. Diabetes Nutr Metab. 2000;13:80–3.

78. Kuhn E, Brodan V, Brodanova M, et al. Metabolic reflection of sleep deprivation. Act Nerv Super (Praha). 1969;11:165–74.

79. Mullington JM, Chan JL, Van Dongen HP, et al. Sleep loss reduces diurnal rhythm amplitude of leptin in healthy men. J Neuroendocrinol. 2003;15:851–4.

80. Schmid SM, Hallschmid M, Jauch-Chara K, et al. Sleep loss alters basal metabolic hormone secretion and modulates the dynamic counterregulatory response to hypoglycemia. J Clin Endocrinol Metab. 2007;92:3044–51.

81. Spiegel K, Leproult R, Van Cauter E. Impact of sleep debt on metabolic and endocrine function. Lancet. 1999;354:1435–9.

82. Buxton OM, Pavlova M, Reid EW, et al. Sleep restriction for 1 week reduces insulin sensitivity in healthy men. Diabetes. 2010;59:2126–33.

83. Darukhanavala A, Booth JN, 3rd, Bromley L, et al. Changes in insulin secretion and action in adults with familial risk for type 2 diabetes who curtail their sleep. Diabetes Care. 2011;34:2259–64.

84. Donga E, van Dijk M, van Dijk JG, et al. A single night of partial sleep deprivation induces insulin resistance in multiple metabolic pathways in healthy subjects. J Clin Endocrinol Metab. 2010;95:2963–8.

85. Leproult R, Van Cauter E. Marked decreased insulin sensitivity and increased evening cortisol levels following one week of partial sleep deprivation. 12th meeting of the European NeuroEndocrine Association (ENEA); 2006; Athens, Greece.

86. Nedeltcheva AV, Kessler L, Imperial J, et al. Exposure to recurrent sleep restriction in the setting of high caloric intake and physical inactivity results in increased insulin resistance and reduced glucose tolerance. J Clin Endocrinol Metab. 2009;94:3242–50.

87. Schmid SM, Hallschmid M, Jauch-Chara K, et al. Disturbed glucoregulatory response to food intake after moderate sleep restriction. Sleep. 2011;34:371–7.

88. Spiegel K, Knutson K, Leproult R, et al. Sleep loss: a novel risk factor for insulin resistance and Type 2 diabetes. J Appl Physiol. 2005;99:2008–19.

89. van Leeuwen WM, Hublin C, Sallinen M, et al. Prolonged sleep restriction affects glucose metabolism in healthy young men. Int J Endocrinol. 2010;2010:108641.

90. Guilleminault C, Powell NB, Martinez S, et al. Preliminary observations on the effects of sleep time in a sleep restriction paradigm. Sleep Med. 2003;4:177–84.

91. Spiegel K, Leproult R, L'Hermite-Baleriaux M, et al. Leptin levels are dependent on sleep duration: relationships with sympathovagal balance, carbohydrate regulation, cortisol, and thyrotropin. J Clin Endocrinol Metab. 2004;89:5762–71.

92. Spiegel K, Tasali E, Penev P, et al. Brief communication: sleep curtailment in healthy young men is associated with decreased leptin levels, elevated ghrelin levels, and increased hunger and appetite. Ann Intern Med. 2004;141:846–50.

93. Bosy-Westphal A, Hinrichs S, Jauch-Chara K, et al. Influence of partial sleep deprivation on energy balance and insulin sensitivity in healthy women. Obes Facts. 2008;1:266–73.

94. Brondel L, Romer MA, Nougues PM, et al. Acute partial sleep deprivation increases food intake in healthy men. Am J Clin Nutr. 2010;91:1550–9.

95. Nedeltcheva AV, Kilkus JM, Imperial J, et al. Sleep curtailment is accompanied by increased intake of calories from snacks. Am J Clin Nutr. 2009;89:126–33.

96. St-Onge MP, Roberts AL, Chen J, et al. Short sleep duration increases energy intakes but does not change energy expenditure in normal-weight individuals. Am J Clin Nutr. 2011;94:410–6.

97. Morselli LL, Balbo M, Van Cauter E, et al. Impact of sleep restriction on the regulation of appetite in middle-aged obese subjects. 4th International World Sleep Congress; 2011. Quebec, Canada; 2011.

98. Tasali E, Broussard J, Day A, et al. Sleep curtailment in healthy young adults is associated with increased ad lib food intake. 23rd Annual Meeting of the Associated Professional Sleep Societies; Seattle, WA, USA. Sleep; 2009. p. Abstract 394.

99. Nedeltcheva AV, Kilkus JM, Imperial J, et al. Insufficient sleep undermines dietary efforts to reduce adiposity. Ann Intern Med. 2010;153:435–41.

100. Tasali E, Leproult R, Ehrmann DA, et al. Slow-wave sleep and the risk of type 2 diabetes in humans. Proc Natl Acad Sci U S A. 2008;105:1044–9.

101. Stamatakis KA, Punjabi NM. Effects of sleep fragmentation on glucose metabolism in normal subjects. Chest. 2010;137:95–101.

102. Wehrens SM, Hampton SM, Finn RE, et al. Effect of total sleep deprivation on postprandial metabolic and insulin responses in shift workers and non-shift workers. J Endocrinol. 2010;206:205–15.

103. Spiegel K, Leproult R, Colecchia EF, et al. Adaptation of the 24-h growth hormone profile to a state of sleep debt. Am J Physiol Regul Integr Comp Physiol. 2000;279:R874–83.

104. Zielinski MR, Kline CE, Kripke DF, et al. No effect of 8-week time in bed restriction on glucose tolerance in older long sleepers. J Sleep Res. 2008;17:412–9.

105. Knutson KL, Leproult R. Apples to oranges: comparing long sleep to short sleep. J Sleep Res. 2010;19:118.

106. Kripke DF, Garfinkel L, Wingard DL, et al. Mortality associated with sleep duration and insomnia. Arch Gen Psychiatry. 2002;59:131–6.

107. Patel SR, Ayas NT, Malhotra MR, et al. A prospective study of sleep duration and mortality risk in women. Sleep. 2004;27:440–4.

108. Shigeta H, Shigeta M, Nakazawa A, et al. Lifestyle, obesity, and insulin resistance. Diabetes Care. 2001;24:608.

109. Singh M, Drake CL, Roehrs T, et al. The association between obesity and short sleep duration: a population-based study. J Clin Sleep Med. 2005;1:357–63.

110. Taheri S, Lin L, Austin D, et al. Short sleep duration is associated with reduced leptin, elevated ghrelin, and increased body mass index. PLoS Med. 2004;1:e62.

111. Vioque J, Torres A, Quiles J. Time spent watching television, sleep duration and obesity in adults living in Valencia, Spain. Int J Obes Relat Metab Disord. 2000;24:1683–8.

112. Vorona RD, Winn MP, Babineau TW, et al. Overweight and obese patients in a primary care population report less sleep than patients with a normal body mass index. Arch Intern Med. 2005;165:25–30.

113. Cappuccio FP, Taggart FM, Kandala NB, et al. Meta-analysis of short sleep duration and obesity in children and adults. Sleep. 2008;31:619–26.

114. Lauderdale DS, Knutson KL, Rathouz PJ, et al. Cross-sectional and longitudinal associations between objectively measured sleep duration and body mass index: the CARDIA Sleep study. Am J Epidemiol. 2009;170:805–13.

115. van den Berg JF, Knvistingh Neven A, Tulen JH, et al. Actigraphic sleep duration and fragmentation are related to obesity in the elderly: the Rotterdam study. Int J Obes (Lond). 2008;32:1083–90.

116. Patel SR, Blackwell T, Redline S, et al. The association between sleep duration and obesity in older adults. Int J Obes (Lond). 2008;32:1825–34.

117. Rao MN, Blackwell T, Redline S, et al. Association between sleep architecture and measures of body composition. Sleep. 2009;32:483–90.

118. Stranges S, Cappuccio FP, Kandala NB, et al. Cross-sectional versus prospective associations of sleep duration with changes in relative weight and body fat distribution: the Whitehall II Study. Am J Epidemiol. 2008;167:321–9.

119. Chaput JP, Despres JP, Bouchard C, et al. Short sleep duration is associated with reduced leptin levels and increased adiposity: results from the Quebec family study. Obesity (Silver Spring). 2007;15:253–61.

120. Watson NF, Harden KP, Buchwald D, et al. Sleep duration and body mass index in twins: a gene-environment interaction. Sleep. 2012;35:597–603.

121. Sanders M. Sleep breathing disorders. In: Kryger M, Roth T, Dement WC, editors. Principles and practice of sleep medicine. Philadelphia: Saunders; 2005. p. 969–1157.

122. Cooper BG, White JE, Ashworth LA, et al. Hormonal and metabolic profiles in subjects with obstructive sleep apnea syndrome and the acute effects of nasal continuous positive airway pressure (CPAP) treatment. Sleep. 1995;18:172–9.

123. Saini J, Krieger J, Brandenberger G, et al. Continuous positive airway pressure treatment. Effects on growth hormone, insulin and glucose profiles in obstructive sleep apnea patients. Horm Metab Res. 1993;25:375–81.

124. Spiegel K, Follenius M, Krieger J, et al. Prolactin secretion during sleep in obstructive sleep apnoea patients. J Sleep Res. 1995;4:56–62.

125. Luboshitzky R, Lavie L, Shen-Orr Z, et al. Pituitary-gonadal function in men with obstructive sleep apnea. The effect of continuous positive airways pressure treatment. Neuro Endocrinol Lett. 2003;24:463–7.

126. Henley DE, Russell GM, Douthwaite JA, et al. Hypothalamic-pituitary-adrenal axis activation in obstructive sleep apnea: the effect of continuous positive airway pressure therapy. J Clin Endocrinol Metab. 2009;94:4234–42.

127. Vgontzas AN, Pejovic S, Zoumakis E, et al. Hypothalamic-pituitary-adrenal axis activity in obese men with and without sleep apnea: effects of continuous positive airway pressure therapy. J Clin Endocrinol Metab. 2007;92:4199–207.

128. Jennum P, Schultz-Larsen K, Christensen N. Snoring, sympathetic activity and cardiovascular risk factors in a 70 year old population. Eur J Epidemiol. 1993;9:477–82.

129. Tiihonen M, Partinen M, Narvanen S. The severity of obstructive sleep apnoea is associated with insulin resistance. J Sleep Res. 1993;2:56–61.

130. Brooks B, Cistulli PA, Borkman M, et al. Obstructive sleep apnea in obese noninsulin-dependent diabetic patients: effect of continuous positive airway pressure treatment on insulin responsiveness. J Clin Endocrinol Metab. 1994;79:1681–5.

131. Morselli LL, Guyon A, Spiegel K. Sleep and metabolic function. Pflugers Arch. 2012;463:139–60.

132. Tasali E, Mokhlesi B, Van Cauter E. Obstructive sleep apnea and type 2 diabetes: interacting epidemics. Chest. 2008;133:496–506.

M.E. Estep and W.C. Orr

List of Abbreviations

ANS	Autonomic nervous system
CNS	Central nervous system
DU	Duodenal ulcer
EMG	Electromyography
GER	Gastroesophageal reflux
GERD	Gastroesophageal reflux disease
GI	Gastrointestinal
H2R	Histamine receptor
IBS	Irritable bowel syndrome
LES	Lower esophageal sphincter
MMC	Migrating motor complex
PSG	Polysomnography
REM	Rapid eye movement

Acid-Related Diseases

Gastric Acid Secretion

The earliest studies of gastric acid and its digestive function were carried out by Dr. William Beaumont around 1830. Dr. Beaumont was a US Army surgeon who attended Alexis St. Martin, who sustained an accidental shotgun wound to the abdomen. St. Martin developed a gastric fistula through which Dr. Beaumont studied the effects of gastric acid on food. Dr. Beaumont's observations led to the important discovery that stomach acid was essential for digestion. Dr. Beaumont also observed the relationship between gastric function and emotional state as the gastric mucosa would become engorged with blood in relation to St. Martin being upset or stressed [1]. Almost a century later, Johnston and Washeim [2] stud-

M. Estep (✉) · W. Orr
Lynn Health Science Institute, 3555 NW 58th, Ste. 800,
Oklahoma City, OK 73112-4703, USA
e-mail: mestep@lhsi.net

W. C. Orr
e-mail: worr@lhsi.net

ied gastric acid secretion during sleep in normal subjects and described a rise in acidity, decrease in volume, and delayed gastric emptying. Later studies of the circadian rhythm of gastric acid secretion in healthy subjects indicated a peak in acid secretion between 10 p.m. and 2 a.m., and minimal acid secretion during wake time [3, 4]. These studies established that gastric acid secretion was very labile and altered not only by emotional state but also by state of consciousness and time of day. These observations laid the groundwork for our understanding of the pathogenesis of gastroesophageal reflux disease (GERD) and duodenal ulcer (DU) disease.

DU and Vagotomy

Prior to the discovery of the important role of *Helicobacter pylori* in the pathogenesis of DU disease, it was felt to be purely an acid-related disease and the healing of DU was felt to be closely related to the suppression of gastric acid secretion [5, 6, 7, 8]. The differential diagnosis and treatment of DU disease was detailed by Moynihan [9], noting that many patients had symptoms of nocturnal abdominal pain which were alleviated by food. The red stippling indicative of a DU was noted by Scudder in 1914 [10]. The stimulus for acid production is related to acid production secondary to vagal nerve stimulation. Vagotomy, or vagal sectioning, was introduced by Dragstedt in the late 1940s as an effective strategy for treating chronic DU disease theoretically caused by excessive vagal stimulation. Initially, the procedure was believed to reduce nocturnal secretion of gastric acid, which is generally elevated [11, 12, 13, 14] in DU patients. This is most likely due to a larger parietal cell mass, producing a larger acid output response to stimuli that provoke gastric secretion. Thus, the greater resting secretion in patients with DU compared to controls is thought to be caused by a normal basal drive acting upon a larger number of normally sensitive parietal cells [15, 16].

Other investigators were not able to support Dragstedt's reasoning that vagotomy reduces basal secretions; instead, it was revealed that the procedure reduces histamine-stimulated secretion [17, 18, 19, 20]. A mechanism whereby vagotomy reduces histamine-stimulated gastric secretion has yet to be fully detailed, although multiple hypotheses have been offered for a sensitization phenomenon [21, 22] or the presence of more than one type of parietal cell responding to either histamine only, or both histamine and insulin (i.e., vagal) stimulation [23]. Nevertheless, Dragstedt's vagotomy initiated decades of careful study of gastric secretory physiology and its effect on the etiology of ulcers, resulting in the notion that vagotomy reduces stimulated gastric secretion, predominately at night, allowing DU to heal.

Esophagitis and Nighttime Heartburn

In 1935, Winkelstein described the clinical entity of esophageal ulcers caused by gastric acid in patients with symptoms of substernal pain and heartburn [24]. Regurgitation of "peptic juice and its stagnation" [25] was demonstrated as the cause for esophagitis in the absence of comorbidities [25]. Subsequent observations have demonstrated that the condition of esophagitis is much more complex than a simple occurrence of acid contact with the esophageal mucosa. The pattern of esophageal acid contact has now been shown to be markedly different during the daytime compared to that during sleep. For example, as early as 1955 Lodge [26] commented on the importance of recumbency in the development of esophagitis.

The notion that sleep-related GER played a role in the development of esophagitis and other complications of GER emerged in the 1970s by the pioneering work of Johnson and DeMeester [27, 28]. Their work, which incorporated the new technology of 24-h esophageal pH monitoring, encouraged further investigation of the effect of sleep on GER and acid contact time. Indeed, these investigators noted that episodes of reflux occurring in the upright position, presumably during the waking state, are rapidly cleared. Episodes of reflux occurring in the recumbent position, presumably during sleep, are associated with markedly prolonged acid clearance. These studies effectively demonstrated the link between prolongation of acid clearance during the sleeping interval and the occurrence of esophagitis [27, 28]. During the same time period, Atkinson and Van Gelder [29] correlated the severity of esophagitis with the duration of nocturnal periods of high esophageal acidity. Collectively, these studies suggested that acid clearance is prolonged during sleep; however, none monitored sleep via polysomnography (PSG) and thus could not confirm this notion.

Orr and colleagues [30] conducted the first PSG study on patients with esophagitis and confirmed that acid clearance from the distal esophagus is prolonged during sleep in both healthy participants and patients with esophagitis, but more so in the esophagitis group. They also provided the additional insight that acid clearance is dependent on a brief awakening from sleep. Thus, patients who reflux during sleep were at greater risk to develop esophagitis [30, 31]. A later study by Robertson and colleagues [32] in which patients were monitored with a 24-h pH probe demonstrated that patients with complications of esophagitis have more severe acid reflux than patients with simple uncomplicated disease, and they concluded that this was likely due to prolonged periods of nighttime acid reflux. With this deeper understanding of the significance of prolonged acid contact time during sleep and its more complicated disease progression, a need for clinically differentiating sleep-related reflux and nighttime heartburn from daytime heartburn has become apparent.

Recognizing nighttime heartburn and associated sleep-related GER as a distinct clinical entity has been suggested in a recent review [33]. Data are reviewed to support the notion that recognizing the presence of nighttime heartburn encourages differential diagnosis and treatment options for GERD patients. Nighttime heartburn and sleep-related GER are considered a distinct clinical entity due to several factors reviewed by Orr [33] including: sleep-related GER is associated with prolonged acid mucosal contact which promotes mucosal injury, patients with nighttime heartburn are at greater risk of developing esophagitis, patients with nighttime heartburn have a higher incidence of extra-esophageal symptoms such as chest pain and cough, and patients with nighttime heartburn have significantly poorer quality of life. Two epidemiological studies have provided similar data which suggest that nighttime heartburn is a more serious and significant manifestation of GER compared to daytime heartburn [34, 35]. Furthermore, the majority of patients with nighttime heartburn (approximately 70 % in both studies) indicated that this symptom disrupted their sleep. Transient lower esophageal sphincter (LES) relaxation is frequently accompanied by GER and occurs postprandially in the daytime and in relation to brief or extended arousals from sleep in the nighttime [36, 37, 38]. Reflux events are less frequent during sleep likely due to inhibition of transient LES relaxation during deep sleep; however, they are typically associated with a marked prolongation in acid clearance [39, 40].

Responses to acid mucosal contact are quite different during sleep compared to responses measured during the waking state. Normal acid mucosal contact produces the waking sensation of heartburn, enhances salivary flow and bicarbonate concentration, and stimulates a higher frequency of swallowing [41]. These responses prevent prolonged acid mucosal contact by effectively removing the refluxate from the distal esophagus and neutralizing the mucosa. However, these responses are suppressed during sleep, resulting in prolonged acid mucosal contact [30, 31]. The subsequent back diffusion of hydrogen ions into the esophageal mucosa is related to the duration of acid mucosal contact [42]. Prolonged acid contact with the esophageal mucosa disrupts the normal barrier to the submucosa by increasing intercellular spaces allowing easier access of hydrogen ions [43, 44]. Thus, the longer reflux episodes noted during sleep carry a greater risk of producing mucosal damage compared to the more rapidly cleared reflux episodes during the waking state. Furthermore, one night of sleep deprivation has been shown to be hyperalgesic in patients with GERD [45]. Sleep-related acid contact time is a critical factor in the pathogenesis of the complications of GER including esophagitis, hiatal hernia, and other respiratory complications [46, 47]. Thus, clinicians may find it useful to assess symptoms of nighttime heartburn in differentiating patients who have a more serious form of GERD and experience more daytime sleepiness and a decline in work productivity [34, 35, 48, 49].

Significance of Nighttime Acid Suppression

The discovery of the important role of *Helicobacter pylori* in the pathogenesis of ulcer disease has markedly changed the treatment of DU disease. However, acid production remains an important factor in the pathogenesis of DU and suppressing acid secretion remains important in the treatment of DU. Historically, vagotomy is credited with eliminating acid reflux for symptomatic relief of ulcers and the subsequent healing [5]. A nonsurgical approach was introduced in the 1970s utilizing histamine receptor (H2R) antagonists to suppress acid secretion [50]. Research in healthy volunteers indicated H2R antagonists inhibited gastric acid secretion [51–53]. Subsequent studies measured gastric secretion volume, pH, and hydrogen-ion concentration in 30-min intervals in patients with DU. A profound inhibition of nocturnal acid secretion was observed in patients with DU given H2R antagonists [54, 55]. Multiple daily doses versus a single bedtime dose of H2R antagonists have indicated the latter to be at least as good as the former in DU healing rates [56, 57, 58]. Maintaining a modest degree of nocturnal acid suppression alone has been shown to prevent the recurrence of DU disease [59]. Ulcers were found to heal and remain dormant with continued use of H2R antagonists, and as a result of this research, nocturnal acid secretion was thought to play a dominant role in the pathogenesis of DU.

Colonic Motility

Colonic Function During Sleep

Fluoroscopic observation was the initial mode for monitoring gastrointestinal (GI) tract motility. Using this noninva-

sive method, Cannon [60] described repetitive constricting activity of the small intestine as "rhythmic segmentation of the intestinal contents" observed in the cat. In order to directly observe intestinal motility, an operation exposing a section of the intact intestine became popular and revealed a wide variation of intestinal activity across different dogs and within the same dog across different days [61]. Results from the indirect and direct methods were in agreement that sleep did not appear to have any effect on intestinal motility. This notion was supported by fluoroscopic observation of the exteriorized human intestine presenting no change in intestinal movement during sleep [62]. Decades later, electronic measuring and recording techniques revealed inconsistent findings with the regard to sleep-related changes in intestinal motility. Specific duodenal recordings in humans during sleep indicated no change in one study [63], while a decrease or an increase in motility were noted during sleep in other studies [64, 65, 66]. Possibly contributing to the conflicting results is that none of these studies used PSG to monitor sleep.

Characterizing intestinal motility using advanced telemetry or electrodes in conjunction with PSG yielded a more comprehensive description of intestinal motor activity in general, and more specifically, during sleep. Electromyographic (EMG) recording of duodenal muscle activity during the various stages of sleep revealed an inhibition of duodenal EMG activity associated with rapid eye movement (REM) sleep and an increase in activity with changes from one sleep phase to another [67]. Deep sleep is associated with decreased motility compared to light sleep, and the motility index for REM sleep is similar to that of light sleep [68], similar to the findings of Tassinari and colleagues [69], who had demonstrated stage 1 sleep to have more duodenal contractions compared to the stages 2, 3, 4, and REM. An overall greater motility found during REM sleep compared to deep sleep resembles the motility of the esophagus [70], stomach [71], and colon [72].

Cyclic motor activity, referred to as the migrating motor complex (MMC), has been observed in human GI tract in the fasting state with a periodicity of 90 min that is significantly altered during sleep compared to wake [73, 74, 75, 76]. These studies found an overall decreased velocity of the MMC and, specifically, phase II (i.e., the phase of irregular contractions) of the MMC to be diminished at night. The physiological significance of the MMC is related to propulsion of intraluminal contents and intestinal absorption of nutrients [77]. Because the human REM/non-REM sleep cycle also has a periodicity of 90 min, hypotheses of the MMC and REM/non-REM cycles being linked initiated several investigations. Finch and colleagues [78] recorded fasting gastroduodenal motility and electroencephalography of nine healthy subjects over 41 nights and concluded the MMC and sleep cycles were linked. However, subsequent studies did not find a correlation between sleep stages and MMC cycling [68, 73, 74, 79], thus providing support for the notion that the MMC cycle is separately regulated by the peripheral enteric nervous system [80, 81], whereas sleep cycling is modulated within the central nervous system (CNS). These studies confirmed that sleep does indeed influence the GI motility, but further research is needed to confirm the details of exactly how intestinal motility is modulated by sleep.

Irritable Bowel Syndrome

Irritable bowel syndrome (IBS) is a functional disorder of intestinal motility [82] which affects women considerably more frequently than men. The definition of IBS relates to three distinguishing characteristics: intermittent abdominal pain, altered bowel habit (constipation or diarrhea), and no obvious organic cause. In the absence of organic abdominal disease, IBS is characterized by abdominal distension and pain, relief of pain with a bowel movement, more frequent and looser stools at the onset of pain, the presence of mucus in the stool, and feelings of incomplete evacuation [83]. Miniature pressure transducers allow for long-term manometric recording in an ambulatory patient including during sleep in order to identify abnormal bowel motility [84, 85]. Striking differences in small bowel motor activity have been observed between waking and sleeping in healthy individuals. A marked increase in contractility recorded in the daytime is notably absent during sleep. Comparatively, patients with IBS experience pain accompanied by propulsive clusters of small bowel contractions with short MMC intervals during the day, and normal MMC propagation velocity during sleep [84, 86]. Although abnormalities associated with IBS are confined to the waking state, sleep disturbances are frequently reported in IBS patients. Nonspecific symptoms of insomnia, nonrestorative sleep, and fatigue have been reported in women with IBS symptoms [87, 88]. This population also reports significantly more awakenings. compared to controls and has been noted to have a significantly longer REM onset latency compared to controls [89, 87, 88]; and it has been reported that poor sleep is associated with subsequent daytimne pain [39]. however, these results have not been confirmed by other studies [78, 90]. Disturbed sleep in IBS patients could also play a role in lowering the visceral sensory threshold similar to the findings of Schey and colleagues [45] in which esophageal hyperalgesia was documented in GERD patients after one night of sleep deprivation.

Although cycling of the MMC has been demonstrated as independent of the REM/non-REM sleep cycle in healthy individuals and IBS patients, Gorard and colleagues [68] hypothesized that a CNS withdrawal during sleep, instead of an independent circadian variation of motility, occurs to differentiate the two biorhythms. Indeed, increased sympathetic nervous system activity among IBS patients was documented in a study of catecholamine and cortisol levels as measures of physiological arousal [91]. In one of very few studies in which PSG data were collected, Kumar and colleagues [79] examined the relationship between PSG sleep patterns and intestinal motility in IBS and controls, documenting subjects with IBS had significantly more REM sleep than the controls. Notably, this increase resulted from prolonged REM episodes rather than an increase in the number of REM episodes or REM latency [79].

Autonomic abnormalities associated with sleep have been highlighted by a study by Heitkemper and colleagues [87] demonstrating significantly lower levels of vagal tone during the sleeping interval in women with IBS compared to women without IBS. Prior to this study, autonomic abnormalities were documented by patient subgroup. Decreased vagal tone (i.e., cholinergic abnormality) was characteristic of patients experiencing constipation-predominant IBS symptoms, whereas patients experiencing diarrhea-predominant IBS symptoms had sympathetic adrenergic dysfunction [92]. Following these observations, Orr and colleagues [93] coupled PSG and autonomic monitoring in IBS patients with alternating symptoms subgroups (i.e., diarrhea- and constipation-predominant patients) to reveal differences in autonomic functioning during sleep. Greater sympathetic activity during wake and greater overall sympathetic dominance during REM sleep was found in patients with IBS. Taken together, these studies support the notion of altered autonomic nervous system activation subserving the pathophysiology of IBS, thus sensitizing the gut to waking stimulation in patients with IBS [93].

Conclusions

Sleep is associated with substantial changes in GI functioning, which has considerable clinical relevance. Acid secretion during sleep and its inhibition plays an important role in the pathogenesis of DU and its effective treatment. Sleep-related GER is now accepted as an important, if not the most important, phenomenon in the pathophysiology of reflux esophagitis. GI motility not only differs between waking and sleeping states but also during REM and non-REM stages of sleep. Further research is needed to better understand the effects of sleep on GI motility and, in turn, effects of functional disorders of GI motility on sleep. This chapter has provided historical and modern evidence-based reasons for gastroenterologists to address sleep symptoms as well as sleep-related changes in physiological functioning, which may have considerable relevance to the pathophysiology of GI diseases.

References

1. Beaumont W. Experiments and observations on the gastric juice and the physiology of digestion. Edinburgh: Maclachlan and Stewart; 1838.
2. Johnstone AS. Peptic ulceration of the oesophagus with partial thoracic stomach. Br J Radiol. 1943;16:357–61.
3. Milton-Thompson GJ, Williams JG, Jenkins DJA, Misiewicz JJ. Inhibition of nocturnal acid secretion in duodenal ulcer by one oral dose of metiamide. Lancet. 1974;1:693–4.
4. Roxburgh JC, Whitfield P, Hobsley M. Parietal cell sensitivity in man: control and duodenal ulcer subjects, smokers and nonsmokers. Europ J Gastroenterol Hepatol. 1994;6:235–40.
5. Card WI, Marks IN. The relationship between the acid output of the stomach following "maximal" histamine stimulation and the parietal cell mass. Clin Sci. 1960;19:147–63.
6. Johnson LF, DeMeester TR, Haggitt RC. Esophageal epithelial response to gastroesophageal reflux, a quantitative study. Am J Dig Dis. 1978;23:498–509.
7. Penzel T, Becker HF, Brandenburg U, Labunski T, Pankow W, Peter JH. Arousal in patients with gastro-oesophageal reflux and sleep apnoea. Eur Respir J. 1999;14:1266–70.
8. Winkelstein A. Peptic esophagitis: new clinical entity. J Am Med Assoc. 1935;104:906–9.
9. Moore JG, Englert E. Circadian rhythm of gastric acid secretion in man. Nature. 1970;226:1261–2.
10. Schey R, Dickman R, Parthasarathy S, Quan SF, Wendel C, Merchant J, et al. Sleep deprivation is hyperalgesic in patients with gastroesophageal reflux disease. Gastroenterol. 2007;133:1787–95.
11. Amdurup E, Jensen H-E. Selective vagotomy of the parietal cell mass preserving innervation of the undrained antrum. Gastroenterology. 1970;59:522–7.
12. Dent J, Dodds WJ, Friedman RH, Sekiguchi T, Hogan WJ, Arndorfer RC, et al. Mechanism of gastroesophageal reflux in recumbent asymptomatic human subjects. J Clin Invest. 1980;65:256–67.
13. Dragstedt LR. Section of vagus nerves to the stomach in the treatment of peptic ulcer. Surgery. 1947;21:144.
14. Faber RG, Hobsley M. Basal gastric secretion: reproducibility and relationships with duodenal ulcers. Gut. 1977;18:57–63.
15. Hobsley M. Pyloric Reflux: a modification of the two-component hypothesis of gastric secretion. Clin Sci Mol Med. 1974; 47:131–41.
16. Robertson D, Aldersley M, Shepherd H, Smith CL. Patterns of acid reflux in complicated oesophagitis. Gut. 1987;28:1484–1488.
17. Dubois RW, Aguilar D, Fass R, Orr WC, Elfant AB, Dean BB, et al. Consequences of frequent nocturnal gastro-oesophageal reflux disease among employed adults: symptom severity, quality of life and work productivity. Aliment Pharmacol Ther. 2007;25:487–500.
18. Farup C, Kleinman L, Sloan S, Ganoczy D, Chee E, Lee C, et al. The impact of nocturnal symptoms associated with gastroesophageal reflux disease on health-related quality of life. Arch Intern Med. 2001;161:45–52.
19. Hines LE, Mead HCA. Peristalsis in a loop of small intestine. Arch Intern Med. 1926;38:539.
20. Hobsley M. Dragstedt, gastric acid and duodenal ulcer. Yale J Biol Med. 1994;67:173–80.
21. Cannon WB. The movements of the intestine studied by means of the Röntgen rays. J Physiol. 1902;6:275–6.
22. Caviglia R, Ribolsi M, Maggiano N, Gabbrielli AM, Emerenziani S, Guarino MP, et al. Dilated intercellular spaces of esophageal epithelium in nonerosive reflux disease patients with physiological esophageal acid exposure. Am J Gastroenterol. 2005;100:543–8.
23. Boulos PB, Faber RG, Whitfield PF, Parkin JV, Hobsley M. Relationship between insulin- and histamine-stimulated secretion before and after vagotomy. Gut. 1981; 24:549–56.
24. Wingate DL. Complex clocks. Dig Dis Sci. 1987;28:1133–40.
25. Scudder CL. The red stippling sign of gastric and duodenal ulcer. Ann Surg. 1914;60:534–534.1.
26. Kumar D, Thompson PD, Wingate DL, Vesselinova-Jenkins CK, Libby G. Abnormal REM sleep in the irritable bowel syndrome. Gastroenterology. 1992;103:12–7.
27. Howden CW, Burget DW, Silletti C, Hunt RH. Single nocturnal doses of pirenzepine effectively inhibit overnight gastric secretion. Hepatogastroenterology. 1985;32:240–2.
28. Johnson LF, Harmon JW. Experimental esophagitis in a rabbit model. Clinical relevance. J Clin Gastroenterol. 1986;8:S26–44.
29. Atkinson M, Van Gelder A. Esophageal intraluminal pH recording in the assessment of gastroesophageal reflux and its consequences. Am J Dig Dis. 1977;22:365–70.
30. Orr WC. Review article: sleep-related gastro-oesophageal reflux as a distinct clinical entity. Aliment Pharmacol Ther. 2010;31:47–56.
31. Orr WC, Robinson MG, Johnson LF. Acid clearance during sleep in the pathogenesis of reflux esophagitis. Dig Dis Sci. 1981;26:423–7.
32. Ritchie HD, Thompson DG, Wingate DL. Diurnal variation in human jejunal fasting motor activity. J Physiol. 1980;305:54–5.
33. Orr WC. Sleep and gastroesophageal reflux disease: a wake-up call. Rev Gastroenterol Disord. 2004;4:S25–32.
34. Farmer DA, Howe CW, Porell WJ, Smithwich RH. The effect of various surgical procedures upon the acidity of the gastric contents of ulcer patients. Ann Surg. 1951;144:319–31.
35. Selye H. The experimental production of peptic haemorrhagic oesophagitis. Can Med Assoc J. 1938;39:447–8.
36. DeMeester TR, Johnson LF, Joseph GJ, Toscano MS, Hall AW, Skinner DB. Patterns of gastroesophageal reflux in health and disease. Ann Surg. 1976;184:459–70.
37. Finch PM, Ingram DM, Henstridge JD, Catchpole BN. Relationship of fasting gastroduodenal motility to the sleep cycle. Gastroenterology. 1982;83:605–12.
38. Orr WC, Elsenbruch S, Harnish MJ. Autonomic regulation of cardiac function during sleep in patients with irritable bowel syndrome. Am J Gastroenterol. 2000;95:2865–71.
39. Buchanan DT, Cain K, Heitkemper M, Burr R, Vitiello MV, Zia J, Jarrett M. Sleep measures predict next-day symptoms in women with irritable bowel syndrome. J Clin Sleep Med 2014;10(9):1003–9.
40. Dean BB, Aguilar D, Johnson LF, McGuigan JE, Orr WC, Fass R, et al. Night-time and day time atypical manifestations of gastro-oesophageal reflux disease: frequency, severity and impact on health-related quality of life. Aliment Pharmacol Ther. 2008;27:327–37.
41. Moynihan BG. A discussion on "The diagnosis and treatment of duodenal ulcer." Proc R Soc Med. 1910;3:69–87.
42. Johnson LF, DeMeester TR. Twenty-four hour pH monitoring of the distal esophageus: a quantitative measure of gastroesophageal reflux. Am J Gastroenterol. 1974;62:325–32.
43. Barlow WJ, Orlando RC. The pathogenesis of heartburn in nonerosive reflux disease: a unifying hypothesis. Gastroenterology. 2005;128:771–8.
44. Castiglione F, Emde C, Armstrong D, Schneider C, Bauerfeind P, Stacher G, et al. Nocturnal oesophageal motor activity is dependent on sleep stage. Gut. 1993;34:1653–9.
45. Sandweiss DJ, Sugarman MH, Podolsky HM, Friedman MHF. Nocturnal gastric secretion in duodenal ulcer: studies on normal subjects and patients, with their bearing on ulcer management. J Am Med Assoc. 1946;130:258–65.
46. Johnston RL, Washeim H. Studies in gastric secretion. Am J Physiol. 1924;70:247–53.
47. Jones MP Sloan SS, Jovanovic B, Kahrilas PJ. Impaired egress rather than increased access: an important predictor of erosive oesophagitis. Neurogastroenterol Motil. 2002;14:625–31.
48. Colin-Jones DG, Ireland A, Gear P, Golding PL, Ramage JK, Williams JG, et al. Reducing overnight secretion of acid to heal duodenal ulcers. Comparison of standard divided dose of ranitidine with a single dose administered at night. Am J Med. 1984;77:116–22.

49. Dragstedt LR. A concept of the etiology of gastric and duodenal ulcers. Gastroenterology. 1956;30:208–220.

50. Black JW, Duncan WAM, Durant GJ, Ganellin CR, Parsons EM. Definition and antagonism of histamine H2-receptors. Nature. 1972;236:385–390.

51. Wood JD. Enteric neurophysiology. Am J Physiol. 1984;247:585–98.

52. Wyllie JH, Hesselbo T. International symposium on histamine H2-receptor antagonists. In: Wood CJ, Simkins MA, editors. elwyn Garden City: Smith Kline and French Laboratories Limited Welwyn Garden City: Smith Kline and French Laboratories Limited 1973; p. 371.

53. Wyllie JH, Hesselbo T, Black JW. Effects in man of histamine H2-receptor blockade by burimamide. Lancet. 1972;2:1117–20.

54. Mathias JR, Sinsky CA, Millar HD, Clench MH, Davis RH. Development of an improved multi-pressure-sensor probe for recording muscle contraction in human intestine. Dig Dis Sci. 1985;30:119–23.

55. Vantrappen G, Janssens J, Hellemans J, Ghoos Y. The interdigestive motor complex of normal subjects and patients with bacterial overgrowth of the small intestine. J Clin Invest. 1977;59:1158–66.

56. Cheng FC, Lam SK, Ong GB. Maximum acid output to graded doses of pentagastrin and its relation to parietal cell mass in Chinese patients with duodenal ulcer. Gut. 1977;18:827–32.

57. Hobsley M, Silen W. Use of an inert marker (phenol red) to improve accuracy in gastric secretion studies. Gut. 1969;10:787–95.

58. Kellow JE, Gill RC, Wingate DL. Prolonged ambulant recordings of small bowel motility demonstrate abnormalities in the irritable bowel syndrome. Gastroenterology. 1990;98:1208–18.

59. Shaker R, Castell DO, Schoenfeld PS, Spechler SJ. Nighttime heartburn is an under-appreciated clinical problem that impacts sleep and daytime function: the results of a Gallup survey conducted on behalf of the American Gastroenterological Association. Am J Gastroenterol. 2003;98:1487–93.

60. Campos GM, Peters JH, DeMeester TR, Oberg S, Crookes PF, Mason RJ. The pattern of esophageal acid exposure in gastro-esophageal reflux disease influences the severity of the disease. Arch Surg. 1999;134:882–7.

61. Barcroft J, Robinson CS. A study of some factors influencing intestinal movements. J Physiol. 1929;67:211–20.

62. Helm JD, Kramer P, MacDonald RM, Ingelfinger FJ. Changes in motility of the human small intestine during sleep. Gastroenterology. 1948;10:135–7.

63. Spire JP, Tassinari CA. Duodenal EMG activity during sleep. Electroencephalogr Clin Neurophysiol. 1971;31:179–83.

64. Adler HF, Atkinson AJ, Ivy AC. A study of the motility of the human colon: an explanation of dysynergia of the colon, or of the unstable colon. Am J Dig Dis. 1941;8:197–202.

65. Bloom PB, Filion RD, Stunkard AJ, Fox S, Stellar E. Gastric and duodenal motility, food intake and hunger measured in man during a 24-hour period. Am J Dig Dis. 1970;15:719–25.

66. Heitkemper M, Charman ABD, Shaver J, Lentz MJ, Jarrett ME. Self-report and polysomnographic measures of sleep in women with irritable bowel syndrome. Nurs Res. 1998;47:270–7.

67. Silvis SE. Final report on the United States Multicenter Trial comparing ranitidine to cimetidine as maintenance therapy following healing of duodenal ulcer. J Clin Gastroenterol. 1985;7:482–7.

68. Furukawa Y, Cook IJ, Panagopoulos V, McEvoy RD, Sharp DJ, Simula M. Relationship between sleep patterns and human colonic motor patterns. Gastroenterology. 1994;107:1372–81.

69. Stanciu C, Bennet J. Gastro-duodenal motility: 24-hour continuous recordings in normal subjects. Med Interne. 1978;16:51–60.

70. Casten DF. Peptic esophagitis, hiatal hernia, and duodenal ulcer: a unified concept. Am J Surg. 1967;113:638–41.

71. Baust W, Rohrwasser W. Gastric motility and pH during natural human sleep. Pflügers Arch. 1969;305:229–40.

72. Freidin N, Fisher MJ, Taylor W, Boyd D, Surratt P, McCallurn RW, et al. Sleep and nocturnal acid reflux in normal subjects and patients with reflux oesophagitis. Gut. 1991;32:1275–9.

73. Kumar D, Wingate D, Ruckebusch Y. Circadian variation in the propagation velocity of the migrating motor complex. Gastroenterology. 1986;91:926–30.

74. Kildebo S, Aronsen O, Bernersen B, Breckan R, Gjellestad A, Johnsen K, et al. Cimetidine, 800 mg at night, in the treatment of duodenal ulcers. Scand J Gastroenterol. 1985;20:1147–50.

75. Peters PM. The pathology of severe digestion oesophagitis. Thorax. 1955;10:269–86.

76. Tassinari CA, Coccagna G, Mantovani M, Dalla Bernardina D, Spire JP, Mancia D, et al. Duodenal EMG activity during sleep in man. In: Jovanovic UJ, editor. The nature of sleep. Stuttgart: Fischer-Verlag; 1973.

77. Barreiro MA, McKenna RD, Beck IT. The physiological significance of intraluminal pressure changes in relation to propulsion and absorption in the human jejunum. Am J Dig Dis. 1968;13:324–51.

78. Fiddian-Green RG, Parkin JV, Faber RG, Russell RCG, Whitfield PF, Hobsley M. The quantification in human gastric juice of duodenogastric reflux by sodium output and by bile-labelling using Indocyanine Green. Klin Wochenschr. 1979;57:815–24.

79. Kumar D, Idzikowski C, Wingate DL, Soffer EE, Thompson P, Siderfin C. Relationship between enteric migrating motor complex and the sleep cycle. Am J Physiol. 1990;259:983–90.

80. Walt RP, Male P-J, Rawling J, Hunt RH, Milton-Thomson GJ, Misiewicz JJ. Comparison of the effects of ranitidine, cimetidine and placebo on the 24 hour intragastric acidity and nocturnal acid secretion in patients with duodenal ulcer. Gut. 1981;22:49–54.

81. Winkelstein A, Wolf BS, Som ML, Marshak RH. Peptic esophagitis with duodenal or gastric ulcer. J Am Med Assoc. 1954;154:885.

82. Gorard DA, Vesselinova-Jenkins CK, Libby GW, Farthing MJ. Migrating motor complex and sleep in health and irritable bowel syndrome. Dig Dis Sci. 1995;40:2383–9.

83. Lodge KV. The pathology of non-specific oesophagitis. J Pathol Bacteriol. 1955;69:17–24.

84. Kellow JE, Phillips SF. Altered small bowel motility in irritable bowel syndrome is correlated with symptoms. Gastroenterology. 1987;92:1885–93.

85. Manning AP, Thompson WG, Heaton KW, Morris AF. Towards positive diagnosis of the irritable bowel. Br Med J. 1978;2:653–4.

86. Kahrilas PJ, Pandolfino JE. Gastroesophageal reflux disease and its complications, including Barrett's metaplasia. In: Feldman M, Friedman LS, Sleisenger MH, editors. Sleisenger and Fordtran gastrointestinal and liver disease. 7th ed. Philadelphia: Saunders; 2002:599–622.

87. Heitkemper M, Jarrett M, Cain K, Shaver J, Bond E, Woods NF, et al. Increased urine catecholamines and cortisol in women with irritable bowel syndrome. Am J Gastroenterol. 1996;91:906–13.

88. Heitkemper M, Burr RL, Jarrett M, Hertiq V, Lustyk MK, Bond EF. Evidence for autonomic nervous system imbalance in women with irritable bowel syndrome. Dig Dis Sci. 1998;43:2093–8.

89. Harvey RF, Salih SY, Read AE. Organic and functional disorders in 2000 gastroenterology outpatients. Lancet. 1983;1:632–4.

90. Orr WC, Johnson LF, Robinson MG. Effect of sleep on swallowing, esophageal peristalsis, and acid clearance. Gastroenterology. 1984;86:814–9.

91. Heitkemper MM, Jarrett M. Pattern of gastrointestinal and somatic symptoms across the menstrual cycle. Gastroenterology. 1992;102:505–13.

92. Aggarwal A, Cutts TF, Abell TL, Cardoso S, Familoni B, Bremer J, et al. Predominant symptoms in irritable bowel syndrome correlate with specific autonomic nervous system abnormalities. Gastroenterology. 1994;106:945–50.

93. Orr WC, Crowell MD, Lin B, Harnish MJ, Chen JD. Sleep and gastric function in irritable bowel syndrome: derailing the brain-gut axis. Gut. 1997;41:390–3.

Impotence and Erectile Problems in Sleep Medicine

Markus H. Schmidt

Introduction

Erection cycles during sleep are often viewed as one of the more unusual physiological events to occur during sleep, yet penile erections are a robust peripheral manifestation of rapid eye movement (REM) sleep in all healthy males. These REM-related erections were previously termed "nocturnal penile tumescence" (NPT), but are now more commonly referred to as "sleep-related erections" (SRE) to reflect the specific association with sleep. The history of SRE testing from its discovery to its clinical role in evaluating male erectile dysfunction is reviewed in this chapter. SRE testing was commonly performed in many sleep laboratories until a decade ago. Although urologists continue to utilize SRE testing using home screening devices, few sleep medicine specialists employ this technique today even though a clear role for formal in-laboratory SRE monitoring remains. Finally, the discovery of an animal model to elucidate some of the basic neural mechanisms of SREs is presented.

Early History of SREs

Prior to any description of SREs in the scientific literature, it had long been known that men commonly awaken out of sleep with an erection or even a nocturnal emission. Awakening with an erection has erroneously been believed a consequence of a full bladder or the need to void. This belief has persisted to this day in the lay public even though SREs have no known association with bladder fullness [1]. From a historical perspective, erections during sleep were commonly viewed by many, and particularly within the religious community, as representing "unhealthy" thoughts or dreams. As a result, efforts were undertaken in some circles to uti-

lize devices designed to prevent erections during wakefulness or sleep. Such devices included "spermatorrhea rings" that comprised a flexible inner ring that was placed around the penis and attached to an inflexible outer ring containing metal teeth that were designed to inflict pain as the penis engorged during an erection when it came in contact with the teeth of the outer ring [1]. Numerous barbaric looking devices were utilized for this purpose, some with electrical switches involving circumferential rings triggered by expansion that would activate buzzers or bells to warn the user or parental guardian of sinful exploits transpiring under the covers. There are reports of adult patients who have been traumatized by such devices during their youth [1].

Although Halverson was the first to report visual observations of erections in infant males during sleep [2], the first systematic evaluation of erections during sleep appearing in the scientific literature was performed by Ohlmeyer et al. in 1944 [3], approximately 10 years prior to the discovery of REM sleep. These authors performed a series of penile erection recordings during sleep in healthy male volunteers using a simple "on–off" type switch that recorded the presence or absence of an erectile event. This recording device included a flexible inner ring placed around the shaft of the penis that was connected to an inflexible outer metal ring (but without the menacing teeth of the "spermatorrhea ring" described above). During an erection, the flexible inner ring came in contact with the outer ring, forming a closed electrical circuit that could be recorded during the night. Using this recording technique, Ohlmeyer and colleagues found that all normal healthy males in the study generally demonstrated three to four erection cycles lasting approximately 25 min each in duration and occurring every 85 min during sleep, similar to the cycling of REM sleep discovered by Aserinsky and Kleitman in 1953 [4].

Several authors, including Aserinsky, were aware of the erection data described by Ohlmeyer and colleagues a decade earlier and speculated that erections may be occurring during REM sleep given the similar cyclicity and duration of these two physiological phenomena during sleep. However,

M. H. Schmidt (✉)
Ohio Sleep Medicine Institute, 4975 Bradenton Ave.,
Dublin, OH 43017, USA
e-mail: mschmidt@sleepmedicine.com

S. Chokroverty, M. Billiard (eds.), *Sleep Medicine,* DOI 10.1007/978-1-4939-2089-1_52,
© Springer Science+Business Media, LLC 2015

it was not until the mid-1960s that Fisher [5] and Karacan [6, 7] independently demonstrated for the first time that erections during sleep are a naturally occurring phenomenon of REM sleep in all healthy males. Early research also demonstrated that women exhibit similar genital activity during REM sleep, including clitoral erections [8], increased vaginal blood flow [9, 10], and increased intrauterine pressures [11] occurring in a cyclical manner during REM sleep as observed in men.

Fisher [5] and Karacan [6, 7] had both utilized an erection recording device involving mercury loop strain gauges. This device involves a mercury-filled silastic tubing that carries a small electrical current passing through the mercury in the loop. During an erection, the silastic tubing stretches as it accommodates the increase in penile circumference, and the column of mercury within the tubing becomes thinner, thus increasing the electrical resistance through the mercury-filled loop. Within a limited range of circumference changes, the gauge is relatively linear in that any given change in circumference relates to a specific change in resistance that may be monitored during sleep with polysomnography [12].

The strain gauge technology became the standard recording method with polysomnography from the 1960s to the present day. Two gauges are typically used for each patient, one placed at the base of the penis and the other just caudal to the glans in the coronal sulcus. Although the strain gauge technology allows for a precise determination of circumference changes during sleep, circumference alone is inadequate for an evaluation of erectile functioning. Some individuals may exhibit a small increase in penile circumference yet demonstrate a maximally rigid erection, whereas others may have a marked increase in circumference with minimal rigidity.

The buckling force device was thus developed to formally evaluate penile rigidity in the sleep laboratory. The patient is awakened during a maximal circumference increase either during or at the end of a REM sleep episode. The technician quickly stabilizes the base of the penis between the thumb and index finger and then presses the buckling force device against the head of the glans along the longitudinal axis of the penis. The pressure at which the penile shaft first bends or buckles is defined as the buckling force pressure. A penis that buckles at less than 500 g of force is generally considered inadequate for vaginal penetration [13]. At least two buckling force measurements are generally performed on every patient.

Other techniques were attempted to monitor erections during sleep in the mid-1960s prior to the strain gauge method becoming the standard of care. Fisher and colleagues in their original publication [5] had also utilized a polyvinyl tube with the size and shape of a doughnut that was filled with water and placed around the base of the penis. During an erection, the increase in circumference of the penis would displace the water in the doughnut-shaped tube and cause a rise in a water-filled column next to the subject's bed. This device, however, was bulky and cumbersome. Finally, temperature monitoring of penis had also been utilized and was found to demonstrate an increase in the temperature of the penis during erection associated with the increase in blood flow during the erection [5], but this technique could not quantify the quality of erectile events during sleep. The ability of the mercury-filled strain gauge to accurately quantify changes in penile circumference and its minimal intrusiveness made this technique the preferred method of monitoring erections during sleep for the several decades that followed.

The Clinical Use of SRE Monitoring

Karacan [14] was the first to suggest that monitoring erections during sleep may provide a clinical tool to differentiate psychogenic from organic erectile dysfunction. Fisher [15, 16] and others also appreciated the clinical value of involuntary erection cycles during sleep, leading to the new development of combining polysomnography with SRE monitoring to evaluate male sexual function. This new technology of SRE monitoring came at a time when erectile dysfunction was poorly understood and provided a new avenue for research opportunities to study sexual function. Masters and Johnson [13] had just published their seminal work suggesting that most male impotence was psychological in origin. However, new interventions were being developed to treat erectile dysfunction, including surgical penile implants, and a greater appreciation of organic or physiological causes of erectile failure were only beginning to be appreciated.

In the mid-1970s and long before the advent of oral medications to treat erectile dysfunction, two primary treatment options were available to men with impotence. Psychotherapy was offered if the impotence was believed to be psychological in origin, whereas a surgical penile prosthesis was considered for men whose erectile failure was thought to be organic or physiological in nature. SRE monitoring with polysomnography provided a new diagnostic technique to guide clinicians to the appropriate treatment option. For example, a patient who complained of difficulty initiating or maintaining an erection but was found to have normally occurring erection cycles during sleep was deemed to have a psychogenic cause of the erectile failure. On the other hand, a patient found to have a decrease or absence in erectile activity during sleep in the presence of adequate REM sleep would suggest that such an individual has an organic etiology of the erectile dysfunction.

SRE monitoring for the clinical evaluation of erectile capability lead to the need of establishing normative data. Karacan and coworkers [7, 17–21], and to a lesser extent Fisher [22], studied penile erections during sleep in normal boys and men of all age groups, demonstrating that erections occur in a tight temporal association with REM sleep in all healthy males tested from infancy to old age. REM-related erections were demonstrated to begin several minutes prior to the onset of REM sleep, and to last several minutes following the termination of REM when detumescence would occur. Later work replicated these findings [23–25]. Although some minor decreases in erection time during sleep are found in men as they age from adolescence to later years, the occurrence of erections as part of the normal physiology of REM sleep is a robust and predictable phenomenon in healthy, potent males, thus establishing SRE monitoring as a valid tool to evaluate erectile function.

Further work established that erections during sleep are generally unaffected by many psychological influences, thus strengthening the clinical value of SRE monitoring as a technique to differentiate psychogenic from organic erectile dysfunction. For example, neither presleep sexual activity nor abstinence appears to alter erections during REM sleep [6, 26–28]. Although the total tumescence time may be decreased in milder forms of depression or anxiety, penile erections persist during REM as a robust phenomenon in these patients with the total tumescence time still exceeding the total REM sleep time [1]. On the other hand, SREs may be adversely affected in some patients with major depressive disorders [29]. It remains to be determined to what extent fragmentation of REM sleep, the proerectile stimulus, in patients with major depression may be the cause of decreased erectile activity during sleep in this select group of patients.

Over the past several decades, a rare disorder has been described in some patients who frequently awaken with painful erections during sleep [30], yet describe no pain associated with erections during sexual intercourse or masturbation [31–34]. Although potential roles for neurovascular compression of the hypothalamus [35] or beta-adrenergic hypersensitivity [32] have been proposed as possible etiological factors, this disorder is poorly understood. Patients typically awaken several times during the night out of REM sleep with a painful erection over a period of many years. Such patients tend to have fragmented REM sleep, which is thought to be secondary to the pain associated with the erection. Patients often have a history of anxiety, but no other clear pathology has been identified. Unfortunately, there are few treatment options for such patients other than some transient relief reported with the beta-blocker propranolol and some sustained benefit with clozapine [32, 36, 37].

SREs and Comorbid Medical Conditions

Many comorbid medical conditions or cardiovascular risks have been found to adversely affect SREs, and many of these same conditions are also known to adversely impact normal, or waking, erectile functioning. For example, SREs have been demonstrated to be decreased in patients with diabetes [38, 39], hypertension [40], smoking [41], alcoholism [42, 43], and intoxication [44]. Men with hypertension and complaints of erectile dysfunction demonstrate significantly less total tumescence time during sleep compared to hypertensive men without erectile complaints. Although many of these comorbid conditions that increase cardiovascular risks are hypothesized to adversely impact erectile capability at the peripheral or end organ level, the impact of such disease states on the central nervous system (CNS) control of erections during wakefulness or sleep has not been adequately examined. Indeed, some evidence has been presented to suggest that diabetes may decrease SREs long before peripheral neurovascular abnormalities are apparent, suggesting that at least some comorbid conditions may impact the CNS control of erections during sleep [45].

Considerable data have been published on SREs with respect to either hypogonadism or the manipulation of androgen levels in males with both low and normal testosterone levels. Although these data show that SREs are adversely affected by low androgen levels, there has been some controversy in the literature over the years as to what extent SREs are "androgen dependent." Testosterone is released during sleep in normal adult males and tends to peak at a time during REM sleep when erections occur [46]. Moreover, testosterone administration has been shown to increase SREs in hypogonadal men [47]. On the other hand, discontinuing testosterone replacement in hypogonadal patients decreases the total tumescence time during sleep, the maximal penile circumference, and the number of tumescence episodes during sleep [48]. These and other data suggest that androgens play an important role in augmenting erections during sleep in adult males [49–52], leading some to suggest that SREs are "androgen dependent" [53]. However, SREs are prominent in infant and prepubescent males [21] in the face of undetectable testosterone levels. Indeed, children exhibit more tumescent time during sleep than adult males secondary to the increase in total REM sleep time in children [21]. Finally, although SREs may be decreased in low androgen states, SREs in hypogonadal males persist and often remain within the normal range [48]. These later data have led to the current view that SREs may be better termed "androgen sensitive" [54, 55] instead of the previously used terminology of "androgen dependent."

One of the major developments in the management of erectile dysfunction has been the growing understanding that obstructive sleep apnea (OSA) may adversely impact erectile functioning during wakefulness. Guilleminault and coworkers reported on an early case series in 1977 that men with OSA had a high prevalence of erectile complaints, and that some men reported improvements in erectile capability following treatment with nasal continuous positive airway pressure (CPAP) [56]. Four years later Schmidt and Wise reported on a series of 15 consecutive patients with impotence presenting to a urology clinic and found that those with organic erectile dysfunction ($n=7$) had a significantly higher prevalence of OSA compared to the group with pscychogenic impotence [57], a finding that was confirmed by Pressman [58] and Hirshkowitz [59]. Karacan and Karatas later reported that one third of patients with OSA demonstrate improved SREs following nasal CPAP therapy [60].

In spite of these early data, it was not until the mid-2000s that the concept of OSA as a potential independent risk factor for the development of erectile dysfunction began to be more seriously entertained. Numerous studies now suggest that sleep apnea patients are at a significantly higher risk for erectile dysfunction and that nasal CPAP may improve erectile capability [61–65], confirming and extending the earlier studies. Finally, intermittent hypoxia during sleep decreases waking erectile functioning in rats [66] and mice [67] using experimental designs that manipulate blood oxygen saturation. Given that OSA has been well documented to be a risk factor for several cardiovascular diseases, as well as a potential independent risk factor for erectile dysfunction during wakefulness, many urology clinics are now screening for OSA in patients presenting with erectile dysfunction as part of a treatment regimen addressing potential modifiable risk factors for impotence [68].

SRE Monitoring Without Polysomnography (Home Screening Devices)

Several techniques have been utilized over the years to evaluate erectile functioning during sleep without involving formal polysomnography. As early as 1980, it was suggested that the cost of erection monitoring during sleep could be reduced from hundreds of dollars in the sleep laboratory to as little as "30 cents" for three nights of home testing using the so-called stamp-ring method [69]. This technique involved using four or five US postage stamps wrapped around the flaccid penile shaft and wetting the overlapping stamp to seal the "stamp ring" prior to bedtime [69]. If the stamp ring was broken the next morning upon awakening, it was presumed that SREs were normal and erectile functioning was intact [70]. However, the validity of this technique was put into question since a breaking of the stamp ring along the perforations between the stamps was found to be an unreliable indicator of normal penile rigidity [71].

These concerns led to the "snap-gauge band," a penile ring that attempted to utilize multiple breakable bands within the ring with varying levels of tension required to break each band in an attempt to quantify the degree of circumferential rigidity obtained during the night of sleep [72–75]. Eventually, similar concerns of reliability were raised with this snap-gauge technique in that some men may have marked

increases in penile circumference during an erection, but with minimal rigidity required for vaginal penetration [76]. A formal comparison of the snap-gauge technique with in-laboratory polysomnography by Allen and Bender [77] also revealed the surprising finding than many men failed to break any of the snap-gauge bands even while demonstrating normal SREs and adequate penile rigidity as measured with the bucking force device. Formal polysomnography was continued to be viewed as the gold standard technique for monitoring SREs [78].

A more advanced screening device was introduced in 1986 called the RigiScan (Endocare, Irvine, CA). Still in use today, it is designed to record erections during sleep at home without monitoring sleep–wake stages [79]. The introduction of the Rigiscan home screening device was in part responsible for a move away from in-laboratory polysomnography as a means of evaluating erectile function during sleep. This recording system utilizes two loop devices placed around the penile shaft, one at the base and the other near the glans, each containing a moveable wire. The loop device has the advantage of being able to simultaneously monitor penile circumference and radial or circumferential rigidity. Increases in circumference of the penis during an erection are monitored via the wire in the loop. In addition, a squeezing force of 283.5 g is applied to the penile shaft at regular intervals during the night by pulling on the wire within the loop. The radial rigidity is measured in arbitrary units so that a 100 % radial rigidity corresponds to no measurable circumferential displacement from the 283.5-g force. For every 0.5-mm loop shortening that is detected, circumferential rigidity decreases by 2.3 %.

The RigiScan has the advantage of monitoring rigidity many times throughout the night, unlike the buckling force that provides only two to three isolated measurements of rigidity. However, circumferential rigidity as measured by the RigiScan device has been shown to be inferior to the buckling force method as a predictor of axial rigidity, which is the rigidity required for vaginal penetration [80]. Moreover, the RigiScan device does not involve the important contribution of patient and technician visual observations of the erection and/or discrepancies in the quality of the erectile event. During buckling force measurements in the sleep lab, both the technician and the patient rate the quality of the erection. Not only may physical abnormalities, such as Peyronie's disease be observed during the nocturnal erection assessment, but also some patients with psychogenic erectile dysfunction tend to underestimate the true capability of erectile function as seen by a discrepancy between the technician and patient rating of the erection.

Urologists have continued to utilize SRE testing even though very few sleep medicine specialists provide this service today. The advent of home screening devices, as well as the introduction of phosphodiesterase inhibitors such as Viagra, has reduced the perceived need for in-laboratory evaluations. Indeed, most SRE monitoring at this time is limited to the RigiScan home screening device [81]. Those who advocate home screening have argued without evidence that monitoring erections at home is more "natural" than in the laboratory, or that in-laboratory testing is not cost effective as a screening tool [81]. However, Schmidt and Schmidt [82] reviewed data demonstrating that a formal in-laboratory SRE evaluation continues to be the "Gold Standard" to evaluate erectile function and may be cost-effective if limited to specific clinical indications such as nonresponders to commonly prescribed medications for erectile dysfunction or those seeking a potential surgical prosthesis as a treatment option, a procedure that would destroy any remaining natural erectile function. Moreover, in-laboratory SRE testing would have particular relevance for medicolegal cases evaluating erectile capability for individuals claiming erectile dysfunction following pelvic injury or when impotence is used as a defense for a male accused of sexual assault [82]. Finally, in-laboratory polysomnography would also identify other potential risk factors contributing to erectile dysfunction, such as OSA. These guidelines for in-laboratory SRE monitoring have been published in detail elsewhere [1, 82].

Potentially contributing to the decreased use of in-laboratory SRE evaluations are several misconceptions within the medical community that continue today regarding erections during sleep. Particular among these is the lack of appreciation that REM sleep is the required stimulus to generate erections during sleep. For example, it is commonly cited in the urology literature that only 80% of all SREs occur during REM, implying that 20% of erections are generated by non-REM sleep (see for example [83]). If one believes that erections may be generated by any stage of well-sustained sleep, then a recording of sleep stages with polysomnography may be viewed as unnecessary by some clinicians. It is often not clarified in such literature that the erection typically begins several minutes prior to the onset of REM sleep and often persists for 10–15 min following the end of the REM period before detumescence is complete. The anticipation or "harbinger" effect of the REM onset, together with the delayed detumescence following the end of REM should help clarify this often-cited statistic. Although 80% of all "erection time" in sleep occurs during REM, each erection cycle requires REM sleep. The strength of the association between REM and the appearance of an erection during sleep should provide even greater interest to evaluate the quantity or quality of the proerection stimulus, REM sleep, when interpreting SRE data [1, 82].

a micro-tip pressure transducer implanted into the bulb of the corpus spongiosum of the penis (CSP) while simultaneously monitoring sleep–wake states with traditional techniques [84]. Penile erections are associated with an increase in baseline erectile tissue pressure within the CSP from 10–15 mm Hg in the flaccid state to a tumescence pressure of 50–70 mmHg. In addition, bursts of electromyographic (EMG) activity in the bulbospongiosus (BS) muscles, which surround and insert onto the bulb of the CSP, are associated with suprasystolic pressure peaks within the bulb exceeding several hundred millimeters of mercury in the rat [85], as has been shown in many other mammalian species during penile erections [86].

Although there were several prior reports of visual observations of erections during sleep in several nonhuman species, these early reports did not clarify if such erections were random events or if they systematically occurred during a specific sleep stage. The recording method developed by Schmidt and colleagues demonstrated for the first time that nonhuman mammals also exhibit penile erections during REM sleep [84], thus establishing a new animal model for SRE research. It still remains to be determined, however, to what extent other mammals may have erections during REM sleep since the armadillo has been shown to instead exhibit erections during non-REM sleep [87].

The rat model was used to elucidate many of the basic mechanisms of SRE neurophysiology. For example, erections during REM sleep are eliminated in the rat following neural transection of the rostral mesencephalon, even though the appearance of REM sleep persists caudal to the transection as seen by the cyclical occurrence of rapid eye movements with muscle atonia [88]. These data demonstrate that although REM-generating mechanisms within the brainstem are sufficient to generate the state of REM, the brainstem is not sufficient to generate erections during REM sleep. A subsequent study using this animal model found that bilateral lesions of the lateral preoptic area (LPOA) using the neurotoxin ibotenic acid eliminated erections during REM sleep while leaving waking-state erections intact [89]. These latter data confirmed the importance of the forebrain in SRE neurophysiology, and localized this control to the LPOA. Schmidt presented the first comprehensive working model on the neural control of SREs in 2000 [90], but little work in this area has been performed since and many questions still remain regarding SRE neurophysiology, such as the role of specific neurotransmitters or the potential role of other brain structures including the amygdala or cortex.

An Animal Model for SRE Research

Schmidt and colleagues in the laboratory of Professor Michel Jouvet in Lyon, France, developed a new animal model in the mid-1990s to monitor erections in freely behaving rats using

Summary

A historical review of SRE testing from its discovery to the present day exposes a major shift in the utilization of this procedure for the clinical management of erectile dysfunction.

After establishing SRE monitoring in combination with in-laboratory polysomnography as the "Gold Standard" in determining male erectile capability, few sleep medicine specialists today have continued the practice. Home monitoring systems and a new generation of medications such as Viagra to treat erectile dysfunction have contributed to the decreased use of in-laboratory SRE testing. However, there persists a need for comprehensive polysomnography with SRE monitoring even in today's "Viagra" era, and revised clinical indications for formal SRE evaluation are discussed. Indeed, REM-related erections are the only type of naturally occurring erections that utilize the entire neuroaxis from the brain and spinal cord to the peripheral end organ level while minimizing psychological influences such as anxiety or lack of libido in the evaluation of male erectile function. Although our understanding of SRE neurophysiology has been much advanced since the original observations of Ohlmeyer, Fisher, and Karacan, more research is needed to further elucidate the neural control of SREs. Such work may not only help to clarify the role of SRE testing in modern medicine but also potentially provide new avenues to treat erectile dysfunction through strategies that are directed to centrally acting mechanisms.

References

1. Hirshkowitz M, Schmidt MH. Sleep-related erections: clinical perspectives and neural mechanisms. Sleep Med Rev. 2005;9(4):311–29.
2. Halverson HM. Genital and sphincter behavior of the male infant. J Genet Psychol. 1940;56:95–136.
3. Ohlmeyer P, Brilmayer H, Hullstrung H. Periodische Vorgange im Schlaf. Pflueger Arch Gesamte Physiol Menschen Tiere. 1944;248:559–60.
4. Aserinsky E, Kleitman N. Regularly occurring periods of eye motility, and concomitant phenomena, during sleep. Science. 1953;118(3062):273–4.
5. Fisher C, Gross J, Zuch J. Cycle of penile erection synchronous with dreaming (Rem) sleep. Preliminary report. Arch Gen Psychiatry. 1965;12:29–45.
6. Karacan I. The effect of exciting presleep events on dream reporting and penile erections during sleep. Unpublished doctoral dissertation, Department of Psychiatry. 1965, Brooklyn, New York: Downstate Medical Center Library, New York University.
7. Karacan I, et al. Erection cycle during sleep in relation to dream anxiety. Arch Gen Psychiatry. 1966;15:183–9.
8. Karacan I, Rosenbloom AL, Williams RL. The clitoral erection cycle during sleep. Sleep Res. 1970;7:338.
9. Fisher C, et al. Patterns of female sexual arousal during sleep and waking: vaginal thermo-conductance studies. Arch Sex Behav. 1983;12:97–122.
10. Cohen HD, Shapiro A. Vaginal blood flow during sleep. Sleep Res. 1970;7:338.
11. Karacan I, et al. Uterine activity during sleep. Sleep. 1986;9(3):393–8.
12. Ware JC. Monitoring erections during sleep. In: Kryger MH, Roth T, Dement WC, editors. Principles and practice of sleep medicine. Philadelphia: Saunders; 1989. pp. 689–95.
13. Masters WH, Johnson VE. Human sexual inadequacy. 1st ed. Boston: Little; 1970. 467 p.
14. Karacan I. Clinical value of nocturnal erection in the prognosis and diagnosis of impotence. Med Aspects Hum Sex. 1970;4:27–34.
15. Fisher C, et al. The assessment of nocturnal REM erection in the differential diagnosis of sexual impotence. J Sex Marital Ther. 1975;1(4):277–89.
16. Fisher C, et al. Evaluation of nocturnal penile tumescence in the differential diagnosis of sexual impotence. A quantitative study. Arch Gen Psychiatry. 1979;36(4):431–7.
17. Karacan I, Hursch CJ, Williams RL. Some characteristics of nocturnal penile tumescence in elderly males. J Gerontol. 1972;27(1):39–45.
18. Karacan I, et al. Some characteristics of nocturnal penile tumescence during puberty. Pediatr Res. 1972;6(6):529–37.
19. Karacan I, et al. Some characteristics of nocturnal penile tumescence in young adults. Arch Gen Psychiatry. 1972;26(4):351–6.
20. Karacan I, et al. Sleep-related penile tumescence as a function of age. Am J Psychiatry. 1975;132(9):932–7.
21. Karacan I, et al. The ontogeny of nocturnal penile tumescence. Waking Sleep. 1976;1:27–44.
22. Kahn E, Fisher C. REM sleep and sexuality in the aged. J Geriatric Psychiatry. 1969;2:181–99.
23. Schiavi RC, Schreiner-Engel P. Nocturnal penile tumescence in healthy aging men. J Gerontol. 1988;43(5):M146–50.
24. Reynolds CF 3rd, et al. Nocturnal penile tumescence in healthy 20- to 59-year-olds: a revisit. Sleep. 1989;12(4):368–73.
25. Ware JC, Hirshkowitz M. Characteristics of penile erections during sleep recorded from normal subjects. J Clin Neurophysiol. 1992;9(1):78–87.
26. Karacan I, Williams RL, Salis PJ. The effect of sexual intercourse on sleep patterns and nocturnal penile erections. Psychophysiology 1970;7:338.
27. Ware JC, et al. Sleep-related erections: absence of change following presleep sexual arousal. J Psychosom Res. 1997;42(6):547–53.
28. Brissette S, et al. Sexual activity and sleep in humans. Biol Psychiatry. 1985;20(7):758–63.
29. Thase ME, et al. Nocturnal penile tumescence in depressed men. Am J Psychiatry. 1987;144(1):89–92.
30. Karacan I. Painful nocturnal penile erections. J Am Med Assoc. 1971;215:1831.
31. Matthews BJ, Crutchfield MB. Painful nocturnal penile erections associated with rapid eye movement sleep. Sleep. 1987;10(2):184–7.
32. Calvet U. Painful nocturnal erection. Sleep Med Rev. 1999;3(1):47–57.
33. Ferini-Strambi L, et al. Sleep-related painful erections: clinical and polysomnographic features. J Sleep Res. 1996;5(3):195–7.
34. Ferini-Strambi L, et al. Cardiac autonomic nervous activity in sleep-related painful erections. Sleep. 1996;19(2):136–8.
35. Szucs A, et al. Sleep-related painful erection is associated with neurovascular compression of basal forebrain. J Neurol. 2002;249(4):486–7.
36. Karsenty G, et al. Sleep-related painful erections. Nat Clin Pract Urol. 2005;2(5):256–60, quiz 261.
37. Steiger A, Benkert O. Examination and treatment of sleep-related painful erections–a case report. Arch Sex Behav. 1989;18(3):263–7.
38. Karacan I, et al. Nocturnal penile tumescence and diagnosis in diabetic impotence. Am J Psychiatry. 1978;135(2):191–7.
39. Hirshkowitz M, et al. Diabetes, erectile dysfunction, and sleep-related erections. Sleep. 1990;13(1):53–68.
40. Rosen RC, Weiner DN. Cardiovascular disease and sleep-related erections. J Psychosom Res. 1997;42(6):517–30.
41. Hirshkowitz M, et al. Nocturnal penile tumescence in cigarette smokers with erectile dysfunction. Urology. 1992;39(2):101–7.
42. Snyder S, Karacan I. Effects of chronic alcoholism on nocturnal penile tumescence. Psychosom Med. 1981;43(5):423–9.

43. Dainoson K. Association between nocturnal penile tumescence (NPT) and sleep of stage 1 with REMs in chronic alcoholics. Kurume Med J. 1991;38(1):25–32.

44. Cooper AJ. The effects of intoxication levels of ethanol on nocturnal penile tumescence. J Sex Marital Ther. 1994;20(1):14–23.

45. Nofzinger EA, Schmidt HS. An exploration of central dysregulation of erectile function as a contributing cause of diabetic impotence. J Nerv Ment Dis. 1990;178:90–5.

46. Luboshitzky R, et al. Relationship between rapid eye movement sleep and testosterone secretion in normal men. J Androl. 1999;20(6):731–7.

47. O'Carroll R, Shapiro C, Bancroft J. Androgens, behaviour and nocturnal erection in hypogonadal men: the effects of varying the replacement dose. Clin Endocrinol (Oxf). 1985;23(5):527–38.

48. Cunningham GR, et al. Testosterone replacement therapy and sleep-related erections in hypogonadal men. J Clin Endocrinol Metab. 1990;70(3):792–7.

49. Carani C, et al. The effects of testosterone administration and visual erotic stimuli on nocturnal penile tumescence in normal men. Horm Behav. 1990;24(3):435–41.

50. Cooper AJ, et al. Medroxyprogesterone acetate, nocturnal penile tumescence, laboratory arousal, and sexual acting out in a male with schizophrenia. Arch Sex Behav. 1990;19(4):361–72.

51. Cooper AJ, Cernovovsky Z. The effects of cyproterone acetate on sleeping and waking penile erections in pedophiles: possible implications for treatment. Can J Psychiatry. 1992;37(1):33–9.

52. Hirshkowitz M, et al. Androgen and sleep-related erections. J Psychosom Res. 1997;42(6):541–6.

53. Carani C, et al. Testosterone and erectile function, nocturnal penile tumescence and rigidity, and erectile response to visual erotic stimuli in hypogonadal and eugonadal men. Psychoneuroendocrinology. 1992;17(6):647–54.

54. Sachs BD. Placing erection in context: the reflexogenic-psychogenic dichotomy reconsidered. Neurosci Biobehav Rev. 1995;19(2):211–24.

55. Schmidt MH. Neural mechanisms of sleep-related penile erections. In: Kryger MH, Roth T, Dement WC, editors. Principles and practice of sleep medicine. Philadelphia: Elsevier Saunders; 2005. pp. 305–17.

56. Guilleminault C, et al. Sleep apnea syndrome due to upper airway obstruction: a review of 25 cases. Arch Intern Med. 1977;137(3):296–300.

57. Schmidt HS, Wise HA 2nd. Significance of impaired penile tumescence and associated polysomnographic abnormalities in the impotent patient. J Urol. 1981;126(3):348–52.

58. Pressman MR, et al. Problems in the interpretation of nocturnal penile tumescence studies: disruption of sleep by occult sleep disorders. J Urol. 1986;136(3):595–8.

59. Hirshkowitz M, et al. Prevalence of sleep apnea in men with erectile dysfunction. Urology. 1990;36(3):232–4.

60. Karacan I, Karatas M. Erectile dysfunction in sleep apnea and response to CPAP. J Sex Marital Ther. 1995;21(4):239–47.

61. Goncalves MA, et al. Erectile dysfunction, obstructive sleep apnea syndrome and nasal CPAP treatment. Sleep Med. 2005;6(4):333–9.

62. Karkoulias K, et al. Does CPAP therapy improve erectile dysfunction in patients with obstructive sleep apnea syndrome? Clin Ter. 2007;158(6):515–8.

63. Margel D, et al. Predictors of erectile function improvement in obstructive sleep apnea patients with long-term CPAP treatment. Int J Impot Res. 2005;17(2):186–90.

64. Perimenis P, et al. The impact of long-term conventional treatment for overlap syndrome (obstructive sleep apnea and chronic obstructive pulmonary disease) on concurrent erectile dysfunction. Respir Med. 2007;101(2):210–6.

65. Margel D, et al. Severe, but not mild, obstructive sleep apnea syndrome is associated with erectile dysfunction. Urology. 2004;63(3):545–9.

66. Schmidt MH, et al. Penile erections are decreased in male rats exposed to intermittent hypoxia. Program No. 663.8. 2004 Neuroscience Meeting Planner. San Diego, CA: Society for Neuroscience, 2004. Online.

67. Soukhova-O'Hare GK, et al. Erectile dysfunction in a murine model of sleep apnea. Am J Respir Crit Care Med. 2008;178(6):644–50.

68. Zias N, et al. Obstructive sleep apnea and erectile dysfunction: still a neglected risk factor? Sleep Breath. 2009;13(1):3–10.

69. Barry JM, Blank B, Boileau M. Nocturnal penile tumescence monitoring with stamps. Urology. 1980;15(2):171–2.

70. Marshall P, et al. Nocturnal penile tumescence recording with stamps: a validity study. J Urol. 1982;128(5):946–7.

71. Marshall PG, et al. Nocturnal penile tumescence with stamps: a comparative study under sleep laboratory conditions. J Urol. 1983. 130(1):88–9.

72. Ek A, Bradley WR, Krane RJ. Nocturnal penile rigidity measured by the snap-gauge band. J Urol. 1983;129(5):964–6.

73. Ek A., Bradley WE, Krane RL. Snap-gauge band: new concept in measuring penile rigidity. Urology. 1983;21(1):63.

74. Morales A, et al. A new device for diagnostic screening of nocturnal penile tumescence. J Urol. 1983;129(2):288–90.

75. Ellis DJ, Doghramji K, Bagley DH. Snap-gauge band versus penile rigidity in impotence assessment. J Urol. 1988;140(1):61–3.

76. Wein AJ, et al. Expansion without significant rigidity during nocturnal penile tumescence testing: a potential source of misinterpretation. J Urol. 1981;126(3):343–4.

77. Allen R, Brendler CB. Snap-gauge compared to a full nocturnal penile tumescence study for evaluation of patients with erectile impotence. J Urol. 1990;143(1):51–4.

78. Condra M, et al. Screening assessment of penile tumescence and rigidity. Clinical test of snap-gauge. Urology. 1987;29(3):254–7.

79. Kaneko S, Bradley WE. Evaluation of erectile dysfunction with continuous monitoring of penile rigidity. J Urol. 1986;136(5):1026–9.

80. Allen RP, et al. Comparison of RigiScan and formal nocturnal penile tumescence testing in the evaluation of erectile rigidity. J Urol. 1993; 149(5 Pt 2):1265–8.

81. Levine LA, Lenting EL. Use of nocturnal penile tumescence and rigidity in the evaluation of male erectile dysfunction. Urol Clin North Am. 1995;22(4):775–88.

82. Schmidt MH, Schmidt HS. Sleep-related erections: neural mechanisms and clinical significance. Curr Neurol Neurosci Rep. 2004;4(2):170–8.

83. Guay AT, Heatley GJ, Murray FT. Comparison of results of nocturnal penile tumescence and rigidity in a sleep laboratory versus a portable home monitor. Urology. 1996;48:912–6.

84. Schmidt MH, et al. Experimental evidence of penile erections during paradoxical sleep in the rat. Neuroreport. 1994;5(5):561–4.

85. Schmidt MH, et al. Corpus spongiosum penis pressure and perineal muscle activity during reflexive erections in the rat. Am J Physiol. 1995; 269(4 Pt 2):R904–13.

86. Schmidt MH, Schmidt HS. The ischiocavernosus and bulbospongiosus muscles in mammalian penile rigidity. Sleep. 1993;16(2):171–83.

87. Affanni JM, Cervino CO, Marcos HJ. Absence of penile erections during paradoxical sleep. Peculiar penile events during wakefulness and slow wave sleep in the armadillo. J Sleep Res. 2001;10(3):219–28.

88. Schmidt MH, et al. The effects of spinal or mesencephalic transections on sleep-related erections and ex-copula penile reflexes in the rat. Sleep. 1999;22(4):409–18.

89. Schmidt MH, et al. Role of the lateral preoptic area in sleep-related erectile mechanisms and sleep generation in the rat. J Neurosci. 2000;20(17):6640–7.

90. Schmidt MH. Sleep-related penile erections. In: Kryger MH, Roth T, Dement WC, editors. Principles and practice of sleep medicine. Philadelphia: Saunders; 2000. pp. 305–18.

Women's Health and Sleep Disorders

Kathryn A. Lee

Development

The development of sleep medicine in relation to women's health issues has lagged behind what has been learned about sleep in general and what has been learned about sleep specifically in men across the lifespan. This lag was primarily a result of two issues. First, most of the pioneering research in the early twentieth century was conducted by male scientists who were focused on basic questions of why we sleep, and how to best measure sleep and its architecture in a controlled laboratory setting. The second issue was the added complexity of the female reproductive cycle, with hormones that fluctuate on a monthly cycle, often in an unpredictable pattern over the monthly cycle. These two issues forced many researchers to limit their animal models to male rats or hamsters, and limit their human research to healthy young males who would voluntarily subject themselves to strange equipment and protocols in clinical laboratory trials over many nights.

In addition to the complexity of studying normal sleep architecture in women while controlling for hormonal fluctuations, there was also fear of doing harm to a potential fetus. This fear was at the forefront of researchers' ethical concerns about involving women of childbearing age in research, regardless of whether it was sleep research or any other type of clinical trial. Even with adequate birth control measures in place, women remained excluded from research participation because of the unknown effects of oral contraceptives on sleep or because of the risk that pregnancy status could change over the course of any longitudinal study.

From studies of gonadal hormones in the first half of the 1900s, we learned how sex steroids function in men and women. Hans Selye (1941) [1, 2], most known for his research on the stress response, was one of the first to note the anesthetic properties of steroid hormones on male and female rats. After Merryman and colleagues (1954) [3] reported that progesterone had soporific properties in humans, there were further supportive studies in both animal models [4-6] and human clinical trials of men and women [7–9]. From these early findings, it was clear that sleep researchers would either need to avoid women of childbearing age, given their fluctuating progesterone levels across the menstrual cycle, or control for these fluctuating hormones in their study design by selecting a particular phase of the menstrual cycle for sleep monitoring in the laboratory setting. As seen in Fig. 53.1, the menstrual cycle is a complex and dynamic endocrine process that occurs monthly, but ovulation is not predictable, and hormonal patterns are not predictable, even in women who do ovulate. If no ovulation occurs (at about day 14 of a 28-day cycle), then hormone levels are flat during the luteal phase [10].

Nathaniel Kleitman and his colleagues (1937) [11] were the first to study human sleep, and their sample of 35 young adults included 11 women, primarily graduate students at the University of Chicago. They described each adult's age, sex, history of smoking and alcohol consumption, and sleep habits, but no mention was made of women's menstrual cycles. In 1966, Williams, Agnew, and Webb published the first report on polysomnography (PSG) sleep characteristics in women. In that study of 16 women, researchers made a point of not monitoring PSG during days of menstrual flow, but exact phase of their cycles were not reported. During menstrual flow, there may be uterine cramping and pain, but all gonadal hormones would be secreted at basal levels, and comparable to levels in men of the same age [12].

A few years later, Williams and colleagues (1974) [13] compiled PSG data in a book format organized by sex and decade of life. These researchers were the first to control for potential menstrual cycle effects by studying women of childbearing age only during their follicular phase. In the follicular phase, before ovulation, progesterone levels remain low. Sample sizes were small (ten women between 20 and 29 years old and ten women between 30 and 39 years old) and

K. A. Lee (✉)
San Francisco Family Health Care Nursing, University of California, 2 Koret Way, Room N411Y, San Francisco, CA 94143-0606, USA

S. Chokroverty, M. Billiard (eds.), *Sleep Medicine,* DOI 10.1007/978-1-4939-2089-1_53,

Fig. 53.1 The menstrual cycle. The menstrual cycle begins day 1 with menses or menstrual bleeding (early follicular phase). In the follicular phase, levels of progesterone and estrogen are low. The mid-follicular phase involves endometrial proliferation and a slow rise in estrogen to the point of ovulation. The follicular phase ends with a burst of luteinizing hormone (LH) if ovulation occurs (about day 14), and the follicle is released from the ovary to begin the luteal phase. At the mid-luteal phase, progesterone is at its peak, and falls until the next cycle begins (about 27–30 days). If ovulation does not occur, there is no luteal phase, progesterone remains flat, and the next cycle may begin earlier than 25 days or later than 35 days [10]. (reprinted with permission from Elsevier Jan 11, 2014)

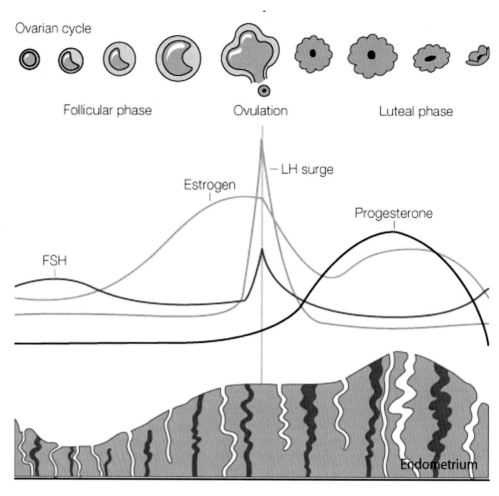

included only healthy females across the lifespan. The small samples of women between 40 and 49 years old and between 50 and 59 years old were likely in various stages of menopausal transition [13]. It was in these comparison studies that older women appeared to have more delta sleep (stages 3 and 4) than men of the same age [13].

Ernest Hartmann (1966) [14] was the first sleep researcher to study women's sleep architecture as it changed during the menstrual cycle. As a psychiatrist, he saw mood disorders in female patients that appeared to fluctuate in severity by phase of the menstrual cycle. He focused on REM sleep and reported PSG findings from four young healthy women and three psychiatric inpatients. Six of these seven women complained of premenstrual symptoms and the seventh was taking hormone therapy and hence not ovulating. He noted differences in rapid eye movement (REM) sleep when the follicular (preovulation) phase was compared to the luteal (postovulation) phase. However, findings from this type of small sample were not particularly generalizable to the population of all young women, and his findings have not been replicated. In the next published study on women's sleep, Ho (1972) [15] reported no changes in REM across three menstrual cycles in her sample of six healthy women. Three

of the women in Ho's study were taking oral contraceptives and had less delta sleep (stages 3 and 4) while the other three women had an increase in delta sleep from their follicular to luteal phase. Ho's (1972) [15] report was published as an abstract and presented at a national sleep conference. More complete details of her dissertation research were also published [16].

Sleep Disorders Associated with the Menstrual Cycle

When published in 1979, the diagnostic classification of sleep and arousal disorders (DCSAD) included a category under excessive somnolence called, "periodic hypersomnia" or "menstrual associated" excessive daytime sleepiness. It was described as "well established" based on three citations ([17], p. 58, 80–81)). However, it was based on one case of a young adolescent with premenstrual hypersomnia [18]. In 1982, another case of periodic hypersomnia was reported involving a 21-year-old with hypersomnia, but her excessive sleepiness occurred during the follicular phase [19]. In an early comparison study of sleep architecture in healthy women at two phases of the menstrual cycle, there were no significant differences in sleep stages that would indicate risk for premenstrual hypersomnia [20].

In the past two decades, there have been some changes and additions to types of sleep disorders associated with the menstrual cycle. Most of these studies involve women with varying levels of premenstrual distress. More severe cases of premenstrual distress are likely to have an underlying mood disorder that may fluctuate on a monthly basis with hormonal fluctuations in phases of the menstrual cycle. In more recent carefully controlled studies of premenstrual dysphoria, researchers have found no particular alterations in sleep architecture when compared to healthy controls [21].

The Diagnostic and Statistical Manual of Mental Disorders (DSM-IV) published by the American Psychiatric Association (APA) includes premenstrual dysphoric disorder (PMDD) and describes disturbed sleep as one of the many symptoms within this disorder [22]. The type of disturbed

sleep is highlighted as subjective reports rather than objective PSG findings, and focuses on complaints about insomnia and increased awakenings during the premenstrual week, rather than hypersomnia. However, DSM-IV research criteria for PMDD diagnosis do not distinguish between insomnia and hypersomnia [22] and the next edition of the DSM, scheduled for publication in 2013, may further refine this disorder.

Today, there is a somewhat better understanding of how progesterone and other hormones affect women's sleep. Whether studies involve natural changes in intrinsic levels of hormone over the menstrual cycle [20] or extrinsic sources of progestins contained in oral contraceptives or hormone replacement therapy, it is critical that sleep researchers attend to the type of hormone and how it is metabolized [23]. Current research on sleep disorders associated with the menstrual cycle continues to focus on premenstrual mood disorders, but women with polycystic ovaries are beginning to be

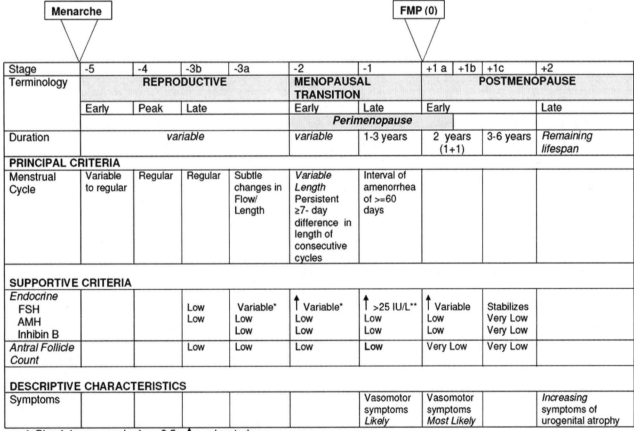

Stage	-5	-4	-3b	-3a	-2	-1	+1 a	+1b	+1c	+2
Terminology	REPRODUCTIVE				MENOPAUSAL TRANSITION		POSTMENOPAUSE			
	Early	Peak	Late		Early	Late	Early			Late
					Perimenopause					
Duration	*variable*				*variable*	1-3 years	2 years (1+1)	3-6 years		*Remaining lifespan*
PRINCIPAL CRITERIA										
Menstrual Cycle	Variable to regular	Regular	Regular	Subtle changes in Flow/ Length	*Variable Length* Persistent ≥7- day difference in length of consecutive cycles	Interval of amenorrhea of >=60 days				
SUPPORTIVE CRITERIA										
Endocrine FSH AMH Inhibin B			Low Low Low	Variable* Low Low	↑ Variable* Low Low	↑ >25 IU/L** Low Low	↑ Variable Low Low	Stabilizes Very Low Very Low		
Antral Follicle Count			Low	Low	Low	Low	Very Low	Very Low		
DESCRIPTIVE CHARACTERISTICS										
Symptoms						Vasomotor symptoms *Likely*	Vasomotor symptoms *Most Likely*			*Increasing symptoms of urogenital atrophy*

* Blood draw on cycle days 2-5   ↑ = elevated
**Approximate expected level based on assays using current international pituitary standard[67-69]

Fig. 53.2 Stages of reproduction and menopausal transition. The stages of women's reproductive aging include reproduction, menopausal transition, and postmenopause. The duration of each stage is variable, but menopausal transition has an early and late phase with endocrine changes noted, particularly in high follicle stimulating hormone (FSH) levels due to the absence of ovarian estrogen. Menopause is defined as no menses for 12 months (FMP = final menstrual period) and occurs at about 50 years of age, on average. Vasomotor symptoms of hot flashes and night sweats are most likely to occur during late perimenopause and early postmenopause stage [38]. (Elsevier journal—reprinted with permission on January 11, 2014)

studied in sleep research because this infertility syndrome includes higher testosterone levels, obesity, and sleep apnea [24].

Sleep Disorders Associated with Pregnancy and Postpartum

The earliest study of women's sleep during the last weeks of pregnancy and first few days after labor and delivery began with Ismet Karacan and his colleagues in Florida, USA. These studies involved only a few women in the hospital setting and results began appearing in published abstracts in 1967 and 1968 [25]. Most notable during those early studies was the researchers' careful control for the newborn's influence on the mother's sleep. Each mother's nocturnal sleep was monitored with PSG during the first few postpartum nights while her newborn was kept in the nursery all night. Since those initial reports, researchers have conducted more carefully controlled laboratory PSG studies with larger samples [26, 27] or focused on the naturalistic setting of the home environment using ambulatory PSG monitoring [28, 29]. Studies of pregnant women using PSG were always limited by small sample sizes and were focused on how maternal sleep disordered breathing might affect the fetus [30] or how pregnancy sleep patterns might predict postpartum depression [25, 31].

Since the normal changes in sleep during pregnancy include primarily less total sleep time due to more discomfort and wake time after sleep onset, rather than substantial changes in sleep architecture, more recent studies have utilized wrist actigraphy measures to objectively describe changes in sleep across pregnancy and transition to motherhood. These newer studies address how infant feeding schedules or breastfeeding influence mother's sleep [32–34] or symptoms of depression [35, 36], and how co-sleeping or bed sharing can influence maternal–infant sleep patterns and sudden infant death syndrome [37].

Sleep Disorders Associated with Menopause

Menopause is defined as the cessation of menstrual periods. Due to irregularities in menstrual cycle lengths during menopausal transition, menopause can only be confirmed after 12 consecutive months without a menstrual period. The mean age of natural menopause is about 50–51 years old, but the ovaries can continue to secrete estrogen in sufficient or insufficient amounts for about 5–8 years prior to the actual onset of menopause. As seen in Fig. 53.2, the perimenopausal transition is variable and occurs over an unpredictable number of years, with irregular menstrual cycles and hormonal fluctuations [38].

Surgical menopause can occur abruptly at any age. The abrupt loss of sex hormones from the ovary results in more severe menopausal symptoms. Without ovarian secretion of estrogen, there is no feedback to the hypothalamus to shut off the secretion of follicle stimulating hormone (FSH). Hence, one biological indicator of menopause is the high level of FSH measured in the blood or urine. Very few researchers report FSH levels in their studies of perimenopausal women's sleep, relying primarily on self-report of menstrual cycle regularity or simply not reporting any criteria for assessing menopausal status in women between 40 and 60 years of age. Furthermore, whether menopause was natural or surgically induced is often not reported for women in these types of research studies.

The first known study of hot flashes during sleep was published in 1981 [39]. In that study, nine postmenopausal women between 30 and 55 years of age underwent three nights of PSG. Given their young age, it is not clear how many had surgical or natural menopause. Skin resistance and temperature were monitored in addition to sleep architecture, and 60 % of the awakenings were associated with a hot flash. A wake episode occurred up to one min before the change in temperature was detected, but lag time in the responsiveness of the temperature measure (rectal thermistor) could explain the time difference between awakening and hot flash. In that study, authors reported that hormone replacement therapy (HRT) reduced the mean number of wake episodes from 1.25 h to only 0.7 h, but there was only one woman who experienced hot flashes [39].

In a randomized clinical trial comparing sleep quality changes with 12 weeks of HRT or placebo, 33 women had PSG one night every other week for 6 weeks and there was no change in wake time over the 6 week protocol [40]. In one survey study of sleep quality conducted on a large sample of employed women, Lee and Taylor (1996) [41] reported that twice as many women taking HRT complained about frequent awakenings due to hot flashes (27 %) than women of the same age not taking HRT (14 %), but this study had no baseline pre-HRT measure and the prevalence of complaints could have been even higher before starting HRT. Finally, 21 postmenopausal women with natural menopause between 45 and 65 years of age, had two nights of PSG at baseline and at 6-month follow-up, and HRT did not change their sleep architecture [42]. That postmenopausal sample had low rates of sleep disordered breathing and periodic leg movements, but each woman was carefully selected using FSH levels, was at least 6 months post natural menopause, had no psychiatric mental health disorders, and was in the normal range for body mass index [42].

Laboratory studies of menopausal women during the 1980s concluded that differences in objective PSG sleep data were minor, primarily small increases in percentage of wake time during the night. These small objective PSG differences did not reflect the type of severity in disturbed sleep that women were self-reporting. Shaver and colleagues (1988) [43] controlled for age and studied 12 perimenopausal women with no symptoms compared to 20 women with menopausal symptoms. Wake time was 10 % in the asymptomatic group and only 13 % in the symptomatic group. These results were supported by later studies as well [44, 45].

When Freedman and Roehrs (2004) [46] studied 12 symptomatic women compared to 8 asymptomatic women between 46 and 51 years of age, they also noted no PSG differences; the symptomatic group averaged 5 hot flashes per night (range 1–18 hot flashes), but interestingly, 6 of the 8 asymptomatic women also had hot flashes during their sleep. Freedman and Roehrs (2006) [47] then studied women over four nights in the sleep laboratory under carefully controlled temperature conditions (30, 23, and 18°C) after a baseline night and reported that hot flashes with arousals were more likely to occur in the first part of the night than in the second half when REM sleep is more prevalent. The hot flashes and arousals were also reduced for the women randomly assigned to sleep in the coldest ambient condition (18°C). Since thermoregulation is absent during REM sleep, and fewer arousals occurred in the second half of the night, the researchers hypothesized that REM sleep may suppress hot flashes [47]. This milestone study on the timing of the hot flashes during the night may begin to explain why subjective sleep complaints are worse than objective PSG recordings summarized over the entire night would indicate. In a follow-up study of over 100 peri and postmenopausal women, they found that objective sleep disturbance was explained by sleep disordered breathing and periodic limb movements rather than hot flashes, while subjective complaints were best explained by hot flashes and higher levels of anxiety [48].

Summary

Many issues related to women and sleep across the lifespan have evolved since the early descriptive studies of the 1960s and 1970s that controlled for healthy lifestyle behaviors and body weight and smoking. Before 2001, many researchers either avoided women as volunteer participants, or failed to describe their reproductive status. With more focus on sleep disorders in the twenty-first century, reproductive status and other health and lifestyle characteristics need to be included in descriptions of the samples that include women. Today, most government sponsors require inclusion of women in research studies, however we are still contending with the smaller samples of women that preclude any statistical analyses by sex, and reconciling the differences between self-reported sleep complaints and objective PSG or actigraphy measures.

References

1. Lee KA, Shaver JF, Giblin EC, Woods NF. Sleep patterns related to menstrual cycle phase and premenstrual affective symptoms. Sleep. 1990;13(5):403–9.
2. Lee K, Taylor DL. Is there a generic midlife woman? The health and symptom experience of midlife women. Menopause. 1996;3(3):154–64.
3. Kawakami M, Sawyer CH. Effects of sex hormones and antifertility steroids on brain thresholds in the rabbit. Endocrinology. 1967;80(5):857–71.
4. Erlik Y, Tataryn IV, Meldrum DR, Lomax P, Bajorek JG, Judd HL. Association of waking episodes with menopausal flushes. JAMA. 1981;245(17):1741–4.
5. Karacan I, Williams RL, Hursch CJ, McCaulley M, Heine MW. Some implications of the sleep patterns of pregnancy for postpartum emotional disturbances. Br J Psychiatry. 1969;115(525):929–35.
6. Papy JJ, Conte-DeVolx B, Sormani J, Porto R, Guillaume V. The periodic hypersomnia and megaphagic syndrome in a young female, correlated with menstrual cycle. Rev Electroencephalogr Neurophysiol Clin. 1982;12(1):54–61.
7. Wolfson AR, Crowley SJ, Anwer U, Bassett JL. Changes in sleep patterns and depressive symptoms in first-time mothers: last trimester to 1-year postpartum. Behav Sleep Med. 2003;1(1):54–67.
8. Lee KA, Zaffke ME, McEnany G. Parity and sleep patterns during and after pregnancy. Obstet Gynecol. 2000;95(1):14–8.
9. Brownell LG, West P, Kryger MH. Breathing during sleep in normal pregnant women. Am Rev Respir Dis. 1986;133(1):38–41.
10. Wilke G, Shapiro CM. Sleep deprivation and the postnatal blues. J Psychosom Res. 1992;36(4):309–16.
11. Selye H. Acquired adaptation to the anesthetic effect of steroid hormones. J Immunol. 1941;41(3):259–68.
12. Williams RL, Karacan I, Hursch CJ. Electroencephalography (EEG) of human sleep: clinical applications. New York: Wiley; 1974.
13. Henderson A, Nemes G, Gordon NB, Roos L. The sleep of regularly menstruating women and of women taking an oral contraceptive. Psychophysiol Abstract. 1970;7:337.
14. Ho A. Sex hormones and the sleep of women. Sleep Res. 1972;1:184.
15. Freedman RR, Roehrs TA. Lack of sleep disturbance from menopausal hot flashes. Fertil Steril. 2004;82(1):138–44.
16. Herrmann WM, Beach RC. Experimental and clinical data indicating the psychotropic properties of progestogens. Postgrad Med J. 1978;54(Suppl. 2):82–7.
17. McKenna JJ, Mosko S, Dungy C, McAninch J. Sleep and arousal patterns of co-sleeping human mother/infant pairs: a preliminary physiological study with implications for the study of sudden infant death syndrome (SIDS). Am J Phys Anthropol. 1990;83(3):331–47.
18. Blumer D, Migeon C. Hormone and hormonal agents in the treatment of aggression. J Nerv Ment Dis. 1975;160(2–1):127–37.
19. Goyal D, Gay C, Lee K. Fragmented maternal sleep is more strongly correlated with depressive symptoms than infant temperament at three months postpartum. Arch Womens Ment Health. 2009;12(4):229–37.
20. Diagnostic Classification of Sleep and Arousal Disorders: DC-SAD. Sleep. 1979 Autumn 2(1):1–154.
21. Yokoyama A, Ramirez VD, Sawyer CH. Sleep and wakefulness in female rats under various hormonal and physiological conditions. Gen Comp Endocrinol. 1966;7(1):10–7.
22. Komisaruk BR, McDonald PG, Whitmoyer DI, Sawyer CH. Effects of progesterone and sensory stimulation on EEG and neuronal activity in the rat. Exp Neurol. 1967;19(4):494–507.

23. Freedman RR, Roehrs TA. Effects of REM sleep and ambient temperature on hot flash-induced sleep disturbance. Menopause. 2006;13(4):576–83.

24. Little BC, Matta RJ, Zahn TP. Physiological and psychological effects of progesterone in man. J Nerv Ment Dis. 1974;159(4):256–62.

25. Williams RL, Agnew HW Jr, Webb WB. Sleep patterns in the young adult female: an EEG study. Electroencephalogr Clin Neurophysiol. 1966;20(3):264–6.

26. Billiard M, Guilleminault C, Dement WC. A menstruation-linked periodic hypersomnia. Kleine-Levin syndrome or new clinical entity? Neurology. 1975;25(5):436–43.

27. Manber R, Armitage R. Sex, steroids, and sleep: a review. Sleep. 1999;22(5):540–55.

28. Purdie DW, Empson JA, Crichton C, McDonald L. Hormone replacement therapy, sleep quality and psychological well-being. Br J Obstet Gynaecol. 1995;102(9):735–9.

29. Selye H. Anesthetic effect of steroid hormones. Exp Biol Med. 1941;46(1):116–21.

30. Young T, Rabago D, Zgierska A, Austin D, Laurel F. Objective and subjective sleep quality in premenopausal, perimenopausal, and postmenopausal women in the Wisconsin Sleep Cohort Study. Sleep. 2003;26(6):667–72.

31. Freedman RR, Roehrs TA. Sleep disturbance in menopause. Menopause. 2007;14(5):826–9.

32. Kleitman N, Mullin FJ, Cooperman NR, Titelbaum S. Sleep characteristics: how they vary and react to changing conditions in the group and the individual. Chicago: University of Chicago Press; 1937.

33. Woodward S, Freedman RR. The thermoregulatory effects of menopausal hot flashes on sleep. Sleep. 1994;17(6):497–501.

34. American Psychiatric Association (APA). Diagnostic and statistical manual of mental disorders: DSM-IV. 4th ed. Washington, DC: American Psychiatric Association; 1994.

35. Baker FC, Sassoon SA, Kahan T, Palaniappan L, Nicholas CL, Trinder J, Colrain IM. Perceived poor sleep quality in the absence of polysomnographic sleep disturbance in women with severe premenstrual syndrome. J Sleep Res. 2012;21(5):535–45.

36. Driver HS, Shapiro CM. A longitudinal study of sleep stages in young women during pregnancy and postpartum. Sleep. 1992;15(5):449–53.

37. Harlow SD, Gass M, Hall JE, Lobo R, Maki P, Rebar RW, Sherman S, Sluss PM, de Villiers TJ, STRAW +10 Collaborative Group. Executive summary of the stages of reproductive aging workshop +10: addressing the unfinished agenda of staging reproductive aging. Fertil Steril. 2012;97(4):843–51.

38. Hartmann E. Dreaming sleep (the D-state) and the menstrual cycle. J Nerv Ment Dis. 1966;143(5):406–16.

39. Shaver J, Giblin E, Lentz M, Lee, KA. Sleep patterns and stability in perimenopausal women. Sleep. 1988;11(6):556–61.

40. Hertz G, Fast A, Feinsilver SH, Albertario CL, Schulman H, Fein AM. Sleep in normal late pregnancy. Sleep. 1992;15(3):246–51.

41. Doan T, Gardiner A, Gay CL, Lee KA. Breast-feeding increases sleep duration of new parents. J Perinat Neonatal Nurs. 2007;21(3):200–6.

42. Coble PA, Reynolds CF, 3rd, Kupfer DJ, Houck PR, Day NL, Giles DE. Childbearing in women with and without a history of affective disorder. II. Electroencephalographic sleep. Comprehensive psychiatry. 1994;35(3):215–24.

43. Merryman W, Boiman R, Barnes L, Rothchld I. Progesterone "anaesthesia" in human subjects. J Clin Endocrinol Metab. 1954;14(12):1567–9.

44. Mokhlesi B, Scoccia B, Mazzone T, Sam S. Risk of obstructive sleep apnea in obese and nonobese women with polycystic ovary syndrome and healthy reproductively normal women. Fertil Steril. 2012;97(3):786–91.

45. Montgomery-Downs HE, Clawges HM, Santy EE. Infant feeding methods and maternal sleep and daytime functioning. Pediatrics. 2010;126(6):e1562–8.

46. Montgomery-Downs HE, Insana SP, Clegg-Kraynok MM, Mancini LM. Normative longitudinal maternal sleep: the first 4 postpartum months. Am J Obstet Gynecol. 2010;203(5):465, e1–7.

47. Montplaisir J, Lorrain J, Denesle R, Petit D. Sleep in menopause: differential effects of two forms of hormone replacement therapy. Menopause. 2001;8(1):10–6.

48. Nillni YI, Toufexis DJ, Rohan KJ. Anxiety sensitivity, the menstrual cycle, and panic disorder: a putative neuroendocrine and psychological interaction. Clin Psychol Rev. 2011;31(7):1183–91.

The Emergence of Pediatric Sleep Medicine

54

Oliviero Bruni and Raffaele Ferri

AASM	American Academy of Sleep Medicine
ADHD	Attention-deficit hyperactivity disorder
AS	Active sleep
CNS	Central nervous system
EEG	Electroencephalography
EPSC	European Pediatric Sleep Club
ESRS	European Sleep Research Society
HVS	High-voltage slow
ICSD	International Classification of Sleep Disorders
IPSA	International Pediatric Sleep Association
OSAS	Obstructive sleep apnea syndrome
PLMS	Periodic limb movements in sleep
QS	Quiet sleep
REM	Rapid eye movement
RLS	Restless legs syndrome
SDB	Sleep-disordered breathing
SIDS	Sudden infant death syndrome

General Overview

Sleep medicine in adults as a scientific field was born in the 1970s, and until the 1980s, the classical pediatric textbooks almost ignored the topics of sleep disturbances with very few parts of the books dedicated to sleep disorders.

The emergence of pediatric sleep medicine started gradually with some important publications that began to raise awareness on the importance of sleep in infancy and childhood development. Richard Ferber in the Boston Children's

O. Bruni (✉)
Department of Developmental and Social Psychology, Center for Pediatric Sleep Disorders, Sapienza University, Rome, Italy
e-mail: oliviero.bruni@uniroma1.it

R. Ferri
Department of Neurology, Sleep Research Centre, I.C., Oasi Institute for Research on Mental Retardation and Brain Aging (IRCCS), Troina, Italy

Hospital wrote the first book for parents entitled *Solve Your Child's Sleep Problems* in 1985 [1], summarizing the behavioral treatment for pediatric insomnia and explaining for the first time the developmental and behavioral aspects of sleep. A hallmark reference for the pediatric sleep research in the following years was the publication of the book *Sleep and Its Disorders in Children,* edited by Christian Guilleminault [2]. The contributions presented in that book provided the basis for the future development of a knowledge base for understanding normal sleep in infants and children [3].

The first comprehensive pediatric sleep textbook *Pediatric Sleep Medicine* was published by Sheldon et al. in 1992 [4], followed by the reference book *Principles and Practice of Sleep Medicine in the Child* by Richard Ferber and Meir Kryger in 1995 [5], and then the revised edition *Principles and Practice of Pediatric Sleep Medicine* by Sheldon et al. in 2005 [6, 7].

Schools of sleep medicine, hospitals, and academic clinics set up training programs, residencies, and fellowships in pediatric sleep medicine and recognized the peculiarity and uniqueness of sleep during human development.

These different approaches led to a gradual and huge increase in pediatric sleep publications and many other books have been published, with special emphasis on respiratory disturbances during sleep, paralleling the amount of publications indexed on PubMed from the 1980s.

Figure 54.1 shows the number of publications that can be found in PubMed with the search word "sleep" limited to humans and all children (01–18 years). There was a steep increase in papers, especially in the past decade.

Over the past 30 years, there has also been an increasing awareness of pediatric pulmonologists and pediatric otolaryngologists on the role of sleep and its disorders in their clinical work, with an increasing understanding of the importance of a comprehensive knowledge of sleep medicine. This awareness led to a proliferation of sleep centers in the USA and in Europe, and more and more countries are still building their own sleep centers. At the same time, the need for the development of specialized centers for children be-

S. Chokroverty, M. Billiard (eds.), *Sleep Medicine,* DOI 10.1007/978-1-4939-2089-1_54,
© Springer Science+Business Media, LLC 2015

Fig. 54.1 Number of publications in PubMed with search word "sleep" limited to humans and all children (0–18 years)

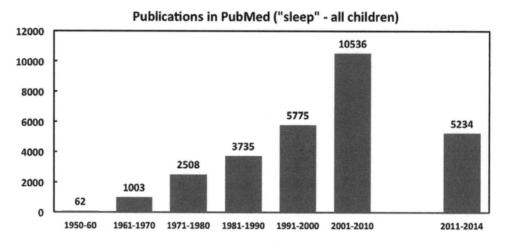

came evident due to the clear differences in sleep physiology and disturbances between adults and infants or children. Finally, at the dawn of the twenty-first century, sleep research began to penetrate into different fields of medicine and social health, with population studies on the effect of sleep on health risks. It became evident that there was a progressive decrease of sleep duration in the modern societies, contributing potentially to ill-health and reduced safety.

In the following sections, we outline the development of pediatric sleep medicine. We first review the clinical picture, analyzing studies on insomnia, parasomnias, respiratory disturbances, narcolepsy, disorders of movements during sleep, and sudden infant death syndrome (SIDS). In the second part, we describe how the initial studies on infant and child sleep helped the discovery of rapid eye movement (REM) sleep and how sleep research led to the definition of sleep structure in newborns, infants, and children. The third part describes the fascinating stories of sleep researchers that made this process possible and that built the history of pediatric sleep medicine. The final section is devoted to the description of the birth of different pediatric sleep associations.

The Unveiling of Infant and Child Sleep Disorders

During the nineteenth century, the first books on infant/child care had been published but sleep in those books was almost completely neglected and was never viewed as a problem. The fact that sleep at night was not consolidated and some activities went on during the night might have led to night awakenings not being considered as disrupting sleep or rest. With the advent of artificial light and the regulation of working and school hours, habits have dramatically changed and sleep has become more and more consolidated into one single bout per night. At the beginning of the twentieth century, the first recommendations for sleep need for infants and children have been published.

The literature of the 1800s includes books by doctors and medical professors that give recommendations about infant sleep and expectations with regard to "normal sleep" (e.g., "newborns don't sleep for more than 2 hours at a time," "children won't sleep through regularly until about 17 months"). Also, in their writings, we can find some useful advice: "by about 6 months of age babies could get used to sleeping at specific times of the day and that mothers should not rush to comfort the baby immediately, but should instead see if it resettles on its own."

Looking at the first scientific publications that can be accessed through PubMed, we found some interesting papers that could give us a picture of how sleep was considered in the first decades of the past century. In one of these papers, "Sleep Requirements of Children" published in the *California State Journal of Medicine* in 1921, there were recommendations for the amount of sleep for each age and several statements of common sense that would have been demonstrated scientifically several years later by the literature [8].

In a lecture at the Section of Diseases of Children at the combined meeting of the British and Canadian Medical Associations, published in 1931, Dr. Cameron categorized sleep disturbances as follows: (1) sleeplessness and continuous crying in young infants, (2) sleeplessness in older children, (3) night terrors, and (4) enuresis. Describing sleeplessness in infants, he identified three causative factors: (a) pain (mainly colic or dyspepsia or aerophagy treated with chloral hydrate 10 min before each feed) or discomfort (nasal obstruction treated with few drops of adrenaline solution in the nostrils before the child is put to the breast), (b) inherited or constitutional neuropathy (that resembles the description of neonatal hyperexcitability), and (c) faulty management that resembles the description of behavioral insomnia of childhood [9]. Dr. Cameron affirmed that most infants who are sleepless and who cry constantly without any specific pain or discomfort do so because the management is faulty: "It is through the mother or the nurse that we must work to get our effects...." Dr. Cameron also suggested some practices to help crying infants, such as the primitive habit in all countries of putting the crying infant in the swaddling clothes and enveloped in the steady pressure of a light and porous shawl, or putting the infant up against the mother's back (as in the African culture), so that he/she takes no part in the expression of her emotions, and divulging her thoughts from the child would lead the restless infant to soundly fall asleep. Interestingly, he finally expounded on a theory by which hypoglycemia or the presence of ketone bodies in the blood leads to enuresis, sleepwalking, and night terrors.

In a paper published in 1936 [10], the causes of disturbances of sleep in children had been classified as: (1) *Constitutional neuropathy:* This included restless children who did not fall asleep easily and who were easily aroused by even trivial environmental stimuli; this was attributed to a calcium deficiency and treated with calcium. (2) *Sleep disturbances accompanying disease:* in infants, painful conditions like otitis media, pain of colic and intestinal disturbances, hunger, teething, and eczema; and in older children, renal colic, rheumatic fever, cardiomyopathies, and respiratory difficulties. Preferred treatments were narcotics (codeine very effective) and the barbiturates were given freely, especially when there was considerable restlessness. (3) *Faulty physical and mental hygiene:* Disturbed sleep or failure to fall asleep may be due to uncomfortable or too much clothing or emotional disturbances. The author suggested that, in infancy, faulty sleeping habits are easily established and difficult to overcome. Overstimulation, as represented by a too-ambitious school program, too many extracurricular activities (dancing, music lessons, etc.), premature and untimely participation in social affairs and pleasures of the adult, and unsuitable movies and radio programs, are not conducive to restful sleep. (4) *Temperatures on the child:* The high temperature would determine a tremendous increase of the child's motor activity. (5) *Heavy meals:* A heavy meal at night is prone to cause not only excessive motor activity but also terrifying dreams, crying out in sleep, and a constant turning in bed.

The famous pediatrician Benjamin Spock, in the late 1940s, made recommendations that have been greatly influential throughout the next several decades. The advice for getting the baby to sleep was: "The cure is simple: Put the baby to bed at a reasonable hour. Say good night affectionately but firmly, walk out of the room, and don't go back…" [11].

In a following paper in *Pediatrics* (1949) [12], Spock stated that chronic resistance to sleep in infancy is a behavior problem which was formerly rare but was becoming more frequent, and its frequency seems to be related to the trend toward self-regulation to babies and to confusion in how to apply this philosophy. The treatment of sleep problem in the baby less than one year of age with the crying-out method showed that most of these babies would cry indignantly from 10 to 20 min the first night and perhaps 5–10 min the second

night, but a great majority of them would be cured of sleep disturbance within two nights. Spock emphasized that this policy of letting the baby "cry it out" is recommended only for chronic resistance to sleep in infants up to the age of 1 or 1.5 years.

In 1949, an interesting paper analyzed for the first time sleep disturbances in 100 children (5–14 years old) with primary behavior and emotional disorders at Rockland State Hospital Children's Group. Sleep disorders were grouped into five categories:

1. Restlessness and minor disturbed states of sleep were found in 46 cases, divided into two subgroups:
(a) restlessness such as rolling, rocking, tossing, and jerky movements and
(b) talking, mumbling, crying, and swearing
2. Nightmares were found in seven cases
3. Night terrors in only two cases
4. Sleepwalking in one case
5. Enuresis in 26 cases

Although no control group was evaluated, the authors state that there is no doubt that a number of these disorders occur more frequently in institutionalized children who suffer from behavior disorders or emotional disturbances. The most frequent disorders were restlessness and minor disturbed states of sleep and enuresis that apparently occurred frequently in rejected children while nightmares, night terrors, and sleepwalking were relatively infrequent [13].

Kleitman in a paper entitled "Mental hygiene of sleep in children" (1949) [14] described perfectly the different aspects of behavioral insomnia of childhood supporting the behavioral approach and stating that "the child is born with certain capacities for learning, including the ability to synchronize, with ease or difficulty, the primitive sleep-wakefulness cycle with diurnal periodicity in his physical and social environment. To establish good sleep habits in children it is necessary to cooperate with the natural tendency to develop a persistent 24-hour rhythm, reinforcing the latter by the customary methods of conditioning." Moreover, he acknowledged the individual variability for the need of sleep and warned about the recommendations on the amount of sleep needed for the infants and children. He affirmed that "the total time spent in sleep, out of each diurnal period, decreases with age, but not uniformly in all children nor in a particular child at different ages. Tables of hours of sleep provided as a guide to parents are misleading in that the figures suggested for all ages are arbitrarily high. Even if more realistic, such figures could stand only for averages, which, by and large, are meaningless when the individual child is considered."

During the period between 1950 and 1970, most papers were devoted to the definition of sleep problems in children during the first 3 years of life. Illingworth published several papers attempting to categorize sleep disturbances in infants and children [15, 16]. Concluding one paper on sleep problems in the first 3 years of age, he stated:

> Enough has been said to indicate the difficulties and complexities of the problem. He who says that he knows all the answers, or suggests that one particular method is infallible, has little experience of children.... It is not enough merely to instruct the parents to discipline the child, to put him to bed at a fixed time, and, if he objects, to leave him to cry or to drug him. The treatment of sleep problems is not nearly so simple.

The treatment of sleep problems at that time was based on common sense and on the beliefs of a single pediatrician. Illingworth suggested that it is wrong to pick a child up at the first whimper but also that it is essential to go immediately to his/her room when a child wakens with a sudden scream because at these times it would be not only cruel but possibly dangerous not to go to the child. He stated that drugs have little place in sleep problems and phenobarbital is useless with these children. The best drug is chloral hydrate given half an hour before bedtime. Regarding early awakenings, it is humorous to read: "By the age of three he can be made to understand that he must not disturb his parents. Before the age of reason, however, one has to accept this behavior as one of the penalties of having children."

Different studies then attempted to define the normative parameters of sleep in children as well as the frequency of sleep disturbances [17]. A paper analyzed the frequency of night awakenings in 1957, finding a prevalence of 17 % at 6 months and 10 % at 12 months [18]. In a longitudinal study, Klackenberg in 1968 defined the sleep behavior of children up to 3 years of age [19].

Recent studies have debated on the global decrease of sleep duration in infants, children, and adolescents. The notion that children are sleeping less than they used to is widespread in both the scientific literature and the popular media. A recent study identified a secular decline of 0.75 min per year in children's sleep duration over the past 100 years, and the greatest rate of decline in sleep occurred for older children and boys, and on school days. This secular decline, variously ascribed to electrification, increased use of technology, and modern lifestyle, is believed to have resulted in many children not getting enough sleep and being chronically sleep deprived [20]. Although there is a lack of consensus regarding what constitutes "adequate" sleep and whether children are in need of more sleep, the results of this study suggest that short sleep duration is associated with different disorders like obesity [21], neurobehavioral and neurocognitive disturbances [22–25], psychiatric disturbances [26], and substance abuse [27].

In the 1980s, the pioneering studies of Mary Carskadon on sleepiness gave impetus to research in children and especially in adolescents. This research paper on sleepiness and adolescent sleep represents another milestone of pediatric

sleep. Adolescence is accompanied by striking changes in sleep behavior and in the phenomenology of sleep, paralleled by changes in adolescent sleep structure. Sleep behaviors change during adolescence in response to maturational changes of sleep regulatory processes and competing behaviors leading to insufficient sleep for many teens on school nights. Sleep reduction results in sleepiness, irritability, distractibility, inattention, and lack of motivation and can also threaten learning by affecting the memory formation process [28]. Following the observation on sleepiness in adolescents, interest rose on the delayed sleep phase syndrome and the first case was reported by Weitzman in 1981 in a medical student at the Montefiore Hospital in New York [29]. Other descriptions of delayed sleep phase syndrome in adolescents have been made by different authors [30] and represented the beginning of the studies on circadian rhythm sleep disorders in pediatrics.

An overview of the discoveries and investigations that led to the identification of the main pediatric sleep disorders is presented below.

Parasomnias

In the late 1960s, the laboratory investigation for parasomnias in children began with the studies by Kales who, at that time, already discovered their occurrence during slow-wave sleep. He suggested that sleepwalking children had bursts of delta rhythms that were not seen in normal children, suggesting a central nervous system (CNS) immaturity factor in sleepwalkers [31].

The landmark publication on parasomnias was published by Broughton in *Science* in 1968. Broughton demonstrated that nocturnal enuresis, somnambulism, nightmares, and sleep terrors occur preferentially during arousal from slow-wave sleep and are virtually never associated with the REM dreaming state. Additionally, he affirmed that they should be considered disorders of arousal and that the slow-wave sleep arousal episode which sets the stage for these attacks is a normal cyclic event [32].

From these historical papers, different types of parasomnias have been more clearly identified and categorized as occurring at sleep onset and during REM sleep or non-REM sleep. Genetic predisposition [33] and an inherent instability of non-REM sleep have been documented [34]. Also the predisposing or triggering role of underlying sleep disturbances such as obstructive sleep apnea or periodic limb movements in sleep (PLMS) has been identified [35]. The differential diagnosis between parasomnias and nocturnal frontal lobe epilepsy has been elucidated, and a specific scheme and scale have been developed to distinguish the two conditions [36].

Obstructive Sleep Apnea Syndrome

For sure, one of the most striking events in the history of sleep medicine was the discovery of sleep apnea. In 1965, Gastaut et al. [37] first described the polygraphic features of the Pickwickian syndrome and then Lugaresi with Coccagna defined more precisely the obstructive sleep apnea syndrome (OSAS), associated with snoring and hypersomnolence [38]. In January 1972, a young French physiologist, Guilleminault, joined the Stanford group and introduced the use of respiratory and cardiac sensors in night sleep studies.

OSAS was clearly described in 1836 by the novelist Charles Dickens who depicted a boy who was obese and always excessively sleepy and whose symptoms of snoring and sleepiness form the basis of the first article to describe the Pickwickian syndrome, published in 1956 [39, 40]. The first professional mention of OSAS in the medical literature was again in a child by William Hill in the *British Medical Journal* in 1889: "The stupid-looking lazy child frequently suffers from headaches at school, breathes through his mouth instead of his nose, snores and is restless at night, and wakes up with a dry mouth in the morning…" [41]. Just a few years later, another complete description of a child with OSAS was made by William Osler: "At night the child's sleep is greatly disturbed; the respirations are loud and snorting, and there are sometimes prolonged pauses, followed by deep, noisy inspirations…the child is very stupid looking, responds slowly to questions and may be sullen and neurocross…. The influence upon mental development is striking…. It is impossible for them to fix the attention for long at a time" [42].

One of the first patients referred to the Stanford sleep clinic for investigation of severe somnolence was a 10-year-old boy. After collecting other patients, Guilleminault published the first paper on OSAS in children in 1976 in *Pediatrics*. He described 8 children of 5–14 years of age who were diagnosed with a sleep apnea syndrome similar to that seen in adults. The clinical picture of the children was similar: They presented with loud snoring interrupted by pauses during sleep, excessive daytime sleepiness, decrease in school performance, abnormal daytime behavior, enuresis, morning headache, abnormal weight, and progressive development of hypertension. Most patients were treated with adenotonsillectomy but one underwent tracheostomy [43].

After this first description, the literature on OSAS in children underwent a huge growth, as witnessed by the number of publications indexed in PubMed that increased from 213 in the decade 1971–1980 to 850 between 1981 and 1990, to 1.145 between 1991 and 2000 and to 3.223 between 2001 and 2012.

The research on OSAS in children began therefore after the mid-1970s when the effects on the cardiovascular func-

tions were initially studied. Successively, the research was oriented toward the effects on growth and development, in the 1980s; the association between sleep-disordered breathing (SDB) and cognitive-behavioral problems, in the 1990s; and, in the past decade, on the relationships with obesity, inflammation, and identification of biomarkers, with the research group led by David Gozal providing a terrific impetus to research [23, 24, 44, 45]. These and other original investigations highlighted the importance of childhood OSAS as a multisystemic disorder that independently increases the risk for neurocognitive deficits, reduced academic performance, and cardiovascular and metabolic morbidities. The development of neuropsychological deficits and cardiovascular morbidity is not present in all children with OSAS, and it has been demonstrated that endothelial dysfunction was highly predictive of the neurocognitive status. Moreover, the role of genetic markers in predicting OSAS vulnerability and the impact of OSAS on the metabolism and the cardiovascular function have been elucidated. The severity of OSAS correlates with both lower adiponectin and increased urinary catecholamines, with inflammatory markers (i.e., C-reactive protein) and with alterations in autonomic cardiovascular parameters [23, 24]. Finally, the strict correlation between obesity and SDB has been elucidated showing that obesity may be an independent risk factor for the metabolic syndrome, mediated by inflammation, and that weight loss is effective in treating obese children with SDB [46].

Narcolepsy

The first systematic description of narcolepsy in children was published by Yoss and Daly. They reported 16 children affected by narcolepsy complaining of excessive sleepiness; cataplectic attacks had occurred in 13 children, sleep paralysis in 3 and hypnagogic hallucinations in 5. The age at onset of symptoms varied from 3 to 14 years. The authors emphasized the problems of misinterpretation of symptoms and erroneous diagnosis [47]. Subsequently, several publications on narcolepsy have been published [48], but only in the past years the group from Bologna led by Plazzi clearly defined the peculiar features of childhood narcolepsy characterizing the cataplectic facies [49], the complex array of "negative" (hypotonia) and "active" (ranging from perioral movements to dyskinetic–dystonic movements or stereotypies) motor disturbances at the onset of the disease [50], as well as the relationships with precocious puberty [51, 52]. New data have shown a robust seasonality of the disease onset in children and the association with *Streptococcus pyogenes,* and influenza A H1N1 infection and H1N1 vaccination [53].

Sudden Infant Death Syndrome (SIDS)

SIDS is still a mystery for sleep researchers and pediatricians. Despite research dating from more than 100 years, the cause of SIDS is still unknown. SIDS is responsible for approximately one third of all infant deaths between the ages of 1 and 6 months and nearly half of infant mortality for children between 4 and 6 months of age. All of these infants die unexpectedly during sleep and investigators focused their research on cardiorespiratory pathophysiology during sleep and on the variations between sleep states and wakefulness without conclusive results. In 1992, the American Academy of Pediatrics initiated the "Back to Sleep" campaign, which recommended supine sleep in all infants when they are placed in bed in an effort to prevent SIDS [54]. The most recent research evidence suggests that all infants should be placed in the supine position; that tobacco exposure pre- and postnatally should be avoided; that room sharing without bed sharing is recommended and overheating should be avoided; and that breast-feeding, the use of pacifiers, and immunization should be encouraged for reduction of the risk of SIDS [55].

Restless Legs Syndrome and Periodic Limb Movements

In the 1600s, sir Thomas Willis described the clinical features of restless legs syndrome (RLS) but this disease was not categorized until 1945 by Ekbom, who described the clinical and pathophysiologic correlates of the condition [56] and also reported that it can occur in children. However, we had to wait until 1994 when the US researchers Walters and Picchietti reported the first five cases of children with RLS with an autosomal dominant mode of inheritance and typical RLS signs of leg discomfort (paresthesias) and motor restlessness prevalent at night and at rest, with temporary relief by activity [57]. At that time, they also pointed out the association with PLMS, with "growing pains" and attention-deficit hyperactivity disorder (ADHD). The complex relationships between RLS, PLMS, and ADHD have been highlighted in the 1996 paper by the same authors [58].

The association of RLS with other disturbances like iron deficiency, insomnia, restless sleep, and daytime sleepiness has been subsequently reported [59–61]. After the standardization of the criteria for the diagnosis of RLS in adults [62], specific criteria for the diagnosis of RLS in children aged 2–12 years were established in 2003 [63]. Currently, the most updated criteria (2011 Revised IRLSSG Diagnostic Criteria for RLS; http://irlssg.org/diagnostic-criteria/) include special mentions for the diagnosis of RLS in children; however, the criteria had undergone a new revision that was published for the inclusion on the new *Diagnostic and Sta-*

tistical Manual of Mental Disorders fifth edition (DSM-V) and the *International Classification of Sleep Disorders third edition* (ICSD-III).

From the last decade of the twenty-first century, several papers have been published involving children with RLS, which highlights the relationships with other medical/psychiatric disorders, such as depression, anxiety, irritability, hyperactivity and oppositional defiant disorder, or other sleep disturbances, such as sleepwalking and sleep terrors, or sleep-related movement disorders such as rhythmical movement disorders, which may be the presenting symptoms in some cases of childhood RLS.

Emerging evidence also suggests that RLS is associated with metabolic dysregulation, autonomic dysfunction, and risk of cardiovascular disease also in children [57, 64, 65].

The Discovery of REM Sleep Through the Infant's Eyes and the Definition of the Sleep Architecture During Development

In 1926, during the Russian Academy of Sciences Congress, the pediatricians Denisova and Figurin presented the results of their first formal pediatric sleep research showing that, several times during sleep, infants presented episodes, lasting for 10–15 min every half an hour, during which respiration and pulse became irregular and fast and small muscles presented numerous twitches. This periodic instability of physiological functions was present in healthy children and the authors concluded that "normal sleep is not a state of rest" [66].

The first description that REMs occur in sleep [67] precedes the landmark study that suggested that REMs represented a "lightening" of sleep and might indicate dreaming, due to the close association with irregular respiration and an increase in heart rate [68].

Before the discovery of REM sleep by Aserinsky and Kleitman in 1953, between 1949 and 1952, Aserinsky observed that sleeping infants exhibited a recurring "motility cycle manifested by ocular and gross bodily activity" paralleling the observation of Denisova and Figurin in 1926 [66].

Aserinsky described "periods of motility" (writhing or twitching of the eyelids) and "periods of no motility." This observation led Aserinsky and Kleitman to look for a similar phenomenon in adults and they discovered REM sleep. The average duration of the periods of quiescence was about 23 min and of the entire motility cycle was approximately 50–60 min [69].

After the description of REM sleep, many researchers applied the methodology for defining the specific sleep electroencephalographic (EEG) patterns of infants as described by the French school of Dreyfus-Brisac and Monod [70, 71] and that by Parmelee [72, 73] who first showed two distinctive

EEG patterns of sleep in infants called "active" sleep (AS) and "quiet" sleep (QS). QS is characterized by preserved chin EMG, few body movements, regular respiration and heart rate, and no eye movements; AS is characterized by REMs, frequent small face and limb movements, irregular respiration and heart rate, and the absence of or minimal chin EMG activity.

The same authors subsequently reported the changes of EEG in infants according to maturation related to conceptional age [74, 75] showing that QS in newborns at term is characterized by one of two EEG patterns: *tracé alternant* or high-voltage slow (HVS) activity.

Tracé alternant is an EEG pattern in which 3–8-s bursts of moderate- to high-voltage 0.5–3.0-Hz slow waves intermixed with 2–4-Hz sharply contoured waveforms alternate with 4–8-s intervals of attenuated mixed frequency EEG activity; because this pattern alternates between activity and much less activity, it is considered to be "discontinuous." In contrast, HVS consists of continuous moderately rhythmic 50–150-μV, 0.5–4-Hz slow activity, without the bursting activity of the *tracé alternant*. HVS represents the more mature pattern of QS in infants.

In 1970, Dreyfus-Brisac observed that active (REM) sleep could be identified in polygraphic tracings by 32 weeks of gestation because of the presence of frequent body movements, irregular respiration, and REMs while the eyes were closed. In 1972, Parmelee and Stern recognized QS or non-REM sleep after 36 weeks of gestation and characterized it by the presence of closed eyes with no eye movements, no body movements, and very regular respiration.

The first description of the ontogenesis of sleep states has been published in *Science* in 1966 by Roffwarg, Muzio, and Dement. Dement and Roffwarg tried to answer the question at what age do humans start having dreams. Observing infants, they confirmed the richness of their REMs; they therefore supposed that REM sleep was fundamental for the optimal development of the CNS. Roffwarg and colleagues found infants spent half of their total sleep time in REM sleep, leading to the theory that REM sleep must play an important role in the development and maturation of the immature brain [76]. At the same time, sleep researchers in Prague described the development of sleep in infancy showing that QS (regular breathing with frequency of 30 min, closed eyes without movements, disappearance of body movements, spindles and slow waves in EEG) alternated with AS (irregular respiration, eyes alternatively closed, half-open or there were movements of bulbus oculi, increased frequency of body movements) in about 50–60-min intervals. These authors stated that the most striking changes took place in the first 12 weeks of life [77].

Soon after the publication of the standards recommended by Rechtschaffen and Kales for the scoring of sleep stages in adults [78], it was clear that they were inappropriate for the scoring sleep stages in newborn infants. Therefore, a committee cochaired by Anders, Emde, and Parmelee worked on the definition of criteria for sleep scoring in infants led to the publication of *A Manual for Standardized Techniques and Criteria for Scoring of States of Sleep and Wakefulness in Newborn Infants* in 1971 [79]. Soon after, Guilleminault and Souquet published a manual on the scoring of sleep and respiration during infancy [80].

Petre-Quadens in 1970 described for the first time a decrease of REM sleep time and of REMs in mentally retarded subjects versus normal children, supporting the hypothesis of the importance of REM sleep for CNS development and learning [81]. This and other observations led the researchers to investigate the relationships between REM sleep and cognition and memory for the next two decades.

Later on, a better definition of the evolution of different physiological parameters during sleep in infants was achieved by Curzi-Dascalova et al. (1988) [82] leading to the publication of a manual of methods for recordings and analyzing sleep–wakefulness states in preterm and full-term infants (1996) [83]. However, standards for evaluating sleep in older infants, toddlers, children, and preadolescents were not addressed until the publication of the new American Academy of Sleep Medicine (AASM) manual in 2007 [84] in which a specific pediatric task force was appointed. Not clearly in the manual, but in the associated papers published in the *Journal of Clinical Sleep Medicine,* a critical review and collection of data defined better the features of the sleep structure during development [85]. Several papers have been published criticizing the new scoring manual especially in children [86], but the new scoring rules have been now widely accepted and will be probably changed again during the next years. A recent fundamental publication defining the sleep structure changes during development and based on the new AASM criteria is the *Polysomnographic Atlas of Sleep-Wake States during Development from Infancy to Adolescence* by Scholle and Feldmann-Ulrich (2012) [87].

Just as the rules for sleep scoring in adults cannot be applied to infants and children without specific adaptation, so also the clinical adult criteria cannot be simply adapted to infant and childhood sleep disorders and several modifications are going to occur in the classifications of pediatric sleep disorders either in the DSM-V or in the ICSD-III.

The Contribution by Researchers from Different Countries

There is no doubt that pediatric sleep medicine received a strong initial input from European researchers 40 years ago. At the beginning, there were different, active groups in Europe publishing on the early development of the sleep cycle, sleep EEG, and sleep behavior in infants. The main contributors in this area were Monod, Dreyfus-Brisac, and Prechtl, and research into neonatal sleep was developed tremendously. The studies by the Italian group of Salzarulo and Fagioli shed light on sleep organization and sleep states during development. The French group (Dreyfus-Brisac, Monod, Curzi-Dascalova) worked on the definition of the features of the sleep EEG and respiratory and cardiovascular parameters in newborns and infants; also, the French research contributed to the characterization of sleep apnea, parasomnias, and narcolepsy (Challamel) together with Nevsimalova, from Prague (Czech Republic). In Belgium, André Kahn and his group (Patricia Franco and José Groswasser) made important advancements in clarifying the mechanisms of the SIDS and infant sleep apnea.

In Germany, Prechtl described sleep patterns before and after birth, emphasizing the concept of "state"; other German groups made a big effort to characterize the features of sleep EEG during development (Schölle), as well as the characterization of infant sleep apnea (Poets). In the UK, Stores investigated mainly sleep in children with mental retardation; other sleep researchers were also involved in the research in pediatric sleep (Wiggs, Gringras, Hill, Fleming, and others).

Halasz from Hungary published several papers on the neurophysiology of sleep and on the relationship between sleep and epilepsy in children.

In Italy, Salzarulo and Fagioli were the pioneers in studying the development of sleep states through the first year of life and its relationship to nutrition, as well as the concept of awakening. Another group of Italian researchers (Bergonzi, Gigli, and Ferri) started to explore sleep neuro- and psychophysiology in children with mental retardation, in an international collaboration with Grubar in France and Petre-Quadens in Belgium. In the 1990s, Oliviero Bruni developed a questionnaire for pediatric sleep disturbances now used in different parts of the world [88]. Giannotti and Cortesi explored the sleep habits in adolescents and the sleep problems in children with neurodevelopmental disabilities such as autism and epilepsy. Bruni and his group, in strict collaboration with Ferri, made a great effort to advance the definition of sleep microstructure of sleep in children, characterizing the alterations of the cyclic alternating pattern in normal children and in those with neurodevelopmental disabilities. In Sicily, Silvestri has contributed to the definition of sleep disorders in children with ADHD. Contributions on sleep apnea in children and on the treatment with orthodontic appliances have been reported by the group of Villa [89].

In Israel, following the input by Lavie, Sadeh began to investigate sleep and developed the algorithm for scoring actigraphic recordings in infants and children [90]. Also his studies on normative sleep data in children and on the relationships between sleep and academic achievement made a great advancement in the pediatric sleep field.

In the USA, pediatric sleep medicine at the beginning was represented by Ferber from the Children' Hospital of Boston, MA, who was the first to structure a comprehensive book for treating behavioral insomnia in infants and children which had an enormous success, so that the acronym "ferberize the child" was invented to indicate that you apply the behavioral technique of extinction to solve your child's sleep problem.

Another pioneer of sleep medicine was Anders, who is considered to be a leading expert in the field of child psychiatry and sleep and his research focused on pediatric sleep patterns, including ontogenesis of sleep–wake states from infancy through early childhood; he was one of the coauthors of the manual for sleep scoring in infants and made several studies on sleep in the first year of life. He classified infants as self-soothers or signalers, depending upon whether they cry following a nighttime awakening, or whether they put themselves back to sleep without signaling to their parents. He also studied sleep disorders in children with autism and other neurodevelopmental disorders.

Guilleminault may be considered to be the one who established the branch of sleep medicine in childhood. With his prolific production, Christian Guilleminault has approached several different aspects of sleep medicine and it can be said that there is no branch of pediatric sleep medicine to which he has not contributed.

Carskadon started her career at the Stanford University and, along with Dement, she developed the Multiple Sleep Latency Test. After leaving Stanford for the Brown University, her research interest was devoted to adolescent sleep/wake behavior and consequences of insufficient sleep in adolescents. These studies raised public health issues and determined some changes in the public policy, such as a later school-start time in secondary schools. She is now one of the most influential persons worldwide in the field of adolescent sleep. Her investigations focus on circadian rhythms and puberty, changes in how sleep pressure functions in adolescents, the role of morning-type or evening-type preference on sleep behaviors, sleep loss, and genetic predictors of depressed mood in college students.

Another giant in the sleep field and especially in the sleep apnea field is David Gozal. His fundamental contributions in the past 20 years have revolutionized the studies on sleep apnea in children, especially the relationships between respiratory sleep disorders and neurobehavioral, cardiovascular, and metabolic disease, the mechanisms that mediate defense responses and that lead to complications from low oxygen levels and disrupted sleep, and long-term health and developmental consequences of chronic sleep and breathing problems during childhood.

Also in the field of sleep apnea, Carole Marcus is a leading expert on the diagnosis and management of childhood OSAS; she headed the publication of several clinical practice guidelines on OSAS and conducted fundamental studies on the use of positive airway pressure therapy in children [91].

In the field of insomnia in childhood, Judith Owens made significant contributions on the pharmacologic treatment of sleep disorders in children and on the interaction between sleep and ADHD, as well as on pediatric insomnia and on the impact of delaying school-start time on adolescent sleep, mood, and behavior. Jodi Mindell, a clinical psychologist specializing in pediatric sleep medicine, has published many papers on the treatment of behaviorally based sleep disorders, on pharmacologic treatment of pediatric sleep disorders, and on cultural issues impacting sleep and on the cultural differences in sleep patterns and behaviors. Together with Owens, she cofounded and cochairs the annual international Pediatric Sleep Medicine Conference.

Ronald Chervin made several important contributions to pediatric sleep medicine, especially on the neurological and behavioral effects of sleep disorders; he developed a Pediatric Sleep Questionnaire showing its utility for clinical research and described an association between inattentive, hyperactive behavior, and symptoms of two primary sleep disorders: OSAS and RLS.

In Canada, Brouillette, over the past 30 years, made major contributions to the understanding of childhood OSAS and other controls of breathing disorders; he also developed a specific scale to assess the clinical severity of OSAS and evaluated the utility of oximetry for the diagnosis of OSAS in children.

More recently, Gruber, from McGill University in Montreal, showed the importance of an adequate sleep duration for optimal functioning in children, demonstrating that even a small sleep deprivation has serious consequences for health and daytime functioning. She also examined the association between sleep and attention in infants, children, and adolescents, and the role of sleep in ADHD.

Also pediatric sleep researchers in Australia in the past years have produced significant and important papers: Horne, Blunden, Matricciani, Lushington, Kennedy, Kohler, and others published on the cardiovascular control during sleep in neonates and children, on the declining trend of sleep duration in children and adolescents, on cognitive functioning in normal children and in children and infants with sleep disordered breathing, and on the behavioral treatment of sleep disorders in children.

In South America, Brazil and Chile had the most prolific researchers: In Chile, Peirano and Algarin conducted several studies on the effect of iron deficiency anemia on sleep in children. In Brazil, several researchers such as Tufik, Lahorgue-Nuñes, Lopes, and Alvés also made substantial contributions.

In Japan, Segawa, in collaboration with Nomura, after the discovery of dopamine-responsive dystonia, also known as hereditary progressive dystonia with diurnal fluctuation or Segawa's disease, explored the body movements during sleep in infancy as indicators for the detection of normal or abnormal CNS development. At the same time, Okawa defined the disorders of the circadian rhythm in brain-damaged children, while other sleep researchers such as Kohyama, Komada, Kato, and many others continued to work in the pediatric sleep medicine field.

Many Asian countries are actually growing in the pediatric sleep medicine field, as acknowledged by the increasing number of publications especially from China, Hong Kong, Taiwan, Singapore, and Thailand, and probably new insights and new developments from other developing countries should be expected.

The Establishment of the Pediatric Sleep Associations

During the first sleep congresses in the 1970s, the pediatric sleep field had a marginal place but it was clear that it would have gradually gained its own place since it was immediately evident that a specific "pediatric sleep knowledge" would have been required in order to identify and treat correctly the different sleep disorders of infants and children. As an example, among the differences between children and adults in specific sleep disorders, we can cite the definition of OSAS and other breathing disorders occurring during sleep, the different pattern of periodic limb movements in children, the linkage between sleep disturbances and daytime neurobehavioral and neurocognitive disorders, the identification of infants at risk for SIDS, etc.

Therefore, starting with small symposia or satellite meetings during the congresses of the main sleep adult societies, such as the European Sleep Research Society (ESRS) and the Associated Professional Sleep Societies (APSS), the question regarding a need to have a "specific pediatric garden" was raised very quickly and the basis for the development of independent associations was acknowledged because of the exponential and huge growth of contributions by pediatric sleep researchers.

The European Pediatric Sleep Club

Pediatric sleep medicine in Europe started within the ESRS and paralleled the development of this society; since the very beginning, the future European Pediatric Sleep Club (EPSC) took an active part in the growth of sleep medicine in Europe. A very small group of pediatricians, child neurologists, psychiatrists, and psychologists interested in sleep during development began to join in informal meetings during the early ESRS congresses. The first studies were mostly led by the French researchers following the pioneering work of Dreyfus-Brisac and Monod. Various basic pediatric sleep scientists such as Curzi-Dascalova, Mirmiran, Paul, Dittrichova, Prechtl, Salzarulo, Fagioli, and Kahn worked together to start the European research of infant sleep [92]. Several other colleagues joined this initial group and began to investigate this new field of research. Just some of them are mentioned here: Navelet, Challamel, Guilleminault, Vecchierini, Gaultier, Stores, Peraita-Adrados, Nevsimalova, Katz Salomon, and Poets, but many other scientists also contributed. After the preliminary informal meetings, this group of scientists subsequently constituted the EPSC, as a part of the ESRS, aimed at consolidating the area of pediatric sleep medicine, in order to bring together clinicians and researchers from different disciplines. The EPSC had his own meeting every year since the first one in 1991 in Paris and joins the ESRS congress every 2 years.

The EPSC meetings were held in Paris (1991), Helsinki (1992), Prague (1993), Firenze (1994), Messina (1995), Brussels (1996), Lyon (1997), Madrid (1998), Dresden (1999), Istanbul (2000), Bled (2001), Reykjavik (2002), Rome (2003), and Prague (2004). Following the efforts by André Kahn, the International Pediatric Sleep Association (IPSA) blossomed in 2005 from the EPSC.

The Pediatric Sleep Medicine Conference

The inaugural Pediatric Sleep Medicine Conference was held in Amelia Island, FL, in February 2005. The meeting was cofounded by Mindell and Owens, with the objective of bringing together pediatric sleep experts from around the world to share their science. The meeting also sought to define priorities for basic and clinical research, patient care, and public policy for the emerging field of pediatric sleep medicine. The inaugural conference had 130 attendees and included pediatricians, pulmonologists, psychologists, psychiatrists, and neurologists, as well as social workers and nurses. The highlights of that first meeting were published in an article in the *Journal of the American Medical Association* and a white paper summarizing the consensus conclusions was published in the *Journal of Clinical Sleep Medicine*. The meeting was held yearly until 2009, at which time it became a biennial meeting offset by biennial meetings of the IPSA. The meeting continues to be held in Amelia Island, FL, and now includes courses on best practices in pediatric sleep medicine and pediatric polysomnography.

The International Pediatric Sleep Association

The story of IPSA begins several years ago when a small group of pediatricians, child neurologists, and psychologists interested in sleep started to join in informal meetings during

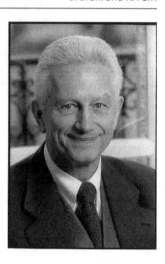

Fig. 54.2 Andrè Kahn

the early ESRS congresses and in 1991 constituted the EPSC, as mentioned above. In 2003, André Kahn and the EPSC started to dream about an international pediatric sleep association. The creation of this international association was the project of André Kahn and was initiated by his efforts and by his dedication to the field of pediatric sleep medicine but, unfortunately, shortly before his 61st birthday, André Kahn abruptly died on September 1, 2004, in Brussels, at the end of his usual karate training session (Fig. 54.2). Thus, during the last EPSC meeting in 2004, it was decided to abandon the EPSC and build up a new international association. This was not an easy step, since there were long debates about the nature of this association which was initially intended as a "clinically oriented" organization. Part of the questions related to the birth of the IPSA was that scientists have too many societies and too many fees to be paid, the fear that founders would not have had the strength and the power to build this association, the uncertainties about who would have really supported this initiative, and the worries about the financial support.

However, the following year, during the World Association of Sleep Medicine (WASM) meeting in Berlin, the IPSA was founded on October 13, 2005, with the crucial contribution of Christian Guilleminault (Fig. 54.3). The bylaws were created stating the mission of IPSA that were: (a) to promote basic and applied research in all areas of sleep in infants, children, and adolescents; (b) to provide topical information to the public about pediatric sleep; (c) to increase the knowledge of pediatric sleep problems and their consequences; (d) to promote teaching programs on pediatric sleep; (e) to hold scientific meetings; and (f) to provide information to the public about perspectives and applications of pediatric sleep research.

The first board was elected and appointed in 2007, with the aim to represent nearly all the countries in the world in which pediatric sleep medicine was pursued, for a 4-year term, consisting of Oliviero Bruni as president, Christian Guilleminault as vice president, and Patricia Franco as sec-

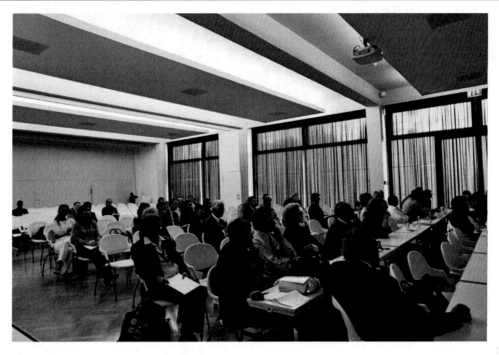

Fig. 54.3 International Pediatric Sleep Association; foundation meeting—Berlin, October 13, 2005

retary. The board of directors comprised Ronald Chervin, David Gozal, Avi Sadeh, Patricio Peirano, Magda Lahorgue-Nuñes, Rosemary Horne, and Daniel Ng.

In 2007, IPSA has been affiliated with Elsevier's journal *Sleep Medicine,* an affiliate of the WASM and, in 2009, it joined the Pediatric Sleep Medicine Conference.

From 2007 to 2009, IPSA meetings were held as part of the WASM congresses but in 2010 the second IPSA congress was organized by Oliviero Bruni in Rome and was the first independent congress of IPSA. The congress was a huge success in terms of participants and high scientific quality, with 203 abstracts, 64 symposia, 1 pediatric sleep course, 1 keynote lecture, and 34 countries represented worldwide.

After this successful meeting, it was decided to continue to have an IPSA meeting every 2 years in different parts of the world. The third IPSA meeting was held in Manchester (UK) in December 2012 and the next IPSA meeting was held in Porto Alegre (Brazil) in 2014.

The goals of the IPSA congresses are and will be to lead to a substantial advancement of pediatric sleep medicine, collecting the most renowned international speakers, and giving to all participants the opportunity to share knowledge in sleep medicine and research.

In 2011, the second election renewed the directors and the current board that will be in charge until 2014.

Finally, in 2012, with the help of Allan O'Bryan (WASM), the IPSA Foundation (a nonprofit organization) has been cre-ated to raise funds from different sources, such as industries and pharmaceutical companies, in order to allow fund-raising for scientific and charity purposes.

Conclusions

This historical overview of the pediatric sleep medicine has several limitations and, most probably, some fundamental researchers have not been cited here or some significant papers not reported. However, the aim was to delineate the evolution of sleep research in infants, children, and adolescents in the past decades. The main important finding is that almost all studies have demonstrated that practically all sleep disorders have a negative impact on the child health. The field of pediatric sleep medicine is a growing field of research with great possibilities of expansion. In a short time, we will contribute to a great technological advancement that will allow us to arrange improved diagnostic equipment and new tools and methods of analysis, specifically for the developmental period. Moreover, the use of new genome-wide approaches will allow us to identify epigenomic profiles associated with specific phenotypes of pediatric sleep disorders, will determine a better understanding of individual risk factors for adverse consequences of sleep disturbance, and will permit us to find the individualized treatment to reduce long-term neurocognitive, cardiovascular, and metabolic consequences.

References

1. Ferber R. Solve your child's sleep problems. New York: Simon & Schuster; 1985.
2. Guilleminault C. Sleep and its disorders in children. New York: Raven Press; 1987.
3. Sheldon SH. Evaluating sleep in infants and children. Philadelphia: Lippincott-Raven; 1996.
4. Sheldon SH, Spire JP, Levy HB. Pediatric sleep medicine. Philadelphia: WB Saunders; 1992. pp. 185–240.
5. Ferber R, Kryger MH. Principles and practice of sleep medicine in the child. Philadelphia: Saunders; 1995.
6. Sheldon SH, Ferber R, Kryger MH. Principles and practice of pediatric sleep medicine. Amsterdam: Elsevier; 2005.
7. Sheldon SH, Ferber R, Kryger MH Gozal D. Principles and Practice of Pediatric Sleep Medicine. 2nd Ed. London: Elsevier Saunders; 2014.
8. No authors listed. Sleep requirements of children. Cal State J Med. 1921;19:418.
9. Cameron HC. Sleep and its disorders in childhood. Can Med Assoc J. 1931;2:239–44.
10. No Authors listed. Disorders of sleep in children. Cal West Med. 1936;45:65–8.
11. Spock B. The common sense book of baby and child care. New York: Duell, Sloan and Pearce; 1946.
12. Spock B. Chronic resistance to sleep in infancy. Pediatrics. 1949;4:89–93.
13. Clardy ER, Hill BC. Sleep disorders in institutionalized disturbed children and delinquent boys. Nerv Child. 1949;8:50–3.
14. Kleitman N. Mental hygiene of sleep in children. Nerv Child. 1949;8:63–6.
15. Illingworth RS. Sleep problems in the first 3 years. BMJ. 1951;1:722–8.
16. Illingworth RS. Sleep problems of children. Clin Pediatr. 1966;5:45–8.
17. Anders TF, Keener M. Developmental course of nighttime sleep-wake patterns in full-term and premature infants during the first year of life: I. Sleep. 1985;8:173–92.
18. Moore T, Ucko LE. Night waking in early infancy. Arch Dis Child. 1957;32:333–42.
19. Klackenberg G. The development of children in a Swedish urban community. A prospective longitudinal study. VI. The sleep behaviour of children up to three years of age. Acta Paediatr Scand Suppl. 1968;187:105–21.
20. Matricciani L, Olds T, Petkov J. In search of lost sleep: secular trends in the sleep time of school-aged children and adolescents. Sleep Med Rev. 2012;16:203–11.
21. Chen X, Beydoun MA, Wang Y. Is sleep duration associated with childhood obesity? A systematic review and meta-analysis. Obesity (Silver Spring). 2008;16:265–74.
22. Ednick M, Cohen AP, McPhail GL, et al. A review of the effects of sleep during the first year of life on cognitive, psychomotor, and temperament development. Sleep. 2009;32:1449–58.
23. Gozal D, Kheirandish-Gozal L, Bhattacharjee R, et al. Neurocognitive and endothelial dysfunction in children with obstructive sleep apnea. Pediatrics. 2010;126:e1161–7.
24. Gozal D, Kheirandish-Gozal L. New approaches to the diagnosis of sleep-disordered breathing in children. Sleep Med. 2010;11:708–13.
25. Hiscock H, Bayer JK, Hampton A, et al. Long-term mother and child mental health effects of a population-based infant sleep intervention: cluster-randomized, controlled trial. Pediatrics. 2008;122:e621–7.
26. Ivanenko A, Johnson K. Sleep disturbances in children with psychiatric disorders. Semin Pediatr Neurol. 2008;15:70–8.
27. Mednick SC, Christakis NA, Fowler JH. The spread of sleep loss influences drug use in adolescent social networks. PLoS One. 2010;5:e9775.
28. Carskadon MA. Sleep's effects on cognition and learning in adolescence. Prog Brain Res. 2011;190:137–43.
29. Weitzman ED, Czeisler CA, Coleman RM, et al. Delayed sleep phase syndrome. A chronobiological disorder with sleep-onset insomnia. Arch Gen Psychiatry. 1981;38:737–46.
30. Thorpy MJ, Korman E, Spielman AJ, et al. Delayed sleep phase syndrome in adolescents. J Adolesc Health Care. 1988;9:22–7.
31. Kales A, Jacobson A, Paulson MJ, Kales JD, Walter RD. Somnambulism: psychophysiological correlates. I. All-night EEG studies. Arch Gen Psychiatry. 1966;14:586–94.
32. Broughton RJ. Sleep disorders: disorders of arousal? Enuresis, somnambulism, and nightmares occur in confusional states of arousal, not in "dreaming sleep". Science. 1968;159:1070–8.
33. Kotagal S. Parasomnias in childhood. Sleep Med Rev. 2009;13:157–68.
34. Bruni O, Ferri R, Novelli L, et al. NREM sleep instability in children with sleep terrors: the role of slow wave activity interruptions. Clin Neurophysiol. 2008;119:985–92.
35. Guilleminault C, Palombini L, Pelayo R, et al. Sleepwalking and sleep terrors in prepubertal children: what triggers them? Pediatrics. 2003;111:e17–25.
36. Derry CP, Harvey AS, Walker MC, et al. NREM arousal parasomnias and their distinction from nocturnal frontal lobe epilepsy: a video EEG analysis. Sleep. 2009;32:1637–44.
37. Gastaut H, Tassinari CA, Duron B. Polygraphic study of diurnal and nocturnal (hypnic and respiratory) episodal manifestations of Pickwick syndrome. Rev Neurol (Paris). 1965;112:568–79.
38. Lugaresi E, Coccagna G, Mantovani M. Hypersomnia with periodic apneas. New York: SP Medical & Scientific Books; 1978.
39. Bickelmann AG, Burwell CS, Robin ED, et al. Extreme obesity associated with alveolar hypoventilation; a Pickwickian syndrome. Am J Med. 1956;21:811–8.
40. Dickens C. Posthumous papers of the Pickwick Club. Philadelphia: Carey, Lea & Blanchard; 1836.
41. Hill W. On some causes of backwardness and stupidity in children. BMJ. 1889;2:771–2.
42. Osler W. The principles and practice of medicine. New York: Appleton; 1892. pp. 335–339.
43. Guilleminault C, Eldridge FL, Simmons FB, et al. Sleep apnea in eight children. Pediatrics. 1976;58:23–30.
44. Beebe DW, Gozal D. Obstructive sleep apnea and the prefrontal cortex: towards a comprehensive model linking nocturnal upper airway obstruction to daytime cognitive and behavioral deficits. J Sleep Res. 2002;11:1–16.
45. Gozal D, Kheirandish-Gozal L. Neurocognitive and behavioral morbidity in children with sleep disorders. Curr Opin Pulm Med. 2007;13:505–9.
46. Van Hoorenbeeck K, Franckx H, Debode P, et al. Weight loss and sleep-disordered breathing in childhood obesity: effects on inflammation and uric acid. Obesity. 2012;20:172–7.
47. Yoss RE, Daly DD. Narcolepsy in children. Pediatrics. 1960;25:1025–33.
48. Nevsimalova S. Narcolepsy in childhood. Sleep Med Rev. 2009;13:169–80.
49. Serra L, Montagna P, Mignot E, et al. Cataplexy features in childhood narcolepsy. Mov Disord. 2008;23:858–65.
50. Plazzi G, Pizza F, Palaia V, et al. Complex movement disorders at disease onset in childhood narcolepsy with cataplexy. Brain. 2011;134:3480–92.
51. Plazzi G, Parmeggiani A, Mignot E, et al. Narcolepsy-cataplexy associated with precocious puberty. Neurology. 2006;66:1577–9.
52. Poli F, Pizza F, Mignot E, et al. High prevalence of precocious puberty and obesity in childhood narcolepsy with cataplexy. Sleep. 2013;36:175–81.

53. Wijnans L, Lecomte C, de Vries C, et al. The incidence of narcolepsy in Europe: before, during, and after the influenza A (H1N1) pdm09 pandemic and vaccination campaigns. Vaccine. 2012. doi:10.1016/j.vaccine.2012.12.015.

54. American Academy of Pediatrics. Task force on infant sleep position and SIDS. Pediatrics. 1992;89:1120–6.

55. Moon RY, Fu L. Sudden infant death syndrome: an update. Pediatr Rev. 2012;33:314–20.

56. Ekbom KA. Restless legs: a clinical study. Acta Med Scand Suppl. 1945;158:1–122.

57. Walters AS, Picchietti DL, Ehrenberg BL, et al. Restless legs syndrome in childhood and adolescence. Pediatr Neurol. 1994;11:241–5.

58. Picchietti DL, Walters AS. Restless legs syndrome and periodic limb movement disorder in children and adolescents comorbidity with attention-deficit hyperactivity disorder. Child Adolesc Psychiatr Clin N Am. 1996;5:729–40.

59. Konofal E, Cortese S, Marchand M, et al. Impact of restless legs syndrome and iron deficiency on attention-deficit/hyperactivity disorder in children. Sleep Med. 2007;7–8:711–5.

60. Kryger MH, Otake K, Foerster J. Low body stores of iron and restless legs syndrome: a correctable cause of insomnia in adolescents and teenagers. Sleep Med. 2002;3:127–32.

61. Picchietti DL, Stevens HE. Early manifestations of restless legs syndrome in childhood and adolescence. Sleep Med. 2008;9:770–81.

62. Walters AS. The International Restless Legs Syndrome Study Group. Toward a better definition of the restless legs syndrome. Mov Disord. 1995;10:634–42.

63. Allen RP, Picchietti D, Henning WA, et al. Restless legs syndrome: diagnostic criteria, special considerations, and epidemiology. A report from the RLS diagnosis and epidemiology workshop at the NIH. Sleep Med. 2003;4:101–19.

64. Angriman M, Bruni O, Cortese S. Does restless legs syndrome increase cardiovascular risk in attention-deficit/hyperactivity disorder? Med Hypotheses. 2013;80:39–42.

65. Walter LM, Foster AM, Patterson RR, et al. Cardiovascular variability during periodic leg movements in sleep in children. Sleep. 2009;32:1093–9.

66. Denisova MP, Figurin NL. Periodic phenomena in the sleep of children. Nov Refl Fiziol Nerv Syst. 1926;2:338–45.

67. De Toni G: I movimenti pendolari dei bulbi oculari dei bambini durante il sonno fisiologico, ed in alcuni stati morbosi. Pediatria. 1933;41:489–98.

68. Aserinsky E, Kleitman N. Regularly occurring periods of eye motility, and concomitant phenomena, during sleep. Science. 1953;118:273–4.

69. Aserinsky E, Kleitman N. A motility cycle in sleeping infants as manifested by ocular and gross bodily activity. J Appl Physiol. 1955;8:11–8.

70. Dreyfus-Brisac C, Fischgold H, Samson-Dollfus D, et al. Veille, sommeil et réactivité sensorielle chez le prématuré, le nouveauné et le nourisson. Clin Neurophysiol. 1957;(Suppl 6):417–40.

71. Monod N, Pajot N. The sleep of the full-term newborn and premature infant. I. Analysis of the polygraphic study (rapid eye movements, respiration and E.E.G.) in the full-term newborn. Biol Neonat. 1965;8:281–307.

72. Parmelee AH, Jr., Schulte FJ, Akiyama Y, et al. Maturation of EEG activity during sleep in premature infants. Electroencephalogr Clin Neurophysiol. 1968;24:319–29.

73. Parmelee A Jr, Akiyama Y, Stern E, et al. A periodic cerebral rhythm in newborn infants. Exp Neurol. 1969;35:575.

74. Dreyfus-Brisac C. Ontogenesis of sleep in human prematures after 32 weeks of conceptional age. Dev Psychobiol. 1970;3:91–121.

75. Parmelee AH, Stern E. Development of states in infants. In: Clemente CD, Purpura DP, Mayer FE, editors. Sleep and the maturing nervous system, New York: Academic Press; 1972. pp. 199–215.

76. Roffwarg HP, Muzio JN, Dement WC. Ontogenetic development of the human sleep-dream cycle. Science. 1966;152:604–19.

77. Dittrichová J. Development of sleep in infancy. J Appl Physiol. 1966;21:1243–6.

78. Rechtschaffen A, Kales A. A manual of standardized terminology, techniques, and scoring system for sleep stages of human subjects. Washington Public Health Service, US Government Printing Office, Washington, DC; 1968.

79. Anders TF, Emde R, Parmelee AH, editors. A manual of standardized terminology, techniques and criteria for scoring of states of sleep and wakefulness in newborn infants. UCLA Brain Information Service, NINDS Neurological Information Network, Los Angeles; 1971.

80. Guilleminault C, Souquet M. Sleep states and related pathology. In: Guilleminault C, Korobkin R, editors. Advances in neonatal neurology. vol. 1. New York: Spectrum Publications; 1979. pp. 225–247.

81. Petre-Quadens O, De Lee C. Eye-movements during sleep: a common criterion of learning capacities and endocrine activity. Dev Med Child Neurol. 1970;12:730–40.

82. Curzi-Dascalova L, Peirano P, Morel-Kahn F. Development of sleep states in normal premature and full-term newborns. Dev Psychobiol. 1988;21:431–44.

83. Curzi-Dascalova L, Mirmiran M. Manual of methods for recordings and analyzing sleep-wakefullness states in preterm and full-term infant. Les Editions INSERM, 1996.

84. Iber C, Ancoli-Israel S, Chesson AL, et al. The AASM manual for the scoring of sleep and associated events: rules, terminology, and technical specifications. 1st ed. Westchester: American Academy of Sleep Medicine; 2007.

85. Grigg-Damberger M, Gozal D, Marcus CL, et al. The visual scoring of sleep and arousal in infants and children. J Clin Sleep Med. 2007;3:201–40.

86. Novelli L, Ferri R, Bruni O. Sleep classification according to AASM and Rechtschaffen and Kales: effects on sleep scoring parameters of children and adolescents. J. Sleep Res. 2010;19:238–47.

87. Scholle, S, Feldmann-Ulrich, E. Polysomnographic atlas of sleepwake states during development from infancy to adolescence. 2nd ed. Landsberg: Ecomed Medizin; 2012. (Polysomnographischer Atlas der Schlaf-Wach-Stadien im Entwicklungsgang vom Säuglings- zum Jugendalter).

88. Bruni O, Ottaviano S, Guidetti V, et al. The sleep disturbance scale for children (SDSC). Construction and validation of an instrument to evaluate sleep disturbances in childhood and adolescence. J Sleep Res. 1996;5:251–61.

89. Villa MP, Bernkopf E, Pagani J, et al. Randomized controlled study of an oral jaw-positioning appliance for the treatment of obstructive sleep apnea in children with malocclusion. Am J Respir Crit Care Med. 2002;165:123–7.

90. Sadeh A, Sharkey KM, Carskadon MA. Activity-based sleepwake identification: an empirical test of methodological issues. Sleep. 1994;17:201–7.

91. Marcus CL, Brooks LJ, Draper KA, et al. American Academy of Pediatrics. Diagnosis and management of childhood obstructive sleep apnea syndrome. Pediatrics. 2012;130:e714–55.

92. Bruni O. Childhood sleep medicine. In: European Sleep Research Society 1972–2012. 40th Anniversary of the ESRS. Claudio L. Bassetti, editor; Knobl B, Schulz H, co-editors. Wecom Gesellschaft für Kommunikation mbH & Co. KG Hildesheim, Germany 2012: pp. 49–50.

Sleep Disorders, Cognition, Accidents, and Performance

Torbjörn Åkerstedt and Pierre Philip

Introduction

Sleep disorders are very common in the adult general population and represent a considerable burden across Western Europe, the USA, and Japan [1]. The prevalence of obstructive sleep apnea syndrome (OSAS) is approximately 5 % in the adult general population [2]. OSAS is not the only disease responsible for excessive daytime sleepiness. Among nonrespiratory sleep disorders, narcolepsy is a major pathology affecting less than 0.1 % of the population [3]. Restless legs syndrome (RLS) and periodic limb movement disorder are frequent pathologies and concern in 5–10 % and 3.9 % of adults, respectively [4]. Insomnia concerns one adult out of five [1].

Sleep disorders affect alertness and cognition and indirectly therefore also affect work performance and safety. But the pattern is complicated and some research is missing. We will here focus mainly on the two major types of sleep disorders—insomnia and OSAS.

The detailed mechanisms linking sleep and performance/accidents have been discussed elsewhere in this volume. However, a brief summary may be appropriate. Thus, the number of hours spent awake will increase sleepiness [5], as will the amount of sleep during the prior night [6]. Over time, sleep shorter than 7 h is associated with increased sleepiness and reduced performance on cognitive and sustained attention tasks [7]. Similarly, sleep fragmentation (>6/h) will increase sleepiness and reduce performance [8]. In addition, the circadian regulation of alertness will be a powerful de-terminant of sleepiness and performance [5], with particularly severe effects in the early morning [5]. The circadian influence applies to sleep disorders that involve circadian misalignment [9], although very few studies exist on the associated performance or safety issues. It is more relevant to work schedules (e.g., shift work) that interfere with sleep, which will cause increased accident risk [10].

Cognition and Performance

Whereas accident risk may be highest in the states in which the individual actually falls asleep and loses contact with the environment, it may also be due to reduced cognitive performance while still being formally awake.

Insomnia

In insomnia, the impairment of cognition and performance has been frequently studied but the results have been variable and often it has been concluded that no impairment is present. Still, subjective ratings indicate quite strong performance impairment. It has been suggested that the cognitive level of insomnia patients may have been so high before the presentation of insomnia symptoms that sleep impairment has only brought down cognitive performance to "normal" levels, perhaps reflected in the subjectively strong impairment in comparison with an earlier higher performance level. Since cognitive performance rarely has been studied before the appearance of symptoms, this hypothesis has never been tested.

However, a recent meta-analysis has shed some light on this issue [11]. Using a sample of 24 adequate studies the authors demonstrated that episodic memory, problem solving, manipulation in working memory, retention in working memory were significantly impaired in insomniacs compared to healthy volunteers. No effects were seen for general cognitive function, perceptual and psychomotor processes,

T. Åkerstedt (✉)
Stockholm University, 10691 Stockholm Sweden
e-mail: torbjorn.akerstedt@stress.su.se

Clinical Neuroscience, Karolinska Institute, 17177 Stockholm, Sweden

P. Philip
Université de Bordeaux, Sommeil, Attention et Neuropsychatrie,
Bordeaux, France
e-mail: pr.philip@free.fr

S. Chokroverty, M. Billiard (eds.), *Sleep Medicine*, DOI 10.1007/978-1-4939-2089-1_55,
© Springer Science+Business Media, LLC 2015

procedural learning, verbal functions, alertness, complex reaction time, speed of information processing, selective attention, sustained attention/vigilance, verbal fluency, and cognitive flexibility. The size of the effect was small, but in some cases moderate. Subjective self-ratings of impairment indicated strong effects.

OSAS

Excessive daytime sleepiness is a key symptom in OSAS and neurocognitive impairment is clearly established, in contrast to the case with insomnia. The relation between sleep apnea and reduced cognitive performance is thus very pronounced. In a recent systematic review Lal et al. [12] found clear effects on inductive and deductive reasoning, attention, vigilance, learning, and memory. The mechanism is not finally determined, but hypoxia, hormonal imbalance, or systemic inflammation are probable causes, either directly or via effects on endothelial dysfunction. It appears that decreased hippocampal volume may be part of the mechanism, as well as focal reductions in gray matter in frontal and parietal areas of the brain.

In contrast to the clear cognitive impairment in OSAS patients, the relation between cognitive performance and quantitative measures of sleep apnea, such as the apnea–hypopnea index (AHI) is usually absent. Clearly, this raises questions as to the mechanism of the apnea/performance dimension.

Sleep Disorders and Traffic Accidents

Transportation is the area where most research on sleep related accidents has been carried out. The awareness of the dangers of drowsy driving appeared rather late. Lisper et al. [13] studied drowsy driving on closed roads by experimental sleep deprivation and reaction time performance while driving.

O'Hanlon reported to the European Economic Community (EEC) (now the European Union—EU) already in 1978 about the dangers of drowsy driving [14]. Among the first studies to address the question of sleepiness or sleep loss on accident risk in driving was a study of temporal patterns of road accidents in Texas, showing increased risk at night for single vehicle accidents [15]. Single-vehicle accidents were seen as closest related to road accident risk since no other object is involved, except exiting the road. Several similar studies followed but the study by Åkerstedt et al. [16] demonstrated an increased risk for *all* types of accidents except for those due to overtaking.

In studies of this type, the causes were assumed to be sleepiness due to a combination of driving at the circadian low, and a long time of prior wakefulness—not specifically due to a sleep disorder per se, but certainly due to impaired sleep of some form. The official recognition of the importance of sleep related accidents (due to a disorder or work schedules) started to arrive with the reports of the National (US) Transportation Safety Board [17] and was followed some years later [18]. Among the first studies to directly link sleepiness to an accident immediately following was that by Connor et al. [19], who interviewed subjects about their sleepiness before the accident. They found quite high levels before the accident compared to controls on the same roads. It was also demonstrated that driving between 02 and 05 in the morning and short sleep were independent risk factors. Another insight from that study and a companion study was that many other accidents were attributed to alcohol [20], simply because blood alcohol levels were exceeded despite the fact that they coincided closely with the timing of sleep related accidents. This is a common procedure in accident investigation and it seems safe to assume that sleep problems also contribute largely to many alcohol-related road accidents.

OSAS and Other Nocturnal Breathing Disorders

OSAS is the most studied pathology with regard to traffic accidents. The first systematic study of accidents in OSAS showed a sevenfold risk in 29 patients compared to controls [21]. The same group also did the first driving simulator test and found poorer performance in (small) patient groups than in controls [22]. Since then, more or less sophisticated driving simulators have been used, some of the simpler ones being nothing more than classical vigilance tests but equipped with a steering wheel or similar devices.

Using a questionnaire on driving habits, Haraldsson et al. [23] reported that the risk of being involved in a single-car accident was about seven times higher for patients with OSAS than for controls and patients with the incomplete triad of symptoms. This result was confirmed by the study of Terán-Santos et al. [24]. The latter authors investigated the relation between OSAS and traffic accidents risk with 152 controls and 102 drivers who received emergency treatment at hospital after an accident. Patients with an AHI of ten or higher had an odds ratio of 6.3 for having a traffic accident as compared to those without sleep apnea. Similarly, in the study of Young et al. [25] patients with the most severe OSAS (AHI >30) presented an accident risk factor higher than controls.

In a meta-analysis on OSAS and driving risk, 23 of 27 studies and 18 of 19 studies with control groups exhibited a statistically significant increased risk, with many of the studies finding a two- to threefold increased risk [26]. However, these studies did not consistently find that the crash risk depended on the severity of the symptoms.

With respect to professional drivers in particular it has been found that truck drivers with sleep-disordered breathing had a twofold higher accident rate per mile than drivers without sleep-disordered breathing [27]. However, accident frequency was, again, not linked to the severity of the sleep-related breathing disorder. In another study comparing long-haul ($N = 184$) and short-haul ($N = 133$) truck drivers, OSAS occurred in about 4 % of the long-haul drivers and in only 2 % of short-haul drivers [28]. Over 20 % of long-haul drivers reported having dozed off at least twice while driving. Near misses due to dozing off had occurred in 17 % of these drivers.

Other disorders like upper airway resistance syndrome have not been studied in terms of responsibility in traffic accidents even if they can generate pathological levels of sleepiness [29].

Taken together, these results indicate clear links between OSAS and driving accidents although the severity of OSAS (measured, for example by the AHI) does not seem to link to accident risk.

Insomnia and Car Accidents

In contrast to the many studies on OSAS and road accidents, there are only few studies on insomnia and road accidents. In one early study, the prevalence of being involved in a car accident was 5 % for individuals suffering from insomnia whereas it was only 2 % for persons without insomnia, thus suggesting that insomnia could potentially be a risk factor for traffic accidents [30].

For the rest, most studies are negative. Thus, Léger et al. [31] found no statistical difference for driving accidents over the past 12 months between severe insomniacs (240) and good sleepers. It was suggested that the insomniacs may have been avoiding driving due to their affliction. Also Lavie et al. [32] failed to find a higher prevalence of driving accidents in insomniacs than in controls. The case was the same for Daley et al. [33], who did not find a different prevalence of driving accidents in insomniacs and normals (935 adults) in the past 6 months. Interestingly, however, insomniacs thought insomnia had played a role in the accidents they had had and would have been involved in other accidents. In another study, Daley et al. [34] again found no relationship between sleep symptoms and the incidence of motor–vehicle accidents. However, this study did find that people with *Diagnostic and Statistical Manual of Mental Disorders-IV* (DSM-IV) categorized insomnia syndrome were twice as likely as good sleepers to have experienced other types of accidents, including work-related incidents and falls, suggesting that the likelihood of having an accident may depend on the demands of the task being completed. Sleep quality may also be affected directly through occupational injury or health problems.

Regarding the effects of treatments on driving ability, it is usually considered that long half-life hypnotics (medium long half-life benzodiazepines (BZD) and antihistamines) may induce a risk of accidents while driving in the morning, and a risk of falls during the night in elderly. In Europe, the vast majority of hypnotics are labeled with a sign indicating the possible risk of accidents due to the treatment. There is little information published on the side effects of common hypnotics on driving ability. However, using a driving simulator, Partinen et al. [35] performed a double-blinded, randomized, placebo-controlled, three-treatment, and three-period crossover study investigating the effects of zolpidem (10 mg) and temazepam (20 mg) vs a placebo in 18 insomniacs, in a real life condition on driving performance. After polysomnography at baseline and at each night of treatment, 5.5 h after drug intake, at 7:30 a.m. on the next morning, patients underwent a driving simulator test. There was no difference between treatments for the primary outcome measure (mean time to collision or for speed deviation or reaction time to tasks). However, lane position deviation was greater after administration of zolpidem.

Using a mathematical model, Menzin et al. [36] calculated the potential effects of sleep medications on motor–vehicle accidents and their cost, and applied the model to France. They used the model of standard deviation of a vehicle's lateral position (SDLP), and hypothesized that compared with zaleplon, the use of zopiclone over 14 days in France would be expected to result in 503 excess accidents per 100,000 drivers.

It should be emphasized that the studies above focus on individuals with some kind of diagnosis of insomnia. In studies of individuals of disturbed sleep in general the links with actual driving accidents is stronger than in controls [19, 37], but may be due to the particular sleep loss on that particular day.

Taken together, the results do not support a link between diagnosed insomnia and driving accidents.

Nonrespiratory and Non-insomnia Sleep Disorders and Traffic Accidents

Among other sleep disorders narcolepsy causes excessive daytime sleepiness and has also been studied as a risk factor for traffic accidents. However, compared to OSAS, only a few studies have investigated this topic.

In the 1960s, it was suggested that due to sleepiness and cataplexy, *narcolepsy* could be considered as a possible cause of automobile accidents [38, 39]. Aldrich [30] compared adults with different sleep disorders (OSAS, narcolepsy, and other sleep disorders with or without excessive sleepiness) and controls. He found that narcoleptics presented a higher risk of accidents than apneics. Moreover, the proportion of adults with sleep-related accidents was 1.5 to 4-fold greater in the hypersomnolent patients than in the control group. Apneics and narcoleptics were involved in 71 % of all sleep-related accidents.

In a study using 21 OSAS patients, 21 controls and 16 narcoleptics, it was found that narcoleptic patients were younger and sleepier than OSAS patients [40]. The performance on a divided-attention driving test (DADT) was worse for both patients groups than for controls.

Philip et al. [41] confirmed that narcolepsy could be a major cause of driving accidents. An internet questionnaire was completed by a large group of regular registered highway drivers (about 35,000 users). Among those users, 5.2 % complained of obstructive OSAS, 9.3 % of insomnia, and 0.1 % of narcolepsy. The results showed that 5.8 % of the reported accidents were sleep-related. Participants suffering from narcolepsy and hypersomnia had the highest risk of accidents (odds ratio 3.16, p <.01) compared to drivers who did not report any sleep or depressive disorders. Aldrich [30] showed that also periodic limb movement disorder (PLMD) and RLS were risk factors for traffic accidents.

Comments

The available information indicates that OSAS is associated with increased risk of driving accidents. The lack of a clear effect of severity, in particular the AHI level, is puzzling, however. It is also remarkable that the number of studies of insomnia and driving accidents are few and inconclusive. This could possibly be related to the lack of reduced cognitive effects in insomnia discussed initially.

Sleep Disorders and Work Accidents

Work accidents has seen much less research in relation to sleep than driving accidents, but the interest may have started during the First World War and with a focus on long work hours as causes of mistakes in the munitions industry [42]. This did not specifically concern disturbed sleep but the long shifts clearly interfered with sleep. Shift work has evoked similar concerns. Bjerner et al. [43] showed that mistakes in taking down reading from displays in a power station reached a peak in the latter part of the night shift, although sleep impairment per se was not addressed.

OSAS and Work Accidents

In the two studies that seem to have been the first to study sleep disorders and safety at work, Lavie et al. [32, 44] showed that workers with excessive daytime sleepiness and

frequent awakenings ran more risk of having occupational accidents than non-complainers. The type of accident was not specified but driving accidents did not seem to have been included. Sleep apneas and "mid-sleep awakenings" seemed to be behind the effects.

The relationship between sleep-disordered breathing and the risk of becoming involved in an occupational accident was studied by Ulfberg et al. [45]. To do this, 704 consecutive patients suffering from sleep-related breathing disorder were compared to 580 controls. The dependent variable was occupational accidents requiring at least one day of absence from work during the previous 10 years. Driving accidents and accidents due to external causes were excluded. The results showed that the risk of being involved in an occupational accident was about twofold among male heavy snorers and increased by 50 % among men suffering from OSAS. Work task and work hours were not controlled for, however.

Insomnia and Work Accidents

Insomnia and work accidents have relatively recently been subjected to a meta-analysis. A total of 11 studies were identified which assessed sleep related accidents [46]. Nine of the eleven studies report significant differences between insomniac and controls.

In one of the studies (with a *prospective* design) a "difficulty sleeping in the past two weeks" ($N = 50.000$) predicted fatal occupational accidents using national registers [47]. This study was controlled for gender, socioeconomic group, work hours, and other factors. In the only other prospective study (of nonfatal) occupational accidents [48], non-refreshing sleep, difficulty initiating sleep, and the presence of any sleep disturbances predicted increased risk of work-related injury in men but not women. However, in this study only injuries followed by a period of sick leave were included in the analysis.

Among the *cross-sectional* studies, the National Sleep Foundation survey [49], for example, found that the risk of accidents and injuries at work was significantly higher among those reporting a sleep latency of >30 min. In a controlled study, those meeting DSM-IV criteria for insomnia reported significantly higher levels of industrial accidents over the past 12 months when compared with good sleepers [31]. Similarly, in a large scale population survey (n. 69,584), an increased odds of work injury was reported for employees reporting poor sleep "most of the time" compared to good sleepers, in both men and women [50]. The same study indicated that both gender and type of job play important roles in the relationship between quality of sleep and accidents. Women in manual jobs or professional occupations (e.g., nursing, teaching) and men working in trades or transportation had the highest odds of work injury.

A cross sectional case-control study of 880 males in the construction industry [51] using logistic regression models, found that workers reporting an occupational injury with subsequent sick leave over the past 2 years were more likely to report shorter (<6 h/day) sleep durations, "not sleeping well," and the consumption of sleeping tablets than controls who had not had an injury. Similar results were found in a study of veterinarians [52] and in a case-control study of 2610 male French railway workers [51] which reported that "sleep disorder" symptoms (defined as a sleep duration of <6 h/day, "not sleeping well," and/or the consumption of sleeping tablets) were specifically related to injuries from physical exertion and pain due to movement.

Using the America Insomnia Survey, Shahly et al. [53] showed that insomnia was related to self-reported work accidents/errors (that entailed a cost of at least $ 500) while controlling for a number of other chronic conditions. Insomnia-related accidents were on the average 50 % more expensive than other accidents. It accounted for 7.2 % of all costly work accidents. The ultimate cost to society was estimated at € 31.1 billion.

In contrast, poor sleep was not shown to be a predictor of workplace accidents in a sample of white-collar telecommunications workers [54], who were desk bound and thus had low risk of accident. Similarly, in a study comparing 785 matched pairs of good sleepers and those meeting DSM-IV criteria for insomnia [49], self-reported minor and major accident rates over a 12 month period showed only nonsignificant elevations of risk among people with insomnia.

Comments

The studies of work accidents in relation to OSAS are few and inconclusive, whereas those involving insomnia are many and indicate a strong relationship. For driving accidents, the situation is the reverse. The reason for the difference in focus in studies of insomniacs and sleep apneics is not clear.

Real-Life Work Performance

Work performance is an area related to work accidents but with a great variety of potential outcome parameters. Still, most occupational areas lack reliable indicators of work performance and there seems to exist no study that has used real life performance measures. However, some studies use scales of work limitation or disability.

OSAS and Work Performance

Mulgrew et al. [55] demonstrated a clear relationship between excessive sleepiness and decreased work productivity in a population referred for suspected sleep-disordered breathing. Using the Epworth Sleepiness Scale (ESS), the work limitations questionnaire (WLQ), and an occupational survey, they studied patients undergoing full-night polysomnography for the investigation of sleep-disordered breathing. Data were collected and analyzed from 498 patients. The first 100 patients to complete the survey were followed up 2 years later. Across the studied group as a whole, there was no significant relationship between the severity of OSAS and the four dimensions of work limitation. However, amongst blue-collar workers, significant differences were detected between patients with mild OSAS (AHI 5–15/h) and those with severe OSAS (AHI > 30/h) regarding time management and mental/personal interactions. In contrast, there were strong associations between subjective sleepiness (as assessed by the ESS) and three of the four scales of work limitation. That is, patients with an ESS of 5 had much less work limitation compared to those with an ESS of 18 in terms of time management, mental–interpersonal relationships and work output.

Accattoli et al. [56] compared 331 workers with OSAS to 100 nonapneics and found that workers with OSAS reported more impairments in work performance than nonapneics, such as difficulties in memory, vigilance, concentration, performing monotonous tasks, responsiveness, learning new tasks, and manual ability.

Sivertsen et al. [57] found that self-reported symptoms of OSAS were an independent risk factor for subsequent long-term sick leave and permanent work disability. Omachi et al. [58] compared work disability in 83 patients with OSAS and excessive daytime sleepiness (OSAS) who were referred to their sleep center, to a group of patients without EDS, and a group without both OSAS and EDS. They created their own work disability questionnaire and found that patients with the combination of OSAS and EDS were at higher risk of both short-term work disability and longer-term work duty modification. However, when examining OSAS independently from EDS, OSAS only contributes to short-term work disability.

Insomnia and Performance at Work

In an early study Johnson and Spinweber [59] identified naval ratings with poor and good sleep and followed up navy performance tests used in their training. The former group had significantly poorer performance.

The other approaches have involved self-report of performance capacity. Leger et al. [31, 60] found performance capacity reduced in people who complained about sleep. Rosekind et al. [61] used work limitation questionnaires in four companies and found that insomnia was associated with reduced performance. Kessler et al. [62] used a national sample, the "America insomnia survey," and a WHO performance questionnaire, and found that insomnia was associated with sickness presenteism (being present at work while ill) corresponding to 11.3 days of "absence" US$ 91 billion in the US population.

Daley et al. [34, 63], with a slightly different approach, asked people to report when their work performance was reduced and then asked for the reason. Fatigue and insomnia dominated as reasons at such times.

Comment

Obviously, there is a lack of objective real life performance data in sleep disorders research. The reason is, very likely, the difficulty of finding suitable performance indicators. The available data on reduction of self-reported work capacity seem to suggest that sleep disorders have pronounced effects on work performance. The suggestion seems reasonable but must be regarded with caution due to the subjectivity of the measures, as well as to the cross-sectional approaches. The latter makes reverse causality highly likely.

Performance Measures

From the discussion above it is obvious that driving simulators have been important performance measures because of their face validity and sensitivity, although largely used only in relation to sleep apnea. However, the simulators vary from the extremely simple, vigilance test type to highly sophisticated high fidelity moving base simulators via the tabletop personal computer (PC) with a steering wheel and pedals attached. In most of these approaches (with steering wheel and pedals) the outcome variables have been the number of line crossings or driving off the road incidents or lateral variability. Also break reaction time has been a popular measure. But, it must be pointed out that even the most sophisticated simulator is not the "real thing" [64], at least not yet. In most studies, the outcome indicators of preference have been lateral variability (the standard deviation in lane position) or number of line crossings, but also reaction time to breaking. Since the advanced driving simulator can provide vast amount of parameters there are many other variables presented in publications, but the ones mentioned appear to be the most popular ones. No absolute criteria for impairment have been agreed on, however.

Real driving with individuals with sleep disorder is extremely rare since it would be illegal in most countries. However, such studies have been carried out with night driving and the effects have been pronounced [65, 66].

Traditional neuropsychological measures have also been used liberally. From traditional sleep loss research favorites have been any measure that requires constant attention. Possibly, the most popular and sensitive measure is the psychomotor vigilance test (PVT) [67] with the emphasis on lapses. An alternative is tracking tests (following the movement of a cursor) but a number of other tests are used, for example, the digit symbol substitution test, letter cancellaton, memory tests, and others [67].

Summary

The most obvious conclusions from the present review are that traffic accidents have been mainly researched in relation to OSAS and work accidents in relation to insomnia. In both cases, the relatively close links have been seen between exposure and outcome. There is clearly a need for more research on work accidents and OSAS as well as on driving accidents and insomnia.

Objective, real life, work performance has not seen any research at all, but the self-reports seem to suggest links with both OSAS and insomnia, even if caution must be exercised due to the lack of prospective studies. Clearly, there is a need for prospective research with objective measures.

References

1. Leger D, Poursain B, Neubauer D, Uchiyama M. An international survey of sleeping problems in the general population. Curr Med Res Opin. 2008;24:307–17.
2. Young T, Evans L, Finn L, Palta M. Estimation of the clinically diagnosed proportion of sleep apnea syndrome in middle-aged men and women. Sleep 1997b;20:705–6.
3. Ohayon MM, Priest RG, Zulley J, Smirne S, Paiva T. Prevalence of narcolepsy symptomatology and diagnosis in the European general population. Neurology. 2002;58:1826–33.
4. Tison F, Crochard A, Léger D, Bouée S, Lainey E, El Hasnaoui A. Epidemiology of restless legs syndrome in French adults: a nationwide survey: the INSTANT Study. Neurology. 2005;65:239–46.
5. Dijk D-J, Czeisler CA. Contribution of the circadian pacemaker and the sleep homeostat to sleep propensity, sleep structure, electroencephalographic slow waves, and sleep spindle activity in humans. J Neurosci. 1995;15:3526–38.
6. Härmä M, Suvanto S, Popkin S, Pulli K, Mulder M, Hirvonen K. A dose-response study of total sleep time and the ability to maintain wakefulness. J Sleep Res. 1998;7:167–74.
7. Van Dongen HP, Maislin G, Mullington JM, Dinges DF. The cumulative cost of additional wakefulness: dose-response effects on neurobehavioral functions and sleep physiology from chronic sleep restriction and total sleep deprivation. Sleep. 2003;26:117–26.

8. Bonnet MH, Arand DL. Clinical effects of sleep fragmentation versus sleep deprivation. Sleep Med Rev. 2003;7:297–310.

9. Zee PC, Manthena P. The brain's master circadian clock: implications and opportunities for therapy of sleep disorders. Sleep Med Rev. 2007;11:59–70.

10. Åkerstedt T, Philip P, Capelli A, Kecklund G. Sleep loss and accident—work hours, life style, and sleep pathology. Prog Brain Res. 2011;190:169–88.

11. Fortier-Brochu E, Beaulieu-Bonneau S, Ivers H, Morin CM. Insomnia and daytime cognitive performance: a meta-analysis. Sleep Med Rev. 2012;16:83–94.

12. Lal C, Strange C, Bachman D. Neurocognitive impairment in obstructive sleep apnea. Chest. 2012;141:1601–10.

13. Lisper HO, Dureman EI, Ericsson S, Karlsson NG. Effects of sleep deprivation and prolonged driving on a subsidiary auditory reaction time. Accid Analys Prevent. 1971;2:335–41.

14. O'Hanlon JF. That is the extent of the driving fatigue problem? In: Driving fatigue in road traffic accidents. Brussels: Commission of the European Communities; 1978.

15. Langlois PH, Smolensky MH, Hsi BP, Weir FW. Temporal patterns of reported single-vehicle car and truck accidents in Texas, USA during 1980–1983. Chronobiol Int. 1985;2:131–46.

16. Åkerstedt T, Kecklund G, Hörte L-G. Night driving, season, and the risk of highway accidents. Sleep. 2001;24:401–06.

17. NTSB. Fatigue, alcohol, other drugs, and medical factors in fatal-to-the-driver heavy truck crashes. National Transportation and Safety Board. Safety Study; 1990. NTST/SS-90/01.

18. NTSB. Evaluation of U.S. Department of Transportation: efforts in the 1990s to address operation fatigue. In: Washington, D.C.: National Transportation Safety Board; 1999. p. 104.

19. Connor J, Norton R, Ameratunga S, Robinson E, Civil I, Dunn R, Bailey J, Jackson R. Driver sleepiness and risk of serious injury to car occupants: population based case control study. Br Med J. 2002;324:1125.

20. Connor J, Norton R, Ameratunga S, Jackson R. The contribution of alcohol to serious car crash injuries. Epidemiology. 2004;15:337–44.

21. Findley LJ, Unverzagt ME, Suratt PM. Automobile accidents involving patients with obstructive sleep apnea. Am Rev Respir Dis. 1988;138:337–40.

22. Findley LJ, Fabrizio M, Thommi G, Suratt PM. Severity of sleep apnea and automobile crashes. N Engl J Med. 1989;320:868–69.

23. Haraldsson P-O, Carenfelt C, Diedrichsen F, Nygren Å, Tingvall C. Clinical symptoms of sleep apnea syndrome and automobile accidents. Otorhinolaryngology. 1990;52:57–62.

24. Terán-Santos J, Jimnénez-Gómez A, Cordero-Guevara J. The association between sleep apnea and the risk of traffic accidents. N Engl J Med. 1999;240:847–51.

25. Young T, Blustein J, Finn L, Palta M. Sleep-disordered breathing and motor vehicle accidents in a population-based sample of employed adults. Sleep. 1997a;20:608–13.

26. Ellen RL, Marshall SC, Palayew M, Molnar FJ, Wilson KG, Man-Son-Hing M. Systematic review of motor vehicle crash risk in persons with sleep apnea. J Clin Sleep Med. 2006;2:193–200.

27. Stoohs RA, Guilleminault C, Itoi A, Dement WC. Traffic accidents in commercial long-haul truck drivers: the influence of sleep-disordered breathing and obesity. Sleep. 1994;17:619–23.

28. Häkkänen H, Summala H. Fatal traffic accidents among trailer truck drivers and accident causes as viewed by other truck drivers. Accid Analys Prevent. 2001;33:187–96.

29. Guilleminault C, Do Kim Y, Chowdhuri S, Horita M, Ohayon M, Kushida C. Sleep and daytime sleepiness in upper airway resistance syndrome compared to obstructive sleep apnoea syndrome. Eur Respir J. 2001;17:838–47.

30. Aldrich MS. Automobile accidents in patients with sleep disorders. Sleep. 1989;12:487–94.

31. Léger D, Guilleminault C, Bader G, Lévy E, Paillard M. Medical and socio-professional impact of insomnia. Sleep. 2002;25:621–25.

32. Lavie P. Sleep habits and sleep disturbances in industry workers in Israel: main findings and some characteristics of workers complaining of excessive daytime sleepiness. Sleep. 1981;4:147–58.

33. Daley ME, Leblance M, Morin CM. The impact of insomnia on absenteeism, productivity and accidents rate. Sleep. 2005;28:A247.

34. Daley M, Morin CM, Leblanc M, Gregoire JP, Savard J. The economic burden of insomnia: direct and indirect costs for individuals with insomnia syndrome, insomnia symptoms, and good sleepers. Sleep. 2009a;32:55–64.

35. Partinen M, Hirvonen K, Hublin C, Halavaara M, Hiltunen H. Effects of after-midnight intake of zolpidem and temazepam on driving ability in women with non-organic insomnia. Sleep Med. 2003;4:553–61.

36. Menzin J, Lang KM, Levy P, Levy E. A general model of the effects of sleep medications on the risk and cost of motor vehicle accidents and its application to France. Pharmacoeconomics. 2001;19:69–78.

37. Stutts JC, Wilkins JW, Scott Osberg J, Vaughn BV. Driver risk factors for sleep-related crashes. Accid Analys Prevent. 2003;35:321–31.

38. Bartels EC, Kusakcioglu O. Narcolepsy: a possible cause of automobile accidents. Lahey Clin Found Bull. 1965;14:21–6.

39. Grubb TC. Narcolepsy and highway accidents. J Am Med Assoc. 1969;209:1720.

40. George CF, Boudreau AC, Smiley A. Comparison of simulated driving performance in narcolepsy and sleep apnea patients. Sleep. 1996;19:711–7.

41. Philip P, Sagaspe P, Lagarde E, Leger D, Ohayon MM, Bioulac B, Boussuge J, Taillard J. Sleep disorders and accidental risk in a large group of regular registered highway drivers. Sleep Med. 2010;11:973–9.

42. Anonymous. Health of Munitions Workers Committee. Final report. Cd 9065. London: HMSO; 1918.

43. Bjerner B, Holm Å, Swensson Å. Diurnal variation of mental perfomance. A study of three-shift workers. Br J Ind Med. 1955;12:103–10.

44. Lavie P, Kremerman S, Wiel M. Sleep disorders and safety at work in industry workers. Accid Analys Prevent. 1982;14:311–14.

45. Ulfberg J, Carter N, Edling C. Sleep-disordered breathing and occupational accidents. Scand J Work Environ Health. 2000;26:237–42.

46. Kucharczyk ER, Morgan K, Hall AP. The occupational impact of sleep quality and insomnia symptoms. Sleep Med Rev. 2012;16:547–59.

47. Åkerstedt T, Fredlund P, Gillberg M, Jansson B. A prospective study of fatal occupational accidents—relationship to sleeping difficulties and occupational factors. J Sleep Res. 2002;11:69–71.

48. Salminen S, Oksanen T, Vahtera J, Sallinen M, Harma M, Salo P, Virtanen M, Kivimaki M. Sleep disturbances as a predictor of occupational injuries among public sector workers. J Sleep Res. 2010;19:207–13.

49. Leger D, Massuel MA, Metlaine A. Professional correlates of insomnia. Sleep. 2006;29:171–8.

50. Kling RN, McLeod CB, Koehoorn M. Sleep problems and workplace injuries in Canada. Sleep. 2010;33:611–8.

51. Chau N, Mur J-M, Touron C, Benamghar L, Dehaene D. Correlates of occupational injuries for various jobs in railway workers: a case-control study. J Occup Health. 2004;46:272–80.

52. Gabel CL, Gerberich SG. Risk factors for injury among veterinarians. Epidemiology. 2002;13:80–6.

53. Shahly V, Berglund PA, Coulouvrat C, Fitzgerald T, Hajak G, Roth T, Shillington AC, Stephenson JJ, Walsh JK, Kessler RC.

The associations of insomnia with costly workplace accidents and errors: results from the america insomnia survey. Arch Gen Psychiatry. 2012;69:1054–63.

54. Doi Y, Minowa M, Tango T. Impact and correlates of poor sleep quality in Japanese white-collar employees. Sleep 2003;26:467–71.

55. Mulgrew AT, Ryan CF, Fleetham JA, Cheema R, Fox N, Koehoorn M, Fitzgerald JM, Marra C, Ayas NT. The impact of obstructive sleep apnea and daytime sleepiness on work limitation. Sleep Med. 2007;9:42–53.

56. Accattoli MP, Muzi G, Dell'omo M, Mazzoli M, Genovese V, Palumbo G, Abbritti G. Occupational accidents, work performance and obstructive sleep apnea syndrome (OSAS). G Ital Med Lav Ergon. 2008;30:297–303.

57. Sivertsen B, Overland S, Pallesen S, Bjorvatn B, Nordhus IH, Maeland JG, Mykletun A. Insomnia and long sleep duration are risk factors for later work disability. The Hordaland Health Study. J Sleep Res, 2009;18:122–8.

58. Omachi TA, Claman DM, Blanc PD, Eisner MD. Obstructive sleep apnea: a risk factor for work disability. Sleep. 2009;32:791–8.

59. Johnson LC, Spinweber CL. Good and poor sleepers differ in Navy performance. Mil Med. 1983;148:727–31.

60. Leger D, Bayon V. Societal costs of insomnia. Sleep Med Rev. 2010;14:379–89.

61. Rosekind MR, Gregory KB, Mallis MM, Brandt SL, Seal B, Lerner D. The cost of poor sleep: workplace productivity loss and associated costs. J Occup Environ Med. 2010;52:91–8.

62. Kessler RC, Berglund PA, Coulouvrat C, Hajak G, Roth T, Shahly V, Shillington AC, Stephenson JJ, Walsh JK. Insomnia and the performance of US workers: results from the America insomnia survey. Sleep. 2011;34:1161–71.

63. Daley M, Morin CM, Leblanc M, Gregoire JP, Savard J, Baillargeon L. Insomnia and its relationship to health-care utilization, work absenteeism, productivity and accidents. Sleep Med. 2009b;10:427–38.

64. Hallvig D, Anund A, Fors C, Kecklund G, Karlsson JG, Wahde M, Akerstedt T. Sleepy driving on the real road and in the simulator—a comparison. Accid Analys Prevent. 2013;50:44–50.

65. Sagaspe P, Taillard J, Akerstedt T, Bayon V, Espie S, Chaumet G, Bioulac B, Philip P. Extended driving impairs nocturnal driving performances. PLoS ONE. 2008;3:e3493.

66. Sandberg D, Anund A, Fors C, Kecklund G, Karlsson JG, Wahde M, Akerstedt T. The characteristics of sleepiness during real driving at night—a study of driving performance, physiology and subjective experience. Sleep. 2011;34:1317–25.

67. Dinges DF. Probing the limits of functional capability: the effects of sleep loss on short-duration tasks. In: Broughton RJ, Ogilvie RD editors. Sleep related disorders and internal diseases. Boston: Birkhauser, 1992. pp. 176–88.

Sleep Deprivation: Societal Impact and Long-Term Consequences

Michael A. Grandner

Introduction: The Issue of Insufficient Sleep

There is substantial debate about the minimum amount of sleep that is required for optimal health and well-being. Traditionally, sleep has been thought of as a relatively passive state of rest—a time for the body to recover from the day's work. This conceptualization has naturally led to the logical conclusion that sleep is for the weak, and functioning in the context of less sleep is a sign of strength and vigor [1]. This idea had generally persisted until the implications of the discovery of complex electroencephalogram (EEG) patterns during sleep [2, 3] were realized. Specifically, the discovery that sleep was associated with an active brain (despite unconsciousness and lack of movement and interaction) suggested that sleep was more than respite. Other discoveries, including that sleep is quite metabolically active [4], further strengthened this notion.

In recent decades, many studies have elucidated many potential functions of sleep [5–12]. These studies have increased our knowledge about benefits of sleep, ranging from the molecular level [12, 13], to functioning [14], and to longevity [15]. It has become clear that sleep represents a biological imperative that is either directly or indirectly related to nearly every physiologic system for which it has been studied. Despite this, there remain two troubling phenomena in the general population. First, there is a perception among many people in the public that sleep is a relatively low priority, compared to other health factors. Second, there is a belief that we live in a "sleep-deprived society," where there are large numbers of people who are achieving suboptimal sleep, which is impairing their health. Although there is accumulating evidence that the degree to which our society is sleep deprived may be sometimes overstated [16], current epidemiologic studies suggest that millions of Americans are coping with insufficient sleep duration, sleep disorders, or other sleep disturbances that are likely detrimental to health.

The Lexicon of Sleep Duration

The Source of the Problem

In any discussion of the societal impact of sleep deprivation, certain terms are used to describe the problem. However, the unclear application (or misapplication) of terms makes this discussion more difficult. For example, the terms "short sleep," "insufficient sleep," "sleep loss," "sleep deprivation," and even "insomnia" are often used interchangeably. For the purpose of this review, we will differentiate among as many of these terms as is feasible, proposing a common lexicon.

Part of the problem is that although the population to which studies addressing this question wish to generalize—the general population—is relatively consistent across studies, there is much heterogeneity among sources of data. In general, there are three categories of data sources. First, laboratory studies maximize precision in measurements and environmental control by typically studying small numbers of young, healthy volunteers for several days or weeks in the laboratory. This approach has many benefits but is limited in generalizability. Second, self-report studies tend to maximize generalizability and clinical utility by frequently recruiting larger samples from the community and measuring common health end points. Major limitations of this approach are generally in the domains of measurement. For example, measurements of sleep often rely on nonvalidated instruments. Third, studies of verified short sleepers are relatively rare. These study individuals are drawn from the population of interest, whose sleep is verified using objective instruments such as actigraphy and polysomnography. Although this is probably the best approach moving forward, there are relatively few studies that use this approach.

M. A. Grandner (✉)
University of Pennsylvania, Philadelphia, PA 19104, USA
e-mail: grandner@upenn.edu

S. Chokroverty, M. Billiard (eds.), *Sleep Medicine*, DOI 10.1007/978-1-4939-2089-1_56,
© Springer Science+Business Media, LLC 2015

Tab. 56.1 Proposed lexicon for sleep duration

Term	Working definition
Habitual sleep duration	Sleep duration that is experienced on a regular basis in real-world situations
Insomnia	A clinical condition that is characterized by pathologically long sleep latency and/or excessive time awake during the night in the context of daytime impairment or distress
Insufficient sleep	Sleep duration that is short enough so that it results in adverse outcomes
Normal sleep	Habitual sleep duration in the normative range (7–8 h)
Partial sleep deprivation	Sleep deprivation in the laboratory setting, where some sleep is obtained (usually lasting multiple days)
Self-reported short sleep	Short sleep assessed using retrospective assessments or prospective assessments that are subjective (e.g., sleep diary)
Short sleep	Habitual sleep duration of 6 h or less. In the context of multiple sleep duration, categories in this range may reflect sleep duration of 5–6 h
Sleep attainment	Habitual sleep duration of adequate quality
Sleep curtailment	Volitional shortening of sleep opportunity, resulting in reduced sleep duration
Sleep deficiency	Habitual experience of insufficient sleep duration and/or inadequate sleep quality (e.g., sleep disturbance)
Sleep deprivation	Sleep curtailment as experienced in a laboratory setting
Sleep disturbance	Experience of clinical or subclinical symptoms of sleep disorders, including insomnia, sleep apnea, or other sleep disorders; often, these are experienced in the context of other clinical conditions such as affective disorders and chronic pain
Sleep duration	The amount of time spent sleeping. Equivalent to "sleep time"
Sleep loss	Decrease in sleep duration over time
Sleep opportunity	The amount of time where sleep is possible; usually this is reflected as time in bed
Sleep restriction	Sleep curtailment (in or out of the laboratory) as part of an experimental protocol, usually lasting multiple days. (In other contexts, sleep restriction therapy is a type of treatment for insomnia.)
Sleep time	The amount of time spent sleeping. Equivalent to "sleep duration"
Total sleep deprivation	Complete lack of sleep during the period of time usually spent asleep; usually refers to in-laboratory experimental protocols lasting at least 24 h
Total sleep time	The amount of time spent sleeping; usually, computed (vs. reported) based on time in and out of bed minus time awake
Verified short sleep	Short sleep that has been verified using objective methods (such as actigraphy or polysomnography)
Very short sleep	Habitual sleep duration of less than 5 h

Another part of the problem is that there exists heterogeneity in how the cultural impact of short sleep is conceptualized. For example, does the definition of sleep duration rely on subjective or objective measures? Sleep diaries tend to underestimate awakenings and overestimate sleep time. Retrospective questionnaires tend to suffer from regression to the mean. Actigraphy tends to overestimate wake after sleep onset, and polysomnography is highly problematic for measuring habitual sleep. All of these approaches have strengths and weaknesses. Comparing a polysomnographic study to a questionnaire study is difficult—it is not that the objective measure is "more correct" but that these estimates of sleep capture different phenomena [17].

Another domain of heterogeneity is the method of exposure to short or shortened sleep duration. In some studies, sleep duration is forced (e.g., in the lab), whereas in others, short duration is volitional (e.g., in the community). Also, the place of study may also play a role. Sleep in the laboratory is known to poorly reflect sleep at home [18–20].

A third domain of heterogeneity lies in the definition of the short sleep exposure. For example, the definition of short sleep varies across studies. Some laboratory studies focus exclusively on total sleep deprivation (no allowed sleep), whereas others use sleep curtailed to 4, 5, or 6 h. Similarly,

in population studies, the short sleep exposure is variably defined. Some studies defined short sleep as 4, 5, 6, or 7 h. Also, the reference group has been variably defined. In some studies, the reference group is 7 h, whereas sometimes it is 8, 7–8, 6–8 h, etc. This also makes comparisons across studies difficult.

A Lexicon of Sleep Duration

Because of the variability in terms used in many studies and reviews that have addressed sleep deprivation, short sleep duration, and insufficient sleep, the present review outlines proposed standard definitions for sleep parameters. These definitions are based on previously published definitions [21] and can be found in Table 56.1. Of particular note, sleep deprivation refers to a state by which sleep is *deprived* across time. This could take place in the laboratory or at home, but for the purposes of this review, sleep deprivation will typically be referred to in terms of experimental studies. Also, "short sleep" will generally refer to habitual sleep duration of <6 h. Any other definition (due to variability in study designs) will be explicitly specified.

Historical Context

Kleitman's classic text [4] describes the earliest studies of sleep deprivation. The first known study of sleep deprivation was performed by Manacéine and published in 1894. In this study, puppies were kept awake until they died several days later. Tarozzi published a study 5 years later of three adult dogs who died after being kept awake for 9, 13, and 17 days. This work was followed by studies in dogs and guinea pigs that identified consequences of sleep deprivation in the brain.

The first programmatic examination of the effects of sleep deprivation was conducted by Legendre and Pièron. These studies involved sleep deprivation of dogs, though not to the point of death. Care was taken to make sure that the animals were well kept and cared for and that they ate well. In these experiments, several changes to behavior and physiology were noted that would presage later findings. These experiments were later followed up by Kleitman, who assessed sleep deprivation in 12 puppies, utilizing a 2-week baseline period and a control group made up of littermates. Over the course of several days, the animals in the experimental group were kept awake and observed. Several notable findings included a replication of findings from earlier work (increased sleep propensity, muscular weakness, etc.) and one of the first observations that the apparent sleepiness could be temporarily alleviated by introducing the control littermate to play—illustrating the social and environmental dimension of sleepiness.

The first sleep deprivation study in humans was performed by Patrick and Gilbert in 1896. In this study, three subjects were kept awake for 90 h. Overall, the most salient findings were psychomotor slowing, slowed reaction time, and impaired cognitive function. Even in this short period, the subjects gained weight. After one night of recovery, subjects appeared normal.

Over the next century, there have been a large number of studies of sleep deprivation. Many reviews have been published [22–46] that have detailed these advances. A few studies in particular are of historical note.

The longest observed sleep deprivation study was published in 1966 by Gulevich, Dement, and Johnson [47]. This case detailed the now famous case of Randy Gardner, a then 17-year-old high school senior who attempted to study the effects of sleep deprivation as a science project over Christmas break. He, along with two friends, set a goal of 264 h, which was 4 h longer than the Guinness World Record at the time. The subject was able to maintain wakefulness for the full duration of the experiment, with several caveats. First, trained researchers were only able to observe the subject for the final 90 h (the rest of the time, he was observed by one or both of the friends who helped design the study). Second, technology was relatively limited—there were no continu-

ous physiological monitors, and, more important, there was no continuous EEG recording, which may have detected short bouts of sleep during apparent wakefulness. Despite these limitations, the findings from this case report were impactful, simply because they tested a condition that could not ethically or reliably be tested in a laboratory. From this report, several important findings emerged. First, during a psychiatric interview at 262 h, the subject was able to demonstrate orientation, logical and coherent thought process, and no detachment from reality (at the time, it was a popular hypothesis that symptoms of schizophrenia would emerge). It was also observed that tolerance to stressful situations was notably diminished, and lack of movement and stimulation resulted in extreme drowsiness. The issue of recovery sleep is also highlighted in this case. He slept 880 min after the deprivation period, and this sleep seemed relatively normal polysomnographically, though long. He then slept for 625 min the next night, 543 min the third night, and, by 1 week after the sleep deprivation period, he slept 424 min.

At around the same time as the case report, another historically significant study had taken place. The longest sleep deprivation to be formally studied in a group of humans was undertaken by Kollar, Pasnau, Rubin, Naitoh, Slater, and Kales at the Neuropsychiatric Institute at the University of California, LA [48]. This study involved four young (age 21–23) males who underwent 205 h of prolonged wakefulness. Unlike the case report, this took place in the well-lit, professional atmosphere of the medical center, and the subjects were attended to by nursing personnel continuously. Perhaps due to the different setting, or slightly higher age, or more intensive monitoring, the findings of this study showed a somewhat different pattern of results. For example, the experimenters noticed that cognitive and perceptual abilities, particularly regarding focus and attention, were dramatically reduced. For example, subjects were unable to maintain sufficient concentration for reading by the third day. Impairments across several measures, including the Minnesota Multiphasic Personality Inventory (MMPI) and a number of neuropsychological tests, were documented.

These classic studies gave rise to the conditions within which current sleep deprivation research is carried out. Studies of total sleep deprivation have been generally replaced with partial sleep deprivation, especially in humans. Most animal studies involve rats or, now more commonly, mice. This chapter will focus on human studies.

Laboratory Studies of Sleep Deprivation

Laboratory studies of sleep deprivation typically involve a small sample of young, healthy adults who stay in the laboratory for days to weeks. These studies typically employ either repeated measures designs that frequently include crossover designs and, less frequently, control groups. These studies typically measure sleep objectively, using polysomnography. The primary question is: When we take healthy, normal-duration sleepers, and artificially curtail their sleep for a short period of time, what happens?

Sleep

In a series of classic studies, Webb and colleagues [49, 50] found that short sleep in the laboratory was associated with less stage 2 and rapid eye movement (REM) sleep but equivalent amount of slow wave sleep (SWS) as compared to normal and long sleep. These findings were later replicated by Benoit and colleagues [51–53], who found that short sleepers do not exhibit different amounts of SWS (whole night) nor do they exhibit cycle by cycle differences in SWS as compared to normal duration sleepers.

Neurobehavioral Performance

Perhaps the most proximal consequence of sleep loss is a resultant increase in "sleepiness" (sleep propensity). Assessment of sleepiness usually involves measurement of sleep in situations in which sleep is not appropriate or desired [54]. Individuals who experience partial or total sleep deprivation demonstrate increased sleepiness [39, 55]. This finding has been replicated across three methods of objective assessment of sleepiness: the multiple sleep latency test, maintenance of wakefulness test, and measurements of oculomotor activity [39, 56–58].

Assessments of neurobehavioral consequences of sleep loss are among the most common outcomes assessed in sleep deprivation studies. This is usually operationalized as sustained attention [38]. The most well-validated measure of sustained attention in this context is the psychomotor vigilance task (PVT) [38, 59]. The PVT has been consistently used to show that sustained attention decreases with sleep restriction in a dose–response manner as sleep opportunity is reduced from 7 to 3 h [38, 39]. Additionally, deficits accumulate across several days [38, 39]. Other work has demonstrated that sleep deprivation is also associated with deficits in executive function [60], learning [61], and memory [62].

There has been significant discussion of the role of impaired functioning due to sleep loss in auto accidents [63–68]. There is a strong evidence that sleepiness is a major factor contributing to automobile accidents [69–71]. Several papers have shown that accidents are related to sleepiness caused by sleep apnea [69, 72, 73] and prolonged wakefulness [71, 74, 75]. Some evidence also suggests that short sleepers may exhibit more sleepiness than average [76, 77], but currently there are very limited data to support the claim

that short sleepers are more likely to experience auto accidents [78], though some evidence exists [79].

Metabolism

In his classic series of studies subjecting rats to extreme sleep deprivation, Rechschaffen and colleagues found that sleep-deprived rats became hyperphagic, even though they demonstrated a depletion of energy reserves [80]. At the time, this was not generally considered in a context of linking sleep with metabolism. However, in a landmark study published in 1991, Van Cauter and colleagues studied metabolic effects of sleep deprivation in eight healthy subjects [81]. This study found that sleep deprivation had a negative impact on glucose tolerance and insulin resistance, but problems resolved with recovery sleep. Since then, several studies have replicated and extended those findings.

Spiegel and colleagues studied 11 young men in the laboratory following a condition of 12 or 4 h in bed [82]. Insulin and glucose measures were obtained during intravenous glucose tolerance test (IVGTT) and after meals 5 and 10 h later. No differences were seen following the meals. However, during the fasting IVGTT, glucose and insulin were both lower, reflected in a lower homeostatic model assessment of insulin resistance value (HOMA-IR—a product of insulin and glucose readings that denote insulin resistance). In a follow-up study, Spiegel and colleagues [83] studied subjects who spent two nights of 10 h in bed (2200–0800), versus two nights of 4 h in bed (0100–0500) in a crossover design. After the second night of each bedtime condition, caloric intake was replaced by an intravenous glucose infusion at a constant rate to avoid fluctuations of hunger and appetite related to meal ingestion. Even though sleep duration was manipulated for only two nights, the glucose and insulin profiles obtained during continuous glucose infusion were consistent with the results obtained using IVGTT in a previous study of six nights. In the early part of the day, after 2 days of short bedtimes, glucose levels were higher and insulin levels were lower than after 2 days of longer bedtimes. These findings have since been replicated in other studies that have shown that sleep deprivation can lead to insulin dysregulation [84–86].

In addition to insulin and glucose, the hormones leptin and ghrelin have also been studied relative to sleep deprivation. Leptin is a hormone that plays a key role in regulating energy intake and energy expenditure. It is secreted by adipose tissue and inhibits appetite at the level of the hypothalamus by counteracting neuropeptide Y (an appetite stimulant) and promoting aMSH (an appetite suppressant). Leptin is generally viewed as an adiposity signal. It decreases with fasting, increases with stress, and decreases with physical activity. Elevated leptin is associated with decreased food consumption, though obese individuals become resistant to its effects. Ghrelin, on the other hand, is a hormone that is frequently considered as the counterpart to leptin. It increases prior to meals and is associated with hunger. It stimulates food intake and activates reward pathways that play a role in the "reward" function of foods. Ghrelin is decreased in obesity, and the normal nocturnal rise in ghrelin is blunted by obesity. Several studies have shown that sleep deprivation is associated with decreased leptin and increased ghrelin [83, 87–89]. If this is the case, a decrease in leptin and an increase in ghrelin (especially in an individual who is obese) would likely lead to an orexigenic eating pattern that could result in weight gain and diabetes over time.

Cardiovascular Function

Cardiovascular end points are usually difficult to measure in short-term human laboratory studies, since only indirect markers of cardiovascular health are possible and these tend to change very slowly. However, there are several laboratory studies that suggest a causal role of sleep deprivation in cardiovascular disease (CVD) risk. Lusardi and colleagues [90] studied ambulatory blood pressure in 18 healthy subjects across a typical night of sleep, and sleep restricted to the second half of the night only, 1 week later. They observed that the sleep restriction condition was associated with elevated systolic and diastolic blood pressure, especially in the early parts of the night (no normal nighttime dipping when the subject was awake). These blood pressure changes may translate into daytime effects as well. Tochikubo and colleagues found that daytime mean systolic and diastolic blood pressure increased after a night of restricted sleep (mean 3.6 h) [91]. The mechanism for this is not clear. One study found that restriction to five nights of <5 h of sleep caused a significant increase in cardiac and peripheral sympathetic modulation, associated with a decrease in endothelial-dependent venodilation, suggesting that acute sleep loss affects endothelial function, potentially through the acetylcholine system [92]. Also, in a study of 27 individuals whose sleep opportunity was less than half of usual, the sleep deprivation condition was associated with a reduction in left atrial early diastolic strain rate in the absence of geometric alterations, suggesting that sleep deprivation may be associated with functional impairments in the left atrium [93].

Sleep deprivation may also interact with cardiovascular responses to stress. For example, sleep deprivation amplified the increased systolic blood pressure associated with psychological stress [94]. Also, 24-h total sleep deprivation was found to amplify heart rate increases in response to mental stress and a cold pressor test, even after recovery [95].

Inflammation

Inflammation is well established as a key mechanism in the development of CVD [96]. Recently, the following pro-inflammatory biomarkers have demonstrated (or suggested) associations with sleep deprivation in the laboratory: tumor necrosis factor α (TNFα); interleukins 1 (IL-1), 6 (IL-6), and 17 (IL-17); and C-reactive protein (CRP).

Regarding TNFα, in a study that evaluated the effects of 12 nights of sleep restriction to 6 h, 24-h TNFα secretion was elevated in men, but not in women [97]. Several laboratory studies have also assessed interleukins. In a study of five nights of sleep restriction to 4 h, 13 healthy young men demonstrated elevated IL-1β at the messenger RNA (mRNA) level but not the protein level [98]. Regarding IL-6, in a study by Haack and colleagues, IL-6 was elevated after 12 days of 4 h of sleep, relative to 8 h. These elevations were associated with increased pain ratings [99]. In another study, after 12 nights of 6 h of sleep, 24-h IL-6 secretion was elevated, relative to 8 h [97]. In a more recent study, after five nights of sleep restriction to 4 h, 13 healthy young men demonstrated elevated IL-6 at the mRNA level but not the protein level [98]. To date, one study has examined sleep restriction in the context of IL-17. After five nights of sleep restricted to 4 h, 13 healthy young men demonstrated elevated IL-17 at the mRNA level and at the protein level [98].

Several studies have investigated whether partial sleep deprivation results in increased CRP levels. Meier-Ewert and colleagues [100] found that during partial sleep deprivation, CRP levels increased significantly. A more recent study by van Leeuwen and colleagues [98] also found that following sleep restriction, CRP was increased compared to baseline (145 % of baseline, $p<0.05$), and continued to increase during recovery (231 % of baseline, $p<0.05$).

Self-Report Studies of Short Sleep Duration

Community-based studies of short sleep duration typically involve a large sample of community-dwelling adults who participate in an observational study (no intervention). These studies typically employ either survey designs or other cohort designs. Sleep is frequently measured using nonvalidated measures (especially in the larger population studies) of sleep or retrospective questionnaires (usually in smaller studies). The primary question is: When we study individuals who self-identify as short sleepers (who obtain the amount of sleep that would be considered sleep deprivation in experimental studies), what impairments do they show?

Sleep

Self-reported short sleepers likely include many individuals who also suffer from sleep disorders or, at least, report significant levels of sleep symptoms. This is important to consider, since sleep duration is often discussed as either a separate construct from sleep disturbance or synonymous with sleep disturbance. These data suggest a more complicated picture, where short sleep findings not only partly reflect effects of duration per se but also partly reflect issues of sleep quality. For example, a study by Grandner and Kripke [101] found that habitual short sleepers are more likely to report difficulty falling asleep, difficulty maintaining sleep, nonrestorative sleep, and daytime sleepiness, compared to 7–8-h sleepers. Although several studies of sleep duration have accounted for some of these issues, it is important to note that many do not.

Mortality

Over 40 years of evidence indicates a strong association between nightly sleep duration and mortality risk [102, 103]. Overall, sleep duration is associated with mortality in a U-shaped fashion, with the highest risk found for short and long sleepers and the lowest risk in individuals who report average sleep durations of 7–8 h. Gallicchio and Kalesan [104] conducted a meta-analysis of 23 studies investigating the association between sleep duration and mortality conducted from 1979 to 2007. Using random-effects meta-analysis, the authors report that the pooled relative risk (RR) for all-cause mortality for short sleep was 1.10 (95 % CI = (1.06, 1.15)), with cardiovascular-related RR at 1.06 (95 % CI = (0.94, 1.30)) and cancer-related RR at 0.99 (95 % CI = (0.88, 1.13)). For long sleep, RR for all-cause mortality was 1.23 (95 % CI = (1.16, 1.30)), with cardiovascular RR at 1.38 (95 % CI = (1.13, 1.69)) and cancer RR at 1.21 (95 % CI = (1.11, 1.32)). In a more recent meta-analysis, including 16 published studies from 1993 to 2009, Cappuccio and colleagues examined whether evidence supports the presence of a relationship between duration of sleep and all-cause mortality and to obtain an estimate of the risk [105]. This meta-analysis demonstrated larger effects, including an RR = 1.12 (95 % CI = (1.06, 1.18)) for short sleep and RR = 1.30 (95 % CI = (1.22, 1.38)) for long sleep. In general, habitual sleep duration is associated with mortality. Specifically, both short and long sleep durations are associated with elevated risk, albeit through potentially different mechanisms [15, 21, 106, 107]. The exact pathways by which this risk is conferred are not well known. One possibility is that both short and long sleep durations are associated with elevated risk of cardiometabolic disease, which could contribute to mortality.

Obesity and Weight Gain

Several dozen studies, in various settings, using various approaches, have documented that short sleep duration (variously defined) is associated with obesity and/or adiposity and/or weight gain [106, 108–120]. As an example of one such study, sleep duration from the 2009 Behavioral Risk Factor Surveillance System (BRFSS) was assessed relative to obesity. In unadjusted analyses, sleep duration of less than 5 h was associated with an additional 2.7 body mass index (BMI) points, and sleep duration of 5–6 h was associated with an additional 0.8 BMI points (relative to 7 h) [121]. In a separate analysis, each day of the week, the participants reported insufficient sleep were associated with 0.2 more BMI points. After adjusting for numerous covariates, relationships for <5 h of sleep and insufficient sleep remained. When insufficient sleep and sleep duration were entered into the same statistical model, along with covariates, the effect for <5 h of sleep remained. This suggests that there is a robust association between very short sleep duration and BMI, which is not accounted for by perceived insufficient sleep.

In addition to cross-sectional studies, several prospective studies have linked short sleep duration with incident weight gain. Data from the Nurse's Health Study found that sleep duration of less than 6 h increased likelihood of gaining > 15 kg over 16 years [122]. In a study of Japanese men, a similar pattern was found, with incident obesity over 1 year significantly higher among 5-h sleepers (odds ratio (OR) = 1.5) and <5-h sleepers (OR = 1.9), relative to 7-h sleepers [123].

Diabetes Mellitus

Several studies have demonstrated population-level associations between short sleep duration and diabetes. There are a number of reviews that summarize many of these studies [108, 109 115, 116, 124, 125]. Since the publication of these reviews, there have been a number of studies that further extend our understanding of this association. Buxton and Marcelli [126] found that sleep duration of <7 h, as assessed using the 2004–2005 National Health Interview Survey (NHIS), was associated with elevated diabetes risk in the American population. Using the 2008 BRFSS, Shankar and colleagues found that self-reported insufficient sleep was positively associated with prevalence of diabetes [127]. However, Vishnu and colleagues note that, in this same sample, the relationship depended on race/ethnicity—it was significant in all groups except non-Hispanic Blacks [128]. In an analysis of the 2005 NHIS, Zizi and colleagues, however, found that both Black and White respondents who were short sleepers (6 h or less) were at increased risk of also reporting diabetes, and that this relationship was significantly stronger in the Black respondents [129]. Complaints of sleep disturbance may also play a role. Using the 2006 BRFSS, Grandner and colleagues showed that sleep disturbances (broadly defined as difficulty initiating or maintaining sleep or sleeping too much) were associated with diabetes prevalence [130, 131]. The extent to which the relationship depends on sleep duration itself or the perceived unmet sleep need is unclear. To address this question, Altman and colleagues used the 2009 BRFSS, which assessed sleep duration and insufficient sleep. This study found that any association is likely driven more by short sleep duration, rather than perceived unmet sleep need [121].

In a study of Japanese men, sleep duration of < 5 h was associated with approximately 63 % elevated risk for diabetes [132]. Another study of Japanese men found that sleep of 5 h or less was associated with greater likelihood of untreated diabetes [133]. Similarly, a study from Iran found that 5 h or less of sleep was associated with impaired fasting glucose [134].

Short sleep duration may also be associated with development of diabetes. In the Western New York Study, Rafaelson and colleagues found that sleep duration < 6 h was associated with development of impaired fasting glucose [135]. This relationship appeared to be partially mediated by insulin resistance. In a study of nondiabetic Japanese government workers, short sleep duration of 5 h or less was associated with a greater than fourfold increased likelihood of developing diabetes [136]. Data from the National Cheng Kung University Hospital in Taiwan showed that short sleepers (< 6 h) were approximately 55 % more likely to present with newly diagnosed diabetes, but not prediabetes. However, a study from New Zealand did find an association between short sleep duration and prediabetes [137]. This study also documented an association between sleep duration at age 32 and HbA_{1C} levels.

Cardiovascular Disease

Hoevenaar-Blom and colleagues [138] conducted a 12-year prospective study of 20,432 men and women in the Netherlands with no history of CVD to investigate the association between short and long sleep duration and total CVD and coronary heart disease (CHD) incidence, independent of other modifiable lifestyle factors. Compared to people who slept 7–8 h, short sleepers (defined as those individuals who slept ≤ 6 h) had a 15 % higher risk of total CVD incidence (hazard ratio (HR): 1.15; 95 % CI: 1.00–1.32) and a 23 % higher risk of CHD incidence (HR: 1.23; 95 % CI: 1.04–1.45). It also appears that the quality of sleep for those people sleeping ≤ 6 h adds additional risk for CVD. When compared to individuals with normal sleep duration and good sleep quality, short sleepers with poor subjective sleep had a 63 % higher risk of CVD (HR: 1.63; 95 % CI: 1.21–2.19) and 79 % higher risk of CHD incidence (HR: 1.79; 95 % CI: 1.24–2.58).

Other recent studies have also demonstrated an association between short sleep duration and CVD. For example, using the Coronary Artery Risk Development in Young Adults (CARDIA) data, Knutson and colleagues found that shorter sleep durations were associated with elevated systolic and diastolic blood pressure, as well as adverse changes in blood pressure over 5 years [139]. Also, Buxton and Marcelli [126] found that short sleep duration is associated with increased prevalence of hypertension and CVD, using the 2004–2005 NHIS data. In a recent analysis of data from the BRFSS, Altman and colleagues [121] found that short sleep duration was associated with elevated prevalence of hypertension, hyperlipidemia, and history of heart attack and stroke. This study also found that the risk was particularly elevated in those reporting < 5 h of sleep (though there was some elevated risk associated with 5–6 h). Also, when self-reported insufficient sleep was assessed, irrespective of sleep duration, days per week of insufficient sleep was also associated with these outcomes. When sleep duration and insufficient sleep were evaluated simultaneously (looking for unique effects of one or the other), insufficient sleep was uniquely predictive of hypertension and hyperlipidemia, whereas sleep duration was uniquely predictive of hypertension, heart attack, and stroke history.

The role of short sleep in predicting cardiovascular mortality has also been assessed via meta-analysis. In a review of 15 studies including 474,684 male and female participants, Cappuccio and colleagues [140] found that short sleep (defined as ≤ 5–6 h) was associated with an RR of 1.48 (95 % CI: 1.22–1.80) and long sleep (defined as > 8–9 h) was associated with an RR of 1.38 (95 % CI: 1.15–1.66) of dying or developing CHD. Similarly, the RR of developing CHD or dying from stroke was 1.15 (95 % CI: 1.00–1.31) for short sleep and 1.65 (95 % CI: 1.45–1.87) for long sleep.

Inflammation

Several studies have assessed inflammatory markers in population samples that assessed self-reported sleep duration. In a study of mothers, sleep duration of < 5 h at 1 year post partum was associated with elevated IL-6 at 3 years post partum [141]. Large epidemiologic cohorts have been leveraged to examine associations between sleep duration and CRP levels in general population samples. Miller and colleagues reported a null association between short and long sleep durations and CRP among men in that cohort after adjusting for covariates. Among women, though, long sleep (≥ 9 h) was associated with a 35 % increase in CRP levels after adjusting for age, marital status, BMI, smoking, systolic blood pressure, and triglyceride levels [142]. Evidence of a significant association between short sleep and CRP among women was also reported in fully adjusted models. A significant relationship between short sleep duration (assessed using polysomnography) and CRP was also found for women enrolled in the Study of Women's Health across the Nation (SWAN) Study [143]. Further analysis showed a significant interaction with race/ethnicity, and post hoc analyses clarified that this relationship only existed among African American women. However, not all studies have documented significant relationships. In the Wisconsin Sleep Cohort ($N=907$), no association was seen between CRP and short or long sleep duration in adjusted models [144]. In this case, investigators examined self-reported as well as polysomnography-assessed sleep duration, and also evaluated quadratic terms in their analysis. This study also did not demonstrate sex-stratified or race-stratified results; however, these findings are based on a sample of predominantly Caucasian participants. Additionally, Suarez and colleagues [145] did not report a significant association between sleep duration and CRP among men, but the small sample size ($N=210$) and younger age group (mean age 28) may account for this.

A recent study utilizing the 2007–2008 National Health and Nutrition Examination Survey (NHANES) cohort aimed to discern relationships between sleep duration and CRP in the American population ($N=5587$), while addressing some of the sample size and generalizability limitations of previous studies. [146] To address issues of low variability of CRP in the population, a polynomial regression analysis examined whether there was a linear trend or a U-shape, even in the absence of any significant elevations among sleep duration groups, relative to 7 h. To address the issue of overly inclusive sleep duration categories (that may obscure effects at the extremes of sleep duration), sleep duration was assessed as <5, 5, 6, 7, 8, 9, and 10+ h, with 7 h as the reference group. To address sex differences, analyses were conducted with men and women both combined and separate. To address race/ethnicity differences, interaction terms and stratified analyses looked at patterns in different groups. Linear and squared terms were significant in all models in the complete sample, with notable differences by sex and ethnoracial group. Overall, in models adjusted for sociodemographics and BMI, different patterns were observed for non-Hispanic White (elevated CRP for <5 h and >9 h), Black/African American (elevated CRP for <5 and 8 h), Hispanic/Latino (elevated CRP for >9 h), and Asian/other (higher in 9 and >9 h and lower in 5 and 6 h) groups. Ethnoracial groups also demonstrated patterning by sex. For example, long sleep effects were more prominent among women.

When fibrin is degraded, one of the products is d-dimer, a biomarker of the formation of thrombotic disorders. Although d-dimer levels are usually very low, elevations have also been seen in other conditions such as liver disease, pregnancy, and post surgery. One previous study found that shorter sleep duration was associated with elevated d-dimer.

In this same study, d-dimer was negatively associated with sleep quality measured with the Pittsburgh Sleep Quality Index [147]. Also, one previous study found that both short sleep duration (<6 h) and long sleep duration (>8 h) were associated with elevated intercellular adhesion molecule (ICAM) in a Taiwanese cohort. [148]

Healthy Behaviors: Diet and Exercise

Several studies have examined associations between self-reported sleep and diet. In a study of adolescents, data from the Healthy Lifestyle in Europe by Nutrition in Adolescence (HELENA) study across several European countries found that short sleepers were less likely to be consuming the recommended levels of fruits, vegetables, fish, skim milk, breakfast cereals, and other foods. Also, shorter sleep duration was associated with increased consumption of pizza, burgers, and pasta [149]. In the Cleveland Children's Sleep and Health Study, short sleep duration was associated with greater energy intake (~200 kcal), greater proportion of calories from fat, lower proportion of calories from carbohydrates, and more calorie consumption in early morning (5:00–7:00) [150].

In adults, data from a study of Japanese factory workers from 1992 to 1998 found that shorter seep duration was associated with more irregular meal timing and eating habits in general, more snacking between meals, more dining out, less consumption of vegetables, more preference for strongly flavored food, and no difference in preference for oily food [151]. Recent data from NHANES examined dietary data gathered from a comprehensive 24-h recall relative to sleep duration. Regarding sleep duration, food variety differentiated groups, with very short (<5 h), short (5 h), and long (9+ h) sleepers, reporting fewer foods in their diet. Regarding macronutrients, after adjusting for overall diet, demographics, socioeconomics, and other health factors, a pattern was found where very short sleepers consumed less protein and carbohydrates than 7–8-h sleepers did. Analysis of micronutrients was done in two ways. First, nutrients were entered into linear regression analyses, adjusting for a number of covariates. From these analyses, very short sleep (<5 h) was associated with less thiamin, folate, phosphorus, iron, zinc, and selenium. Short sleep (5–6 h) was associated with less water, and long sleep (9+ h) was associated with less phosphorus and more alcohol. In a stepwise regression analysis (which accounts for intercorrelations among nutrients), very short sleep (<5 h) was associated with less water and lycopene; short sleep (5–6 h) was associated with less vitamin C, water, and selenium, and more lutein/zeaxanthin; and long sleep (9+ h) was associated with less theobromine and choline, and more alcohol [152].

Neurobehavioral Performance

Few studies have assessed whether habitual short sleepers exhibit any neurobehavioral performance impairments. A recent study showed that among an epidemiologic sample in the USA, short sleepers were more likely to report nodding off or falling asleep at the wheel. Overall, 3.6 % of the population reported drowsy driving. Self-identified short sleepers reported drowsy driving more often, and long sleepers, less often. For example, compared to those reporting sleeping 7–8 h, those reporting 5 h or less per night were over 3.5 times as likely to report nodding off or falling asleep at the wheel and those reporting 6 h were nearly twice as likely. Participants in this study were also asked how often they experience insufficient sleep. Among those who reported insufficient sleep 7 nights/week, effects were greater. Compared to those reporting 7–8 h of sleep, those reporting less than 5 h were more than four times as likely and those reporting 6 h were more than three times as likely to report nodding off. Surprisingly, when analyses were restricted to only those who report 0 nights/week of insufficient sleep, significant differences remained. Compared to those reporting 7–8 h of sleep, those who reported less than 5 or 6 h were more than 2.5 times as likely to report nodding off at the wheel [79]. Although other research suggests that short sleepers may not be at higher risk for driving accidents [78], the above findings suggest that some cognitive impairments may exist due to inability to maintain vigilance.

Conceptualizing Societal Impact

The societal impact of sleep deprivation is difficult to characterize but is imperative to understand. In 2006, the Institute of Medicine released a report entitled, "Sleep Disorders and Sleep Deprivation: An Unmet Public Health Problem" [153]. This report detailed research and recommendations regarding how sleep loss, experienced in and outside of the context of sleep disorders, plays a major role in many public health issues, and that these relationships need to be better understood and addressed. The Institute of Medicine issued another report in 2010 on "Resident Duty Hours," which focused on the public health implications of the many medical residents who are working at hours that predispose them to health and safety risks [154]. This report led to major changes in rules regarding medical residencies [155–163]. Other safety critical industries have also begun to recognize the importance of sleep. For example, new or proposed regulations for commercial drivers, air traffic controllers, pilots, and rail workers aim to mitigate health and safety concerns associated with insufficient sleep. Finally, in 2010, adequate sleep has been included, for the first time, in the US Federal program that delineates national health priorities and targets: Healthy People [164].

Understanding how to translate this recognition of the importance of sleep for health into effective change at the societal level will require a better understanding of the societal impact of sleep on health, and the social and environmental factors that contribute to poor sleep. Several studies (outlined below) have begun to address these questions. In the context of specific studies, a framework is needed to provide guiding principles to the conceptualization of sleep and health in society. Other domains of health behavior have adopted social–ecological models to account for the complex relationship of the individual to embedded social systems [165]. These models describe how individual-level factors, dubbed the "microsystem" (e.g., health and behavior), are embedded within social networks that exist beyond the individual, dubbed the "mesosystem" (e.g., family, neighborhood), and how these relate to each other, separate from the individual, dubbed the "exosystem," and how these are all embedded in societal networks, dubbed the "macrosystem" (e.g., public policy, technological progress).

Recently, a social–ecological model was proposed by Grandner, Hale, Moore, and Patel [15] that adapts this perspective to sleep and health. This model proposes that sleep is associated with mortality through proposed health consequences of sleep loss (e.g., cardiovascular, metabolic, psychological, and other effects) that are all interrelated. Further, this model proposes that sleep loss is a consequence of individual factors (e.g., behavior, genetics) that exist within social networks that play a role in determining sleep (e.g., home and work responsibilities, neighborhoods, culture), and these are themselves embedded in societal contexts that also play a role in sleep (e.g., policy, globalization, population characteristics). When brought together, this model is a comprehensive representation of the causes and effects of sleep loss in society. However, many of the potential determinants of sleep have yet to be studied in detail. In this way, the proposed model theorizes relationships that have yet to be established. Although much work is still needed, several studies have examined a number of societal determinants of sleep loss, described below.

Social and Societal Determinants

Race/Ethnicity

Several studies have examined associations between sleep duration and race/ethnicity in cohort studies. Hale and Do found that, compared to White adults, Black, non-Mexican Hispanic, and other non-Hispanic minorities were more likely to be short sleepers, and Black adults were more likely to be long sleepers [166]. In a study by Nunes and colleagues that analyzed data from the NHIS, Black Americans were more likely than White Americans to sleep 5 or less, 6, and

9 h or more [167]. These data are supported by a meta-analysis, in which Ruiter and colleagues demonstrated that African Americans slept less than White Americans, whether sleep was assessed objectively or subjectively [168].

This relationship is complex in the consideration of differential experience of sleep difficulties. For example, Grandner and colleagues [169] assessed >150,000 American respondents to the 2006 BRFSS and found that Black/African American, Hispanic/Latino, and Asian/other women were less likely than White women to report sleep disturbances, and Asian/other men were less likely than White men to report sleep disturbances. This finding may be partially due to response biases to the survey items. To illustrate this, in a more recent study, Grandner and colleagues [170] evaluated sleep symptoms asked as part of the 2007–2008 NHANES. Difficulty falling asleep was assessed via an elicited complaint (asking for how often respondents have difficulty) and by asking for a typical sleep latency (and dichotomizing around 30 min). When respondents were asked if they had difficulty falling asleep, those in minority groups generally reported fewer complaints than White respondents. However, when the question was asked in a nonjudgmental way (just asking for sleep latency, without any indication of what is a complaint of a problem), minority groups were more likely to report sleep latencies greater than 30 min. This suggests that assessing subjective sleep across racial/ethnic groups is complicated by how the question is asked.

Socioeconomics

In an analysis of NHIS data by Krueger and Friedman [171], sleep duration was associated with household income, such that the shortest and longest sleep durations were associated with the lowest household income. Similarly, Stamatakis and colleagues demonstrated that those in the lowest income quintile are 54% more likely to report short sleep duration [172], and this likelihood declines in higher income categories in a dose–response manner. In a recent analysis of the 2009 BRFSS data, increased amounts of self-reported insufficient sleep were associated with decreased household income; however, these relationships were completely accounted for by other demographic, social, and health factors, suggesting that it is these factors that link income with insufficient sleep [173]. Other socioeconomic factors are also related to sleep difficulties. For example, Grandner and colleagues [170] showed that (in adjusted analyses) lower education is associated with long sleep latency, snorting/gasping during sleep, and snoring; lack of access to private health insurance is associated with long sleep latency; and food insecurity is associated with long sleep latency, difficulty falling asleep, difficulty maintaining sleep, early morning awakenings, nonrestorative sleep, sleepiness, snorting/

gasping during sleep, and snoring. Although these relationships were adjusted for racial/ethnic variables, other studies have shown that the relationship between sleep quality and socioeconomics depends on race [174].

Home and Family

Several studies have shown that marital status and relationship quality are associated with sleep. For example, compared to married adults, those who are single, part of an unmarried couple, divorced, and separated are more likely to report sleep disturbance in general [169]. Being divorced is also associated with increased likelihood of early-morning awakenings, nonrestorative sleep, and daytime sleepiness [170]. A comprehensive review of research relating relationship quality to sleep is provided by Troxel and colleagues [175].

Work and Occupation

Analysis of the American Time Use Survey (ATUS) by Basner and colleagues demonstrated that Americans in general do not trade sleep for more leisure time—they tend to trade sleep for work [176]. In separate analyses for both weekday and workday time, there is a marked negative linear relationship between time spent in work activities and time spent sleeping. No such relationship exists for other time use categories. One of the ways that individuals cope with work-related sleep loss is to sleep in on weekends. In a recent study by Kubo and colleagues [177], a weekend sleep extension intervention assessed performance gains in the subsequent workweek. No improvements were found for drowsiness or blood pressure. On the Monday following the intervention, there was a slight improvement in neurobehavioral performance (using the PVT), but this was followed by a systematic worsening of PVT performance on that Thursday. Therefore, the short-term benefits of sleeping in on weekends are not clear.

Neighborhood and Geography

Living in an inner-city area is associated with a 24% increased risk of habitual short sleep duration [178]. Further, neighborhoods perceived as unclean, noisy, and crime-ridden are associated with poorer health and psychological distress. Hale and colleagues have shown that sleep quality partially mediates the relationship between living in this type of neighborhood and both physical and mental health [179].

Two studies have assessed geographic aspects of sleep. McKnight-Eily and colleagues [180] assessed the prevalence of insufficient sleep using the 2008 BRFSS. Their analysis showed that among the 48 continental US states and Washington, DC, the states with the highest rates of insufficient sleep every night were (in order), West Virginia (19.3%), Tennessee (14.8%), Kentucky (14.4%), Oklahoma (14.3%), Florida (13.5%), Georgia (13.4%), Missouri (13.4%), Alabama (13.2%), Mississippi (13.1%), Louisiana (13.0%), and North Carolina (13.0%). Using the 2006 BRFSS, Grandner and colleagues [181] examined state-level prevalence of general sleep disturbance (which included difficulty falling asleep, difficulty maintaining sleep, or sleeping too much), as well as daytime tiredness/fatigue. This analysis also found that the states with the highest concentrations of both sleep disturbance and daytime/fatigue included West Virginia, Alabama, Mississippi, Missouri, and Oklahoma. This study found that variation in sleep disturbance at the census region level was driven by regional differences in mental health, race/ethnicity, access to health care, socioeconomics, smoking, and weather patterns.

Physical Environment

Aspects of the physical environment may also affect sleep. One of the most powerful environmental influences may be light. Environmental light is the primary external stimulus to the circadian pacemaker [182]. Light in the morning advances circadian phase and light in the evening delays circadian phase [183]. This effect is heightened using light in the blue-green spectrum, which is around the peak of sensitivity of the melanopsin-containing retinal ganglion cells that project to the suprachiasmatic nucleus [184–187]. In addition to light, environmental noise may disturb sleep. Several recent studies have demonstrated that loud noises at night interfere with sleep [188–195]. For example, Basner and colleagues found that sound at 45 dBA increased the likelihood of sleep state change by about 50% and EEG arousal by about 85%, and noise at 65 dBA was associated with an approximately fourfold increase in the likelihood of a sleep state change or EEG arousal, as well as awakenings. Temperature may also play a role. Perhaps because of the coupling of the body temperature rhythm to sleep [196], environmental temperature can impact sleep if it is too warm or too cool (the ideal seems to be between 60 and 72 degrees).

Future Research Directions

The scientific study of sleep deprivation has a long history and is currently being assessed in many contexts. Studies are examining effects on the molecular level, effects in invertebrates, effects in nonhuman mammals, effects in humans of both total and partial sleep deprivation, and effects at the community and population level. Studies are examining causes and consequences of sleep deprivation at both the physiologic and environmental levels. Conceptualizing sleep as a domain of healthy behavior (alongside diet and physical activity), rather than simply a physiologic process or aspect of health that may be disordered, affords sleep researchers many new opportunities and contexts for the study of sleep and its impact on health.

References

1. Henry D, McClellen D, Rosenthal L, Dedrick D, Gosdin M. Is sleep really for sissies? Understanding the role of work in insomnia in the US. Soc Sci Med. 2008 Feb; 66(3):715–26.
2. Loomis AL, Harvey EN, Hobart G. Further observations on the potential rhythms of the cerebral cortex during sleep. Science. 1935 Aug; 82(2122):198–200.
3. Loomis AL, Harvey EN, Hobart G. Potential rhythms of the cerebral cortex during sleep. Science. 1935 Jun; 81(2111):597–8.
4. Kleitman N. Sleep and wakefulness. Chicago: University of Chicago Press; 1939.
5. Hartmann EL. Experiments in nature: variable sleepers. In: Hartmann EL, editor. The functions of sleep. New Haven: Yale University Press; 1973. p. 71–81.
6. Hartmann EL. Experiments in nature: long and short sleepers. In: Hartmann EL, editor. The functions of sleep. New Haven: Yale University Press; 1973. p. 53–70.
7. Horne J. Why we sleep: the functions of sleep in humans and other mammals. Oxford: Oxford University Press; 1988.
8. Siegel JM. Sleep phylogeny: clues to the evolution and function of sleep. In: Luppi PH, editor. Sleep circuits and functions. Boca Raton: CRC Press; 2005.
9. Tononi G, Cirelli C. Sleep function and synaptic homeostasis. Sleep Med Rev. 2006 Feb; 10(1):49–62.
10. Rattenborg NC, Lesku JA, Martinez-Gonzalez D, Lima SL. The non-trivial functions of sleep. Sleep Med Rev. 2007 Oct; 11(5):405–9. (author reply 411–7).
11. Rial RV, Nicolau MC, Gamundi A, et al. The trivial function of sleep. Sleep Med Rev. 2007 Aug; 11(4):311–25.
12. Mackiewicz M, Naidoo N, Zimmerman JE, Pack AI. Molecular mechanisms of sleep and wakefulness. Ann N Y Acad Sci. 2008;1129:335–49.
13. Mackiewicz M, Shockley KR, Romer MA, et al. Macromolecule biosynthesis: a key function of sleep. Physiol Genomics. 2007 Nov; 31(3):441–57.
14. Achermann P. The two-process model of sleep regulation revisited. Aviat Space Environ Med. 2004 Mar; 75(3 Suppl):A37–43.
15. Grandner MA, Patel NP, Hale L, Moore M. Mortality associated with sleep duration: the evidence, the possible mechanisms, and the future. Sleep Med Rev. 2010;14:191–203.
16. Knutson KL, Van Cauter E, Rathouz PJ, DeLeire T, Lauderdale DS. Trends in the prevalence of short sleepers in the USA: 1975–2006. Sleep. 2010 Jan; 33(1):37–45.
17. Smith LJ, Nowakowski S, Soeffing JP, Orff HJ, Perlis M. The measurement of sleep. In: Perlis ML, Lichstein KL, editors. Treating sleep disorders: principles and practice of behavioral sleep medicine. Hoboken: Wiley; 2003. p. 29–73.
18. Van de Water AT, Holmes A, Hurley DA. Objective measurements of sleep for non-laboratory settings as alternatives to polysomnography—a systematic review. J Sleep Res. 2011 Mar; 20(1 Pt 2):183–200.
19. Agnew HW Jr, Webb WB, Williams RL. The first night effect: an EEG study of sleep. Psychophysiology. 1966 Jan; 2(3):263–6.

20. Buysse DJ, Ancoli-Israel S, Edinger JD, Lichstein KL, Morin CM. Recommendations for a standard research assessment of insomnia. Sleep. 2006 Sep; 29(9):1155–73.

21. Grandner MA, Patel NP, Gehrman PR, Perlis ML, Pack AI. Problems associated with short sleep: bridging the gap between laboratory and epidemiological studies. Sleep Med Rev. 2010 Nov; 14:239–47.

22. Solarz DE, Mullington JM, Meier-Ewert HK. Sleep, inflammation and cardiovascular disease. Front Biosci. (Elite Ed). 2012;4:2490–501.

23. Aldabal L, Bahammam AS. Metabolic, endocrine, and immune consequences of sleep deprivation. Open Respir Med J. 2011;5:31–43.

24. Benedetti F, Colombo C. Sleep deprivation in mood disorders. Neuropsychobiology. 2011;64(3):141–51.

25. Heatherley SV. Caffeine withdrawal, sleepiness, and driving performance: what does the research really tell us? Nutr Neurosci. 2011 May; 14(3):89–95.

26. Okifuji A, Hare BD. Do sleep disorders contribute to pain sensitivity? Curr Rheumatol Rep. 2011 Dec; 13(6):528–34.

27. Faraut B, Boudjeltia KZ, Vanhamme L, Kerkhofs M. Immune, inflammatory and cardiovascular consequences of sleep restriction and recovery. Sleep Med Rev. 2012 Apr; 16(2):137–49.

28. Kronfeld-Schor N, Einat H. Circadian rhythms and depression: human psychopathology and animal models. Neuropharmacology. 2012 Jan; 62(1):101–14.

29. McCoy JG, Strecker RE. The cognitive cost of sleep lost. Neurobiol Learn Mem. 2011 Nov; 96(4):564–82.

30. Majekodunmi A, Landrigan CP. The effect of physician sleep deprivation on patient safety in perinatal-neonatal medicine. Am J Perinatol. 2012 Jan; 29(1):43–8.

31. Motivala SJ. Sleep and inflammation: psychoneuroimmunology in the context of cardiovascular disease. Ann Behav Med. 2011 Oct; 42(2):141–52.

32. Kopasz M, Loessl B, Hornyak M, et al. Sleep and memory in healthy children and adolescents—a critical review. Sleep Med Rev. 2010 Jun; 14(3):167–77.

33. Roux FJ, Kryger MH. Medication effects on sleep. Clin Chest Med. 2010 Jun; 31(2):397–405.

34. Poe GR, Walsh CM, Bjorness TE. Cognitive neuroscience of sleep. In: Kerkhof GA, Van Dongen HPA, editors. Human sleep and cognition, Part I: basic research. Amsterdam: Elsevier; 2010. p. 1–19.

35. Reynolds AC, Banks S. Total sleep deprivation, chronic sleep restriction and sleep disruption. In: Kerkhof GA, Van Dongen HPA, editors. Human sleep and cognition, Part I: basic research. Amsterdam: Elsevier; 2010. p. 91–103.

36. Mullington JM, Haack M, Toth M, Serrador JM, Meier-Ewert HK. Cardiovascular, inflammatory, and metabolic consequences of sleep deprivation. Prog Cardiovasc Dis. 2009 Jan–Feb; 51(4):294–302.

37. Clark SL. Sleep deprivation: implications for obstetric practice in the United States. Am J Obstet Gynecol. 2009 Aug; 201(2):136. e1–4.

38. Lim J, Dinges DF. Sleep deprivation and vigilant attention. Ann N Y Acad Sci. 2008;1129:305–22.

39. Banks S, Dinges DF. Behavioral and physiological consequences of sleep restriction. J Clin Sleep Med. 2007 Aug; 3(5):519–28.

40. Dinges DF. The state of sleep deprivation: from functional biology to functional consequences. Sleep Med Rev. 2006 Oct; 10(5): 303–5.

41. Durmer JS, Dinges DF. Neurocognitive consequences of sleep deprivation. Semin Neurol. 2005 Mar; 25(1):117–29.

42. Van Dongen HP, Vitellaro KM, Dinges DF. Individual differences in adult human sleep and wakefulness: leitmotif for a research agenda. Sleep. 2005 Apr; 28(4):479–96.

43. Dinges DF. Critical research issues in development of biomathematical models of fatigue and performance. Aviat Space Environ Med. 2004 Mar; 75(3 Suppl):A181–91.

44. Mallis MM, Mejdal S, Nguyen TT, Dinges DF. Summary of the key features of seven biomathematical models of human fatigue and performance. Aviat Space Environ Med. 2004 Mar; 75(3 Suppl):A4–14.

45. Rogers NL, Dorrian J, Dinges DF. Sleep, waking and neurobehavioural performance. Front Biosci. 2003 Sep; 8:s1056–67.

46. Rogers NL, Szuba MP, Staab JP, Evans DL, Dinges DF. Neuroimmunologic aspects of sleep and sleep loss. Semin Clin Neuropsychiatry. 2001 Oct; 6(4):295–307.

47. Gulevich G, Dement W, Johnson L. Psychiatric and EEG observations on a case of prolonged (264 hours) wakefulness. Arch Gen Psychiatry. 1966 Jul; 15(1):29–35.

48. Kollar EJ, Pasnau RO, Rubin RT, Naitoh P, Slater GG, Kales A. Psychological, psychophysiological, and biochemical correlates of prolonged sleep deprivation. Am J Psychiatry. 1969 Oct; 126(4):488–97.

49. Webb WB, Friel J. Sleep stage and personality characteristics of "natural" long and short sleepers. Science. 1971 Feb; 171(971):587–8.

50. Webb WB, Agnew HW Jr. Sleep stage characteristics of long and short sleepers. Science. 1970 Apr; 168(927):146–7.

51. Benoit O, Foret J, Merle B, Bouard G. Diurnal rhythm of axillary temperature in long and short sleepers: effects of sleep deprivation and sleep displacement. Sleep. 1981;4(4):359–65.

52. Benoit O, Foret J, Bouard G. The time course of slow wave sleep and REM sleep in habitual long and short sleepers: effect of prior wakefulness. Hum Neurobiol. 1983;2(2):91–6.

53. Benoit O, Foret J, Merle B, Reinberg A. Circadian rhythms (temperature, heart rate, vigilance, mood) of short and long sleepers: effects of sleep deprivation. Chronobiologia. 1981 Oct–Dec; 8(4):341–50.

54. Kryger MH, Roth T, Dement WC. Principles and practice of sleep medicine. 4th ed. Philadelphia: Elsevier; 2005.

55. Pack AI, Dinges DF, Gehrman PR, Staley B, Pack FM, Maislin G. Risk factors for excessive sleepiness in older adults. Ann Neurol. 2006 Jun; 59(6):893–904.

56. Dinges DF, Pack F, Williams K, et al. Cumulative sleepiness, mood disturbance, and psychomotor vigilance performance decrements during a week of sleep restricted to 4–5 hours per night. Sleep. 1997 Apr; 20(4):267–77.

57. Guilleminault C, Powell NB, Martinez S, et al. Preliminary observations on the effects of sleep time in a sleep restriction paradigm. Sleep Med. 2003 May; 4(3):177–84.

58. Banks S, Dinges DF. Is the maintenance of wakefulness test sensitive to varying amounts of recovery sleep after chronic sleep restriction? Sleep. 2005;28(Abstract Supplement):A136.

59. Dinges DF, Powell JW. Microcomputer analysis of performance on a portable, simple visual RT task during sustained operations. Beh Res Methods Instrum Comput. 1985;17:652–5.

60. Boonstra TW, Stins JF, Daffertshofer A, Beek PJ. Effects of sleep deprivation on neural functioning: an integrative review. Cell Mol Life Sci. 2007 Apr; 64(7–8):934–46.

61. Curcio G, Ferrara M, De Gennaro L. Sleep loss, learning capacity and academic performance. Sleep Med Rev. 2006 Oct; 10(5):323–37.

62. Chee MW, Chuah LY, Venkatraman V, Chan WY, Philip P, Dinges DF. Functional imaging of working memory following normal sleep and after 24 and 35 h of sleep deprivation: correlations of fronto-parietal activation with performance. Neuroimage. 2006 May; 31(1):419–28.

63. Radun I, Ohisalo J, Radun JE, Summala H, Tolvanen M. Fell asleep and caused a fatal head-on crash? A case study of multidisciplinary in-depth analysis vs. the court. Traffic Inj Prev. 2009 Mar; 10(1):76–83.

64. Anund A, Kecklund G, Vadeby A, Hjalmdahl M, Akerstedt T. The alerting effect of hitting a rumble strip—a simulator study with sleepy drivers. Accid Anal Prev. 2008 Nov; 40(6):1970–6.

65. Ingre M, Akerstedt T, Peters B, Anund A, Kecklund G, Pickles A. Subjective sleepiness and accident risk avoiding the ecological fallacy. J Sleep Res. 2006 Jun; 15(2):142–8.

66. MacLean AW, Davies DR, Thiele K. The hazards and prevention of driving while sleepy. Sleep Med Rev. 2003 Dec; 7(6):507–21.

67. McConnell CF, Bretz KM, Dwyer WO. Falling asleep at the wheel: a close look at 1269 fatal and serious injury-producing crashes. Behav Sleep Med. 2003;1(3):171–83.

68. Varughese J, Allen RP. Fatal accidents following changes in daylight savings time: the American experience. Sleep Med. 2001 Jan; 2(1):31–6.

69. Pizza F, Contardi S, Mondini S, Trentin L, Cirignotta F. Daytime sleepiness and driving performance in patients with obstructive sleep apnea: comparison of the MSLT, the MWT, and a simulated driving task. Sleep. 2009 Mar; 32(3):382–91.

70. Powell NB, Schechtman KB, Riley RW, Guilleminault C, Chiang RP, Weaver EM. Sleepy driver near-misses may predict accident risks. Sleep. 2007 Mar; 30(3):331–42.

71. Philip P, Akerstedt T. Transport and industrial safety, how are they affected by sleepiness and sleep restriction? Sleep Med Rev. 2006 Oct; 10(5):347–56.

72. Gurubhagavatula I, Nkwuo JE, Maislin G, Pack AI. Estimated cost of crashes in commercial drivers supports screening and treatment of obstructive sleep apnea. Accid Anal Prev. 2008 Jan; 40(1):104–15.

73. Al-Barrak M, Shepertycky MR, Kryger MH. Morbidity and mortality in obstructive sleep apnea syndrome 2: effect of treatment on neuropsychiatric morbidity and quality of life. Sleep Biol Rhythms. 2003;1:65–74.

74. Sagaspe P, Taillard J, Akerstedt T, et al. Extended driving impairs nocturnal driving performances. PLoS ONE. 2008;3(10):e3493.

75. Scott LD, Hwang WT, Rogers AE, Nysse T, Dean GE, Dinges DF. The relationship between nurse work schedules, sleep duration, and drowsy driving. Sleep. 2007 Dec; 30(12):1801–7.

76. Aeschbach D, Postolache TT, Sher L, Matthews JR, Jackson MA, Wehr TA. Evidence from the waking electroencephalogram that short sleepers live under higher homeostatic sleep pressure than long sleepers. Neuroscience. 2001;102(3):493–502.

77. Aeschbach D, Cajochen C, Landolt H, Borbely AA. Homeostatic sleep regulation in habitual short sleepers and long sleepers. Am J Physiol. 1996 Jan; 270(1 Pt 2):R41–53.

78. Kripke DF, Rex K. Short sleepers are not at higher risk for driving accidents or other violations. Sleep. 2002;25(Abstract Supplement):A284–5.

79. Maia Q, Grandner MA, Findley J, Gurubhagavatula I. Short sleep duration associated with drowsy driving and the role of perceived sleep insufficiency. Accid Anal Prev. 2013;59:618–22.

80. Rechtschaffen A, Bergmann BM. Sleep deprivation in the rat: an update of the 1989 paper. Sleep. 2002 Feb; 25(1):18–24.

81. Van Cauter E, Blackman JD, Roland D, Spire JP, Refetoff S, Polonsky KS. Modulation of glucose regulation and insulin secretion by circadian rhythmicity and sleep. J Clin Invest. 1991 Sep; 88(3):934–42.

82. Spiegel K, Leproult R, Van Cauter E. Impact of sleep debt on metabolic and endocrine function. Lancet. 1999 Oct; 354(9188):1435–9.

83. Spiegel K, Tasali E, Penev P, Van Cauter E. Brief communication: sleep curtailment in healthy young men is associated with decreased leptin levels, elevated ghrelin levels, and increased hunger and appetite. Ann Intern Med. 2004 Dec; 141(11):846–50.

84. Donga E, van Dijk M, van Dijk JG, et al. A single night of partial sleep deprivation induces insulin resistance in multiple metabolic pathways in healthy subjects. J Clin Endocrinol Metab. 2010 Jun; 95(6):2963–8.

85. Donga E, van Dijk M, van Dijk JG, et al. Partial sleep restriction decreases insulin sensitivity in type 1 diabetes. Diabetes Care. 2010 Jul; 33(7):1573–7.

86. Buxton OM, Pavlova M, Reid EW, Wang W, Simonson DC, Adler GK. Sleep restriction for 1 week reduces insulin sensitivity in healthy men. Diabetes. 2010 Sep; 59(9):2126–33.

87. Benedict C, Hallschmid M, Lassen A, et al. Acute sleep deprivation reduces energy expenditure in healthy men. Am J Clin Nutr. 2011 Jun; 93(6):1229–36.

88. Everson CA, Crowley WR. Reductions in circulating anabolic hormones induced by sustained sleep deprivation in rats. Am J Physiol Endocrinol Metab. 2004 Jun; 286(6):E1060–70.

89. Mullington JM, Chan JL, Van Dongen HP, et al. Sleep loss reduces diurnal rhythm amplitude of leptin in healthy men. J Neuroendocrinol. 2003 Sep; 15(9):851–4.

90. Lusardi P, Vanasia A, Mugellini A, Zoppi A, Preti P, Fogari R. Evaluation of nocturnal blood pressure by the Multi-P analysis of 24-hour ambulatory monitoring. Z Kardiol. 1996;85(Suppl 3):121–3.

91. Tochikubo O, Ikeda A, Miyajima E, Ishii M. Effects of insufficient sleep on blood pressure monitored by a new multibiomedical recorder. Hypertension. 1996 Jun; 27(6):1318–24.

92. Dettoni JL, Consolim-Colombo FM, Drager LF, et al. Cardiovascular effects of partial sleep deprivation in healthy volunteers. J Appl Physiol. 2012 Jul; 113(2):232–6.

93. Acar G, Akcakoyun M, Sari I, et al. Acute sleep deprivation in healthy adults is associated with a reduction in left atrial early diastolic strain rate. Sleep Breath. 2013 Sep; 17(3):975–83.

94. Franzen PL, Gianaros PJ, Marsland AL, et al. Cardiovascular reactivity to acute psychological stress following sleep deprivation. Psychosom Med. 2011 Oct; 73(8):679–82.

95. Yang H, Durocher JJ, Larson RA, Dellavalla JP, Carter JR. Total sleep deprivation alters cardiovascular reactivity to acute stressors in humans. J Appl Physiol. 2012 Sep; 113(6):903–8.

96. Ross R. Atherosclerosis—an inflammatory disease. N Engl J Med. 1999 Jan; 340(2):115–26.

97. Vgontzas AN, Zoumakis E, Bixler EO, et al. Adverse effects of modest sleep restriction on sleepiness, performance, and inflammatory cytokines. J Clin Endocrinol Metab. 2004 May; 89(5):2119–26.

98. van Leeuwen WM, Lehto M, Karisola P, et al. Sleep restriction increases the risk of developing cardiovascular diseases by augmenting proinflammatory responses through IL-17 and CRP. PLoS ONE. 2009;4(2):e4589.

99. Haack M, Sanchez E, Mullington JM. Elevated inflammatory markers in response to prolonged sleep restriction are associated with increased pain experience in healthy volunteers. Sleep. 2007 Sep; 30(9):1145–52.

100. Meier-Ewert HK, Ridker PM, Rifai N, et al. Effect of sleep loss on C-reactive protein, an inflammatory marker of cardiovascular risk. J Am Coll Cardiol. 2004 Feb; 43(4):678–83.

101. Grandner MA, Kripke DF. Self-reported sleep complaints with long and short sleep: a nationally representative sample. Psychosom Med. 2004 Mar–Apr; 66(2):239–41.

102. Grandner MA, Drummond SP. Who are the long sleepers? Towards an understanding of the mortality relationship. Sleep Med Rev. 2007 Oct; 11(5):341–60.

103. Youngstedt SD, Kripke DF. Long sleep and mortality: rationale for sleep restriction. Sleep Med Rev. 2004 Jun; 8(3):159–74.

104. Gallicchio L, Kalesan B. Sleep duration and mortality: a systematic review and meta-analysis. J Sleep Res. 2009;18(2):148–58.

105. Cappuccio FP, D'Elia L, Strazzullo P, Miller MA. Sleep duration and all-cause mortality: a systematic review and meta-analysis of prospective studies. Sleep. 2010 May; 33(5):585–92.

106. Grandner MA, Patel NP. From sleep duration to mortality: implications of meta-analysis and future directions. J Sleep Res. 2009;18(2):145–7.

107. Bliwise DL, Young TB. The parable of parabola: what the U-shaped curve can and cannot tell us about sleep. Sleep. 2007 Dec; 30(12):1614–5.

108. Morselli LL, Guyon A, Spiegel K. Sleep and metabolic function. Pflugers Arch. 2012 Jan; 463(1):139–60.

109. Knutson KL. Does inadequate sleep play a role in vulnerability to obesity? Am J Hum Biol. 2012 May–Jun; 24(3):361–71.

110. Klingenberg L, Sjodin A, Holmback U, Astrup A, Chaput JP. Short sleep duration and its association with energy metabolism. Obes Rev. 2012 Jul; 13(7):565–77.

111. Chaput JP. Short sleep duration as a cause of obesity: myth or reality? Obes Rev. 2011 May; 12(5):e2–3.

112. Beccuti G, Pannain S. Sleep and obesity. Curr Opin Clin Nutr Metab Care. 2011 Jul; 14(4):402–12.

113. Reiter RJ, Tan DX, Korkmaz A, Ma S. Obesity and metabolic syndrome: association with chronodisruption, sleep deprivation, and melatonin suppression. Ann Med. 2012 Sep; 44(6):564–77.

114. Nielsen LS, Danielsen KV, Sorensen TI. Short sleep duration as a possible cause of obesity: critical analysis of the epidemiological evidence. Obes Rev. 2011 Feb; 12(2):78–92.

115. Knutson KL. Sleep duration and cardiometabolic risk: a review of the epidemiologic evidence. Best Pract Res Clin Endocrinol Metab. 2010 Oct; 24(5):731–43.

116. Knutson KL, Van Cauter E. Associations between sleep loss and increased risk of obesity and diabetes. Ann N Y Acad Sci. 2008;1129:287–304.

117. Marshall NS, Glozier N, Grunstein RR. Is sleep duration related to obesity? A critical review of the epidemiological evidence. Sleep Med Rev. 2008 Aug; 12(4):289–98.

118. Taheri S, Thomas GN. Is sleep duration associated with obesity—where do U stand? Sleep Med Rev. 2008 Aug; 12(4):299–302.

119. Van Cauter E, Knutson K. Sleep and the epidemic of obesity in children and adults. Eur J Endocrinol. 2008 Aug; 159(Suppl 1):S59–66.

120. Patel SR, Hu FB. Short sleep duration and weight gain: a systematic review. Obesity (Silver Spring). 2008 Mar; 16(3):643–53.

121. Altman NG, Izci-Balserak B, Schopfer E, et al. Sleep duration versus sleep insufficiency as predictors of cardiometabolic health outcomes. Sleep Med. 2012 Dec; 13(10):1261–70.

122. Patel SR, Malhotra A, White DP, Gottlieb DJ, Hu FB. Association between reduced sleep and weight gain in women. Am J Epidemiol. 2006 Nov; 164(10):947–54.

123. Watanabe M, Kikuchi H, Tanaka K, Takahashi M. Association of short sleep duration with weight gain and obesity at 1-year follow-up: a large-scale prospective study. Sleep. 2010;33(2):161–7.

124. Bopparaju S, Surani S. Sleep and diabetes. Int J Endocrinol. 2010;2010:759509.

125. Zizi F, Jean-Louis G, Brown CD, Ogedegbe G, Boutin-Foster C, McFarlane SI. Sleep duration and the risk of diabetes mellitus: epidemiologic evidence and pathophysiologic insights. Curr Diab Rep. 2010 Feb; 10(1):43–7.

126. Buxton OM, Marcelli E. Short and long sleep are positively associated with obesity, diabetes, hypertension, and cardiovascular disease among adults in the United States. Soc Sci Med. 2010 Sep; 71(5):1027–36.

127. Shankar A, Syamala S, Kalidindi S. Insufficient rest or sleep and its relation to cardiovascular disease, diabetes and obesity in a national, multiethnic sample. PLoS ONE. 2010;5(11):e14189.

128. Vishnu A, Shankar A, Kalidindi S. Examination of the association between insufficient sleep and cardiovascular disease and diabetes by race/ethnicity. Int J Endocrinol. 2011;2011:789358.

129. Zizi F, Pandey A, Murrray-Bachmann R, et al. Race/ethnicity, sleep duration, and diabetes mellitus: analysis of the National Health Interview Survey. Am J Med. 2012 Feb; 125(2):162–7.

130. Grandner MA, Jackson NJ, Pak VM, Gehrman PR. Sleep disturbance is associated with cardiovascular and metabolic disorders. J Sleep Res. 2012 Aug; 21(4):427–33.

131. Grandner MA, Patel NP, Perlis ML, et al. Obesity, diabetes, and exercise associated with sleep-related complaints in the American population. J Public Health. 2011 Oct; 19(5):463–74.

132. Hsieh SD, Muto T, Murase T, Tsuji H, Arase Y. Association of short sleep duration with obesity, diabetes, fatty liver and behavioral factors in Japanese men. Intern Med. 2011;50(21):2499–502.

133. Kachi Y, Ohwaki K, Yano E. Association of sleep duration with untreated diabetes in Japanese men. Sleep Med. 2012 Mar; 13(3):307–9.

134. Najafian J, Toghianifar N, Mohammadifard N, Nouri F. Association between sleep duration and metabolic syndrome in a population-based study: Isfahan Healthy Heart Program. J Res Med Sci. 2011 Jun; 16(6):801–6.

135. Rafalson L, Donahue RP, Stranges S, et al. Short sleep duration is associated with the development of impaired fasting glucose: the Western New York Health Study. Ann Epidemiol. 2010 Dec; 20(12):883–9.

136. Kita T, Yoshioka E, Satoh H, et al. Short sleep duration and poor sleep quality increase the risk of diabetes in Japanese workers with no family history of diabetes. Diabetes Care. 2012 Feb; 35(2):313–8.

137. Hancox RJ, Landhuis CE. Association between sleep duration and haemoglobin A1c in young adults. J Epidemiol Community Health. 2012 Oct; 66(10):957–61.

138. Hoevenaar-Blom MP, Spijkerman AM, Kromhout D, van den Berg JF, Verschuren WM. Sleep duration and sleep quality in relation to 12-year cardiovascular disease incidence: the MORGEN study. Sleep. 2011;34(11):1487–92.

139. Knutson KL, Van Cauter E, Rathouz PJ, et al. Association between sleep and blood pressure in midlife: the CARDIA sleep study. Arch Intern Med. 2009 Jun; 169(11):1055–61.

140. Cappuccio FP, Cooper D, D'Elia L, Strazzullo P, Miller MA. Sleep duration predicts cardiovascular outcomes: a systematic review and meta-analysis of prospective studies. Eur Heart J. 2011 Jun; 32(12):1484–92.

141. Taveras EM, Rifas-Shiman SL, Rich-Edwards JW, Mantzoros CS. Maternal short sleep duration is associated with increased levels of inflammatory markers at 3 years postpartum. Metabolism. 2011 Jul; 60(7):982–6.

142. Miller MA, Kandala NB, Kivimaki M, et al. Gender differences in the cross-sectional relationships between sleep duration and markers of inflammation: Whitehall II study. Sleep. 2009 Jul; 32(7):857–64.

143. Matthews KA, Zheng H, Kravitz HM, et al. Are inflammatory and coagulation biomarkers related to sleep characteristics in mid-life women? Study of women's health across the nation sleep study. Sleep. 2010 Dec; 33(12):1649–55.

144. Taheri S, Austin D, Lin L, Nieto FJ, Young T, Mignot E. Correlates of serum C-reactive protein (CRP)—no association with sleep duration or sleep disordered breathing. Sleep. 2007 Aug; 30(8):991–6.

145. Suarez EC. Self-reported symptoms of sleep disturbance and inflammation, coagulation, insulin resistance and psychosocial distress: evidence for gender disparity. Brain Behav Immun. 2008 Aug; 22(6):960–8.

146. Grandner MA, Buxton OM, Jackson N, Sands MR, Pandey AK, Jean-Louis G. Extreme sleep durations and increased C-reactive protein: effects of sex and ethnoracial group. Sleep. 2013;36(5):769–79E.

147. von Kanel R, Ancoli-Israel S, Dimsdale JE, et al. Sleep and biomarkers of atherosclerosis in elderly Alzheimer caregivers and controls. Gerontology. 2010;56(1):41–50.

148. Dowd JB, Goldman N, Weinstein M. Sleep duration, sleep quality, and biomarkers of inflammation in a Taiwanese population. Ann Epidemiol. 2011 Nov; 21(11):799–806.

149. Garaulet M, Ortega FB, Ruiz JR, et al. Short sleep duration is associated with increased obesity markers in European adolescents: effect of physical activity and dietary habits. The HELENA study. Int J Obes (Lond). 2011 Oct; 35(10):1308–17.

150. Weiss A, Xu F, Storfer-Isser A, Thomas A, Ievers-Landis CE, Redline S. The association of sleep duration with adolescents' fat and carbohydrate consumption. Sleep. 2010 Sep; 33(9):1201–9.

151. Imaki M, Hatanaka Y, Ogawa Y, Yoshida Y, Tanada S. An epidemiological study on relationship between the hours of sleep and life style factors in Japanese factory workers. J Physiol Anthropol Appl Human Sci. 2002 Mar; 21(2):115–20.

152. Grandner MA, Jackson N, Gerstner JR, Knutson KL. Dietary nutrients associated with short and long sleep duration. Data from a nationally representative sample. Appetite. 2013 May; 64:71–80.

153. Colten HR, Altevogt BM, Institute of Medicine Committee on Sleep Medicine and Research. Sleep disorders and sleep deprivation: an unmet public health problem. Washington, DC: Institute of Medicine: National Academies Press; 2006.

154. Ulmer C, Wolman DM, Johns MME, Institute of Medicine Committee on Optimizing Graduate Medical Trainee (Resident) Hours and Work Schedules to Improve Patient Safety. Resident duty hours: enhancing sleep, supervision, and safety. Washington, D.C.: National Academies Press; 2009.

155. Zohar D, Tzischinsky O, Epstein R, Lavie P. The effects of sleep loss on medical residents' emotional reactions to work events: a cognitive-energy model. Sleep. 2005 Jan; 28(1):47–54.

156. Weinger MB, Ancoli-Israel S. Sleep deprivation and clinical performance. JAMA. 2002 Feb; 287(8):955–7.

157. Borman KR, Biester TW, Jones AT, Shea JA. Sleep, supervision, education, and service: views of junior and senior residents. J Surg Educ. 2011 Nov; 68(6):495–501.

158. Borman KR, Fuhrman GM. "Resident duty hours: enhancing sleep, supervision, and safety": response of the Association of Program Directors in Surgery to the December 2008 Report of the Institute of Medicine. Surgery. 2009 Sep; 146(3):420 7.

159. Britt LD, Sachdeva AK, Healy GB, Whalen TV, Blair PG. Resident duty hours in surgery for ensuring patient safety, providing optimum resident education and training, and promoting resident well-being: a response from the American College of Surgeons to the Report of the Institute of Medicine, "resident duty hours: enhancing sleep, supervision, and safety". Surgery. 2009 Sep; 146(3):398–409.

160. Lewis FR. Comment of the American Board of Surgery on the recommendations of the Institute of Medicine Report, "resident duty hours: enhancing sleep, supervision, and safety". Surgery. 2009 Sep; 146(3):410–9.

161. Sataloff RT. Resident duty hours: concerns and consequences. Ear Nose Throat J. 2009 Mar; 88(3):812–6.

162. Blatman KH. The Institute of Medicine resident work hours recommendations: a resident's viewpoint. J Clin Sleep Med. 2009 Feb; 5(1):13.

163. Meinke L. The Institute of Medicine resident work hours recommendations: a program director's viewpoint. J Clin Sleep Med. 2009 Feb; 5(1):12.

164. Office of Disease Prevention and Health Promotion. Healthy people 2020 objective topic areas. Washington, DC: US Department of Health and Human Services; 2011.

165. Bronfenbrenner U. Toward an experimental ecology of human development. Am Psychol. 1977;32:513–31.

166. Hale L, Do DP. Racial differences in self-reports of sleep duration in a population-based study. Sleep. 2007 Sep; 30(9):1096–103.

167. Nunes J, Jean-Louis G, Zizi F, et al. Sleep duration among black and white Americans: results of the National Health Interview Survey. J Natl Med Assoc. 2008 Mar; 100(3):317–22.

168. Ruiter ME, Decoster J, Jacobs L, Lichstein KL. Normal sleep in African-Americans and Caucasian-Americans: a meta-analysis. Sleep Med. 2011 Mar; 12(3):209–14.

169. Grandner MA, Patel NP, Gehrman PR, et al. Who gets the best sleep? Ethnic and socioeconomic factors related to sleep disturbance. Sleep Med. 2010;11:470–9.

170. Grandner MA, Ruiter Petrov ME, Jackson N, Rattanaumpawan P, Patel NP. Sleep symptoms, race/ethnicity, and socioeconomic position. J Clin Sleep Med. 2013;9(9):897–905, 905A–905D.

171. Krueger PM, Friedman EM. Sleep duration in the United States: a cross-sectional population-based study. Am J Epidemiol. 2009 May; 169(9):1052–63.

172. Stamatakis KA, Kaplan GA, Roberts RE. Short sleep duration across income, education, and race/ethnic groups: population prevalence and growing disparities during 34 years of follow-up. Ann Epidemiol. 2007 Dec; 17(12):948–55.

173. Grandner MA, Lang RA, Jackson NJ, Patel NP, Murray-Bachmann R, Jean-Louis G. Biopsychosocial predictors of insufficient rest or sleep in the American population. Sleep. 2011;34(Abstract Supplement):A260.

174. Patel NP, Grandner MA, Xie D, Branas CC, Gooneratne N. "Sleep disparity" in the population: poor sleep quality is strongly associated with poverty and ethnicity. BMC Public Health. 2010 Aug; 10(1):475.

175. Troxel WM, Robles TF, Hall M, Buysse DJ. Marital quality and the marital bed: examining the covariation between relationship quality and sleep. Sleep Med Rev. 2007 Oct; 11(5):389–404.

176. Basner M, Fomberstein KM, Razavi FM, et al. American time use survey: sleep time and its relationship to waking activities. Sleep. 2007 Sep; 30(9):1085–95.

177. Kubo T, Takahashi M, Sato T, Sasaki T, Oka T, Iwasaki K. Weekend sleep intervention for workers with habitually short sleep periods. Scand J Work Environ Health. 2011 Sep; 37(5):418–26.

178. Hale L, Do DP. Sleep and the inner city: how race and neighborhood context relate to sleep duration. Population Association of America Annual Meeting Program. 2006.

179. Hale L, Hill TD, Burdette AM. Does sleep quality mediate the association between neighborhood disorder and self-rated physical health? Prev Med. 2010 Sep–Oct; 51(3–4):275–8.

180. McKnight-Eily LR, Liu Y, Perry GS, et al. Perceived insufficient rest or sleep among adults—United States, 2008. MMWR Morb Mortal Wkly Rep. 2009;58(42):1175–9.

181. Grandner MA, Jackson NJ, Pigeon WR, Gooneratne NS, Patel NP. State and regional prevalence of sleep disturbance and daytime fatigue. J Clin Sleep Med. 2012;8(1):77–86.

182. Guido ME, Garbarino-Pico E, Contin MA, et al. Inner retinal circadian clocks and non-visual photoreceptors: novel players in the circadian system. Prog Neurobiol. 2010 Dec; 92(4):484–504.

183. Sack RL. Clinical practice. Jet lag. N Engl J Med. 2010 Feb; 362(5):440–7.

184. Hatori M, Panda S. The emerging roles of melanopsin in behavioral adaptation to light. Trends Mol Med. 2010 Oct; 16(10):435–46.

185. La Morgia C, Ross-Cisneros FN, Hannibal J, Montagna P, Sadun AA, Carelli V. Melanopsin-expressing retinal ganglion cells: implications for human diseases. Vision Res. 2011 Jan; 51(2):296–302.

186. Lall GS, Revell VL, Momiji H, et al. Distinct contributions of rod, cone, and melanopsin photoreceptors to encoding irradiance. Neuron. 2010 May; 66(3):417–28.

187. Bailes HJ, Lucas RJ. Melanopsin and inner retinal photoreception. Cell Mol Life Sci. 2010 Jan; 67(1): 99–111.

188. Elmenhorst EM, Pennig S, Rolny V, et al. Examining nocturnal railway noise and aircraft noise in the field: Sleep, psychomotor performance, and annoyance. Sci Total Environ. 2012 May; 424:48–56.

189. Agarwal S, Swami BL. Road traffic noise, annoyance and community health survey—a case study for an Indian city. Noise Health. 2011 Jul–Aug; 13(53):272–6.

190. Omlin S, Bauer GF, Brink M. Effects of noise from non-traffic-related ambient sources on sleep: review of the literature of 1990–2010. Noise Health. 2011 Jul–Aug; 13(53):299–309.

191. Ndrepepa A, Twardella D. Relationship between noise annoyance from road traffic noise and cardiovascular diseases: a meta-analysis. Noise Health. 2011 May–Jun; 13(52):251–9.

192. Kawada T. Noise and health: sleep disturbance in adults. J Occup Health. 2011 Dec; 53(6):413–6.

193. Pirrera S, De Valck E, Cluydts R. Nocturnal road traffic noise: a review on its assessment and consequences on sleep and health. Environ Int. 2010 Jul; 36(5):492–8.

194. Fyhri A, Aasvang GM. Noise, sleep and poor health: Modeling the relationship between road traffic noise and cardiovascular problems. Sci Total Environ. 2010 Oct; 408(21):4935–42.

195. Hong J, Kim J, Lim C, Kim K, Lee S. The effects of long-term exposure to railway and road traffic noise on subjective sleep disturbance. J Acoust Soc Am. 2010 Nov; 128(5):2829–35.

196. Basner M, Glatz C, Griefahn B, Penzel T, Samel A. Aircraft noise: effects on macro- and microstructure of sleep. Sleep Med. 2008 May; 9(4):382–7.

Sleep Models

Mitsuyuki Nakao, Akihiro Karashima and Norihiro Katayama

Introduction

In human sleep research, interactions between homeostasis and circadian control or those between multiple circadian oscillators have long been investigated, which were embodied as the mathematical models at a behavioral level in the 1970s and 1980s [1–3]. Although 30 years have passed since the models were developed, at least their concepts still survive to provide perspective and integrative view of sleep-wake regulation. On the other hand, at a neurophysiological level, the reciprocal interaction model between monoaminergic and cholinergic systems is a first conceptualization of REM (rapid eye movement sleep)-NREM (non-REM sleep) regulation [4]. Thereafter, neurophysiological knowledge concerning REM regulatory system in the brainstem has been accumulated [5, 6]. A possibility of involvement of orexin neurons in canine narcolepsy and ventrolateral preoptic (VLPO) neurons in sleep regulation leads us to flip-flop models of sleep/wake and NREM/REM regulations [7–9].

The study of regulatory mechanisms of sleep-wake rhythm using mathematical modeling has been done concerning cooperative/competitive interactions between homeostasis and circadian control. The two process model is one of the most widely accepted models [3, 10]. It integrates the two processes of homeostatic and circadian control of sleep-wake rhythm in a simple and elegant way, schematized in Fig. 57.1a. Recent models generally share the same framework of the two process model, although the interaction between the homeostatic and the circadian regulations (homeostasis-rhythm interaction) are differently expressed [3, 11, 12]. Borbély and his colleagues have been attempting to extend the applicability of the two process model by including a process of vigilance state and REM-NREM ultradian rhythm whose period is much shorter than 24 h [13, 14].

In spite of its appeal, the framework of homeostasis-rhythm interaction is not necessarily applicable for all aspects of the sleep-wake rhythm. Circadian rhythms often behave like a multioscillator system, which leads to another trend of modeling [2, 15–18]. This multioscillator framework is schematized as Fig. 57.1b (see also the following sections). In addition, as neurophysiological knowledge including the anterior and posterior hypothalamic areas and the brainstem becomes newly available, detailed neural network models of sleep-wake rhythm have formed a new trend of modeling [19–22].

In this chapter, model constructions based on the frameworks shown above and their characteristics are reviewed comparatively. Then, recently acquired knowledge of neural regulatory mechanisms of sleep-wake rhythm is summarized. The detailed neural network models of sleep-wake regulation are also reviewed. These models constructed within various frameworks could serve for testing reality of a physiologist's idea and for exploring a possible mechanism at various levels underlying pathological states of sleep-wake rhythm.

Human Sleep Models

Models Based on Interactions Between Homeostatic and Circadian Control of Sleep-Wake Rhythm

Homeostatic control of sleep-wake rhythm can be intuitively understood; because it is usually experienced that sleep deficit is compensated by a deeper and/or longer recovery sleep. This intuition is well embodied in the two process model [3, 10], which consists of periodic C processes and an exponentially rising-decaying S process. C process works as a reflecting boundary against S process: the S process rebounds when it reaches the C process. As many reviews of the two process model have already been written by Borbély and his colleagues (e.g., [23]), here we summarize aspects of the model not typically covered elsewhere. The two process

M. Nakao (✉) · A. Karashima · N. Katayama
Biomodeling Lab, Graduate School of Information Sciences, Tohoku University, Sendai 980-8579, Japan
e-mail: nakao@ecei.tohoku.ac.jp

S. Chokroverty, M. Billiard (eds.), *Sleep Medicine*, DOI 10.1007/978-1-4939-2089-1_57,
© Springer Science+Business Media, LLC 2015

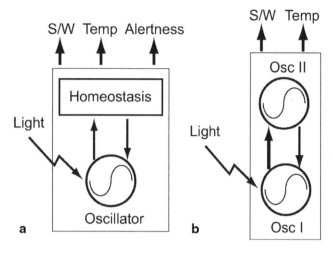

Fig. 57.1 Major frameworks for modeling sleep-wake rhythms [37]. S/W and Temp denote sleep-wake and temperature rhythms, respectively. **a** Two process framework integrating homeostatic and circadian regulations. **b** Multioscillator framework consists of interacting multiple oscillators, where line thickness indicates strength of coupling. For more detail explanation, see the text

model was developed based on the empirical data obtained under short-term sleep deprivations [3]. Namely, the S process represents a build-up of slow wave electroencephalographic activity (SWA) during wake, and its decay during sleep. The shape of C process is determined by a level of SWA and sleep-onset/wake-onset timing [3, 10]. The two process model provides an intuitively tractable structure that enables researchers to test their ideas by manipulating the parameters and model operations: changing the gap between C processes (short and long sleeper), skipping the reflection of S process at the intersection of two processes (sleep deprivation and shift work), reducing build-up of S process (napping), and so on [23]. For 30 years after the development of the two process model, its simplicity and utility have led to its extensive acceptance as a symbolic conceptualization of the integration of homeostatic and circadian controls.

One possible modeling framework of homeostatic control is a negative feedback control. According to the physiological finding that thermoregulation and sleep control may be integrated in the preoptic/anterior hypothalamic area [24], a thermoregulatory model of sleep control was developed. In this context, the mathematical model consists of two circadian oscillators and two negative feedback loops for thermoregulation, one of which is mediated by sleep-wake rhythm [25, 26]. This model has variables mimicking "sleepiness" in addition to sleep-wake patterns, the hypothalamic temperature, and a set-point of thermoregulation. This model can predict behavior of sleepiness and temperature under various situations such as sleep deprivation and shift work [25, 26]. A possible physiological origin of biphasic sleepiness was explored in light of this model structure [27]. This is another

mathematical modeling of the interactions between homeostatic and circadian controls of sleep-wake rhythm.

Prediction of alertness and cognitive performance under various environments is one of major targets of recent modeling [11, 12, 28]. Most of the models generally share the framework of the two process model, although the interactions between the homeostatic and circadian regulations are differently expressed. In addition, another component such as sleep inertia (transitional state of lowered arousal occurring immediately after awakening) can be included as in a three process model [11, 29]. The distinct structure in these models is nonlinear mutual interactions between the homeostatic and circadian regulations, in contrast with a unidirectional effect of C process on S process in the original two process model. The nonlinear interactions were added to reflect results from the forced desynchronization protocol which attempts to separately evaluate the homeostatic and circadian regulations of wide variety of physiological and cognitive variables [30–32]. Borbély and his colleagues have been extending the structure of the two process model by including circadian and ultradian REM-NREM oscillators in a composite form [13], or by implementing a REM-NREM regulatory mechanism [33]. Daytime vigilance can also be simulated by the extended model [14, 34].

The two process model also has a sophisticated structure as a nonlinear oscillator [35]. Due to this structure, it can easily accommodate a wide variety of behavior in sleep-wake rhythm. Actually, the different types of internal desynchronizations can be understood as a bifurcation of the dynamics of the two process model [35, 36]. The beauty of the two process model may be in its simple and abstract structure with no redundancy, which deserves more investigation [37].

Models Based on Interacting Multiple Oscillators

Discovery of dissociation between temperature/melatonin and sleep-wake rhythms (internal desynchronization) in a situation without any time cues such as light and feeding (free-run) prompted development of multioscillator models [1, 2, 15, 18]. As shown in Fig. 57.1b, the fundamental framework of a multioscillator model is two mutually interacting oscillators: one drives temperature and melatonin rhythms (tentatively called Osc I), generally reflecting the actions of the suprachiasmatic nucleus (SCN), and the other controls the sleep-wake rhythm (tentatively called Osc II) that is often represented by plural oscillators [16, 18]. In addition, Osc I is photo-responsive, and exerts a stronger effect on Osc II than the opposite direction. This organization is assumed because of the robustness of Osc I relative to Osc II. These models simulate the behavior of circadian rhythms in a free-run situation including the internal desynchronization and the non-monotonic relationship between the sleep-onset phase and the corresponding sleep length [38].

The physiological reality of the multioscillator framework and the homeostasis-rhythm interaction framework has been disputed [39]. Currently, prediction of alertness and cognitive performance prefers the latter framework. However, it is still argued how homeostatic and circadian regulations interact with each other [11, 34]. It should be noted that the rigid experimental and theoretical separations between homeostatic and circadian regulations are difficult to be done, because a stable limit cycle, which is a general model of circadian oscillator, is characterized by an ability to restore its oscillatory orbit against external perturbations just like homeostasis.

In the multioscillator framework, a physiological origin of Osc II has not yet been identified, in contrast with Osc I (which represents the SCN). This fact may weaken its physiological reality. Honma and his colleagues have tried to map Osc II onto a physiologic process or structure, and to clarify its dynamics [40]. In their experiment, the rest-activity cycle (schedule) of a subject was advanced by 8 h relative to the spontaneous sleep-wake rhythm under the free-run condition, and the reentrainment of the melatonin rhythm was traced after release from the schedule. It took several days for the sleep-wake rhythm to be reentrained to the melatonin rhythm after an 8-day advanced schedule. In contrast, after a 4-day schedule, the sleep-wake rhythm immediately caught up with the melatonin rhythm in most subjects. These results suggest that the sleep-wake rhythm is underlain by an oscillator (presumably Osc II), which could be entrained by the rest-activity schedule (i.e., a nonphotic entrainment). The nonphotic entrainment of Osc II was found to take 4 days or longer; implying that there is a critical period for the entrainment of Osc II. In other words, an adaptive feedback mechanism from the rest-activity cycle to the circadian oscillators is suggested to exist. There is physiological evidence supporting such adaptive feedback mechanisms [41–44].

Existence of the nonphotic as well as photic entrainment mechanisms leads to the multioscillator model with feedbacks [17, 18, 45]. This model can simulate behavior of sleep-wake rhythm under transmeridian flight and shift work where the photic and nonphotic entrainment mechanisms should interact with each other. Incorporating the thermoregulatory model of sleep control the multioscillator model could raise its applicability under diverse situations [46].

Neural Network Models of Sleep-Wake Rhythm

Most of the aforementioned models have abstract structures in which the details of mechanisms at neural and molecular levels are not explicitly represented. Their applicability in understanding the mechanisms underlying the pathologi-

cal states of sleep-wake rhythm is therefore confined to the behavioral level. Therefore, a microscopic level model of sleep-wake rhythm is needed.

The reciprocal interaction model which McCarley and Hobson [4] proposed initiated modeling studies of ultradian rhythm of REM/NREM alternation. Their model is based on the concept that a prey-predator-like interaction between cholinergic and monoaminergic neurons in the brainstem induces the ultradian rhythm, and their later work extended the prey-predator model to the limit cycle model [47, 48]. However, since then knowledge of the neural mechanism regulating sleep and wake states is continuously being updated.

Overview of Recent Neurophysiological Knowledge

Examples of such updates include findings of the involvement of neurons in the ventrolateral preoptic hypothalamic area (VLPO), the extended VLPO (VLPOe), and the median preoptic nucleus (MnPN) in the regulation of NREM as well as REM [8, 9, 49]. The interactions of these neuron groups with those regulating wakefulness and REM in the perifornical/posterior hypothalamic nuclei and the brainstem have been suggested to underlie the physiological mechanisms for maintenance and alternation of sleep and wakefulness [50, 51]. In addition, possible involvement of the glutamatergic and GABAergic neuron groups in the brainstem adds new aspects to regulatory mechanisms of REM [52–54]. So to speak, more light has been shed on glutamatergic neurons in sublaterodorsal nucleus (SLD) in rats (peri-LCα in cats) as an essential physiological substrate of regulatory mechanism of REM [5, 52, 54]. As the recent glutamatergic-GABAergic stories are mainly based on the *c-fos* studies, Sakai's studies [5] provide a part of their evidence in terms of neuronal activities [52, 54]. Nevertheless, they have not yet reached a unified story. There are some discrepancies in involvement of forebrain structure in REM regulation and possible contribution of GABAergic inputs toward formation of REM-off activities [5, 52, 54]. Mathematical models could contribute to providing an integrative view to neural regulatory mechanism of sleep-wake rhythm.

Flip-Flop Models of Sleep Regulatory Mechanism

Thus recently accumulated knowledge has prompted sleep researchers to update the prey-predator framework of REM-NREM regulation so that it involves GABAergic systems [55–57]. For the switching mechanisms between wakefulness and sleep as well as NREM and REM, conceptual "double flip-flop" models have recently been proposed [50, 58–60],

Fig. 57.2 Double flip-flop
regime underlying regulation
of sleep-wake states. Mutual
interactions between them
are likely

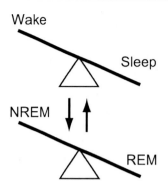

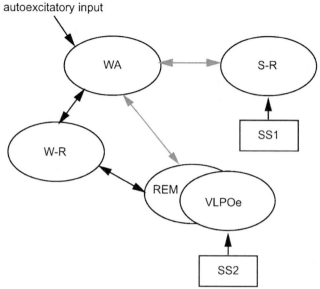

Fig. 57.3 Reduced minimal configuration of the network model of regulatory mechanism of sleep-wake states, which is composed of neuron
groups, WA, S-R, REM, VLPOe, and W-R under the control of sleep-
promoting substances, SS1 and SS2 [61]. Definition of each neuron
group is described in the text. *Black* and *gray arrows* indicate excitatory
and inhibitory effects, respectively. Note that the model is constructed
roughly by the mutual inhibitions between the neural groups and the
auto-excitation in each group

where the flip-flop is a metaphor of mechanism that each of
possible two states is alternatively activated (Fig. 57.2).

Although its implementations are different from each
other, the flip-flop concept is shared in the recently proposed
models [19–22]. Tamakawa et al. proposed one of starting
mathematical models based on the recent findings of VLPO
and orexinergic neurons, which has been updated so far
[19, 22, 61]. Their current model consists of quartet neuron groups: (1) sleep-active preoptic/anterior hypothalamic
neurons (S-R group); (2) wake-active hypothalamic and
brainstem neurons exhibiting the highest rate of discharge
during wakefulness and the lowest rate of discharge during
paradoxical sleep or REM (WA group); (3) brainstem and
extended VLPO (VLPOe) neurons exhibiting the highest
rate of discharge during REM (REM group); and (4) basal
forebrain, hypothalamic, and brainstem neurons exhibiting a higher rate of discharge during both wakefulness and
REM than during NREM (W-R group). This model can be
regarded as a "multi-flip-flop" model in which a flip occurs
by accumulation and dissipation of two kinds of sleep-promoting substances, SS1 and SS2: SS1 is accumulated during
wakefulness, activates S-R neurons, and is dissipated during
sleep. SS2 is accumulated during wakefulness and NREM,
activates VLPOe neurons and is dissipated during REM. The
reduced minimal configuration of their model is shown in
Fig. 57.3. One of novel features of their model is involvement of cholinergic W-R neuron group, which is assumed
to contribute toward induction of wakefulness as well as
REM by selectively mediating autocatalytic activation with
the WA or REM neurons. Through activity of this neuron
group, the wakefulness-sleep flip-flop and the REM-NREM
flip-flop interact with each other in the model. The model
successfully reproduces the normal sleep-wake patterns and
those under pathological states [22, 61]. In addition, Phillips and Robinson implemented a flip-flop between arousal
system and sleep-promoting system, which consists of the
reciprocal interaction between monoaminergic and cholinergic neuron groups involving the mutual inhibition with
VLPO neurons [21]. Their model provides a framework
accommodating sophisticated dynamical analysis of sleep-
wake rhythm and its pathological state such as narcolepsy.

The flip-flop mechanism is further investigated by simulating neurophysiological effects exerted by microinjections on
sleep-wake rhythms [20], where the model is constructed by
referring to the recent knowledge including VLPO sleep promoting GABAergic neurons, brainstem arousal monoaminergic neurons, and brainstem cholinergic REM-on neurons.

How a Flip-Flop Cycle?

Essential structure of bistable system, i.e., flip-flop, consists of two elements which have auto-excitatory/external
activations and mutually suppressive interactions as shown
in Fig. 57.4. Analogous structure can be found in the neural network models explained in the preceding section. In
addition, for switching between the alternative states, there
should be a system unstabilizing each state. A neural flip-
flop seems to be a sufficient regime underlying regulations
of sleep-wake states and NREM-REM ultradian rhythm.
However, switching intervals up to minutes or longer is too
long for the dynamics of neural interaction. Slower unstabilizing mechanisms are expected to exist. In the conceptual
models, plausible mechanisms underlying state-switching
with longer time scales are not concerned [59]. In most of the
mathematical models based on flip-flop mechanisms, accumulation and dissipation of somnogens are assumed to be an

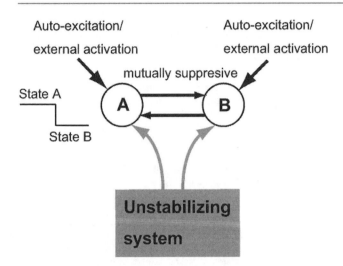

Fig. 57.4 Essential structure of bistable (flip-flop) system incorporated with unstabilizing system for cyclic state alternations

unstabilizer [19–20], although the somnogens under concern are still hypothetical ones. Actually, molecular processes involving some genes and signaling could work as an unstabilizing mechanism (e.g., McCarley and Massaquoi mentioned to intracellular signals of cyclic AMP and cyclic GMP [47]). Possible neurochemical and molecular unstabilizing systems remain unidentified, which will be an essential future target for sleep physiology and modeling.

Concluding Remarks

A recent objective of modeling sleep-wake rhythm is to predict alertness and cognitive performance rather than focusing on the behavior of circadian rhythms. Although these models have provided a close fit to the time courses of alertness and cognitive performance observed experimentally, still to be modeled are the age-dependence and/or the pathological alternation of the phase relationships between the sleep-wake and the temperature rhythms, and between the temperature rhythm and the clock time [44]. On the other hand, a detail model is required to link the findings at molecular as well as neural level to disorders of sleep-wake rhythm. Mathematical models will continue to play key roles in the study and conceptualization from molecular to behavioral levels of sleep-wake regulations.

Acknowledgments This work is supported in part by Ministry of Education, Science, Sports, and Culture, Grant-in-Aid for Scientific Research (C) 24500368, for Young Scientists (B) 23700464, and for Scientific Research on Innovative Areas.

References

1. Wever RA. The circadian system of man. Results of experiments under temporal isolation. New York: Springer; 1979.
2. Kronauer RE, Czeisler CA, Pilato SF, Moore-Ede MC, Weitzman ED. Mathematical model of the human circadian system with two interacting oscillators. Am J Physiol. 1982;242:R3–17.
3. Daan S, Beersma DG, Borbély AA. Timing of human sleep: recovery process gated by a circadian pacemaker. Am J Physiol. 1984;246:R161–78.
4. McCarley RW, Hobson JA. Neuronal excitability modulation over the sleep cycle: a structural and mathematical model. Science. 1975;189:58–60.
5. Sakai K, Crochet S. A neural mechanism of sleep and wakefulness. Sleep Biol Rhythms. 2003;1:29–42.
6. Pace-Schott EF, Hobson JA. The neurobiology of sleep: genetics, cellular physiology and subcortical networks. Nature Rev Neurosci. 2002;3:591–605.
7. Lin L, Faraco J, Li R, Kadotani H, Rogers W, Lin X, Qiu X, de Jong PJ, Nishino S, Mignot E. The sleep disorder canine narcolepsy is caused by a mutation in the hypocretin (orexin) receptor 2 gene. Cell. 1999;98:365–76.
8. Sherin JE, Shiromani PJ, McCarley RW, Saper CB. Activation of ventrolateral preoptic neurons during sleep. Science. 1996;271:216–9.
9. Lu J, Bjorkum AA, Xu M, Gaus SE, Shiromani PJ, Saper CB. Selective activation of the extended ventrolateral preoptic nucleus during rapid eye movement sleep. J Neurosci. 2002;22:4568–76.
10. Borbély AA. A two process model of sleep regulation. Hum Neurobiol. 1982;1:195–204.
11. Jewett ME, Kronauer RE. Interactive mathematical models of subjective alertness and cognitive throughput in humans. J Biol Rhythms. 1999;14:588–97.
12. Kronauer RE, Jewett ME, Dijk D-J, Czeisler CA. A model for reduced circadian modulation of alertness at extremes of homeostatic influence. J Sleep Res. 1996;5(Suppl. 1):113.
13. Achermann P, Borbély AA. Simulation of human sleep: Ultradian dynamics of electroencephalographic slow-wave activity. J Biol Rhythms. 1990;5:141–57.
14. Achermann P, Borbély AA. Simulation of daytime vigilance by additive interaction of a homeostatic and a circadian process. Biol Cybern. 1994;71:115–21.
15. Strogatz SH. Human sleep and circadian rhythms: a simple model based on two coupled oscillators. J Math Biol. 1987;25:327–47.
16. Nakao M, Yamamoto K, Katayama N, Yamamoto M. A phase dynamics model of human circadian rhythms. J Biol Rhythms. 2002;17:476–89.
17. Nakao M, Yamamoto K, Honma K, Hashimoto S, Honma S, Katayama N, Yamamoto M. Modeling interactions between photic and nonphotic entrainment mechanisms in transmeridian flights. Biol Cybern. 2004;91:138–47.
18. Kawato M, Fujita K, Suzuki R, Winfree AT. A three oscillator model of the human circadian system controlling the core temperature rhythm and the sleep-wake cycle. J Theor Biol. 1982;98:369–92.
19. Tamakawa Y, Karashima A, Koyama Y, Katayama N, Nakao M. A quartet neural system model orchestrating sleep and wakefulness mechanisms. J Neurophysiol. 2006;95:2055–69.
20. Diniz Behn CD, Booth V. Simulating microinjection experiments in a novel model of the rat sleep-wake regulatory network. J Neurophysiol. 2010;103:1937–53.
21. Phillips AJK, Robinson PA. A quantitative model of sleep-wake dynamics based on the physiology of the brainstem ascending arousal system. J Biol Rhythms. 2007;22:167–79.

22. Karashima A, Tamakawa Y, Koyama Y, Katayama N, Nakao M. Neural modeling for cooperative/competitive regulation of REM sleep with NREM sleep and wakefulness. In: Mallick BN, Pandi-Perumal SR, McCarley RW, editors. REM sleep: regulation and function. Cambridge: Cambridge University Press; 2011. pp. 437–49.

23. Borbély AA, Achermann P. Sleep homeostasis and models of sleep regulation. J Biol Rhythms. 1999;14:557–68.

24. McGinty D, Szymusiak R. Keeping cool: a hypothesis about the mechanisms and functions of slow-wave sleep. Trends Neurosci. 1990;13:480–7.

25. Nakao M, McGinty D, Szymusiak R, Yamamoto M. A thermoregulatory model of sleep control. Jpn J Physiol. 1995;45:291–309.

26. Nakao M, McGinty D, Szymusiak R, Yamamoto M. Thermoregulatory model of sleep control: losing the heat memory. J Biol Rhythms. 1999;14:547–56.

27. Nakao M, Nishiyama H, McGinty D, Szymusiak R, Yamamoto M. A model-based interpretation of the biphasic daily pattern of sleepiness. Biol Cybern. 1999;81:403–14.

28. Åkerstedt T, Folkard S. The three-process model of alertness and its extension to performance, sleep latency, and sleep length. Chronobiol Int. 1997;14:115–23.

29. Åkerstedt T, Folkard S. Validation of the S and C components of the three-process model of alertness regulation. Sleep. 1995;18:1–6.

30. Dijk D, Duffy JF, Czeisler CA. Circadian and sleep/wake dependent aspects of subjective alertness and cognitive performance. J Sleep Res. 1992;1:112–17.

31. Dijk D, Czeisler CA. Contribution of the circadian pacemaker and the sleep homeostat to sleep propensity, sleep structure, electroencephalographic slow waves, and sleep spindle activity in humans. J Neurosci. 1995;15:3526–38.

32. Dijk D, Jewett ME, Czeisler CA, Kronauer RE. Nonlinear interactions between circadian and homeostatic processes: models or metrics? Reply to Achermann. J Biol Rhythms. 1999;14:602–3.

33. Achermann P, Borbély AA. Combining various models of sleep regulation. J Sleep Res. 1992;1:144–7.

34. Achermann P. The two process model of sleep regulation revisited. Aviat Space Environ Med. 2004;75:A37–43.

35. Nakao M, Sakai H, Yamamoto M. An interpretation of the internal desynchronizations based on dynamics of the two process model. Methods Inform Med. 1997;36:282–5.

36. Nakao M, Yamamoto M. Bifurcation properties of the two process model. Psych Clin Neurosci. 1998;52:131–3.

37. Nakao M, Karashima A, Katayama N. Mathematical models of regulatory mechanisms of sleep-wake rhythms. Cell Mol Life Sci. 2007;64:1236–43.

38. Zulley J, Wever R, Aschoff J. The dependence of onset and duration of sleep on the circadian rhythm of rectal temperature. Pflüger Arch. 1981;391:314–8.

39. Moore-Ede MC, Czeisler CA, editors. Mathematical models of the circadian sleep-wake cycle. New York: Raven Press; 1984.

40. Hashimoto S, Nakamura K, Miyazaki T, Honma S, Honma K. Nonphotic entrainment of human rest-activity rhythm independently of the circadian pacemaker. Sleep Biol Rhythms. 2004;2:29–36.

41. Carrier J, Monk TH, Buysse DJ, Kupfer DJ. Amplitude reduction of the circadian temperature and sleep rhythms in the elderly. Chronobiol Int. 1996;13:373–86.

42. Nakamura K, Hashimoto S, Honma S, Honma K, Tagawa Y. A sighted man with non-24-hour sleep-wake syndrome shows damped plasma melatonin rhythm. Psych Clin Neurosci. 1997;51:115–9.

43. Souetre E, Salvati E, Belugou JL, Pringuey D, Candito M, Krebs B, Ardisson JL, Darcourt G. Circadian rhythms in depression and recovery: evidence for blunted amplitude as the main chronobiological abnormality. Psych Res. 1989;28:263–78.

44. Dijk D-J, Lockley SW. Integration of human sleep-wake regulation and circadian rhythmicity. J Appl Physiol. 2002;92:852–62.

45. Nakao M, Yamamoto K, Honma K, Hashimoto S, Honma S, Katayama N, Yamamoto M. Modeling photic and nonphotic entrainment mechanisms in human circadian system. In: Columbus F, editor. Trends in chronobiology research. New York: Nova Science Publishers; 2005. pp. 157–212.

46. Ishiura D, Karashima A, Katayama N, Nakao M. Integrated model incorporating circadian phase dynamics and the thermoregulatory mechanism of sleep. Sleep Biol Rhythms. 2007;5:259–70.

47. McCarley RW, Massaquoi SG. A limit cycle mathematical model of the REM sleep oscillator system. Am J Physiol. 1986;251:1011–29.

48. Massaquoi SG, McCarley RW. Extension of the limit cycle reciprocal interaction model of REM cycle control. An integrated sleep control model. J Sleep Res. 1992;1:138–43.

49. Suntsova N, Szymusiak R, Alam MN, Guzman-Marin R, McGinty D. Sleep-waking discharge patterns of median preoptic nucleus neurons in rats. J Physiol. 2002;543:665–77.

50. Saper CB, Chou TC, Scammell TE. The sleep switch: hypothalamic control of sleep and wakefulness. Trends Neurosci. 2001;24:726–31.

51. McGinty D, Szymusiak R. Hypothalamic regulation of sleep and arousal. Frontiers Biosci. 2003;8:1074–83.

52. Fuller PM, Saper CB, Lu J. The pontine REM switch: past and present. J Physiol. 2007;584:735–41.

53. Gvilia I, Turner A, McGinty D, Szymusiak R. Preoptic area neurons and the homeostatic regulation of rapid eye movement sleep. J Neurosci. 2006;26:3037–44.

54. Luppi P-H, Gervasoni D, Verret L, Goutagny R, Peyron C, Salvert D, Leger L, Fort P. Paradoxical (REM) sleep genesis: the switch from an aminergic–cholinergic to a GABAergic–glutamatergic hypothesis. J Physiol Paris. 2007;100:271–83.

55. McCarley RW, Greene RW, Rainnie DG, Portas CM. Brainstem neuromodulation and REM sleep. Neuroscience. 1995;7:341–54.

56. Pal D, Mallick BN. Role of Noradrenergic and GABA-ergic inputs in pedunculopontine tegmentum for regulation of rapid eye movement sleep in rats. Neuropharmacology. 2006;51:1–11.

57. McCarley RW. Neurobiology of REM and NREM sleep. Sleep Med. 2007;8:302–30.

58. McGinty D, Szymusiak R. The sleep-wake switch: a neuronal alarm clock. Nat Med. 2000;6:510–1.

59. Lu J, Sherman D, Devor M, Saper CB. A putative flip-flop switch for control of REM sleep. Nature. 2006;441:589–94.

60. Saper CB, Fuller PM, Pedersen NP, Lu J, Scammell TE. Sleep state switching. Neuron. 2010;68:1023–42.

61. Nakao M. From flip-flop to cycles: neural regulation mechanism of sleep-wake states. World sleep 2011; 2011. pp. ES-3–4.

Arthur J. Spielman and Paul B. Glovinsky

The theoretical and clinical foundations of the nonpharmacological treatment of insomnia were for the most part laid down a generation ago, making this an opportune moment to recap the history of the field while still benefitting from the personal recollections of early participants in its growth.[1] The treatment of insomnia is rendered problematic not only by the subjective nature of the disorder but also by the complex interactions between diverse factors that produce chronic sleeplessness. In the eight decades since progressive muscle relaxation (PMR) first targeted insomnia's somatic inputs, cadres of researchers and clinicians have approached the task of treating it a bit like the blind men treat their elephant, each finding a distinctive feature on which to obtain a grasp.

In the 1960s, research began on arousal mechanisms underlying insomnia, a line of work that continues to prove fruitful. The sleep stages were codified, and efforts made to understand good and poor sleep using a shared guide to its polysomnographic features. The 1970s brought work on the psychopathological correlates of chronic insomnia, compilation of everyday behaviors, and practices that improve sleep under the rubric of "sleep hygiene," the parsing of insomnia subtypes in the first official sleep nosology and understanding of insomnia as the consequence of maladaptive conditioning. This latter effort led to the first nonpharmacological treatment expressly formulated for insomnia, now known as stimulus control therapy. The 1980s introduced the insomnia community to the critical role that the circadian regulation of sleep plays in their field. This demonstration of the importance of a factor *intrinsic* to sleep (akin to and taken together with the then well-known homeostatic enhancement of subsequent sleep following sleep loss) sparked the development of sleep restriction therapy.

The 1990s saw the incorporation of general cognitive principles into a systematic and focused treatment for insomnia. This work was quickly joined with behavioral approaches to form cognitive behavioral treatment for insomnia (CBT-I), which assumed first-line status among nonpharmacological treatments for the disorder. By the turn of the century, the effectiveness of CBT-I was evidenced in a wide range of populations, and was gaining increasing recognition among the primary-care providers who treat the vast majority of patients with insomnia. Current initiatives include extending the delivery of CBT-I beyond traditional clinical settings, for example, using web-based models or therapists drawn from outside the sleep community. Entirely new treatments have also been developed. The field of behavioral sleep medicine has grown vibrant, with recognized textbooks, a journal, an annual conference, and a certifying examination.

There is a general convention among historians that reliable history cannot be written on the heels of events. Various degrees of restraint are recommended; for major upheavals, these boil down to the prescription that major protagonists should have passed on. While no one is suggesting that advances in the CBT-I have been cataclysmic, still some might wonder if a sufficient interval has transpired to gain the perspective necessary to write their history. What's the rush, they might ask?

We would reply that it is not so much of a rush. Thirty to forty years have passed since many of the works we will be discussing here were first published. While this thankfully remains too short a spell to satisfy the dictum mentioned above, it does confer some urgency on a particular task: writing a history that is informed by personal accounts of

---

[1] We mourn the passing of our esteemed colleague and teacher Peter Hauri in the interval between the writing of this paper and its publication, but at the same time take solace in the fact that we were able to benefit from his wisdom and generosity almost to the last.

A. J. Spielman (✉) · P. B. Glovinsky
Department of Psychology, The City College of the City University of New York, New York, NY, USA
e-mail: artspielman@gmail.com

Center for Sleep Medicine, Weill Cornell Medical College, Cornel University, New York, NY, USA

P. B. Glovinsky
St. Peter's Sleep Center, Albany, NY, USA

S. Chokroverty, M. Billiard (eds.), *Sleep Medicine,* DOI 10.1007/978-1-4939-2089-1_58,
© Springer Science+Business Media, LLC 2015

the major developments that spurred growth in our field. For with the exception of PMR, the components of CBT-I are still represented by their originators, evaluators, disseminators, and early practitioners. We therefore surveyed a number of our colleagues with the aim of obtaining their first-hand perspectives on key developments and early controversies, as well as other contributions that might enliven this brief account.

We thus acknowledge that without the gracious contributions of Richard Bootzin, Colin Espie, Peter Hauri, Charles Morin, Michael Perlis, Howard Roffwarg, and Tom Roth, including useful citations and helpful comments beyond their personal reminiscences, we would have had very little chance of meeting even our limited objectives for this chapter. Finally, we apologize to the many deserving researchers and clinicians whose important contributions could not be included in this brief survey due to space limitations.

We also must state at the outset that we do not present here a comprehensive survey of insomnia treatments. We will leave it to those who played a central role in the development of hypnotic medications to tell that fascinating story. Similarly, the particular challenges faced by pediatric behavioral sleep specialists as they worked with both children and parents to devise effective interventions deserve an insider's account.

Challenges in Defining Insomnia

The complaint of unsatisfactory sleep and consequent daytime impairment compose the essential features of insomnia from the patient's perspective. The advent of objective electrophysiological recording of sleep and the definition of sleep stages in 1968 have added surprisingly little to these defining characteristics over the years. According to one theorist, this state of affairs is also not surprising—given that the precise function of sleep is unknown, "How can we say when we have had enough of it?" [1]. Furthermore, the electrophysiological, brain imaging, or quantitative electroencephalogram (EEG) correlates of insomnia may reflect the mechanisms of the sleep disturbance, the consequences of insomnia, or the compensatory response to insomnia (adapted from [2]). Just as the sleep disturbance in insomnia in the end remains a subjective assessment, its associated daytime complaints, such as fatigue, lack of interest, or performance deficits, are also susceptible to subjective interpretation. A hypochondriac, for example, may well exaggerate minor sleep disturbance, whereas a hearty individual's vital engagement with life could minimize the effects of significant sleep loss. These unresolved issues along with other conceptual problems have contributed to changes in the definition of insomnia (see below).

Progress in understanding insomnia from an objective basis has likely been limited because polysomnography (PSG) is not a regular component of the workup in sleep disorders centers. Both insurance reimbursement issues and the decision in 2000 by the Practice Parameter Committee of the American Academy of Sleep Medicine (AASM) to recommend that PSG not be part of the routine assessment of chronic insomnia has limited the potential contribution of objective recording to this common health problem (for an example of the contribution of PSG to insomnia, see [3, 4]).

Given the difficulties of defining insomnia beyond the simple subjective notions stated above, we have opted for an indirect approach—gaining understanding of this elusive malady by reviewing efforts to treat it: Specifically, we review historical developments in the nonpharmacological treatments of insomnia. This viewpoint highlights historical changes in the conceptual understanding of insomnia, along with changing rationales for emerging therapies and shifts in nosological schemes.

First-Generation Approaches to Insomnia

PMR [5] can fairly be taken as the start of the modern era of nondrug approaches to insomnia. PMR was expressly intended as a treatment for stress-related problems including insomnia and continues to be used as such. In addition, PMR spawned a range of self-management techniques to address insomnia, including biofeedback (muscle, body temperature, sensory-motor rhythm, heart rate), patterned breathing, and autogenic training. While many studies have demonstrated the effectiveness of relaxation for insomnia (e.g., [6]), in at least one [7], this effectiveness was not apparent, while in others, self-report measures [8] showed a greater degree of change compared to EEG measures [9]. Relaxation continues to be included in multicomponent interventions of demonstrated effectiveness (for a review, see [10]).

In the 1960s, much of the systematic research on arousal mechanisms producing insomnia, such as the effects of presleep activities and the physiological differences between good and poor sleepers, was guided by Rechtschaffen and his students [11, 12] . Physiological hyperarousal in insomnia patients has been (e.g., [13]) and continues to be (see [14]) a prominent etiological mechanism.

In investigating the psychological character structure typical of individuals with insomnia, Kales and colleagues theorized that a relatively small set of neurotic character styles was responsible for the disorder [15]. A series of studies (first major study was [16]) found that the majority of insomnia sufferers exhibit a concurrence of elevated Minnesota Multiphasic Personality Inventory (MMPI) profiles (Hy, D, Pt, and Hs) that indicate the presence of hysteria, depression, obsessional anxiety, fatigue, and hypochondriasis [17]. On the basis of these test profiles, it was concluded that insomnia resulted from arousal secondary to the internalization of psychological conflict. Considerable empirical evidence demonstrated a high prevalence of this typology in insomnia. In addition, these investigators emphasized the clinical observation that worrying about sleeplessness contributes to the exacerbation of sleep problems, i.e., that insomnia can be the result of a self-fulfilling prophecy. This observation was *une forme fruste* of an aspect of the cognitive theory of insomnia that has blossomed in recent years (see below).

Nearly contemporaneous with Kales' psychopathological conception of the origins of insomnia was Bootzin's view that insomnia is a product of maladaptive conditioning, and that just a few instructions to correct this conditioning are sufficient for effective treatment. Stimulus control instructions (now called stimulus control therapy; SCT, [18]) was the first nondrug treatment specifically designed to treat insomnia. Bootzin did not embrace the psychopathological conceptualization of Kales and colleagues, which was the dominant understanding of insomnia at the time. Rather, his approach viewed insomnia squarely from a behavioral perspective, as resulting from the repeated pairing of (a) the experience of insomnia—agitated tossing and turning, worrying, and sleeplessness—with (b) bedroom cues including the bed.

SCT comprises the following:

1. Use the bed only for sleep and sex. Do not get into bed until you are ready for sleep.
2. If you are not asleep within about 20 min, get out of bed.
3. Return to bed when sleepy (or ready to go to sleep).
4. Repeat steps 2 and 3 if necessary.
5. Get up and out of bed the same time every day.
6. Do not nap.

Permission for sex in bed was a later addition to the SCT instructions, perhaps prompted by feedback, whether of restraint or inventiveness, from those who would follow the original directions to the letter.

SCT is rated as a standard of care as both a stand-alone treatment and a component of CBT in the AASM's practice parameters and clinical guidelines for the management of insomnia [19, 20]. SCT is now always a component of CBT-I (see below). SCT recently inspired a new treatment called intensive sleep retraining ([21, 22]; for a commentary, see [23]). Harris and colleagues have shown that chronic insomnia can be effectively addressed and treatment gains maintained with just a single 25-h treatment, using a behavioral scheme based on learning theory along with the aid of sleep laboratory technology.

After SCT was introduced, an influential monograph on sleep disorders by Hauri included the claim that good sleep was promoted with good "sleep hygiene" [24]. As Hauri has pointed out, recommendations with face validity that would later be called sleep hygiene have been with us for quite a long time. We can recall Hauri's refrain each time a colleague asked for a name change to something less tinged with a moralistic tone: "Make a suggestion and we'll change it!" No new name has emerged to denote sleep hygiene.

The list of what constitutes good sleep hygiene practice has not undergone rigorous development, but is rather a free-form compilation of dos and don'ts based on evidence, anecdote, and theory. It has changed over the years but in general prescribes some behaviors and practices, such as going to bed and getting out of bed the same time every day and keeping the room dark and quiet, while proscribing others, such as excessive napping, looking at the clock during the night, consuming caffeine after noon, or exercising close to bedtime.

Research studies have not demonstrated reliable and robust effectiveness of sleep hygiene as a treatment for insomnia [25]. However, one can trace the origins of multicomponent treatments as in CBT-I to sleep hygiene. The list reminds insomnia sufferers that it may be necessary to change a number of behaviors concurrently to address sleep disturbance, and that changes are required across diverse aspects of our experience, both by day and by night. In addition, good sleep hygiene can be seen as a preparatory phase that is useful in eliminating or limiting egregious practices (for example, napping before bedtime) that could undermine the effectiveness of insomnia therapy of any kind.

In addition to focusing on practices and habits that contribute to insomnia, Hauri and colleagues conducted a series of studies showing that different types of biofeedback were effective for its treatment. In one of these studies, assessment of certain patient characteristics predicted whether a particular intervention would be effective [26]. Although the current state of the art does not focus on the proper matching of treatment intervention to patient for good outcomes, Hauri's early search for such a match was laudable, and is in keeping with multifactorial models of insomnia genesis.

The publication [27] of the first stand-alone sleep disorders nosology, under the guidance of Roffwarg for the now distant forebear of the present AASM, was a major step in the development in the field. While the delineation of eight distinct insomnia disorders remains controversial, there is no doubt that some of the insomnia presentations emerging from obscurity received their rightful attention.

Psychophysiological insomnia, for example, became the first insomnia entity that was not defined as "associated with" other conditions and situations. Psychophysiological insomnia was seen as a sleep disturbance that was *learned*. It was the unfortunate result of *normal* psychological and physiological processes, such as the ability of arousal to be heightened or of worry to be somatized. Prior to this, most clinicians understood insomnia to be a symptom of underlying psychiatric and medical disorders or a reaction to painful or stressful conditions. The refrain that echoed constantly in their training was "insomnia is a symptom, not a disorder." The groundbreaking notion that insomnia could be "primary," that is, not necessarily due to another disorder, was formally restated in the Diagnostic and Statistical Manual (DSM) IV [28].

As clinical psychologists, the authors well remember being taught to search for the psychopathology that must somewhere be underlying insomnia complaints. (Such a search is still useful today even if just to rule out psychopathology, since sleep-related complaints of course figure prominently in the clinical description of a number of mood and anxiety disorders.) In trying to win our patients' cooperation in this search, we often resorted to the medical model. We might offer the analogy for example that, just as complaints of breathing difficulty could signal underlying disease of various sorts and prompt a wide-ranging workup prior to treatment, disturbed sleep might reflect psychological issues that would have to be uncovered and addressed to optimize treatment.

The advent of psychophysiological insomnia as a diagnosis prompted clinicians to reset their expectations to appreciate that some individuals with insomnia may be somewhat "wound up" or sad but not clinically anxious or depressed. In fact, they might be beset by worries no bigger than how the night's sleep would go. This new conceptualization of insomnia also challenged clinicians and theoreticians to focus attention on a more diverse set of factors contributing to insomnia, such as physiological and cognitive hyperarousal, maladaptive habits and practices, and learning mechanisms. No longer would psychopathology conveniently serve as the default cause of insomnia.

While this reconceptualization of insomnia eventually proved a watershed, the change was not without turbulence. The dominant view, as agreed upon at the first Consensus Development Conference of the National Institutes of Health (NIH) [29], remained that insomnia was often secondary to psychiatric and medical conditions, as suggested by the following:

> The first obligation of the practitioner is to search for a specific psychiatric or medical disease as the underlying cause. [29]

Resolution of the underlying psychiatric and medical causes of the insomnia continued to be the recommended approach, which promised an optimistic prognosis:

> Treatment should be directed toward the medical or psychiatric condition and, if treatment is successful, the insomnia ordinarily responds concomitantly. [29]

It would be 22 years before this view was changed at a succeeding NIH conference [30]. The recently published DSM V in 2013 uses the new term "insomnia disorder" to replace both "primary insomnia and insomnia(s) associated with...." It is the latest step in this conceptual evolution.

Another diagnosis that appeared for the first time in the 1979 nosology, pseudo-insomnia, pertained to individuals complaining of sleep problems who nevertheless had no sleep disturbance when studied in the laboratory. Hauri (personal communication) recalls heated controversy concerning the inclusion of this diagnosis in the nosology. One charter member of the field argued that pseudo-insomnia was clearly not an authentic disturbance of sleep and therefore should not be included. This prompted another to counter that perhaps obsessive-compulsive disturbance should not be classified as a disorder either, since that problem also had no demonstrable physiological substrate. This type of disagreement is of course to be expected when a new field is trying to establish its legitimacy. Many studies have subsequently demonstrated that, compared to good sleepers, sufferers of insomnia in general (not only those whose complaints form the basis of a pseudo-insomnia diagnosis) show a greater discrepancy between subjective and objective measures of their sleep.

The disputatious legacy of pseudo-insomnia can be traced through discussions of sleep state misperception and, most recently, paradoxical insomnia. The diagnosis of sleep state misperception was explicitly based on demonstration of an exaggerated discrepancy between subjective estimates of sleep with objective PSG findings, with the PSG considered the gold standard. Dissenters from this view noted that the existence of sleep state misperception could just as well be taken as evidence of the inadequacy of the PSG with regard to capturing the varieties of subjective sleep experience. Brain imaging and animal studies have been added to this longstanding controversy. Nofzinger and colleagues have demonstrated that insomniacs have heightened neuronal activation, relative to good sleepers, in brain areas subserving arousal and emotion during EEG-scored sleep [31]. Cano and colleagues have developed an animal model of insomnia and shown concurrent activation of both sleep and arousal centers ([32], see also [33] for a relevant model).

Rapid advances in understanding the circadian regulation of sleep and its disorders in humans had a number of ramifications for thinking about insomnia. Czeisler, Weitzman, and colleagues' papers on delayed sleep phase syndrome (DSPS) carved out a new entity that presented as sleep-onset insomnia but was newly conceived of as a biological rhythm disorder [34, 35]. Clinicians were made aware of entirely new factors to consider, such as the endogenous period length of a biological rhythm, the phase response of that rhythm to external stimuli, and the timing, duration, and, more recently, hue of light exposure as influences on sleep.

A typology of morningness and eveningness, so-called larks and owls [36], was constructed, suggesting that endogenous clock mechanisms could predispose some individuals to sleep onset problems and others to early-morning awakenings. Taking into account such contributions from chronobiology, clinicians no longer would reflexively diagnose early-morning awakening insomnia as a depressive symptom, for example. They began to give consideration to the timing of the endogenous circadian phase (in this case, an advance) as a possible cause of early awakenings. Chronotherapy, a purely behavioral approach, was devised as a treatment for DSPS [34, 35]. Timed exposure to light as a treatment for circadian rhythm sleep disorders (most notably DSPS) in addition to seasonal affective disorder was established. While preliminary work has shown some promise, more research is needed to determine how useful bright light treatment will be in the management of cases of sleeplessness that do not primarily reflect a circadian rhythm disorder.

The early clinical practice of one of the authors (AJS), together with experience gained in the effort to formulate new treatments, led to a greater appreciation of the chronic nature of insomnia and especially how the disorder often grew over time to become "functionally autonomous from its origins" [37]. In particular, it was observed that initial conditions and events that had apparently triggered an ongoing, raging insomnia were often long past and seemingly of marginal significance by the time of clinical presentation. Furthermore, it was noted that significant improvements in sleep could often be obtained with behavioral adjustments that did not take into account the etiology of the condition.

Motivated to highlight behaviors and thoughts that were currently active and amenable to modification, we developed a conceptualization that, while acknowledging vulnerability to insomnia (predisposing factors) and salient triggers of insomnia (precipitating factors), focused attention on what maintained the insomnia (perpetuating factors). What became the 3P model was originally described in an early report [37]. Fleshed out with a graphic depiction [38], it became a leading model and oft-employed heuristic for our field (Fig. 58.1).

The 3P model's appeal may have been due to its offering a theoretical footing for all stakeholders. The model does not propose particular mechanisms responsible for insomnia but rather assigns processes to different stages in the development of insomnia. Clinicians who see insomnia developing out of vulnerability to stress, psychopathological predilection, or based on physiological hyperarousal can locate the early origins of insomnia within the predisposing factors. Others who see the salience of triggering factors, such as illness, psychopathology, or acute worry, will emphasize their importance as precipitating factors. Yet others who focus on conditioning, sleep habits, practices of daily living, and maladaptive thinking may view these processes as either precipitating or perpetuating factors. The 3P model results in a historical narrative of determinants that offer an explanatory model as well as directs intervention strategies.

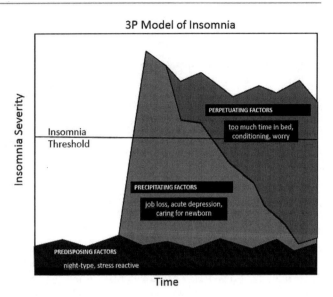

Fig. 58.1 3P Model of Insomnia

A number of threads led to the development of sleep restriction therapy (SRT) ([38, 39], see also [40]. In no small part, SRT was based on the documented and near-universal experience of sleep loss producing a compensatory enhancement of subsequent sleep. In addition, by inducing patients to fall asleep quickly from the start of the treatment, SRT aimed to break the vicious cycle of anticipatory anxiety of sleeplessness leading to actual sleeplessness leading to even more anticipatory anxiety that perpetuates insomnia.

At the time SRT was developed, three behavioral approaches to trouble sleeping were models for the success of nondrug treatments. Bootzin and Hauri's treatments (see above) were widely applied. These treatments issued from solid rationales (conditioning and principles of sleep regulation, respectively) and provided encouragement that innovative behavioral methods could be useful. Furthermore, one of us (AJS) had participated in the first treatment trial of chronotherapy [35] and was chastened that his pet theory regarding the etiology of DSPS (schizoidal and oppositional personality structure) was clearly not a necessary requirement for rapid and effective treatment. To his mind, the success of chronotherapy prompted a radical rethinking: The historical perspective with its focus on psychopathology no longer seemed central to understanding the genesis of insomnia. Instead, focus shifted to a current behavioral analysis. This prompted both a reconceptualization of insomnia determinants (see 3P model above) and the origin of SRT.

The rules for conducting SRT are as follows:
1. Determine average time asleep from sleep diary
2. Set time in bed = time asleep

3. Set a consistent wake-up time
4. No daytime naps
5. If 5-day average sleep efficiency is equal to or greater than 90 % (85 % in > 65 year olds), then increase time in bed (15–30 min)
6. If 5-day average sleep efficiency is less than 85 % (80 % in > 65 year olds), then decrease time in bed (15–30 min)

For convenience, we now recommend determining if a change in time in bed is warranted every 7 days rather than every 5 days. Subtleties in deciding what particular time to use for the initial time in bed are discussed elsewhere (e.g., setting the "lights out," retiring time later for sleep-onset sufferers and setting the "lights on," out-of-bed time earlier for early-morning awakening sufferers [41]). Alternatives to the SRT rules have been used, for example, setting the initial time in bed to 30 min above reported sleep time; or gradually reducing time in bed from its initial duration ("sleep compression," developed in the late 1980s and 1990s, see [42]). Inherent in the process of SRT is a trade-off between sleep efficiency and total sleep time. At the extremes, high sleep efficiency comes at the price of total sleep time and conversely high total sleep time degrades sleep efficiency (see [40] for a discussion of cost–benefit ratio in SRT). The SRT method titrates time in bed over the course of 6–8 weeks to yield a new habitual time in bed. Ultimately, how the patient feels and functions must be balanced against sleep efficiency and the long-term stability of sleep when deciding on a final recommendation.

Similar to the cognitive approach to insomnia treatment (see below), SRT has had limited empirical tests as a stand-alone treatment (for a list of citations, see [40]). SRT quickly became a component of CBT-I and is now more common than relaxation (see [10, 40]) as the third part of CBT-I (joining SCT and cognitive therapy). The latest AASM practice parameter for the psychological and behavioral treatment of insomnia [19] as well as the AASM clinical guidelines for the evaluation and management of chronic insomnia [20] include SRT as part of CBT, which is rated as a standard of care. SRT as a stand-alone treatment is rated as a guideline.

Current Generation of Approaches to Insomnia

While other precursors to the cognitive theory of insomnia can be found, the insights of Aaron Beck and Albert Ellis regarding maladaptive thought processes clearly form its foundation. Cognitive principles provided the underpinning of early treatments such as paradoxical intention and self-management ([43], for a review, see [44, 45]). However, the field awaited Morin to develop a systematic, empirically based approach to insomnia treatment that drew comprehensively from the cognitive theory that had by then been flour-

ishing for nearly a generation [46]. The view that thought content and the thinking process were important in insomnia development or maintenance received no direct test as a stand-alone treatment until recently [47, 48]. The early work by Morin and colleagues [46, 49], Edinger and colleagues [50, 51, 52], and others [53, 54, 55] combined cognitive interventions with behavioral approaches in the treatment of insomnia.

The addition of cognitive approaches to insomnia treatment proved very fruitful, with distortions in thinking about sleep, cognitive hyperarousal (whether due to worrying, working, or entertainment), and catastrophizing about the effects of sleeplessness on health or daily functioning all identified as etiological agents and targets for intervention. In this new zeitgeist (spirit of the time), the perennial complaint of many patients that the only thing they were worried about was their sleep and daytime fatigue garnered new respect, and was directly addressed with strategies aiming to dampen the hyperarousal that attended such worries. The publication of a scale that identified specific erroneous beliefs often held by sufferers of insomnia [56] led to greater appreciation of the wide range of maladaptive thoughts that contribute to disturbed sleep.

The cognitive domain continued to spark new conceptualizations of the mechanisms of insomnia [57, 58, 59, 60] and a new approach which comprehensively targets the full complement of cognitive mechanisms [48]. Currently, cognitive contents and processes are as central to the understanding of insomnia as are physiological hyperarousal, stress, learning, maladaptive habits and practices, and medical and psychopathological conditions. The cognitive approach has been bundled into a multicomponent treatment known as CBT-I with demonstrable effectiveness. The components of CBT-I vary somewhat between studies. They invariably include cognitive interventions and SCT, and often include SRT or relaxation.

CBT-I has been the subject of many studies including randomized clinical treatment trials (for reviews see [10, 49, 61]) and meta-analyses [54, 60]. Its effectiveness has been explored in different insomnia populations (e.g., sleep disorders center patients, community dwellers, young and old) with various comorbidities (e.g., psychopathology, pain, cancer), with different modes of delivery (e.g., individual, group, mail, and web based), with different number of sessions, and in comparison with pharmacotherapy (see [62]).

Throughout 25 years, CBT-I has been shown to be robustly effective. As mentioned above, CBT-I has been established as a standard of care by the AASM. The most recent state of the science NIH conference concluded that CBT-I is as effective as hypnotic medications and more durable [63]. In this conference, psychological models of insomnia were no longer eclipsed by presumed medical and psychiatric causes:

Evidence supports both psychological and physiological models in the etiology of insomnia. Psychological models include the concepts of conditioning, hyperarousal, stress response, predisposing personality traits, and attitudes and beliefs about sleep. [63]

Systematic reviews [10, 61, 64, 65], NIH consensus conferences ([29], [63]), and the development of practice parameters [19, 66] and practice guidelines [20] for the assessment and treatment of insomnia helped establish nonpharmacological treatment as an effective approach recognized by physicians, psychologists, and other clinicians both within and outside the field of sleep.

A new development is the creation of web-based treatment programs for administration of CBT-I [37]. From our perspective, a number of the demonstrations were engaging, well-thought out, and presented a sophisticated approach to the application of CBT-I in an interactive program. Time will tell if the potential of online therapy is realized in empirical studies.

Insomnia Treatment Within Behavioral Sleep Medicine

The development of CBT-I, while unfolding over two generations, still woefully outpaced clinical practice. As the new millennium dawned, just hundreds of therapists had been trained in the application of these techniques, while millions of individuals suffering from insomnia continued to have few treatment options besides sleeping pills. At the same time, experimental, epidemiological, and population-based research showed that short or impaired sleep adversely affects basic physiological processes such as glucose metabolism as well as overall morbidity and mortality, strengthening the case for the health significance of good sleep.

This challenge was taken up by an array of organizational, professional, and educational initiatives broadly described as behavioral sleep medicine. We are limited here to briefly listing some of the signal achievements of this nascent movement. These include publication of the first textbook of the principles and practices of behavioral sleep medicine [68], a CBT-I manual [69], and establishment of the Journal of Behavioral Sleep Medicine under the stewardship of Lichstein.

A process of credentialing practitioners as certified in behavioral sleep medicine was developed under the auspices of the AASM by a committee of senior researchers and clinicians. This process included mandating training requirements as well as an examination. The preparation of nurse practitioners to deliver CBT-I in community settings [53] and the large-scale systematic training in CBT-I of veterans administration clinicians [70] are significant milestones in making the knowledge gained through two generations of research and practice of the behavioral treatment of insomnia finally available to the public.

References

1. Rechtschaffen A, Monroe, LJ. Laboratory studies of insomnia. p. 159. In: Kales A, editor. Sleep: physiology and pathology. Philadelphia: Lippincott; 1969. pp. 158–69.
2. Rechtschaffen A. The function of sleep: Methodological issues. In: Drucker-Colin R, Shkurovich M, Sterman MB, editors. The functions of sleep. New York: Academic; 1979. pp. 1–17.
3. Krakow B, Romero E, Ulibarri VA, Kikta S. Prospective assessment of nocturnal awakenings in a case series of treatment-seeking chronic insomnia patients: a pilot study of subjective and objective causes. Sleep. 2012;35(12):1685–92.
4. Pigeon WR, Sateia MJ. Is insomnia a breathing disorder? Sleep. 2012;35(12):1589–90.
5. Jacobson, E. You Must Relax. New York and London: Whittlesey-House; 1934.
6. Borkovec T, Fowles D. Controlled investigation of the effects of progressive and hypnotic relaxation on insomnia. J Abnorm Psychol. 1973;82(1):153–8.
7. Nicassio PM, Boylan MB, McCabe TG. Progressive relaxation, EMG biofeedback and biofeedback placebo in the treatment of sleep-onset insomnia. Br J Med Psychol. 1982;55(Pt 2):159–66.
8. Nicassio PM, Bootzin RR. A comparison of progressive relaxation and autogenic training as treatments for insomnia. J Abnorm Psychol. 1974;83(3):253–60.
9. Borkovec T, Weerts T. Effects of progressive relaxation on sleep disturbance: An electroencephalographic evaluation. Psychosomat Med. 1976;38(3):173–80.
10. Morin CM, Bootzin RR, Buysse DJ, et al. Psychological and behavioral treatment of insomnia: Update of the recent evidence (1998–2004). Sleep. 2006;29(11):1398–414.
11. Monroe LJ. Psychological and physiological differences between good and poor sleepers. J Abnorm Psychol. 1967;72(3):255–64.
12. Hauri PJ. Effect of evening activity on early night sleep. Psychophysiology. 1968;4(3):267–77.
13. Bonnet MH, Arand DL. 24-hour metabolic rate in insomniacs and matched normal sleepers. Sleep. 1995;18(7):581–8.
14. Pejovic S, Vgontzas AN. Neurobiological disturbances in insomnia: Clinical utility of objective measures of sleep. In: Sateia MJ, Buysse DJ, editors. Insomnia: diagnosis and treatment. London: Informa; 2010. pp. 65–76.
15. Kales A. and Kales, JD. Evaluation and treatment of insomnia. New York: Oxford University Press; 1984.
16. Kales A, Caldwell AB, Preston TA, Healey S, and Kales, JD. Personality patterns in insomnia. Arch Gen Psychiatry. 1976; 33: 1128–34. 70.
17. McCrae CS, Lichstein KL. Secondary insomnia: diagnostic challenges and intervention opportunities. Sleep Med Rev. 2001;5(1):47–61.
18. Bootzin RR. Stimulus control treatment for insomnia. Proc Am Psychol Assoc. 1972;7(6):395–6.
19. Morgenthaler T, Kramer M, Alessi C, et al. Practice parameters for the psychological and behavioral treatment of insomnia: an update. An American Academy of Sleep Medicine Report. Sleep. 2006;29(11):1415–9.
20. Schutte-Rodin S, Broch L, Buysse D, Dorsey C, Sateia M. Clinical guideline for the evaluation and management of chronic insomnia in adults. J Clin Sleep Med. 2008;4(5):487–504.
21. Harris J, Lack L, Wright H, Gradisar M, Brooks A. Intensive Sleep Retraining treatment for chronic primary insomnia: a preliminary investigation. J Sleep Res. 2007;16(3):276–84.
22. Harris J, Lack L, Kemp K, Wright H, Bootzin R. A randomized controlled trial of intensive sleep retraining (ISR): a brief conditioning treatment for chronic insomnia. Sleep. 2012;35(1):49–60.
23. Spielman AJ, Glovinsky PB. What a difference a day makes. Sleep. 2012;35(1):11–2.

24. Hauri PJ. The sleep disorders. Current concepts. Kalamazoo: Scope Publications, The Upjohn Co; 1977.
25. Stepanski EJ, Wyatt JK. Use of sleep hygiene in the treatment of insomnia. Sleep Med Rev. 2003;7(3):215–25.
26. Hauri PJ. Treating psychophysiologic insomnia with biofeedback. Arch Gen Psychiatry. 1981;38(7):752–8.
27. Association of Sleep Disorders Centers. Diagnostic classification of sleep and arousal disorders, prepared by the Sleep Disorders Classification Committee, Roffwarg HP, Chairman. Sleep. 1979;2(1):1–137.
28. American Psychiatric Association. Diagnostic and statistical manual of mental disorders. 4th edn. Washington, DC: American Psychiatric Association; 1994.
29. Drugs and Insomnia: The Use of Medications to Promote Sleep. NIH Consensus Statement Online; 5–17 Nov 1983;4(10):1–19.
30. Morin CM. Inventory of beliefs and attitudes about sleep: preliminary scale development. Behav Ther. 1994;17:163–4.
31. Nofzinger EA, Buysse DJ, Germain A, Price JC, Miewald JM, Kupfer DJ. Functional neuroimaging evidence for hyperarousal in insomnia. Am J Psychiatry. 2004;161(11):2126–9.
32. Cano, G, Mochizuki T, Saper C. Neural circuitry of stress-induced insomnia in rats. J Neurosci. 2008;28(40):10167–84.
33. Buysse DJ, Germain A, Hall M, Monk TH, Nofzinger EA. A neurobiological model of insomnia. Drug Discov Today Dis Models. 2011;8(4):129–37.
34. Czeisler CA, Richardson GS, Coleman RM, Zimmerman JC, Moore-Ede MC, Dement WC, Weitzman ED. Chronotherapy: resetting the circadian clocks of patients with delayed sleep phase insomnia. Sleep. 1981;4(1):1–21.
35. Weitzman ED, Czeisler CA, Coleman R, Spielman AJ, Zimmerman J, Dement WC, et al. Delayed sleep phase syndrome: a chronobiological disorder with sleep onset insomnia. Arch Gen Psychiatry. 1981;38(7):737–46.
36. Horne JA, Östberg OA. Self-assessment questionnaire to determine morningness-eveningness in human circadian rhythms. Int J Chronobiol. 1976;4(2):97–110.
37. Spielman AJ. Assessment of insomnia. Clin Psychol Rev. 1986;6:11–25.
38. Spielman, AJ, Caruso L, Glovinsky PB. A behavioral perspective on insomnia treatment. Psychiatric Clin N Am. 1987a;10(4):541–53.
39. Spielman AJ, Saskin P, Thorpy MJ. Treatment of chronic insomnia by restriction of time spent in bed. Sleep. 1987b;10(1):45–56.
40. Spielman AJ, Yang CM, Glovinsky PB. Sleep restriction therapy. In: Sateia MJ, Buysse DJ, editors. Insomnia: diagnosis and treatment. London: Informa; 2010. pp. 277–89.
41. Spielman AJ, Yang CM, Glovinsky PB. Sleep restriction therapy. In: Perlis M, Aloia M, Kuhn B, editors. Behavioral treatments for sleep disorders. Academic, Elsevier; 2011. pp. 9–19.
42. Lichstein KL, Riedel BW, Wilson NM, Lester KW, Aguillard RN. Relaxation and sleep compression for late-life insomnia: a placebo controlled trial. J Consult Clin Psychol. 2001;69(2):227–39.
43. Borkovec T. Insomnia. J Consult Clin Psychol. 1982;50:880–95.
44. Espie CA. The psychological treatment of insomnia. Chichester: Wiley; 1991.
45. Espie CA, Lindsay WR, Brooks DN, Hood EM, Turvey T. A controlled comparative investigation of psychological treatments for chronic sleep-onset insomnia. Behav Res Ther. 1989;27(1):79–88.
46. Morin CM. Insomnia; psychological assessment and management. New York: Guilford; 1993.
47. Harvey, AG. The attempted suppression of presleep cognitive activity in insomnia. Cognit Ther Res. 2003;27(6):593–602.
48. Harvey AG, Sharpley AL, Ree MJ, Stinson K, Clark DM. An open trial of cognitive therapy for chronic insomnia. Behav Res Ther. 2007;45(10):2491–501.

49. Morin CM, Colecchi C, Stone J, Sood R. Behavioral and pharmacological therapies for late-life insomnia: a randomized controlled trial. JAMA. 1999b;281(11):991–9.
50. Edinger JD, Hoelscher TJ, Marsh GR, Lipper S, Ionescue-Pioggia M. A cognitive–behavioral therapy for sleep-maintenance insomnia in older adults. Psychol Aging. 1992;7(2):282–9.
51. Edinger JD, Wohlgemuth WK, Radtke RA, Marsh GR, Quillian RE. Cognitive behavioral therapy for treatment of chronic primary insomnia: a randomized controlled trial. JAMA. 2001;285(14):1856–64.
52. Hoelscher TJ, Edinger JD. Treatment of sleep-maintenance insomnia in older adults: Sleep period reduction, sleep education, and modified stimulus control. Psychol Aging. 1988;3(3):258–63.
53. Espie CA, Inglis SJ, Tessier S, Harvey L. The clinical effectiveness of cognitive behaviour therapy for chronic insomnia: implementation and evaluation of a sleep clinic in general medical practice. Behav Res Ther. 2001;39(1):45–60.
54. Jacobs G, Benson H, Friedman R. Home-based central nervous system assessment of a multifactor behavioral intervention for chronic sleep-onset insomnia. Behav Ther. 1993;24(1):159–74.
55. Perlis ML, Aloia M, Millikan A, Boehmler J, Smith M, Greenblatt D, Giles D. Behavioral treatment of insomnia: a clinical case series study. J Behav Med. 2000;23(2):149–61.
56. Morin CM, Culbert J, Schwartz S. Nonpharmacological treatments of insomnia: a meta-analysis of treatment efficacy. Am J Psychiatry. 1994;151(8):1172–80.
57. Espie CA. Insomnia: Conceptual issues in the development, persistence, and treatment of sleep disorder in adults. Annu Rev Psychol. 2002;53:215–43.
58. Espie CA, Broomfield NM, MacMahon KMA, Macphee LM, Taylor LM. The attention-intention-effort pathway in the development of Psychophysiologic Insomnia: a theoretical review. Sleep Med Rev. 2006;10(4):215–45.
59. Harvey AG. A cognitive model of insomnia. Behav Res Ther. 2002;40(8):869–93.
60. Perlis ML, Giles DE, Mendelson WB, Bootzin RR, Wyatt JK. Psychophysiological insomnia: the behavioural model and a neurocognitive perspective. J Sleep Res. 1997;6(3):179–88.
61. McCurry SM, Logsdon RG, Teri L, Vitiello MV. Evidence-based psychological treatments for insomnia in older adults. Psychol Aging. 2007;22(1);18–27.
62. Smith MT, Perlis ML, Park A, Smith MS, Pennington J, Giles DE, Buysse DJ. Comparative meta-analysis of pharmacotherapy and behavior therapy for persistent insomnia. Am J Psychiatry. 2002;159(1):5–11.
63. NIH State-of-the-Science Conference on Manifestations and Management of Chronic Insomnia in Adults. Bethesda, Maryland: 13–15 June 2005.
64. Morin CM, Hauri PJ, Espie CA, Spielman AJ, Buysse DJ, Bootzin RR. Nonpharmacologic treatment of chronic insomnia. Sleep. 1999a; 22(8);1134–56.
65. Sateia MJ, Doghramji D, Hauri PJ, Morin CM. Evaluation of chronic insomnia. Sleep. 2000;23(2):243–308.
66. Chesson AL, Anderson WM, Littner M, Davila D, Hartse K, Johnson S, et al. Practice parameters for the nonpharmacologic treatment of chronic insomnia. Sleep. 1999;22(8):1–5.
67. Manber R, Morin CM. Co-Chairs, Internet based interventions and other self help therapies for insomnia. Panel at Sleep 2012, 12 June 2012; Boston, MA.
68. Perlis ML, Lichstein KL, editors. Treating sleep disorders: Principles and practice of behavioral sleep medicine. Hoboken: Wiley; 2003.
69. Perlis ML, Jungquist C, Smith M, Posner D. Cognitive behavioral treatment of insomnia: a session-by-session guide. New York: Springer; 2005.
70. Manber R, Carney C, Edinger J, Epstein D, Friedman L, Haynes PL, et al. Dissemination of CBTI to the non-sleep specialist: protocol development and training issues. J Clin Sleep Med. 2012;8(2):209–18.

The Pharmacological Treatment of Sleep Disorders

Jaime M. Monti

Abbreviations

CNS	Central nervous system
EDS	Excessive daytime sleepiness
GABA	γ-hydroxybutyric acid
NREMS	Non-rapid-eye movement sleep
OSAS	Obstructive sleep apnea syndrome
REMS	Rapid-eye movement sleep

Sleep is closely related to every facet of daily life. In this respect, disturbed sleep affects not only our health and well-being but also our quality of life. Dement and Kleitman [10] and Rechtschaffen and Kales [32] provided a description of sleep cycles and a classification system of sleep stages that comprised four non-rapid-eye movement sleep (NREMS) stages and rapid-eye movement sleep (REMS). In 2007, the American Academy of Sleep Medicine [13] introduced new guidelines to score all-night polysomnographic recordings, which seem to differ from those obtained after visual scoring following the Rechtschaffen and Kales rules in that light sleep (S1 vs. N1) and deep sleep (S3 + S4 vs. N3) are significantly increased while intermediate sleep (S2 vs. N2) is reduced [27].

Here, I will consider the evolution of the treatment of insomnia and excessive daytime sleepiness defined according to clinical and all-night polysomnographic recordings. Insomnia is a complaint characterized by difficulty in falling asleep, insufficient sleep, numerous nocturnal awakenings, and early morning awakening with inability to resume sleep, or non-restorative sleep. Common daytime complaints include somnolence, fatigue, irritability, and difficulty concentrating and performing everyday tasks. In addition, subjects with a diagnosis of insomnia are at risk of injury,

drowsiness while driving, and illness. Before the advent of modern sleep medicine only two of these variables were usually considered by the physician when interacting with the patient, namely prolonged sleep-onset latency and reduced total sleep time. The severity and duration of insomnia have been considered important guides to its evaluation and treatment. With respect to patterns of insomnia, an effective program of pharmacological therapy must take into account all of the changing dynamics of the sleep disturbance, including both the difficulties of sleep initiation as well as that of sleep maintenance. As a chronic disorder insomnia affects about 10 % of the population. Sleep professionals know now that its treatment is often challenging, and moreover, it is associated with a substantial number of comorbid symptoms [28]. Chronic insomnia can manifest as primary or comorbid insomnia. The American Psychiatric Association [3] considers primary insomnia as a complaint of difficulty initiating and maintaining sleep or nonrestorative sleep that lasts for at least one month and causes clinically significant distress in several areas. The determinants of comorbid insomnia include mental disorders, neurological diseases, medical conditions, another sleep disorder, and substance-induced sleep disorders.

Excessive daytime sleepiness (EDS) is defined by the International Classification of Sleep Disorders as "the inability to stay awake and alert during the day, resulting in lapses of drowsiness or sleep" [2]. The most common causes of EDS are obstructive sleep apnea syndrome (OSAS), narcolepsy, restless legs syndrome, periodic limb movement disorder, idiopathic hypersomnia and hypersomnia due to medical conditions, and drug or substance intake.

Drugs Used for the Treatment of Insomnia

Ethyl Alcohol

Ethyl alcohol has been used since the dawn of history for the treatment of insomnia. It is still widely employed to induce

J. M. Monti (✉)
Department of Pharmacology and Therapeutics,
School of Medicine, Clinics Hospital,
J. Zudanez Street 2833/602, Montevideo 11600, Uruguay
e-mail: jmonti@mednet.org.uy

S. Chokroverty, M. Billiard (eds.), *Sleep Medicine*, DOI 10.1007/978-1-4939-2089-1_59,
© Springer Science+Business Media, LLC 2015

Table 59.1 Drugs used in the past and presently for the pharmacological treatment of insomnia

Drug	Chemical structure	Mechanism of action	Therapeutic use(s)
Ethyl alcohol	–	Increase of GABA	Insomnia activity
Chloral hydrate	Conversion to trichloroethanol	–	Insomnia
Paraldehyde	Polymer of acetaldehyde	–	Insomnia
Barbiturates	Oxybarbiturate derivatives	Activation of GABA-A receptor	Insomnia
Benzodiazepines		Allosteric modulation of GABA-A receptor	Insomnia
Zopiclone and eszopiclone	Cyclopyrrolones	Allosteric modulation of GABA-A receptor	Primary and comorbid insomnia
Zolpidem	Imidazopyridine	Allosteric modulation of GABA-A receptor	Primary and comorbid insomnia
Zaleplon	Pyrazolopyrimidine	Allosteric modulation of GABA-A receptor	Insomnia
Melatonin	Acetyl-methoxytryptamine	Activation of melatonergic receptors	Insomnia
Ramelteon	Indenofuran derivative	Agonist at MT1 and MT2 receptors	Insomnia

sleep by lay persons. Chronic use of alcohol produces tolerance, physical dependence, and withdrawal phenomena (Table 59.1).

Potassium Bromide

The sedative action of potassium bromide was recognized more than 150 years ago. In adequate doses the compound was found to cause sedation, drowsiness, and sleep. However, the sleep induced by the bromide salt was neither as deep nor as "refreshing" as that produced by chloral hydrate or paraldehyde, and hangover was frequent. In addition, single doses sufficient to cause sedation and sleep were very difficult to retain without vomiting, which led to its displacement by the barbiturates and benzodiazepines for the treatment of insomnia.

Chloral Hydrate

The compound was synthesized by Liebig in 1832, and introduced into medicine by Liebreich in 1869 [19]. By that time ethyl alcohol, opium, and cannabis were mainly used for the treatment of insomnia. In small doses the compound induces sedation, whereas greater doses, in the order of 1–2 mg, taken in a quiet environment induce sleep accompanied by dreams. Sleep usually starts after a latency of 60 min and lasts for at least 5 h. Greater amounts of chloral hydrate have been shown to increase the duration of sleep, but also to augment the incidence of hangover. Habituation, tolerance, and addiction were described with some frequency in patients taking the derivative for long periods of time.

Paraldehyde

The drug was discovered by Wiedenbusch in 1829 and introduced into medicine by Cervello in 1882 [8]. Administration of a dose of 4–8 ml by oral route was reported to induce sleep in 10–15 min which persisted for only 2–3 h, and was accompanied with some frequency by after effects. Paraldehyde was considered an efficacious hypnotic drug but its penetrating odor and burning taste led to its withdrawal for the treatment of insomnia.

Barbiturates

Barbital (veronal), the oldest barbiturate was introduced into medicine by Fisher and von Mering in 1903. About 10 years later Loewe [20] brought into use phenobarbital (luminal). An additional number of derivatives with shorter duration of action were synthesized during the next few years including secobarbital, amobarbital, and pentobarbital. Barbiturates became the drugs of choice for the treatment of insomnia, and this practice persisted until the introduction of the benzodiazepine derivatives in the 1970s. Almost all available barbiturates were shown to be effective for the treatment of "simple insomnia" (presently called primary insomnia) after administration of appropriate oral doses. They differed mainly in speed of onset of action and in duration of action. Sleep usually started with a latency of 20–60 min and, depending on the elimination half-life of the derivative, lasted from 2 to 8 h. In the absence of sleep laboratory studies, it was initially proposed that the sleep induced by barbiturates closely resembled physiological sleep. Notwithstanding this, patients reported that their sleep was dreamless. Tolerance and addiction were shown to develop during the chronic use of barbiturates. Of interest, depending on the dose administered, all the barbiturates used for the treatment of insomnia were known to produce a broad range of effects, extending from sedation to deep coma and death, which can explain the relatively high incidence of suicide attempts with these drugs.

Benzodiazepines

The 1,4-benzodiazepine derivatives were synthesized by Sternbach et al. in the late 1950s [34, 35]. Soon after, Randall et al. characterized the sedative property of chlordiazepoxide and diazepam in laboratory animals [31]. A few years later several other benzodiazepine derivatives were introduced for the selective treatment of insomnia, and became for almost 20 years the most frequently prescribed group of hypnotics, because of their efficacy and relative safety compared with the barbiturates and chloral hydrate. According to their elimination half-life they were divided into short- (midazolam, triazolam), intermediate- (flunitrazepam, temazepam), and long-acting (flurazepam, nitrazepam) derivatives. The evaluation of the effect of benzodiazepine hypnotic drugs on sleep induction and maintenance was carried out mainly in patients with primary chronic insomnia, and was based on sleep laboratory studies and subjective data from clinical trials. Oswald and Priest [29] evaluated for the first time a benzodiazepine hypnotic (nitrazepam) in the sleep laboratory in the year 1965. A few years later, Kales et al. [15] and Monti et al. [25] examined the effects of flurazepam and flunitrazepam, respectively, on sleep variables in patients with a diagnosis of insomnia. It was found that the sleep induced by benzodiazepine hypnotics was characterized by a shortened sleep-onset latency, decreased number of nocturnal awakenings, reduced time spent awake, an increase in stage 2 NREMS, a consistent reduction in slow wave sleep, a dose-dependent suppression of REMS, and an improvement in the subjective quality of sleep compared with no treatment. Thus, from the point of view of sleep architecture, they did not induce a physiological sleep. It was learned also that the short-acting benzodiazepine derivatives were effective predominantly in patients with a prolonged sleep-onset latency, and that rebound insomnia occurred upon their sudden withdrawal. The benzodiazepines, irrespective of their eliminations half-life, showed to be effective hypnotics when administered over a relatively short period of time (4–6 weeks) in patients with chronic insomnia. In addition, dependence was described in patients who were given large doses over a prolonged period of time.

Non-Benzodiazepine Derivatives

In addition to the benzodiazepine hypnotics, a structural dissimilar group of non-benzodiazepine derivatives has become available for the treatment of insomnia. They include zopiclone, eszopiclone, zolpidem, and zaleplon that belong to the cyclopyrrolone, imidazopyridine, and pyrazolopyrimidine classes, respectively. Together with the benzodiazepine derivatives they act as GABA-A receptor allosteric modulators. Melatonin and the melatonin receptor agonist ramelteon are being used also for the treatment of insomnia.

Zopiclone and Eszopiclone

After the introduction in 1960 of chlordiazepoxide by Hoffmann-La Roche, Basel, Switzerland, the number of benzodiazepine derivatives available for the treatment of insomnia grew steadily. During the same period of time Rhône Poulenc Pharma, France started searching for a new family of compounds possessing pharmacological properties similar to those of the benzodiazepines. The studies led to the synthesis of about 500 compounds from which zopiclone (RP-27267) was selected. The effects of zopiclone on sleep and wakefulness were described for the first time by Bardone et al. in 1978 [4]. During the next year, Duriez et al. [12] published a study in the journal Therapy on the effects of zopiclone in patients with insomnia, which was followed by numerous reports on the effects of the hypnotic drug in patients with difficulty falling asleep or having insufficient sleep. In this respect, studies in transient and chronic insomnia, both in adult and in elderly patients, showed that clinically significant hypnotic effects (reduction of sleep-onset latency and of the number of nocturnal awakenings, and increase of total sleep time) could be obtained with a 3.75–7.5 mg dose of zopiclone. Zopiclone was as effective as the benzodiazepine hypnotics triazolam, temazepam, flunitrazepam, and flurazepam in the treatment of insomnia. In healthy volunteers zopiclone reduced stage 1 sleep and increased stage 2 and stage 3 sleep. However, in adult and elderly patients with insomnia, zopiclone decreased or had no effect on slow wave sleep [14]. No development of tolerance was observed in studies of zopiclone that lasted up to 17 weeks, and in contrast to the benzodiazepines, very little rebound was reported following its withdrawal. Dependence and abuse to zopiclone have been described in a small number of drug abusers.

Zopiclone is available as a racemic mixture. In addition, the (S)-isomer of zopiclone (eszopiclone) is now available for the treatment of insomnia. The (S)-isomer of zopiclone is responsible for the hypnotic effect of zopiclone, whereas the (R)-isomer has no hypnotic properties. Sleep laboratory studies of the effects of eszopiclone have confirmed the drug's clinical efficacy in subjects with chronic primary insomnia and in patients with comorbid insomnia. Three mg doses of eszopiclone administered for a period of up to 12 months was associated with a sustained beneficial effect on sleep induction and maintenance, with no occurrence of tolerance.

Zolpidem

The Laboratoires d'Etudes et de Recherches Synthélabo (LERS) of Paris, France, also considered to develop a hypnotic agent of clinical interest possessing a pharmacological and clinical profile with potential benefits over the benzodiazepines, including a rapid onset, short duration of action, and the absence of active metabolites. In that respect, Kaplan and George [16] characterized a group of imidazopyridines that possessed hypnotic activity in laboratory animals. Among them zolpidem was found to combine the above mentioned properties. Soon after, it was shown in middle-aged normal subjects that zolpidem 10 and 20 mg reduced the number of awakenings and total wake time without significantly modifying slow wave sleep and REMS [21]. In addition, administration of zolpidem 10 mg to patients with chronic primary insomnia significantly decreased stage 2 sleep latency and the number of nocturnal awakenings. Total sleep time increase was related to greater amounts of stage 2 whereas slow wave sleep and REMS remained unchanged [22]. All these findings led to the recognition of its therapeutic potential for the treatment of sleep disorders [24]. Notwithstanding this, more recent studies have indicated that plasma levels of zolpidem immediate release frequently decline too quickly for effective sleep maintenance. To address this problem zolpidem extended release was developed. At age-specific dosages, it increases, in middle-aged and elderly patients, total sleep time and reduces the number of nocturnal awakenings. Both zolpidem immediate release and extended release have favorable toxicological profiles. Adverse effects are moderate, and less frequent and severe than those of benzodiazepines. Both variants of zolpidem are practically devoid of next-day hangover effects, and only infrequently cause rebound insomnia of usually short duration. In addition, they have a limited potential for dependence and abuse [26].

Zaleplon

Zaleplon was synthesized by American Cyanamid Co. in the 1980s, and showed sedative and hypnotic effects in preclinical evaluation studies [1]. Polysomnographic and subjective assessments carried out during the years 1998–2000 tended to indicate that zaleplon significantly reduces the time required to fall asleep in adult and elderly patients with chronic insomnia. Estimates of total sleep time and number of awakenings showed no significant differences between placebo and zaleplon. Moreover, the hypnotic agent did not affect NREMS stages or REMS. Zaleplon was approved in September 1999 by the Food and Drug Administration (FDA) of the USA for the treatment of insomnia. It has been also available in Denmark, Sweden, and Germany to treat sleep disorders since 1999.

Melatonin and Ramelteon

Initial studies addressing the effects of melatonin on sleep made use of the intravenous or the intranasal route or administered very large doses of the methoxyindole by the oral route [9, 18]. From these early studies it was concluded that melatonin reduces sleep latency and induces sleepiness and fatigue. More recently, the effects of lower pharmacologic or physiologic doses of melatonin were examined in different laboratories. Melatonin administration reduced sleep-onset latency, and increased total sleep time and sleep efficiency [23]. However, some studies reported an absence of effects, which was attributed mainly to the short elimination half-life of the compound. This led to the development of prolonged-release melatonin which was approved in Europe in 2007 for the treatment of patients aged 55 years and older with primary insomnia. Prolonged-release melatonin has been shown to improve sleep latency and total sleep time during long-term administration with no rebound or withdrawal symptoms following its discontinuation [36]. Two melatonin receptors, MT1 and MT2, have been characterized that exhibit subnanomolar binding affinity for melatonin. This led to the development of ramelteon (Takeda Pharmaceuticals, Japan, 1996), a melatonin receptor agonist that binds with high affinity to MT1 and MT2 receptors. In all clinical studies undertaken so far to evaluate the efficacy and safety of ramelteon in patients with chronic primary insomnia, it has been shown that the compound reduces sleep-onset latency and moderately increases total sleep time [33]. Moreover, tolerance or abuse have not been described during its administration, and rebound insomnia does not occur on sudden withdrawal.

Drugs used for the Treatment of Daytime Sleepiness

Central nervous system (CNS) stimulants used for the treatment of diseases where EDS is an important symptom have included caffeine, ephedrine, amphetamine and dextroamphetamine, methylphenidate, and modafinil. Sodium

Table 59.2 Drugs used for the pharmacological treatment of excessive daytime sleepiness

Drug	Chemical structure	Mechanism of action	Therapeutic use(s)
Caffeine	Methyl-xanthine derivative	Antagonist at adenosine receptors	Sleepiness
Amphetamine d-amphetamine	β-phenylisopropyl-amine derivatives	Release of biogenic amines and blockade of their reuptake	Narcolepsy, idiopathic hypersomnia
Methylphenidate	Piperidine derivative	Release of biogenic amines	Narcolepsy
Modafinil Armodafinil	Diphenylmethyl-sulfinyl acetamides	Dopamine reuptake inhibitors	Narcolepsy, idiopahic hypersomnia, refractory sleepiness in OSAS, and shift work disorder
Sodium oxybate	Sodium salt of γ-hydroxybutyrate	Agonist at GABA and γ-hydroxybutyrate receptors	EDS and cataplexy in narcolepsy

oxybate, an hypnotic drug, is also indicated for the treatment of EDS and cataplexy in narcolepsy.

OSAS was initially treated with chronic tracheostomy. In the 1980s it was replaced by the procedures called uvulo-palatopharyngoplasty and continuous positive nasal airway pressure technique.

Caffeine

As early as 1672, coffee was prescribed for disorders associated with sleepiness. The effect of coffee is related to the presence of caffeine which was officially discovered in 1819. Caffeine is present in soft drinks, coffee, tea, and over-the-counter drugs. In some countries it is available also in a tablet form; the usual dose amounts to 100 mg twice daily. The stimulatory effect of the xanthine derivative is rather mild, and tolerance occurs frequently during its administration (Table 59.2).

Ephedrine

The drug was introduced in the USA by Doyle and Daniels in 1931 for the treatment of narcolepsy [11]. Ephedrine taken orally in doses of 10–50 mg, three times daily, afforded symptomatic relief from the narcoleptic and cataplectic attacks. It was reported also that the compound improved nocturnal sleep and suppressed terrifying dreams and hypnagogic hallucinations. However, the rather high incidence of side effects and rapid occurrence of tolerance led to its discontinuation for the treatment of narcolepsy.

Amphetamines

Prinzmetal and Bloomberg [30] were the first to administer the compound for the treatment of narcolepsy. Amphetamine and dextro-amphetamine showed greater CNS stimulation effects as compared to ephedrine. In addition, the d-isomer had less peripheral effects. By the 1940s the amphetamines became the treatment of choice for EDS related to narcolepsy. In this respect, the drugs were shown to prevent attacks of sleep in most patients, and cataplexy was often much improved. However, amphetamines are no longer marketed in many countries because of the risk of abuse and dependence.

Methylphenidate

The piperidine derivative was introduced in the 1950s for the treatment of narcolepsy [37]. It is a mild CNS stimulant that shares the pharmacological actions of amphetamines including potential for abuse. Because of its short duration of action, a sustained-release form has been made available to treat narcolepsy symptoms.

Modafinil

The compound was originally developed in France. It was approved in France in 1994 and in the USA in late 1998. Of note, the R isomer of modafinil (armodafinil) has a longer elimination half-life, and was approved by the FDA in 2007 for the treatment of narcolepsy. Modafinil at doses of 200–400 mg has been shown to decrease EDS in narcolepsy; however, it does not reduce cataplexy [5, 6]. The drug is useful also for the treatment of idiopathic hypersomnia and EDS related to Parkinson's disease, multiple sclerosis, and myotonic distrophy. Interestingly, modafinil has been administered with success as adjunctive therapy for refractory sleepiness in patients with OSAS, treated with continuous positive nasal airway pressure technique.

Sodium Oxybate

The sodium salt of γ-hydroxybutyrate, sodium oxybate, is a sedative-hypnotic drug that exerts a favorable effect on EDS and cataplexy in narcoleptics [7]. Its mechanism of action is partly related to the activation of GABA-B and γ-hydroxybutyrate receptors at central sites. Sodium oxybate was registered for the treatment of narcolepsy in Europe in the year 2005 [17]. It should be mentioned that the compound has the potential to induce dependence and abuse.

References

1. Abel MS, Day I. Screening for a new anxiolytic. Correlations of TBPS binding in vitro and degree of sedative-hypnotic effects in vivo. Pearl River, New York: American Cyanamid CNS Department. Research Seminars; 1990.

2. American Academy of Sleep Medicine. The international classification of sleep disorders: diagnostic and coding manual. 3rd ed. Darien, IL: American Academy of Sleep Med; 2014.

3. American Psychiatric Association. Diagnostic and Statistical Manual of Mental Disorders. 4th ed. Washington, DC: American Psychiatric Press; 1994.

4. Bardone MC, Ducrot R, Garret C, Julou L. Benzodiazepine-like central effects of R.P: 27267, a dihydro-7-oxo-5 H-pyrrolo[3,4-b]pyrazine derivative. 7th Int Congr Pharmacol, Paris. London: Pergamon Press; 1978.

5. Billiard M. Narcolepsy: current treatment options and future approaches. Neuropsychiat Dis Treat. 2008;4:557–66.

6. Billiard M, Besset A, Montplaisir J, Laffont F, Goldenberg F, Weill JS et al. Modafinil: a double-blind multicentric study. Sleep. 1994;17(Suppl 8):S107–12.

7. Broughton R, Mamelak M. The treatment of narcolepsy-cataplexy with nocturnal gamma-hydroxybutyrate. Can J Neurol Sci. 1979;6:1–6.

8. Cervello V. Sull'Azione Fisiologica della Paraldeide e Contributo Allo Studio del Cloralio Idrato. Ricerche. Arch per le sc Med. 1882;6:177–214. Italian.

9. Cramer H, Rudolph J, Consbruch U, Kendel K. On the effects of melatonin on sleep and behavior in man. Adv Biochem Psychopharmacol. 1974;11:187–91.

10. Dement W, Kleitman N. The relation of eye movements during sleep to dream activity: an objective method for the study of dreaming. J Exp Psychol. 1957;53:284–7.

11. Doyle JB, Daniel LE. Symptomatic treatment for narcolepsy. JAMA. 1931;96:1370–2.

12. Duriez R, Barthélémy CI, Rives H, Courjaret J, Gregoire J. Traitement des troubles du sommeil par la zopiclone. Essais cliniques en double insu contre placébo. Thérapie. 1979;34:317–25. French.

13. Iber C, Ancoli-Israel S, Chesson A, Quan SF, editors. The AASM manual for the scoring of sleep and associated events: rules, terminology, and technical specifications. 1st ed. Westchester: American Academy of Sleep Medicine; 2007.

14. Jovanovic UJ, Dreyfuss JF. Polygraphical sleep recording in insomniac patients under zopiclone or nitrazepam. Pharmacology. 1983;27:136–45.

15. Kales A, Kales JD, Scharf M, Tan TL. Hypnotics and altered sleep-dream patterns. II. All-night EEG studies of chloral hydrate, flurazepam, and methaqualone. Arch Gen Psychiat. 1970;23:219–25.

16. Kaplan JP, George P. Imidazo[1,2-a]pyridine derivatives and their therapeutic use. European Patent 0050663;1982.

17. Lammers GJ, Bassetti C, Billiard M, Black J, Broughton R, Dauvilliers Y et al. Sodium oxybate is an effective and safe treatment for narcolepsy. Sleep Med. 2010;11:105–6; author reply 106–8.

18. Lieberman HR, Waldhauser F, Garfield G, Lynch HJ, Wurtman RJ. Effects of melatonin on human mood and performance. Brain Res. 1984;323:201–7.

19. Liebreich O. Das chloralhydrat ein neues Hypnoticum und Anastheticum. Berlin: Otto Muller's Verlag; 1869. German

20. Loewe S. Klinische Erfahrungen mit Luminal. Deutsche med Wchnschr. 1912;38:947–8. German.

21. Lund R, Rüther E, Wober W, Hippius H. Effects of zolpidem (10 and 20 mg), lormetazepam, triazolam and placebo on night sleep and residual effects during the day. In: Savanet JP, Langer SZ, Morselli PL, editors. Imidazopyridines in sleep disorders. New York: Raven Press;1988. p. 193–203.

22. Monti JM. Effects of zolpidem on sleep in insomniac patients. Eur J Clin Pharmacol. 1989;36:461–6.

23. Monti JM, Cardinali D. A critical assessment of the melatonin effect on sleep in humans. Biol Signals Recept. 2000;9:328–39.

24. Monti JM, Monti D. Overview of currently available benzodiazepine and nonbenzodiazepine hypnotics. In: Pandi-Perumal SR, Monti JM, editors. Clinical Pharmacology of Sleep. Basel: Birkhäuser; 2006. p. 207–23.

25. Monti JM, Trenchi HM, Morales F. Flunitrazepam (RO 5–4200) and sleep cycle in insomniac patients. Acta Neurol Lat-Amer. 1971;17:5–11.

26. Monti JM, Spence DW, Pandi-Perumal SR, Langer SZ, Hardeland R. Pharmacotherapy of insomnia: Focus on zolpidem extended release. Clin Med Ther. 2009;1:123–40.

27. Moser D, Anderer P, Gruber G, Parapatics S, Loretz E, Boeck M, et al. Sleep classification according to AASM and Rechtschaffen & Kales: Effects on sleep scoring parameters. Sleep. 2009;32:139–49.

28. National Institutes of Health. NIH statement regarding the treatment of insomnia. State of the Science Conference Statement: Manifestations and management of chronic insomnia in adults. Sleep. 2005;28:1049–57.

29. Oswald I, Priest RG. Five weeks to escape the sleeping-pill habit. Br Med J. 1965;2:1093–9.

30. Prinzmental M, Bloomberg W. Use of benzedrine for the treatment of narcolepsy. JAMA. 1935;105:2051–4.

31. Randall LO, Kappell B. Pharmacological activity of some benzodiazepines and their metabolites. In: Garattini S, Mussini E, Randall LO, editors. The benzodiazepines. New York: Raven Press; 1973. p. 27–51.

32. Rechtschaffen A, Kales A, editors. A manual of standardized terminology, techniques and scoring system of sleep stages in human subjects. Los Angeles: Brain Information Service/Brain Research Institute, University of California; 1968.

33. Srinivasan V, Zakaria R, Othaman Z, Brzezinski A, Prasad A, Brown GM. Melatoninergic drugs for therapeutic use in insomnia and sleep disturbances of mood disorders. CNS Neurol Disorders Drug Targets. 2012;11:180–9.

34. Sternbach LH. United States patent 2893–992. 1959.

35. Sternbach LH, Fryer RI, Keller O, Metlesics W, Sach G, Steiger N. Quinazolines and 1,4-benzodiazepines. X. Nitro-substituted 5-phenyl-1,4-benzodiazepine derivatives. J Med Chem. 1963;6:261–5.

36. Wade AG, Crawford G, Ford I, McConnachie A, Nir T, Laudon M et al. Prolonged release melatonin in the treatment of primary insomnia: evaluation of the age cut-off for short- and long-term response. Curr Med Res Opinion. 2011;27:87–98.

37. Yoss RE, Daly DD. Treatment of narcolepsy with Ritalin. Neurology. 1959;9:171–3.

Psychological Treatment of Insomnia: The Evolution of Behavior Therapy and Cognitive Behavior Therapy

60

María Montserrat Sánchez-Ortuño and Jack D. Edinger

Introduction: The Behavior Therapy Movement

Since various forms of psychopathology (e.g., mood disorders, anxiety disorders) are commonly associated with sleep disturbance, insomnia was long considered a symptom of such conditions. As such, it was generally assumed that psychotherapeutic interventions which effectively treat the primary psychiatric condition would be needed to alleviate the associated insomnia symptoms. Many of the early insomnia interventions proposed entailed complex and time consuming psychotherapies (e.g., psychoanalysis) that were of limited availability due to the special training and expertise they required. Moreover, the usefulness of these approaches for insomnia management remained questionable, due to the general lack of properly controlled studies to demonstrate their efficacy [1].

The emergence of behavioral therapies in the 1950s represented a shift in this orientation, not only for the treatment of psychopathology in general, but also for the treatment of insomnia. Indeed, the behavior therapies are designed to directly correct presenting problems, instead of exploring and understanding their psychological origins (e.g., psychological conflicts) [2]. Admittedly, one of the main features distinguishing behavioral therapy from other forms of psychotherapy is that it defines problems in terms of identifiable behavioral excesses and deficits[1]. Therefore, compared to prior psychotherapeutic approaches, this goal-oriented form

of psychotherapy treatment takes a more hands-on, practical approach to problem-solving. As a consequence, behavior therapy is much quicker and less costly. Furthermore, and of utmost importance, a strong scientific orientation is a hallmark of behavior therapy. These distinctive features have contributed to its success through the years, leading in the development of empirically validated behavioral treatment approaches for a variety of conditions including chronic insomnia. In fact, the behavior therapy movement has produced the majority of the empirically validated non-drug treatments for insomnia currently available to clinicians.

First-Generation Behavioral Therapies for the Treatment of Insomnia: Targeting Somatic Arousal

The evolution of behavioral insomnia therapies was aided by both empirical and clinical identification of physiological, emotional, and behavioral factors that serve to perpetuate sleep disturbance. One such factor that received early attention in this evolution was that of somatic arousal. In an early study comparing good and poor sleepers, Monroe [3] noted that poor sleepers showed greater autonomic arousal (i.e., higher body temperature and faster heart rate) prior to and during sleep than did good sleepers. This observation led to the early speculation that a heightened state of somatic arousal prior to and during sleep might serve to sustain insomnia. This speculation, in turn, led to the supposition that treatments designed to reduce this somatic arousal would be effective for ameliorating insomnia.

Early insomnia treatments designed to target sleep disruptive somatic arousal have their roots in the work of Edmund Jacobson, who was the first to propose a formal structured behavioral therapy for reducing such arousal. In the 1930s Jacobson first proposed the use of a structured exercise involving the alternate tensing and relaxing of major skeletal muscle groups so as to promote a reduction in generalized somatic arousal [4]. Applications of this sort of approach to

---

[1] Here, the use of the term behavior refers to any and all activities of the integrated organism. Therefore, since thinking, feeling, and imagining are things people do, they would be considered behavior along with publicly observable behaviors.

M. M. Sánchez-Ortuño (✉)
Facultad de Enfermería, Campus de Espinardo, Universidad de Murcia, 30100 Murcia, Spain
e-mail: montses@um.es

J. D. Edinger
National Jewish Health, 1400 Jackson Street, Denver, CO 80206, USA
e-mail: EdingerJ@njhealth.com

S. Chokroverty, M. Billiard (eds.), *Sleep Medicine*, DOI 10.1007/978-1-4939-2089-1_60,

insomnia management first appeared in the form of single case and case-series studies in the 1950s and 1960s [5, 6]. Perhaps among the more notable of these early studies was a case series study by Kahn et al. [7] who used an imagery-based variant of relaxation training called autogenic training to treat a series of 16 college students complaining of insomnia. In another early study, Geer et al. [8] used a variant of desensitization therapy in which a patient was instructed in relaxation and then instructed to visualize being at home in bed falling asleep while being relaxed. Although wrought with methodological limitations, such early studies provided encouraging results in regard to the potential efficacy of relaxation approaches for insomnia management.

It was not until the 1970s when behavioral treatments for insomnia gained popularity and researchers began conducting more well-controlled and convincing insomnia treatment studies. The first series of controlled studies tested a host of relaxation procedures whose focus was mainly on reducing bedtime physiological arousal presumed to maintain the sleep difficulties. These therapies included progressive muscle relaxation training, autogenic training, imagery training, and hypnosis [9, 10]. Of these, progressive relaxation was probably the most thoroughly tested [11]. However, researchers also tested alternate approaches, such as frontalis electromyograph (EMG) biofeedback [12, 13], in the belief that achieving frontalis muscle relaxation will generalize to other muscle groups, resulting in a global relaxation effect that would facilitate sleep. Although individuals participating in these early tests of relaxation and biofeedback did improve their sleep, findings of these studies did not produce convincing evidence that elevated arousal was a major factor in insomnia. Indeed, a study by Borkovec et al. [9] reported that reduction in arousal during therapy was unrelated to sleep outcome measures. In the same vein, Hauri [13] showed the amount of EMG reduction achieved during treatment did not correlate with improvement in sleep. Furthermore, this author noted that not all the insomnia sufferers are necessarily tense. Collectively these various findings suggested that procedures aimed at reducing somatic arousal at bedtime may be essential for some but not all insomnia sufferers.

First-Generation Behavioral Therapies for the Treatment of Insomnia: Targeting Cognitive Arousal

A closer look at the findings of the studies cited above raised the possibility that a process other than the reduction of somatic arousal could explain the sleep improvements observed in the insomnia sufferers studied. Borkovec et al. [9] believed that the self-generated monotonous stimulation inherent in relaxation training may be the crucial variable. Indeed, it had been noted that a frequent complaint in insomnia sufferers was excessive cognitive activity after retiring [8], that is, they complain of "racing thoughts". In a classic study by Lichstein et al. [14] the authors asked a series of 296 insomnia sufferers whether cognitive or somatic arousal was the main determinant of their insomnia. The largest number of subjects (55%) perceived cognitive arousal to be the cause of their sleep problems, whereas another 35% claimed that their insomnia was caused by both somatic and cognitive arousal. Thus, 90% of these individuals implicated cognitive arousal in their insomnia. Such findings suggest that instruction and training in a method of attention focusing that is incompatible with that cognitive activity may serve to facilitate sleep.

Based on this assumption, a number of investigators started testing interventions designed to reduce cognitive arousal so as to improve the sleep of insomnia sufferers. With the goal of teaching patients to concentrate on non-arousing thoughts, some of the earlier cognitive interventions consisted of a number of attention focusing techniques, such as meditation [15] and guided imagery [16]. Although limited in number, these early studies yielded favorable results, pointing out that reducing cognitive arousal, per se, is an important component for the overall management of insomnia [11].

As the focus on cognitive arousal grew, the importance of the exact nature, content, and focus of insomnia sufferers' pre-sleep cognitions became increasingly apparent [17]. In this regard, it was commonly observed that individuals complaining of sleep onset difficulties go to bed preoccupied with getting to sleep quickly and that, in fact, exacerbates their problem by this heightened intention to directly control their sleep processes. Therefore, it was hypothesized that this pre-sleep concern might be an important therapy target for those with sleep-onset insomnia. To address this sleep-defeating mentation, Turner et al. [18] developed a creative treatment for insomnia named paradoxical intention. They argued that performance anxiety over sleep could be reduced if patients were encouraged to focus upon trying not to fall asleep. Therefore, if the patient complies and genuinely tries to remain awake in bed, performance anxiety over not sleeping is alleviated and sleep becomes less difficult to initiate. In their classical study, Turner et al. [18] found good success rates for paradoxical intention, equivalent to that achieved with other promising first generation interventions. However, results have been less consistent across subsequent studies [19], with several suggesting an exacerbation of sleep problems in some patients following this therapy [20].

First-Generation Behavioral Therapies for the Treatment of Insomnia: Targeting Sleep-Disruptive Habits

Paralleling the early proliferation of studies devoted to relaxation interventions for insomnia was a growing recognition that bedtime arousal and associated sleep difficulties is often, if not usually, sustained by sleep-disruptive habits. This recognition, in turn, led to the development of a variety of insomnia therapies designed to improve sleep primarily by eliminating patients' sleep-disruptive practices. Among these therapies, stimulus control therapy (SCT) has been the most studied and proven technique. SCT, developed by Bootzin in 1972 [21], is based on the observation that, for many insomnia sufferers, the bed and bedroom are not cues for drowsiness and the onset of sleep. Instead, they become strong signals or discriminative stimuli for alertness, sleeplessness, and frustration through their repeated association with unsuccessful sleep attempts. The resulting conditioned arousal at bedtime, thus, serves to sustain insomnia. Therefore, SCT's main goal is to teach the patient to reassociate the bed and the bedroom with rapid and successful sleep onset. This is done by instructing the insomnia sufferer to curtail all sleep-incompatible behaviors in the bedroom that serve as cues for staying awake (e.g., watching TV, talking on the phone). In addition, the patient is explicitly asked to go to bed only when sleepy and to get out of bed when lying in bed awake for an extended period unable to fall asleep. The conditioning theory from which this technique derives implies that, by following these recommendations, the individual will learn again to associate the bed and the bedroom with the rapid onset of sleepiness [22]. However, it should be noted that SCT also includes such recommendations as adhering to a standard rise time and avoiding daytime napping. These additional recommendations may also have sleep promoting effects by eliminating habits that respectively disrupt the circadian timing of sleep and reduce sleep drive at bedtime. Hence, this therapy actually addresses several putative mechanisms that serve to perpetuate insomnia over time. This fact likely explains the relative efficacy and consequent popularity of SCT when compared to other first generation treatments [23]. Indeed this treatment has arguably proven among the more efficacious first-generation behavioral insomnia therapies [24], and as will be discussed later, earned a role in the more current-day insomnia treatments [25].

A few years after the emergence of SCT, Hauri [26] proposed another approach for the management of insomnia called sleep hygiene therapy (SHT). In contrast to SCT, SHT generally targets global lifestyle and environmental factors that serve as sleep inhibitors. SHT is basically an educational intervention, which includes general guidelines about health-related practices, such as exercise, substance use, etc., and environmental factors, such as light, noise, and uncomfortable temperatures, which may affect sleep. Although the success of this approach to treat insomnia, when used in isolation, has not been strongly documented [24, 27], this primarily "educational" intervention has remained an important and fundamental part of overall insomnia management [25].

Following the emergence of SCT and SHT, Spielman et al. [28] introduced sleep restriction therapy (SRT), a form of therapy that addressed one of the factors that they believed commonly perpetuated insomnia, namely excessive time in bed (TIB). SRT, thus, involved restricting available sleep time and making changes in TIB contingent upon the patient's clinical response. It was thought that this approach would help to restore normal (homeostatic) sleep drive that was markedly reduced by the practice of spending excessive time in bed each night. Like SCT, SRT proved to be relatively effective for insomnia management and thus has enjoyed wide popularity through the years since it was first proposed [24, 29].

Despite their proven efficacy, each of the first-generation behavioral therapies had their limitations. Indeed, none of these interventions in itself addressed all mechanisms thought to perpetuate insomnia. Whereas relaxation approaches target bedtime arousal and sleep-related anxiety, they largely ignore other mechanisms commonly involved in insomnia, such as circadian, homeostatic, and sleep-inhibitory (i.e., conditioned arousal) factors. In contrast, these latter factors were addressed more directly by SCT and SRT, yet these therapies did not deal with cognitive factors sustaining many sleep-disruptive attitudes and beliefs seen in insomnia sufferers. On the other hand, whereas SHT directly addresses some inhibitory mechanisms (e.g., use of caffeine, nicotine) and indirectly may alter some dysfunctional sleep-related beliefs, this educational intervention, when used alone, seemed to have little impact on sleep outcome.

It should also be mentioned that much of the early research with the first generation therapies was rather limited in focus. In fact, the majority of studies testing the efficacy of these interventions focused on correcting sleep-onset insomnia [30]. Studies examining the efficacy of these interventions for sleep-maintenance insomnia were rare and often less promising. This lack of attention given to sleep-maintenance insomnia was particularly surprising, particularly when one considers that it is a more common complaint than sleep-onset insomnia, especially in middle-aged and older populations. Due to the limitations of these first-generation approaches, a more omnibus multi-component approach for the management of insomnia started to gain popularity by the end of the 1980s.

Second-Generation Behavioral Therapy for the Treatment of Insomnia: Cognitive-Behavior Therapy

In an effort to overcome the limitations of the narrowly targeted first-generation insomnia therapies, and especially their shortcomings for the treatment of sleep-maintenance insomnia, researchers turned their attention to the use of behavioral treatment packages. It was assumed that a better treatment response would be attained if the range of insomnia perpetuating mechanisms could be addressed during the course of therapy.

In a collection of three case studies published in 1981, Thoresen et al. [31] reported on the use of a behavioral treatment package consisting of relaxation training, cognitive restructuring, and problem solving to address both sleep-onset and sleep-maintenance insomnia. A few years later, Hoelscher et al. [30], based on the assumption that sleep-maintenance insomnia may be more refractory to behavioral treatments than sleep-onset insomnia, developed a more "aggressive" form of behavioral treatment, comprising three components: sleep period reduction (i.e., SRT), sleep education, and stimulus control, and tested this "package" with four chronic insomnia sufferers. Their findings, although preliminary, were encouraging and called for further controlled evaluations of the efficacy of a behavioral treatment package addressing behavioral and cognitive targets for sleep-maintenance insomnia.

Over the following decade, the 1990s, various renditions of a multi-component approach for the management of insomnia were described and tested [32]. Although the core behavioral components, SCT and SRT, have been included in the majority of the so-called CBT treatments, the cognitive arm has varied across studies. To correct common dysfunctional attitudes and beliefs about sleep, some interventions have used formal cognitive restructuring [33] whereas others have employed a standardized sleep education package [34].

Soon after the emergence of these CBT protocols, various carefully designed studies were conducted to test their efficacy, mainly with individuals suffering from primary insomnia. The findings from these studies suggested that CBT produces significantly greater subjective and objective sleep improvements than: no treatment [32, 35], pharmacologic and psychological placebo interventions [36], and progressive relaxation therapy [34]. These studies also demonstrated that sleep improvements resulting from CBT tend to endure across extended post-treatment follow-up periods varying between 6 months and 2 years in duration. Furthermore, one study combining CBT with pharmacotherapy suggested that a combined treatment may produce slightly greater short-term sleep improvements than does CBT alone [36]. Yet, advantages of this combined approach over the long-term seemed less clear. In fact, findings from this study indicate that those receiving CBT alone showed better maintenance of their sleep improvements at the end of a 2-year follow-up than did those receiving combined CBT and pharmacotherapy.

Most of the early investigations conducted with CBT are best characterized as tightly controlled efficacy studies that included highly screened insomnia sufferers who arguably do not represent the typical insomnia patient seen in clinical venues. However, these efficacy studies were soon accompanied by various effectiveness studies, conducted in more traditional clinical venues with less carefully screened "real-world" patients. Results from these studies generally corroborated those obtained in the more tightly controlled efficacy trials [37] and encouraged the broader application of CBT for insomnia. Further buttressing these effectiveness trials were two meta-analytic studies that were published by the mid-1990s. These studies concluded that CBT was broadly effective in the treatment of primary insomnia [38, 39]. Finally, a task-force report published in 1999 and sponsored by the American Academy of Sleep Medicine (AASM) [40], concluded that there is compelling evidence that CBT is a lastingly effective treatment for chronic insomnia.

Hence, by the end of the previous millennium, CBT had become established as a viable and well-supported intervention for insomnia management.

Contemporary Research on Cognitive-Behavioral Therapy for Insomnia

Research testing CBT during the first decade of the current millennium has buttressed the findings obtained in previous years, casting little doubt about the benefits of CBT for the management of primary insomnia [41], benefits that were, in some instances, superior to those obtained with pharmacotherapies [42]. Yet, despite the evolution of CBT insomnia interventions in the 1980s, it has not been until after beginning of this millennium that most research applications of this intervention with comorbid insomnia have been conducted [43]. As a consequence, it was as recently as 2006 when the utility of CBT for comorbid/secondary insomnia was first officially recognized. In that year, a second AASM taskforce report concerning practice parameters for the psychological and behavioral treatment of insomnia first recommended the use of CBT for secondary (comorbid) forms of insomnia [44]. Since the publication of the 2006 AASM report, there has been a slow, albeit steady, progression of research assessing the efficacy of CBT for insomnia occurring as comorbid to various forms of mental and medical disorders [45]. Collectively, these studies are providing additional encouragement for applications of CBT to insomnia associated with medical and psychiatric disorders.

Furthermore, although the behavioral arm of CBT has not changed substantially over time, including primarily a combination SCT and SRT, somewhat more refined cognitive approaches have been proposed as this therapy has been extended to comorbid populations. Further theoretical and empirical work highlighting the contribution of cognitive processes to insomnia, summarized in the work by Harvey published in 2002 [46], have fueled this evolution of cognitive interventions. Among those, interventions facilitating the emotional processing of concerns prior to sleep onset, such as the Pennebaker-style writing intervention [47], have been proposed. This technique requires patients to engage in writing with the aim of processing emotional material on a day by day basis. It is expected that this activity will reduce pre-sleep worry and intrusive thinking. In a related vein, a recent study has included a constructive worry intervention combined with SCT and SRT for the management of insomnia [48]. This relatively new cognitive intervention assumes that training people to set aside concerns earlier in the evening, by asking them to record problems and worries having the greatest likelihood of keeping them awake at bedtime, as well as strategies that could contribute to their resolution, would result in less cognitive arousal in the pre-sleep period.

Further developments of the cognitive arm of CBT for insomnia include the addition of mindfulness meditation to the core behavioral interventions used for insomnia, SCT and SRT [49]. It is hypothetized that this treatment component will help insomnia sufferers to manage their emotional reactions to sleep disturbance and daytime fatigue that commonly arise during the course of chronic insomnia. Preliminary work testing this relatively new form of CBT for insomnia has yielded promising results.

Yet, despite the formidable progress and accomplishments obtained with the use of CBT for chronic insomnia, it has been argued that the field is not, as yet, at a point where patients can be offered a maximally effective treatment [50]. Indeed, it has been noted that while the effect size for CBT for insomnia is moderate, it is lower than the effect sizes reported for CBT for a range of other psychological disorders [51]. This suggests that there is still room for improvement. With this goal, more innovative studies are trying to ascertain, for example, whether combining CBT with sleep medication could represent a superior strategy, not only in regard to short and long-term effectiveness, but also in regard to costs and patient satisfaction [52]. Furthermore, work now in progress is trying to disentangle the specific benefits and therapeutic mechanisms of the cognitive and behavioral arms of CBT.

Finally, a promising research venue concerns the dissemination of CBT. In this regard, it has been argued that, at this point, "the challenge for CBT is no longer to prove its credentials, but to punch its weight" [53]. Indeed, CBT still has very little impact on the high volume of insomnia patient care field that is still dominated by the prescription of medication. Indeed, widespread use of CBT for insomnia is limited by the number of specialty-trained clinicians and by the duration, intensity, and initial cost of 6–8 individual treatment sessions. Strategies to enhance the delivery of CBT on a whole population basis include the CBT for insomnia dissemination training program currently underway in the Veterans Affairs (VA) nation-wide healthcare system [54]. This program is training VA healthcare providers (e.g., psychologists, psychiatrists, social workers, nurse practitioners) in the delivery of basic cognitive and behavioral insomnia treatment techniques. Other CBT dissemination strategies include developing briefer and more straightforward renditions of CBT [29, 55] and training paraprofessionals to administer these simplified versions of CBT in 'real world' primary care settings [56].

Furthermore, as technology increasingly pervades the health-care world, more than ever there is a call to develop innovative ways of improving the reach of CBT using tools such as the Internet and mobile phones. In this line, recent studies using Web-based applications for CBT delivery in insomnia sufferers are yielding interesting results [57, 58]. Currently, most of these efforts are in their early developmental stages so their outcomes will have to await future reports. Nonetheless, early findings of these efforts have been encouraging so it is likely that CBT's reach will be greatly enhanced in the foreseeable future.

References

1. Kales A, Kales JD. Evaluation and treatment of insomnia. New York: Oxford University Press; 1984.
2. Wilson KG. Science and treatment development: Lessons from the history of behavior therapy. Behav Ther. 1997;547–58.
3. Monroe LJ. Psychological and physiological differences between good and poor sleepers. J Abnorm Psychol. 1967;72:255–64.
4. Jacobson E. Progressive relaxation; a physiological and clinical investigation of muscular states and their significance in psychology and medical practice. 2nd ed. Chicago: University of Chicago Press; 1938.
5. Schultz JH, Luthe W. Autogenic training; a psychophysiologic approach in psychotherapy. New York: Grune & Stratton; 1959.
6. Evans DR, Bond IK. Reciprocal inhibition therapy and classical conditioning in the treatment of insomnia. Behav Res Ther. 1969;7:323–5.
7. Kahn M, Baker BL, Weiss JM. Treatment of insomnia by relaxation training. J Abnorm Psychol. 1968;73:556–8.
8. Geer JH, Katkin ES. Treatment of insomnia using a variant of systematic desensitization: A case report. J Abnorm Psychol. 1966;71:161–4.
9. Borkovec TD, Fowles DC. Controlled investigation of the effects of progressive and hypnotic relaxation on insomnia. J Abnorm Psychol. 1973;82:153–8.
10. Nicassio P, Bootzin R. A comparison of progressive relaxation and autogenic training as treatments for insomnia. J Abnorm Psychol. 1974;83:253–60.

11. Lacks P. Behavioral treatment for persistent insomnia. 1st ed. New York: Pergamon Press; 1987.

12. Surwit RS, Keefe FJ. Frontalis EMG feedback training: an electronic panacea? Behav Ther. 1978;9:779–92.

13. Hauri P. Treating psychophysiologic insomnia with biofeedback. Arch Gen Psychiatry. 1981;38:752–8.

14. Lichstein KL, Rosenthal TL. Insomniacs' perceptions of cognitive versus somatic determinants of sleep disturbance. J Abnorm Psychol. 1980;89:105–7.

15. Woolfolk RL, Carr-Kaffashan L, McNulty TF, Lehrer PM. Meditation training as a treatment for insomnia. Behav Ther. 1976;359–65.

16. Woolfolk RL, McNulty TF. Relaxation treatment for insomnia: A component analysis. J Consult Clin Psychol. 1983;51:495–503.

17. Borkovec TD, Lane TW, VanOot PH. Phenomenology of sleep among insomniacs and good sleepers: Wakefulness experience when cortically asleep. J Abnorm Psychol. 1981;90:607–9.

18. Turner RM, Ascher LM. Controlled comparison of progressive relaxation, stimulus control, and paradoxical intention therapies for insomnia. J Consult Clin Psychol. 1979;47:500–8.

19. Lacks P, Bertelson AD, Gans L, Kunkel J. The effectiveness of 3 behavioral treatments for different degrees of sleep onset insomnia. Behav Ther. 1983;14:593–605.

20. Espie CA, Lindsay WR. Paradoxical intention in the treatment of chronic insomnia: six case studies illustrating variability in therapeutic response. Behav Res Ther. 1985;23:703–9.

21. Bootzin R. Stimulus control treatment for insomnia. Proceedings of the 80th Annual Convention of the American Psychological Association; 1972; p. 395–6.

22. Zwart CA, Lisman SA. Analysis of stimulus control treatment of sleep-onset insomnia. J Consult Clin Psychol. 1979;47:113–8.

23. Morin CM, Azrin NH. Stimulus control and imagery training in treating sleep-maintenance insomnia. J Consult Clin Psychol. 1987;55:260–2.

24. Morin CM, Hauri PJ, Espie CA, Spielman AJ, Buysse DJ, Bootzin RR. Nonpharmacologic treatment of chronic insomnia. An American academy of sleep medicine review. Sleep. 1999;22:1134–56.

25. Edinger JD, Carney C. Overcoming insomnia: A cognitive-behavioral therapy approach therapist guide. Oxford, New York: Oxford University Press; 2008.

26. Hauri P. The sleep disorders. 2nd ed. Kalamazoo: Upjohn; 1982.

27. Schoicket SL, Bertelson AD, Lacks P. Is sleep hygiene a sufficient treatment for sleep-maintenance insomnia? Behav Ther. 1988;19:183–90.

28. Spielman AJ, Saskin P, Thorpy MJ. Treatment of chronic insomnia by restriction of time in bed. Sleep. 1987;10:45–56.

29. Buysse DJ, Germain A, Moul DE, Franzen PL, Brar LK, Fletcher ME, et al. Efficacy of brief behavioral treatment for chronic insomnia in older adults. Arch Intern Med. 2011;171:887–95.

30. Hoelscher TJ, Edinger JD. Treatment of sleep-maintenance insomnia in older adults: sleep period reduction, sleep education, and modified stimulus control. Psychol Aging. 1988;3:258–63.

31. Thoresen CE, Coates TJ, Kirmil-Gray K, Rosekind MR. Behavioral self-management in treating sleep-maintenance insomnia. J Behav Med. 1981;4:41–52.

32. Morin CM, Kowatch RA, Barry T, Walton E. Cognitive-behavior therapy for late-life insomnia. J Consult Clin Psychol. 1993;61:137–46.

33. Morin CM. Insomnia: Psychological assessment and management. New York: Guilford Press; 1993.

34. Edinger JD, Hoelscher TJ, Marsh GR, Lipper S, Ionescu-Pioggia M. A cognitive-behavioral therapy for sleep-maintenance insomnia in older adults. Psychol Aging. 1992;7:282–9.

35. Mimeault V, Morin CM. Self-help treatment for insomnia: Bibliotherapy with and without professional guidance. J Consult Clin Psychol. 1999;67:511–9.

36. Morin C, Colecchi C, Stone J, Sood R, Brink D. Behavioral and pharmacological therapies for late-life insomnia: a randomized controlled trial. JAMA. 1999;281:991–9.

37. Morin CM, Sonte J, McDonald K, Jones S. Psychological management of insomnia—a clinical replication series with 100 patients. Behav Ther. 1994;25:291–309.

38. Morin CM, Culbert JP, Schwartz SM. Nonpharmacological interventions for insomnia—a metaanalysis of treatment efficacy. Am J Psychiatry. 1994;151:1172–80.

39. Murtagh DRR, Greenwood KM. Identifying effective psychological treatments for insomnia——a metaanalysis. J Consult Clin Psychol. 1995;63: 79–89.

40. Chesson AL, Anderson WM, Littner M, Davila D, Hartse K, Johnson S, et al. Practice parameters for the nonpharmacologic treatment of chronic insomnia. An American academy of sleep medicine report. Standards of practice committee of the American academy of sleep medicine. Sleep. 1999;22:1128–33.

41. Edinger JD, Wohlgemuth WK, Radtke RA, Marsh GR, Quillian RE. Cognitive behavioral therapy for treatment of chronic primary insomnia—A randomized controlled trial. JAMA. 2001;285:1856–64.

42. Smith MT, Perlis ML, Park A, Smith MS, Pennington J, Giles DE, et al. Comparative meta-analysis of pharmacotherapy and behavior therapy for persistent insomnia. Am J Psychiatry. 2002;159:5–11.

43. Stepanski EJ, Rybarczyk B. Emerging research on the treatment and etiology of secondary or comorbid insomnia. Sleep Med Rev. 2006;10:7–18.

44. Morgenthaler T, Kramer M, Alessi C, Friedman L, Boehlecke B, Brown T, et al. Practice parameters for the psychological and behavioral treatment of insomnia: an update. An american academy of sleep medicine report. Sleep. 2006;29:1415–9.

45. Edinger JD, Olsen MK, Stechuchak KM, Means MK, Lineberger MD, Kirby A, et al. Cognitive behavioral therapy for patients with primary insomnia or insomnia associated predominantly with mixed psychiatric disorders: a randomized clinical trial. Sleep. 2009;32:499–510.

46. Harvey AG. A cognitive model of insomnia. Behav Res Ther. 2002;40:869–93.

47. Pennebaker JW. Writing about emotional experiences as a therapeutic process. Psychol Sci. 1997;8:162–6.

48. Jansson-Frojmark M, Lind M, Sunnhed R. Don't worry, be constructive: A randomized controlled feasibility study comparing behaviour therapy singly and combined with constructive worry for insomnia. Brit J Clin Psychol. 2012;51:142–57.

49. Ong J, Sholtes D. A mindfulness-based approach to the treatment of insomnia. J Clin Psychol. 2010;66:1175–84.

50. Espie CA, Inglis SJ, Harvey L. Predicting clinically significant response to cognitive behavior therapy for chronic insomnia in general medical practice: Analyses of outcome data at 12 months posttreatment. J Consult Clin Psychol. 2001;69:58–99.

51. Harvey AG, Tang NKY. Cognitive behaviour therapy for primary insomnia: Can we rest yet? Sleep Med Rev. 2003;7:237–62.

52. Morin C, Vallières A, Guay B, Ivers H, Savard J, Mérette C, et al. Cognitive behavioral therapy, singly and combined with medication, for persistent insomnia: a randomized controlled trial. JAMA. 2009;301:2005–15.

53. Espie CA. « Stepped care »: A health technology solution for delivering cognitive behavioral therapy as a first line insomnia treatment. Sleep. 2009;32:1549–58.

54. Manber R, Carney C, Edinger J, Epstein D, Friedman L, Haynes PL, et al. Dissemination of CBTI to the non-sleep specialist: protocol development and training issues. J Clin Sleep Med. 2012;8:209–18.

55. Edinger JD, Sampson WS. A primary care "friendly" cognitive behavioral insomnia therapy. Sleep. 2003;26:177–82.

56. Espie CA, MacMahon KM, Kelly HL, Broomfield NM, Douglas NJ, Engleman HM, et al. Randomized clinical effectiveness trial of nurse-administered small-group cognitive behavior therapy for persistent insomnia in general practice. Sleep. 2007;30:574–84.

57. Espie CA, Kyle SD, Williams C, Ong JC, Douglas NJ, Hames P, et al. A randomized, Placebo-controlled trial of online cognitive behavioral therapy for chronic insomnia disorder delivered via an automated media-rich web application. Sleep. 2012;35:769–81.

58. Ritterband LM, Thorndike FP, Gonder-Frederick LA, Magee JC, Bailey ET, Saylor DK, et al. Efficacy of an Internet-based behavioral intervention for adults with insomnia. Arch Gen Psychiatry. 2009;66:692–8.

Modafinil: Development and Use of the Compound

61

Michel Billiard and Serge Lubin

Modafinil is a wake promoting drug which has transformed the treatment of excessive daytime sleepiness associated with narcolepsy. In this chapter we will consider three successive periods in the history of modafinil. The 1974–1992 period corresponds to the development of the compound and the first clinical trials in France, as well as the first studies on the mechanism of action in France and in Stanford. The 1993–2006 is the time of the large clinical trials performed in Canada and the USA, of the discovery of the prominent role of the dopamine transporter (DAT) in the mechanism of action of modafinil, and of the expansion of the indications of modafinil other than narcolepsy. The last period is initiated by the arrival of armodafinil, the R-enantiomer, as a complement in the armamentarium against narcolepsy.

1974–1992

The history of modafinil dates back to 1974 in France. As they were screening molecules in search of analgesics, two chemists from Lafon Ltd., a pharmaceutical company based in Maisons-Alfort, near Paris, Assous and Gombert, identified a new molecule, adrafinil [benzhydryl sulfinyl-2 acetohydroxamic acid], later passed on to two pharmacologists, Duteil and Rambert, also from Lafon Ltd. These pharmacologists observed that mice treated with this molecule were hyperactive [1] and foresaw a potential interest for it. Following further tests in mice and rats, and more refined pharmacology in dogs, the molecule was given to Jouvet for evaluation in the cat and to Milhaud and Klein for evaluation in the monkey. Interestingly, a decrease of sleep and an

increase of wakefulness were found by the first group and an increase of nocturnal activity by the second group. Eventually, in 1977–1978, Jouvet prescribed adrafinil to narcoleptic patients subjects with inconsistent results.

Meanwhile, in 1976, the kinetic of adrafinil led to the identification of an active metabolite, modafinil (2-[diphenylmethyl] sulfinyl] acetamide). Modafinil went through the same steps of development leading to the demonstration of a dose-dependent increase of locomotor activity in mice [2], an increase of wakefulness and a decrease of sleep in the cat [3], and an increase in nocturnal activity and in behavioural arousal without stereotyped behaviour in rhesus monkeys [4]. As soon as early 1983, Jouvet prescribed modafinil to narcoleptic patients and the results outdid the expectations. From then on, Jouvet continued to use modafinil with success in both narcoleptic and idiopathic hypersomnia patients subjects. In 1984, Lafon Ltd. decided to start clinical trials in both healthy volunteers [5, 6] and narcoleptic and idiopathic hypersomnia patients [7] under the leadership of Lubin and Weil, medical and clinical directors at Lafon Ltd.

As the Gulf War (August 1990–February 1991) was breaking out and French troops were to be sent to Iraq, the French Ministry of Defense demanded that Lafon Ltd. provide the French Army with modafinil, in view of testing the drug in normal military subjects before a possible use in military operations. The drug was tested in eight normal military subjects undergoing sleep deprivation for 60 h. Modafinil 200 mg or a placebo was given every 8 h for 3 days [8]. Results on cognitive tests were positive and no consistent adverse effect was recorded. In January 1991, the military doctors accompanying the "Daguet" operation (the name given to the French participation in the international coalition) were allowed to prescribe modafinil and the drug was used on 24–28 February 1991, during the Operation Desert Storm, mainly by military pilots and mechanics. Unfortunately, the prescriptions were not scientifically conducted, neither in terms of dosage nor in terms of timing, an aerial and ground combat zone not being the best environment to test a novel compound.

M. Billiard (✉)
Department of Neurology, Gui de Chauliac Hospital, 80, Avenue Augustin Fliche, 34295 Montpellier cedex 5, France
e-mail: mbilliard@orange.fr

S. Lubin
Former Medical Director of L. Lafon Laboratory, Maisons-Alfort, France

S. Chokroverty, M. Billiard (eds.), *Sleep Medicine*, DOI 10.1007/978-1-4939-2089-1_61,
© Springer Science+Business Media, LLC 2015

Following further open label studies conducted in different French sleep centres, the first multicenter, randomized, placebo-controlled trial of modafinil in hypersomnia patients subjects (33 men and 17 women) was performed [9]. Modafinil was administered in a double-blind cross-over design, at a dosage of 300 mg versus placebo and results judged through questionnaire on therapeutic effects, sleep log, polysomnography and MWT. An overall clinical benefit was noted by physicians as well as by subjects. Above all there was a significant improvement in the results of the MWT for patients on modafinil in comparison with placebo ($p < 0.05$).

Modafinil was officially registered for narcolepsy in France in June 1992 and became commercially available, also in France in September 1994.

After oral administration the maximal concentration of the product was reached within 2–4 h. The elimination half-life was 10–13 h. The adverse effects were relatively limited and not significant. These included headaches, irritability and insomnia, particularly at the onset of treatment. The compound was judged effective in 60–70 % of narcoleptic patients. It was prescribed at a dose of 100 mg in the morning and 100 mg at noon up to 400 mg/day.

Mechanism

Initially, it was thought that modafinil involved the stimulation of alpha-1 adrenergic mechanisms due to the ability of central alpha-1 antagonists such as prazosin or phenoxybenzamine to antagonize the modafinil-induced increase motor activity in mice [2] and wakefulness in cats [3]. However, the compound did not bind alpha-1 receptors in vitro and did not modify canine cataplexy, although canine cataplexy is very sensitive to compounds acting on adrenergic transmission [10].

On the other hand a systematic receptor screening revealed that modafinil did not bind to adenosine, choline, GABA, dopamine, norepinephrine and serotonin, but bound to the DA transporter (DAT) with low affinity [11]. This binding affinity was low, but not negligible, since modafinil did not bind to any other known receptor and since clinical doses of modafinil were high (up to several mg/kg in humans). At this stage it was not yet clear whether the binding of modafinil to the dopamine transporter had any functional effect on dopamine uptake [11].

1993 –2006

Clinical research in the USA on modafinil began in 1993 when Cephalon, Inc., a Pennsylvania-based biotechnology firm, licensed the rights to modafinil in the USA from its developer, Lafon Ltd.

From that time, Cephalon conducted preclinical and phase I studies on pharmacokinetics and mechanism of action that supplemented previous French research in these areas, while large scale clinical trials were performed. The first one was a Class II evidence study in 70 patients in Canada. It showed a significant decrease in the likelihood of falling asleep measured by the Epworth Sleepiness Scale, a reduction of severe excessive daytime sleepiness and irresistible episodes of sleep as assessed by the sleep log, and a significant improvement in maintaining wakefulness measured with the MWT, with both 200 and 400 mg/day [12]. The following ones were two Class I evidence studies in 285 and 273 patients respectively, which showed consistent improvements in subjective measures of sleepiness (ESS) and in clinical-assessed changes in the patient's condition (Clinical Global Impression), and significant improvement in maintaining wakefulness (MWT) and in decreasing sleepiness judged on the MSLT with both the 200 and the 400 mg/day doses [13, 14]. Overall modafinil exhibited a favourable adverse event profile in these studies, the most common adverse effects consisting of headache, nausea, nervousness and rhinitis.

The use of modafinil was approved by the Food and Drug Administration in 1998.

Three further studies dealt with open-label extension which showed positive treatment effects sustained for periods of 40 weeks [15]; 16 weeks [16] and 40 weeks [17]. As in previous trials modafinil was generally well tolerated in these studies. Moreover, abuse potential was low and post-marketed surveillance did not detect interest in modafinil as a drug of abuse.

Exceptional cases of serious or life-threatening rashes have been reported in adults and children in worldwide post-marketing experience. Teratology studies performed in animals did not show any evidence of harm to the foetus.

In 2004, the USA's indication for modafinil was expanded to include residual excessive daytime sleepiness in patients with obstructive sleep apnea/hypopnea syndrome, treated with nasal continuous positive airway pressure and sleepiness in shift work sleep disorder.

Mechanism

During this period a study measuring c-fos expression in the cat showed that amphetamines and methylphenidate produced diffuse activation of the striatum, the cortex and accumbens nuclei, whereas modafinil led to a relatively specific activation of the anterior hypothalamic sites which may be involved in the mechanisms of sleep and wakefulness [18]. But the most striking advance was a study using polygraphic recordings and caudate micro-dialysate measurements in narcoleptic dogs, which showed that modafinil and amphetamine increase extracellular dopamine [19]. Moreover DAT knock-out mice were completely unresponsive to the wake-promoting effects of amphetamines, DAT reuptake inhibitors and modafinil, confirming the critical role of DAT in mediating the wake-promoting effects of amphetamines and modafinil [19].

2007–2013

In 2007, a longer-acting form of modafinil, armodafinil, the R-enantiomer, was approved for the treatment of excessive sleepiness associated with narcolepsy, residual OSA and shift work disorder.

Armodafinil has a half-life of 10–14 h, whereas the S-enantiomer has a half-life of 3–4 h [20]. Modafinil has equal amounts of R and S-enantiomers, but the S-enantiomer is eliminated three times faster than the R-enantiomer and therefore most of the circulating compound is armodafinil. Armodafinil is well absorbed and peak levels are obtained after 2 h.

Doses of 150 mg and 250 mg of armodafinil, and placebo, were tested in 196 patients with narcolepsy. The MWT was the main endpoint. Significant improvements were seen at all time points for the 150 mg dose while statistical significance was not reached at 8 and 12 weeks for the 250 mg dose [21].

Mechanism

In 2009 and 2010 it was found that modafinil administered at wake-promoting doses can displace DAT positron emission tomography ligands in vivo, putting an end to the debate on its mechanism of action [22, 23], not meaning that other mechanisms of action of modafinil may not be involved.

Prescribing Modafinil/Armodafinil

A typical treatment with modafinil, (racemic mixture) in an adult with narcolepsy starts with 100 mg in the morning, and generally a second 100 mg dose at noon. The total dose can increase up to 400 mg/day. For R-modafinil, as the potency is approximately twice, the initial dose may be 50 mg or 100 mg in the morning to increase to as much as 250 mg in the morning. Occasionally it is helpful to add a short-acting drug, such as methylphenidate, in addition to modafinil, when modafinil needs to be supplemented at a specific time of the day, or in situations were maximum alertness is required. Modafinil and armodafinil are category C for pregnancy. The general recommendation is for patients to avoid taking modafinil or armodafinil during pregnancy unless the risk-benefit ratio suggests otherwise.

In conclusion, modafinil is a drug of choice to treat excessive daytime sleepiness associated with narcolepsy, residual sleepiness in obstructive sleep apnea syndrome and sleepiness in shift work disorder. It has also been tried on disease-related fatigue, attention-deficit disorder, age-related memory decline, depression. One of the present issues is whether modafinil should be used in healthy individuals to enhance their alertness or to mitigate fatigue.

References

1. Duteil J, Rambert FA, Pessonnier J, et al. A possible α-adrenergic mechanism for drug (CRL 40028)—induced hyperactivity. Eur J Pharmacol. 1979;59:121–23.
2. Duteil J, Rambert FA, Pessonnier J, et al. Central α-1-adrenergic stimulation in relation to the behaviour stimulating effect of modafinil: studies with experimental animals. Eur J Pharmacol. 1990;180:49–58.
3. Lin J, Roussel B, Akakoa H, et al. Role of catecholamines in the modafinil and amphetamine induced wakefulness, a comparative pharmacological study in the cat. Brain Res. 1992;591:19–26.
4. Hermant JF, Rambert FA, Duteil J. Awakening properties of modafinil effect on nocturnal activity in monkeys (Macaca mulatta) after acute and repeated administration. Psychopharmacology. 1991;103:28–32.
5. Goldenberg F, Weil JS, Von Frenckeel R. Effects of modafinil on diurnal variation of objective sleepiness in normal subjects. Sleep Res. 1987;16:91.
6. Saletu B, Frey R, Krupka M, et al. Differential effects of a new central adrenergic agonist modafinil and d-amphetamine on sleep and early morning behaviour in young healthy volunteers. Int J Clin Pharm Res. 1989;9:183–95.
7. Bastujji H, Jouvet M. Successful treatment of idiopathic hypersomnia and narcolepsy with modafinil. Prog Neuropsychopharmacol Biol Psychiatry. 1988;12:695–700.
8. Lagarde D, Batejat D, Van Beers P, et al. Interest of modafinil, a new psychostimulant, during a sixty-hour sleep deprivation experiment. Fundam Clin Pharmacol. 1995;9:271–79.
9. Billiard M, Besset A, Montplaisir J, et al. Modafinil: a double blind multicenter study. Sleep. 1994;17:S107–S112.
10. Shelton J, Nishino S, Vaught J, et al. Comparative effects of amphetamine and modafinil on cataplexy and daytime sleepiness in narcoleptic canines. Sleep Res. 1994;23:3.
11. Mignot E, Nishino S, Guilleminault C, et al. Modafinil binds to dopamine uptake carrier site with low affinity. Sleep. 1994;17:436–37.
12. Broughton RJ, Fleming JAE, George CFP, et al. Randomized, double-blind, placebo-controlled crossover trial of modafinil in the treatment of excessive daytime sleepiness in narcolepsy. Neurology. 1997;49:444–51.
13. U.S. Modafinil in Narcolepsy Multicenter Study Group. Randomized trial of modafinil for the treatment of pathological somnolence in narcolepsy. Ann Neurol. 1998;43:88–97.
14. U.S. Modafinil in Narcolepsy Multicenter Study Group. Randomized trial of modafinil as a treatment for the excessive daytime somnolence of narcolepsy. Neurology. 2000;54:1166–75.
15. Beusterien KM, Rogers AE, Walsleben JA, et al. Health-related quality of life effects of modafinil for treatment of narcolepsy. Sleep. 1999;22:557–65.
16. Moldofsky H, Broughton RJ, Hill JD. A randomized trial of the long-term, continued efficacy and safety of modafinil in narcolepsy. Sleep Med. 2000;1:109–16.

17. Mitler MM, Hirsh J, Hirshkowitz M, et al. Long-term efficacy and safety of modafinil (PROVIGIL®) for the treatment of excessive daytime sleepiness associated with narcolepsy. Sleep Med. 2000;1:231–43.

18. Lin JS, Hou Y, Jouvet M. Potential brain neuronal targets for amphetamine, methylphenidate, and modafinil-induced wakefulness, evidence by *c-fos* immunocytochemistry in the cat. Proc Nat Acad Sci U S A. 1996;93:1428–33.

19. Wisor JP, Nishino S, Sora I, et al. Dopaminergic role in stimulant-induced wakefulness. J Neurosci. 2001;21:1787–94.

20. Robertson P Jr, Hellriegel ET. Clinical pharmacokinetic profile of modafinil. Clin Pharmacokinet. 2003;42:123–37.

21. Harsh JR, Hayduk R, Rosenberg R, et al. The efficacy and safety of armodafinil as treatment for adults with excessive sleepiness associated with narcolepsy. Curr Med Res Opin. 2006;22:159–67.

22. Volkow ND, Fowler JS, Logan J, et al. Effects of modafinil on dopamine and dopamine transporters in the male human brain: clinical implications. JAMA. 2009;301:1148–54.

23. Spencer TJ, Madras BK, Bonab AA, et al. A positron emission tomography study examining the dopaminergic activity of armodafinil in adults using [11C] altropane and [11C] raclopride. Biol Psychiatry. 2010;68:964–70.

Phylogeny in Sleep Medicine

62

Kristyna M. Hartse

The "witchery of sleep" has historically been a topic of inquiry for many diverse scientific disciplines as well as a source of personal fascination for most people.

> The cry for sleep is ever greater than the cry for bread. Existence depends on both; but we eat to sleep, while we sleep to live. Sleep is of far greater importance than food for the preservation of life. [1, p. 21]

This mysterious brew of an as-yet-undeciphered formula of genetic, electrophysiological, psychological, neurochemical, and molecular events has been implicated in determining mortality and morbidity; in affecting mental and physical health; and in altering memory, cognition, and quality of life. The study of sleep, once confined almost exclusively to the scientific laboratory, has cultivated an entire specialized field of sleep disorders medicine. However, despite dramatic increases in knowledge about basic sleep mechanisms and human sleep disorders, the function and purpose of sleep still continue to remain touched by the diaphanous veil of witchery.

The universality of sleep, in fact, suggests that sleep serves an important biological function. Sleep has now been studied both behaviorally and electrophysiologically in a wide variety of organisms. The majority of sleep studies have been performed on familiar mammals such as mice, rats, cats, dogs, and humans. However, the phylogenetic study of sleep also encompasses nonmammalian organisms with wide variations in habitat, electrophysiology, and behavior. Insects, invertebrates, fish, birds, reptiles, amphibians, and monotremes (platypus and echidna) as well as more unusual mammals such as sloths, elephants, and cetaceans (whales and dolphins) have been studied behaviorally and in several cases electrophysiologically (for recent reviews, see [2–6]). By examining living organisms which have a long history represented in the fossil record, clues to the contribution of sleep in the survival of a species as well as the func-tion of sleep in living species might be determined. Here, we discuss specific findings which have emerged from phylogenetic studies, drawing primarily on nonmammalian organisms, and which have significance for unraveling human sleep disorders.

The Definition of Sleep

The behavioral criteria for defining sleep are well known, and the application of these criteria permits the identification of sleep in diverse species. These criteria include: (1) a species-specific posture, (2) behavioral quiescence, (3) elevated arousal thresholds, (4) state reversibility to distinguish sleep from coma or torpor, and (5) a homeostatic response to sleep deprivation [4]. There is well-known electrophysiology which occurs in conjunction with these behavioral criteria. Nonrapid eye movement sleep (NREM), defined by the presence of high-amplitude slow waves, occurs in cyclic alteration with rapid eye movement (REM) or paradoxical (PS) sleep, defined by the presence of REMs, skeletal muscle atonia, increases in brain temperature, male penile erections, and, in humans, mental activity. Since there is a close relationship between behavior and electrophysiology in mammals, electrophysiology substitutes for visual observations of the sleeping state in virtually all mammalian studies.

The high-amplitude slow waves of mammalian NREM sleep are not a well-defined electrophysiological feature during behavioral quiescence in nonmammalian vertebrates with the exception of birds [7]. This is not surprising given the absence of the thick neocortical layer responsible for generating slow waves in nonmammalian vertebrates. Additionally, REM sleep has not been convincingly demonstrated in nonmammalian organisms with the exception of brief REM sleep bouts, usually lasting less than 10 s, in birds. There have been relatively few electrophysiological recordings, with the exceptions of birds and reptiles, performed during behavioral quiescence in nonmammalian vertebrates. However, in contrast to the reliable expression of REM sleep

K. M. Hartse (✉)
Sonno Sleep Centers, El Paso, TX, USA

S. Chokroverty, M. Billiard (eds.), *Sleep Medicine,* DOI 10.1007/978-1-4939-2089-1_62,
© Springer Science+Business Media, LLC 2015

545

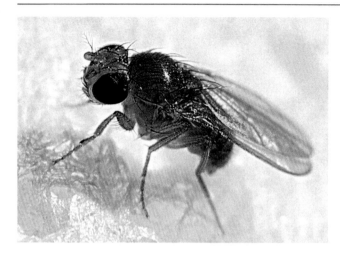

Fig. 62.1 A model organism for the study of sleep, *Drosophila mela-nogaster*. (Photo used with permission of Max Westby on Flickr)

in mammals, a wide spectrum of electrophysiology during behavioral sleep has been reported in nonmammals. These variations include an absence of electrical activity during behavioral wakefulness and isolated spikes or spike trains during behavioral quiescence in the octopus [8]; spikes during behavioral wakefulness and slower waves of 15–20 Hz in the crayfish [9]; a decline in local field potentials during behavioral quiescence in the fruit fly [10, 11]; high-amplitude spikes during behavioral sleep which disappear during behavioral waking in turtles, tortoises, lizards, and caimans [12–15]; and recently spindle-like activity during behavioral quiescence in the frog [16]. These differences from mammalian sleep electrophysiology have raised the issue of whether nonmammalian organisms exhibit "true" sleep. This debate has been particularly vigorous with respect to reptilian sleep [17, 18] since various investigators have reported the presence of slow waves characteristic of NREM sleep [19], the presence of REM sleep [20], the presence of slow waves during waking [21], and the presence of high-amplitude spikes during behavioral sleep which appear analogous to spikes recorded in the ventral hippocampus of mammals during slow-wave sleep (SWS) [14, 22]. These specific controversies are not reviewed here, but rather we examine those findings from phylogenetic studies which can provide insight into human sleep disorders.

Model Systems in the Study of Sleep

Studying sleep in new or unusual nonmammalian organisms is of intrinsic interest for understanding the diversity of behavioral and electrophysiological expressions which sleep can take in the animal world. Unfortunately, most nonmammalian phylogenetic studies have not substantially advanced our understanding of the specific genetic or molecular mech-

anisms which control the presence or absence of sleep. A recent extensive review by Toth and Bhargava [23] underlines the fact that mammals, including rats, mice, cats, and dogs, have most commonly served as subjects to study sleep. However, nonmammalian organisms, specifically the fruit fly (*Drosophila melanogaster*), the zebrafish (*Danio rerio*), and the nematode roundworm (*Caenorhabditis elegans*), share a large number of genetic homologues with humans, and they have provided powerful biological models for unraveling the complex molecular and genetic mechanisms which control not only human disease but also sleep mechanisms [24–27].

Drosophila (Fig. 62.1), which has arguably been used more than any other model organism for evaluating the genetics and neurochemistry of sleep, offers several practical advantages [28]. Flies, which have a well-studied genome, are readily available experimental organisms, and large colonies can be maintained in a relatively small space with cost efficiency as compared to most mammals. Furthermore, the life span and reproductive cycle are short, allowing for timely analysis of multiple genetic and molecular interventions, and the resulting large populations which can be generated increase statistical power in evaluating the effects of manipulations. Most major neurotransmitter systems including serotonin, dopamine, and epinephrine, which have been identified as having key roles in human sleep and waking, have also been identified in *Drosophila*. Zebrafish offers similar advantages as a model organism [29], and a recent detailed, quantified behavioral analysis of the roundworm (*C. elegans*) during the quiescent periods accompanying lethargus reinforces the use of this organism as a model for studying sleep [30].

Although there may be striking genetic similarities between these organisms and humans, a "model system" is a useful model only if the behavior of interest, sleep, is convincingly demonstrated to exist in these creatures. There are several lines of evidence which strongly suggest that the behavioral quiescence observed in *Drosophila* is analogous to sleep in humans and other mammals [28, 31]. First, the behavioral criteria for sleep are met in flies including a stereotypic posture during behavioral quiescence and elevated arousal thresholds. Deprivation of the quiescent state resulted in a homeostatic response, i.e., an increase in quiescence following deprivation of quiescence. The presence of sleep is also regulated by circadian clock genes. That this quiescent state following deprivation represents a sleep state different from a permutation in circadian clocks is indicated by a homeostatic response to rest deprivation in flies which were absent in the central clock gene, *period*. However, mutation of *timeless*, a second clock gene, did not result in a homeostatic response to deprivation [28, 31]. Further evidence comes from the response to drugs, including caffeine, modafinil, and methamphetamine, all of which produce alerting responses in *Drosophila*, similar to patterns of wakefulness in humans [32–34]. Antihistamines increase sleep amounts [31]. Finally, patterns of quiescence vary across the life span with age-related changes in sleep [35]. Thus, despite the apparent dissimilarity between *Drosophila* and humans, the fruit fly appears to be a good candidate for studying molecular and genetic sleep mechanisms potentially impacting sleep disorders.

There are several areas in which phylogenetic studies have provided new insights into sleep and the effects of sleep in humans.

Mortality/Aging/Insomnia

The connection between character and bedtime which grew up from association when human life was less complex than now has some counterpart in the world of butterflies and insects. The industrious bees go to bed much earlier than the roving wasps. The latter, which have been out stealing fruit and meat, and foraging on their own individual account, "knock in" at all hours til dark, and may sometimes be seen in a state of disgraceful intoxication, hardly able to find the way in at their own front door. The bees are all asleep by then in their communal dormitory. [36, p. 49]

It is well known that there are significant variations in sleep times throughout the animal kingdom [37]. The significance of these variations for determining life span or aging in various species or for promoting the survival of the species, however, is unclear. An important question, the answer to which is universally sought, is whether sleep duration has an impact on life span and mortality and whether life span can be extended by an optimal amount of sleep. In humans, there are now numerous epidemiological studies which suggest extremes of sleep length confer increased risk for mortality (for reviews, see [38–40]). Both short and long sleep times have been associated with increased mortality, and the best survival curves appear to be associated with a sleep duration of about 7 h per night. Somewhat surprisingly, in contrast to common recommendations for many years, 8 h or more of sleep per night has been reported to be associated with increased mortality [41]. Both short and long sleep has also been associated with the development of obesity, diabetes, hypertension, and cardiovascular disease [42]. The specific factors which produce these variations in mortality at both ends of the U-shaped spectrum are unknown. Although a causal relationship between sleep and mortality derived from epidemiological studies is an appealing one, a recent review raises the issue of whether variable methodologies and assumptions preclude any definitive conclusions about the relationship between sleep and mortality [43]. Of note is that very few polysomnographic studies have been performed over a prolonged period of time in a large number of subjects which suggest a relationship between mortality and sleep. In one study in adults followed up for a mean of 12.8 years, sleep latencies of greater than 30 min were associated with a 2.14 times greater mortality risk, and sleep efficiencies of less than 80 % were associated with a 1.93 times greater mortality risk [44]. More recently, polysomnographically determined sleep efficiency in subjective long sleepers with chronic heart failure predicted mortality [45]. To add to this mix on mortality and sleep duration, a dose–response relationship between hypnotics commonly used for insomnia treatment and an increased risk of death as well as an increased cancer risk for the most frequent hypnotic users has been reported [46]. Model systems may be excellent substrates to evaluate the significance of these findings on mortality.

Genetic mutants have been developed in the fruit fly to elucidate the molecular effects of sleep on mortality and aging. It would, of course, be of considerable interest to determine whether measures of sleep duration or sleep quality predict life span. *Minisleep* (*mns*), *Hyperkinetic* (*Hk*), *insomnia-like* (*ins-l*), and *Sleepless* (*sss*) are genetically engineered insomnia mutants which are each associated with marked reductions in total daily sleep time as compared to wild-type flies [47–51]. Even more striking is the finding that life span is reduced in short-sleeping flies, suggesting that sleep duration does, in fact, have a direct impact on longevity. It has been demonstrated that these mutations are mediated by *Shaker*, a gene which codes for the voltage-dependent potassium channel. In contrast to these findings, another short-sleeping mutant fly strain, *Fumin* (*fmn*), which has alterations in the dopamine transporter gene (DAT), has normal longevity, and *fmn* mutants do not exhibit a homeostatic response to sleep deprivation, suggesting that dopamine transporter activity is a critical element in sleep homeostasis [52]. Also of interest are the findings that a high-calorie diet in *fmn* mutants produces even further reductions in already-shortened sleep and markedly reduces longevity, suggesting that accelerated aging and shortened sleep are strongly influenced by elevated caloric intake [53]. Other studies also demonstrate that pharmacological and genetic manipulation of the dopaminergic system in *Drosophila* affects sleep and arousal [32]. Finally, mutations of the fragile X mental retardation gene (*Fmr1*) in *Drosophila* reveal that overexpression of *dFmr1* results in increased sleep amounts, and complete loss of *dFmr1* expression results in flies with significantly longer sleep amounts as compared to controls. Relevant to the short and long sleep associated with increased mortality in humans, both short- and long-sleeping flies had shortened life span [54]. Similar to *fmn* mutants, flies with both *dFmr1* overexpression and loss of expression did not exhibit a homeostatic rebound in sleep following 24 h of sleep deprivation.

These studies appear to be consistent with much of the data obtained from human studies and provide new insights into the specific genetic mechanisms which are responsible for short sleep. However, the literature has still not answered the specific question of how much sleep is required for a maximal life span. Some of this ambiguity is likely to be the result of technical issues in both human and *Drosophila* studies. For example, subtle differences in survey questioning presented by different investigators may lead to human over- or underestimation of sleep time [43]. In the case of the *Drosophila*, there may be significant variations in experimental conditions which produce inconsistent results relative to estimating life span [55, 56]. Seemingly minor factors, including the type of food and social isolation, can interact with genetic background to affect sleep variability in *Drosophila* [57]. Furthermore, the commonly studied Canton-S strain of flies obtained from different sources exhibits marked differences in total amounts of nighttime sleep depending upon the source of origin, and wild-caught flies from different climates and altitudes also show differences in sleep fragmentation with age [58]. Other nonmammalian studies suggest that various environmental conditions can significantly affect the expression of sleep. For example, differing electrophysiological manifestations of behavioral sleep in *Caiman sclerops* were found under differing environmental recording conditions, and indeed at least part of the differences in these studies may be directly traced to inadequate environmental adaptation [12, 19]. Social influences and diet can also affect sleep amounts, interact with genetic makeup, and potentially affect longevity in *Drosophila* [57, 59]. Changes in environmental conditions can improve sleep consolidation in old flies [60]. Finally, one of the most commonly used technologies in determining amounts of *Drosophila* sleep, the Drosophila Activity Monitoring System (DAMS), substantially overestimates amounts of fly sleep in comparison to more detailed digital video analysis [61].

The genetically and neurochemically engineered sleeplessness of fruit flies and zebrafish raises the issue of whether this sleeplessness is functionally comparable to sleepless-

ness as it occurs in nature. Recent studies in the Mexican cave fish (*Astyanax mexicanus*) shed new light on evolutionarily derived sleeplessness and provide new insights into the effect of habitat on the development of sleep and arousal systems ([62, 63]; Fig. 62.2). Surface- and cave-dwelling populations of these fish differ significantly in daily amounts of sleep with surface fish averaging more than 800 min and three different cave-dwelling populations averaging 110–250 min per day. Blockade of B-adrenergic receptors with propranolol produced a dose-dependent increase in total sleep time, an increase in sleep bout length, and a decrease in sleep bout number in cave fish without any effect at any dose on the sleep of surface-dwelling fish. B-1-, B-2-, and B-3-adrenergic antagonists did not affect sleep in surface dwellers, but cave fish sleep increased significantly in response only to the B-1 antagonist atenolol with a near statistically significant sleep increase in response to the B-3 antagonist SR59203A. Neuroanatomical studies demonstrated that the number of catecholamine neurons was conserved in cave fish as compared to surface-dwelling fish. These findings suggest that evolution has resulted in an increase in the adrenergic arousal system in the cave fish as compared to surface dwellers. Other recent studies in the killifish (*Nothobranchius korthausae*) and the three-spot wrasse (*Halichoeres trimaculatus*) provide evidence for the improvement in the circadian rhythmicity of aging fish and in the induction of quiescence by melatonin [64, 65].

In summary, human epidemiological studies suggest that sleep duration is associated with life span, and *Drosophila* studies indicate that this relationship is probably not as straightforward as determining a golden standard for nightly sleep duration, independent of other factors, for the maximization of life span. Genetics, social influences, and environmental factors, largely uncontrolled in human studies, clearly have a powerful influence on sleep amounts and, potentially, longevity. Furthermore, new studies in cave fish may provide a natural model of ecologically distinct sleeping and waking behaviors. Although there are methodological issues which contribute substantially to the findings on mortality and sleep in humans and even with findings from the *Drosophila* studies, an unambiguous answer to the question of how much sleep is necessary for maximum longevity still remains unanswered.

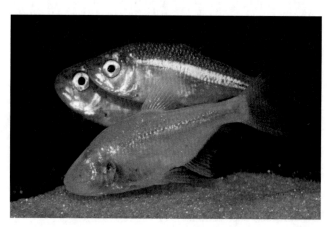

Fig. 62.2 Mexican cave fish (*Astyanax mexicanus*) surface dwelling (*top*) and cave dwelling (*bottom*). (Photo used with permission of Richard L. Borowsky, Ph.D.)

Pharmacological Development

The genetic correspondence between human disease genes and *Drosophila* genes offers a unique substrate for studying not only human disease processes but also sleep disorders [26]. Similarly, approximately 70 % of human genes have at least one zebrafish orthologue, and, as a result, zebrafish have been extensively used in developing human disease models [25, 66]. These correspondences between human genes and genes of model systems suggest that model organisms may be of importance in developing in vivo drug treatments at a molecular level for modifying or treating human sleep disorders. Screening of a large number of compounds utilizing behavioral measures of waking and quiescence in larval zebrafish have revealed important insights into mechanisms of drug action including the similar effects on waking and quiescence produced by major neurotransmitter pathways in both zebrafish and mammals, better prediction of the differential effects of poorly understood compounds on waking and quiescence, and identification of additional pathways of drug action on quiescence not previously known [67]. In *Drosophila*, amylase is a biomarker of increased sleep drive following sleep loss, and an increase in human salivary amylase demonstrates similar properties following sleep deprivation [34]. Furthermore, two *Drosophila* genes identified in *ins-l* mutants were modulated in their human homologues following human sleep deprivation [51].

These findings suggest that *Drosophila* could be effectively used to evaluate the effects of or to be utilized in the development of medications with alerting or sleep-inducing properties. In addition, pharmacological studies in other nonmammalian vertebrates, for example, fish [63–65] and reptiles [68, 69], suggest that these organisms may provide clues about the phylogenetic development of neurochemical mechanisms in the control of sleeping and waking. Although molecular studies in model systems suggest the development of more effective treatments for insomnia, this promise has not been fully realized in the development of safe, effective, widely used, well-tolerated treatments for humans.

Sleep Disorders

Narcolepsy

There has been remarkable progress in understanding the underlying causes of narcolepsy which has resulted directly from animal research (for recent reviews, see [70] and [71]). The discovery of orexin (hypocretin) deficiency resulting from the loss of orexigenic neurons in narcoleptic dogs and mice and the subsequent discovery of the human leukocyte antigen DQB1*0602 and DQA1*0102 in almost all patients with narcolepsy have led to the conclusion that narcolepsy is an autoimmune disease. However, the mechanism or mechanisms by which orexin depletion occurs is still unknown, although upper airway infections and H1N1 flu vaccination in genetically susceptible individuals have been identified as potential environmental triggers in this process [72, 73].

Potentially effective treatments for narcolepsy arising out of animal studies appear to be within the closest reach. Gene replacement therapy in orexin-deficient mice restores sleep consolidation and the timing of REM sleep, but does not improve cataplexy [74], whereas gene transfer into the zona incerta in orexin-deficient mice improved cataplexy, but did not improve sleep fragmentation [75]. In humans, an orexin antagonist has recently been demonstrated to improve sleep in insomniac humans [76]. Gene therapy clinical trials are now being performed worldwide for a number of human diseases including, for example, cancer, cardiovascular diseases, Parkinson's disease, and cystic fibrosis [77]. Unlike current narcolepsy drug treatments which target symptom improvement in excessive daytime sleepiness, the results of gene transfer therapy in animal models suggest that this approach has the potential to produce a treatment which targets the molecular and cellular deficits in human narcolepsy.

It does not seem likely that nonmammalian models of narcolepsy are on the horizon, in large part because, with the exception of birds which have very brief bouts of REM sleep, REM sleep has not been convincingly demonstrated. Although the zebrafish does not exhibit behavioral characteristics of narcolepsy per se, the overexpression of hypocretin/orexin as well as null mutations for hypocretin/orexin produce increases in locomotor activity, decreases in arousal thresholds, and shortened, fragmented sleep in the dark [78, 79]. Also of interest is that Yokogawa and colleagues [79], during the course of evaluating hypocretin receptor mutants, demonstrated that normal adult zebrafish maintained under constant light conditions exhibit an almost complete suppression of sleep. There was no homeostatic rebound in response to this sleep suppression, but a progressive return to sleep occurred after 1–2 weeks. Similarly, following sleep deprivation with electrical stimulation, no sleep rebound occurred upon release into light, but release into darkness resulted in a homeostatic sleep rebound. Exposure to light alone during the last 6 h of the biological night resulted in a marked suppression of sleep without a subsequent rebound upon release into darkness. These findings raise the issue of whether these anomalies in sleep homeostasis and sleep suppression in response to light are factors which may decrease the usefulness of the zebrafish as a model organism for the study of human disorders such as narcolepsy. Additionally, both the absence of behaviors such as cataplexy in the zebrafish and the absence of REM sleep suggest that this model system is unlikely to offer significant advantages beyond the current mammalian models in exploring narcolepsy.

Sleep Apnea

Insomnia is the most common sleep complaint, typically occurring in about one third of the population, but sleep apnea has more visibly alarming and recognizable symptoms including loud snoring, periods of observable breath holding, vigorous movements, and excessive daytime sleepiness. Often, these symptoms are not recognized as having direct links to cardiovascular disease, metabolic disorders, and cognitive deficits, thus increasing the potential medical complications related to sleep apnea. A familial, and possibly a genetic, component to sleep apnea has been recognized for several years [80–82]. A naturally occurring model of sleep apnea has been described in the English bulldog which has crowded upper airway anatomy similar to human sleep apnea patients [83], and sleep apnea has been reported in obese miniature pigs [84]. However, sleep apnea has not been described in nonmammalian organisms.

Through artificial occlusion of the airway and exposure to repetitive hypoxemia, induced sleep apnea in dog, rat, and mice preparations has been used to demonstrate the physiologic effects of sleep apnea [85–88]. These mammalian studies have shed new light on, for example, the cardiovascular and neurochemical consequences of sleep apnea [89, 90], but model organisms have not been forthcoming in determining the genetic basis for the mechanisms of this disorder. Given the myriad of factors which impact the expression of sleep apnea including age, obesity, gender, and factors such as alcohol consumption in addition to influences on cardiovascular, metabolic, and respiratory systems, it seems likely that a different animal model will be required. No genome-wide association studies (GWAS) which involve scanning the DNA of a large population to determine specific genetic markers of a particular disease, in this case sleep apnea, have been performed. The gene encoding the allele APOE e4, which plays a critical role in cholesterol metabolism and transport, has been associated with obstructive sleep apnea in both adults and children, but a meta-analysis of studies examining APOE and sleep apnea concluded that the evidence for this association is weak [91]. In an additional meta-analysis of sleep apnea, genetic association studies revealed only one association, TNFA rs1800629, which was significantly associated with obstructive sleep apnea [92]. Thus, the molecular basis of sleep apnea remains murky in humans, and animal studies or model systems have not, to date, added significant clarification to the genetic or neurochemical basis of this disorder.

Restless Legs Syndrome

There have been substantial advances in understanding the genetic underpinnings of restless legs syndrome in humans, largely as the result of large-scale GWAS. Genetic loci have been identified at *MEIS1, BTBD9,* and *MAP2K5/SKOR1* which are associated with increased risk for restless legs syndrome [93–95]. Naturally occurring restless legs or periodic limb movements have not been described in either the mammalian or nonmammalian animal literature. However, the identification of these human genetic loci has stimulated

the development of a *Drosophila* model of restless legs syndrome [96].

The criteria for identifying restless legs syndrome are well known, and include an overwhelming urge to move the legs, an improvement in the sensations of discomfort with movement, a worsening of the sensation with inactivity, and a worsening of the sensation in the evening hours [97]. Patients with restless legs syndrome typically have difficulty falling asleep, experience fragmented nighttime sleep, and as a result complain of daytime fatigue. Iron deficiency is thought to be a major factor in the expression of restless legs, and dopamine agonists, including pramipexole and ropinirole, are now the recommended treatments for restless legs syndrome [98].

The sensation of restlessness and discomfort, a key feature of restless legs syndrome, cannot, of course, be communicated by *Drosophila*. However, since these uncomfortable sensations in humans are accompanied by vigorous movements of the legs, the measurement of movement can be operationally used to evaluate such an animal model of restless legs. Following genetic alterations of the fly homologue (*dBTBD9*) which corresponds to human *BTBD9*, mutant dBTBD9 flies revealed, in comparison to controls, significant disruptions in sleep and an increase in movement time. Average sleep bout lengths decreased, the number of bouts increased, and the amount of wake after sleep increased, mirroring features of the disturbed sleep in restless legs syndrome. When mutant flies were enclosed in a restricted space, they became hyperactive with longer bouts of walking in comparison to controls, similar to the motor restlessness present in human subjects during immobility. Although *dBTBD9* expression could not be determined in *Drosophila* dopaminergic neurons similar to the *BTBD9* expression in dopaminergic neurons located in the substantial nigra of the human brain, there was a 50 % reduction in total dopamine levels in dBTBD9 in *Drosophila* brains as compared to controls, suggesting that BTBD9 plays a role in dopamine synthesis. Additional manipulations suggest that BTBD9 regulates ferritin levels via an iron regulatory protein. Finally, the dopamine agonist, pramipexole, which is an effective treatment for human restless legs syndrome, restored bout number, bout length, and wake after sleep onset to control levels in these *Drosophila* mutants.

The results of this study provides evidence for the first molecular interventions into the expression of restless legs syndrome. It would be of interest, for example, to determine if these mutants with a specific alteration of BTBD9 resulting in a model restless legs syndrome exhibit shortened life span in conjunction with their shortened sleep. These new insights into the gene expression of restless legs syndrome and the role of dopamine agonists are clearly a major advance in potentially elaborating upon effective treatments in humans.

Unusual Sleep Disorders

Another less well-understood category of sleep disorders, the parasomnias, are also associated with sleep disruption. However, in these disorders, which include sleepwalking and REM sleep behavior disorder (RBD), complex, vigorous, undesirable violent or dramatic motor activity, and vocalizations can intrude into sleep [99]. However, little is known about the prevalence or the mechanisms which trigger the development of these behaviors. Recent epidemiological studies suggest that some parasomnias, specifically sleepwalking and RBD, may be somewhat more common than previously suspected. In adults 18 years of age or older, the lifetime prevalence of sleepwalking has been estimated at 29.2 % [100], and it has been recently estimated, based upon interview and attended polysomnography with simultaneous video monitoring, that the prevalence of RBD in a Korean elderly population is 2.01 % and subclinical RBD is 4.95 % [101].

There has been very little animal research in this area, although pontine tegmental brain-stem lesion studies in cats result in "dream enacting" behavior suggestive of the more recently described RBD in humans [102, 103]. Not surprisingly, there does not appear to be a naturally occurring model of parasomnias in the animal world. There are, however, clues from phylogenetic studies which may provide insight into the incongruous behavior of persons who are electrophysiologically asleep, but who exhibit apparent waking behavior.

There are interesting variations in both nonmammalian and mammalian sleep which do not fit the typical concept of sleep as a global state, i.e., an organism is either exclusively awake or exclusively asleep. These variations might be most accurately described as "nonquiescent" or literally "active" sleep, suggesting the temporal coexistence of both sleep and waking in the same neural substrate. For example, nocturnal "sleep-swimming fish" which occupy coral reefs in the Red Sea vigorously move the dorsal, pectoral, and caudal fins during fixed body positions. The frequency of fin strokes is approximately twice the rate occurring with daytime swimming outside the coral reef, suggesting that this behavior aerates the reef and ensures healthy corals [104]. Killer whale and bottlenose dolphin neonates as well as their mothers do not exhibit signs of behavioral sleep for several months post partum [105]. Perhaps the most striking example of coexisting waking and sleep occurs during unihemispheric sleep, a state in which one hemisphere of the brain exhibits waking electroencephalographic (EEG) activity simultaneously with sleeping EEG activity in the other hemisphere. Unihemispheric sleep has been recorded in dolphins [106], whales [107], fur seals [108], and birds [7], and the ability to experience unihemispheric sleep may offer significant advantages, for example, during migration over long distances [109].

Unihemispheric sleep is probably not simply a physiological oddity of nature in a restricted number of nonhuman species. Recent human electrophysiological studies utilizing scalp, intracerebral EEG, and unit recordings support the regionality of sleep electrophysiology [110]. A majority of slow waves, 85 %, were detected in less than 50 % of recording sites as were 75.8 % of spindles, indicating that both of these waveforms were represented locally rather than globally across the entire spectrum of the brain. The regionality of human sleep waveforms in addition to those examples of nonhuman unihemispheric sleep suggests that the comingling of waking and sleep in the same organism may have an electrophysiological basis which could help explain parasomnias such as sleepwalking or RBD. Other recent reports in humans support this possibility. In patients undergoing evaluation for pharmacoresistant focal epilepsy and who had no reported sleep disorders, simultaneous periods of cortical activation lasting from 5 to more than 60 s as recorded from intracerebral electrodes in the motor cortex occurred simultaneously with an increase in slow-wave activity in the dorsolateral prefrontal cortex EEG [111]. Further electrophysiological evidence for this comingling of waking and sleep comes from a single subject with confusional nocturnal arousals [112]. The neurological and magnetic resonance imaging (MRI) findings were normal, and antiepileptic drugs had failed to resolve the episodes. Stereotaxically implanted electrodes revealed localized activation of the motor, cingulate, insular, temporopolar, and amygdalar cortices in the presence of slow waves recorded from the frontal and parietal dorsolateral cortices as well as spindles in the hippocampal cortex during these episodes.

It could be speculated that these human electrophysiological studies provide hints that the behavior and brain activity during some parasomnias might represent a variation on nonhuman unihemispheric sleep. They also suggest that the temporal coexistence of electrophysiologically identified brain activation and sleep is possible in humans. Of course, further study of both unihemispheric sleep and the electrical activity of the human brain during unusual arousal disorders will be required before any analogies between regional brain activity in animals and humans can be made. Nonetheless, colloquial reports of sleeping with "one eye open" may have a basis in electrophysiology.

Conclusions

To know something of that condition in which we spend one-third of our lives, is not an unworthy inquiry. *And* yet the thought may at first occur to you,—What can be better known than *sleep?*—a thing of which we have all of us common experience. But simple *and* obvious as it may seem to be, we shall find that the more we investigate it, the more is it productive of topics for interesting *and* curious speculation, *and* of questions not very easily answered. [113]

Phylogenetic sleep studies have provided striking new insights into the mechanisms and importance of sleep in many different animals. An important question is whether studies in nonmammalian organisms have added to our understanding of why we sleep and whether our understanding of human sleep disorders has been, if not clarified, enriched by these studies. At the forefront in today's research are the model sleep systems, most notably the fruit fly and the zebrafish, which allow for sophisticated genetic and molecular manipulations. These studies have allowed the field to move from inference and deduction about the mechanisms controlling sleep to a much more precise understanding of specific elements controlling sleep. Importantly, these studies have emphasized the importance of scientific rigor in understanding sleep mechanisms beyond careful behavioral observation and electrophysiological investigations which characterized the early studies in phylogeny. Although it is undoubtedly the case that our understanding of sleep genetics and molecular control have been advanced by model systems, there are significant areas of discussion which arise as a result of these studies.

Are model systems truly "models" for understanding human sleep disorders? Similar molecular and neurochemical systems are present in humans and model organisms. However, a collection of genes and molecules is not equivalent to a complex disease process with psychological or psychiatric overlays as, for example, in many cases of persistent insomnia. The behavior and environment of fruit flies, zebrafish, or worms obviously do not mimic or even approach the complexity of environmental, psychological, and social factors which impact human sleep. In addition, the diagnosis of human sleep disorders is heavily dependent upon patient and bed-partner descriptions of symptoms. Although neurochemistry and genetics have clearly been invaluable in elucidating mechanisms, this approach will not necessarily produce a model equivalent of a human sleep disorder such as, for example, restless legs syndrome. Other data suggest possible fundamental differences between human sleep and model organisms, suggesting that there may be an incomplete modeling of some aspects of sleep. The absence of homeostatic rebounds in some short-sleeping *Drosophila* following deprivation of quiescence or the marked suppression of sleep by light in the zebrafish suggest that these models do not, in fact, model all aspects of most mammalian sleep. The concept of a "partial model" may be worthy of consideration. Another issue, particularly in regard to sleep disorders, is that the effects of molecular and genetic manipulations in model systems cannot be examined with respect to either electrophysiological influences on NREM and REM sleep. The question still remains as to whether the measurement of sleep by behavioral measures alone can be meaningfully extrapolated to elucidating the causes for human sleep prob-

lems or whether the detailed gene manipulations which are currently not possible in humans are powerful enough to nullify this concern.

Does information about detailed molecular and genetic sleep mechanisms translate into more effective treatments for human sleep disorders? A further, and arguably more important, issue is whether the results of nonhuman studies in fact translate into effective treatments for management of sleep disorders. To date, routine, effective, safe treatments have not emerged, even in the case of narcolepsy which has been more thoroughly studied than any other sleep disorder in animals. Ideally, the detailed understanding of sleep mechanisms will be used to deploy more effective treatments. Genetic screens for sleep disorders might also be another potential beneficial outcome of nonhuman studies.

What do phylogenetic studies tell us about both normal and disturbed human sleep? Nonmammalian organisms frequently challenge our concept of what constitutes normal sleep. Unihemispheric sleep, for example, which has been considered to be somewhat of an oddity in a limited number of animals may, in fact, provide a substrate for further exploration of arousal disorders during human sleep. Nonquiescent behavior during sleep such as in sleep-swimming fish, or the presence of unusual sleep-related EEG waveforms such as reptilian spikes, suggests that there is potentially great diversity in both the behavior and electrophysiology of sleep which may still be undiscovered in nonmammalian organisms and which may be of benefit in understanding the diversity of sleep in humans. New techniques in phylogenetic sleep studies continue to develop and hold promise for elaborating upon the diversity of sleep. Ostriches have been behaviorally and electrophysiologically evaluated in their natural habitat [114] as have rain-forest-dwelling sloths [115]. Technical improvements in tracking *Drosophila* activity utilizing green fluorescent protein with three-dimensional (3-D) video monitoring hold promise for more refined analyses of behavior, and a new technique utilizing an array of aqueous droplets, rather than an agar surface, for studies in the roundworm, *C. elegans,* suggests a more efficient technique for evaluation of manipulations [116, 117].

Phylogenetic sleep studies have, without a doubt, increased our understanding of genetic, molecular, and environmental factors governing the expression of sleep in humans. More broadly, they have enriched our understanding of the diverse behavioral and electrophysiological aspects of sleep in living organisms. However, the answer to the question of why we sleep is still unanswered by these studies, even though there are clearly answers to multiple niches of this question. The "witchery of sleep" will continue to propel research forward in the search for the answer.

Referrences

1. Moyer W. The witchery of sleep. New York: Ostermoor; 1903.
2. Allada R, Siegel J. Unearthing the phylogenetic roots of sleep. Curr Biol. 2008;18:R670–8.
3. Crocker A, Sehgal A. Genetic analysis of sleep. Genes Develop. 2010;24:1220–35.
4. Hartse KM. The phylogeny of sleep. In: Montagna P, Chokroverty S, volume editors. Handbook of clinical neurology, vol 98 (3rd series) sleep disorders part I. New York: Elsevier B.V.; 2011. pp. 97–109.
5. McNamara P, Barton RA, Nunn CL, editors. Evolution of sleep. Phylogenetic and functional perspectives. New York: Cambridge University Press; 2010.
6. Tobler I. Phylogeny of sleep regulation. In: Kryger MH, Roth T, Dement WC, editors. Principles and practice of sleep medicine, 5th edn. St. Louis: Elsevier Saunders; 2011. pp. 112–25.
7. Rattenborg NC, Amlaner CJ. A bird's eye view of the function of sleep. In: McNamara P, Barton RA, Nunn CL, editors. Evolution of sleep. Phylogenetic and functional perspectives. New York: Cambridge University press; 2010. pp. 145–71.
8. Brown ER, Piscopo S, DeStefano R, Gioditta A. Brain and behavioural evidence for rest-activity cycles in *Octopus vulgaris*. Behav Brain Res. 2006;172:335–9.
9. Mendoza-Angeles K, Hernandez-Falcon J, Ramon F. Slow waves during sleep in crayfish. Origin and spread. J Exp Biol. 2010;213:2154–64.
10. Nitz DA, Van Swinderen B, Tonono G, Greenspan RJ. Electrophysiological correlates of rest and activity in *Drosophila melanogaster*. Curr Biol. 2002;12:1934–40.
11. Van Alphen B, Yap MHW, Kirszenblat L, Kottler B, van Swindern B. A dynamic deep sleep stage in *Drosophila*. J Neurosci. 2013;33:6917–27.
12. Flanigan WF. Sleep and wakefulness in iguanid lizards, *Ctenosaura pectinata and Iguana iguana*. Brain Behav Evol. 1973;8:401–36.
13. Flanigan WF. Sleep and wakefulness in chelonian reptiles. II. The red-footed tortoise, *Geochelone carbonaria*. Arch Ital Biol. 1974;112:253–77.
14. Flanigan WF, Wilcox RH, Rechtschaffen A. The EEG and behavioral continuum of the crocodilian, *Caiman sclerops*. Electroenceph Clin Neurophys. 1973;34:521–38.
15. Flanigan WF, Knight CP, Hartse KM, Rechtschaffen A. Sleep and wakefulness in chelonian reptiles. I. The box turtle, *Terrapene carolina*. Arch Ital Biol. 1974;112:227–52.
16. Fang G, Chen Q, Cui J, Tang Y. Electroencephalogram bands modulated by vigilance states in an anuran species: a factor analysis approach. J Comp Physiol A. 2012;198:119–27.
17. Rattenborg NC. Evolution of slow-wave sleep and palliopallial connectivity in mammals and birds: a hypothesis. Brain Res Bull. 2006b;69:20–9.
18. Rial RV, Nicolau MC, Gamundi A, Akaarir M, Garau C, Aparicio S. et al. Letter to the editor. Comments on evolution of slow wave sleep and palliopallial connectivity in mammals and birds: a hypothesis. Brain Res Bull. 2007;72:183–6.
19. Warner BF, Huggins SE. An electroencephalographic study of sleep in young caimans in a colony. Comp Biochem Physiol. 1978;59A:139–44.
20. Ayala-Guerrero F, Mexicano G. Sleep and wakefulness in the green iguanid lizard (*Iguana iguana*). Comp Biochem Physiol A Mol Integr Physiol. 2008;151:305–12.
21. DeVera L, Gonzalez J, Rial RV. Reptilian waking EEG: slow waves, spindles and evoked potentials. Electroenceph Clin Neurophysiol. 1994;90:298–303.
22. Hartse KM, Eisenhart SF, Bergmann BM, Rechtschaffen A. Hippocampal spikes during sleep, wakefulness, and arousal in the cat. Sleep. 1979;1:231–46.
23. Toth LA, Bhargova P. Animal models of sleep disorders. Comp Med. 2013;63:91–104.
24. Bier E. *Drosophila*, the golden bug, emerges as a tool for human genetics. Nat Rev Genet. 2005;6:9–23.
25. Howe K, Clark MD, Torroja CF, Torrance J, Berthelot C, Muffato M, Collins JE, et al. The zebrafish reference genome sequence and its relationship to the human genome. Nature. 2013;496:498–503.
26. Reiter LT, Potocki L, Chien S, Gribskov M, Bier E. A systematic analysis of human disease associated gene sequences in *Drosophila melanogaster*. Genome Res. 2013;11:1114–25.
27. Rubin, GM, Yandell MD, Wortman JR, Gabor Miklos GL, Nelson CR, Hariharan IK, et al. Comparative genomics of the eukaryotes. Science. 2000;287:2204–15.
28. Hendricks JC, Finn SM, Panckeri KA, Chavkin J, Williams JA, Sehgal A, Pack AI. Rest in *Drosophila* is a sleep-like state. Neuron. 2000;25:129–38.
29. Zhdanova IV. Sleep and its regulation in zebrafish. Rev Neurosci. 2011;22:27–36.
30. Iwanir S, Tramm N, Nagy S, Wright C, Ish D, Biron D. The microarchitecture of *C. elegans* behavior during lethargis: homeostatic bout dynamics, a typical body posture, and regulation by a central neuron. Sleep. 2013;36:385–95.
31. Shaw PJ, Cirelli C, Greenspan RJ, Tononi G. Correlated of sleep and waking in *Drosophila melanogaster*. Science. 2000;287:1834–7.
32. Andretic R, Van Swindern B, Greenspan RJ. Dopaminergic modulation of arousal in *Drosophila*. Curr Biol. 2005:15:1165–75.
33. Hendricks JC, Kirk D, Panckeri KA, Miller MS, Pack AI. Modafinil maintains waking in the fruit fly *Drosophila melanogaster*. Sleep. 2003;26:139–46.
34. Seugnet L, Boera J, Gottschalk L, Duntley S, Shaw PJ. Identification of a biomarker for sleep drive in flies and humans. Proc Natl Acad Sci U S A. 2006;103:19913–8.
35. Koh K, Evans JM, Hendricks JC, Sehgal A. A *Drosophila* model for age-associated changes in sleep-wake cycles. Proc Nat Acad Sci U S A. 2006;103:13843–7.
36. Cornish CJ. The naturalist on the Thames. London: Seeley and Col. Ltd; 1902.
37. Zeplin H, Siegel JM, Tobler I. Mammalian sleep. In Kryger MH, Roth T, Dement WC, editors. Principals and practice of sleep medicine (4th edition). Philadelphia: WB Saunders; 2005. pp. 91–100.
38. Cappuccio FP, D'Ela L, Strazzullo P, Miller MA. Sleep duration and all cause mortality: a systematic review and meta-analysis of prospective studies. Sleep. 2010;33:585–92.
39. Grandner MA, Drummond SPA. Who are the long sleepers? Towards an understanding of the mortality relationship. Sleep Med Rev. 2007;11:341–60.
40. Grandner MA, Hale L, Moore M, Patel NP. Mortality associated with short sleep duration: the evidence, the possible mechanisms, and the future. Sleep Med Rev. 2010;14:191–203.
41. Kripke DF, Garfinkel L, Wingard DL, Klauber MR, Marler MR. Mortality associated with sleep duration and insomnia. Arch Gen Psychiatry. 2002;59:131–6.
42. Buxton OM, Marcelli E. Short and long sleep are positively associated with obesity, diabetes, hypertension, and cardiovascular disease among adults in the United States. Social Sci Med. 2010;71:1027–36.
43. Kurina LM, McClintock MK, Chen J-H, Waite LJ, Thisted RA, Lauderdale DS. Sleep duration and all-cause mortality: a critical review of measurement and associations. Ann Epidem. 2013;23:361–70.

44. Dew MA, Hoch CC, Buysse DJ, Monk TH, Begley AE, Houck PR, et al. Healthy older adults' sleep predicts all-cause mortality at 4 to 19 years of follow up. Psychosom Med. 2003;65:63–73.

45. Reinhard W, Plappert N, Zeman F, Hengstenberg C, Riegger G, Novack V, Maimon N, Pfeifer M, Arzt M. Prognostic impact of sleep duration and sleep efficiency on mortality in patients with chronic heart failure. Sleep Med. 2013;14:502–9.

46. Kripke DF, Langer RD, Kline LE. Hypnotic association with mortality or cancer: a matched cohort study. BMJ Open. 2012;2:e00850.

47. Bushey D, Huber R, Tononi G, Cirelli C. *Drosophila* hyperkinetic mutants have reduced sleep and impaired memory. J Neurosci. 2007;270:5384–93.

48. Bushey D, Hughes KA, Tononi G, Cirelli C. Sleep, aging and lifespan in *Drosophila*. BMC Neurosci. 2010;11:1471–2202.

49. Cirelli C, Bushey D, Hill S, Huber R, Kreber R, Ganetzky B, Tonono G. Reduced sleep in *Drosophila* Shaker mutants. Nature. 2005;434:1087–92.

50. Koh K, Joiner WJ, Wu MN, Yue Z, Smith CJ, Sehgal A. Identification of SLEEPLESS, a sleep-promoting factor. Science. 2008;321:372–6.

51. Seugnet L, Suzuki Y, Thimgan M, Donlea J, Gimbel SI, Gottschalk L, et al. Identifying sleep regulatory genes using a *Drosophila* model of insomnia. J Neurosci. 2009;29:7148–57.

52. Kume K, Kume S, Park SK, Hirsh J, Jackson FR. Dopamine is a regulator of arousal in the fruit fly. J Neurosci. 2005;25:7377–84.

53. Yamazaki M, Tomita J, Takahama K, Ueno T, Mitsuyoshi M, Sakamoto E, Kume S, Kume K. High calorie diet augments age-associated sleep impairment in *Drosophila*. Biochem Biophy Res Comm. 2012;417;812–816.

54. Bushey D, Tononi G, Cirelli C. The drosophila Fragile X mental retardation gene regulates sleep need. J Neurosci. 2009;29:1948–61.

55. Burnett C, Valentini S, Cabreiro P, Goss M, Somogyvari M, Piper MD, et al. Absence of effects of SIR2 overexpression on lifespan in *C. elegans* and *Drosophila*. Nature. 2011;477:482–6.

56. Linford NJ, Bilgir C, Ro J, Pletcher SD. Measurement of lifespan in *Drosophila melanogaster*. J Vis Exp. 2013;71:e50068.

57. Zimmerman JE, Chan MT, Jackson N, Maislin G, Pack AI. Genetic background has a major impact on differences in sleep resulting from environmental influences in *Drosophila*. Sleep. 2012;35:545–57.

58. Koudounas S, Green EW, Clancy D. Reliability and variability of sleep and activity as biomarkers of ageing in *Drosophila*. Biogerontol. 2012;13:489–99.

59. Ganguly-Fitzgerald I, Donlea J, Shaw PJ. Waking experience affects sleep need in *Drosophila*. Science. 2006;313:1775–80.

60. Luo W, Chen W-F, Yue Z, Chen D, Sowick M, Sehgal A, Zheng X. Old flies have a robust central oscillator but weaker behavioral rhythms that can be improved by genetic and environmental manipulations. Aging Cell. 2012;11:428–38.

61. Zimmerman JE, Raizen DM, Maycock MH, Maislin G, Pack AI. A video method to study *Drosophila* sleep. Sleep. 2008;31:587–98.

62. Duboue ER, Keene AC, Borowsky RL. Evolutionary convergence on sleep loss in cavefish populations. Curr Biol. 2011;21:671–6.

63. Duboue ER, Borowsky RL, Keene AC. B-adrenergic signaling regulates evolutionarily derived sleep loss in the Mexican cavefish. Brain Behav Evol. 2012;80:233–43.

64. Hur SP, Takeuchi Y, Itoh H, Uchimura M, Takahashi K, Kang H-C, Lee Y-D, Kim S-J, Takemura A. Fish sleeping under sandy bottom: interplay of melatonin and clock genes. Gen Comp Endocrinol. 2012;177:37–44.

65. Lucas-Sanchez A, Almaida-Pagan PF, Martinez-Nichols A, Madrid JA, Mendiola P, de Costa J. Rest-activity circadian rhythms in aged *Nothobranchius korthausae*. The effects of melatonin. Exp Gerontol. 2013;48:507–16.

66. Santoriello C, Zon LI. Hooked! Modeling human disease in zebrafish. J Clin Investiga. 2012;122:2337–43.

67. Rihel J, Prober DA, Arvanites A, Lam K, Zimmerman S, Jang S, et al. Zebrafish behavioral profiling links drugs to biological targets and rest/wake regulation. Science. 2010;327:348–51.

68. Ayala-Guerrero F, Uuitron-Resendiz S, Mexicano G. Effect of a depleter of cerebral monoamines on sleep patterns of a Chelonian reptile. Drug Dev Res. 1996;39:115–20.

69. Hartse KM, Rechtschaffen A. The effect of amphetamine, nembutal, alpha-methyl-tyrosine, and parachlorophenylalanine on the sleep-related spike activity of the tortoise, *Geochelone carbonaria* and on the cat ventral hippocampus spike. Brain Behav Evol. 1982;21:199–222.

70. De la Herran-Arita AK, Guerra-Crespo M, Drucker-Colin R. Narcolepsy and orexins: an example of progress in sleep research. Frontiers Neurol. 2011;2:1–8.

71. Faraco J, Mignot E. Immunological and genetic aspects of narcolepsy. Sleep Med Res. 2011;2:2–9.

72. Dauvilliers Y, Montplaisir J, Cochen V, Desautels A, Einen M, Lin I, et al. Post-H1N1 narcolepsy-cataplexy. Sleep. 2010;33:1428–30.

73. Koepsell TD, Longstreth WT, Ton TG. Medical exposures in youth and the frequency of narcolepsy with cataplexy: a population-based case-control study in genetically predisposed people. J Sleep Res. 2010;19:80–6.

74. Cantor S, Mochizuki T, Lops SN, Ko B, Clain E, Clark E, Yamamoto M, Scammell TE. Orexin gene therapy restores the timing and maintenance of wakefulness in narcoleptic mice. Sleep. 2013;36;1129–38.

75. Liu M, Blanco Centuron C, Konadhode RR, Begum S, Pelluru D, Gerashchenko D, Sakurai T, Yanagisawa M, van den Pol AN, Shiromani PJ. Orexin gene transfer into zona incerta neurons suppresses muscle paralysis in narcoleptic mice. J Neurosci. 2011;31:6028–40.

76. Bettica P, Squassante L, Zamuner S, Nucci G, Danker-Hopfe H, Ratti E. The orexin antagonist SB-649868 promotes and maintains sleep in men with primary insomnia. Sleep. 2012;35:2012.

77. Ginn SL, Alexander IE, Edelstein ML, Abedi MR, Wion J. Gene therapy clinical trials worldwide to 2012—an update. J Gene Med. 2013;15:65–77.

78. Prober DA, Rihel J, Onah AA, Sung R-J, Schier AF. Hypocretin/orexin overexpression induces an insomnia-like phenotype in zebrafish. J Neurosci. 2006;26:13400–10.

79. Yokogawa T, Marin W, Faraco J, Pezeron G, Appelbaum L, Zhang J, Rosa F, Mourrain P, Mignot E. Characterization of sleep in zebrafish and insomnia in hypocretin receptor mutants. Plos Biol. 2007;5:e277.

80. Ovchinsky A, Rao M, Lotwin I, Goldstein NA. The familial aggregation of pediatric obstructive sleep apnea syndrome. Arch Otolaryngol Head Neck Surg. 2002;128:815–8.

81. Redline S, Tosteson T, Tishler PV, Carskadon MA, Millman RP. Familial aggregation of symptoms associated with sleep related breathing disorders. Am Rev Respir Dis. 1992;145:440–4.

82. Strohl KP, Saunders NA, Feldman NT, Halett M. Obstructive sleep apnea in family members. N Engl J Med. 1978;299:969–73.

83. Hendricks JC, Kline LR, Kovalski JA, O'Brien JA, Morrison AR, Pack AI. The English bulldog: a natural model of sleep-disordered breathing. J Appl Physiol. 1987;63:1344–50.

84. Lonergan RP, Ware JC, Atkinson RL, Winter WC, Suratt PM. Sleep apnea in obese miniature pigs. J Appl Physiol. 1998;84:531–6.

85. Farre R, Nacher M, Serrano-Mollar A, Galdiz JB, Alvarez FJ, Navajas D, Montserrat JM. Rat model of chronic recurrent airway obstructions to study the sleep apnea syndrome. Sleep. 2007;30:930–3.

86. Kimoff RJ, Makino H, Horner RL, Kozar LF, Lue F, Slutsky AS, Phillipson EA. Canine model of obstructive sleep apnea:

model description and preliminary application. J Appl Physiol. 1994;76:1810–7.

87. Kimoff RJ, Brooks D, Horner RL, Kozar LF, Render-Teixeira CL, Champagne V, Mayer P, Phillipson EA. Ventilatory and arousal responses to hypoxia and hypercapnia in a canine model of obstructive sleep apnea. Am J Respir Crit Care Med. 1997;156:886–94.

88. Simpson JA, Brunt KR, Iscoes S. Repeated inspiratory occlusion acutely impairs myocardial function in rats. J Physiol. 2008;586:2345–55.

89. Dumitrascu R, Heitmann J, Seeger W, Weissmann N, Schulz R. Obstructive sleep apnea, oxidative stress and cardiovascular disease: lessons from animal studies. Oxid Med Cell Longev. 2014;234631.

90. Zhu Y, Fenik P, Zhan G, Mazza E, Kelz M, Aston-Jones G, Veasseys C. Selective loss of catecholaminergic wake-active neurons in a murine sleep apnea model. J Neurosci. 2007;27:10060–71.

91. Thakret P, Mamtani MR, Kulkami H. Lack of association of the APOEe4 allele with the risk of obstructive sleep apnea: metaanalysis and meta-regression. Sleep. 2009;32:1507–11.

92. Varvarigov V, Dahabreh IJ, Malhotra A, Kales SN. A review of genetic association studies of obstructive sleep apnea: field synopsis and meta analysis. Sleep. 2011;34:1461–8.

93. Stefansson H, Rye DB, Hicks A, Petursson H, Ingason A, Thorgeirsson TE, et al. A genetic risk factor for periodic limb movements in sleep. N Engl J Med. 2007;357:639–47.

94. Winkelmann J, Czamara D, Schormair B, Knauf F, Schulte E, Trenkwalder C, et al. Genome-wide association study identifies novel restless legs syndrome susceptibility loci on 2p14 and 16Q12.1. Plos Genet. 2011;7:e1002171.

95. Yang Q, Li L, Chen Q, Foldvary-Schaefer N, Ondo WG, Wang QK. Association studies of variants in *MES1, BTBD9,* and *MAP2K5/SKOR1* with restless legs syndrome in a US population. Sleep Med. 2011;12:800–4.

96. Freeman A, Pranak E, Miller RD, Radmard S, Bernhard D, Jinnah H, et al. Sleep fragmentation and motor restlessness in a *Drosophila* model of restless legs syndrome. Curr Biol. 2012;22:1142–8.

97. Allen RP, Picchietti D, Hening WA, Trenkwalder C, Walters AS, Montplaisir J. Restless legs syndrome: diagnostic criteria, special considerations, and epidemiology. A report from the restless legs syndrome diagnosis and epidemiology workshop at the National Institutes of Health. Sleep Med. 2003;4:101–19.

98. Auora RN, Kristo DA, Bista SR, Rowley JA, Zak RS, Casey KR, Lamm CI, Tracy SI, Rosenberg RS. The treatment of restless legs syndrome and periodic limb movement disorder in adults—an update for 2012: practice parameters with an evidence-based systematic review and meta-analyses. Sleep. 2012;35:1039–62.

99. Mahowald MW, Schenk CH, Cramer Bornemann MA. Violent parasomnias: forensic implications. In: Montagna P, Chokroverty S, volume editors. Handbook of clinical neurology, vol 98 (3rd series) sleep disorders part II. New York: Elsevier B. V.; 2011. pp. 1149–50.

100. Ohayon MM, Mahowald MW, Dauvilliers Y, Krystal AD, Leger D. Prevalence and comorbidity of nocturnal wandering in the US adult general population. Neurology. 2012;72:1583–9.

101. Kang H-H, Yoon I-Y, Lee SD, Han JW, Kim TH, Kim KW. REM sleep behavior disorder in the Korean elderly population: prevalence and clinical characteristics. Sleep. 2013;36:1147–52.

102. Jouvet M, Delorme F. Locus coeruleus et sommeil paradoxal. C R Séances Soc Biol Fil. 1965;159;895–9.

103. Schenck CH, Bundlie SR, Ettinger MG, Mahowald M. Chronic behavioral disorders of human REM sleep: a new category of parasomnias. Sleep. 1986;9:293–308.

104. Goldschmid R, Holzman R. Aeration of corals by sleep-swimming fish. Limmol Oceanogr. 2004;49:1832–9.

105. Lyamin O, Pryaslova J, Lance V, Siegel J. Continuous activity in cetaceans after birth. Nature. 2005;435:1177.

106. Mukhametov LM, Supin Ay, Polyakova IG. Interhemispheric asymmetry of the electroencephalographic sleep patterns in dolphins. Brain Res. 1977;134:581–4.

107. Lyamin OI, Mukhametov LM, Siegel JM, Nazarenko EA, Polyakova IG, Shpak OV. Unihemispheric slow wave sleep and the state of the eyes in a white whale. Behav Brain Res. 2002;129:125–9.

108. Lyamin OI, Lapierre JL, Kosenko PO, Mukhametov LM, Siegel JM. Electroencephalogram asymmetry and spectral power during sleep in the northern fur seal. J Sleep Res. 2008;17:154–65.

109. Rattenborg NC. Do birds sleep in flight? Naturwissenschaften. 2006a;93:413–25.

110. Nir Y, Staba RJ, Andrillon T, Vyazovskly V, Cirelli C, Fried I, Tononi G. Regional slow waves and spindles in human sleep. Neuron. 2011;70:153–69.

111. Nobili L, Ferrara M, Moroni F, DeGennaro L, LoRusso G, Campus C, Cardinale F, DeCarli F. Dissociated wake-like and sleep-like electro-cortical activity during sleep. Neurolimage. 2011;58:612–9.

112. Terzaghi M, Sartori I, Tassi L, Rustioni V, Proserpio P, L'Orusso G, Manni R, Nobili L. Dissociated local arousal states underlying essential clinical features of non-rapid eye movement arousal parasomnias: an intracerebral stereo-electroencephalographic study. J Sleep Res. 2012;21:502–6.

113. Symonds, JA. Sleep and dreams: two lectures. Albermarle Street: John Murray; 1851.

114. Lesku JA, Meyer LCR, Fuller A, Maloney SK, Dell'Omo G, Vyssotski AL, Rattenborg NC. Ostriches sleep like platypuses. Plos ONE. 2011;6:e23203.

115. Rattenborg NC, Voirin B, Vyssotski AL, Kays RW, Spoelstra K, Kuemmeth F, Heidrich W, Wikelski M. Sleeping outside the box: electroencephalographic measures of sleep in sloths inhabiting a rainforest. Biol Lett. 2008;4:402–25.

116. Ardekani R, Huang YM, Sancheti P, Stanciauskas R, Tavare S, Tower J. Using GFP video to track 3-D movements and conditional gene expression in free-moving flies. Plos ONE. 2012;7:e40506.

117. Belfer SJ, Chuang H-S, Freedman BJ, Yuan J, Norton M, Bau HH, Raizen DM. Caenorhabditis-in-drop array for monitoring *C. elegans* quiescent behavior. Sleep. 2013;36:689–98.

Gamma-Hydroxybutyrate (Sodium Oxybate): From the Initial Synthesis to the Treatment of Narcolepsy–Cataplexy and Beyond

63

Roger Broughton

Fragmented sleep with consequent daytime sleepiness and some impairment of cognitive ability characterizes many sleep disorders, especially those of neurological and psychiatric origin [1]. The failure of hypnotics that are commonly used to improve sleep quality and/or duration relates in large part to their inability to induce, or reproduce, natural physiological sleep. Most tend to suppress both rapid eye movement (REM) and slow-wave sleep (SWS, now stage N3). Moreover, their hypnotic effect tends to wane over time with the development of tolerance [2].

In the 1960s, Henri Laborit (Fig. 63.1) and his colleagues searched for a way to deliver gamma-aminobutyric acid (GABA) across the blood–brain barrier into the brain. With this objective, they synthesized gamma-hydroxybutyrate (GHB) as a precursor to GABA [3–5]. Soon afterwards, it was shown that GHB is a normal metabolite, rather than a precursor, of GABA [6]. It later became recognized as a normal constituent of virtually all life forms whether bacteria, protozoa, plants or animals. Early studies showed that, in normal doses, GHB had anaesthetic and hypnotic properties in man and animals [3, 5, 7]. Moreover, in animal and human [8] studies, GHB induced both REM sleep and SWS [9] without development of tolerance to its hypnotic effects [7].

First Clinical Trials

These seemingly unique properties led initially to the use of GHB in the treatment of patients suffering from major depressive disorders and bipolar disorder. In both, there is severe insomnia that, in the latter, it usually precedes the periods of hypomania or mania. It was hoped that GHB would restore a normal sleep architecture, prolong the duration and continuity of sleep, correct the timing of REM sleep and increase the duration of SWS. But, in early clinical trials in patients with these conditions, GHB unexpectedly reversed the normal sequence of sleep states and radically altered the architecture of sleep [10] by further shortening the already brief REM sleep latency and even inducing sleep-onset REM sleep periods that could last close to an hour and were then followed by almost equally prolonged periods of SWS. GHB appeared, in retrospect, to have partially induced the polysomnographic (PSG) features of narcolepsy.

Discovery of GHB Efficacy in Narcolepsy

The pathogenesis of narcolepsy at that time was poorly understood, in part because the integrating functions of the hypocretins (orexins) had not as yet been discovered [11–13]. In PSG studies of narcolepsy, the orchestration of sleep/wake states appeared to have broken down and the different states of sleep and their components to have become dissociated from one another and gone adrift around the 24-h. Others had shown that cataplexy reflects the selective activation in wakefulness by emotional stimuli of the motor atonic component of REM sleep, and that sleep paralysis represents continuation of REM atonia mechanisms with those of cerebral REM sleep being replaced by wakefulness. These features had led me [14] to define narcolepsy as a disease of state boundary control.

Concerning sleep distribution across the 24-h, the then current belief was that the daytime sleep and drowsiness/sleepiness in narcolepsy-cataplexy reflected a homeostatic "make-up" of the highly fragmented and reduced amount of night sleep. Much later this was shown not to be the case, as 24-h ambulatory sleep/wake recordings in narcolepsy–cataplexy found that there was no correlation between the amount of night sleep and that of subsequent day sleep [15]. The evidence much more strongly supported a weak circadian arousal rhythm as being the cause [16].

R. Broughton (✉)
Division of Neurology, Department of Medicine, University of Ottawa, 1001-20 Driveway, Ottawa, Ontario, Canada
e-mail: rjbroughton78@gmail.com; rbrough@uottawa.ca

S. Chokroverty, M. Billiard (eds.), *Sleep Medicine,* DOI 10.1007/978-1-4939-2089-1_63,

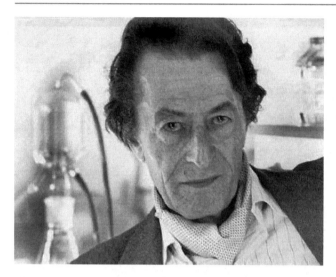

Fig. 63.1 Henri Laborit (1914-1995). GHB discoverer and synthesizer

Given GHB's proven capacity to promote both REM and SWS, I proposed to Mortimer Mamelak that we use it to try and consolidate sleep into the night-time period. GHB in its sodium form was imported into Canada from Laboratoire Égic in France. Our open-label studies began in 1974/5 [17]. GHB was given in two or three doses with the objective to induce as continuous a night of sleep as possible. The first dose was 1.5–2.25 g (10–15 ml) at bedtime, followed by one or two further doses of 1.0–1.5 g with awakenings, if at least

2.5 h had passed since the previous dose. The total dosage ranged from 3.75 to 6.0 g corresponding on average to some 50 mg/kg. GHB alleviated daytime sleep attacks, drowsiness and sleepiness measured by the Stanford Sleepiness Scale [18] and virtually eliminated cataplexy [17, 19–21]. Nighttime sleep on GHB became consolidated with increased SWS and REM sleep, a decreased number of stage shifts per 100 min for both non-REM (NREM) and REM sleep, increased REM period efficiency, shortened REM latency and decreased stage N1 drowsiness (Figs. 63.2 and 63.3). Daytime stage N1 drowsiness, sleep attacks and naps were markedly reduced. A few patients no longer had any daytime sleep on nocturnal GHB (Fig. 63.4). Some nocturnal electroencephalography (EEG) delta waves on GHB were of extreme duration of 1.5–2.0 s (Fig. 63.5) and this appeared to be a direct drug effect.

The positive clinical effects on subjective and objective quality of night sleep, daytime improvement of alertness, reduced sleep, and suppression of cataplexy plus the other REM-based symptoms including sleep paralysis, hypnagogic hallucinations and nightmares, was seen in all patients. This was true even in four very severe patients who had not been improved on prior traditional combinations of stimulants for daytime somnolence and sleep, antidepressants for REM-based symptoms, and hypnotics for nocturnal insomnia. Tolerance did not develop in any patients on GHB and side effects were few in number and generally short-lived.

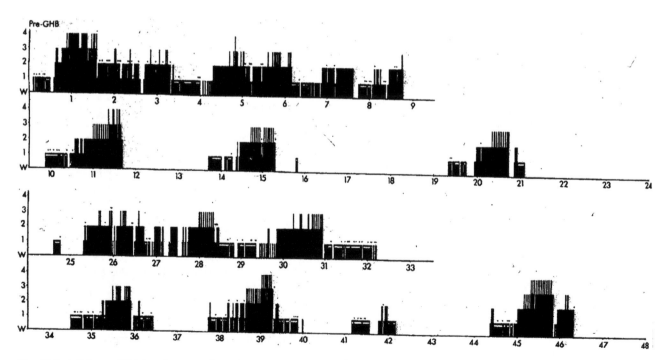

Fig. 63.2 A 48-h pre-GHB baseline recording of a patient with narcolepsycataplexy shows frequent awakenings in night sleep, multiple night and day sleep onset REM sleep periods, and fragmented REM periods. Vertical axis shows NREM stages 1, 2, 3 and 4. REM sleep is shown as a white horizontal bar at the same level as NREM stage 1 (i.e., drowsiness). Major movements are shown as small triangles above the vertical stage lines. Time zero was between 10:30 and 11:00 pm in both Figs. 63.2 and 63.3 [from 21]

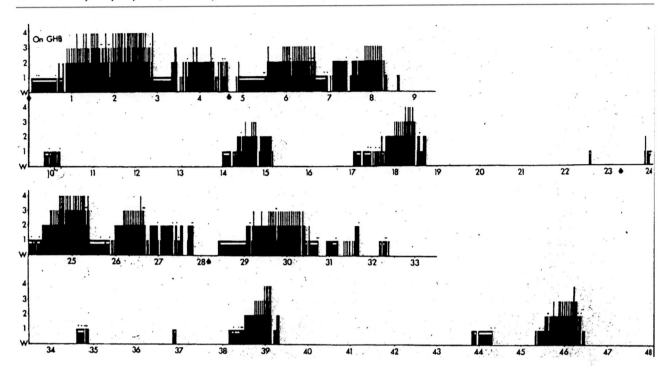

Fig. 63.3 On-GHB. Same patient but on days 9 and 10 of nocturnal GHB. Times of GHB administration pre-sleep and within the night sleep periods are shown as arrows below the horizontal time line. Night sleep has more SWS and is more continuous, as are the REM periods.

Day sleep is greatly reduced. Patient slept on hospital bed with long wire electrodes for both studies. Ambulatory monitoring studies allowing normal movement showed less day sleep. From[21]

Fig. 63.4 24-h clocks of sleep/wake patters pre-GHB and on the 5th consecutive day of nocturnal GHB in a young patient with narcolepsy-cataplexy. GHB greatly consolidated night sleep and both REM and NREM during the nighttime sleep period, Daytime reduction of stage N1 (drowsiness), sleep attacks and voluntary naps was marked, daytime sleep being virtually abolished. Such dramatic effects were seen in only a few patients. The majority of patients showed some degree of residual drowsiness (N1) and some daytime NREM and REM sleep

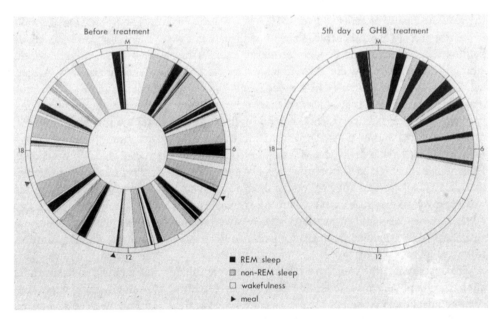

These findings of efficacy of GHB in the treatment of narcolepsy–cataplexy were soon confirmed by investigators in the USA and Europe in double-blind, placebo-controlled studies [22–24]. Other clinicians collected large case series and also found that tolerance failed to develop to GHB's therapeutic efficacy. This was in stark contrast to the effects of the then conventional treatment using hypnotics, stimulants and antidepressants all of which too often required

increasing doses to suppress the symptoms of the disease [25–27]. I have followed patients with narcolepsy-cataplexy treated with GHB for over 30 years without seeing a single patient develop tolerance to the drug.

Studies have shown that patients with narcolepsy–cataplexy, compared to normal controls, have broad negative effects on work, income, education, driving, accidents and many other parameters of quality of life [28], and that these

Fig. 63.5 Some of the nocturnal EEG delta waves on GHB were of extreme duration of 1.5–2.0 s and this appeared to be a direct drug effect

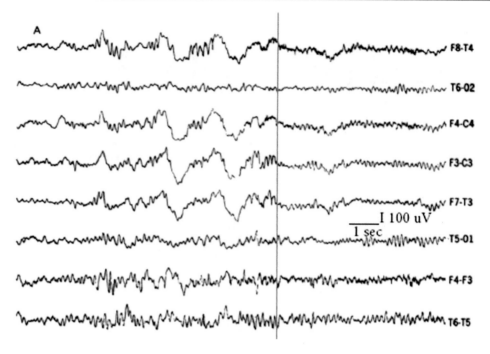

are seen equally in North American, Asian and European patients [29]. These effects are even more pervasive and greater than those of the well-documented life effects in epilepsy patients without significant organic brain disease [30]. The treatment of narcolepsy with GHB has been shown to vastly improve the quality of patient's lives [31].

In response to these benefits, patients with narcolepsy petitioned the orphan drug division of the Food and Drug Administration (FDA) in the USA to undertake the clinical trials required to abolish GHB's experimental status and make it a prescription drug. Martin Scharf must be given particular credit for his persistent advocacy on behalf both of these patients and of GHB. Orphan Medical, under the remarkable leadership of its chief medical officer, William Houghton, undertook the task of bringing GHB to market. In 2002, GHB in its sodium form as sodium oxybate (Xyrem®) was approved in the USA for the treatment of cataplexy. In 2005, approval was granted for GHB in excessive daytime sleepiness (EDS). Similar approvals for its use in EDS soon followed in Canada and Europe.

The marketing of Xyrem® on prescription began only after the completion of a series of necessary large multicentre clinical trials in the USA, Canada and Europe. In the first of these trials [32], 136 patients with narcolepsy and cataplexy remained on their stable dose of stimulant medication and then were gradually withdrawn from their anticataplectic and hypnotic medication. Following a washout period, patients were assigned to receive either placebo or 3, 6 or 9 g of GHB for 4 weeks in equally divided doses at bedtime and again 2.5–4.0 h later. The findings revealed that the magnitude of the anticataplectic effect was dose related

and was greatest in the 9-g group. This was true as well for measures of EDS that, in a number of patients, actually fell into the normal range. There was a significant decrease in the number of inadvertent sleep attacks and voluntary naps during the day in the 6- and 9-g groups, and a significant decrease in nocturnal awakenings in the 9-g group.

One hundred and eighteen of the patients who participated in the initial 4-week trial agreed to join a 12-month extension trial [33]. All patients began treatment at 6 g per night in equally divided doses, as before. Based on the clinical response, the investigators could choose to decrease the total nightly dose to 3 or 4.5 g or increase it to 7.5 or 9 g. Data from this open-label study revealed that all doses between 3 and 9 g produced significant long-term reductions in the frequency of cataplexy. This improvement was rapid and progressive during the first month of treatment; and the incidence of cataplexy fell further during the course of the year. There was also a significant reduction in daytime sleepiness for all treatment groups. Patients who were also on stimulants felt even more alert and better able to concentrate with the added use of GHB. The quality of sleep at night was significantly improved. There was no dose escalation to indicate the development of tolerance.

Another US Xyrem® multi-center study found that abrupt withdrawal of GHB from patients with narcolepsy who had received nightly doses of 3–9 g for 7 to 44 months led to a gradual return of the symptoms of the disease [34]. As in the first studies [20, 21], there was no rebound increase in cataplexy, or appearance of status catiplecticus, as often occurs in withdrawal of antidepressants [35].

The effects of GHB on sleep architecture were further examined [36] in a study on 25 patients using the Maintenance of wakefulness test (MWT) [37] and the Epworth Sleepiness Scale (ESS) [38] to determine the effects on daytime sleepiness. Subjects were maintained on their usual daytime stimulant dose. All subjects received 4.5 g of GHB each night in divided doses for 4 weeks followed by escalating doses of 6, 7.5 and 9 g at subsequent 2-week intervals. Bedtime GHB initially further reduced the already short REM latency and increased the duration of REM sleep in 4 h that followed. After 4 weeks, this effect was no longer evident and, in fact, increasing doses of GHB then progressively depressed the duration of REM sleep and increased that of SWS. Curiously, total sleep time in this study was not increased even at the highest dose, although the number of nocturnal awakenings declined significantly with increasing doses. Despite its failure to increase total sleep time, GHB showed a dose-related improvement in alertness on MWT. At the highest (9 g) dose, a number of subjects rated their sleepiness in the normal range, an effect objectively confirmed by MWT.

The beneficial effect of GHB on MWT at the 9-g dose was again demonstrated in a multi-centre placebo-controlled parallel group trial that involved 228 patients [39, 40]. The reasons for the improvement of daytime alertness on GHB have yet to be determined, but they may be related to the provision of energy to the brain by GHB or a metabolite, to its antioxidant effect or to a rebound increase in the activity of various neurotransmitter systems engaged in the induction and maintenance of wakefulness as the effects of GHB wear off in the morning [25].

Another double-blind controlled trial was undertaken on 270 patients with narcolepsy in order to compare the impact on daytime drowsiness of GHB alone with that of modafinil. GHB was studied in doses up to 9 g at bedtime [41]. MWT testing demonstrated that GHB alone was as effective in maintaining daytime alertness as was modafinil alone. But again even greater alertness was achieved when modafinil and GHB were combined, suggesting a synergistic effect. GHB alone also produced a significant decrease in the ESS rating. When GHB at night was combined with daytime modafinil, a greater reduction in the ESS occurred.

A study of the effects of GHB treatment on such psychosocial variables as level of activity, vigilance and personal productivity in 285 patients, [31] reported several very significant findings. A dose response was demonstrated with the greatest benefit found at 9 g. The authors commented that the findings were not only statistically significant but also clinically important. GHB substantially improved daytime functioning even further in the 50 % of the subjects who also received the stimulant modafinil. The levels of excessive daytime drowsiness then often fell into the normal ranges.

Narcolepsy–cataplexy and GHB in Childhood and Adolescence

The first report of GHB in childhood narcolepsy with cataplexy [42] involved a group of eight children with a severe form of the disease documented by history, nocturnal polysomnography, a modified Epworth Sleepiness Scale and the multiple sleep latency test (MSLT) [43]. On GHB all patients but one improved significantly and had marked reduction of cataplexy frequency and severity, and improved ESS ratings.

Aran et al. [44] retrospectively studied a cohort of 51 children divided into those in whom narcolepsy–cataplexy appeared before (53 %), around (29 %) or after (18 %) puberty. The only clinical difference between the three age groups was an increased occurrence of sleep paralysis with age. Weight gain was common prior to the development of the disease and puberty occurred earlier than for other family members. Streptococcus throat infections within 6 months of disease onset were reported in 20 % of the patients. PSG features were similar in all three groups. Three pre-pubertal children did not meet the usual MSLT diagnostic criteria for the diagnosis despite pathognomonic symptoms. Patients were treated with a variety of drugs including modafinil (84 %), GHB (79 %) and venlafaxine (68 %). Other drugs tried including methylphenidate, tricyclic antidepressants and SSRIs; but these were rarely continued. GHB was effective for all symptoms, modafinil for EDS and sleep attacks alone and venlafaxine for cataplexy alone. At the end of the study, half of the children were on GHB either alone or with the addition of one of the other two drugs. Older children were often maintained on more than two drugs.

Peraita-Adrados et al. [45] reported a series of nine children with narcolepsy–cataplexy treated with a variety of medications including either methylphenidate or modafinil combined with an antidepressant or, in two cases, by GHB. The children also had scheduled naps. The two children on GHB responded particularly well.

In a retrospective study of 15 paediatric patients (children and adolescents, aged 3–17 years) treated for narcolepsy–cataplexy with GHB supplemented by any prior medication for sleepiness or cataplexy [46], the supplementation of GHB improved ESS scores, reduced the number of cataplexy episodes reported by parents and reduced cataplexy severity. Three patients discontinued GHB: one for insurance reasons, another for constipation plus dissociative feelings, and the third (only temporarily) for dizziness plus body aches and pains that did not reappear after return to GHB therapy. The dosage of GHB was 5.0 ± 2.5 g per night and no tolerance developed. Lecendreux et al. [47] reported a multi-centre study that retrospectively studied 27 children treated off-label in a clinical setting. It found a good clinical and laboratory response to GHB which was well tolerated by all patients.

Unfortunately, to date there are no randomized double-blind controlled trials of GHB efficacy in narcolepsy with cataplexy during childhood or adolescence.

Obstructive Sleep Apnea Syndrome (OSAS) with Excessive Sleepiness

The positive response of EDS to GHB in narcolepsy–cataplexy led to attempts to see whether sleepiness in the more common disorder of obstructive sleep apnea would respond equally well. A main concern was that GHB at higher doses is an anaesthetic and there is a potential risk of suppression of the brainstem centres controlling respiration. The results have been mixed.

Charles George and collaborators at the University of Western Ontario have published two safety trials of the effects of GHB on respiratory function. In the first study George et al. [48] noted that OSAS often coexisted with narcolepsy–cataplexy. Sixty patients with mild-to-moderate OSA received one of four treatments: (a) 9 g of GHB in the evening, (b) 200 mg modafinil in the daytime, (c) 10 mg zolpidem before retiring or (d) placebo, as part of a randomized crossover design involving four nights with overnight PSG. The apnea-hypopnea index and the mean SaO_2 did not change significantly on GHB. Patients showed an increase in central apneas and three had significant oxygen desaturations. There were some adverse clinical effects, mainly headache and nausea. The authors concluded that in OSAS, with or without coexistent narcolepsy, GHB in some patients may cause central respiratory depression with central apneas and oxygen desaturation, and that it should therefore be used with caution.

In their second study George et al. [49] performed a 2-week assessment of GHB at 4.5 g nightly versus placebo in patients with OSAS. Compared with placebo, GHB increased reduction in the apnea–hypopnea index and also increased SWS. There was no difference in SaO_2 levels, central respiratory events or in other respiratory measures. Headache was noted in a third of patients and was the only significant side effect. They concluded that short-term use of GHB at 4.5 g per night was well tolerated but that longer usage needed study, and that the drug should be used with caution in such patients. Neither study assessed the impact of GHB on daytime function.

There does appear to be some respiratory risk in this usage of GHB. Seeck-Hirschner et al. [50] reported two patients with narcolepsy-cataplexy and OSAS treated with GHB in whom there was an increase in sleep-related breathing disturbances.

Fibromyalgia and Chronic Fatigue Syndromes

Since the original report of Moldofsky [51] describing the efficacy of GHB to alleviate the characteristic widespread pain, tender points in specific anatomical regions, and non-restorative sleep of the rheumatological condition of fibromyalgia, there has been a cavalcade of confirmatory studies. Russell et al. [52] using the standard criteria of the American College of Rheumatology treated [53] a large series of 188 patients with 4.5 or 6.0 g or matching placebo once per night for 8 weeks. Patients filled in the Fibromyalgia Impact Questionnaire, the Patient Global Impression of Change, and the Jenkins Scale of Sleep of subjective sleep quality. All three scales showed improvement. GHB was well tolerated other than for occasional dose-related nausea and dizziness with both tending to resolve with continued treatment. In a study in which the majority of patients had chronic fatigue syndrome and a minority fibromyalgia, Spitzer and Broadman [54] found GHB improved 60 % those of the symptoms of pain and 75 % those of fatigue.

The first double-blind, randomized, placebo-controlled study of the efficacy of the effects of GHB on fibromyalgia was by Moldofsky et al. [55] who studied 304 patients diagnosed by the standard criteria. Polysomnography was done in 200 patients and 195 patients were randomized with 151 completing a double-blind, cross-over, placebo-controlled protocol at doses of 4.5 and 6.0 g per night. Pretreatment assessments showed high amounts of alpha intrusion in the sleep EEG (66 % of subjects), periodic leg movements in sleep (20.1 %) and moderate-to-severe obstructive sleep apnea (15.3 %). Compared to placebo, there was a significant improvement in the ESS, the Jenkins Scale of Sleep quality, the Functional Outcome of Sleep Questionnaire, the SF-36 Vitality Scale, and the Fibromyalgia Impact Questionnaire. Polysomnography showed decreased wakefulness after sleep onset with increases in stage N2 sleep, SWS (N3) and total non-REM sleep. Some side effects encountered included nausea, pain in the extremities, dizziness, restlessness and occasional urinary incontinence. Similar findings using a comparable crossover, double-blind, placebo-controlled design were reported by Russell et al. [56]. Subsequent confirmatory studies are those of Staud [57, 58], Crawford et al. [59], and an international phase 3 trial [60].

Neurodegenerative Diseases

Another promising area of GHB clinical usage is that of neurodegenerative diseases. It is now well documented that REM sleep behaviour disorder (RBD), in which the atonia of REM sleep is absent permitting complex behaviours while asleep, is often a harbinger of Parkinson disease (PD), as in some 33–65 % of cases RBD is either followed several years later by the appearance of PD or accompanies diagnosed PD [61–66]. There is a single report of GHB successfully treating RBD. The patient's symptoms had persisted for 5 years uncontrolled on other drugs, including clonazepam. GHB at low doses led to cessation of all nocturnal events, an effect sustained during a one-year follow-up period [67].

PD has been treated with GHB with the intention of reducing the excessive sleepiness that often is a part of the disease along with the tremor, rigidity, cognitive problems and other characteristic symptoms. As reported by Arnulf and Leu-Semenescu [68], EDS in about a third of PD patients and may even be accompanied by sleep attacks without prodroma. These sleep attacks, like those of narcolepsy-cataplexy, often contain REM sleep with sleep-onset REM periods sometimes associated with hypnagogic hallucinations or frank dreams. The authors noted that modafinil is only partially effective and that patients respond much better to either GHB or anti-histamine-3 drugs. Ondo et al. also reported an improvement of EDS when PD patients are treated with GHB [69].

Stroke may also be considered a neurodegenerative disorder given the neuronal loss resulting from an ischemic or hemorrhagic event. There are no clinical reports of stroke treated by GHB. However, in an experimental study in which the middle cerebral artery was occluded [70], those mice receiving intra-peritoneal GHB (100 mg per kg, twice a day, given 8 h apart) recovered much more rapidly than those treated with saline. Recovery was assessed behaviourally by grip strength, and histologically using cresyl violet and neuronal staining. Similar results are by MacMillan [71], Ottani et al. [72] and Sadasivan et al. [73].

Alzheimer's dementia is characterized amongst other things by oxidative stress, limited neuronal energy resources, excitotoxicity and vascular endothelial pathology. GHB has been shown experimentally to reduce the tissue damage resulting from oxidative stress. It has been proposed [74, 75] that GHB might be able to buttress this protective process which ends with the release of beta-amyloid and the formation of neurofibrillary tangles that together are the pathological hallmarks of the disease. No clinical trials have been reported.

Side Effects of GHB

GHB has repeatedly shown itself to have very few deleterious side effects. Table 63.1 summarizes those side effects reported in the already cited open-label and double-blind crossover studies in narcolepsy. Further side effects have been the focus of individual case reports. These effects are in general much more rare than those already well documented in the clinical trial studies. To date few such seemingly idiosyncratic drug reactions have been published.

Husain et al. [76] reported weight loss averaging 3.4 kg in a series of 54 patients with narcolepsy being treated with GHB. Wallace et al. [53] described a patient on GHB who experienced a single instance of drug-induced sleep-driving and two episodes of sleep-eating.

Patients experiencing psychological side effects independent of clinical trials have also been reported. Rossetti et al. [77] described the occasional rapid appearance of depression when GHB was added to modafinil. Langford and Gross [78] noted that, when taken as a drug of abuse, GHB can produce serious psychiatric side effects and also withdrawal symptoms, whereas in patients taking recommended doses, such effects have never been reported. They described a single patient with narcolepsy treated with the recommended doses of GHB who showed initial altered mental status and later became psychotic on abrupt discontinuation of the medication.

Table 63.1 Side effects reported by the main clinical trials

	First symptom	Second symptom	Third symptom	Fourth symptom	Other	Other, or a note
Broughton and Mamelak [20, 21]	Thick head	Ocular discomfort	Enuresis	Confusion	Hangover	
Scrima et al. [23, 24]	Nausea with emesis	Dizziness	Weakness and fatigue	Urinary urgency	Morning sluggishness	Morning stiffness
Lammers [22]	Sleep paralysis + hallucination	Weight loss				Very few side effects
US Xyrem® [32]	Nausea	Dizziness	Enuresis	Somnolence	Feeling drunk	Confusion
US Xyrem® [33]	Headache	Nausea	Nasopharyngitis	Vomiting	Somnolence	
US Xyrem® [34]	No differences from controls					
Mamelak et al. [36]	Confusion if resist effects	Enuresis	Induced sleep paralysis	Sleepwalking	Weight loss	
Xyrem® Inter [39]	Nausea	Dizziness	Enuresis	Confusion	Somnolence	Attentional problems
Xyrem® Inter [40]	Various minor					
Black and Houghton [41]	Headache	Nausea	Dizziness	Nasopharyngitis	Vomiting	Somnolence

In an early study, Bèdard et al. [79] found that GHB in narcolepsy–cataplexy can be associated with an increase in periodic leg movements in sleep that have the potential of opposing the sleep consolidation effect of the substance.

Extremely rarely, GHB has been reported to induce a form of parasomnia. Poli et al. [80] describe a series of narcolepsy patients treated with GHB, some with associated OSAS, in whom 14 % developed catathrenia. This condition consists of groaning and an abnormal respiratory pattern in sleep confirmed by PSG recordings. No worsening of respiratory measures occurred in the narcolepsy-cataplexy patients with OSAS, and the catathrenia was considered benign.

Four deaths have been reported in patients taking GHB. Akins et al. [81] reported a 53-year old woman with narcolepsy-cataplexy who was also taking tramadol, gabapentin, cetirizine, carisoprodol and modafinil and who had well documented significant OSAS. The combination of central nervous system (CNS) depressants and OSAS, both of which are contraindications for GHB treatment, was considered the cause of death which itself was believed to be accidental. Zvosec et al. [82] reported a further three patients who died on GHB. One was associated with GHB abuse and had post-mortem blood GHB levels that were extremely high. Concurrent use of sedative hypnotics, OSAS and obesity were in volved in the two other patients, both of whom took GHB in the recommended doses. In two of the three patients, post-mortem GHB levels were assessed and were only 141 and 110 mg/L, i.e. within the expected post-mortem range for GHB. The third case was a patient with a history of intentional drug overdose, and whose actual cause of death remained uncertain.

Zvosec et al. [83] investigated 226 deaths attributed to GHB. These included 213 from cardiorespiratory arrest and 13 fatal accidents. Seventy-one instances (34 %) had no related intoxicants. Post-mortem blood GHB was 18–4400 mg/L (median = 347) in those deaths negative for co-intoxicants.

Lammers et al. [84] emphasized the fact that there are no reported deaths in patients with narcolepsy-cataplexy, or indeed with other medical conditions, who are treated with the recommended doses of GHB. Moreover, it must be said that the reports of GHB usage in "date-rape" episodes, especially since the death of Kurt Cobain, a GHB abuser, has had an overblown negative press. Surely for each GHB-associated date-rape episode, there were a 100 or more rapes associated with amphetamines (especially methylamphetamine, Ecstasy), sedative-hypnotics (especially flunitrazepam, Rohypnol), esketamine (Ketamine), more alcohol, or other CNS active agents slipped into the drinks of the unfortunate victims. The excessive negative press coverage for GHB affected government officials, policy makers and the public to the point that it took years to have this useful medication available on prescription.

In summary, the objective evidence after worldwide experience involving several thousands of patients on GHB is that clearly GHB (sodium oxybate), when taken at the recommended dosage levels, and in the absence of significant OSAS and respiratory depressants such as sedative-hypnotics, tranquilizers and alcohol, is one of the safest prescription drugs on the market. Moreover, in experimental animal studies, the LD-50 of GHB is some 20 times the therapeutic sleep-inducing dose. A UK parliamentary committee's commissioned report found the use of GHB to be less dangerous than tobacco and alcohol in social harms, physical harm, and addiction [85].

Mechanisms of Action

What then is the mechanism, or rather what are the mechanisms, of GHB in delivering its clinical benefits? First, it must be said that a full description of the mechanisms of action and the neurochemical pathways of GHB is beyond the scope of this mainly clinical chapter. An excellent recent review is that of Xie et al. [86].

Given orally, GHB readily crosses the blood-brain barrier and is converted to a number of metabolites before entering the Krebs cycle and becoming CO_2 and water. GHB is also endogenously produced in cells as a metabolite of GABA-B. There are many downstream metabolites of GHB, but the biological roles of these remain in general unknown. A summary of the main GHB pathways is presented in Fig. 63.6.

As discussed above, the main biological effects of GHB needing explanation include: the deepening sleep as measured by the increase in number of slow waves and increase in total SWS (stage N3); the suppression of arousals in sleep thereby leading to increased sleep period efficiency. Unlike most other sleep-inducing compounds including traditional hypnotics, it reduces neither SWS nor REM sleep [19, 21, 87]. Moreover, by yet unknown mechanisms, GHB appears to increase the strength of state boundary control with the consolidation of both major sleep states. This is evidenced by the fact that the number of stage shifts within, and in and out of, both NREM and REM sleep is markedly reduced, as first reported by Broughton and Mamelak [21].

Particularly noteworthy is GHB's effect on REM sleep which in narcolepsy-cataplexy is both fragmented in its continuity within individual REM periods [21, 88] and shows dissociations of the sub-components of REM state seen most dramatically as cataplexy, narcolepsy's pathognomonic symptom, as well as the replacement of the ascending mechanisms for REM sleep by those of wakefulness giving an EEG associated with REM atonia, as occurs in sleep paralysis. With GHB treatment, REM periods become more continuous and the REM state more integrated with the suppression of these state component dissociations and their as-

Fig. 63.6 A summary of the main GHB pathways

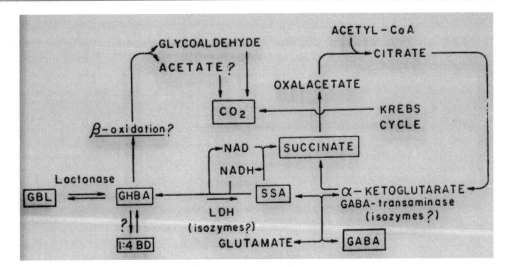

sociated clinical symptoms. The latency of REM sleep from sleep onset is also shortened by GHB.

From a physiological point of view, there is evidence that the greater the nocturnal fragmentation of REM sleep (i.,e the lower the REM sleep state efficency) the higher the number of daytime cataplexy attacks [89]. GHB's effect of increasing REM sleep efficiency [21] may therefore diminish the pressure for REM state dissociations in general, thereby reducing the frequency of cataplexy, sleep paralysis, hallucinations, and nightmares.

Less easily explained is how this effect may work at neurochemical, molecular and possibly genetic levels. How can nocturnal GHB that has a serum and CSF half-life of only 1.5–2 h [112] create a durable suppression of cataplexy across the much longer following waking period? If hypocretin (orexin) is the main neurotransmitter which integrates the REM sleep state, as I propose, then perhaps GHB somehow increases the functionality of the reduced number of hypocretin cells that remain in narcolepsy with cataplexy. After GHB withdrawal, suppression of cataplexy can continue for several days which suggests the induction of a very slow and long-lasting process which may involve gene activation and the production of proteins which help re-establish REM state integrity. It has, in fact, been shown that GHB can activate CNS C-fos expression localized in many hypothalamic nuclei (paraventricular, supraoptic, median proptic, ventral premammillary), the central nucleus of the amygdala, Edinger–Westphal nucleus, parabrachial nucleus, locus coeruleus and the nucleus of the solitary tract [90]. The study of Zeitzer et al. [91] in squirrel monkeys analysing time-dependent patterns of CSF hypocretin, serum cortisol and activity levels in baseline sleep/wake and sleep deprivation conditions shows a large increase in hypocretin levels during the wake period and a secondary smaller increase during sleep. This bimodal distribution suggests that hypocretin may help consolidate the components not only of wake but also of REM sleep.

The dissociations of REM sleep components can also be usefully considered in the context of increasing evidence that in man, as in lower animals, so-called "local sleep" can occur in parts of the intact brain while other are awake [92–94]. This can readily be considered the case in, for example, cataplexy during which REM sleep's neural sub-systems controlling motor atonia and paralysis are selectively triggered into their REM sleep state during the wake state by emotional stimuli.

We now know a very great deal about the neurochemical mechanisms of all three basic mammalian biological states: wakefulness, NREM sleep and REM sleep. For example, it is become evident that wakefulness is created and sustained by at least five distinct neurochemical–anatomical sub-systems, each of which has ascending activating properties to maintain aspects of arousal. They are: dopaminergic, originating in the striatum; cholinergic, located in a number of subcortical nuclei of the ascending reticular activating system; noradrenergic; mainly originating in the locus coeruleus; histaminergic, originating in the posterior hypothalamus; and hypocretinergic, also originating in the hypothalamus but more laterally with widespread ascending and descending connections throughout the CNS and, in particular, diffuse connections to the neocortex. How in normal persons do these multiple sub-systems create and maintain aspects of wakefulness? How they interact to create the variations in intensity and quality of wakefulness remains unknown and requires investigation.

One such mechanism, however, seems to be clear. To date, the evidence strongly indicates that, the onset of narcolepsy–cataplexy, i.e., the appearance of cataplexy, closely approximates that of the disappearance of normal levels of CSF hypocretin (orexin) [95]. This implies that hypocretin is a strong candidate for the neurochemical basis of integrating the sub-components of REM sleep into the fully developed REM state. Weakened hypocretin cell function in the circadian arousal systems seems to be a main mechanism of the daytime excessive somnolence and sleep. There is much evidence that the treatment of PD with L-dopa and dopamine agonists may lead to, or increase, EDS and sleep attacks.

Unfortunately, we know almost nothing about the biological basis of the mechanisms that integrate the multiple subcomponents of wakefulness, NREM sleep or REM sleep. Until these mechanisms are better understood we will make little progress in understanding those fundamental processes by which these states can be decomposed to produce sleep paralysis, cataplexy and other dissociative symptoms including so called "double consciousness" (i.e., simultaneous consciousness of mental activity or dreaming and of the outside world) [96].

These neurochemical considerations concerning GHB's hypocretin-related mechanisms of action in narcolepsy-cataplexy do not appear very relevant to its action in improving other very different clinical conditions such as fibromyalgia or chronic fatigue syndrome, nor GHB's apparent efficacy in treating the EDS affecting many patients with PD. Other biological effects of GHB may be the basis of improving these symptoms. For example, it has long been known that GHB reduces muscle tone and inhibits the monosynaptic H-reflex [97]. This may be part of the series of events which leads to fewer body movements and to a more continuous sleep giving, in turn, rise to a more restful and more recuperative sleep.

There is a strong suggestion that immune functions may be involved in GHB's therapeutic effects. Evidence exists that an autoimmune dysfunction underlies the triggering of the onset symptoms of narcolepsy-cataplexy, as first proposed by Parkes et al. [98] and reviewed by Mignot et al. [99]. This is supported by the efficacy at disease onset, as signalled by the appearance of cataplexy, of intravenous injections of immunoglobulins [100]. As well, fibromyalgia and chronic fatigue syndrome, which are also improved by GHB, are currently considered as being, at least in part, autoimmune diseases.

That GHB is so effective in controlling the range of symptoms of narcolepsy-cataplexy, fibromyalgia and chronic fatigue syndrome each with their attendant insomnia raises the possibility that a significant part of its therapeutic action is through strengthening immune functions. In narcolepsy-cataplexy, this may be the basis of the improved sleep efficiencies of NREM and REM sleep and the relief of REM-based symptoms. In fibromyalgia and chronic fatigue syndrome, the mechanism may well be through the deepening of sleep and the increased efficiency of both NREM and REM sleep with a consequent decrease in daytime mental and physical fatigue, as well as by the reduction of the hyperalgesia that many studies confirm develops with sleep loss [101–103].

What then are the fundamental mechanisms of this effect on immune function? Good sleep that is associated with a normal circadian sleep-wake/temperature/neuroendocrine pattern strengthens the immune system by increasing interleukin-1 (IL-1) activity and to a lesser extent also IL-2, natural killer (NK) cell and mitogen response shortly after sleep onset and timed closely with the onset of SWS [104–106]. In contrast, sleep loss or sleep fragmentation is associated with changes in immunological, neuroendocrine and thermal body functions that contribute to pathological processes such as infections. The altered immune status feeds back on the CNS sleep-regulating mechanisms [107]. These interactions between the circadian/sleep/wake brain systems and the cytokine/immune/endocrine systems are reciprocal and integral to sustaining homeostasis and health.

Conversely, sleep deprivation for 40 h affects human immune functions and leads to increased nocturnal plasma IL-1 and IL-2 like activities [108]. Sleep deprivation also delays the normal nocturnal response of lymphocytes to pokeweed mitogen stimulation. With return to natural night sleep, there is a prolonged reduction in nocturnal NK activity and a return of an increased response to pokeweed mitogen. These effects appear to be independent of the circadian rhythm of cortisol, which in this study was unchanged.

Injection of bacterial endotoxin in humans has been used to model the numerous effects of infections including the release of inflammatory cytokines. Small amounts of endotoxin that do not affect body temperature or neuroendocrine measures, but which mildly stimulate release of inflammatory cytokines, lead to an increase in NREM sleep amount and intensity [109]. By contrast, febrile host responses to higher doses are associated with marked sleep changes, the most probable mediator of this effect being the cytokine inflammatory factor tumour necrosis factor-alpha [110]. It has been suggested by Mullington et al. [111] that the debilitating fatigue in fibromyalgia, chronic fatigue syndrome and similar conditions may be related to altered cytokine profiles.

It is now apparent that the human circadian/sleep/wake systems and the immune systems have a bidirectional communication interaction that is altered in diseases having an immune dysfunction component such as narcolepsy with cataplexy, fibromyalgia and chronic fatigue syndrome [112–114]; and that these pathological disturbances are reduced even totally suppressed by GHB therapy with a resultant improvement in clinical symptoms of insomnia, sleepiness, fatigue, cataplexy, and pain. So how does this occur?

Concerning the altered immune function in narcolepsy-cataplexy, the postulated immune-mediated mechanism could either be autoimmune alone or also involve epigenetics. It is well documented that there is a genetic component to the etiology of narcolepsy, the solid evidence for which has been comprehensively summarized by Mignot [115]. Epigenetic mechanisms pair such a genetic predisposition with either endogenous factors or external environmental, behavioural or other factors which reflect the epigenetic interaction between genetic and nongenetic factors. There are several candidates.

Significant sleep loss and irregular sleep such as in rotating shift work often precedes the onset of narcolepsy [116, 117] and would lead to the immune disturbances described earlier. Moreover, in narcolepsy-cataplexy, there is a misalignment of the circadian clock which is phase advanced compared to the timing of night sleep [118]. This may be an equally important factor as sleep loss, because as there is evidence that circadian timing problems alone predispose to suppression of immune function [119].

Exposure to certain infections appears also to be a facilitator of the initiation of the immune process leading to the appearance of narcolepsy. A first association with infection was reported at the same conference by Billiard et al. [120] and Montplaisir et al. [121]. Both studies showed elevated antibodies to streptococcal antigens around the time of onset of narcolepsy-cataplexy and, in the Montplaisir et al. study, also of idiopathic hypersomnia. This association has been confirmed by Mueller-Eckhardt et al. [112], Longstreth et al. [123] and Aran et al. [124]. Infections by streptococci are, however, not the only infectious trigger, as the swine flu (H1N1) epidemic was also associated with an increase in new cases of narcolepsy-cataplexy [125].

The mechanism by which infection induces an autoimmune process leading to widespread loss of hypocretin (orexin) cells in the CNS [126], which is the fundamental etiology of the disease, is complex. These authors propose that either autoantigen-specific CD4* T cells or superantigen stimulated CD8* T cells [127], through the activation of DQB1*0602 signalling, activates microglia and macrophages leading to release of neurotoxic molecules, such as quinolinic acid, known to cause selective destruction of hypocretin cells in the hypothalamus. The finding that narcolepsy-cataplexy is strongly associated with the T-cell receptor alpha locus [128] is compatible with this proposed mechanism. How GHB apparently halts or may even reverse, this destructive process remains to be established.

The Future

What does the future hold now that GHB has become the drug of choice in the symptomatic treatment of narcolepsy-cataplexy and has also been shown to be effective in other neurological and in psychiatric sleep disorders? Because of GHB's short duration of action, the drug must be given more than once during the night. Although most patients rapidly adapt to this treatment regimen, a formulation using a longer duration of action should improve the acceptability of GHB and broaden its use. Sleepwalking and sleep-eating between the two nightly doses are not uncommon and are possibly related to the rebound release of dopamine at this time [129].

They could be eliminated with a longer acting formulation of GHB. A longer half-life might make it possible for sleep to smoothly run its full 6–8-h nightly course and this, in turn, reduce the need for daytime stimulants. A longer half-life with a better pharmacokinetic profile would also make GHB more acceptable for the treatment of other various types of insomnia [56].

Research continues on the diverse pharmacological actions of GHB and on its natural function in cells throughout the biological kingdom. For example, there is now increasing reason to believe that muscarinic cholinergic super-sensitivity is a key pathological feature common to both depression and narcolepsy. That GHB was able in depression to induce both sleep-onset REM periods and sleep paralysis is, perhaps, because it inhibits dopamine release, and this in-turn enables the release of acetylcholine which then acts on sensitized receptors primed to induce REM sleep. Repeated application of GHB and the recurrent release of acetylcholine reduce this sensitivity and raise the threshold for the induction of cataplexy [25, 130]. Might GHB have a similar mechanism in the treatment of depression? Could the elimination of cholinergic super-sensitivity in depression stabilize this recurrent mood disorder [131]?

GHB is in all life forms and appears to be a component of a metabolic system that comes into play when cellular structures are under stress. Under those conditions, GHB may serve as a source of carbon, energy and antioxidant power and act to protect the endangered cells. These properties suggest that GHB may find widespread use in the treatment of many different types of human disease [75,132, 133].

Approaches other than GHB to treat narcolepsy-cataplexy are also being proposed and investigated. These include for narcolepsy-cataplexy, developing antagonists of the presynaptic histaminergic H3 receptors and the replacement of the lost CNS hypocretin (orexin) cells by nasal inhalation of hypocretin or by the stem cell transplant approach [134].

References

1. Benca RM, Obermeyer WH, Thisted RA, Gillin JC. Sleep and psychiatric disorders. meta-analysis. Arch Gen Psychiatry. 1992;49(8):651–68.
2. Charney DS, Mihic SJ, Harris RA. Hypnotics and sedatives. In: Brunton LL, Lazo JS, Parker KL, editors. The pharmacological basis of therapeutics. 11th ed. New York: McGraw-Hill; 2006. pp. 401–23.
3. Laborit H-M. Sodium-4-hydroxybutyrate. Int J Neuropharmacol. 1964;3:433–52.
4. Laborit H, Jouany JM, Gerard J, Fabiani F. Generalities concerning the experimental study and clinical use of gamma hydroxybutyrate of Na [Article in French]. Agressologie. 1960;1:387–406.
5. Muyard J, Laborit H-M. Gammahydroxybutyrate psychotherapeutic drugs: Part-II. In: Usdin E, Forrest J, editors. Applications: psychopharmacology. New York: Marcel-Dekker; 1977. pp. 1339–75.

6. Roth RH, Giarman NJ. Conversion in vivo of gamma-aminobu-tyric to gamma-hydroxybutyric acid in the rat. Biochem Pharmacol. 1969;18(1):247–50.

7. Vickers MD. Gammahydroxybutyric acid. Int Anesthesiol Clin. 1969;7(1):75–89.

8. Mamelak M, Escriu JM, Stokan O. The effects of gamma-hydroxybutyrate on sleep. Biol Psychiatry. 1977;12(2):273–88.

9. Godbout R, Montplaisir J. Effects of γ-hydroxybutyrate on sleep. In: Tunnicliff G, Cash CD, editors. Gammahydroxybutyrate: molecular, functional and clinical aspects. London: Taylor and Francis; 2002. pp. 120–32.

10. Mamelak M, Escriu JM, Stokan O. Sleep-inducing effects of gammahydroxybutyrate. Lancet. 1973;2(7824):328–9.

11. Nishino S, Kanbayashi T. Symptomatic narcolepsy, cataplexy and hypersomnia, and their implications in the hypothalamic hypocretin/orexin system. Sleep Med Rev. 2005;9(4):269–310.

12. Sakurai T. Roles of orexin/hypocretin in regulation of sleep/wakefulness and energy homeostasis. Sleep Med Rev. 2005;9(4):231–41.

13. Sakurai T. The neural circuit of orexin (hypocretin): maintaining sleep and wakefulness. Nat. Rev. Neurosci. 2007;8:171–81.

14. Broughton R, Valley V, Aguire M, Roberts J, Suwalski W, Dunham W. Excessive daytime sleepiness and the pathophysiology of narcolepsy-cataplexy: a laboratory perspective. Sleep 1986;9(1):205–15.

15. Broughton R, Dunham W, Weiskopf M, Rivers M. Night sleep does not predict day sleep in narcolepsy. Electroenceph Clin Neurophysiol. 1994;91:67–70.

16. Broughton RJ, Krupa S, Boucher B, Rivers M, Mullington J. Impaired circadian waking arousal in narcolepsy-cataplexy. Sleep Res Online. 1998;1(4):159–65. http://www.sro.org/1988/broughton/159/.

17. Broughton R, Mamelak M. Gamma-hydroxy-butyrate in the treatment of compound narcolepsy. Sleep Res. 1975;4:211.

18. Hoddes E, Zarcone V, Smythe H, Philips R, Dement WC. Quantification of sleepiness: a new approach. Psychophysiol. 1973;10:431–6.

19. Broughton R, Mamelak M. Gammahydroxybutyrate in the treatment of narcolepsy: a preliminary report. In: Guillemmault C, Dement WC, Passouant P, editors. Narcolepsy. Advances in sleep research. New York: Spectrum; 1976. pp. 659–67.

20. Broughton R, Mamelak M. The treatment of narcolepsy-cataplexy with nocturnal gamma-hydroxybutyrate. Can J Neurol Sci. 1979;6(1):1–6.

21. Broughton R, Mamelak M. Effects of nocturnal gamma-hydroxybutyrate on sleep/waking patterns in narcolepsy-cataplexy. Can J Neurol Sci. 1980;7(1):23–31.

22. Lammers GJ, Arends J, Declerck AC, Ferrari MD, Schouwink G, Troost J. Gammahydroxybutyrate and narcolepsy: a double-blind placebo-controlled study. Sleep. 1993;16(3):216–20.

23. Scrima L, Hartman PG, Johnson FH Jr, Hiller FC. Efficacy of gamma-hydroxybutyrate versus placebo in treating narcolepsy-cataplexy: double-blind subjective measures. Biol Psychiatry. 1989;26(4):331–43.

24. Scrima L, Hartman PG, Johnson FH Jr, Thomas EE, Hiller FC. The effects of gamma-hydroxybutyrate on the sleep of narcolepsy patients: a double-blind study. Sleep. 1990;13(6):479–90.

25. Mamelak M. Narcolepsy and depression and the neurobiology of gammahydroxybutyrate. Prog Neurobiol. 2009;89(2):193–219.

26. Mamelak M, Scharf MB, Woods M. Treatment of narcolepsy with gamma-hydroxybutyrate. A review of clinical and sleep laboratory findings. Sleep. 1986; 9(1 Pt 2):285–9.

27. Scharf MB, Brown D, Woods M, Brown L, Hirschowitz J. The effects and effectiveness of gamma-hydroxybutyrate in patients with narcolepsy. J Clin Psychiatry. 1985;46(6):222–5.

28. Broughton R, Ghanem Q, Hishikawa Y, Sugita Y, Nevsimalova S, Roth B. Life effects of narcolepsy in 180 patients from North-America, Asia and Europe compared to matched controls. Can J Neurol Sci. 1981;8:299–304.

29. Broughton R, Ghanem Q, Hishikawa Y, Sugita Y, Nevsimalova S, Roth B. Life effects of narcolepsy: relationships to geographic origin (North American, Asian or European and to other patient and illness variables. Can J Neurol Sci. 1983;10:100–4.

30. Broughton R, Guberman A, Roberts J. Comparison of psychosocial effects of epilepsy and of narcolepsy-cataplexy: a controlled study. Epilepsia. 1984;25:423–33.

31. Weaver TE, Cuellar N. A randomized trial evaluating the effectiveness of sodium oxybate therapy on quality of life in narcolepsy. Sleep. 2006;29(9):1189–94.

32. US Xyrem Multicenter Study Group. A randomized double blind, placebo controlled multicenter trial comparing the effects of three doses of orally administered sodium oxybate with placebo for the treatment of narcolepsy. Sleep. 2002;25:42–9.

33. US Xyrem Multicenter Study Group. A 12 month, open label, multicenter extension trial of orally administered sodium oxybate for the treatment of narcolepsy. Sleep. 2003;26:31–5.

34. US Xyrem Multicenter Study Group. Sodium oxybate demonstrates long term efficacy for the treatment of cataplexy in patients with narcolepsy. Sleep Med. 2004;5:119–23.

35. Martinez-Rodriguez J, Iranzo A, Santamaria J, Genis D, Molins A, Silva Y, et al. Status cataplecticus induced by abrupt withdrawal of clomipramine. Neurologia. 2002;17(2):113–6.

36. Mamelak M, Black J, Montplaisir J, Ristanovic R. A pilot study on the effects of sodium oxybate on sleep architecture and daytime alertness in narcolepsy. Sleep. 2004;27(7):1327–34.

37. Mitler MM, Gujavarty S, Browman CP. Maintenance of wakefulness test: a polysomnographic technique for evaluating treatment efficacy in patients with excessive somnolence. Electroenceph Clin Neurophysiol. 1982;53:658–61.

38. Johns MW. A new method for measuring daytime sleepiness: The Epworth sleepiness scale. Sleep 1991;14:540–5.

39. Xyrem International Study Group. Further evidence supporting the use of sodium oxybate for the treatment of cataplexy: a double blind placebo-controlled study in 228 patients. Sleep Med. 2005a;6:415–21.

40. Xyrem International Study Group. A double blind, placebo controlled study demonstrates sodium oxybate is effective for the treatment of excessive daytime sleepiness in narcolepsy. J Clin Sleep Med. 2005b;1:391–7

41. Black J, Houghton WC. Sodium oxybate improves excessive daytime sleepiness in narcolepsy. Sleep 2006;29(7):939–46.

42. Murali H, Kotagal S. Off-label treatment of severe childhood narcolepsy-cataplexy with sodium butyrate. Sleep. 2006;29(8):1025–9.

43. Richardson GS, Carskadon MA, Flagg W, van den Hoed J, Dement WC, Mitler MM. Excessive daytime sleepiness in man: multiple sleep latency measurements in narcoleptic and control subjects. Electroencephalogr Clin Neurophysiol. 1978;45: 621–7.

44. Aran A, Einen M, Lin L, Plazzi G, Nishino S, Mignot E. Clinical and therapeutic aspects of childhood narcolepsy-cataplexy: a retrospective study of 51 children. Sleep. 2010;33(11):1457–64.

45. Peraita-Adrados R, Garcia-Peñas JJ, Ruiz-Falco L, Gutiērrez-Solana L, Lopez-Esteban P, Vicario JL, Miano S, Aparicio-Meix M, Martinez-Sopena MJ. Clinical, polysomnographic and laboratory characteristics of narcolepsy-cataplexy in a sample of chidren and adolescents. Sleep Med. 2011;12:24–7. (Epub 2010 Nov 2).

46. Mansukhani MP, Kotagal S. Sodium oxybate in the treatment of childhoon narcolepsy-cataplexy: a retrospective study. Sleep Med. 2012;13(6):606–10. (Epub 2012 Mar 24).

47. Lecendreux M, Poli F, Oudiette D, Benazzouz F, Doniacour CE, Franceschini C, Finotti E, Pizza F, Bruni O, Piazzi G. Tolerance and efficacy of sodium oxybate in childhood narcolepsy with cataplexy: a retrospective study. Sleep. 2012;35(5):709–11.

48. George CF, Feldman N, Inhaber N, Steininger TL, Greschik SM, Lai C, Zheng Y. A safety trial of sodium oxybate in patients with obstructive sleep apnea: acute effects on sleep-disordered breathing. Sleep Med. 2010;11(1):38–42.

49. George CF, Feldman N, Zheng Y, Steininger TL, Grzeschik SM, Lai C, Inhaber N. A 2-week, polysomnographic safety trial of sodium oxybate in obstructive sleep apnea syndrome. Sleep Breath. 2011;15(1):13–20. (Epub 2010 Jan 18).

50. Seeck-Hirschner M, Baier PC, von Freier A, Aldenhoff J, Göder R. Increase in sleep-related breathing disturbances after treatment with sodium oxybate in patients with narcolepsy and mild obstructive sleep apnea syndrome: two case reports. Sleep Med. 2009;10(1):154–5. (Epub 2008 Jan 28).

51. Moldofsky H. The significance of the sleeping-waking brain for the understanding of the widespread musculoskeletal pain and fatigue in fibromyalgia and allied syndromes. Joint Bone Spine. 2008;75(4):397–402. (Epub 2008 May 5).

52. Russell IJ, Perkins AT, Michalek JE. Oxybate SXB-26 fibromyalgia study group. Arthritis Rheum. 2009;60(1):299–309.

53. Wallace DM, Maze T, Shafazand S. Sodium oxybate-induced sleep driving and sleep-related eating disorder. J Clin Sleep Med. 2011;7(3):310–1.

54. Spitzer AR, Broadman M. Treatment of the narcoleptiform sleep disorder in chronic fatigue syndrome and fibromyalgia with sodium oxybate. Pain Pract. 2010;10(1):54–9.

55. Moldofsky M, Inhaber NH, Guintya DR, Alvarez-Horine SB. Effects of sodium oxybate on sleep physiology and sleep/wake related symptoms in patients with fibromyalgia syndrome: a double-blind, randomized, placebo-controlled study. J Rheumatol. 2010;37(10):2156–66. (Epub 2010 Aug 3).

56. Russell IJ, Holman AJ, Swick TJ, Varez-Horine S, Wang YG, Guinta D. Sodium oxybate reduces pain, fatigue, and sleep disturbance and improves functionality in fibromyalgia: results from a 14-week, randomized, double-blind, placebo-controlled study. Pain. 2011;152(5):1007–17.

57. Staud R. Pharmacological treatment of fibromyalgia syndrome: new developments. Drugs. 2010;70(1)1–14.

58. Staud R. Sodium oxybate for the treatment of fibromyalgia. Expert Opin Pharmacother. 2011;12(11):1789–98. (Epub 2011 June 16).

59. Crawford BK, Piault EC, Lai C, Bennett RM. Assessing fibromyalgia-related fatigue: content validity and psychometric performance of the fatigue visual analog scale in adult patients with fibromyalgia. Clin Exp Rheumatol. 2011;29(6 Suppl 69):S34–63. (Epub 2012 Jan 3).

60. Spaeth M, Bennett RM, Benson BA, Wang YG, Lai C, Choy EH. Sodium oxybate therapy provides multidimensional improvement in fibromyalgia: results of an international phase 3 trial. Ann Rheum Dis. 2012;71(6):935–42.

61. Boeve BF, Silber MH, Ferman TJ, Kokmen E, Smith GE, Ivnik RJ, Parisi JE, Olson EJ, Petersen RC. REM sleep behaviour disorder and degenerative dementia: an association likely reflecting Lewy body disease. Neurology. 1998;51(2):363–70.

62. Boeve BF, Silber MH, Saper CB, Ferman TJ, Dickson DW, Parisi JE, Benarroch EE, Ahiskog JE, Smith GE, Caselli RC, Tipppman-Peikert M, Olson EJ, Lin S-C, Young T, Wszolek Z, Schenck CH, Mahowald MW, Catillo PR, Del Tredici K, Braak H. Pathophysiology of REM sleep behaviour disorder and relevance to neurodegenerative disease. Brain 2007;130:2770–88.

63. Gagnon J-F, Bédard M-A, Fantini ML, Petit D, Panisset M, Rompré S, Carrier J, Montplaisir J. REM sleep behavior disorder and REM sleep without atonia in Parkinson's disease. Neurology. 2002;59(4):585–9.

64. Olson EJ, Boeve BF, Silber MH. Rapid eye movement behavior disorder: demographic, clinical and laboratory findings in 93 cases. Brain. 2000;123:331–9.

65. Schenck C, Bundlie SR, Mahowald MW. Delayed emergence of a parkinsonian disorder in 38 % of 29 older men initially diagnosed with idiopathic rapid eye movement sleep behaviour disorder. Neurology 1996;46(2):388–93.

66. Sixel-Döring F, Trautmann E, Mollenhauer B, Trenkwalder C. Associated factors for REM sleep behavior disorder in Parkinson disease. Neurology. 2011;77(11):1048–54.

67. Shneesen JM. Successful treatment of REM sleep behaviour disorder with sodium oxybate. Clin Neuropharm. 2009;32(3):158–9.

68. Arnulf I, Leu-Semenescu S. Sleepiness in Parkinson's disease. Parkinsonism Relat Disord. 2009;15(Suppl. 3):S101–4.

69. Ondo WG, Perkins T, Swick T, Hull KL, Jiminez JE, Garrir TS, Pardi D. Sodium oxybate for excessive daytime sleepiness in Parkinson disease. Arch Neurol. 2008;63(10):1337–40.

70. Gao B, Kilic E, Baumann CR, Hermann DM, Bassetti CL. Gamma-hydroxybutyrate accelerates functional recovery after focal cerebral ischemia. Cerebrovasc Dis. 2008;26(4):413–9. (Epub 2008 Aug 28).

71. MacMillan V. Effects of gamma-hydroxybutrate and gamma-butyrolactone on cerebral energy metabolism during exposure and recovery from hypoxemia-oligemia. Stroke. 1080;11(3):271–7.

72. Ottani A, Saltini S, Bartiromo M, Zaffe D, Renzo-Botticelli A, Ferrari A, Bertolini A, Genedani S. Effect of gamma-hydroxybutyrate in two rat models of focal cerebral damage. Brain Res. 2003;986(1/2):181–90.

73. Sadasivan S, Maher TJ, Quang LS. Gamma-hydroxybutyrate (GHB), gamma-butyrolactone (GBL) and 1,4-butanedio (1,4-BD) reduce the volume of cerebral infarction in rodent transient middle cerebral artery occlusion. Ann N Y Acad Sci. 2006;1074:537–44

74. Mamelak M. Alzheimer's disease, oxidative stress and gamma-hydroxybutyrate. Neurobiol Aging. 2007;28(9):1340–60. (Epub 2006 Jul 11).

75. Mamelak M. Sporadic Alzheimer's disease: the starving brain. J Alzheimers Dis. 2012;31(3):459–74.

76. Husain Am, Ristanovic RK, Bogan RK. Weight loss in narcolepsy patients treated with sodium oxybate. Sleep Med. 2009;10(6):661–3. (Epub 2008 Nov 17).

77. Rossetti AQ, Heinzer RC, Tafti M, Buclin T. Rapid occurrence of depression following addition of sodium oxybate to modafinil. Sleep Med. 2010;11(5):500–1. (Epub 2010 Feb 4).

78. Langford J, Gross WL. Psychosis in the context of sodium oxybate therapy. J Clin Sleep Med. 2011;7(6):665–6.

79. Bédard MA, Montplaisir J, Godbout R, Lapierre O. Nocturnal gamma-hydroxybutyrate. Effect on periodic leg movements and sleep organization of narcoleptic patients. Clin Neuropharmacol. 1989;12(1):29–36.

80. Poli F, Ricotta L, Vandi S, Franceschini C, Pizza F, Palaia V, Moghadam KK, Banal D, Vetrugno R, Thorpy MJ, Plazzi G. Catathrenia under sodium oxybate in narcolepsy with cataplexy. Sleep Breath. 2012;16(2):427–34. (Epub 2011 Apr 12).

81. Akins BE, Miranda E, Lacy JM, Logan BK. A multi-drug intoxication fatality involving Xyrem (GHB). J Forensic Sci. 2009;54(2):495–6. (Epub 2009 Jan 29).

82. Zvosec DL, Smith SW, Hall BJ. Three deaths associated with use of Xyrem. Sleep Med. 2009;10(4):490–3. (Epub 2009 Mar 9).

83. Zvosec DL, Smith SW, Porrata T., Strobl AQ, Dyer JE. Case series of 226 gamma-hydroxybutyrate-associated deaths: lethal toxicity and trauma. Am J Emerg Med. 2011;29(3):319–32.

84. Lammers GJ, Bassetti C, Billiard M, Black J, Broughton R, Dauvilliers Y, Ferini-Strambi L, Garcia-Borreguero D, Goswami M, Högl B, Iranzo A, Jennum P, Khatami R, Lecendreux M, Mayer G, Mignot E, Montplaisir J, Nevsimalova S, Peraita-Adrados R, Plazzi G, Scammell T, Silber M, Sonka K, Tafti M, Thorpy M. Sodium oxybate is an effective and safe treatment for narcolepsy. Sleep Med. 2010;11:105–8.

85. House of Commons, Science and Technology Committee. Fifth Report of Session 2005–05. 2006. http://news.bbc.co.uk/1/shared/bsp/hi/pdfs/31_07_06_drugsreport.pdf. Accessed 31 Jul 2006.

86. Xie XS, Pardi D, Black J. Molecular and cellular actions of γ-hydroxybutyric acid: possible mechanisms underlying GHB efficacy in narcolepsy. In: Bassetti CL, Billiard M, Mignot E, editors. Narcolepsy and hypersomnia. New York: Informa Healthcare; 2007. pp. 583–620.

87. Lapierre O, Montplaisir J, Lamarre M, Bedard MA. The effect of gamma-hydroxybutyrate on nocturnal and diurnal sleep of normal subjects: further considerations on REM sleep-triggering mechanisms. Sleep. 1990;13(1):24–30.

88. Passouant P. Problemes physiopathologiques de la narcolepsie et periodicité du sommeil rapide au cours du nycthemère. In: Gastaut H, Lugaresi E, Berti Ceroni G, Coccagna G, editors. The abnormalities of sleep in man. Bologna: Aulo Gaggi Editore; 1968. p. 177–190.

89. Montplaisir J, Godbout R. Nocturnal sleep of narcoleptic patients: revisited. Sleep. 1986; 9(1 Pt 2):159–61.

90. Van Nieuwenhuijzen PS, McGregor IS, Hunt GE. The distribution of gamma-hydroxybutyrate-induced Fos expression in rat brain: comparison with baclofen. Neurosci. 2009;158(2):441–55. (Epub 2008 Oct 17).

91. Zeitzer JM, Buckmaster CL, Parker KL, Hauck CM, Lyons DM, Mignot E. Circadian and homeostatic regulation of hypocretin in a primate model: implications for the consolidation of wakefulness. J Neurosci. 2003;23(8):3555–60.

92. Huber R, Ghilardi F, Massimini M, Tononi G. Local sleep and learning. Nature 2004;430:78–81.

93. Lesku A, Vyssotski AL, Martinez-Gonzalez D, Wilzeck C, Rattenborg NC. Local sleep homeostasis in the avian brain: convergence of sleep function in mammals and birds? Proc Biol Soi. 2011;278(1717):2419–28. (Epub 2011 Jan 5).

94. Vyazovskiy VV, Olcese U, Hanlon E, Nir Y, Cirelli C, Tononi G. Local sleep in awake rats. Nature. 2011;472(7344):443–7.

95. Mignot E. CSF hypocretin-1/orexin-A in narcolepsy: technical aspects and clinical experience in the United States. In: Bassetti CL, Billiard M, Mignot E. Narcolepsy and hypersomnia. New York: Informa Healthcare; 2007. pp. 287–99.

96. Broughton R. Human consciousness and sleep/waking rhythms: a review and some neuropsychological considerations. J Clin Neuropsychol. 1982;4:193–218.

97. Mamelak H, Snowden K. The effect of gammahydroxybutyrate on the H-reflex. Neurology. 1983;33(11):1497–500.

98. Parkes D, Langdon N, Lock C. Narcolepsy and immunity. BMJ. 1986;292(6517):359–60.

99. Mignot E, Tafti M, Dement WC, Grumet FC. Narcolepsy and immunity. Adv Neuroimmunol. 1995;5(1):23–37.

100. Dauvillier Y, Carlander B, Rivier F, Touchon J, Tafti M. Successful management of cataplexy with intravenous immunoglobulins at narcolepsy onset. Ann Neurol. 2004;56:905–8.

101. Lavigne GJ. Effect of sleep restriction on pain perception: towards greater attention! Pain. 2010;148(1):6–7. (Epub 2009 Nov 14).

102. Onen SH, Alloui A, Gross A, Eschallier A, Dubray C. The effects of total sleep deprivation, selective sleep interruption and sleep recovery on pain tolerance threshold in healthy subjects. J Sleep Res. 2001;10(1):35–42.

103. Roehrs T, Hyde M, Blaisdell B, Greenwald M, Roth T. Sleep loss and REM sleep loss are hyperalgesic. Sleep. 2006;29(2):145–51.

104. Moldofsky H. Sleep, neuroimmune and neuroendocrine functions in fibromyalgia and chronic fatigue syndrome. Adv Neuroimmunol. 1995;5(1):39–56.

105. Moldofsky H, Lue FA, Eisen J, Keystone E, Gorczynski RM. The relationship of interleukin-1 and immune functions to sleep in humans. Psychosom Med. 1986;48(5):309–18.

106. Moldofsky H, Lue FA, Davidson JR, Gorczynski R. Effects of sleep deprivation on human immune functions. FASEB. 1989;3(8):1072–7.

107. Pollmächer T, Mullington J, Korth C, Hinze-Selch D. Influence of host defense activation on sleep in normal. Adv Neuroimmunol. 1995;5(2):155–69.

108. Dickstein JB, Moldofsky H. Sleep, cytokines and immune function. Sleep Med Rev. 1999;3(3):219–28.

109. Mullington J, Korth C, Hermann DM, Orth A, Galanos C, Holsboer F, Pollmächer T. Dose-dependent effects of endotoxin on human sleep. Am J Physiol Regulatory Integrative Comp Physiol. 2000;278:R947–55.

110. Pollmächer T, Schuld A, Kraus T, Haack M, Hinze-Selch D, Mullington J. Experimental immunomodulation, sleep, and sleepiness in humans. Ann N Y Acad Sci. 2000;917:488–99.

111. Mullington JM, Hirze-Selch D, Pollmächer T. Mediators of inflammation and their interaction with sleep: relevance for chronic fatigue syndrome and related conditions. Ann N Y Acad Med. 2001;933:201–10

112. Lorton D, Lubahn CL, Estus C, Millar BA, Carter JL, Wood CA, Bellinger DL. Bidirectional communication between the brain and the immune system: implications for physiological sleep and disorders with disrupted sleep. Neuroimmunomodulation. 2006;13(5/6):357–74. (Epub 2007 Aug 6).

113. Schuld A, Haack M, Hinze-Salch D, Mullington J, Pollmächer T. Experimental studies on the interaction between sleep and the immune system in humans. Psychother Psychosom Med Psychol. 2005;55(1):29–35.

114. Wrona D. Neural-immune interactions: an integrative view of the bidirectional relationship between the brain and immune systems. J Neuroimmunol. 2006;172(1/2):38–58. (Epub 2006 Jan 10).

115. Mignot E. Behavioral genetics '97: genetics of narcolepsy and other sleep disorders. Am J Hum Genet. 1997;60:1289–302.

116. Broughton R. Narcolepsy (letter to the editor). Can Med Assoc J. 1974;110:1007.

117. Mitchell S, Dement WC. Narcolepsy syndromes: antecedent, contiguous and concomitant sleep disordering and deprivation. Psychophysiology. 1968;4:398.

118. Mullington J, Newman J, Dunham W, Broughton RJ. Phase timing and duration of naps in narcolepsy-cataplexy: preliminary findings. In: Horne J, editor. Sleep '90. Bochum: Pontenagel; 1990. pp. 158–60.

119. Castanon-Cervantes O, Wu M, Ehlen JC, Paul K, Gamble KL, Johnson RL, Besing RC, Menaker M, Gewirtz AT, Davidson AJ. Dysregulation of inflammatory responses by chronic circadian disruption. J Immunol. 2010;185(10):5796–805. (Epub 2010 Oct 13).

120. Billiard M, Laaberki M, Reygrobellet C, Seignalet J, Brissaud L, Besset A. Elevated antibodies to streptococcal antigens in narcoleptic subjects. Sleep Res. 1989;18:201.

121. Montplaisir J, Poirier G, Lapierre O, Montplaisir S. Streptococcal antibodies in narcolepsy and idiopathic hypersomnia. Sleep Res. 1989;18:271.

122. Mueller-Eckhardt G, Meier-Ewert K, Schiefer HG. Is there an infectious origin of narcolepsy? Lancet. 1990;17(8686):424.

123. Longstreth WT Jr, Ton TG, Koepsell TD. Narcolepsy and streptococcal infections. Sleep. 2009;32(12):1548.

124. Aran A, Lin L, Nevsimalova S, Plazzi G, Chul Hong S, Weiner K, Zeitzer J, Mignot E. Elevated anti-streptococcal antibodies in patients with recent narcolepsy onset. Sleep. 2008;32(8):979–83.

125. Dauvillier Y, Montplaisir J, Cochen V, Desautels A, Einen M, Lin L, Kawashima M, Barard S, Monaca C, Tiberge M, Filipini D, Tripathy A, Hong Nouven B, Kotagal S, Mignot E. Post-H1N1 narcolepsy-cataplexy. Sleep. 2010;33(11):1428–30.

126. Fontana A, Gast H, Reith W, Recher M, Birchler T, Bassetti CL. Narcolepsy: autoimmunity, effector T cell activation due to in-

fection, or T cell independent histocompatibility complex class II induced neuronal loss. Brain. 2010;133:1300–11.

127. Bollinger T, Bollinger A, Skrum L, Dimitrov S, Lange T, Solbach W. Sleep-dependent activity of T cells and regulatory T cells. Clin Exp Immunol. 2009;155(2):231–8. (Epub 2008 Nov 24).

128. Hallmayer J, Faraco J, Lin L, Hesselson S, Winkelmann J, Kawashima M, Mayer G, Plazzi G, Nevsimalova S, Bourgin P, Hong S-C, Honda Y, Honda M, Högl B, Longstreth WT, Monplaisir J, Kemlink D, Einen M, Chen J, Musone SL, Akana M, Miyagawa T, Duan J, Desautels A, Erhardt C, Hesla PE, Poli F, Frauscher B, Jeong J-H, Lww A-P, Ton TGN, Kvale M, Kolestar L, Dobrovolna M, Nepom GT, Salomon D, Wichmann H-E, Rouleau GA, Gieger C, Levinson DF, Gejman PV, Meitinge T, Young T, Peppard P, Tokunaga K, Kwok P-Y, Rissch N, Mignot E. Narcolepsy is strongly associated with the T-cell receptor alpha locus. Nat Genet. 2009;41(6):708–11.

129. Redgrave P, Taha EB, White L, Dean P. Increased food intake following the manipulation of intracerebral dopamine levels with gamma-hydroxybutyrate. Psychopharmacology (Berl). 1982;76(3):273–7.

130. Giorgi O, Rubio MC. Decreased 3H-L-quinuclidinyl benzilate binding and muscarine receptor subsensitivity after chronic gamma-butyrolactone treatment. Naunyn Schmiedebergs Arch Pharmacol. 1981;318(1):14–8.

131. Janowsky DS, el-Yousef MK, Davis JM, Sekerke HJ. A cholinergic-adrenergic hypothesis of mania and depression. Lancet 1972;2(7778):632–5.

132. Mamelak M. Neurodegeneration, sleep and cerebral energy metabolism: a testable hypothesis. J Geriatr Psychiatry Neurol. 1997;10(1):29–32.

133. Mamelak M, Hyndman D. Gamma-hydroxybutyrate and oxidative stress. In: Tunnicliff G, Cash C, editors. Gamma-hydroxybutyrate: molecular, functional and clinical aspects. London: Taylor and Francis; 2002. pp. 218–35.

134. Dauvilliers Y. Narcolepsie. In: Billiard M, Dauvilliers Y, editors. Les Troubles du Sommeil. France: Elsevier Issy-les-Moulineaux; 2012. pp. 201–14.

Julien Q. M. Ly, Sarah L. Chellappa and Pierre Maquet

Introduction

During the last two decades, neuroimaging techniques have been applied to sleep studies and contributed to a better understanding of sleeping process and its disorders. These techniques can provide information about both brain structure and function. This chapter reviews both aspects in the field of sleep research. At first, we will give an overview of the different imaging techniques and findings they brought in normal human sleep. A short paragraph will then be dedicated to imaging studies of sleep and memory. Finally, we will finish with a section on neuroimaging in sleep disorders. Further information can be found in previous reviews on the same topic.

1. Maquet P. Functional neuroimaging of normal human sleep by positron emission tomography. J Sleep Res. 2000 Sept;9(3):207–31.
2. Desseilles M, Dang-Vu T, Schabus M, Sterpenich V, Maquet P, Schwartz S. Neuroimaging insights into the pathophysiology of sleep disorders. Sleep. 2008 Jun;31(6):777–94.
3. Dang-Vu TT, Schabus M, Desseilles M, Sterpenich V, Bonjean M, Maquet P. Functional neuroimaging insights into the physiology of human sleep. Sleep. 2010 Dec;33(12):1589–603.
4. Jedidi Z, Rikir E, Muto V, Mascetti L, Kussé C, Foret A, Shaffii-Le Bourdiec A, Vandewalle G, Maquet P. Functional neuroimaging of the reciprocal influences between sleep and wakefulness. Pflugers Arch. 2012 Jan;463(1).

Neuroanatomical Assessments

Structural brain imaging is clinically relevant for two reasons. First, it is widely available and second, it requires a limited collaboration from the patient. The objective is usually to characterize regional-specific modifications in brain structure between healthy participants and patients suffering from certain sleep disorders. These cerebral changes are supposed to be relatively persistent and thus can be observed independently from the patient's state of vigilance during the examination. It does not necessarily require the patient to be sleeping (or performing a task).

Within this type of neuroanatomical ways of assessment, the two basic techniques are *Voxel-based morphometry* (VBM) and *magnetic resonance spectroscopy* (MRS).

VBM is becoming the standard way of analyzing structural brain data. Based on high resolution scans, VBM allows between-group, statistical comparisons of tissue composition (gray and white matter) across all brain regions. Usually built on a general linear model, it tests for voxel-wise differences in signal between patients and controls or for linear regression between structural brain aspects and specific explanatory variables (age, duration of disease…).

MRS allows obtaining biochemical information about regional brain tissue composition by measuring absolute and relative rate of different compounds such as choline (Cho), creatinine (Cr), N-acetyl aspartate (NAA).

As VBM and MRS exclusively concern pathological sleep research we will reserve illustrations of their applications for the last section dedicated to neuroimaging in sleep disorders.

Sleep Functional Neuroimaging

In contrast to structural imaging, functional imaging offers a dynamical approach to probe behavioral states, such as sleep and wakefulness. As it confers a better and faster temporal resolution, it tracks down fluctuations in the global and/or

P. Maquet (✉) · J. Q. M. Ly · S. L. Chellappa
Cyclotron Research Centre, University of Liège,
Allée du 6 Août, 8, 4000 Liège, Belgium
e-mail: pmaquet@ulg.ac.be

S. Chokroverty, M. Billiard (eds.), *Sleep Medicine*, DOI 10.1007/978-1-4939-2089-1_64,
© Springer Science+Business Media, LLC 2015

regional brain activity. Sleep functional neuroimaging by definition implies the assessment of a concomitant state of vigilance, and consequently requires simultaneous EEG recordings.

Initially, sleep functional imaging studies used positron emission tomography (PET) and single photon emission computed tomography (SPECT). However, during the last decade, functional magnetic resonance imaging (fMRI) has emerged as the "gold" technique to probe regional brain activity during sleep, despite the difficulty inherent to simultaneous EEG and fMRI acquisitions [1].

Global Metabolism Level During Sleep: First Studies Using 18-FDG PET

Glucose metabolism, determined by [^{18}F] fluorodeoxyglucosed (18-FDG), was the 1980s most popular marker of brain activity measured by PET. Buchsbaum et al. and Maquet et al. were the first to apply this method in sleep research by two pioneering studies, carried out in 1989 and 1990 respectively. They showed that global glucose metabolism was lower during slow wave sleep (SWS), while it was sustained during REM sleep as compared to wakefulness [2, 3].

18-FDG PET studies rapidly found their limits in sleep research. The poor spatial resolution of this method (~5 mm) and the absence of voxel-wise analysis techniques limited an in-depth characterization of regional brain function. However, an activation of left temporal and occipital areas during REM sleep and a bilateral thalamic deactivation during slow wave sleep (SWS) were already reported [3, 4].

Another 18-FDG drawback is its very limited time resolution. Its long time acquisition (45 min) restricts studies to long lasting effects such as wakefulness, REM and NREM sleep episodes, although the long half-life of 18-FDG (108 min) limits the repetition of measurements in the same subject in a single session [5]. The latter advent of 15-oxygen labeled water (H$_2$^{15}O) in PET studies came as a major progress.

First Assessments of Regional Cerebral Activity: PET with Infusions of H$_2$^{15}O

After using 18-FDG PET, sleep researchers, including Hofle (1997), Andersson (1998), and Maquet and Phillips (1998), started to investigate regional cerebral activity by means of PET with infusions of 15-oxygen labeled water (H$_2$^{15}O). In contrast to 18-FDG PET, H$_2$^{15}O studies do not measure glucose metabolism, but rather the regional cerebral blood flow (rCBF). The reduced time acquisition (1.5 min) and labeled

compounds/shorter half-life (123 s) significantly improved time resolution [5].

During *NREM sleep* (NREMS), H$_2$^{15}O PET studies showed a global but also regional reductions of brain activity in cortical (prefrontal, anterior cingulate, precuneus, associative parietal, and mesial aspect of temporal lobe) and subcortical (brainstem, thalamus, basal ganglia, hypothalamus, basal forebrain) regions [6, 7]. These areas include neuronal populations involved in arousal and awakening, which are among the most activated regions during wakefulness.

Using H$_2$^{15}O PET, *REM sleep* has been associated with the activation of pontine tegmentum, basal forebrain, thalamus, limbic areas (amygdala, hippocampus, anterior cingulate cortex), and temporo-occipital cortices whereas associative prefrontal and parietal areas were deactivated. This pattern can readily be associated with dream features, which mostly occur during REM sleep. Visual and auditory dream perception can be, respectively, correlated to occipital and temporal activations, while affect and emotional intensification can be related to limbic and paralimbic system activation. Conversely, the quiescence of prefrontal areas may account for temporal distortions, weakening of self-reflecting control, or amnesia on awakening [8–11].

Despite the advantages brought on by H$_2$^{15}O, *PET temporal resolution could not directly capture changes in brain activity during transient events,* such as a spindle or a slow wave. However, attempts were made to correlate rCBF variations with EEG spectral activity in sigma (spindles) and delta (slow wave activity) ranges. Accordingly, *sigma power* (12–16 Hz) was negatively correlated to rCBF in the thalamus bilaterally [12] indicating its central role in spindle generation. In a similar vein, *delta power* (0.5–4 Hz) was negatively correlated with rCBF in several brain areas such as thalamus, cerebellum, anterior and posterior cingulate gyrus, precuneus, orbitofrontal cortex, ventro medial prefrontal cortex (vMPFC), basal forebrain, striatum (putamen), and insula [13]. This mapping shows striking similarities with the distribution of deactivated brain areas during NREM sleep, as compared to wakefulness, suggesting a similar neural network in the regulation of NREM sleep and slow waves. The strongest association with delta power was found in vMPFC correlating with the prefrontal predominance of slow wave activity observed in EEG recordings.

Functional Magnetic Resonance Imaging

Functional MRI describes neural activity by assessing the blood oxygen level-dependent (BOLD) signal, a non-linear mix of changes in local brain vascular volume, blood flow, and level of deoxy-hemoglobin. Its success benefits from better spatial and temporal resolution, relative to emission

Table 64.1 As indicated in Table 64.1, each technique has its own advantages and drawbacks in terms of spatial and temporal resolutions but feasibility, accessibility, safety, and cost

	PET	fMRI
What it shows	Distribution of compounds labeled with positron-emitting isotopes	Variations in brain perfusion related to neural activity by assessing the blood oxygen level-dependent signal (BOLD)
Time resolution	Depends on labeled compounds with which vary the biological half-life (HF) and the required exam time acquisition (TA)	~10 s
	FDG	
	TA: 45 min: description restricted to long lasting changes	
	long half-life (108 min): restrict the repetition of measurements of a same subject in a single session	
	H2 15O	
	shorter half-life (123 s)	
	time acquisition (1–2 min)	
Spatial resolution	~5 mm	~2–3 mm
Comfort	Require catheterism	Narrow space and noise hamper
Safety	Infectious risk due to catheterism,; radioactive agent injection, X-ray exposition	Totally non invasive, no injection of a radioactive agent, no irradiation; respect of ferromagnetic contra-indications and precautions
Cost	Important infrastructure required (cyclotron and chemists for radioactive compound production, ...)	
EEG combining	No compatibility or artifacts problems	Requires an MRI compatible EEG cap and amplifier Post processing necessary to remove scan gradient and cardio ballistic artifacts

tomography. The improvement of the latter compared to PET has enabled the direct observation of changes in brain activity for short-lasting events, such as a spindle or a slow wave. In contrast to PET, fMRI is X-ray free and completely non-invasive since it requires neither catheter nor radioactive compound injection. However, the high noise level and exiguity of the device make the environment rather unfavorable to sleep. The EEG recording is also made difficult by the magnetic environment, resulting mainly in gradient scan and pulse-related artifacts which have required the development of MRI compatible EEG caps and artifacts rejecting processes [14]. For comparison between PET and fMRI refer to Table 64.1.

Spatial patterns of regional brain activity described in fMRI during NREMS were globally consistent with those reported by PET sleep studies. However, fMRI allowed to address NREMS phasic activity and was thus able to report transient brain activations while PET studies consistently reported decreased brain activity [15].

NREM phasic activities, as assessed by fMRI studies, are associated with increased (but not decreased) brain responses. For instance, *spindles* are positively correlated with increased activity in lateral and posterior aspects of the thalamus, paralimbic (anterior cingulate cortex, insula), and neocortex (superior temporal gyrus). This confirms the thalamic involvement in spindles generation and suggests the participation of specific cortical areas in their modulation [16]. Likewise, *slow waves* are associated with significantly increased activity in inferior and medial frontal cortices, parahippocampal gyrus, precuneus, posterior cingulate

cortex, ponto-mesencephalic tegmentum, and cerebellum. These results contrast with the classical view of brainstem nuclei promoting vigilance and wakefulness, because it suggests that several pontine structures including the locus coeruleus might be active during NREM sleep concomitant with SWA [15]. Cortical responses during slow wave occur in brain areas which are now known as major hubs in cortical structural connectivity and are also the most active during wakefulness [17]. These results have now been replicated [18] and are supported by source reconstruction of slow waves [19]. Altogether, these data underline that simple reduction of NREMS to a state of global and regional brain activity decrease is no longer defensible. See Fig. 64.1 for fMRI neural correlates of NREM sleep oscillations.

To date, *REM sleep* has been much less investigated by fMRI studies. Positive correlation between BOLD signal and density of REM was reported in thalamus, pons, and primary visual cortex, which is the main recording site of ponto-geniculo-occipital (PGO) activity. Activations described in the anterior cingulate cortex, parahippocampal gyrus, and amygdala make these regions potentially involved in REM sleep modulation [20, 21].

Sleep and Memory

Sleep is considered to have life-sustaining functions. In particular, it is now suggested that sleep intimately results from the energy metabolic demands implied by synaptic transmission induced by wakefulness [22]. It has also been associ-

Fig. 64.1 Neural correlates of NREM sleep oscillations as assessed by EEG/fMRI

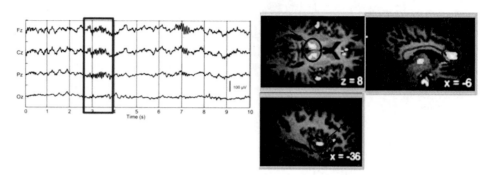

a. FMRI correlates of spindles. Left panel shows a NREM sleep epoch (stage 2) with spindles recorded by scalp EEG. Right panel illustrates the neural correlates associated to spindles during NREM sleep. Significant increases of brain activity are observed in the **a** thalamus (T), anterior cingulate cortex (AC) and insula (I). (16)

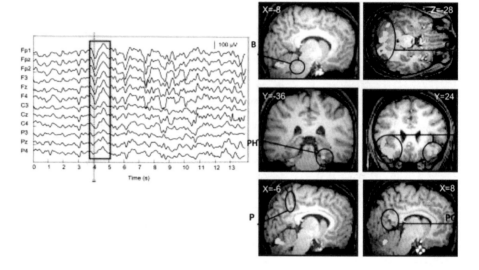

FMRI correlates of slow waves. Left panel shows a NREM sleep epoch (stage 4) with slow waves recorded by scalp EEG. Right panel illustrates the neural correlates associated to spindles during NREM sleep. Significant increases of brain activity are observed in the **b** brainstem (B), cerebellum (C), parahippocampal gyrus (PH), inferior frontal gyrus (IF), precuneus (P) and posterior cingulate gyrus (PC). (15)

ated with consolidation of recent memories. Recent reviews are available on these topics [23–25]. This very brief section aims to illustrate the interest of functional neuroimaging in better understanding these processes.

PET and fMRI have shown that waking experience influences regional brain activity during subsequent NREM and REM sleep. Indeed, a number of studies have demonstrated specific regional reactivations during post-learning sleep. For instance, a $H_2{}^{15}O$ PET study showed that several areas activated during procedural motor sequence learning were significantly more active during subsequent REM sleep [10]. The same lab also showed that hippocampal and parahippocampal gyrus previously recruited during a spatial memory task were reactivated during post-training SWS and, interestingly, the amount of this reactivation was positively correlated with overnight spatial navigation improvement [26]. Finally, an fMRI study demonstrated a significant reactivation in primary visual cortex during NREM sleep after intensive visual perceptual learning [27].

Sleep also seems to provide the special conditions needed to transfer and transform fresh memories. In an fMRI study, a declarative memory using word pairs was shown to initially recruit hippocampus-dependent memories. 6 months after learning, memory recall was associated with activation of the MPFC but not the hippocampus. This activation was more pronounced when subjects were initially allowed to sleep after learning [28]. Recall networks are reorganized during sleep. Fresh memory after having transiently been stored in hippocampus is then transferred to neocortical areas by a process which is especially supported by consolidation during sleep.

Neuroimaging in Sleep Patholophysiology

Sleep disorders are highly prevalent among the general population. Their consequences are being revealed in terms of morbidity and quality of life. However, sleep disorders remain poorly identified and treated. [29]. Neuroimaging currently remains a research tool to better understand the causes and brain consequences of sleep disruption. The objective of this section is to provide some illustrative examples of how neuroimaging can contribute to a better understanding of the neural correlates of sleep impairments, and possibly hinting to a diagnosis and therapeutic improvement. We will stay focused on the three most frequently studied intrinsic sleep disorders: primary insomnia, obstructive sleep apnea syndrome, and narcolepsy.

Primary Insomnia

Primary insomnia is characterized by difficulty in initiating sleep, maintaining sleep, or non-restorative sleep, which result in clinically significant distress or impairment in social, occupational, or other important areas of functioning [30]. It represents about 20% of insomniac patients seen at sleep disorders centers, and comprises the most prevalent sleep disorder as approximately one third of the general population complain of insomnia [29]. According to the International Classification of Sleep Disorders (ICSD-2), primary insomnia "*is a lifelong inability to obtain adequate sleep that is presumably due to an abnormality of the neurological control of the sleep-wake system.*" It is thought to reflect an imbalance between arousal and sleep promoting systems, which results in a global cortical hyperactivity. This theory coined as "hyperarousal hypothesis" is evidenced by EEG studies showing increased beta/gamma activity at sleep onset and during NREM sleep [31] and later confirmed by 18-FDG PET studies. The reduction in relative CMRglu from waking to NREM sleep was smaller in insomniac patients than in healthy controls in ascending reticular activating system, hypothalamus, insular cortex, amygdala, hippocampus, anterior cingulate, and medial prefrontal cortices. Conversely, during wakefulness, a decreased metabolism was observed in subcortical (thalamus, hypothalamus, brainstem reticular formation) and cortical (prefrontal bilaterally, left superior temporal, parietal, and occipital cortices) areas [32]. These results suggest abnormally high regional brain activity during sleep states, associated with reduced brain metabolism during wakefulness.

Obstructive Sleep Apnea Syndrome (OSAS)

Obstructive sleep apnea syndrome (OSAS) is a cluster of clinical features, such as snoring, cessations of breathing, excessive daytime sleepiness, and so forth, due to repetitive episodes of upper airway obstructions during sleep, with reduction in blood oxygen saturation and increased microarousals. These features considerably disturb sleep archi-

tecture and may lead to an almost complete deprivation of REM sleep and deep NREM sleep. Both sleep disturbances and hypoxemia contribute to excessive daytime sleepiness, a common symptom of the syndrome. OSAS is becoming a major health hazard in our society as it concerns 2–4% of the general population [29]. This number, probably underestimated [33], is still growing with increasing prevalence of obesity. OSAS is associated with significant morbidity, such as hypertension, cardiovascular disease, stroke, and motor vehicle accidents. Alterations of cognitive processes and mood disorders, especially depression, are also commonly reported in OSAS patients. Both hypoxemia and fragmented sleep are proposed as the main factors leading to neurocognitive impairments during wakefulness.

Structural brain alterations have been reported in OSAS patients as compared to healthy subjects. VBM studies indicated gray matter losses in multiple sites, including frontal and parietal cortex, temporal lobe, anterior cingulate, hippocampus, and cerebellum [34, 35]. Biochemical brain changes have also been described. A MRS study showed lower N-acetyl aspartate/choline (NAA/Cr), choline/creatinine (Cho/Cr) ratios and absolute concentrations of NAA and Cho measured by spectroscopy in prefrontal and parieto-occipital cortices, and frontal periventricular white matter of OSAS patients [36].

These structural and/or biochemical regional alterations in OSAS imply involvement of several brain areas responsible for upper airway motor as well as in cognition and mood regulation.

Functional neuroimaging provided evidence of autonomic dysfunction and impaired ventilatory control in OSAS patients. Several fMRI studies reported abnormal brain responses to cardiovascular [37, 38] or respiratory [39, 40] stresses in regions (e.g., cerebellum, cingulate, frontal motor cortex, and insula) known to play an important role in autonomic regulation. Interestingly, mandibular advancement in OSAS, was also found to decrease hyperactivation induced by resistive inspiratory loading in the left cingular and bilateral prefrontal cortices which are involved in the respiratory control [41]. Cognition has also been explored with functional neuroimaging in OSAS. Using fMRI, impaired performance during a working memory task in OSAS patients was associated with a relative deactivation of the dorsolateral prefrontal cortex [42]. For the same level of performance as controls in a 2-back-memory task, another fMRI research showed over-recruitment of several brain regions, possibly a compensatory mechanism due to sleep deprivation. After CPAP therapy, normalization in prefrontal and hippocampal activities was observed compared to baseline concomitant with improvement of cognitive and functional deficits, including depressive symptoms [43].

Narcolepsy

Narcolepsy, despite its rare prevalence affecting around 0.045% [44] of the general population, is one of the most well-known sleep-wake disorders with its clinical tetrad of excessive daytime sleepiness, sudden loss of muscle tone (cataplexy), sleep paralysis, and hypnagogic hallucinations. It has been associated with several biological markers such as higher prevalence of human leukocyte antigen (HLA) subtype DQB1*0602 positivity (mainly in cataplexy subgroup) and sleep onset REM periods (SOREMPs) in multiple sleep latency tests (MSLT). Reduced cerebrospinal fluid hypocretin (orexin) level is a useful diagnosis tool [45, 46].

VBM studies have described loss of gray matter in several regions including hypothalamus and pontine tegmentum in narcoleptic patients relative to healthy individuals, which may reflect secondary neuronal losses due to the destruction of specific hypocretin projections [47]. MRS studies reported reduced brain N-acetyl aspartate (NAA) in the ventral pontine [48] and the hypothalamus [49], possibly due to neuronal dysfunction in addition to neuronal loss. These results should be taken cautiously, since they were weakly reproducible. A further VBM study found no differences in global gray or white matter volumes between patients particularly, in the hypothalamus suffering from hypocretin-deficient narcolepsy and controls [50]. At present, there is no clear-cut evidence for structural changes in narcoleptic patients.

Functional neuroimaging, PET, and SPECT studies, indicate decreased metabolism and blood flow in the hypothalamus in idiopathic narcolepsy, which would be consistent with the suspected pathophysiology of the affection [51]. A further SPECT study on two patients during a cataplexy episode reported increased perfusion in the amygdala and anterior cingulate regions compared with REM sleep or wakefulness [52]. An fMRI study showed that humorous pictures elicited, reduced hypothalamic response together with enhanced amygdala response in narcoleptic patients [53].

Taken together, these observations suggest that cataplexy, which is well known to be triggered by emotion, might involve impaired hypothalamic/amygdala interactions.

Conclusion

In the past two decades, diverse neuroimaging techniques, particularly fMRI, have provided a fine-grained description of brain activity across different states of vigilance. Earlier studies using PET unraveled specific brain networks associated with both NREM and REM sleep. The advent of fMRI combined with EEG enabled the characterization of phasic events occurring within sleep, such as sleep oscillations. Taken together, these neuroimaging techniques bring interesting insights on the cerebral correlates of sleep regulation

and memory consolidation. Within the framework of sleep disorders, functional neuroimaging enhances the capacity to explore brain function during pathological sleep. Despite the current state-of-the-art neuroimaging techniques, wide gaps of uncertainty still remain concerning the neurophysiological mechanisms involved in sleep disorders, particularly in those mechanisms that play a causal role in their pathophysiology. Future studies using brain imaging will shed light on the functional and structural effects of sleep disorders, and may be valuable for the diagnosis and therapeutic management of these sleep pathologies.

References

1. Duyn JH. EEG-fMRI methods for the study of brain networks during sleep. Front Neurol. 2012; 3:100.
2. Buchsbaum MS, et al. Regional cerebral glucose metabolic rate in human sleep assessed by positron emission tomography. Life Sci. 1989;45(15):1349–56.
3. Maquet P, et al. Cerebral glucose utilization during sleep-wake cycle in man determined by positron emission tomography and [18F]2-fluoro-2-deoxy-D-glucose method. Brain Res. 1990;513(1):136–43.
4. Maquet P, et al. Cerebral glucose utilization during stage 2 sleep in man. Brain Res. 1992;571(1):149–53.
5. Maquet P, Phillips C. Functional brain imaging of human sleep. J Sleep Res. 1998;7(Suppl 1):42–7.
6. Maquet P, et al. Functional neuroanatomy of human slow wave sleep. J Neurosci. 1997;17(8):2807–12.
7. Andersson JLR, et al. Brain networks affected by synchronized sleep visualized by positron emission tomography. J Cereb Blood Flow Metab. 1998;18(7):701–715.
8. Kusse C, et al. Neuroimaging of dreaming: state of the art and limitations. Int Rev Neurobiol. 2010;92:87–99.
9. Maquet P, et al. Functional neuroanatomy of human rapid-eye-movement sleep and dreaming. Nature. 1996;383(6596):163–6.
10. Maquet P, et al. Experience-dependent changes in cerebral activation during human REM sleep. Nat Neurosci. 2000;3(8):831–6.
11. Hobson JA, et al. To dream or not to dream? Relevant data from new neuroimaging and electrophysiological studies. Curr Opin Neurobiol. 1998;8(2):239–44.
12. Hofle N, et al. Regional cerebral blood flow changes as a function of delta and spindle activity during slow wave sleep in humans. J Neurosci. 1997;17(12):4800–8.
13. Dang-Vu TT, et al. Cerebral correlates of delta waves during non-REM sleep revisited. Neuroimage. 2005;28(1):14–21.
14. Leclercq Y, et al. fMRI artefact rejection and sleep scoring toolbox. Comput Intell Neurosci. 2011;2011:598206.
15. Dang-Vu TT, et al. Spontaneous neural activity during human slow wave sleep. Proc Natl Acad Sci U S A. 2008;105(39):15160–5.
16. Schabus M, et al. Hemodynamic cerebral correlates of sleep spindles during human non-rapid eye movement sleep. Proc Natl Acad Sci. 2007;104(32):13164–69.
17. Maquet P. Functional neuroimaging of normal human sleep by positron emission tomography. J Sleep Res. 2000;9(3):207–31.
18. Andrade KC, et al. Sleep spindles and hippocampal functional connectivity in human NREM sleep. J Neurosci. 2011;31(28):10331–9.
19. Murphy M. et al. Source modeling sleep slow waves. Proc Natl Acad Sci U S A. 2009;106(5):1608–13.
20. Wehrle R, et al. Rapid eye movement-related brain activation in human sleep: a functional magnetic resonance imaging study. Neuroreport. 2005;16(8):853–7.

21. Miyauchi S, et al. Human brain activity time-locked to rapid eye movements during REM sleep. Exp Brain Res. 2009;192(4):657–67.
22. Tononi G, Cirelli C. Sleep and synaptic homeostasis: a hypothesis. Brain Res Bull. 2003;62(2):143–50.
23. Tononi G, Cirelli C. Sleep function and synaptic homeostasis. Sleep Med Rev. 2006;10(1):49–62.
24. Diekelmann S, Born J. The memory function of sleep. Nat Rev Neurosci. 2010;11(2):114–26.
25. Muto V, et al. Reciprocal interactions between wakefulness and sleep influence global and regional brain activity. Curr Top Med Chem. 2011;11(19):2403–13.
26. Peigneux P, et al. Are spatial memories strengthened in the human hippocampus during slow wave sleep? Neuron. 2004;44(3):535–45.
27. Yotsumoto Y, et al. Location-specific cortical activation changes during sleep after training for perceptual learning. Curr Biol. 2009;19(15):1278–82.
28. Gais S, et al. Sleep transforms the cerebral trace of declarative memories. Proc Natl Acad Sci U S A. 2007;104(47)18778–83.
29. Ohayon MM, et al. [Prevalence and comorbidity of sleep disorders in general population]. Rev Prat. 2007;57(14):1521 8.
30. Cortoos A, Verstraeten E, Cluydts R. Neurophysiological aspects of primary insomnia: implications for its treatment. Sleep Med Rev. 2006;10(4):255–66.
31. Perlis ML, et al. Beta EEG activity and insomnia. Sleep Med Rev. 2001;5(5):363–374.
32. Nofzinger EA, et al. Functional neuroimaging evidence for hyperarousal in insomnia. Am J Psychiatry. 2004;161(11):2126–8.
33. Fuhrman C, et al. Symptoms of sleep apnea syndrome: high prevalence and underdiagnosis in the French population. Sleep Med. 2012;13(7):852–8.
34. Macey PM, et al. Brain morphology associated with obstructive sleep apnea. Am J Respir Crit Care Med. 2002;166(10):1382–7.
35. Morrell MJ, et al. Changes in brain morphology in patients with obstructive sleep apnoea. Thorax. 2010;65(10):908–14.
36. Alchanatis M, et al. Frontal brain lobe impairment in obstructive sleep apnoea: a proton MR spectroscopy study. Eur Respir J. 2004;24(6):980–6.
37. Harper RM, et al. fMRI responses to cold pressor challenges in control and obstructive sleep apnea subjects. J Appl Physiol. 2003;94(4):1583–95.
38. Henderson LA, et al. Neural responses during Valsalva maneuvers in obstructive sleep apnea syndrome. J Appl Physiol. 2003;94(3):1063–74.
39. Macey PM, et al. Functional magnetic resonance imaging responses to expiratory loading in obstructive sleep apnea. Respir Physiol Neurobiol. 2003;138(2–3):275–90.
40. Macey KE, et al. Inspiratory loading elicits aberrant fMRI signal changes in obstructive sleep apnea. Respir Physiol Neurobiol. 2006;151(1):44–60.
41. Hashimoto K, et al. Effects of mandibular advancement on brain activation during inspiratory loading in healthy subjects: a functional magnetic resonance imaging study. J Appl Physiol. 2006;100(2):579–86.
42. Thomas RJ, et al. Functional imaging of working memory in obstructive sleep-disordered breathing. J Appl Physiol. 2005;98(6):2226–34.
43. Castronovo V, et al. Brain activation changes before and after PAP treatment in obstructive sleep apnea. Sleep. 2009;32(9):1161–72.
44. Ohayon MM. From wakefulness to excessive sleepiness: what we know and still need to know. Sleep Med Rev. 2008;12(2):129–41.
45. Mignot E, et al. The role of cerebrospinal fluid hypocretin measurement in the diagnosis of narcolepsy and other hypersomnias. Arch Neurol. 2002;59(10):1553–62.
46. Baumann CR, Bassetti CL. Hypocretins (orexins): clinical impact of the discovery of a neurotransmitter. Sleep Med Rev. 2005;9(4):253–68.
47. Draganski B, et al. Hypothalamic gray matter changes in narcoleptic patients. Nat Med. 2002;8(11):1186–8.
48. Ellis CM, et al. Proton spectroscopy in the narcoleptic syndrome. Is there evidence of a brainstem lesion? Neurology. 1998; 50(2 Suppl 1):23–6.
49. Lodi R, et al. In vivo evidence of neuronal loss in the hypothalamus of narcoleptic patients. Neurology. 2004;63(8):1513–5.
50. Overeem S, et al. Voxel-based morphometry in hypocretin-deficient narcolepsy. Sleep. 2003;26(1):44–6.
51. Joo EY, et al. Glucose hypometabolism of hypothalamus and thalamus in narcolepsy. Ann Neurol. 2004;56(3):437–40.
52. Hong SB, Tae WS, Joo EY. Cerebral perfusion changes during cataplexy in narcolepsy patients. Neurology. 2006;66(11):1747–9.
53. Schwartz S, et al. Abnormal activity in hypothalamus and amygdala during humour processing in human narcolepsy with cataplexy. Brain. 2008;131:514–22.

Index

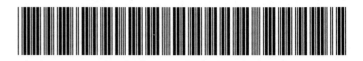